PERIPHERAL VASCULAR DISEASES

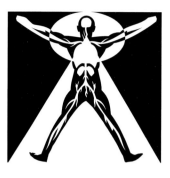

PERIPHERAL VASCULAR DISEASES

SECOND EDITION

Edited by

JESS R. YOUNG, M.D.
Chairman, Department of Vascular Medicine
The Cleveland Clinic Foundation
Cleveland, Ohio

JEFFREY W. OLIN, D.O.
Department of Vascular Medicine
The Cleveland Clinic Foundation
Cleveland, Ohio

JOHN R. BARTHOLOMEW, M.D.
Department of Vascular Medicine
The Cleveland Clinic Foundation
Cleveland, Ohio

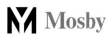 Mosby

St. Louis Baltimore Boston
Carlsbad Chicago Naples New York Philadelphia Portland
London Madrid Mexico City Singapore Sydney Tokyo Toronto Wiesbaden

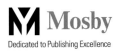

Mosby

Dedicated to Publishing Excellence

A Times Mirror
Company

Editor: Stephanie Manning
Developmental Editors: Laura Berendson, Carolyn Malik
Project Manager: Linda Clarke
Production Editor: Julie Cullen
Designer: Carolyn O'Brien
Manufacturing Supervisor: Andrew Christensen

2nd EDITION

Printed in the United States of America
Composition by Graphic World Inc.
Printing/binding by The Maple–Vail York Book Manufacturing Group

Mosby–Year Book, Inc.
11830 Westline Industrial Drive
St. Louis, Missouri 63146

Library of Congress Cataloging in Publication Data

Peripheral vascular diseases / edited by Jess R. Young, Jeffrey W.
 Olin, John R. Bartholomew. — 2nd ed.
    p. cm.
  Includes bibliographical references and index.
  ISBN 0-8151-9785-3
  1. Peripheral vascular diseases. I. Young, Jess R., 1928–
II. Olin, Jeffrey W.   III. Bartholomew, John R.
  [DNLM: 1. Peripheral Vascular Diseases.   WG 500 P445 1996]
RC694.P487 1996
616.1'31—dc20
DNLM/DLC
for Library of Congress   95-48133
                                                              CIP

96 97 98 99 00 / 9 8 7 6 5 4 3 2 1

CONTRIBUTORS

Walid Arrabi, M.D.
Fellow
Department of Vascular Medicine
Cleveland Clinic Foundation
Cleveland, Ohio

J. Michael Bacharach, M.D.
Head
Section of Vascular Medicine and Peripheral
    Vascular Intervention
North Central Heart and Vascular Institute
Sioux Falls, South Dakota

Edwin G. Beven, M.D.
Department of Vascular Surgery
Cleveland Clinic Center
Cleveland, Ohio

Earl Z. Browne Jr., M.D.
Head
Section of Plastic Surgery Research
Department of Plastic and Reconstructive Surgery
Cleveland Clinic Foundation
Cleveland, Ohio

Leonard H. Calabrese, D.O.
Vice-Chairman
Department of Rheumatic and Immunologic
    Diseases
Cleveland Clinic Foundation
Cleveland, Ohio

Guy M. Chisolm, III, Ph.D.
Department of Cell Biology
Cleveland Clinic Foundation
Cleveland, Ohio

Richard W. Chitwood, M.D.
Fellow
Division of Vascular Surgery
Henry Ford Hospital
Detroit, Michigan

John D. Clough, M.D.
Department of Rheumatology and Immunology
Chairman
Division of Health Affairs
Cleveland Clinic Foundation
Cleveland, Ohio

Jay D. Coffman, M.D.
Professor of Medicine
Chief
Vascular Medicine Section
Department of Medicine
Boston University Medical Center
Boston, Massachusetts

Anthony J. Comerota, M.D.
Professor of Surgery
Chief of Vascular Surgery
Department of Surgery
Temple University School of Medicine
Philadelphia, Pennsylvania

Michael D. Cressman, D.O.
Director
Hypertension Treatment Program
Associate Professor of Medicine
Center for Clinic Pharmacology
University of Pennsylvania Medical Center
Pittsburgh, Pennsylvania

William J. Davros, Ph.D.
Diagnostic Medical Physicist
Department of Radiology
Cleveland Clinic Foundation
Cleveland, Ohio

Ralph G. De Palma, M.D., F.A.C.S.
Professor of Surgery
Vice Chairman
Department of Surgery
Associate Dean, University of Nevada
Department of Surgery
University of Nevada
Reno, Nevada

Paul E. DiCorleto, Ph.D.
Chairman
Department of Cell Biology
Cleveland Clinic Foundation
Cleveland, Ohio

Bart Dolmatch, M.D.
Head
Section of Vascular and Interventional Radiology
Cleveland Clinic Foundation
Cleveland, Ohio

David Driscoll, M.D.
Professor of Pediatrics
Head, Section of Pediatric Cardiology
Mayo Medical School
Mayo Clinic
Rochester, Minnesota

L. Allen Ehrhart, Ph.D.
Department of Cell Biology
Cleveland Clinic Foundation
Cleveland, Ohio

Calvin B. Ernst, M.D.
Clinical Professor of Surgery
University of Michigan Medical School
Ann Arbor, Michigan
Head, Division of Vascular Surgery
Henry Ford Hospital
Detroit, Michigan

Peter Gloviczki, M.D.
Consultant
Section of Vascular Surgery
Mayo Clinic
Rochester, Minnesota

Bruce H. Gray, D.O.
Co-Director
Intervention Laboratory
Department of Vascular Medicine
Cleveland Clinic Foundation
Cleveland, Ohio

Thomas M. Grist, M.D.
Assistant Professor of Radiology
Chief of MRI
University of Wisconsin
Madison, Wisconsin

Russell N. Harada, M.D.
Fellow, Vascular Surgery
Department of Surgery
Temple University School of Medicine
Philadelphia, Pennsylvania

Norman R. Hertzer, M.D.
Chairman
Department of Vascular Surgery
Cleveland Clinic Foundation
Cleveland, Ohio

Henry F. Hoff, Ph.D.
Department of Cell Biology
Cleveland Clinic Foundation
Cleveland, Ohio

Gary S. Hoffman, M.D.
Chairman
Department of Rheumatic and Immunologic
    Diseases
Cleveland Clinic Foundation
Cleveland, Ohio

Byron J. Hoogwerf, M.D.
Department of Endocrinology
Cleveland Clinic Foundation
Cleveland, Ohio

Michael R. Jaff, D.O.
Director
Vascular Medicine and the Non-Invasive Vascular
    Laboratory
Milwaukee Heart & Vascular Clinic
Milwaukee, Wisconsin

John W. Joyce, M.D.
Professor of Medicine
Division of Cardiovascular Diseases and Internal
    Medicine
Mayo Medical School, Mayo Clinic
Rochester, Minnesota

Kandice Kottke-Marchant, M.D., Ph.D.
Director
Hemostasis and Thrombosis Laboratory
Department of Clinical Pathology
Cleveland Clinic Foundation
Cleveland, Ohio

Leonard P. Krajewski, M.D.
Department of Vascular Surgery
Cleveland Clinic Foundation
Cleveland, Ohio

Marvin E. Levin, M.D.
Professor of Clinical Medicine
Department of Medicine
Division of Metabolism
Washington University School of Medicine
St. Louis, Missouri

Thomas H. Marwick
Director
Cardiac Stress Imaging
Department of Cardiology
Cleveland Clinic Foundation
Cleveland, Ohio

Alvin J. Mathe, D.O.
Assistant Professor of Medicine
University of North Texas Health
    Service Center
Fort Worth, Texas

Kevin M. McIntyre, M.D.
Associate Clinical Professor of Medicine
Harvard Medical School
Attending Physician
Brockton/West Roxbury Veterans Affairs
    Medical Center
West Roxbury, Massachusetts

Douglas S. Moodie, M.D., M.S.
Chairman
Division of Pediatrics
Cleveland Clinic Foundation
Cleveland, Ohio

Richard E. Morton, Ph.D.
Department of Cell Biology
Cleveland Clinic Foundation
Cleveland, Ohio

Felipe Navarro, M.D.
Interventional Fellow
Department of Vascular Medicine
Cleveland Clinic Foundation
Cleveland, Ohio

Andrew C. Novick
Chairman
Department of Urology
Cleveland Clinic Foundation
Cleveland, Ohio

Thomas F. O'Donnell, Jr., M.D.
Professor and Chairman
Surgeon-in-Chief
Chief
Division of Vascular Surgery
Department of Surgery
Tufts University School of Medicine
Boston, Massachusetts

Patrick J. O'Hara, M.D.
Department of Vascular Surgery
Cleveland Clinic Foundation
Cleveland, Ohio

Malcolm O. Perry, M.D.
Professor
Department of Surgery
Texas Tech University Health Sciences Center
Lubbock, Texas

Henry H. Roenigk Jr., M.D.
Professor
Department of Dermatology
Northwestern University Medical School
Chicago, Illinois

Thom W. Rooke, M.D.
Associate Professor of Medicine
Director, Gonda Vascular Center
Department of Cardiovascular Diseases
Mayo Medical Center
Rochester, Minnesota

William F. Ruschhaupt, III, M.D.
Department of Vascular Medicine
Cleveland Clinic Foundation
Cleveland, Ohio

Dawn Salvatore, M.D.
Fellow
Division of Pediatrics
Cleveland Clinic Foundation
Cleveland, Ohio

Arthur A. Sasahara, M.D.
Senior Medical Director
Thrombolytic Medicine
Pharmaceutical Products Division
Abbott Laboratories
Abbott Park, Illinois
Professor of Medicine, Emeritus
Harvard Medical School
Senior Physician (on leave)
Department of Medicine
Brigham and Women's Hospital
Boston, Massachusetts

Alexander Schirger, M.D.
Consultant in Medicine
Mayo Clinic Professor of Medicine
Division of Cardiovascular Diseases and Division
    of Hypertension
Mayo Medical School
Rochester, Minnesota

G.V.R.K. Sharma, M.D.
Associate Professor of Medicine
Harvard Medical School
Associate Chief, Cardiology Section
Brockton/West Roxbury Veterans Affairs Medical
    Center
West Roxbury, Massachusetts

Anthony W. Stanson, M.D.
Associate Professor
Diagnostic Radiology
Mayo Clinic
Rochester, Minnesota

D. Eugene Strandness, Jr., M.D.
Professor and Chief
Division of Vascular Surgery
Department of Surgery
University of Washington
Seattle, Washington

Timothy M. Sullivan, M.D.
Department of Vascular Surgery
Cleveland Clinic Foundation
Cleveland, Ohio

Donald G. Vidt, M.D.
Department of Nephrology and Hypertension
Cleveland Clinic Foundation
Cleveland, Ohio

Cheryl E. Weinstein, M.D.
Department of General Internal Medicine
Cleveland Clinic Foundation
Cleveland, Ohio

Harold J. Welch, M.D.
Assistant Professor of Surgery
Staff Vascular Surgeon
Department of Surgery
Tufts University School of Medicine
Boston, Massachusetts

AFFECTIONATELY DEDICATED TO OUR PATIENT AND
UNDERSTANDING WIVES AND OUR CHILDREN

PREFACE

This is the second edition of a text first published in 1991. In the interval, knowledge and technology in the field of peripheral vascular disease continue to advance rapidly. Diagnostic techniques, medical therapies, nonsurgical interventional procedures, and surgical procedures are increasingly complex and sophisticated. There have been some significant philosophical changes in the management of certain vascular diseases such as symptomatic and asymptomatic severe carotid artery stenosis. Rapid advances in thrombolytic therapy include the development of new agents and the refinement of dosing regimens and modes of administration. Research in the field of vascular biology continues at an accelerated rate, providing great potential for new insights into the diseases we treat as clinicians. Particular emphasis has been placed on the biology of the endothelium and the vascular wall, and on gene therapy.

Each chapter of this second edition has been revised and updated. The growing importance of the field of antithrombotic therapy has been emphasized by dedicating a full chapter to this subject. We have added two new chapters, one on angiography and one on vascular diseases in infancy and childhood. Color plates have been added to enhance our appreciation of some of the conditions that we see in the field of peripheral vascular disease.

We wish to thank and commend our contributors for their fine efforts. We are indebted to each of these collaborators for providing current and balanced information for their assigned topics.

Our goal is to cover the various vascular disorders in a practical and topical manner. We continue to try to keep this text clinically oriented, written mainly by practicing clinicians. We hope that it will prove useful for all physicians caring for patients with vascular diseases, including family physicians, internists, cardiologists, dermatologists, vascular surgeons, general surgeons, interventional radiologists, and podiatrists.

Jess R. Young
Jeffrey W. Olin
John R. Bartholomew

CONTENTS

PERIPHERAL
VASCULAR
DISEASES

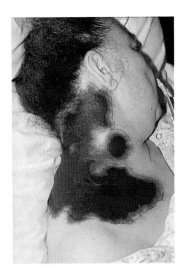

Plate 1. Warfarin (coumarin) skin necrosis in a patient being treated for a deep venous thrombosis.

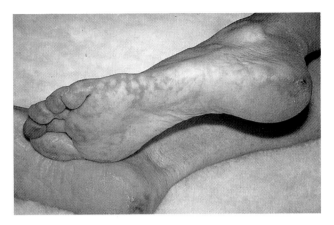

Plate 2. Classic appearance of atheromatous emboli with a livedo reticularis pattern on the toes, lateral aspect of the foot, and heel.

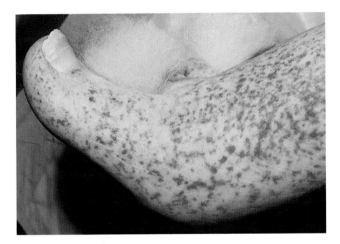

Plate 3. Palpable purpura leukocytoclastic vasculitis in a patient with a drug reaction to antibiotics.

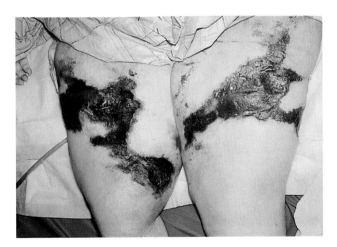

Plate 4. Cutaneous calciphylaxis lesions of the thigh in a patient undergoing long-term hemodialysis for chronic renal failure.

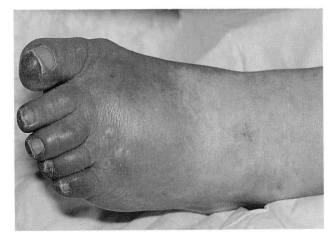

Plate 5. Phlegmasia cerulea dolens (venous gangrene) in a patient with ovarian carcinoma.

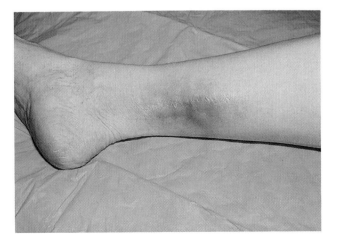

Plate 6. Chronic, indurated, sterile, stasis cellulitis in a patient with chronic venous insufficiency.

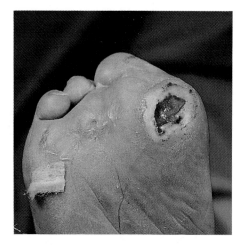

Plate 7. Neurotrophic ulcer over the head of the first metatarsal in a patient with diabetes mellitus. Note the typical callus surrounding the ulcer.

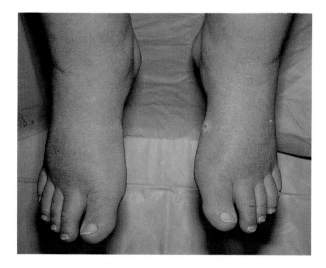

Plate 8. Red, warm, swollen, painful feet of a 26-year-old woman with primary erythermalgia.

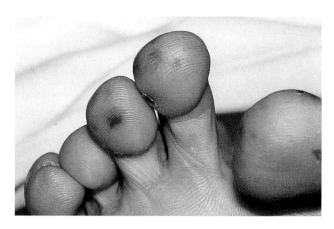

Plate 9. Typical yellow-brown discoloration with shallow ulcers on the toes of a patient with chronic pernio.

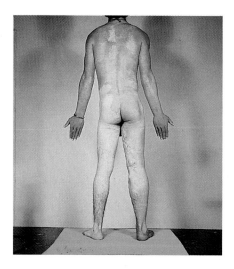

Plate 10. Klippel-Trenaunay syndrome with a port-wine stain of the trunk and extremities, and muscular hypertrophy and varicose veins of the right leg.

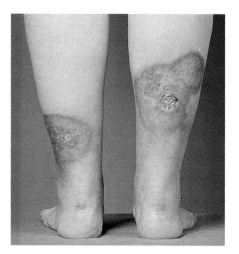

Plate 11. Necrobiosis lipoidica diabeticorum with ulcerati on in a patient with diabetes mellitus. Typical orange or yellow indurated lesions with telangiectasias, demarcated from the surrounding skin by a violet border.

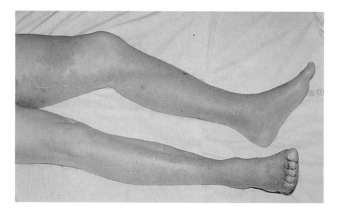

Plate 12. Cellulitis of the left leg with skipped areas of involvement of the calf and thigh.

PART I

BASIC CONSIDERATIONS

CLINICAL CLUES TO PERIPHERAL VASCULAR DISEASE

Jess R. Young

Physicians are not well acquainted with peripheral vascular diseases. Vascular medicine is a field that is poorly taught in medical schools and in postgraduate programs. The signs and symptoms of vascular disease can therefore be quite confusing to most physicians. However, vascular medicine is a specialty that lends itself to solving problems by using the powers of observation. The clinical clues to vascular disease are usually there for the trained clinician to discover.

ARTERIAL DISEASE

Cold hands and cold feet are not good indicators of arterial insufficiency. Tense patients and patients with an overactive sympathetic nervous system can have impressively cold hands and feet in spite of excellent arterial circulation to the extremities. Some of these tense patients may also have vasomotor instability with cyanosis or mottling of the hands and feet during exposure to cold or with increased tension.

Poor hair growth, poor skin condition, and deformed or slowly growing toenails are frequently mentioned as signs of arterial insufficiency. However these are not reliable signs. *Ischemic fissures* of the feet (Fig. 1-1), *decubitus ulcers* of ankles (Fig. 1-2) and heels (Fig. 1-3), and *ischemic ulcers* (Fig. 1-4) are much more reliable signs of arterial insufficiency.

Tendinous (Fig. 1-5) *and tuberous* (Fig. 1-6) *xanthomas* may be clues that the patient has hypercholesterolemia and therefore may have an increased tendency to develop arteriosclerosis obliterans. *Xanthelasma* of the eyelids (Fig. 1-7) is associated with hypercholesterolemia in approximately 50% of the persons who have xanthelasma. The other 50% cannot be considered to have a benign disorder, however, since Bates and Warren[1] found that 94% of their patients with xanthelasma had less than mean levels of high-density lipoprotein (HDL) cholesterol and 69% of the patients had documented cardiovascular disease.

Intermittent claudication is a classic and usually reliable symptom of arteriosclerosis obliterans. Unless the ischemia is severe, the patient is typically distressed only with walking and is relieved within 1 or 2 minutes by stopping and standing in place. The distance that the patient can walk before he must stop varies little from day to day, and he does not need to sit down to get relief from his symptoms.

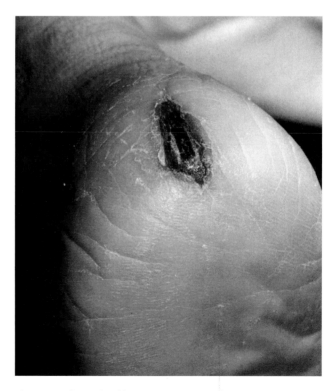

Fig. 1-1. Ischemic heel fissure in a patient with arteriosclerosis obliterans. This is often a precursor of a heel ulcer.

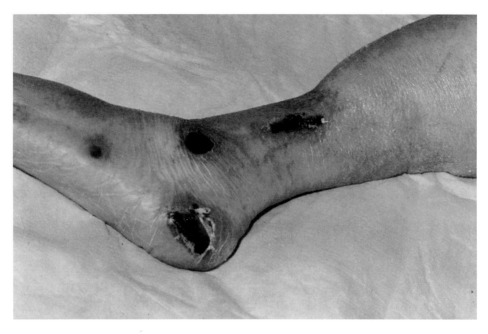

Fig. 1-2. Necrotic areas over the lateral leg and foot in a patient with impaired arterial circulation. The lesions occurred secondary to prolonged pressure while lying in bed.

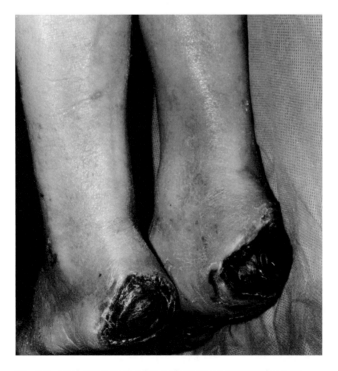

Fig. 1-3. Heel pressure decubitus ulcers in a patient with arteriosclerosis obliterans.

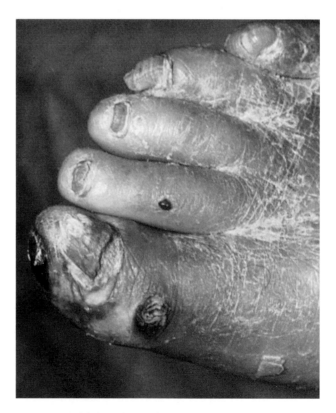

Fig. 1-4. Painful dry ischemic digital ulcers in a patient with severe arterial insufficiency.

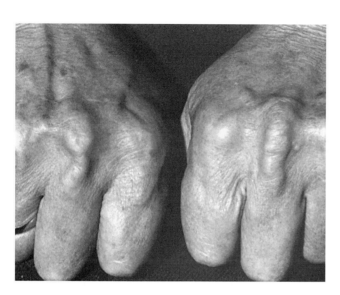

Fig. 1-5. Tendinous xanthomas in a patient with type IIA hyperlipidemia.

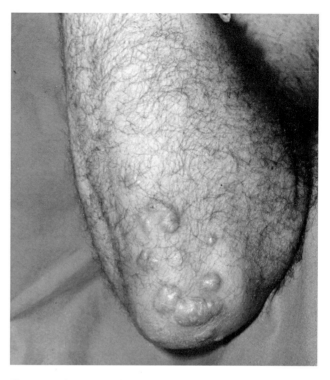

Fig. 1-6. Tuberous xanthomas of the elbow in a patient with type IIA hyperlipidemia.

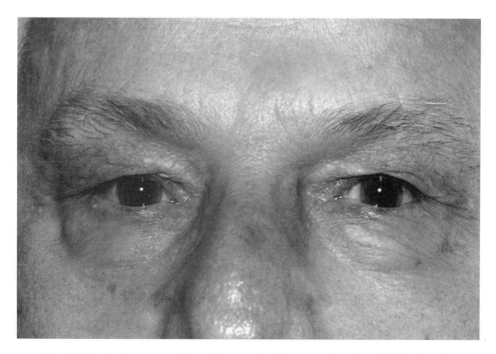

Fig. 1-7. Xanthelasma in a patient with normal total cholesterol and low HDL cholesterol.

Increasing numbers of patients are being seen who have *pseudoclaudication* (see Chapter 11) associated with the cauda equina syndrome. This syndrome occurs when there is pressure on the lower spine as a result of lumbar canal stenosis, herniated disk, or hypertrophic ridging. Although the clinical picture can closely mimic true claudication, the distress in a patient with pseudoclaudication may also occur when he straightens his back, either while in bed, standing, or walking. Often the patient will stand or walk slightly bent over in a "gorilla position." The distance that a patient with pseudoclaudication can walk before stopping varies considerably from time to time. The distress is often described with some neurologic component such as a tingling, weakness, incoordination, or clumsiness, as well as the classic symptoms of aching or cramping. A final differentiating point is that the patient usually must sit or lie for at least 5 or 10 minutes to obtain relief, whereas the patient with true claudication is usually relieved within 2 or 3 minutes of standing in place.

Ischemic rest pain is usually worse at night and may be difficult to differentiate from the pain of peripheral neuropathy. In general, patients with peripheral neuropathy have equal pain in both extremities, and the discomfort is not relieved by dependency. They have signs of peripheral neuropathy with absent or decreased deep tendon reflexes and loss of touch and vibratory sensation. The patient with ischemic rest pain usually does not have symmetric discomfort, does get some relief with dependency, and has no signs of peripheral neuropathy. In addition, the patient with ischemic rest pain has other evidence of marked ischemia, including marked pallor on elevation of the legs, marked rubor on dependency, and delayed venous filling time (see Chapter 2).

Ischemic ulcers are painful lesions found distally on the toes or on pressure points of the feet (Fig. 1-8). A patient with ischemic lesions often sits with his legs dangling over the side of the bed (Fig. 1-9) or sits in a chair all night because the dependent position gives him the best possible blood supply to the painful extremities. As a result of prolonged dependency, the extremities can become quite edematous.

The *peripheral gangrene* of severe arterial insufficiency (Fig. 1-10) may be difficult to differentiate from that of venous gangrene (phlegmasia cerulea dolens) (Fig. 1-11). In a patient with venous gangrene marked swelling in the extremity usually occurs early before the onset of frank ischemic changes. In a patient with arterial ischemia the severe ischemic changes usually occur first, followed by edema because the limb is kept in a constant dependent position. If the patient is a poor observer and is seen after ischemia and edema are well established, there may be great difficulty in differentiating these two entities.

Thromboangiitis obliterans (Buerger's disease) (see Chapter 21) usually occurs in young adults less than 40 years of age, but older patients can also be affected. In the past it was thought that only men were afflicted, but recent reports show that 20% to 30% of the patients are women. All patients with thromboangiitis obliterans either smoke tobacco or are exposed to nicotine in some form. The first symptom may be intermittent claudication, but more commonly the more distal arteries are involved so that ulceration and gangrenous changes of the digits may be the initial presentation. The upper extremities are involved in at least 40% of patients with thromboangiitis obliterans. An Allen test should be done to test the patency of the radial and ulnar arteries in anyone suspected of having this condition (see Chapter 2). Thrombophlebitis—usually superficial thrombophlebitis (Fig. 1-12)—occurs at some stage of the disease in approximately 40% of the cases.

Arterial embolism (see Chapter 15) is a fairly common

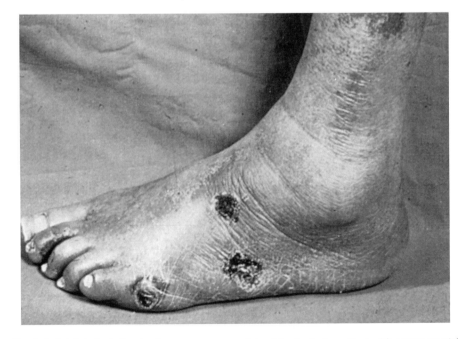

Fig. 1-8. Painful, dry ischemic ulcers on pressure points of the foot of a patient with severe arterial insufficiency.

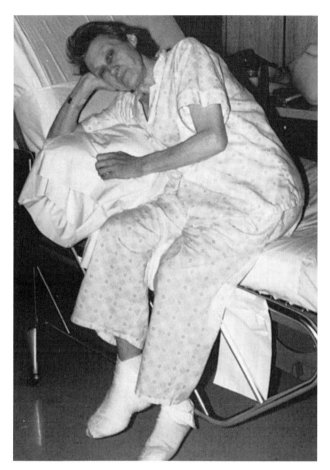

Fig. 1-9. Typical position assumed by a patient with severe arteriosclerosis obliterans and rest pain. The legs are dangled in an attempt to relieve the pain.

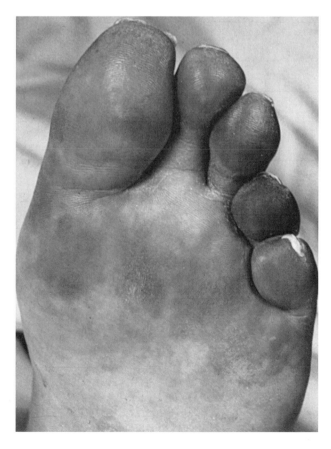

Fig. 1-10. Distal gangrene in a patient with severe arteriosclerosis obliterans.

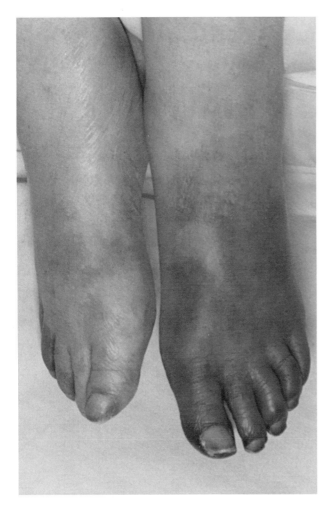

Fig. 1-11. Phlegmasia cerulea dolens (venous gangrene) in a patient with carcinoma of the lung.

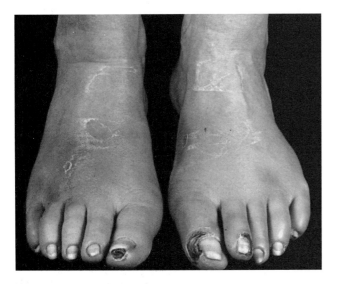

Fig. 1-12. Ischemic lesions of the toes and superficial thrombophlebitis of the dorsum of the feet in a 38-year-old man with thromboangiitis obliterans (Buerger's disease).

cause of occlusion of both large and small arteries of the extremities. The changes produced are often dramatic and at times pathognomonic of embolism, with either acutely ischemic limbs or scattered areas of well-demarcated ischemia (Fig. 1-13). Approximately 90% of large emboli originate in the heart. The cardiac causes include atrial fibrillation, myocardial infarction with mural thrombus, infective or marantic endocarditis, ventricular aneurysm, atrial myxoma, cardiomyopathy, and valve prosthesis. Another 5% of emboli originate in aneurysms of the more proximal arteries. Embolism should be suspected in the patient with an ischemic limb who has a potential source for emboli, who has no previous history of intermittent claudication, and who has good pulses in the uninvolved limb.

Atheromatous embolization (see Chapter 14) is a fairly common problem and produces multiple scattered areas of cyanosis or gangrene in the toes and feet (Fig. 1-14) and occasionally in the calves, thighs, and buttocks. A livedo reticularis pattern, representing emboli to the dermal vessels, can be seen at times in the involved areas. Extensive embolization can result in ischemic ulcers and gangrene. Atheromatous emboli may also cause myocardial

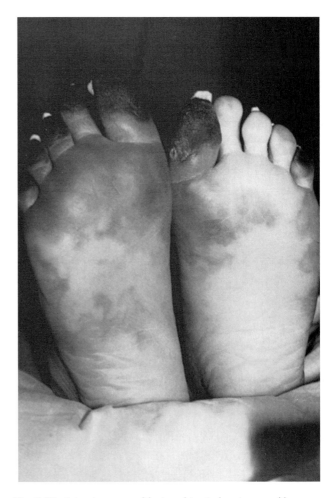

Fig. 1-13. Extensive areas of foot and toe ischemia caused by emboli from an abdominal aortic aneurysm.

infarctions, transient ischemic attacks, strokes, pancreatitis, renal infarctions and failure, gastrointestinal bleeding, and bowel ischemia.

The scattered areas of fixed mottling in the toes associ-

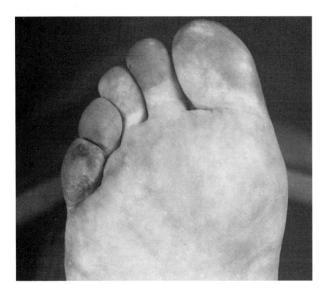

Fig. 1-14. Scattered areas of ischemia in a patient with atheromatous emboli from an atheromatous abdominal aorta.

ated with atheromatous embolization must be differentiated from the lesions of *chronic pernio* (chilblains) (see Chapter 35). These lesions typically begin as reddish-blue or violet blisters on the toes or dorsum of the feet, then later form superficial painful ulcers (Fig. 1-15). Pernio lesions appear in the fall at the onset of cold weather and usually disappear in the spring in warm weather.

Aneurysms (see Chapter 19) may initially be seen clinically as one of three complications: rupture, thrombosis, or embolization. Uncomplicated aneurysms may be seen as a visible or palpable pulsating mass (Fig. 1-16) or be detected as a result of pressure on surrounding structures, including long bones, vertebrae, nerves, veins, or ureters.

Abdominal aortic aneurysms can rupture into the intraabdominal cavity and become evident as sudden abdominal pain and shock. They can rupture in the retroperitoneal area and result in severe back pain, pain of renal colic, or hypotension. Rupture into the inferior vena cava can produce sudden edema of the extremities and acute congestive failure. Rupture into the gastrointestinal tract can produce an acute gastrointestinal bleed. *Mycotic aneurysms* or a secondarily infected aneurysm can give the clinical picture of a pulsating mass in a patient with a fever of unknown origin.

Aneurysms of the carotid arteries are rare. In some patients, especially middle-aged women with hypertension, the carotid or innominate arteries may be elongated

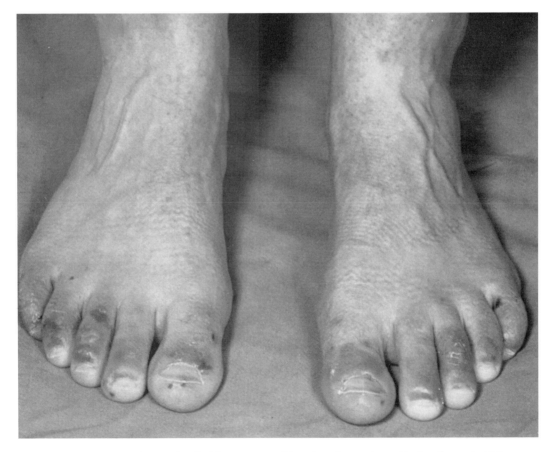

Fig. 1-15. Reddish-blue and violet blisters, some with eschars, in a patient with chronic pernio (chilblains).

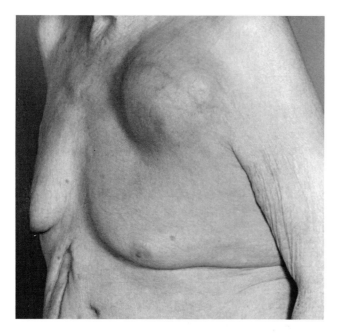

Fig. 1-16. False aneurysm of the anterior chest wall caused by a disruption of the suture line of an axillofemoral bypass graft.

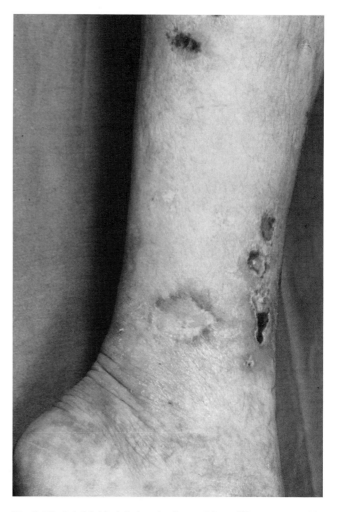

Fig. 1-17. Painful, black ischemic ulcers of the calf in a patient with lupus erythematosus.

and tortuous. This S-shaped curve of the artery may at first feel like an aneurysm. Careful palpation or duplex ultrasound scanning will confirm that this is a *tortuous carotid, subclavian, or innominate artery* and is not an aneurysm. This "buckling" is far more common than true aneurysms in this area. Another condition that can be mistaken for a carotid aneurysm is a *carotid body tumor.* It usually appears as a mass at the common carotid artery bifurcation and can be diagnosed by arteriography or by duplex ultrasound scan.

The clinical picture seen in a patient with an *aortic dissecting aneurysm* is extremely variable. The event usually starts as severe chest pain, often described as a "tearing" pain. This discomfort may begin in the anterior or posterior chest and may migrate downward. Depending on which arteries and structures are involved, the patient can also have a myocardial infarction if the coronary arteries are involved, congestive failure if the aortic valve is affected, cardiac tamponade, stroke, renal failure, mesenteric ischemia, paraplegia, or ischemia of the extremities. With rupture, death usually results, often as a result of cardiac tamponade. Because of these many clinical manifestations, the diagnosis is often missed because it was never considered.

Vasculitis can produce patterns of change in the extremities varying from palpable purpura to ischemic ulcers in atypical locations or to frank gangrene. Typical locations for ischemic ulcers with arteriosclerosis obliterans or thromboangiitis obliterans would be distally on the toes or on pressure points of the foot, including the ankles, heels, and tarsal-metatarsal joint areas. Vasculitic ulcers not uncommonly are found higher up on the calf or thigh (Fig. 1-17). In addition to vasculitis, these ischemic ulcers in atypical locations can also be caused by atheromatous emboli or by trauma to an already ischemic limb.

The patient with *Raynaud's phenomenon* (Fig. 1-18) should be examined closely for signs of underlying causes (see Chapter 23). The Allen test (see Chapter 2) may show an occluded radial or ulnar artery that may be a clue to scleroderma, thromboangiitis obliterans, or vasculitis with associated Raynaud's phenomenon. Thickening of the skin of the hands and fingers in patients with scleroderma may be difficult to detect early. An attempt should be made to pinch the skin between the middle and distal knuckles of the fingers (Fig. 1-19). Early in the course of scleroderma the skin at this site is thickened so that it cannot be pinched between the thumb and index finger of the examiner. Superficial, small open or healed ulcerations on the tips of the fingers (Fig. 1-20) or spider angioma (telangiectasia) (Fig. 1-21) can also be early signs of scleroderma.

VENOUS DISEASE

Varicose veins (Fig. 1-22) usually develop because of a hereditary weakness in the structures of the vein walls or valves or both. Contributing factors include pregnancy, obesity, and occupations requiring long periods of standing. When varices appear early in life and without obvious

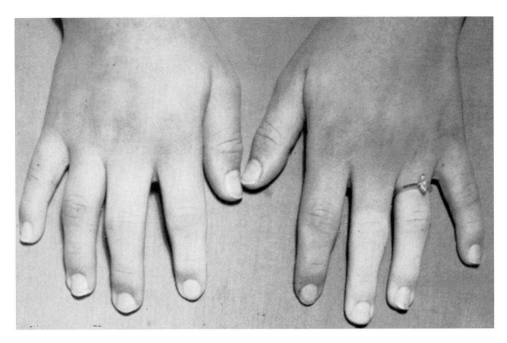

Fig. 1-18. Pallor phase of Raynaud's phenomenon in a young woman with primary Raynaud's disease.

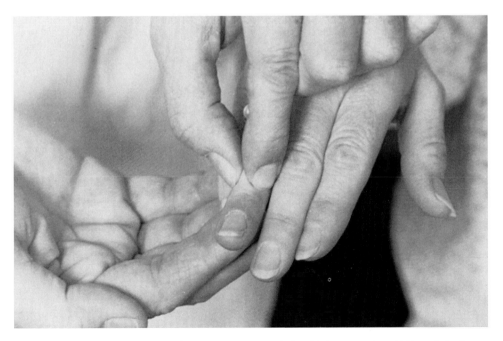

Fig. 1-19. Testing for scleroderma by attempting to pinch the skin between the middle and distal knuckles of a patient with Raynaud's phenomenon.

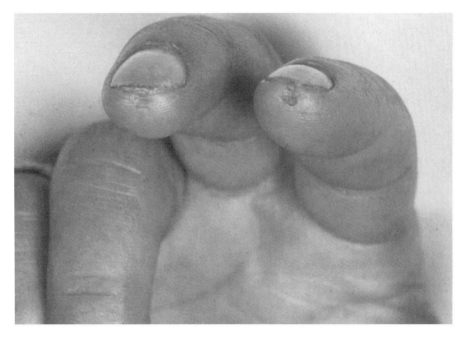

Fig. 1-20. Small healed fingertip ulcers in a patient with scleroderma.

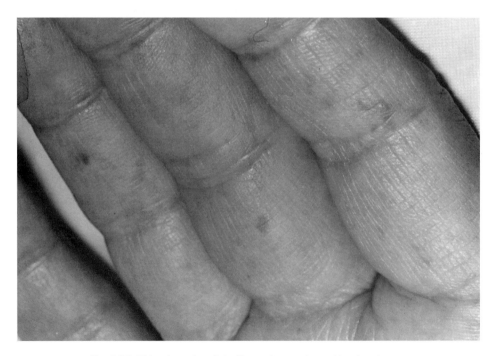

Fig. 1-21. Telangiectasias of the fingers in a patient with scleroderma.

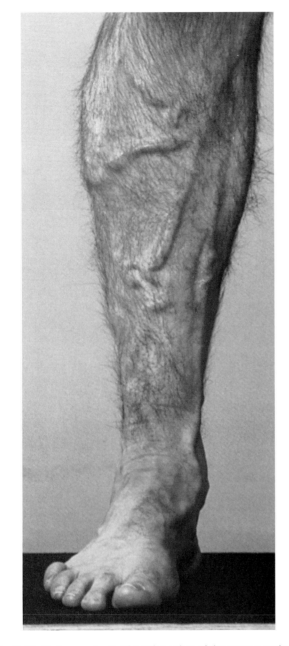

Fig. 1-22. Varicose veins involving branches of the greater saphenous vein.

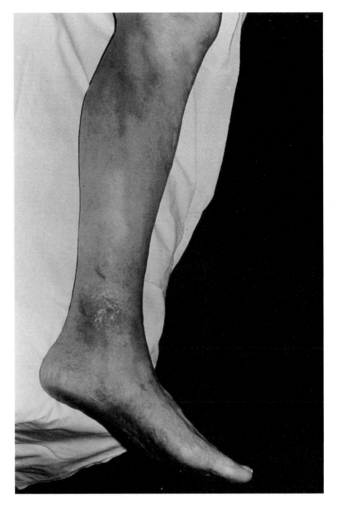

Fig. 1-23. Superficial phlebitis of the greater saphenous vein, presenting as a raised, red, tender, indurated cord.

cause, particularly when they are unilateral, arteriovenous fistulas should be suspected. This is especially true if the varices are in an unusual location or are associated with ulceration, a birthmark, elongation of a limb, or distal gangrene.

Superficial thrombophlebitis (see Chapter 26) is usually an easily diagnosed condition. A raised, red, slightly indurated, warm tender cord is usually present along the course of the involved vein (Fig. 1-23). Erythema nodosum or lymphangitis can produce a somewhat similar picture, although lymphangitis is usually associated with cellulitis and sepsis.

Deep vein thrombosis (DVT) (see Chapter 26) may be present with no clinical signs or symptoms in 50% to 80% of patients. Therefore in a proper setting any change at all in an extremity should be considered venous thrombosis until proven otherwise. Swelling is the most common sign, but any new discomfort in a leg or any increased temperature, any change in color, ranging from pink to reddish-blue, or any increased prominence of the superficial veins (Fig. 1-24) should raise the possibility of DVT. A temperature up to 38° C is compatible with DVT, but a higher temperature or the appearance of shaking chills is not associated with venous thrombosis unless the patient has septic thrombosis. The higher temperature and shaking chills usually indicate that the patient has *cellulitis and lymphangitis*. Localized areas of erythema would also suggest cellulitis (Fig. 1-25) rather than deep venous thrombosis. Erythema of the skin in venous thrombosis should be generalized in the extremity and not localized.

Patients with *phlegmasia cerulea dolens* (venous gangrene) (see Chapter 26) usually present a striking clinical picture (Fig. 1-26). The involved extremity may be markedly swollen, at least distally. The skin is taut, shiny, and deeply cyanotic. Superficial gangrene is followed by more extensive gangrene. Distal pulses are decreased or absent.

Chronic venous insufficiency (see Chapter 28) is most commonly the result of venous valvular damage secondary to remote deep thrombophlebitis. The first sign of venous insufficiency is edema. Prominent superficial veins may also be present. Later, pigmentation, induration, and

dermatitis may occur. A painful, tender, red area of chronic indurated cellulitis can develop up and down the lower calf on the medial side. Venous stasis ulcers usually occur in the region of the ankle in the vicinity of the malleoli, especially the medial malleolus (Fig. 1-27). There is usually brown pigmentation in the surrounding skin, and the leg is often edematous. The ulcers may be moderately painful but are never as painful as ischemic ulcers. The differential diagnosis of leg ulcer is covered in Chapter 37.

LYMPHATIC DISEASE

Lymphedema usually occurs gradually over a period of weeks, months, or even years. It starts as a slight hump of swelling on the dorsum of the foot and swelling around the ankle (Fig. 1-28), then later involves the leg itself. Stasis pigmentation is not present, and usually no superficial veins are visible in the lymphedematous leg. If lymphedema is extensive and long-standing and has been neglected as far as elastic supports are concerned, the tissue may be firm and resistant to pitting because of extensive fibrosis. In this stage the skin may be thickened and verrucous.

Lymphedema should be differentiated from *lipedema*, a painless, symmetric, bilateral deposition of fat in the lower extremities that affects women almost exclusively. The buttocks may also be involved. There is often a history of lipedema in other female members of the family. The distinguishing feature in lipedema is that the adipose tissue, which does not pit, always stops at the ankle thus sparing the foot (Fig. 1-29). For a more extensive differential diagnosis of the swollen leg, see Chapter 38.

A yellow discoloration of the fingernails and/or toenails in a patient with lymphedema may indicate the presence of *"yellow nail syndrome"* (see Chapter 29) with associated chylothorax or chylous ascites.

Patients with lymphedema have an increased suscepti-

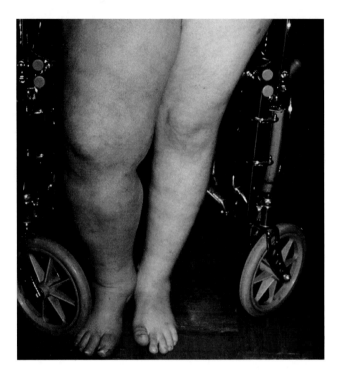

Fig. 1-24. Edema, reddish cyanotic color, and dilated superficial veins in a patient with acute deep venous thrombosis involving the iliac and femoral veins.

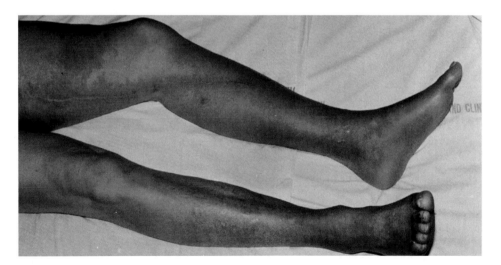

Fig. 1-25. Cellulitis of the left leg with edema and localized areas of erythema, heat, and tenderness. Note the sparing of areas in the thigh.

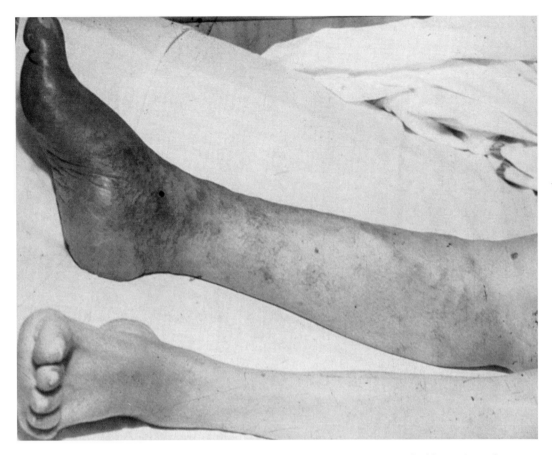

Fig. 1-26. Marked swelling of the leg with severe distal ischemia in a patient with phlegmasia cerulea dolens.

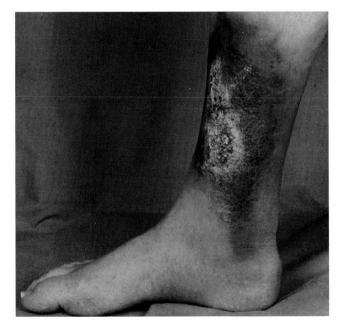

Fig. 1-27. Stasis pigmentation, dermatitis, and ulcerations in a patient with chronic venous insufficiency.

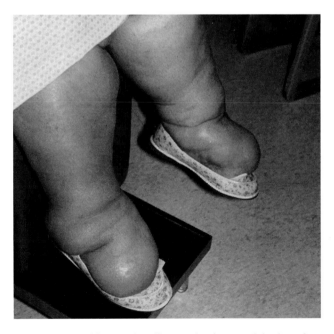

Fig. 1-28. Typical hump of swelling on the dorsum of the feet of a woman with lymphedema praecox.

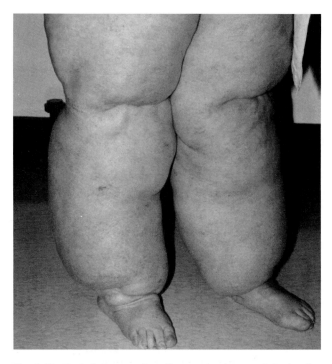

Fig. 1-29. Typical absence of swelling on the dorsum of the feet in this patient with lipedema.

bility to episodes of cellulitis. The portals of entry include fissured skin from athlete's foot, ingrown toenails, or trauma to the skin or nails. Typically the patient suddenly experiences a severe shaking chill with a fever of 38° C to 41° C. This may be preceded by a short period of distress in the involved extremity or proximal lymph nodes. Soon a localized area of erythematous, inflamed skin appears on the extremity and rapidly increases in size. Reddened streaks may occur along the course of inflamed lymphatic vessels, and the proximal lymph nodes are often enlarged, tender, and painful. The response to antibiotic therapy is usually rapid.

ARTERIOVENOUS FISTULAS

Arteriovenous fistulas that affect the limbs (see Chapter 33) can be either congenital or traumatic in origin. A traumatic arteriovenous fistula may be associated with edema of the extremity, prominent veins, and congestive heart failure if the fistula is large enough. Thrills and bruits are common. Congenital arteriovenous fistulas are usually associated with the presence of varicose veins. Thrills and bruits are usually not present. The involved limb may have an increased length and increased muscular development. The temperature of the skin is usually higher than that of the normal extremity. Ulcerations and gangrene may affect the distal parts of the limb.

Birthmarks are present in approximately half the patients with congenital arteriovenous fistulas involving the extremities. They are either port-wine stains (nevus flammeus) or more diffuse hemangiomas. The *Klippel-*

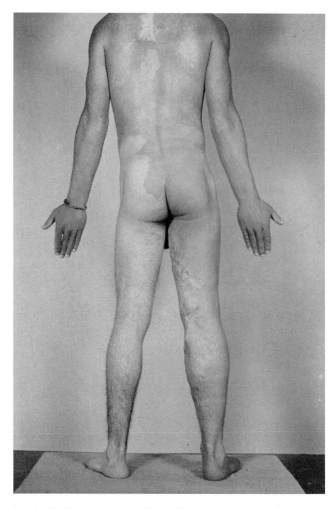

Fig. 1-30. Young man with Klippel-Trenaunay-Weber syndrome, demonstrating the triad of muscular hypertrophy, varicose veins, and port-wine stain.

Trenaunay-Weber syndrome comprises a triad of port-wine stain, muscular hypertrophy, and varicose veins (Fig. 1-30). The patients may also have congenital arteriovenous fistulas or localized areas of agenesis of the deep venous system.

THORACIC OUTLET SYNDROME

The great majority of patients who have evidence of arterial compression during thoracic outlet maneuvers has no symptoms at all. However, symptoms can be produced by compression of the artery, vein, nerves, or combinations of them (see Chapter 31).

Neurologic symptoms are the most common clinical manifestations of thoracic outlet syndrome. Numbness, tingling, or weakness of the fingers, hand, and arm may be intermittent or constant and may or may not be associated with position of the arms above the shoulder level. Arterial symptoms associated with thoracic outlet syndrome include intermittent claudication when working with the

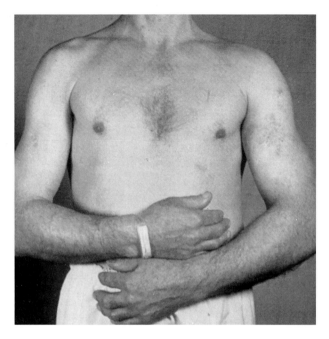

Fig. 1-31. Edema and dilated veins of left arm in a patient with subclavian vein thrombosis secondary to thoracic outlet syndrome.

arms above shoulder level, Raynaud's phenomenon, and distal ischemia caused by emboli from a mural thrombosis of the subclavian artery. A subclavian artery aneurysm can be caused by trauma at the thoracic outlet and can, in turn, cause ischemia as a result of an embolism or thrombosis-.Finally, ischemia can be caused by thrombosis of the subclavian artery itself. Cerebral embolism secondary to retrograde extension of a subclavian artery thrombosis can occur. Venous compression can produce intermittent obstruction of the subclavian vein with intermittent swelling and cyanosis of the arm. Subclavian venous thrombosis, the so-called "effort" thrombosis, can also occur and is the most common cause, other than iatrogenic, of subclavian and axillary venous thrombosis. Clinically this thrombosis can result in edema of the involved arm and dilated superficial veins and venules (Fig. 1-31).

REFERENCE

1. Bates MC and Warren SG: Xanthelasma: clinical indicator of decreased levels of high-density lipoprotein cholesterol, South Med J 82:570, 1989.

CHAPTER TWO

PHYSICAL EXAMINATION

Jess R. Young

Despite new developments in the noninvasive vascular laboratory, new imaging techniques with ultrasound duplex studies, and new arteriographic and venographic techniques, the basic foundation for diagnosis in vascular disease remains a good history and a thorough physical examination. Unfortunately these skills are rarely adequately taught in medical schools and in residency programs. In this chapter the basic examination of the patient with vascular disease is reviewed.

HEAD AND NECK

In checking for arterial disease of the head and neck, the eyes must also be examined carefully. Xanthelasma of the lids may be an indicator that the patient has either hypercholesterolemia or a low level of high-density lipoprotein (HDL) and therefore may be prone to develop atherosclerosis. An arcus senilis in a younger patient may be a sign of premature atherosclerosis. The fundi may reveal evidence of severe hypertension, diabetes mellitus, extensive atherosclerosis, or atheromatous embolization.

Pulse palpation should begin with the temporal artery. The pulsation is always found just anterior to the tragus of the ear (Fig. 2-1). The strength of the pulse should be gauged, and the artery should be examined for the thickening or inflammation found in temporal arteritis. Aneurysms of the temporal artery are also occasionally found.

When palpating for the carotid arteries, the carotid bifurcation area high in the neck should be avoided. Palpation in this area can cause dislodgment of atheromatous emboli that most commonly develop at the bifurcation. Palpation near the carotid sinus at the bifurcation may also produce marked bradycardia or asystole if a hypersensitive carotid sinus reflex is present. The carotid artery can be palpated low in the neck by hooking the fingers or thumb of the examining hand around in front of the sternocleidomastoid muscles (Fig. 2-2). The subclavian artery pulse is most easily appreciated by palpation with the thumb, with the remaining fingers braced behind the neck (Fig. 2-3). As with pulses elsewhere, the strength of the

pulsation on one side of the body should be compared with the pulse on the other side.

Bruits can best be heard with the bell of the stethoscope. The bell fits better in the various areas of the neck and the globe of the eye that will be examined, and low rumbling bruits are heard better with the bell. Bruits heard over the eyeball may indicate intracranial carotid artery stenosis. As much care and detail should be given in describing the bruits as is given in describing heart murmurs. The bruit should be rated as to severity, with either four or six

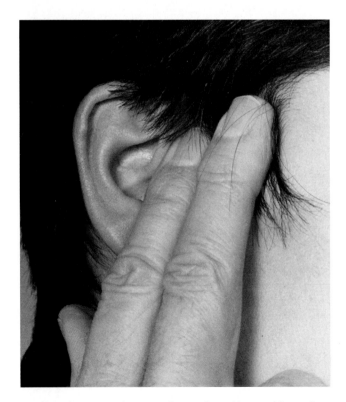

Fig. 2-1. The temporal artery pulse is palpated just anterior to the tragus of the ear.

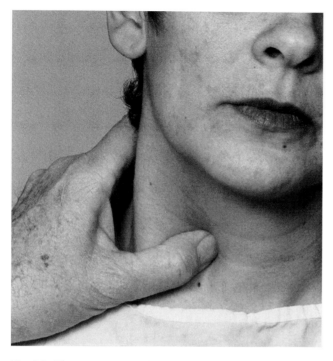

Fig. 2-2. The common carotid pulse should be palpated low in the neck.

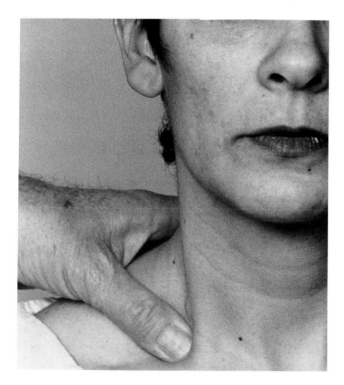

Fig. 2-3. Subclavian artery palpation.

categories. The location of the bruit should be described, whether it is low in the neck, in the midneck, at the angle of the mandible, or over the subclavian artery. The quality of the bruit should be described, whether it is low and rumbling, blowing, or high pitched and musical. Notation should be made as to whether the bruit is purely systolic or whether it extends into diastole.

The examination for carotid artery bruits should begin as high in the neck as possible, getting up under the mandible as far as the bell of the stethoscope can reach (Fig. 2-4). After noting the presence or absence of bruits at this location, the examiner moves the stethoscope slowly down the course of the common carotid artery to the base of the neck (Fig. 2-5), noting whether the bruit is increasing or decreasing in intensity. After the base of the neck is reached, the stethoscope is moved into the supraclavicular area over the subclavian artery (Fig. 2-6), and any bruits in this location are noted. Vertebral artery bruits should be looked for in the area posterior to the sternocleidomastoid muscles (Fig. 2-7). Arteriovenous malformations are sometimes heard more posteriorly in the neck and occipital areas (Fig. 2-8). Finally, auscultation at the aortic and pulmonic valve areas over the upper chest (Fig. 2-9) is done to determine whether or not the neck bruits might be transmitted from the heart. Usually a murmur from an aortic stenosis or sclerosis will be transmitted up into all four neck vessels, the subclavian and the common carotid

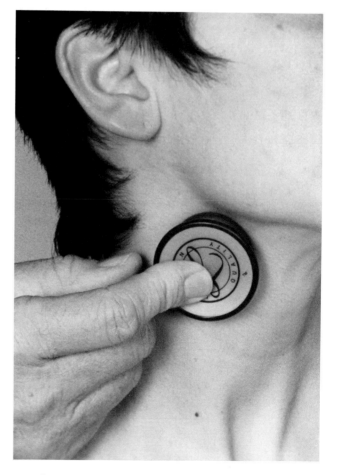

Fig. 2-4. Auscultation for bruits at the carotid bifurcation.

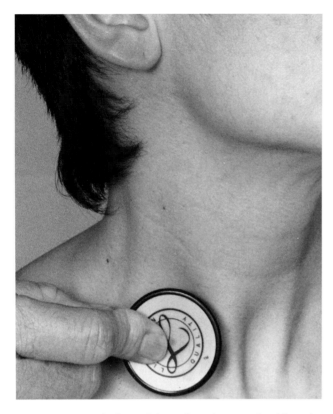

Fig. 2-5. Bruits at the base of the neck can be transmitted from the heart or from carotid, innominate, or subclavian stenosis.

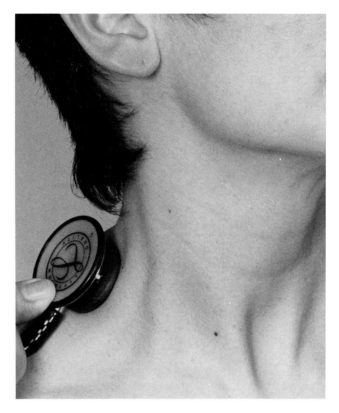

Fig. 2-7. Vertebral artery bruits may be loudest at the posterior cervical triangle area.

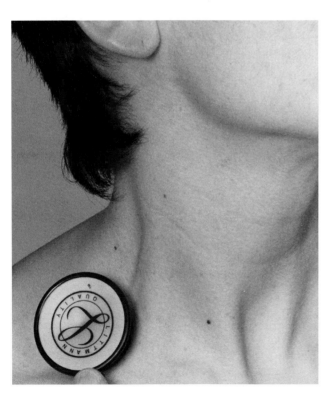

Fig. 2-6. Subclavian artery bruits are usually loudest at the supraclavicular area.

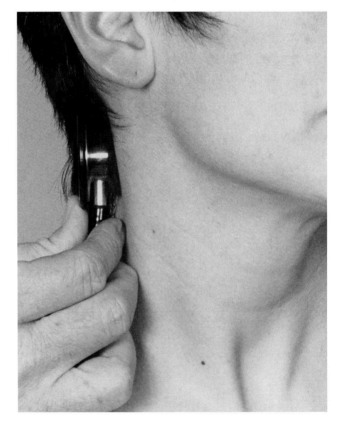

Fig. 2-8. Bruits of arteriovenous malformations may be loudest posteriorly in the neck and occipital areas.

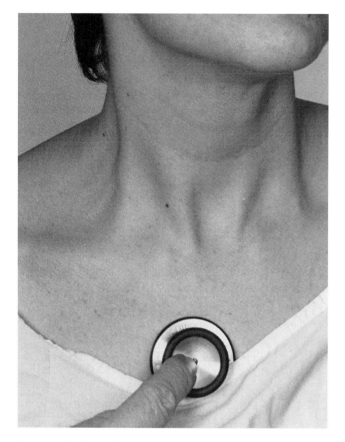

Fig. 2-9. The heart should be checked for murmurs, a possible cause of bruits transmitted to the neck.

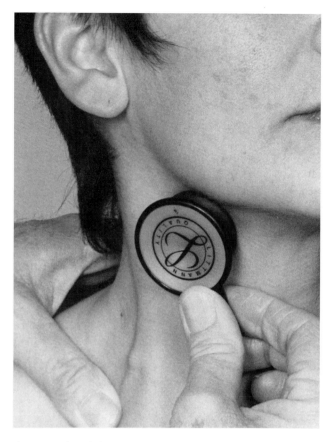

Fig. 2-10. If a subclavian artery bruit is transmitted to the carotid artery area, it will disappear with digital compression of the subclavian artery.

arteries, equally, and the intensity of the bruits will diminish as the stethoscope is moved up the neck.

To determine whether a bruit over the carotid artery is transmitted from a stenosis of the subclavian artery, the examiner compresses the subclavian artery (Fig. 2-10) while listening to the bruit over the carotid. If the bruit disappears, the stenosis is in the subclavian artery and not the carotid artery.

A bruit that is heard during both systole and diastole may indicate a severe arterial stenosis, an arteriovenous malformation, an arteriovenous fistula, or a venous hum. The systolic-diastolic bruit caused by severe carotid stenosis is usually heard at the carotid bifurcation area high in the neck. An important point in this situation is that either a severe stenosis or a complete occlusion of the contralateral internal carotid artery is present in more than 60% of patients.[1] Arteriovenous fistulas are often traumatic in origin. The bruit of an arteriovenous fistula may often be heard in other areas of the head and neck, including the back of the neck and the temple areas. A venous hum is usually heard at the base of the neck. It can be easily detected by lightly compressing the external jugular vein with a finger (Fig. 2-11), thus stopping venous flow and immediately eliminating the continuous bruit.

Dilated jugular veins may indicate an arteriovenous fistula (Fig. 2-12), congestive heart failure, or venous occlusion proximal to the dilated vein. If both sides of the

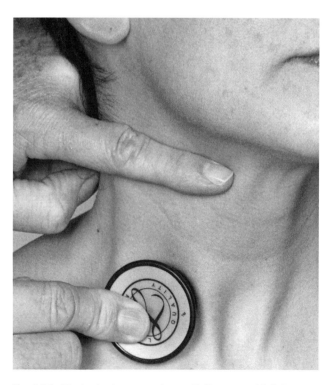

Fig. 2-11. The bruit of a venous hum will disappear with light compression of the external jugular vein.

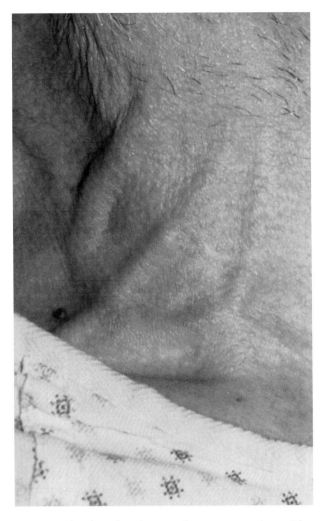

Fig. 2-12. Dilated jugular veins secondary to a traumatic carotid-jugular arteriovenous fistula.

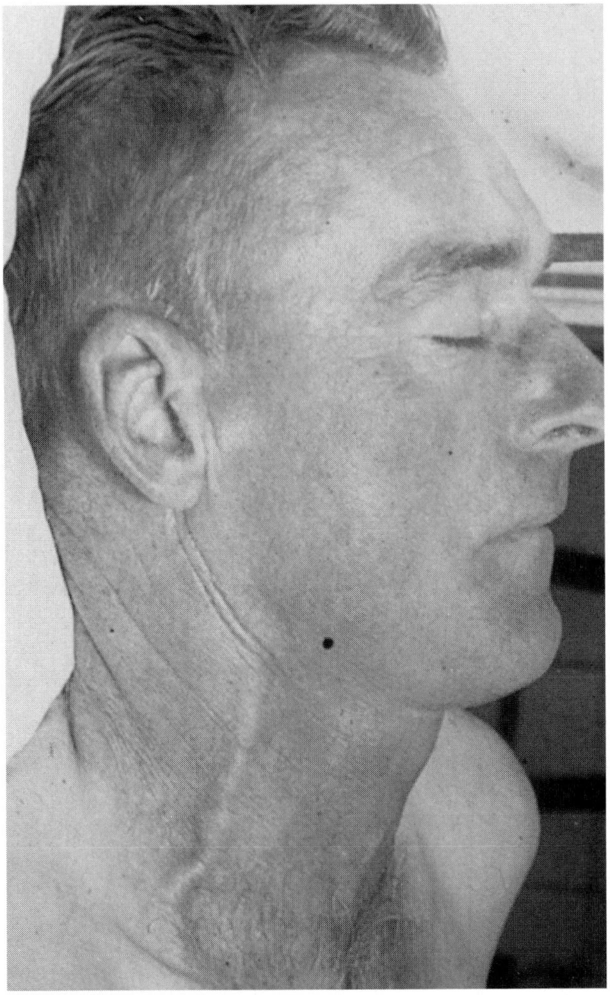

Fig. 2-13. Dilated jugular veins and facial plethora secondary to an acute superior vena caval syndrome caused by an acute dissecting aneurysm.

neck and both arms have dilated veins, a superior vena caval syndrome can be suspected (Fig. 2-13).

UPPER EXTREMITIES

A blood pressure check should be made in both arms to see if there is a significant difference in pressures. A significant difference (more than 10 mm of mercury) would suggest that one of the subclavian arteries or the innominate artery is narrowed or occluded.

The arms should be examined for symmetry. Asymmetry could indicate congenital hypertrophy or atrophy on one side, previous neurologic disease, an arteriovenous fistula on one side, or edema secondary to lymphedema or venous insufficiency. Edema and dilated superficial veins would suggest a previous deep venous thrombosis on that side.

The axillary (Fig. 2-14), brachial (Fig. 2-15), radial (Fig. 2-16), and ulnar pulses (Fig. 2-17) should be palpated. The presence or absence of aneurysms of these arteries should be noted (Fig. 2-18). Auscultation of the arm for bruits that

might suggest arterial stenosis or an arteriovenous fistula should be done. The temperature of the skin of the two arms should be compared.

When indicated, thoracic outlet maneuvers should be done. They are best performed by bracing the patient's shoulder with one hand while the other hand abducts and externally rotates the patient's arm (Fig. 2-19). If the pulse does not obliterate or if symptoms are not produced, further checking would include having the patient look first to one side and then to the other with the chin extended (Fig. 2-20). If the test is still negative, the patient should perform a Valsalva maneuver while looking first to the right and then to the left with the chin extended. A thoracic outlet maneuver is positive when the patient's symptoms are reproduced. As a rule, the pulse will also disappear when the patient's symptoms are reproduced, but this is not necessary for a positive test.

If occlusion of the arteries distal to the wrist are suspected, an Allen test should be done. The patient is instructed to make a tight fist, which will empty most of the blood from the hand and fingers except for the thenar

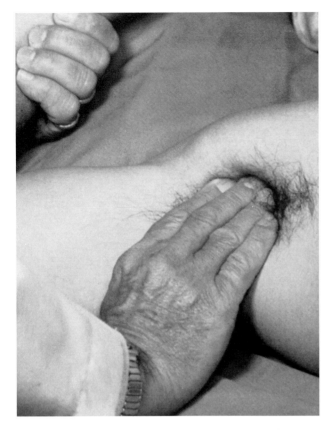

Fig. 2-14. The axillary pulse is felt deep in the axilla.

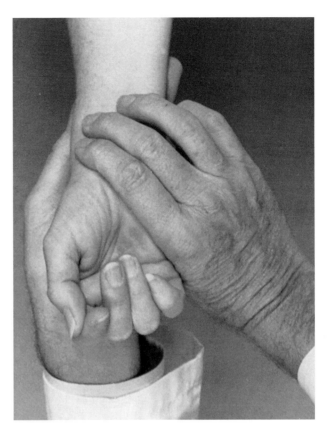

Fig. 2-16. Radial pulse palpation.

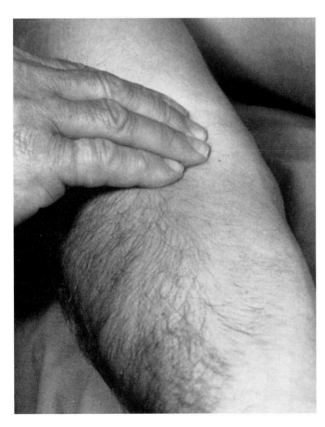

Fig. 2-15. Brachial pulse palpation.

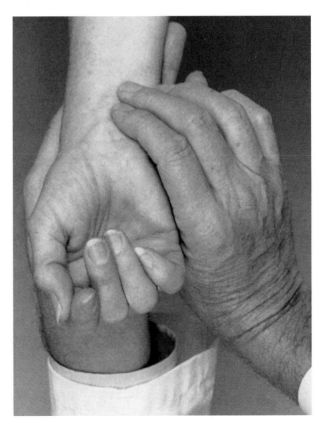

Fig. 2-17. Ulnar pulse palpation.

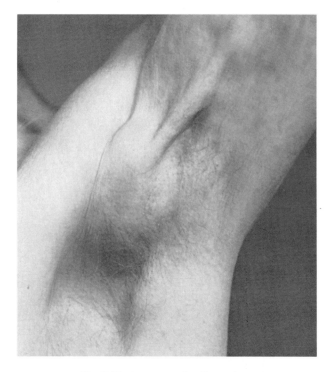

Fig. 2-18. Aneurysm of axillary artery.

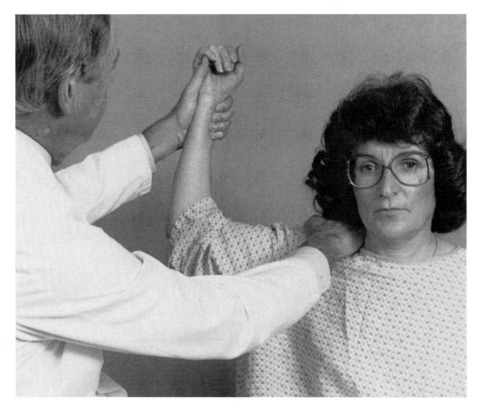

Fig. 2-19. Thoracic outlet maneuver. The patient's shoulder is braced by the examiner's right hand while the left hand abducts and externally rotates the patient's arm. The patient's radial pulse is monitored by the fingers of the examiner's left hand.

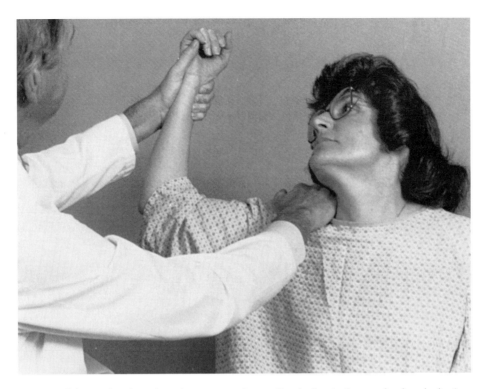

Fig. 2-20. If the routine thoracic outlet maneuver is negative, further testing can be done by having the patient turn the head to one side or the other while extending the chin.

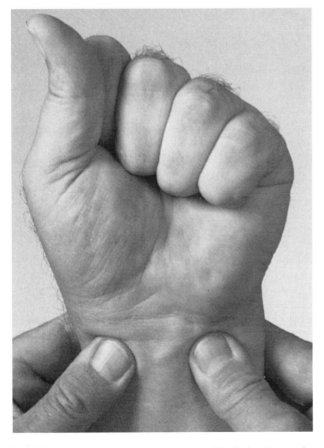

Fig. 2-21. Allen test, showing compression of both the ulnar and radial arteries by the examiner's thumbs.

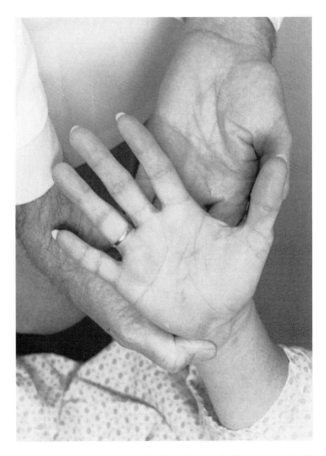

Fig. 2-22. Hyperextension of the hand when the fist is opened will result in no arterial filling of the hand, giving a false-positive Allen test.

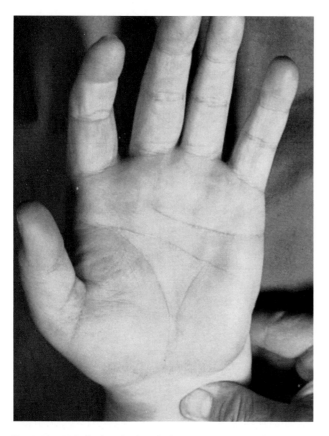

Fig. 2-23. With the hand relaxed, there is rapid arterial filling via the radial artery, with rapid return of color.

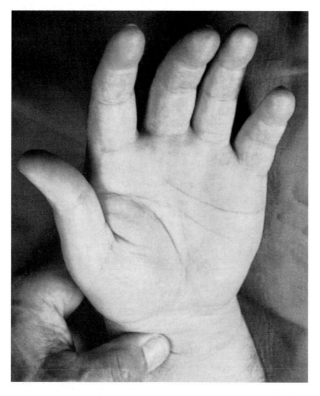

Fig. 2-24. Normal Allen test with rapid return of color when pressure on the ulnar artery is released.

and hypothenar eminences. These eminences are drained of blood by the examiner's swiping his thumbs down across the eminences to the wrist and then with the same motion occluding both the radial and ulnar arteries with his thumbs (Fig. 2-21). The patient then opens his hand, making sure that he does not overextend his fingers. Overextension will cause a false-positive Allen's test (Fig. 2-22). After opening the hand for a few seconds, making sure that the hand stays blanched, one artery is released (Fig. 2-23), either the radial or the ulnar. If there is prompt filling from that artery with a prompt return of color to the hand, the maneuver is repeated; then the second artery is released (Fig. 2-24). Thus the patency of the radial and ulnar arteries are determined. A positive test results when there is no return of color to the blanched hand when the occluded artery is released (Fig. 2-25).

CHEST

The chest reveals little about the patient with vascular disease. Occasionally a large aneurysm of the ascending aorta may be felt as a pulsation high in the chest near the sternum. The sudden appearance of a murmur of aortic insufficiency may be a clue to the presence of a dissecting aneurysm. The presence of dilated veins on the chest may suggest the presence of an axillary or subclavian venous thrombosis (Fig. 2-26) or a superior or inferior vena caval occlusion.

ABDOMEN

In the abdomen a careful check for bruits should be carried out (Fig. 2-27). A systolic-diastolic bruit may indicate a severe stenosis of a renal artery or the presence of an arteriovenous fistula. Bruits are common over atherosclerotic plaques or over aneurysms.

A real attempt should be made to feel the abdominal aorta in all patients. This can be difficult in the obese patient and in the patient with a low pain threshold. The patient must relax his abdominal muscles as much as possible to allow the examiner to feel deep in the abdomen. The aorta should be sought just left of the midline and in the area between the umbilicus and the costal margin. An attempt should be made to measure the width of the abdominal aorta. One hand should try to locate the lateral border of the aorta and the other hand the medial border. Both borders should then be palpated at the same time (Fig. 2-28), using a ruler to get an accurate measurement between the fingertips of the palpating hands. Another maneuver that often is helpful in determining whether the patient has an aneurysm or whether there is merely a tortuous, normal-sized aorta is to roll the aorta back and forth under the fingertips (Fig. 2-29).

A check should be made in the right lower quadrant and left lower quadrant for aneurysms of the iliac arteries.

LOWER EXTREMITIES

The pulse examination of the legs and feet is not difficult, but it takes some practice to develop these skills. While palpating the pulses, the presence or absence of aneurysmal dilation should also be noted.

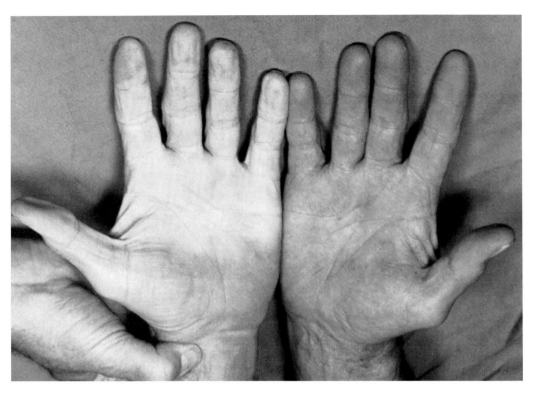

Fig. 2-25. Positive Allen test with no filling via the left ulnar artery.

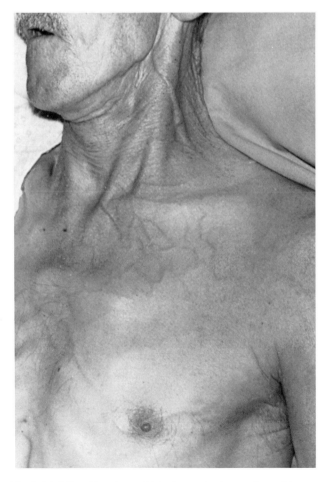

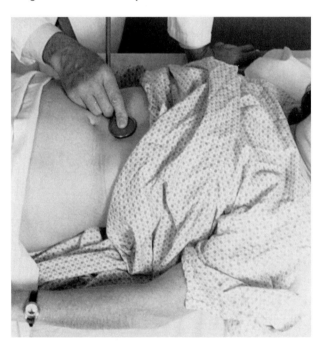

Fig. 2-27. Listening for abdominal bruits, using light pressure on the bell of the stethoscope.

Fig. 2-26. Dilated jugular and left chest veins in a patient with a left subclavian vein occlusion.

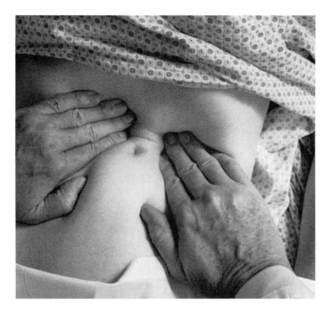

Fig. 2-28. Checking the size of the abdominal aorta.

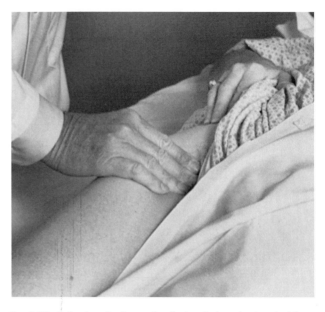

Fig. 2-30. Palpating the femoral pulse just below the inguinal ligament.

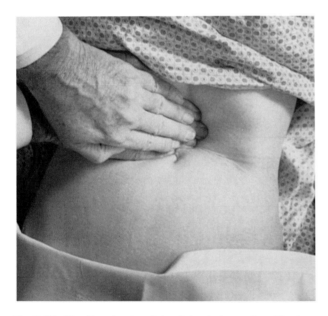

Fig. 2-29. Checking the size of the abdominal aorta by rolling it under the fingertips of the examiner's hand.

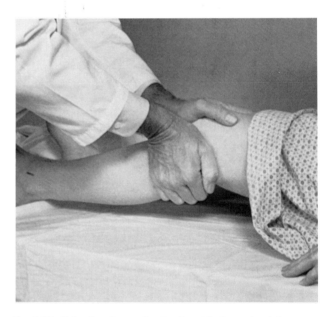

Fig. 2-31. Palpating the popliteal pulse with the patient's knee slightly flexed.

The femoral pulse is palpated just below the inguinal ligament and approximately midway across this ligament (Fig. 2-30). Firm pressure must be applied to feel the pulse, which is rather deep in the groin in most patients.

Physicians have great difficulty in palpating the popliteal pulse. Generally there are three major errors in technique. One is that the location of the popliteal artery is unknown to the examiner. Normally the pulse should be felt directly below the lateral aspect of the patella. The second error is in bending the knee too much at the time of the examination. The knee should be flexed only approximately 10 degrees (Fig. 2-31). The third error is in not palpating deep enough. Firm pressure must be applied

to allow the fingers to go deep in the popliteal space. The pulse should be sought with the pads of the fingers and not the tips of the fingers.

The usual sites for palpating foot pulses are demonstrated in Fig. 2-32. The posterior tibial pulse has quite a variable course posterior to the medial malleolus. Once the skills to palpate the femoral and popliteal pulse are honed, the posterior tibial pulse is one of the more difficult ones to find. The patient's right posterior tibial pulse should be sought with the examiner's left hand, for the curvature of the fingers of the left hand fits well into the curve behind the malleolus (Fig. 2-33). The fingers of the examiner's hand should be spread slightly to minimize the possibility

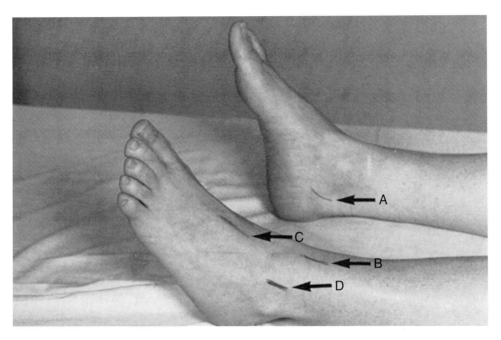

Fig. 2-32. Usual sites for pedal pulse palpation. **A,** Posterior tibial artery. **B,** Anterior tibial artery. **C,** Dorsalis pedis artery. **D,** Perforating branch of peroneal artery.

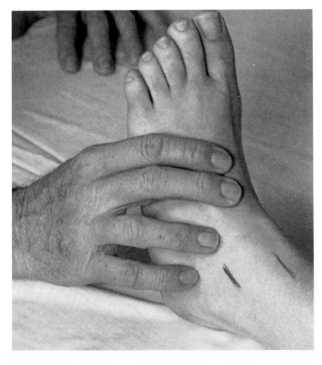

Fig. 2-33. Palpating the posterior tibial artery with the examiner's fingers held slightly apart. The examiner's right hand is used to adjust the angle of the ankle.

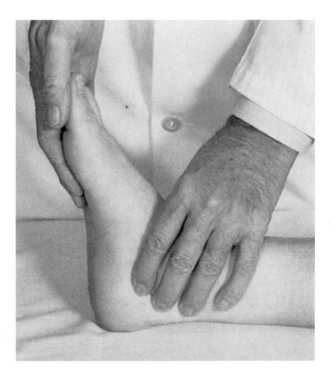

Fig. 2-34. Palpating the dorsalis pedis pulse with a light touch of the pads of the fingers.

of the examiner feeling his own digital pulse and mistaking it for the patient's pulse. The examiner's right hand should be used to adjust the angle of the ankle (Fig. 2-33), for these adjustments may at times be necessary to feel the pulse more easily. The patient's left posterior tibial pulse should be examined by the examiner's right hand, using the left

hand to adjust the angle of the ankle. The dorsalis pedis pulse is usually felt along the line of the second metatarsal bone and is best appreciated by light touch of the pads of the fingers (Fig. 2-34). If the dorsalis pedis pulse cannot be felt, the anterior tibial pulse should be sought (Fig. 2-35). Firm pressure with the pads of the fingers is necessary to

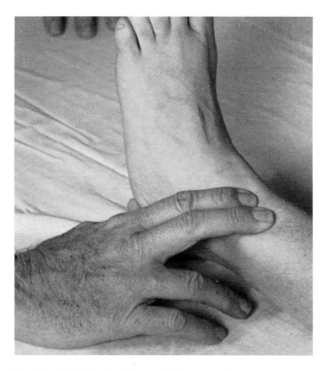

Fig. 2-35. Palpating the anterior tibial pulse with a firm pressure on the pads of the fingers.

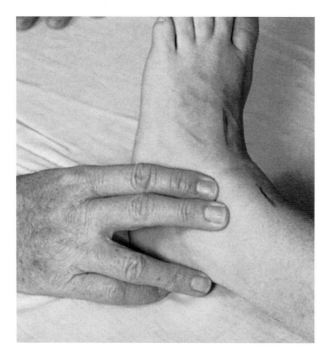

Fig. 2-36. Palpating the perforating branch of the peroneal artery, just anterior to the lateral malleolus.

detect this pulse. If neither the dorsalis pedis pulse nor the anterior tibial pulse can be felt, the perforating branch of the peroneal artery should be sought. This artery usually runs just anterior to the lateral malleolus (Fig. 2-36).

If arterial insufficiency is suspected, the amount of pallor of the feet on elevation should be determined. Both

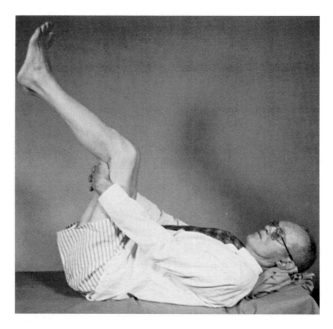

Fig. 2-37. To check for pallor on elevation, the feet must be elevated above the level of the heart.

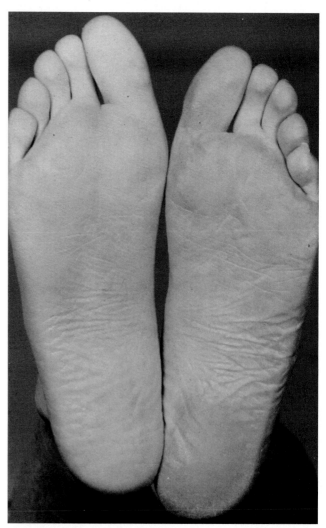

Fig. 2-38. Pallor on elevation is noted in the right foot.

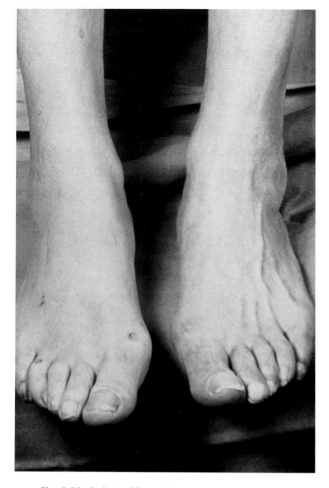

Fig. 2-39. Delay in filling of the veins of the right foot.

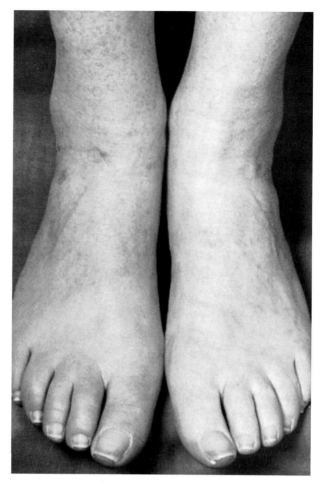

Fig. 2-40. Rubor on dependency is obvious in the right foot.

of the patient's legs and feet should be elevated above the heart level (Fig. 2-37). The color should then be milked from the soles of the feet by gentle pressure; then after approximately 30 seconds the amount of color that reappears is noted. If the patient has significant arterial disease, he will have significant persistent pallor on elevation (Fig. 2-38). This can be graded between 0 and 4+, with 4+ indicating marked pallor.

Following this determination, the patient sits up quickly, and the length of time that it takes the first vein to fill on the dorsum of the foot is recorded (Fig. 2-39). This is the venous filling time, and with normal arterial circulation the first veins should fill within 10 to 15 seconds. In a patient with significant arterial disease there will be a delay in venous filling time up to 30 to 60 seconds or more. After recording the venous filling time, the amount of rubor in the feet after 2 or 3 more minutes should be noted. With significant arterial disease there will be significant rubor on dependency (Fig. 2-40).

For examiners who are not sure of their ability to feel pulses, the investment in a pocket Doppler device (Fig. 2-41) is advisable if patients with vascular disease are being seen in the office. The Doppler systolic pressure at the ankle should be equal to the brachial Doppler systolic pressure. Any decrease in pressure indicates some narrowing of the

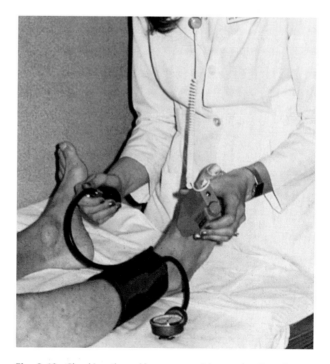

Fig. 2-41. Checking the ankle pressure with a pocket Doppler instrument.

arteries. A decrease of more than 50% at the ankle as compared to the brachial pressure would indicate quite significant narrowing. If the ankle pressure is less than 20% of the brachial pressure, severe narrowing of the arteries is usually present.

As with the upper extremities, the lower extremities should be examined closely for asymmetry, edema, dilated veins, signs of inflammation, and stasis pigmentation. Although the condition of the skin, the hair, and the nails is not always a good indicator of arterial insufficiency, this observation should be noted. The presence or absence of dermatophytosis should be determined, for the fissures associated with dermatophytosis are often the portals of entry for recurrent cellulitis and lymphangitis.

REFERENCE

1. Graor RA, deWolfe VG, and Elliott I: A clinical vignette: the clinical significance of systolic-diastolic bruits in the carotid arteries, Cleve Clin Q 51:155, 1984.

CHAPTER THREE

NONINVASIVE VASCULAR LABORATORY AND VASCULAR IMAGING

D. Eugene Strandness, Jr.

The objective evaluation of diseases of the circulatory system has been best approached by routine clinical appraisal combined with methods of documenting the site(s) of involvement and the functional significance of the disorder. This is best done by combining the information obtained from the history and the physical examination with that obtained from both noninvasive and invasive diagnostic procedures. With the evolution of the vascular diagnostic laboratory, we no longer have to rely entirely on the information obtained by the invasive diagnostic tests to both plan and predict the likelihood of success. In addition, objective evaluation of the outcome of interventional procedures can now regularly be achieved by the proper application of noninvasive vascular testing.

Although the importance of the history and the physical examination cannot be doubted, they should serve as just the starting point in the evaluation. Often it was the practice to proceed directly with angiography to outline the site(s) of disease; however, such an approach should be used only if some form of intervention is being considered. In addition, there are now areas where angiographic studies may be avoided entirely, resulting in considerable savings for the health care system without any adverse effects on the outcome of therapy. This practice will continue and grow as we gain more experience.

I became convinced of the need for good noninvasive testing when I tried to assess the outcome of arterial procedures through a review of hospital records. It soon became apparent that it was often difficult to tell from a review of the hospital record whether a patient was indeed improved after surgical therapy and it was difficult to determine the extent of improvement. This led to a search for better methods of evaluation that would provide objective evidence that could be used, not only for evalu-

ating the initial event, but also for follow-up purposes as well.[1] The evolution of the methods of evaluation described in this chapter serves as a suitable outline of the status of the field and what we may anticipate in the future.

To maintain some continuity, the discussion focuses on areas of clinical interest, dealing with the patients as they appear and how the available testing procedures may be of value.

PERIPHERAL ARTERIAL SYSTEM

Those diseases that affect the arterial supply of the upper and lower extremity are discussed in this section. Although the majority of the diseases affects the large- and medium-sized arteries (those with proper names), other disorders that involve the microcirculation also benefit from referral to the vascular laboratory. For the large- and medium-sized arteries the most common disorders include atherosclerosis, aneurysmal disease, and thromboangiitis obliterans. The level and extent of involvement of atherosclerosis and thromboangiitis obliterans are somewhat different, and the questions that need answers are also different. In general, atherosclerosis is a disease of branch points and bifurcations, but for unknown reasons it spares those arteries distal to the origin of the subclavian artery.[2] Thromboangiitis obliterans involves the distal medium-sized arteries of the legs and the palmar and digital arteries of the hand.[3,4] Although a history of instep claudication and cold sensitivity may suggest the diagnosis of thromboangiitis obliterans and serve to distinguish it from atherosclerosis, noninvasive testing may be of some value in making this distinction. Although trauma to the major arteries is common, it is considered under the category of "acute ischemia" since its important clinical manifestations are usually in this area.

For most patients the diagnosis of arterial narrowing and occlusion is made on the basis of a history of intermittent claudication, the presence of arterial bruits, and the detection of pulse deficits. The typical patient with atherosclerosis will have disease that involves major proximal arterial segments (popliteal to aorta), with thromboangiitis involving the arteries of the distal leg, and in approximately half of cases, the arteries of the distal arm and hand. A very important subset of patients are those with diabetes mellitus (particularly the type II, non–insulin-dependent patients) who have a different pattern and distribution of atherosclerosis.[5,6] These patients have less involvement of the aortoiliac segment with equal occurrence in the femoropopliteal segment but more extensive occlusions in the tibial and peroneal arteries. In addition, it is not at all unusual for medial calcification (Mönckeberg's medial sclerosis) to be present in the arteries below the knee. However, medial calcification (while unique to patients with diabetes) bears no relationship to the arteriosclerosis obliterans that frequently involves the same arterial segments.[2]

The information that may be obtained from a referral to the vascular laboratory depends on the patient presentation and the issues to be resolved. The testing procedures used vary in complexity, with each providing information that may or may not be necessary or complementary for the diagnosis and planning of therapy. It is thus important to know what type of information can be obtained and how the data may be of assistance. These tests can be considered in the categories of screening and planning of therapy.

Screening Tests

If one assumes that the diagnosis can be made on the basis of the history and physical examination alone, under what circumstances would further testing be needed? The noninvasive tests are done to confirm the diagnosis and provide an estimate of the extent of the involvement. Screening tests include three basic procedures of value: measurement of limb blood pressure, exercise testing, and assessment of velocity patterns.

LIMB BLOOD PRESSURE. The measurement of blood pressure is the most commonly applied noninvasive test of cardiovascular function. It is primarily done for detecting high blood pressure but is also of value in evaluating hypotensive states. It may be the best single indicator of how well perfusion is being maintained. Although not often thought of in this manner, acute and chronic arterial occlusion produces regional hypotension, the magnitude of which is determined by the extent of the disease and the status of the collateral circulation. If anything is done to improve the circulation by removing or bypassing the areas of obstruction, this action would be immediately recognized by an increase in the intraarterial pressure distal to the site of involvement.

One of the impediments to the measurement of arterial pressure distal to sites of occlusion is that the usual auscultatory method is not applicable. It is necessary to use sensors distal to a pneumatic cuff that can detect when flow is restored during cuff deflation.[7,8] These methods are able to measure systolic pressure but not diastolic pressure.

This is not a major problem since it is the systolic pressure that is the first to fall with arterial narrowing and is the most sensitive to changes in resistance to flow. The most commonly available sensors include the continuous wave Doppler flowmeter, photoplethysmography, and strain-gauge plethysmography. The most common method in use is the Doppler device, which has the advantage of being able to measure pressure in any artery in which flow can be detected.

The measurements of pressure with the Doppler device can be done at the time the patient is first seen. However, the physician, nurse, or technician must know how to do the test properly. For the test to be reliable and useful it must be done in the following manner: (1) the arm systolic pressure should always be measured with the Doppler device as well, for the value obtained by the auscultatory method is not adequate; (2) the pressure must be recorded in both arms and both tibial arteries at the ankle; (3) the systolic pressure is taken at that point at which flow is first detected during cuff deflation and not at the point it disappears during cuff inflation; and (4) both the absolute levels of pressure and the ankle/arm (A/A) index are recorded.[9]

What is normal? The systolic pressure in the arterial system increases from the central aorta to the periphery.[9,10] This is due to the fact that the arteries toward the periphery become stiffer. In addition, reflections from the branch points, bifurcations, and arterioles amplify the systolic pressure. The mean pressure, on the other hand, is decreasing, permitting flow to occur toward the distal limb. Given the fact that the systolic pressure is being amplified, the A/A index is 1.0 or greater in healthy patients. Since there may be some variability in the measurement, we have elected to use a value of greater than 0.95 as normal.

Since patients with diabetes mellitus often have medial calcification in their tibial and peroneal arteries, the measurement of the A/A index may not be possible or result in artifactually high ankle pressures. To take this fact into account, a workshop was held in 1992 to make recommendations concerning the assessment of arterial circulation in diabetic patients.[11] The recommendations can be summarized as follows:

1. If the A/A index is less than 0.90, occlusive arterial disease should be considered present.
2. The variability in the measurement is ±0.15.
3. When medial calcification is present or suspected, the systolic pressure must be measured from the toe either with a photoplethysmograph or by the strain-gauge technique.
4. The toe systolic pressure can also be compared with that of the arm—the toe systolic pressure index (TSPI). This should normally be greater than 0.60. The variability in this measurement is ±0.17.

When an area of narrowing exceeds 50% in terms of diameter reduction or occlusion, the systolic pressure will fall beyond the site of involvement (Fig. 3-1). The magnitude of the pressure fall is a reflection of two things—the magnitude of the resistance offered by the stenosis (occlusion) and that offered by the collateral arteries bypassing

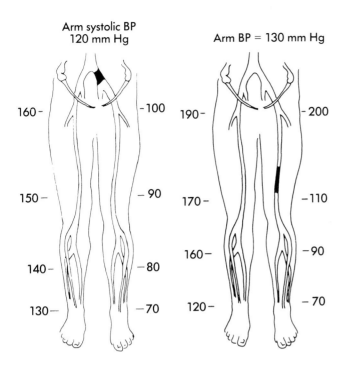

Arm systolic BP
120 mm Hg

Arm BP = 130 mm Hg

Fig. 3-1. Systolic pressures recorded from two patients with arterial occlusions in the common iliac artery and superficial femoral artery. There is a large drop in systolic pressure across the areas of obstruction. *(From Strandness DE Jr: Peripheral arterial disease, Boston, 1969, Little, Brown & Co.)*

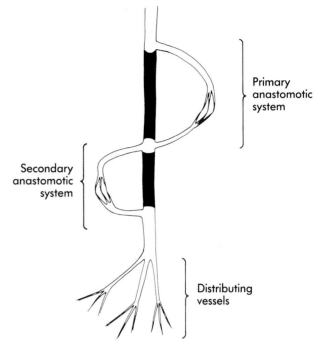

Fig. 3-2. With multiple levels of occlusion the resistance to flow offered by collateral arteries is additive. This explains why the ankle systolic pressures distal to multiple levels of involvement are lower than found with single occlusions.

the area of involvement. If there are multiple levels of stenosis or occlusion, the systolic pressure level measured distal to the last area of involvement will reflect the additive resistances offered by the collateral circuits, which are in series[12] (Fig. 3-2). In general terms, in patients with chronic occlusive arterial disease an A/A index of greater than 0.5 is seen with single segments of occlusion. With levels below this value, it is likely that multiple levels of involvement are present.

The absolute levels of pressure at the ankle and the digits may also be useful in providing a rough estimate of the extent of the perfusion. It has been my experience that levels greater than 50 mm Hg are consistent with normal tissue perfusion, whereas levels below this become worrisome, particularly if an open lesion is present and the prospects for healing without intervention become important.

The TSPI can also be of help in predicting healing of open lesions. If the TSPI is less than 30 mm Hg, healing is very unlikely to occur unless more blood is brought to the extremity.[13]

In addition to measuring the blood pressure at the ankle and digits, it is possible to estimate the pressure at the level of the calf and at the low and high thigh.[9,14] This is done by placing the pneumatic cuffs at these levels and inflating them to suprasystolic levels to interrupt flow. The Doppler sensor is placed in the same locations at the ankle that are used to measure ankle pressure. The pressures that are recorded by this method will be artifactually high, and this fact must be taken into account when this procedure is used. This is due to the fact that the cuffs used may not

Table 3-1. Summary of Systolic Blood Pressures in the Limbs and Their Interpretation

Measurement Site	Range of Values
Ankle pressure	Normally greater than brachial pressure
Ankle pressure index	Normally 1.0-1.2; hemodynamically significant <0.95
Ankle pressure after exercise	Normally drops <20% of baseline; returns to preexercise levels in 3 minutes or less
Proximal thigh pressure	Normally 30-40 mm Hg higher than brachial pressure
Segmental pressures	Normally <20 mm Hg difference between two levels of limb
Toe pressure	Normally >60% of brachial pressure
Toe indexes	Normally >0.60; hemodynamically significant lesion, <0.60; rest pain, <0.15

effectively transmit the pressure to the vessels deep in the leg. Those interested in reviewing this problem further are urged to review the work of Carter,[9] who has examined this issue in great detail. The results of measuring systolic limb pressures and their interpretation are summarized in Table 3-1.

Another method used to assess the perfusion at various

levels of the limb is the pulse-volume recorder (PVR). This device records the pulsatile volume changes that occur in the limb with each heartbeat. The pneumatic cuffs used for this purpose are the same as used for the measurement of limb blood pressures and in the same locations. A measured quantity of air is injected into the cuff until a preset pressure is reached. As the limb expands with each heartbeat, the pressure in the cuff changes, and this can be recorded on a strip chart. In general, a 1 mm Hg pressure change in the cuff will produce a 20 mm chart deflection. The waveform by its phasic characteristics can provide information concerning the nature of the arterial system at that level. Extensive studies have been done establishing PVR categories based on the magnitude of the deflection noted at each level of the limb. They in turn can be related to the location of the occlusive disease, giving rise to the finding. For more complete information the reader is urged to review the work of Raines[15] who was the person who developed this method for clinical use.

ASSESSMENT OF VELOCITY PATTERNS. Vascular laboratory studies may include a survey with the continuous wave Doppler flowmeter at the following standard sites: (1) external iliac–common femoral artery; (2) proximal, mid, and distal superficial femoral artery; (3) popliteal artery; and (4) tibial arteries at the ankle. By such scanning it is possible roughly to localize the areas of involvement because the method is used without imaging; thus one cannot always be certain the intended vessel is being evaluated. Nonetheless, it does serve a useful purpose for screening. As is discussed shortly, more definitive information can be obtained with duplex scanning of the arterial supply to the lower limbs.

The normal arterial velocity patterns have characteristic features that are altered by the presence of arterial stenoses that exceed 50% (diameter reduction) and total occlusion. The normal patterns from the level of the abdominal aorta to the arteries at the ankle are similar, with three separate and distinct phases easily seen on a hard-copy spectral display of the waveform.[16] They include the forward-flow velocity associated with myocardial contraction, the reverse-flow component that occurs in late systole and early diastole, and a secondary forward-flow component that is seen in late diastole (Fig. 3-3). When there is a high-grade stenosis or total occlusion, blunting of the systolic peak occurs, with loss of the reverse-flow component resulting in a monophasic waveform. If the normal triphasic waveform is noted, it is very unlikely that significant disease is proximal to the recording site. The finding of a monophasic waveform is *certain* evidence of disease proximal to the recording site.

The upper extremity can be assessed in a similar fashion. The waveforms from the subclavian artery commonly show the three components seen in the lower-extremity arteries. However, those recorded from the brachial, radial, and ulnar arteries may not show the reverse-flow component in up to one half of healthy individuals. This may be due to the fact that the resistance to flow is less than that seen uniformly in the lower limbs in which the reverse-flow component is always normally seen. It is also possible to survey the hand's flow patterns in the palmar arch, the digital arteries, and the tip of the fingers. In fact, the most accurate way to determine the status of the palmar arch is to use the continuous wave Doppler sensor. This can be done by listening over the radial and ulnar sides of the

Blood velocities in the lower extremities

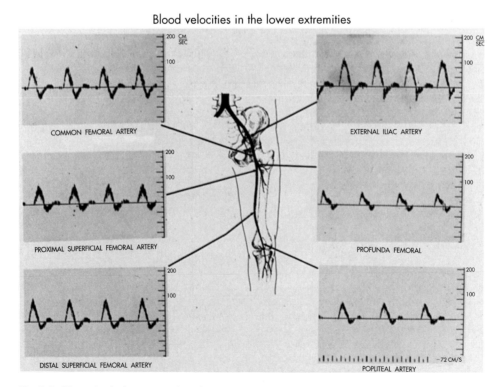

Fig. 3-3. Normal velocity patterns found in peripheral arteries. The triphasic component is seen at all levels.

palmar arch while the two arteries are sequentially occluded. This is a much better method than using Allen's
test, which depends on the appearance of the hand, with
clenching and release of the hand when the arteries at the
wrist are sequentially occluded. With arterial stenosis and
occlusion, the velocity patterns observed are similar to
those seen in the lower limbs.

EXERCISE TESTING. The typical patient with intermittent claudication has a history of pain in the leg with
exercise that is relieved with rest. The major diagnostic
features are a walk-pain-rest cycle that is constant from day
to day.[17] In addition, the pain is always made worse by an
activity that increases the work load such as going up a hill
or stairs. When this history is obtained and combined with
pertinent physical findings, the diagnosis is nearly certain,
with the only remaining questions concerning its severity
and how much it interferes with the patient's life-style.

An increasing problem in our society is the aging patient
who may develop neurospinal problems that produce pain
in the limbs with exercise that may be confused with
intermittent claudication.[18,19] The neurospinal problem
has several characteristic features that can be recognized
on the basis of the history alone. The walk-pain-rest cycle
is not constant from day to day; these patients have good
days and bad days. In addition, the pain may be brought on
by sitting or standing. Some patients also have to lie down
for pain relief—something never required for patients who
have true claudication.

Stress testing is commonly used for evaluation of cardiac performance because it is recognized that it provides a
much better index of myocardial perfusion. The principles
are similar for the legs. There are differences in how the test
is done and how the performance is estimated. In this

regard performance is gauged in two ways: (1) the duration
of the walking time and (2) the ankle systolic blood
pressure response to the walk.

The work load to which the patient is subjected is
modest. The speed and elevation of the treadmill used for
this purpose vary in different laboratories. In general, the
walking speed is 1½ to 2 miles per hour, with an elevation
grade of 10% to 12%. Using this walking speed and
elevation, most people can perform the test unless they
have significant cardiac, rheumatologic, or pulmonary
problems. We limit the amount of time the patient walks
to 5 minutes. If he can walk this long, he is mildly symptomatic and should rarely be considered for interventional
therapy. On the other hand, we have found that walking
times less than 1 minute represent severely limiting claudication. For walking times of 3 to 5 minutes, the impact
depends on the patient's needs and daily activities. If, for
example, the patient is a postman and needs to walk for a
living, even mild claudication may be a problem.

To estimate the hemodynamic response to walking, the
changes in the ankle systolic blood pressure must be
measured, as must the response of the pulse-volume
recorder, if used, after the patient resumes the supine
position. A healthy person walking at this rate and elevation for 5 minutes will sustain little or no drop in ankle
systolic pressure after the exercise is completed.[20] However, if the patient has true claudication and it was the basis
for the initial symptoms, there will be a large drop in ankle
pressure and flattening of the pulse volume recording with
a very delayed recovery to the preexercise levels[21] (Fig. 3-4).
True intermittent claudication cannot occur without a
drop in the ankle systolic blood pressure and a diminution
of the pulse volume amplitude. This is true even if the

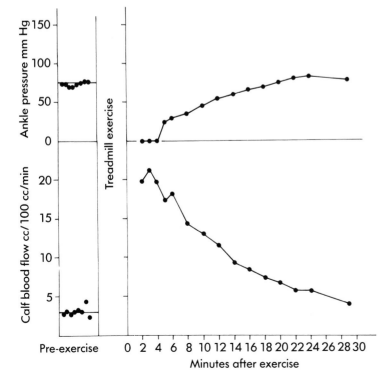

Fig. 3-4. Ankle systolic blood pressure as compared with calf
blood flow in a patient with intermittent claudication. The
abnormal response is characterized by a large fall in the
blood pressure with a very delayed recovery time.

patient's walking time is less than 1 minute. What this means is that if the pressure does not fall, other causes for the leg pain must be sought.[22]

What of the circumstance in which the patient has arterial disease and also suffers from an associated condition such as spinal canal stenosis? When this occurs and when the nonvascular problem is responsible for the leg discomfort, it is this problem that usually prevents the patient from continued walking, and there is usually a disparity between the magnitude of the ankle blood pressure fall and its recovery time. For example, if a patient with true claudication is forced to stop in less than 1 minute of walking because of ischemic pain, the ankle systolic pressure often will fall to unrecordable levels and require in excess of 30 minutes of recovery. Conversely, in a patient with pseudoclaudication the pressure decrease—if any occurs—will not be of the magnitude seen with true intermittent claudication.

One or more of the above diagnostic tests may supply most of the answers to questions that may arise at the time the patient is first seen, providing enough data to confirm the initial impression and to provide the necessary information about what must be done next. The clinical presentation, along with the results of this screening procedure, will determine the course of action to follow.

Duplex Scanning

Since duplex scanning potentially can evaluate the location and extent of disease for all levels of supply to the lower limbs, it may serve as a useful planning study for the direction of therapy.[16,23] Under what circumstances might it provide definitive data? Nine circumstances are described.

1. Since angioplasty has become the standard method of treating isolated stenoses in the aortoiliac segment, being able to predict who may need the procedure would be a great help. Given these considerations, we scan patients who may well fit into this category; and if they have a stenosis, they are scheduled for angioplasty. If they are occluded, some form of direct arterial surgery is planned after arteriography has been performed. Although we continue to use preoperative arteriography to define the location and extent of the arterial disease, it is becoming clear that duplex scanning can provide functional information that is useful not only in planning therapy but in monitoring its outcome as well.

2. For patients with severe occlusive disease (A/A index of less than 0.5) it is likely there are multiple levels of disease. In this situation it is essential to define the location and extent of involvement in planning therapy. Questions always arise when there is a stenosis in the aortoiliac area combined with femoropopliteal disease. It is important to know to what extent the proximal disease contributes to the ischemia.

3. The saphenous veins of patients who will undergo femoropopliteal or femorotibial bypass grafting are scanned and measured before any procedure.[24] It is possible to define the dimensions of the vein and also

to identify anomalous branches or duplications that might compromise the procedure, thus removing the uncertainty often present at the time of the operation in defining the proximal and distal sites of insertion.

4. Any patient who has had an interventional procedure, be it angioplasty or surgery, and then is seen with new complaints should be scanned with the duplex scanner.[25] This procedure will nearly always define the location and extent of the problem and permit in some cases a direct approach to the involved segment without the need for arteriography.

5. All patients with suspected aortic or peripheral aneurysms should be scanned to permit an estimate of the size and extent of the lesion. If the patient also has occlusive arterial disease, this procedure will permit locating it and estimating its extent.

6. Those patients initially seen with microemboli to the foot will benefit from a scan since it may identify the source of the embolic material. This information may then be used to direct the arteriographer to those segments in which the offending source may be found.

7. With the common use of coronary arteriography and angioplasty, it is not unusual for groin masses to develop for which one considers the diagnosis of false aneurysm versus hematoma. Duplex scanning is the ideal method for making this distinction. In addition, the transducer used in duplex scanning can often be used to compress the aneurysm, halting flow into it and permitting thrombosis to occur. This can be curative.[26]

8. Another indication for duplex scanning is for the patient in the intensive care unit who has a balloon pump in place. The measurement of the A/A index along with a scan of the limb may be necessary to verify both the status of the inflow to that limb and any compromise of the outflow arteries.

9. There is increasing use of duplex scanning in the operating room to immediately verify the outcome of arterial reconstruction. This may be particularly important for cases in which an operative failure could be disastrous for the patient. For example, when renal artery reconstructions are carried out, loss of the graft could mean loss of the kidney. Dougherty et al[27] reported on their experience in 35 cases in which technical problems were discovered by duplex scanning in 10.9%. Correction of these problems resulted in a satisfactory outcome.

What Information Is Available?

To assess the contribution of arterial lesions to the clinical picture properly, it is necessary both to localize the disease and estimate its hemodynamic significance. Ultrasonic duplex scanners combine imaging of the underlying blood vessel with the capability of estimating the velocity changes at that site by the use of a pulsed Doppler device. Although the image resolution of the modern systems has greatly improved, it is still not sufficient to permit an estimate of the degree of narrowing on the basis of the image alone. It is also necessary to measure the velocity change in an involved segment to estimate the degree of narrowing. Although the use of an absolute velocity change in centimeters per second would be helpful, there is so much variability even in healthy individuals that it is preferable to relate the velocity changes from one segment of the artery to the next as the most reliable method of documenting the extent of diameter reduction.[16,23] As the artery becomes narrowed, the velocity increase in the stenosis will increase in a predictable fashion, permitting a reasonable estimate of the degree of narrowing at the site where the velocity increase is recorded.

In documenting such changes by duplex scanning it was necessary to develop the diagnostic criteria and compare the results to those with arteriography and/or to the variability found in arteriographic estimates of the degree of stenosis. Jager, Ricketts, and Strandness[16] carried out such a study and found the following criteria suitable for documentation of the status of the arterial system:

1. The normal velocity patterns in all peripheral arteries are monotonously similar with the three phases: forward flow, a prominent reverse-flow component, and a secondary late forward-flow component (Fig. 3-3). If the velocity is recorded from a center stream site of the artery, no spectral broadening will be present.
2. When the arterial wall becomes roughened, the most prominent changes are seen in the development of spectral broadening without an increase in peak systolic velocity. The reverse flow component is preserved. These patients are labeled as having a 1% to 19% narrowing (Fig. 3-5).

3. The next category of stenosis is a 20% to 49% diameter reduction that is not hemodynamically significant at resting levels of flow. For this category an increase in the peak systolic velocity is greater than 30% but less than 100% from the preceding arterial segment, with preservation of the reverse-flow component (Fig. 3-5).
4. For the hemodynamically significant lesions (greater than 50%) the increase in peak velocity is greater than 100% in the stenosis, with loss of reverse flow and the presence of marked spectral broadening (Fig. 3-5).
5. For total occlusions there is no detectable flow within a visualized segment.

Using these criteria, the results of duplex scanning as compared to arteriography are summarized in Table 3-2. The results when two radiologists review the same films are shown in Table 3-3. The results of these studies are important in several ways, with the very high negative predictive value of particular note.[16,23] This is important because it shows that if the duplex scan predicts that a particular segment is normal "hemodynamically" (has a less than 50% stenosis), it is likely to be accurate.

Legemate et al[28] used slightly different criteria for the detection of a greater than 50% diameter–reducing stenosis. They used an increase of more than 150% in peak systolic velocity from one segment to another. For the aortoiliac area this resulted in a sensitivity of 92% with a specificity of 98%. In the femoropopliteal area the sensitivity was 90% with a specificity of 100%.

Edwards et al[29] tested the accuracy of duplex scanning

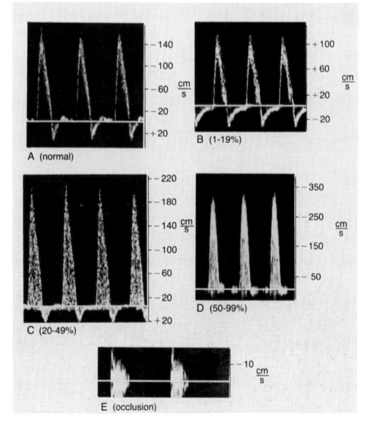

Fig. 3-5. Velocity pattern seen with varying degrees of involvement with atherosclerosis. *(From Moneta GL and Strandness DE Jr: Peripheral arterial duplex scanning, J Clin Ultrasound 15:645, 1987.)*

Table 3-2. Comparison of Duplex Scanning with Arteriography

Arterial Segment	n	Sensitivity	Specificity	PPV	NPV
Aortic*	25	1.00	1.00	1.00	1.00
Iliac	110	0.89	0.90	0.75	0.96
Common femoral	50	0.67	0.98	0.80	0.96
Superficial femoral	123	0.84	0.93	0.90	0.88
Popliteal	37	0.75	0.97	0.86	0.93
All segments	393	0.82	0.92	0.80	0.93

*No aortic segments had >50% stenosis. *PPV*, Positive predictive value; *NPV*, negative predictive value.

Table 3-3. Accuracy of Duplex Scanning for Various Categories of Disease Compared to Reading of the Same Film by Two Radiologists

Disease Grade (% Stenosis)	Arteriography vs Duplex Scanning (% Agreement)	Radiologists' Arteriographic Reading, 1 vs 2 (% Agreement)
Normal	81	68
1-19	83	58
16-49	83	57
50-95	60	70
Occlusion	94	100

for predicting which patients with occlusive disease might be candidates for angioplasty. There were 110 arteriograms performed that were preceded by duplex studies. In 50 cases (45%) the duplex studies suggested that angioplasty would be feasible. This was successfully performed in 47 of the cases (94%). An example of the type of case in which duplex studies are helpful is shown in Fig. 3-6. The demonstration of a stenotic common iliac artery is good evidence that angioplasty should be done and should be successful.

Follow-up Care

Since patients with occlusive arterial disease are not cured by any form of intervention, it is only natural that noninvasive methods would be used during the follow-up phases of a patient's care (Fig. 3-7). Those who deal with these patients have come to realize that long-term monitoring of the outcome is important both for preserving function and avoiding complications or failure of the initial reconstruction, be it by angioplasty or direct arterial surgery. Since the follow-up protocol will vary somewhat depending on the initial therapy, it is important to consider these therapies separately.

TRANSLUMINAL ANGIOPLASTY

Angioplasty achieves restoration of function by splitting the intima longitudinally adjacent to the plaque into the media and up to the adventitia, permitting the arterial lumen to increase in size.[30] If this procedure is successful, the cross-sectional area of the vessel increases, and the velocity changes across the stenotic segment will improve and in some cases return to normal. The major problem with this therapy is the development of myointimal hyperplasia, which occurs in up to 20% to 30% of the segments. The recurrence rate appears lowest for the iliac arteries and highest for the smaller peripheral arteries such as the superficial femoral and popliteal arteries. These arterial segments can be restudied early after the procedure and followed over time to monitor the long-term results.[31] If the patient becomes symptomatic, it is a simple matter to reassess the situation and determine the basis for the return in symptoms.

SAPHENOUS VEIN GRAFTS

One of the more common methods of correcting lesions involving the femoropopliteal segment is to use the greater saphenous vein either by the in situ approach or by reversing the vein. These conduits, which can provide very good long-term benefit, may develop problems—particularly during the first year—that, if detected, can be corrected before graft failure occurs. The lesions that develop and can influence both graft patency and long-term function may occur in the inflow and outflow arteries and within the body of the graft itself. There is now good evidence that graft patency can be greatly extended by frequently performed duplex studies, particularly during the first year. Although there is some variation in the study intervals that may be employed, we use the following protocol:

1. At the time of each study the A/A index and the velocity changes along the body of the graft are assessed.
2. The first study should be done on the day of discharge (some investigators are recommending intra-operative studies as well), and after discharge the study intervals should be no longer than 6 weeks during the first year.
3. If the A/A index falls more than 0.15, the cause must be found since this is significant hemodynamically.
4. Although there is some disagreement about the

Abdominal aorta stenosis:>50%

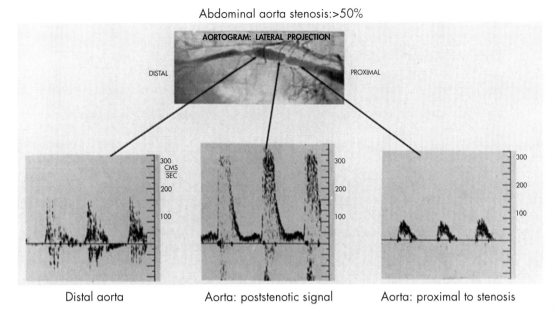

Distal aorta   Aorta: poststenotic signal   Aorta: proximal to stenosis

Fig. 3-6. Duplex scanning findings in a patient with a stenosis of the abdominal aorta. *(From Strandness DE Jr: Duplex scanning for diagnosis of peripheral arterial disease, Herz 13:372, 1988.)*

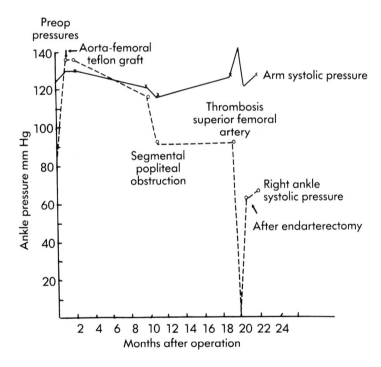

Fig. 3-7. Ankle systolic pressures recorded during 2 years following an aortobifemoral graft. With the development of new areas of disease, the ankle pressure decreased.

criteria used to document the degree of stenosis in a vein graft, it is clear that the tighter stenoses are those most likely to lead to thrombosis and graft failure.[32-34] Most investigators have used the peak systolic velocity at the site of narrowing divided by that immediately proximal to the lesion. If this ratio exceeds 2 to 2.5, it is likely that the stenosis is greater than 50%. If the ratio exceeds 3.5, it is likely that the stenosis exceeds 75% in terms of diameter reduction.

By using these types of studies and intervening early after detection of high-grade lesions with or without a fall

in the A/A index, the primary assisted patency can be extended to 85% at 5 years.

The use of the A/A index is based on the observation that when a lesion that is hemodynamically significant develops within the venous graft, the A/A index will decrease. It is well established that a fall greater than 0.15 is significant and should prompt an aggressive examination for the basis of the observed fall. In this setting it is also possible to use exercise testing to document the deterioration in graft function, but this is not a necessary routine study for most cases of graft surveillance.

What about monitoring prosthetic arterial grafts?

When these conduits fail, they do so at one of the anastomotic sites. For aortofemoral grafts it is the distal anastomosis that is the site of greatest concern since failure at the proximal end is very uncommon. For femoropopliteal grafts the problem may develop at either union, with the cause usually myointimal hyperplasia. We have not found the surveillance intervals as helpful in this case, but it is clear that follow-up with the assessment of the A/A index and the study of the anastomotic sites may detect problems before complete occlusion occurs.

ANEURYSMAL DISEASE

The most lethal vascular disorder is the abdominal aortic aneurysm that if untreated may lead to rupture and death. Even if the patient survives the initial bleeding episode to arrive at the hospital, the mortality rate will be high, in the range of 50% to 80%. Since most of these lesions are not noticed by the patient until he becomes symptomatic, it is important to define objectively the relationships between size of the aneurysm, its location, and its outcome.

What is the magnitude of the problem and how can these lesions be detected and followed? A study by Collins et al[35] screened 426 men between the ages of 65 and 74 with ultrasound to assess the prevalence of aneurysms of the abdominal aorta. An aneurysm was discovered in 5.4% of the men, with the aneurysm 4 cm or greater in size in 2.3% of them. It was found that men with evidence of occlusive arterial disease were the most likely to have lesions found on scanning. In fact, these patients accounted for 20% of the aneurysms discovered. These studies have pointed out that aneurysms are not uncommon and should be considered in any patient who is being evaluated for occlusive arterial disease.

Any patient considered at risk or who has a ''palpable aorta'' suggesting dilation or the presence of an aneurysm should have an ultrasound examination. As Bernstein, Harris, and Leopold[36] have shown by repeat studies, there is very little variation (2 to 3 mm) in the assessment of size when this method is used. The other option available is computed axial tomographic (CT) scanning, which appears to be more precise but should only be done when the ultrasound is deemed inadequate or inconclusive.

As previously noted, the value of such a study is the determination of aneurysm size, which is important for determining which lesion should be removed. Although it is not the purpose of this chapter to discuss indications for therapy, it is clear that ultrasound is the best method for documenting changes in size over time. In the study by Bernstein, Harris, and Leopold[36] the changes in size noted during follow-up were evaluated in 110 poor-risk patients followed for a mean period of almost 4 years. The expansion rate for this group of patients was 0.4 cm/yr. In this group of patients were 46 who underwent resection because their lesions reached 6 cm or more. Thirty-six patients died of causes unrelated to the aneurysms. Six patients died of aortic rupture, with three not undergoing an operation because of serious coexisting disease. Using this method of long-term study, the mortality rate from aortic rupture was 7.5%.

The most controversial area relates to the treatment of the smaller aneurysms (less than 5 cm). It appears that rupture of aneurysms of this size is an uncommon event.[37] The most common cause of death in this group of patients is myocardial infarction. However, as previously noted, enlargement does occur and can be detected by repeat ultrasound studies. For lesions greater than 4 cm, we restudy these patients every 3 months as recommended by Bernstein, Harris, and Leopold.[36]

The problems that develop with peripheral aneurysms (femoral and popliteal) are different. These lesions rarely rupture but are known to undergo thrombosis and/or to be the site of emboli to the lower limbs.[38] Although peripheral aneurysms can occur in isolation, they are more common in patients who have aneurysms of the abdominal aorta. They can be diagnosed by both physical examination and ultrasound. However, the criteria as to size and the potential danger posed for limb survival have not been worked out. In general, the criterion for making the diagnosis has related to the dimension of the artery proximal to the suspicious area. The most frequently used guideline is that a vessel that is 1½ to 2 times the diameter of the artery immediately proximal to the suspicious area should be considered aneurysmal. Patients who are candidates for screening are those with very prominent popliteal pulses and/or any elderly patient who has sudden onset of ischemia to the limb.

EXTRACRANIAL ARTERIAL DISEASE

With the publication of the results of the North American Carotid Endarterectomy Trial (NASCET) and the European Carotid Surgery Trial (ECST), we now have some guidelines regarding management of patients with carotid artery disease who are symptomatic.[39,40] Both of these trials published results showing that if the degree of diameter reduction exceeds 70%, these patients are best treated by carotid endarterectomy. However, as will be discussed, the method of assessing the degree of narrowing was different for the two trials—a fact that has created considerable confusion.

The remaining area of concern deals with the asymptomatic patient with carotid artery disease. The two major studies in this area—the Veterans Affairs Cooperative Study and the National Institutes of Health (NIH)–supported Asymptomatic Carotid Atherosclerosis Study (ACAS)—have reported their results.[41,42] Although the latter was reported as a clinical alert in October 1994, the data are of sufficient importance to merit attention. In the Veterans Affairs Cooperative Study, patients with a greater than 50% diameter–reducing lesion had greater benefit from surgery than medical therapy for the prevention of strokes and transient ischemic attacks (TIAs). In the ACAS trial the patients with a greater than 60% diameter reduction of the carotid bulb showed a relative risk reduction for stroke of 55%. These two trials, and the NASCET study, arrived at different cutoff points for the degree of stenosis that needs attention. This complicates the screening method.

Screening Tests

A host of tests have been developed to permit assessment of the extracranial arteries. These can be divided into indirect and direct tests. The more commonly used indirect tests include those that derive their information at a point away from the carotid bulb itself. They include periorbital directional Doppler[43] and oculoplethysmography.[44,45] Both methods use information about the arterial inflow to the eye through the ophthalmic artery as an index of the hemodynamic changes that occur as the carotid artery becomes progressively narrowed. At some time in the progression of a plaque, the diameter of the artery will reach a point at which a pressure gradient will develop along with a drop in flow across the involved area. When this occurs, the pressure in the ophthalmic artery will fall, and the collateral blood supply to the ipsilateral cortex will be activated. In the case of the carotid artery, the most common input collateral artery that is easily studied is the external carotid artery and its communications with the ophthalmic artery through the medial frontal and supraorbital arteries. When the carotid artery is significantly narrowed, the direction of flow in the medial frontal and supraorbital arteries will be reversed.

The directional changes in flow induced by the tight stenoses of the carotid bulb can be detected using a direction-sensing continuous wave Doppler sensor placed over the medial frontal and supraorbital arteries[43] (Fig. 3-8). It is also possible to test the effect of temporal artery compression on the flows being recorded. Although this has been widely tested, the method has serious limitations that are readily apparent. It cannot distinguish a tight stenosis from a total occlusion and cannot be used for monitoring the progression of disease in the carotid bulb.

The oculoplethysmographic system developed by Gee[45] is an elegantly simple method that uses cups applied to the sclera of the eye that are placed under a negative pressure sufficient to stop blood flow to the eye. As the pressure in the system is gradually reduced, there will be a point at which the ocular pulsations return. It is possible to relate this pressure to that which is present in the ophthalmic artery on that side. This test, which is much like the periorbital Doppler method, is most useful in detecting those lesions that are pressure and flow reducing. It also has the problem of being unable to distinguish a tight stenosis from a total occlusion. The only advantage this method has over the use of duplex scanning is that it could depict a siphon lesion that would be missed by scanning in the neck. This is, however, a very unusual occurrence in my experience.

Although these methods have been used extensively, they have been largely superseded by the use of the direct methods of investigating not only the carotid bifurcation but also the vessels at the level of the arch and the vertebral arteries as well. More recently, with the advent of the transcranial Doppler, a new method of examining the arteries inside the skull is available.

What Information Is Available?

When patients with suspected carotid artery disease are first seen, there is no way based on the clinical presentation alone to estimate either the location or extent of the arterial involvement. Although bruits are markers of disease of the bulb, they are little else. Except for arteriography, there is no way short of the use of duplex scanning to determine the degree of narrowing that is producing the noise in the neck.

Duplex scanning has been widely applied and tested in this area and has been found the best single method of screening for bifurcation disease.[46,47] It provides information about the site and extent of disease, using categories that are of clinical value. Depending on one's clinical practice and bias, it is possible to eliminate most patients from consideration for arteriography. The categories of disease that are used with minor variations from center to center are as follows:

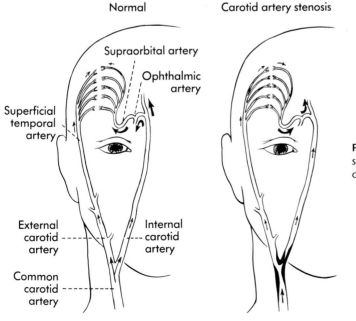

Fig. 3-8. Direction of flow in the supraorbital arteries in normal subjects and patients with a high-grade stenosis of the internal carotid artery.

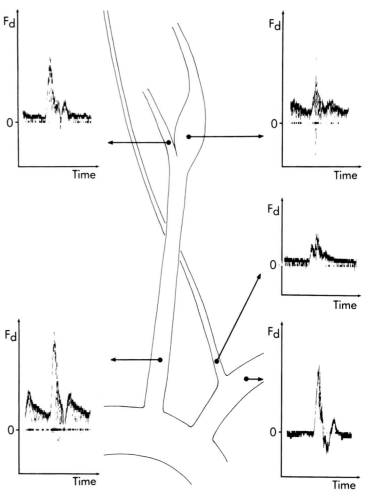

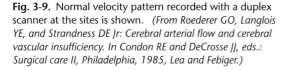

Fig. 3-9. Normal velocity pattern recorded with a duplex scanner at the sites is shown. *(From Roederer GO, Langlois YE, and Strandness DE Jr: Cerebral arterial flow and cerebral vascular insufficiency. In Condon RE and DeCrosse JJ, eds.: Surgical care II, Philadelphia, 1985, Lea and Febiger.)*

1. *Normal.* Finding a normal carotid bulb with boundary layer separation is nearly certain evidence that the bifurcation is not the cause of either transient ischemic events and/or strokes (Fig. 3-9).
2. *Minimal wall disease—1% to 15% narrowing.* This is rarely significant clinically except in the *very unusual* case in which this type of lesion may be the site of ulceration. In our experience with patients undergoing an operation for carotid artery disease only 3% of the patients had disease in this category (Fig. 3-10).
3. *16% to 49% stenosis.* These lesions are generally considered of moderate severity and are not associated with a pressure gradient or a reduction in flow. They can be the cause of TIAs and strokes, which also are not very common. In my experience only approximately 10% of patients with either a TIA or stroke will have this degree of stenosis.
4. *50% to 79% narrowing.* Once the artery is narrowed to this extent, there is a marked increase in velocity within the stenotic segment, and there may be an associated pressure drop. When this degree of stenosis is found, the lesions are more complex pathologically and can be the cause of symptoms. These lesions account for approximately 42% of patients who undergo carotid endarterectomy (Fig. 3-10).

5. *80% to 99% stenosis.* This is often referred to as the "preocclusive" lesion because of its propensity to progress to a total occlusion of the internal carotid artery. The plaques that produce this degree of narrowing are also of the complicated variety, with loss of surface covering, necrosis, calcification, and intraplaque hemorrhage (Fig. 3-10).
6. *Total occlusion.* The finding of a total occlusion is important because it removes the patient from consideration for surgical therapy. However, even if the artery occludes and does not lead to an event at the time of the occlusion, there is an ongoing stroke rate in the range of 5%/yr.

The type of information available through duplex scanning is important not only for planning therapy but also for serving as the baseline study for long-term follow-up (Fig. 3-11). Although there is and will continue to be some controversy about the significance of these lesions, particularly in asymptomatic patients, guidelines exist with which most investigators can agree. Those lesions that narrow the artery by less than 80% can be safely followed with a very low incidence of ischemic events (1% to 4%/yr).[48,49] For those that narrow the artery by greater than 80% the occlusion and event rate is much higher, in the range of 5% to 10%/yr, which has led us to be more

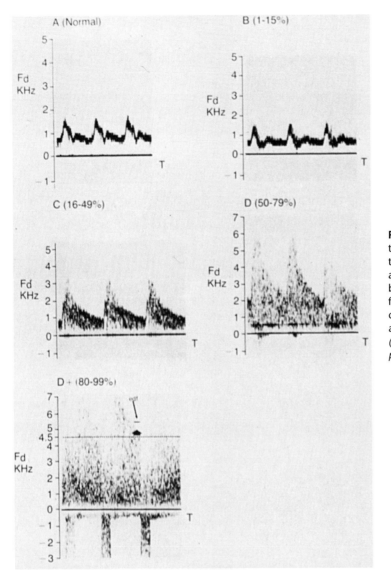

Fig. 3-10. Spectral analysis of velocity changes noted at the site of the lesion for the categories of involvement. For the 16%-49% stenosis, the main diagnostic features are a peak frequency below 4 kHz (125 cm/sec) and spectral broadening. For the 50%-79% stenosis, the peak systolic frequency is >4 kHz. For the 80%-99% stenosis, the main diagnostic features are a peak systolic frequency >4 kHz and an end-systolic frequency >4.5 kHz (145 cm/sec). *(From Taylor DC and Strandness DE Jr: Carotid artery duplex scanning, J Clin Ultrasound 15:635, 1987.)*

aggressive in treating this degree of involvement.

To estimate the degree of narrowing of the carotid bulb, the NASCET group used the internal carotid artery distal to the bulb as the "normal" reference artery. In the ECST study all of the measurements were made directly from the bulb itself. Thus a 70% diameter reduction, which both trials suggest is best treated by endarterectomy, is not the same. To further confuse the issue, how can one relate the results of the ultrasound studies to determine if the lesion does, in fact, reach the 70% diameter-reducing cutoff point? Moneta et al[50] and Edwards et al[51] have established criteria that can be obtained from a standard duplex study as previously outlined to estimate whether an apparent lesion is above the 70% cutoff point. This can be done by taking the ratio of the peak systolic velocity at the site of narrowing to that measured from the common carotid artery proximal to the lesion. If that ratio is greater than 4.0 it will have a positive predictive value of 77%, a negative predictive value of 95%, and overall accuracy of 88%. This simple adaptation of the standard ultrasound study should

be used in assessing symptomatic patients with carotid artery disease.

What of the 60% lesion found by ACAS as being significant in asymptomatic patients? What should one use for determining this degree of stenosis? Edwards et al[52] also have examined this issue and arrived at guidelines that can be used by the vascular diagnostic laboratory. If one uses a ratio of 3.2 for the peak systolic velocity at the site of the narrowing divided by that from the common carotid artery, a sensitivity of 92% and a specificity of 86% can be achieved. This gives a positive predictive value of 85%, a negative predictive value of 93%, with an overall accuracy rate of 89%.

These values do not take into account the variability associated with arteriography. This is not insignificant, and even in carefully done studies any single value for the degree of narrowing is probably in the range of ±20% of the reported value. This ultimately leaves the therapeutic decision to be based on multiple factors, of which the degree of diameter reduction is only one.

JB 59   Right ICA

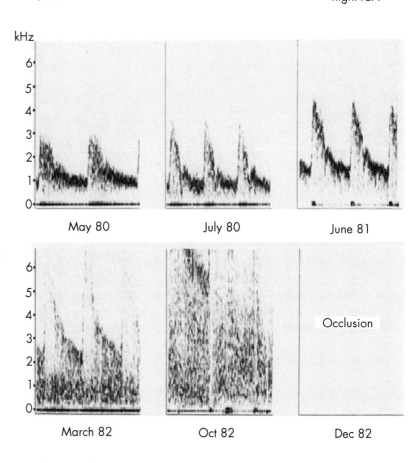

Fig. 3-11. Serial duplex velocity readings from the right internal carotid artery (ICA) in a 59-year-old white male. At the time of the first study in May 1980, the ICA was narrowed to the 16%-49% category of stenosis. *(From Roederer GO et al: The natural history of carotid arterial disease in asymptomatic patients with cervical bruits, Stroke 15:605, 1984, by permission of the American Heart Association.)*

We now have information on the rate of progression for moderate carotid artery stenosis (less than 80% diameter reduction) in asymptomatic patients followed up to 7 years with repeat ultrasonic duplex scans.[53] Progression in the degree of narrowing was noted in 23% of 232 patients (136 males, 96 females) with nearly half progressing to a greater than 80% diameter-reducing lesion. The risk of progression was greatest for those patients whose lesions were in the 50% to 79% diameter range at time of entry into the study. The cumulative stroke risk for patients with a less than 50% stenosis at entry was 6%, compared with 11% for those who entered the study with a 50% to 79% lesion. Regular follow-up will permit detection of those patients who are progressing and at risk for an ischemic event.

Another major advantage of duplex scanning for the carotid circulation is for the evaluation of the patient who has undergone surgery and returns for evaluation. This evaluation can be divided into the following phases:

1. *The perioperative period—first 24 hours.* If an ischemic event occurs within this time frame, the duplex scan can be quickly done to establish patency of the reconstruction but should not be used in an attempt to define lesser degrees of involvement.
2. *The postoperative period.* Although it is possible to study patients during the early period after discharge, usually on the third hospital day, it is not wise to attempt to do a detailed examination of the

bulb region until the healing process is mature and the region is stable. We have arbitrarily set this time at 3 months after the operation. After this period of time, the most common lesion that develops is myointimal hyperplasia, a process that is largely benign and not responsible for recurrent ischemic episodes.[54] Annual visits are in order to monitor the status of the carotid bulb. After the first 2 years the lesions that develop are most likely to represent new atherosclerotic plaques.

VERTEBROBASILAR INSUFFICIENCY

One of the less satisfying areas to evaluate in the vascular laboratory is ischemia of the posterior circulation. The major problems are the nonspecific nature of the patient's symptoms and the difficulty in identifying the specific arterial lesions responsible for its development. The most common syndrome is that associated with reversal of flow in the vertebral artery (the subclavian steal syndrome).[55] This is thought to occur as a result of "siphoning" blood away from the posterior fossa when there is a hemodynamically significant lesion in the ipsilateral subclavian artery. This results in reverse flow in the vertebral artery that now serves as an important collateral artery for the arm. When this syndrome was first described, it was thought that exercise of the arm on the side of the subclavian occlusion would further increase the reverse flow in the vertebral artery and lead to brainstem ischemia. However, most patients with subclavian artery stenosis and/or occlusion with reverse flow in the vertebral artery never develop symptoms either at rest or with exercise of the arm on the side of the occlusion.[56] The fully developed subclavian steal syndrome is rare.

However, it is feasible to study patients suspected of having the problem to document the presence of reverse flow in the vertebral artery. A subset of patients who have oscillatory flow (forward-reverse) in the vertebral artery are apt to be more symptomatic than those who have reverse flow at all times.[57] It is possible that the use of transcranial Doppler may help shed some light on this difficult clinical problem.

INTRACRANIAL HEMODYNAMICS

Although the skull has been considered an impenetrable barrier to the use of ultrasound, it has been shown by Aaslid, Markwaider, and Nornes[58] that it is possible to obtain velocity data from the basal cerebral arteries using 2 MHz pulsed Doppler systems to gain access to the arteries inside the skull. It appears that there are three sites that can be used to gain access to the arteries that comprise the circle of Willis: the eye, the temporal bone "window" just above the zygomatic arch, and the foramen magnum. These positions provide access to the intracranial internal carotid, the middle cerebral, and the vertebral and basilar arteries. The assumption is made that the angle of insonation of these arteries is 0 degrees. If it is assumed that the angle of insonation is 0 degrees, the maximum error that would occur if this were off by 20 degrees would be 6%. The data that can be obtained for analysis are the peak systolic velocity or the mean velocity (time-averaged maximum velocity). If an additional assumption is made that the vessel's diameter remains constant, then the method would be suitable for monitoring changes in volume flow.[59] This is an assumption that may not be correct, and one would have to define carefully the circumstances in which the measurements are being made. For example, one of the more common uses of this technique is to monitor flow in the middle cerebral artery after an episode of subarachnoid bleeding. It is well-known that cerebral vasospasm occurs, so any relationship between the velocity changes and flow to the cortex would have to take this fact into account.

What is the role of transcranial Doppler at the present time? More work will be needed to determine its place. Some of the areas in which it could be helpful are as follows:

1. *Evaluation of the circle of Willis.* In theory it is possible to monitor flow and its direction in all major components of the circle of Willis with the exception of the posterior communicating artery. It should then be possible to estimate the risk of events such as thrombosis of the internal carotid artery in terms of the likelihood that an ischemic event might occur. However, some problems have not been resolved. Although it is feasible to test the adequacy of the circle with compression of the common carotid artery, this is not the same as would occur with involvement of the internal carotid artery alone. In addition, if an ischemic event occurred because of the extension of a thrombus intracranially to block the middle cerebral artery, the effect of this event could not be predicted by transcranial Doppler. It is also possible to monitor flow in the middle cerebral artery during endarterectomy. The results are promising, but more study is needed.[60]

2. *Detection of intracranial lesions involving the middle cerebral artery.* There is no doubt that this method has the potential for discovering such lesions by virtue of the increase in velocity that occurs when a stenotic segment is located.[61] On the other hand, the absence of flow that might signify a total occlusion must be interpreted with caution. There are patients who do not have an acoustic window in the temporal bone. The problem would appear to be less severe with the vertebral and basilar arteries in which there is no problem with regard to an acoustic window.

3. *Subarachnoid hemorrhage.* The one application that has been tested and found of value is in this area. It is possible to monitor the time course of cerebral artery vasospasm by using transcranial Doppler.[62]

4. *Documentation of cerebral arterial response to carbon dioxide inhalation.* This is a potentially exciting area of research. It appears there are some patients whose vascular reactivity is severely limited, and this limitation can be uncovered by this method. Perhaps identification of these patients will provide an idea of which patients are likely to suffer when an occlusion of the internal carotid artery occurs.[63]

5. *Evaluation of vertebrobasilar insufficiency.* As noted in an earlier section, this is one area that is very confusing and difficult to evaluate. Perhaps the ability to study directly not only the vertebral but basilar artery as well will give a better idea about the role of reverse flow in these arteries as the basis for ischemic symptoms.

Vertebrobasilar insufficiency can be difficult to evaluate regardless of the etiology. Although disease of the subclavian and vertebral arteries with resulting reverse flow in the vertebral arteries is always a consideration, positional ischemia of the brainstem can also account for symptoms.[64] Transcranial Doppler can be helpful because it allows examination of flow in the posterior cerebral artery with the head in various positions. If the flow in the posterior cerebral artery decreases and coincides with the appearance of symptoms, this is strong presumptive evidence as to the cause. When found, this should be followed by arteriographic confirmation.

RENOVASCULAR HYPERTENSION

Hypertension affects approximately 10% of the U.S. population. Within this very large group of patients it has been estimated that 1% to 6% will have renal artery disease as the cause of the problem.[65] This occurs in two forms—

atherosclerosis and fibromuscular hyperplasia. When atherosclerosis is the inciting disorder, it is more likely to affect people over the age of 50. The proximal renal artery is the most common site of involvement. With fibromuscular hyperplasia the involvement can be at all levels of the renal artery, but it is unusual for the orifice of the artery to be involved.[66] Since these disorders can be treated by either transluminal angioplasty or direct arterial surgery, it is important that they be detected if at all possible.

Over the years several screening methods have been tested to determine if they might be suitable for noninvasive detection of renal artery stenosis. The most common methods developed included intravenous urography and radionuclide studies. Both of these methods had unacceptably high false-positive and false-negative rates, making them unsuitable for screening purposes. The urographic and nuclear scans have a sensitivity of only approximately 70% for the diagnosis of significant renal artery stenosis.[67] They have a false-positive rate that can be as high as 20%. In addition, the screening tests are unreliable in the presence of bilateral renal artery disease, which is a common occurrence. For a screening test to be of great value it must have a very high specificity to avoid unnecessary application of invasive studies such as arteriography.[68]

Although intravenous digital subtraction arteriography was introduced as a possible method for screening purposes, it has not turned out to be a useful method. The method requires large volumes of contrast material, and the images obtained do not have the resolution necessary to permit reliable detection of most renal artery lesions.

Ultrasonic duplex scanning provides a useful alternative since it is possible to examine the renal arteries directly and to detect areas of narrowing.[69,70] It is known that when there is a fall in pressure and flow across the renal artery, the renin-angiotensin system will be activated. It has been shown experimentally and clinically that this usually occurs at the level of a 60% reduction in the diameter of the renal artery.

Patients who are candidates for this study include the following: (1) young patients with hypertension; (2) patients with rapidly accelerating hypertension; (3) those with malignant hypertension; (4) patients who have hypertension and renal failure; and (5) hypertensive patients with an abdominal bruit. The algorithm we currently use is shown in Fig. 3-12.

Ultrasonic duplex scanning studies are designed to provide the following information: (1) the status of the renal arteries from the level of the aorta to the renal hilum; (2) renal size; (3) blood flow patterns in the upper, middle, and lower poles of the kidney; and (4) information on the gross morphology of the kidney.

To obtain the maximal amount of information, it is necessary to study the patient in the fasting state—preferably for 12 hours. It is also beneficial to study the patient in the early morning before much air swallowing has occurred. Air in the bowel is one of the major problems encountered in carrying out these studies because it interferes with the transmission of ultrasound to the area of interest. When proper preparation has been done, we can study adequately approximately 90% of the patients referred for the procedure.

In developing this method we used two parameters to detect renal artery stenoses.[71] The first is the peak systolic velocity at suspected sites of narrowing with the second being the ratio of the peak systolic velocity at the site of narrowing to that recorded from the abdominal aorta (renal aortic ratio [RAR]). For lesions that narrow the artery by less than 60%, the peak systolic velocity will be greater than 180 cm/sec, but the RAR will be less than 3.5. If the RAR is greater than 3.5, the degree of narrowing will be greater than 60% (Fig. 3-13).

Occlusions of the renal artery can be difficult to detect unless one is always aware of this possibility. Occlusions of the renal artery are commonly associated with a kidney less than 9 cm in length. In a series of 58 renal arteries scanned that also had arteriographic studies, total occlusions were

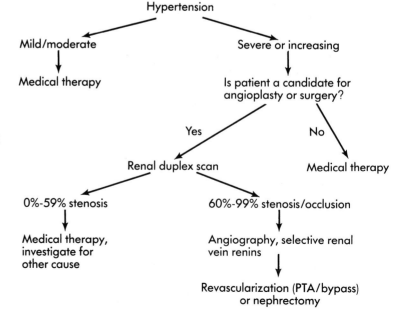

Fig. 3-12. Algorithm illustrates the proposed use of renal artery duplex scanning. *(From Taylor DC et al: Duplex ultrasound scanning in the diagnosis of renal artery stenosis: a prospective study, J Vasc Surg 7:363, 1988.)*

found in five instances. This was verified by duplex scanning in four cases. In the remaining case the degree of disease was classified in the greater than 60% stenosis category.[70]

Another much more difficult problem for duplex scanning is the patient with multiple renal arteries. In the series of 58 renal arteries prospectively studied, there were four instances in which multiple arteries were present, and we were able to detect only one of them. It is certainly possible for there to be a lesion in an accessory renal artery causing hypertension, and it would be missed by this method. To date we have not encountered such a patient, but this is clearly a possibility that must be considered.

How good is such screening in detecting significant renal artery lesions? Our data suggest that with this method one can expect to obtain a sensitivity of 84%, with a specificity of 97% and an overall accuracy of 93%.[69,70] Is this good enough? The very high specificity is important for the use of a screening test applied to a population with a low prevalence of disease such as the hypertensive population in this country. It would be unacceptable to perform unnecessary arteriograms on a large number of healthy individuals.

It is important to understand that the finding of atherosclerotic renal artery disease may well be a marker for disease in other arterial beds. Louie et al[72] studied 60 patients with renal artery stenosis to assess the prevalence of atherosclerosis in the carotid and peripheral arteries. If a high-grade (greater than 60%) renal artery stenosis was found, 46% of the patients had a greater than 50% diameter reduction of one or both carotid arteries, and 73% had an abnormal A/A index. This suggests that the finding of renal artery disease should also prompt investigation of these other vascular beds.

Follow-up Studies

One of the major problems encountered in patients with renal arterial disease is the lack of suitable methods for sequential study of lesions, regardless of the treatment used. Because of this, the end point most commonly used in defining success or failure is control of the blood pressure. If the patient after transluminal angioplasty or surgery does not require drugs for therapy, it is assumed, probably rightly, that the therapy has been successful. However, most patients do not fall into this "cured" category, and assessment of the reconstructed segment is important. In addition, the largest group of patients with renal vascular disease will not have any intervention other than medical therapy. The major question that has never been answered for this group of patients is what happens to the lesions over time and in particular what effect will progression of disease have on renal function.

Once a patient with renal arterial disease has been studied successfully, the procedure can almost always be repeated to document any change that may have occurred. This is also true of those patients who have had direct intervention, be it angioplasty or surgery. It is not a difficult matter to repeat the evaluation to document the outcome both early and late. In the long-term studies we have done to date, it has been possible to document the

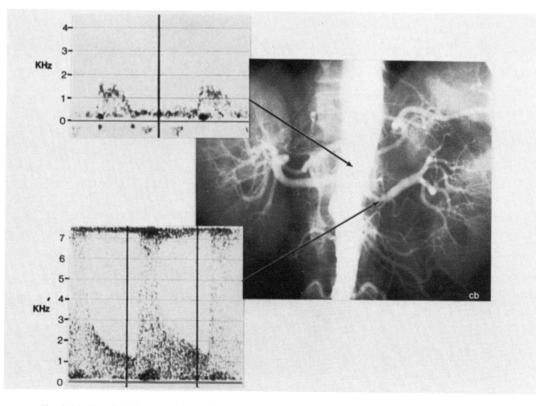

Fig. 3-13. Renal duplex scan in a patient with a >60% stenosis of the left renal artery. The renal aortic ratio was 9.4. *(From Taylor DC et al: Duplex ultrasound scanning in the diagnosis of renal artery stenosis. A prospective study, J Vasc Surg 7:363, 1988.)*

results, thus removing any uncertainty as to outcome. Three groups of patients have been examined.[73]

1. Five patients underwent angioplasty; there was documented improvement by duplex scanning in two. Both of these patients had relief of their hypertension. In the other three patients there was no improvement in the stenotic segments revealed by duplex scanning, and in each patient the hypertension persisted. The great advantage of duplex scanning is that it can be applied immediately after the procedure to determine the status of the arterial segment. Furthermore, if at any time later a problem with blood pressure control becomes evident, the study can be repeated.

2. In the surgical group of patients there were 10 stenotic arteries in seven patients studied after the procedure. At a mean follow-up period of 9 months, there was continued patency in eight arteries and unexpected occlusion in two bypasses (Fig. 3-14). Thus this approach has been very helpful in documenting the basis for the failure and will have increasing applications for those cases in which the bypass has been done to a small kidney. The fate of bypass grafts to small kidneys (7 cm in length or less) is an important area that needs study.

3. A most important group of patients to follow are those with a greater than 60% diameter reduction who have not had any form of intervention. We evaluated two aspects of this problem: (1) the changes in renal length that occurred over time, and (2) the changes in the degree of narrowing of the renal artery.[74,75] In 49 renal arteries with a greater than 60% diameter-reducing stenosis, 26% showed a greater than 1-cm decrease in renal length with an average follow-up of 14.4 months. The estimated risk for a decrease of 1 cm in length was 19% at 1 year. Renal length did not decrease in the patients with a normal renal artery or one with a less than 60% decrease in diameter.

Renal artery disease progression was assessed in 95 arteries followed for at least 6 months, 70 arteries followed for 24 months, 48 arteries followed for 18 months, and 19 arteries followed for 24 months. None of the normal arteries developed new disease, but 7 of the 35 arteries with a less than 60% stenosis at entry progressed to a greater than 60% lesion. The cumulative incidence of progression was $23 \pm 9\%$ at 12 months and $42 \pm 14\%$ at 24 months. Four renal arteries progressed to total occlusion and in each case had a greater than 60% stenosis at time of entry into the study. The cumulative incidence of progression to occlusion was $5 \pm 3\%$ at 12 months and $11 \pm 6\%$ at 24 months.

TRANSPLANTED KIDNEY

Duplex scanning is also of benefit in examining the transplanted kidney, both in the early period after its placement and for the long-term. In the early postoperative period a question that frequently arises is the issue of rejection vs reversible ischemic injury.[76,77] It has been

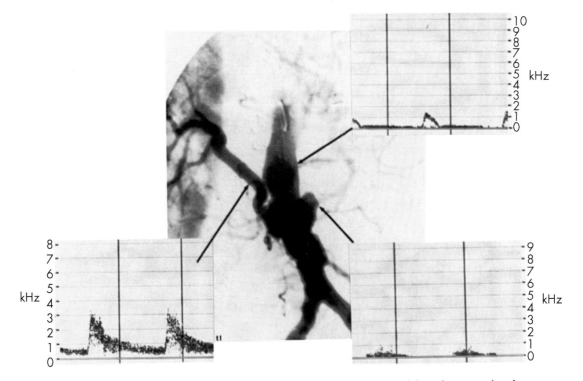

Fig. 3-14. Postoperative duplex scanning study in a patient who underwent bilateral aortorenal grafting. The graft to the left kidney was visualized, but there was no flow. *(From Taylor DC, Moneta GL, and Strandness DE Jr: Follow-up of renal artery stenosis by duplex ultrasound, J Vasc Surg 9:410, 1989.)*

postulated that the process associated with rejection dramatically increases resistance to flow and that is in turn reflected in the pattern of the velocities detected both in the renal artery and the parenchyma of the kidney.[78] Slightly different algorithms have been used to describe this finding, but they all have taken into account the degree to which the end-diastolic frequency approaches zero. We have preferred to use the end-diastolic ratio (EDR), which is the end-diastolic velocity divided by the peak systolic velocity. The normal value for the EDR is 0.35 or less.

Other investigators have used the resistive index (RI), which is the peak systolic velocity minus the end-diastolic velocity divided by the peak systolic velocity. Both the EDR and the RI reflect the resistance to flow offered by the small vessels in the kidney. The experience with this type of analysis as a predictor of rejection remains unsettled at the moment. Fleischer et al[78] did show differences between the rejecting kidney vs controls. As the RI moved toward a value of 1.0, it appeared likely that this reflected rejection. However, Genkins, Sanflippo, and Carroll[79] showed that, although changes in the RI did reflect pathologic changes within the allograft, they did not specifically identify the cause of the transplant dysfunction. This problem will clearly require more study with more cases in which the pathologic basis for change in the RI has been documented.

One area in which duplex scanning can be of great value is in the chronic renal transplant patient who has developed hypertension or renal failure.[80] It is important to know if the renal artery supplying the patient's kidney has developed a stenotic lesion. Since the transplanted kidney is in an easily accessible location, it is a relatively simple matter to scan the renal artery from its origin to detect any areas of narrowing that may be present. This is very important since many of these narrowings may be corrected by transluminal angioplasty.

MESENTERIC CIRCULATION

Since atherosclerosis is a disease of branch points and bifurcations, it is not unexpected that the major suppliers to the small and large bowel, the superior and inferior mesenteric arteries, would also be affected. The other arteries of great importance to this region are the celiac and hypogastric arteries that can serve as important collateral sources when the mesenteric arteries become narrowed and occluded. In fact, the collateral potential is extremely good for this region and is the major reason that chronic lesions do not often lead to the development of intestinal ischemia.

The major clinical problems involving the small bowel are acute and chronic mesenteric ischemia. In acute ischemia the superior mesenteric artery becomes occluded either by emboli or by a thrombosis on a preexisting atherosclerotic plaque. When this occurs, the presentation is often dramatic, with acute and severe abdominal pain, very hyperactive bowel tones, and a nearly normal abdominal examination. If the diagnosis is not made promptly and therapy instituted quickly, bowel death rapidly ensues, and the patient will die. There is rarely time to do an ultrasound scan of the patient's abdomen to assess the inflow to the gut. In fact, such studies should be discouraged since they only delay the opportunity to correct the underlying problem.

In a patient with chronic ischemia the involvement has occurred gradually, and the clinical presentation will reflect the inability of the superior mesenteric artery to supply the blood flow needs to the gut during digestion, resulting in the syndrome commonly referred to as mesenteric angina. When this occurs, the patient when eating will develop abdominal pain that is often followed by diarrhea and progressive weight loss. Such a patient soon finds that food intake is always followed by pain, so he will markedly limit his intake. The weight loss will be profound if the lesions producing the problem are not relieved.

It is well established that the celiac, superior mesenteric, and perhaps the inferior mesenteric arteries must be involved to produce chronic mesenteric angina because the collateral supply is so rich that normal levels of blood flow, even after eating, can be provided by these alternate routes. In clinical practice the only method that has proved satisfactory in making the diagnosis is arteriography with its lateral views of the abdominal aorta to demonstrate the celiac, superior mesenteric, and inferior mesenteric arteries. Arteriography is necessary to confirm the diagnosis and is mandatory before any procedure designed to correct the situation, direct arterial surgery, or angioplasty.

Since many pain syndromes in the aging patient may suggest the diagnosis, it is only natural that duplex scanning would be used as a screening test and also as a method for monitoring the long-term results with therapy. The celiac and the superior mesenteric arteries are readily available to this modality and are relatively easy to study by virtue of their position in the upper abdomen where these vessels originate (Fig. 3-15).

The velocity patterns recorded in the normal celiac and superior mesenteric arteries reflect the resistance of the organs they supply.[81,82] The liver and spleen have low vascular resistance, similar to that of the brain and the kidneys. The low resistance means that there should always be a high mean flow level, no reverse flow, and a high end-diastolic velocity. The superior mesenteric artery supplies an organ of variable resistance with wide ranges of blood flow, depending mainly on the time of day and the relationship to eating and what the patient has ingested.[83]

In the fasting state the velocity pattern in the superior mesenteric artery is often triphasic, with a definite but brief period of reverse flow seen in late systole. The end-diastolic flow will be quite variable. However, with eating some dramatic changes occur that reflect the decrease in resistance as the small arteries and arterioles in the bowel dilate to promote the increase in flow that is needed for digestion (Fig. 3-16). This begins within 1 minute after eating, reaching a maximal level 40 minutes after the meal is completed. The magnitude of the response depends to a large degree on what has been eaten.[84] The normal range of values is shown in Tables 3-4 and 3-5.

Moneta et al[85] tested the accuracy of using absolute velocity values for predicting the presence of a greater than 70% diameter-reducing lesion in the celiac and superior mesenteric arteries. They found that by using a cutoff peak

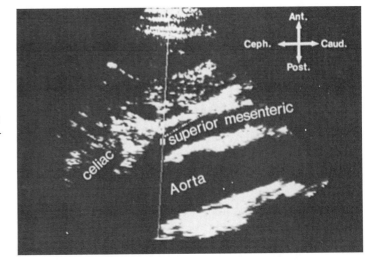

Fig. 3-15. Longitudinal B-mode scan showing the aorta, the origin of the celiac, and the first 4 cm of the superior mesenteric artery.

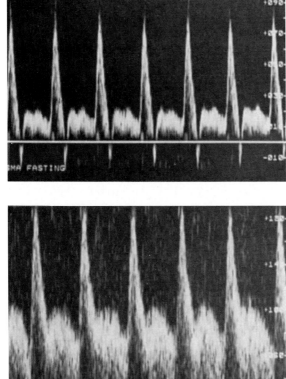

Fig. 3-16. In the fasting state **(A)** flow in the superior mesenteric shows a brief reverse flow component and a low end-diastolic velocity. After eating **(B)** there is an increase in both the peak systolic and end-diastolic velocities. *(From Taylor DC and Moneta GL: Duplex ultrasound scanning of the renal and mesenteric circulation, Semin Vasc Surg 1:23, 1988.)*

Table 3-4. Range of Values for Blood Flow in the Celiac and Superior Mesenteric Arteries*

Artery	Peak Systolic Velocity (cm/sec)	End-diastolic Velocity (cm/sec)	Volume Flow (ml/min)
Celiac	101 ± 3.5	33 ± 1.4	1083 ± 75
Superior mesenteric	113 ± 3.9	15 ± 1.1	538 ± 37

*Mean and standard error of the mean.

Table 3-5. Maximal Percentage Increases in the Celiac and Superior Mesenteric Arteries after a Mixed Meal*

Artery	Peak Systolic Velocity (cm/sec)	End-diastolic Velocity (cm/sec)	Volume Flow (ml/min)
Celiac	20 ± 6	24 ± 9	18 ± 4
Superior mesenteric	42 ± 4	321 ± 100	164 ± 30

*Mean and standard error of the mean.

systolic value of greater than 200 cm/sec for the celiac and greater than 275 cm/sec for the superior mesenteric artery, the following results were obtained when compared with lateral aortograms: (1) for the superior mesenteric artery there was a sensitivity of 92% and a specificity of 96%, a positive predictive value of 80% with a negative predictive value of 99%, and an overall accuracy of 96%; and (2) for

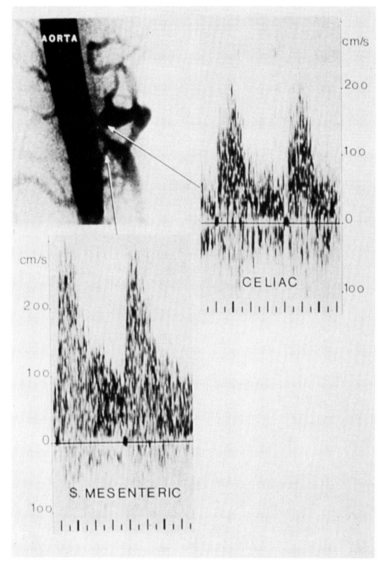

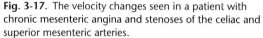

Fig. 3-17. The velocity changes seen in a patient with chronic mesenteric angina and stenoses of the celiac and superior mesenteric arteries.

the celiac artery there was a sensitivity of 87% with a specificity of 80%, a positive predictive value of 63% with a negative predictive value of 94%, and an overall accuracy of 82%.

These should be considered to be guidelines only since there is some variability in making these estimations by arteriography. As noted later, in our experience patients who have chronic mesenteric ischemia have all had extensive narrowing or occlusion of both the celiac and superior mesenteric arteries.

In the six patients encountered with chronic mesenteric angina, the diagnosis has been readily made on the basis of the duplex scan results alone. In each case there have been high-grade (greater than 50%) diameter-reducing lesions in both the celiac and the superior mesenteric arteries (Fig. 3-17). We have not yet seen a patient with a chronic stenosis or occlusion of the superior mesenteric artery alone who had the syndrome.

Since the inferior mesenteric artery can serve as an excellent collateral for the entire small bowel, it would be important to evaluate this vessel in the course of screening patients suspected of having chronic mesenteric angina. Because of its size and location, the inferior mesenteric artery has been difficult to study until recent advances in technology have made it possible. With color flow Doppler it is often possible to identify the origin of the artery and then assess its status. In our preliminary studies we have been able to show that flow in this artery does not increase in response to the type of material ingested by the patient to study flow patterns in the superior mesenteric and celiac arteries. On the other hand, if the subject ingests a material such as lactulose, which is metabolized in the colon, flow in the inferior mesenteric artery will increase when the material reaches that portion of the gut. This is shown in Fig. 3-18.

Another important function of the duplex studies is that they can be applied to the postoperative patient to document the results. We have found this to be very useful after angioplasty and direct arterial surgery. An example of these studies is shown in Fig. 3-19.

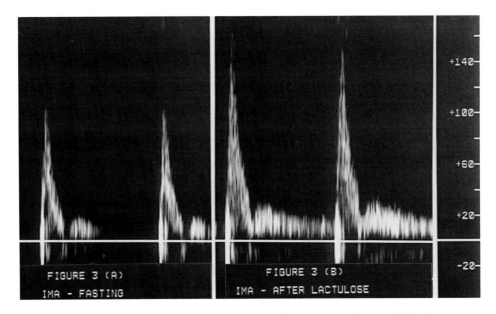

Fig. 3-18. The flow is the inferior mesenteric artery (IMA) during fasting *(left panel)*. After ingesting lactulose, flow in the IMA increases. This can be seen as an increase in the peak systolic and end-diastolic velocity. (See text.)

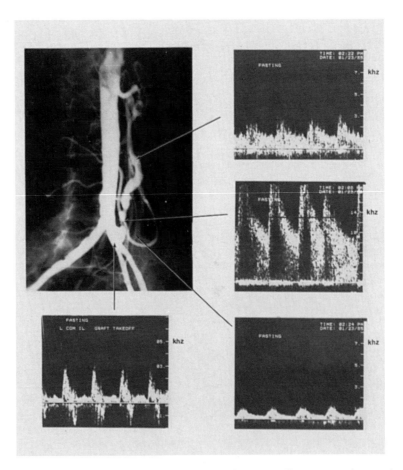

Fig. 3-19. This patient had a vein graft placed from the left common iliac artery to the superior mesenteric artery. Nine months after the operation, symptoms returned and a stenosis at the origin of the vein graft was discovered. This was treated by transluminal angioplasty.

ACUTE VENOUS THROMBOSIS

Whereas diseases of the arterial system have dominated the attention of the American medical community, thrombosis of the deep veins with all of the potential sequelae remains a constant and ongoing problem that is not likely to diminish in numbers or importance. In fact, any patient who sustains an injury to the lower limb, be it surgical or outside the hospital, is always at risk. In addition, any patient who is hospitalized for nearly any reason is also at risk for developing the problem. A major problem that continues to face the medical profession is when to suspect the diagnosis and how to confirm it effectively. There are few areas in clinical medicine in which the need to disregard one's impression based on clinical findings can be more important. Physicians must stop trying to make a definitive diagnosis at the bedside since they will be correct only one half the time.[86] The key point to make is that if the diagnosis is entertained, it must be either established or ruled out by some objective test that has proved to be both sensitive and specific for the problem.

The one diagnostic approach that has stood the test of time is phlebography.[87] This procedure permits an objective assessment of the major deep veins at all points at which the contrast material can be found. It is usually performed by injecting contrast material in a vein on the dorsum of the foot, inserting enough volume to fill the major deep veins and follow the course of the dye to the level of the inferior vena cava. In theory this is the best possible test, but there are the following limitations: (1) the test is painful; (2) it should be done bilaterally; (3) there is always the risk of a contrast allergy occurring; (4) in a small percentage of cases (less than 10%) the dye may induce a chemical phlebitis that must be treated[88]; (5) the iliac veins and inferior vena cava will not be seen well in 20% of cases; (6) the deep femoral vein will not be seen in one half of the cases studied; (7) it is difficult to repeat the test to document changes that might have occurred; and (8) it is costly.

Because of the inaccuracy of the bedside diagnosis and the problems associated with phlebography, noninvasive methods were developed to fill this gap in the approach to this common problem. Since the 1970s a variety of methods have been developed that can satisfy the needs of the practicing community when faced with this problem. Deep venous thrombosis produces changes in flow at the site(s) of involvement, with redirection of flow through the collateral circulation that develops. It was only natural that the initial efforts would be directed at measuring these changes in flow.

Before considering the tests currently in use and their accuracy, it is necessary to review the common sites of involvement and how they affect both the clinical presentation and the methods used to detect them. Most of the knowledge about localization of deep venous thrombi has come from the studies done with the labeled fibrinogen introduced by Hobbs.[89] This method uses the injection of iodine 125–labeled fibrinogen, which is incorporated into the evolving thrombus, setting up a site of increased radioactivity that can be detected externally by scintillation detectors. These studies were designed to detect early thrombi and to permit the findings to be a marker for documenting the natural history of the disorder. This method was also used to monitor prophylactic methods designed to prevent the deep venous thrombosis from occurring.[90] These studies, which have been numerous, have shown that the site for the earliest development of thrombi is within the sinuses of the soleus muscle. If left untreated, up to 80% of the thrombi will resolve, but the remaining 20% will propagate to the deep veins of the calf and extend to the level of the popliteal vein.[91] Unfortunately, the iodine 125 test is relatively insensitive to thrombi that develop in the superficial femoral, common femoral, and iliac veins and the inferior vena cava. The labeled fibrinogen test is no longer in use because of the potential problems associated with the use of blood products.

One theory is that all thrombi originate in the calf and secondarily involve the more proximal deep veins. This is too simplistic a view since thrombi may develop de novo at the more proximal sites. For example, it is known that the sinuses of the venous valves are a site from which the thrombi may develop and then extend into the lumen, setting the stage for complete occlusion to occur.[90] In addition, the left iliofemoral segment is a site where there is usually compression by the right common iliac artery, producing some element of "stasis." Also, other factors that may be responsible for the development of deep venous thrombosis may predispose the patient to the development of deep venous thrombosis. It must also be recognized that the most dangerous thrombi are those that involve the large proximal veins since they can lead to the development of serious and, on occasion, fatal pulmonary emboli.[91] In this regard, thrombi that remain confined to the calf region rarely if ever result in serious and clinically evident pulmonary emboli.

Given these considerations it is important to review the current diagnostic methods and how they can be applied to the patient who is suspected of having the problem.

Continuous Wave Doppler

Since ultrasound penetrates the skin, it is only natural that the availability of such a method can be used to monitor the blood flow in those veins accessible to this form of energy.[92] When this modality is used alone, it cannot distinguish with certainty the vessels being interrogated. It is therefore necessary to use the companion artery to identify the vein of interest. For example, to evaluate the common femoral vein one first locates the common femoral artery as the landmark. The same applies to the other veins distal to the inguinal ligament. It is not possible to identify with certainty the iliac veins and the inferior vena cava, so one must infer on the basis of the flow patterns in the external iliac vein whether or not there is some proximal obstruction.

Below the knee it is possible to study the tibial and peroneal veins, but this has proven difficult in our laboratory because the veins are small and there are many of them, compounding the problem. There is hope that with the use of duplex scanning and color it may be possible to expedite the examination and permit a more comprehensive review of the vessels in this area.

Even with the problems of localization, several aspects of the Doppler findings are of clinical use.[93] The first is that the absence of flow from a major deep vein is certain evidence of its occlusion. This is particularly true for the proximal veins (popliteal to external iliac). Other bits of information can be obtained from veins that are patent by observing the flow patterns. Normally flow in the deep veins of the leg is very dependent on the pressure changes associated with each respiratory cycle. For example, as the diaphragm descends, the increase in intraabdominal pressure exceeds that found in the major deep veins of the leg. This results in a transient cessation in blood flow during inspiration that can normally be observed to the level of the popliteal vein. Below the knee these spontaneous flow patterns may not be detected, and one may be forced to compress the leg in an attempt to augment flow to assess patency of the venous segment. One factor that has been of assistance in documenting the presence of thrombi is to examine the velocity patterns below areas of thrombosis. It is well known both from the early studies done with continuous wave Doppler and, more recently, duplex scanning that flow in this circumstance is often continuous and not responsive to the intraabdominal pressure changes that occur with respiration.

When the Doppler method is compared with phlebography, the results are quite good. Overall the sensitivity should be in the range of 87% with a specificity of 88%.[92] The successful use of this method requires a very experienced technologist who understands both the principle of Doppler ultrasound and the physiologic basis for the changes that occur when the deep venous system becomes occluded. A major problem with the method is the subjective nature of the test and the interpretation of the results. One has to depend entirely on the skill of the person performing the test.

Venous Outflow Plethysmography

Since venous thrombi reduce outflow through the involved venous segment(s), it is only natural that a method be used that could assess the rate of venous outflow in the limbs. Flow—in the presence of venous occlusion—is diverted through collateral channels that have a higher resistance to flow than do the normal unobstructed veins. Thus one would expect that at least early after the onset of the event that the rate of venous emptying would be reduced. To this end, the strain-gauge method,[94,95] impedance plethysmography,[96] and air plethysmography have been used to make this measurement. All of these methods use a cuff placed around the thigh that is inflated to 50 mm Hg to impede venous outflow temporarily. During the phase of venous occlusion venous volume in the limb increases to reach a maximal level in approximately 2 minutes. When the maximal limb volume has been reached and is stabilized, the cuff is suddenly deflated, and the rate at which the venous blood is emptied is assessed. When the strain-gauge method is used, the volume change that occurs can be expressed in terms of centimeters per 100 cc of tissue per minute. The impedance and air plethysmographic methods cannot be quantitated in a similar manner but do permit a similar

estimate that is related to the volume increase that occurs during cuff inflation.

Although the sensor is placed around the calf, the methods are only sensitive to the development of proximal venous thrombosis (popliteal to inferior vena cava). The methods are totally insensitive to thrombi in the calf region.

The venous outflow approach has been widely tested as a screening procedure and has been compared to phlebography. For proximal venous thrombosis the test has a sensitivity of 93% and a specificity of 94%.[96] It is accepted that this method is satisfactory as a screening method since a positive test is highly likely to be associated with acute deep venous thrombosis. A negative test can be used to withhold treatment with minimal risk of an unheralded pulmonary embolus occurring.

Although this method has been extensively tested, it does have problems of concern. It does not permit localization of the disease and cannot be reliably used as a method for documenting changes that occur with therapy. As the collateral circulation improves, venous outflow tends to normalize, and as the venous thrombi themselves begin to lyse, the vessels recanalize. Although new episodes or extension of the process will be reflected in a worsening of the venous outflow, it is not possible to define the basis for the change without some anatomic confirmation.

Duplex Scanning

Since duplex scanning provides both an image of the vein and the ability to assess flow, it is only natural that the method would also be applied to the venous system.[97] As the technology has improved with the availability of different transmitting frequencies and the ability to access vessels at greater depths, it has become possible to study all major veins that are the sites of venous thrombosis.

The value of this method is the combined anatomic and physiologic information that can be obtained. The imaging component is used in three ways: (1) to identify the vein of interest with certainty; (2) to identify the presence of an occluding thrombus (Fig. 3-20); and (3) to permit selective sampling of flow in the imaged vessels.

Although there have been reports of using imaging systems alone only to the level of the external iliac veins, this is not sufficient.[98] With the availability of low-frequency scan heads (2 to 3.5 MHz), one can see the entire iliac venous system and the inferior vena cava.[99] Anything less than this would constitute an inadequate examination. It is possible to study all the major veins below the inguinal ligament regularly to the level of the popliteal vein. The veins below the knee are more difficult, but with the addition of color to the system, it may be feasible to study these segments with regularity.

Imaging is used in two ways to identify the presence or absence of thrombi. Although the answers are not yet complete with regard to the echogenicity of thrombi, they apparently are most echogenic early.[100,101] As time passes, the lesion will become less echogenic. Seeing a thrombus is certain evidence that the vein is involved. However, failure to see a thrombus does not rule out the presence of the problem. For example, in our studies the visualization of

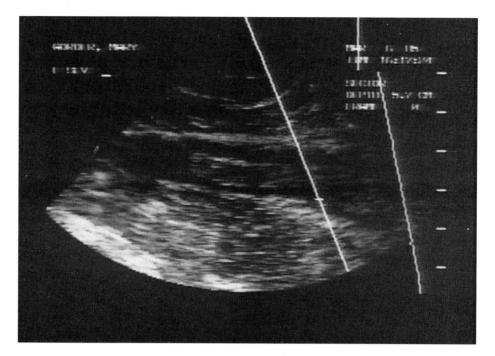

Fig. 3-20. Ultrasonic duplex scan of a superficial femoral vein shows the presence of a large thrombus.

thrombus had a positive predictive value of 95% with a negative predictive value of 50%.[99]

The other element of the imaging component that is used is the inability to compress the vein being visualized. The presumption is that a vein occluded by a thrombus will not be compressible when pressure is applied to the skin surface. Our experience is that compression is not as useful a tool as some investigators would imply, primarily because there are sites that are difficult to compress even in normal individuals. These sites include the iliac veins, the inferior vena cava, and the superficial femoral vein in the adductor canal. In our studies incompressibility had a positive predictive value of 88% with a negative predictive value of 50%.[99]

Surprisingly, the use of velocity parameters was more sensitive and specific in arriving at a diagnosis. The absence of phasicity of flow in a visualized segment had a positive predictive value of 97% and a negative predictive value of 79%. The inability to detect spontaneous flow in a venous segment had a positive predictive value of 100% and a negative predictive value of 57%. In the studies we performed, all of the false-negative cases were secondary to isolated calf vein thrombi.[99] Because of the difficulty of studying the veins of the calf, we recommend that when disease not found on the initial study is suspected in this area, the procedure should be repeated in 3 days to reassess the situation.

CHRONIC VENOUS INSUFFICIENCY

The patient who is initially seen with chronic venous problems generally falls into two categories: (1) those suspected of having primary varicose veins and (2) those whose presentation suggests the presence of underlying deep venous occlusion or valvular incompetence.[102,103] The distinction becomes important in terms of management and long-term prognosis.[104]

Patients with varicose veins as the presenting complaint generally are aware of the problem primarily in terms of the appearance of the limb, the cosmetic deformity, and the symptoms that may be associated with prolonged standing and sitting. When these patients are seen, the major question that must be answered is whether the varicose veins are secondary to defects in the superficial venous system or whether they occurred because of venous valvular incompetence of the deep veins and their communicators with the superficial system. Historically, patients with no deep venous involvement are classified into the primary category and can be treated either by the use of support hose, injection therapy, or surgical means.[102] Although these patients can be suspected because of a strong family history of the problem and no previous history of deep venous thrombosis, it is important to verify this suspicion through some noninvasive testing procedures such as screening with continuous wave Doppler or duplex scanning. Patients with varices secondary to deep venous and perforator incompetence are classified as having secondary varices.

The key issues to address in the noninvasive testing is the patency of the deep veins and the competence of the major deep veins.[99] Competence of the deep veins is noted by the failure to induce reflux when the pressure gradient proximal to the valves is reversed by procedures such as a Valsalva maneuver, limb compression or release of the pressure in a pneumatic cuff placed around the limb.[105] The purpose is to document the status of the valves at all levels from the iliac veins to the region below the knee.

The most common methods of inducing reflux in the lower limb veins is to use a Valsalva maneuver and limb compression. Both will in theory induce a reverse transvalvular pressure gradient, which would encourage reverse flow through the venous valves. Several problems associated with these maneuvers can be summarized as follows:

1. One intact valve proximal to the site of valvular incompetence renders the testing procedure invalid.
2. It is difficult to generate sufficient pressure in some limbs to promote reflux even when valves are incompetent.
3. The results cannot be quantitated. In some cases with gross reflux, quantitation is not necessary, but in borderline cases it might be difficult.

Van Bemmelen et al[105] developed the pneumatic cuff test for quantitating reflux in the upright position. This technique, which uses cuffs at the thigh, calf, and ankle, can be used to study both the superficial and deep veins at all levels. When this test is used, the valve closure time is 0.5 seconds or less in 95% of normal subjects. Many laboratories do not have the expertise to do this test, so some compromise must be sought. We recommend that patients be studied in a −10 degrees Trendelenburg's position to encourage venous filling. When studied in this fashion, the Valsalva maneuver can be used to test proximal venous competence (superficial femoral vein to inferior vena cava) with limb compression best for the venous segments below the knee.

When the deep venous system has been damaged by the presence of deep venous thrombosis, there are changes occurring that explain the subsequent course of events.[106] They are as follows:

1. Production of chronic venous occlusion
2. Destruction of the venous valves at single or multiple sites
3. Lysis of the thrombi with preservation of valve function and venous patency
4. Lysis with recanalization of the involved segments but with destruction of the venous valves

The clinical problems that occur because of the above changes are well known. They include edema, pain, hyperpigmentation, and in the late stages, ulceration. In rare instances the patient may complain of pain in the involved limb that occurs with vigorous exercise and is relieved by rest.[107] We classify these patients as having *postthrombotic syndrome*, even though the more common terminology in use is *postphlebitic syndrome*. We believe this latter terminology is incorrect because it implies that the process that led to the problem had an inflammatory component, which it does not. The patient with exercise-induced leg pain secondary to chronic venous disease is termed as having *venous claudication.*

The testing procedures that might be applied are the same as those used for the patient with varicose veins except for the patient who has symptoms suggestive of venous claudication. The pathophysiology of this problem is related primarily to chronic venous obstruction and the inability of the involved limb to empty itself of the marked increase in venous volume that occurs in response to the stimulus of vigorous exercise. When this is suspected, the abnormality can be documented by carrying out measurements of venous outflow before and after a period of vigorous exercise.[108]

Another method that has been applied quite widely to assess the status of the venous valves is photoplethysmography.[109] This method uses infrared light to assess changes in the venous volume of the dermis. Its application to the study of venous disease is based on the observation that the changes in the venous volume of the dermis are similar in terms of both magnitude and time as those that occur when venous pressures are measured after a period of walking. As is well known, when a healthy individual begins to walk, there is a dramatic fall in the venous pressure measured at the level of the foot. This fall occurs with even a single step. After the walking is stopped, there is a very slow return in the pressure to the preexercise level. Although the skin blood volume change recorded with the photoplethysmograph cannot be quantitated, the directional and time-related changes can be quantitated and used as an index of venous valvular function.

The test can be performed in a variety of ways, the most widely used way has the patient sitting on the edge of a bed or examining table. The patient then dorsiflexes the foot five times, following which the changes in skin blood volume are recorded. Because it is difficult to standardize this method, we prefer to simulate exercise by inflating a pneumatic cuff to 60 mm Hg at the calf level. This inflation-deflation cycle is repeated in rapid succession five times. The variable we have found most useful is the venous recovery time.[108] This is the time required for the dermal blood volume to return to the baseline level. The normal venous recovery time in our laboratory is 24 ± 12 seconds. In patients with valvular incompetence these values are greatly shortened. If there is valvular damage, the venous recovery times are in the range of 9 seconds. This method does not permit any conclusions about the level at which the valvular incompetence is occurring. This can be sorted out to some degree by placing a tourniquet around the calf to occlude the superficial veins and then repeating the test. If the incompetence is confined to the superficial veins, the test results will normalize.

VASOSPASTIC DISORDERS

One of the more common types of patients referred to the vascular laboratory is one who, when exposed to cold, will note the development of color changes in his digits, usually the fingers but in some cases the toes as well. The clinical dilemma is to determine if the changes are of the harmless type associated with Raynaud's disease or secondary to some underlying associated disorder such as scleroderma.[110] Although the history is often useful in making this distinction, a referral to the vascular laboratory can provide useful confirmatory information concerning the status of the digital circulation. If the patient has primary Raynaud's disease, the digital arteries will be patent but hyperresponsive when exposed to cold. When the problem is secondary to an underlying disease, it is common to find the digital arteries occluded in one or more of the affected digits. This can be determined by measurement of the digit blood pressure, which can be done by the use of either strain-gauge plethysmography or photoplethysmography.[111] In addition, it is possible by examining the digit-pulse waveform to document the status of the digital vessels.[112] Normally, the digital systolic blood pressure should be greater than 80% of that recorded from the upper arm. These values are commonly seen in patients with Raynaud's disease. This gradient in pressure will not change significantly with heating.

When the digital arteries are occluded, the pressure gradient between the upper arm and the digit will widen. In addition, the shape of the digit-volume pulse will change from one with a sharp systolic peak and a dicrotic wave to one with a rounded contour in which the upslope and downslope times equalize (a damped waveform). It is also possible to study the digit blood pressure response to cooling.[111] If the patient has true cold sensitivity, the digit blood pressure will fall as the digits are cooled. This response is useful in confirming the clinical suspicion but is not helpful in defining the basis for the problem.

THORACIC OUTLET SYNDROME

When patients complain of pain, dysesthesias, and numbness in various positions of their arms, they are often referred to the vascular laboratory for screening purposes. Testing is done to assess whether or not the patient is able to diminish or completely shut off blood flow to the arm in various positions. This is done by using either a continuous wave Doppler device over the radial or brachial artery or by duplex scanning. It can also be done by checking Doppler systolic pressures or through pulse-volume recordings using the air plethysmograph. The testing is simple but does not provide any diagnostic information that cannot be obtained by a carefully performed physical examination. The problem is that there is a large number of healthy people without symptoms who can reduce or shut off blood flow in various positions of the arm. The only time the testing may be useful is when the results show no compression. Under these circumstances it is at least possible to determine that arterial compression is not the basis for the problem.

A very small number of patients will develop problems within the vessel secondary to intimal injury because of thoracic outlet compression of the subclavian artery. When this occurs, local thrombosis or embolization to the hand may take place. A duplex scan may provide some information, but in most cases an arteriogram will be needed to sort out the problem.

THE FUTURE

Although it is dangerous to attempt to predict the future of the noninvasive laboratory and its place in the field of peripheral vascular diseases, the rapid developments of the last 10 years are impressive. There has been concern about the costs of the instrumentation, particularly duplex scanning equipment, but no other diagnostic system in medicine currently offers the versatility and scope of applications that this method permits. It is remarkable to think

that it is possible with this device to study every major organ system that is affected by atherosclerosis, the most common vascular disease we treat. The systems are even being modified to permit their use as a method of obtaining transcranial information—one of the new applications that is under intense study. Where will this type of study go in the future? Many of the applications of duplex scanning mentioned in this chapter are not yet in general use in the United States. The reasons are quite clear and include the following: (1) the tests in some cases require further study to document their relevance, accuracy, and cost-effectiveness in addressing the problems at hand; (2) the tests in some cases are quite time-consuming, raising the question about the costs of the procedures and the numbers of examinations that can be performed on a daily basis; (3) as the applications expand, the skills required of the technologists also increase (it is apparent that the noninvasive laboratory is only as good as the technologists who are involved); (4) the time required to train a technologist to do the entire battery of examinations is increasing because of the complexity of the testing procedures; and (5) the concern that the use of these tests does not in reality represent a saving of money for the health care delivery system but simply adds to it.

Are some of these tests performed in the noninvasive laboratory going to eliminate some of the more costly and dangerous invasive methods? The answer to this is yes if one is willing to accept certain assumptions. Some examples in which this has occurred and will continue to do so are as follows:

1. *Screening for carotid artery disease.* With the publication of the results of the many clinical trials examining the role of carotid endarterectomy in the prevention of stroke, it will be increasingly necessary to develop guidelines for screening and follow-up as well. Since arteriography is not and will not be a suitable screening test, ultrasonic duplex scanning will remain the test of choice. However, it will be necessary for the testing to be accurate enough to determine which patients should be considered for carotid endarterectomy. Once the screening is done and the patient's course of therapy is determined, what should the follow-up consist of and how often should the studies be repeated if at all? To answer this, it is necessary to determine the outcome as it relates to both the rate of progression and the degree of narrowing that is commonly associated with the development of a stroke. We have conducted such a study, which spanned 10 years with enough data for a 7-year life table analysis. In brief, we noted the following:[113] (a) in 232 patients with a greater than 80% stenosis, 23% were found to have progression of the lesion; (b) of those who progressed, nearly half progressed to a greater than 80% narrowing of the carotid bulb; (c) the risk of progression to severe stenosis and occlusion was greater for those whose initial lesion was in the 50% to 79% range; (d) the cumulative stroke risk for patients with mild stenosis (less than 50%) was 6%, compared with 11% for those with a 50% to 79% narrowing after 7 years; (e)

there were 12 strokes in this cohort of patients, and in 8 of these the stroke occurred in relationship to progression of the lesion.

Given these results, we concluded that the follow-up of patients with detected carotid artery disease should be an annual study. This is particularly true for those patients who have a 50% to 79% lesion when first studied. For patients with a less than 50% stenosis at the time of entry, studies done every 2 years would be sufficient. For lesions that progress, one should give serious consideration to carotid endarterectomy, particularly when they progress to the moderately severe and severe lesions.

2. *Diagnosis of deep venous thrombosis.* Without the availability of noninvasive testing this most common vascular disorder could be diagnosed by only one test, venography. With the extensive studies done using the Doppler and plethysmographic methods, it is clear that most patients with this problem can be spared the invasive procedure. The more recent application of duplex scanning has further reduced the need for venography. It is certain that this will become the definitive test of the future for this problem and for the evaluation of the patient with chronic venous insufficiency.

3. *Documentation of therapeutic outcome.* In the past most therapies for vascular disease were gauged by the subjective responses of the patient and the effects noted by the physician on the status of the variables that could be evaluated on physical examinations. The mysteries surrounding this type of evaluation process are no longer a problem. The outcome for practically all therapies can now be objectively and repeatedly tested by a variety of noninvasive tests.

As the technology has improved, there is increasing interest in eliminating arteriography before carotid endarterectomy.[113] The concerns with this approach have been the fear of missing lesions of the carotid siphon and inside the skull that might compromise the outcome of the procedure. It is now clear that lesions of the carotid siphon do not play a role in affecting the outcome of endarterectomy.[114] To investigate the role of endarterectomy without arteriography, we prospectively studied this in 111 consecutive cases. The surgeons involved had to indicate before the arteriogram whether they would be willing to proceed on the basis of the duplex findings alone. Sixteen patients were excluded because arteriography was not done or was performed before the surgeon's evaluation. The duplex scans were diagnostic in 88 cases (95%). Of the remaining seven cases the following was found: (1) the disease was not limited to the distal common carotid artery or bulb in four cases, (2) anatomic or pathologic features limited the study in one case, and (3) an internal carotid occlusion could not with certainty be distinguished from a tight stenosis in two cases.

Arteriography affected strategy in only one case. This patient had a middle cerebral artery occlusion in addition to the high-grade stenosis. Endarterectomy was not performed; this patient's internal carotid artery went on to

occlude and he suffered a fatal stroke. In retrospect this patient should have undergone the operative procedure. Based on these results we now will proceed with operation without arteriography as long as the duplex scan is diagnostic of the problem.

For reconstructions of the limb arteries the question of eliminating arteriography is more difficult because of the total length of the arteries that must be surveyed and the type of information that vascular surgeons need to make judgments about the surgical approaches most likely to lead to a good outcome. On the other hand, vascular surgeons have known for many years that arteriography tends to underestimate the degree of involvement, particularly in the estimation of stenotic lesions. This is due to the fact that it is the posterior wall of the arteries that is most frequently involved and not seen well on arteriography, particularly when the views shown are not biplanar. What type of information is necessary to proceed with an interventional procedure? This can be summarized as follows:

1. *The location and hemodynamic significance of stenotic lesions, particularly in the aortoiliac and femoropopliteal segments.* Prospective studies done to compare the accuracy of duplex scanning to arteriography have shown that the duplex method is as accurate as the invasive method in defining the significance of such lesions. In fact, the variability that is found when two radiologists read the same arteriograms is at least as great as that encountered when duplex scanning is compared to the results of a single angiographer.[16]

2. *The status of the run-off vessels.* How are these vessels defined? In general, they are all the arteries distal to the point at which the reconstruction ends. For example, in the case of aortoiliac reconstructions it would be the femoropopliteal and below-the-knee arteries. For femoropopliteal and femorotibial reconstructions it is those arteries distal to the lowermost anastomosis. At the moment there is evidence that duplex scanning can be used to predict accurately the status of the femoropopliteal segments and also to assess the patency of the tibial arteries.

To test the hypothesis that the duplex scanning results can be adequate in predicting the type of reconstruction that would be needed, we provided both duplex scanning and arteriographic data, along with pertinent clinical data, to six experienced vascular surgeons in a blinded fashion to determine what the form of therapy would be.[115] The information on the location and extent of involvement was presented on anatomic charts along with an estimate of the degree of narrowing. It was clear that in most cases the duplex data were accurate enough to permit making a reasonable decision about the surgical procedure to use.

To replace arteriography with a combination of indirect tests such as obtaining ankle pressures, exercise testing, and duplex scanning represents such a departure from conventional thinking that it will require considerable study, but it is a direction that needs further investigation. We have in fact found that duplex scanning results can be sufficient for the planning of transluminal angioplasty, particularly for patients with aortoiliac disease. The finding of a hemodynamically significant stenotic lesion in this area is sufficient evidence that we can proceed with the angioplasty as the planned procedure.

Are there new technologies that may affect the role of the noninvasive laboratory and its use in the evaluation of vascular disease? The two methods that might fall into this area are CT scanning and magnetic resonance imaging (MRI). CT scanning has had its greatest impact in the evaluation of aneurysmal disease, particularly as it relates to the evaluation of thoracoabdominal lesions that are difficult to evaluate by ultrasound alone. MRI, with its potential for not only anatomic but flow information, is under intensive study.

How can MRI be of value in vascular disease evaluation? Its value can be summarized as follows:

1. *Anatomy of the vascular system.* It remains to be determined if it will be better when applied in a fashion similar to that for CT scanning.[116,117] There is evidence that the method is able to detect thrombi, but it is also true that turbulent flow may give images that are similar, making the distinction a difficult one at the moment.
2. *MRI angiography.* There is evidence that arteriograms, particularly of the thoracoabdominal vessels, can be generated that are very similar to those obtained with conventional arteriographic means.[118] Resolution with smaller arteries such as the carotid and femoropopliteal segments remains a very serious problem. The resolution currently available is similar to that seen with intravenous digital subtraction arteriography, which most clinicians find inadequate for clinical purposes. Even if it had the same resolution as standard contrast studies, we are faced with very serious logistic problems that will continue to plague the use of this method. Disregarding the costs of such systems, the demands placed on them is such that it makes MRI an impractical method at the moment. For example, it is very likely that such systems would have to be used for this purpose alone to justify their application. The cost of the systems and the cost associated with installation and maintenance make it very unlikely that the current health care delivery system could afford such expense.
3. *Measurement of volume flow.* Such measurement with the system is possible.[119,120] In fact, prototype MRI systems designed for just this purpose are under study. At the moment attention has been directed to the lower limbs in which it appears the method may have some promise. However, before such a method is applied clinically, it must be shown that such information is of clinical value. All of the studies done in the past to examine the value of volume flow measurements have been disappointing. Whether the same type of information gathered by this new modality will be any better or any more useful is definitely open to question.
4. *Potentially, the study of the metabolic activity of skeletal muscle in the normal and ischemic state.* At the moment this is a research tool with some promise and should be pursued. Whether it will have an impact on the clinical appraisal of vascular disease remains to be demonstrated.

REFERENCES

1. Strandness DE Jr: Peripheral arterial disease: a physiological approach, Boston, 1969, Little, Brown & Co, Inc.
2. Lindbom A: Arteriosclerosis and arterial thrombosis in the lower limb. A roentgenological study, Acta Radiol Suppl 80:1, 1950.
3. McKusick VA et al: Buerger's disease: a distinct clinical and pathologic entity, JAMA 181:5, 1962.
4. Strandness DE Jr: Thromboangiitis obliterans. In Peripheral arterial disease: a physiologic approach, Boston, 1969, Little, Brown & Co, Inc.
5. Gensler SW et al: Study of vascular lesions in diabetic, nondiabetic patients, Arch Surg 9:617, 1965.
6. Strandness DE Jr, Priest RE, and Gibbons GE: A combined clinical and pathologic study of diabetic and nondiabetic peripheral arterial disease, Diabetes 13:366, 1964.
7. Winsor TA: Influence of arterial disease on the systolic blood pressure gradients of the extremity, Am J Med Sci 220:117, 1950.
8. Strandness DE Jr, McCutcheon EP, and Rushmer RF: Application of a transcutaneous Doppler flowmeter in the evaluation of occlusive arterial disease, Surg Gynecol Obstet 122:1039, 1966.
9. Carter SA: Role of pressure measurements in vascular disease. In Bernstein EF, ed.: Noninvasive diagnostic techniques in vascular disease, St Louis, 1978, The CV Mosby Co.
10. Taylor MG: Wave travel in arteries and design of the cardiovascular system. In Attinger EO, ed.: Pulsatile blood flow, New York, 1964, McGraw-Hill Book Co.
11. Orchard TJ and Strandness DE Jr: Assessment of peripheral vascular disease in diabetes, Circulation 88:819, 1993.
12. Strandness DE Jr and Sumner DS: The effect of geometry on arterial blood flow. In Strandness DE Jr and Sumner DS, eds.: Hemodynamics for surgeons, New York, 1975, Grune & Stratton, Inc.
13. Holstein P and Lassen NA: Healing of ulcers on the feet correlated with distal blood pressure measurements in occlusive arterial disease, Acta Orthop Scand 51:995, 1980.
14. Strandness DE Jr and Bell JW: Peripheral vascular disease: diagnosis and objective evaluation using a mercury strain gauge, Am Surg 161(suppl):1, 1965.
15. Raines JK: Use of pulse volume recorder in peripheral arterial disease. In Bernstein EF, ed.: Noninvasive diagnostic techniques in vascular disease, ed 3, St Louis, 1985, The CV Mosby Co.
16. Jager KA, Ricketts HJ, and Strandness DE Jr: Duplex scanning for the evaluation of lower limb arterial disease. In Bernstein EF, ed.: Noninvasive diagnostic techniques in vascular disease, ed 3, St Louis, 1985, The CV Mosby Co.
17. Strandness DE Jr: Intermittent claudication. In Gifford R, ed.: Peripheral vascular disease, Philadelphia, 1971, FA Davis Co.
18. Silver RA et al: Intermittent claudication of neurospinal origin, Arch Surg 98:523, 1969.
19. Kavanaugh GJ et al: "Pseudoclaudication" syndrome produced by compression of the equina, JAMA 206:2477, 1968.
20. Stahler C and Strandness DE Jr: Ankle blood pressure response to graded treadmill exercise, Angiology 18:237, 1967.
21. Sumner DS and Strandness DE Jr: The relationship between calf blood flow and ankle blood pressure in patients with intermittent claudication, Surgery 65:763, 1969.

22. Strandness DE Jr and Zierler RE: Exercise ankle pressure measurements in arterial disease. In Bernstein EF, ed.: Noninvasive diagnostic techniques in vascular disease, ed 3, St Louis, 1985, The CV Mosby Co.

23. Kohler TR et al: Duplex scanning for diagnosis of aortoiliac and femoropopliteal disease, Circulation 5:1074, 1987.

24. Leather RP and Kupinski AM: Preoperative evaluation of the saphenous vein as a suitable graft, Semin Vasc Surg 1:51, 1988.

25. Bandyk DF: Monitoring functional patency of vascular grafts, Semin Vasc Surg 1:40, 1988.

26. Cox GS et al: Ultrasound guided compression of traumatic pseudoaneurysms, J Vasc Surg 19:683, 1994.

27. Dougherty MJ et al: Optimizing technical success of renal revascularization: does intraoperative color flow duplex ultrasonography enhance results? J Vasc Surg 17:849, 1993.

28. Legemate DA et al: The potential for duplex scanning to replace aortoiliac and femoropopliteal angiography, Eur J Vasc Surg 3:49, 1989.

29. Edwards JM et al: The role of duplex scanning in the selection of patients for transluminal angioplasty, J Vasc Surg 13:69, 1991.

30. Katzen BT: Percutaneous transluminal angioplasty in peripheral vascular disease. In Haimovici H et al, eds.: Vascular Surgery, ed 3, Norwalk, Conn, 1989, Appleton & Lange.

31. Yao JST: Surgical uses of pressure studies in peripheral arterial disease. In Bernstein EF, ed.: Noninvasive diagnostic techniques in vascular disease, ed 3, St Louis, 1985, The CV Mosby Co.

32. Idu MM et al: Impact of color-flow duplex surveillance program on infrainguinal vein graft patency, J Vasc Surg 17:42, 1993.

33. Mattos MA et al: Does correction of stenoses identified by color duplex scanning improve infrainguinal graft patency? J Vasc Surg 17:54, 1993.

34. Bandyk DF et al: Monitoring functional patency of in-situ saphenous vein bypasses: the impact of a surveillance protocol and elective revision, J Vasc Surg 9:286, 1989.

35. Collins J et al: Oxford screening program for abdominal aortic aneurysm in men 65-74 years, Lancet:613, 1988.

36. Bernstein EF, Harris R, and Leopold GR: Noninvasive evaluation of abdominal aortic aneurysm by ultrasonic imaging and computed tomography scanning. In Bernstein EF, ed.: Noninvasive diagnostic techniques in vascular disease, ed 3, St Louis, 1985, The CV Mosby Co.

37. Nevitt MP, Ballard DJ, and Hallett JW Jr: Prognosis of abdominal aortic aneurysms, N Engl J Med 321:1009, 1989.

38. Haimovici H: Peripheral arterial aneurysms. In Haimovici H et al, eds.: Vascular surgery, ed 3, Norwalk, Conn, 1989, Appleton & Lange.

39. North American Carotid Endarterectomy Trial Collaborators: Beneficial effect of carotid endarterectomy in symptomatic patients with high-grade carotid stenosis, N Engl J Med 325:445, 1991.

40. European Carotid Surgery Trialist's Collaborative Group: MRC European carotid surgery trial. Interim results for symptomatic patients with severe (70-99%) or with mild (0-29%) stenosis, Lancet 337:1235, 1991.

41. Hobson RW et al: Efficacy of carotid endarterectomy for asymptomatic carotid stenosis, N Engl J Med 328:221, 1993.

42. Clinical Advisory, Carotid Endarterectomy for Patients with Asymptomatic Internal Carotid Artery Stenosis. National Institutes of Health, September 28, 1994.

43. Barnes RW et al: The Doppler cerebrovascular examination: Improved results with refinements in technique, Stroke 8:468, 1977.

44. Kartchner MM, McRae LP, and Morrison FD: Noninvasive detection and evaluation of carotid occlusive disease, Arch Surg 106:528, 1973.

45. Gee W: Carotid physiology with ocular pneumoplethysmography, Stroke 5:666, 1982.

46. Langlois YE et al: Evaluation of carotid artery disease. The concordance between pulsed Doppler spectrum analysis and angiography, Ultrasound Med Biol 9:51, 1983.

47. Langlois YE, Roederer GO, and Strandness DE Jr: Ultrasonic evaluation of the carotid bifurcation, Echocardiography 4:141, 1987.

48. Roederer GO et al: The natural history of carotid arterial disease in asymptomatic patients with cervical bruits, Stroke 15:605, 1984.

49. Moneta GL et al: Operative versus nonoperative management of asymptomatic high-grade internal carotid artery stenosis: improved results with endarterectomy, Stroke 18:1005, 1987.

50. Moneta GL et al: Correlation of North American Symptomatic Carotid Endarterectomy Trial (NASCET): angiographic definition of 70-99% carotid stenosis with duplex scanning, J Vasc Surg 17:152, 1993.

51. Edwards JM et al: Duplex criteria for 70-99% internal carotid stenosis, Stroke 25:359, 1994.

52. Edwards JM et al: Duplex ultrasound criteria for determining ≥50% and ≥60% internal carotid stenosis: implications for screening examinations (in preparation).

53. Johnson BF et al: Clinical outcome in patients with mild and moderate carotid stenosis, J Vasc Surg 21 (in press), 1995.

54. Nicholls SC et al: Carotid endarterectomy: relationship of outcome to early restenosis, J Vasc Surg 2:375, 1985.

55. Reivich M et al: Reversal of blood flow through the vertebral artery and its effects on cerebral circulation, N Engl J Med 265:878, 1961.

56. Bornstein NM and Norris JW: Subclavian steal? A harmless hemodynamic phenomenon? Lancet 2:303, 1986.

57. Nicholls SC, Koutlas T, and Strandness DE Jr: Unpublished data.

58. Aaslid R, Markwaider TM, and Nornes H: Noninvasive transcranial Doppler ultrasound recording of flow velocity in basal cerebral arteries, J Neurosurg 57:769, 1982.

59. Kirkham FJ et al: Transcranial measurement of blood velocities in the basal cerebral arteries using pulsed Doppler ultrasound: velocity as index of flow, Ultrasound Med Biol 12:15, 1986.

60. Padayachee TS et al: Monitoring middle cerebral artery blood velocity during endarterectomy, Br J Surg 73:98, 1986.

61. Hennerici M, Rautenberg W, and Schwartz A: Transcranial Doppler ultrasound for assessment of intracranial artery occlusive disorders, Surg Neurol 27:523, 1987.

62. Harders AG and Gilsbach JM: Time course of blood velocity changes related to vasospasm in the circle of Willis measured by transcranial Doppler ultrasound, J Neurosurg 66:718, 1987.

63. Harper AM and Glass HE: Effect of alterations in the arterial carbon dioxide tension in the blood flow through the cerebral cortex at normal and low arterial blood pressures, J Neurol Neurosurg Psychiatry 28:449, 1966.

64. Sturtznegger M et al: Dynamic transcranial Doppler assessment of positional vertebrobasilar ischemia, Stroke 25:1776, 1994.

65. Gifford RW: Epidemiology and clinical manifestation of renovascular hypertension. In Stanley J, Ernst C, and Fry W, eds.: Renovascular hypertension, Philadelphia, 1984, WB Saunders Co.

66. Ernst CB: Renal artery reconstruction. In Haimovici H et al, eds.: Vascular surgery, ed 3, Norwalk, Conn, 1989, Appleton & Lange.

67. Treadway KK and Slater EE: Renovascular hypertension, Ann Rev Med 35:665, 1984.

68. Vaughan ED: Renovascular hypertension, Kidney Int 27:811, 1985.

69. Kohler TR et al: Noninvasive diagnosis of renal artery stenosis by ultrasonic duplex scanning, J Vasc Surg 4:450, 1986.

70. Taylor DC et al: Duplex scanning in the diagnosis of renal artery stenosis: a prospective evaluation, J Vasc Surg 7:363, 1988.

71. Hoffman U et al: Role of duplex scanning for the detection of atherosclerotic renal artery disease, Kidney Int 39:1232, 1991.

72. Louie J et al: Prevalence of carotid and lower extremity arterial disease in patients with renal artery stenosis, Am J Hypertens 7:436, 1994.

73. Taylor DC, Moneta GL, and Strandness DE Jr: Follow-up of renal artery stenosis by duplex ultrasound, J Vasc Surg 9:410, 1989.

74. Guzman RP et al: Renal atrophy and arterial stenosis: a prospective study with duplex ultrasound, Hypertension 23:346, 1994.

75. Zierler RE et al: Natural history of atherosclerotic renal artery stenosis: a prospective study with duplex ultrasonography, J Vasc Surg 19:250, 1994.

76. Rigsby CM et al: Doppler signal quantitation in renal allografts. Comparison in normal and rejecting transplants, with pathologic correlation, Radiology 162:31, 1987.

77. Reinite ER et al: Evaluation of transplant renal artery blood flow by Doppler sound-spectrum analysis, Arch Surg 118:415, 1983.

78. Fleischer AC et al: Duplex Doppler sonography of renal transplants. Correlation with histopathology, J Ultrasound Med 8:89, 1989.

79. Genkins SM, Sanflippo FD, and Carroll BA: Duplex sonography of renal transplants: lack of sensitivity and specificity in establishing pathologic diagnosis, AJR 152:535, 1989.

80. Taylor DC: Evaluation of mesenteric and renal vascular disease. In Strandness DE Jr and Taylor KW, eds.: Duplex doppler ultrasound, New York, 1989, Churchill Livingstone, Inc.

81. Jager KA et al: Noninvasive diagnosis of intestinal angina, J Clin Ultrasound 12:588, 1984.

82. Jager K et al: Measurement of mesenteric blood flow by duplex scanning, J Vasc Surg 3:462, 1986.

83. Nicholls SC et al: Use of hemodynamic parameters in the diagnosis of mesenteric insufficiency, J Vasc Surg 3:507, 1986.

84. Moneta GL et al: Duplex ultrasound measurement of postprandial intestinal blood flow: effect of meal composition, Gastroenterology 95:1294, 1988.

85. Moneta GL et al: Mesenteric duplex scanning: a blinded prospective study, J Vasc Surg 17:79, 1993.

86. Haeger K: Problem of acute deep venous thrombosis. The interpretation of symptoms and signs, Angiology 20:219, 1969.

87. Rabinov K and Paulin S: Roentgen diagnosis of venous thrombosis, Arch Surg 104:134, 1972.

88. Athanasoulis CA: Phlebography for diagnosis of deep leg vein thrombosis and pulmonary embolism, DHEW Pub (NIH) No. 76-866, Washington DC, 1975.

89. Hobbs JT: External measurement of fibrinogen uptake in experimental venous thrombosis and other pathological states, Br J Exp Pathol 43:48, 1962.

90. Nicolaides AN, Kakkar VV, and Renney JTG: Soleus sinuses and stasis, Br J Surg 58:307, 1971.

91. Kakkar VV et al: Natural history of deep vein thrombosis, Lancet 2:230, 1969.

92. Strandness DE Jr and Thiele BL: Venous thrombosis and pulmonary embolism. In Selected topics in vascular disorders, Mt Kisco, NY, 1981, Futura Publishing Co.

93. Sumner DS: Doppler evaluation of the venous circulation. In Rutherford RB, ed.: Vascular surgery, Philadelphia, 1977, WB Saunders Co.

94. Barnes RW et al: Noninvasive quantitation of maximum venous outflow in acute thrombophlebitis, Surgery 72:971, 1973.

95. Sumner DS: Strain gauge plethysmography. In Bernstein EF, ed.: Noninvasive diagnostic techniques in vascular disease, ed 3, St Louis, 1985, The CV Mosby Co.

96. Wheeler HB and Anderson FA: The diagnosis of venous thrombosis by impedance plethysmography. In Bernstein EF, ed.: Noninvasive diagnostic techniques in vascular disease, ed 3, St Louis, 1985, The CV Mosby Co.

97. Sullivan ED, Peter DJ, and Cranely JJ: Real-time B-mode venous ultrasound, J Vasc Surg 1:465, 1984.

98. Lensing AWA et al: Detection of deep-vein thrombosis by real-time B-mode ultrasonography, N Engl J Med 320:342, 1989.

99. Killewich LA et al: Diagnosis of deep-venous thrombosis: a prospective study comparing duplex scanning to contrast venography, Circulation 79:810, 1989.

100. Coehlo JCV et al: B-mode ultrasonography of blood clots, J Clin Ultrasound 10:323, 1982.

101. Alanen A and Kormand M: Correlation of the echogenicity and structure of clotted blood, J Ultrasound Med 4:421, 1985.

102. Strandness DE Jr and Thiele BL: Varicose veins. In Selected topics in venous disorder, Mt Kisco, NY, 1981, Futura Publishing Co, Inc.

103. Strandness DE Jr and Thiele BL: Postthrombotic venous insufficiency. In Selected topics in venous disorders, Mt Kisco, NY, 1981, Futura Publishing Co, Inc.

104. Strandness DE Jr et al: Long-term sequelae of acute venous thrombosis, JAMA 250:1289, 1983.

105. van Bemmelen PS et al: Quantitative segmental evaluation of venous valvular reflux with ultrasonic duplex scanning, J Vasc Surg 10:425, 1990.

106. Killewich LA et al: Spontaneous lysis of deep venous thrombosis. Rate and outcome, J Vasc Surg 9:89, 1989.

107. Killewich LA et al: Pathophysiology of venous claudication, J Vasc Surg 1:507, 1984.

108. Killewich LA et al: An objective assessment of the physiologic changes in the postthrombotic syndrome, Arch Surg 120:424, 1985.

109. Flinn WR et al: The use of photoplethysmography in the assessment of chronic venous insufficiency. In Kempczinski RF, ed.: Practical noninvasive vascular diagnosis, Chicago, 1982, Year Book Medical Publishers.

110. Carter SA: Clinical problem in peripheral arterial disease: is the clinical diagnosis adequate? In Bernstein EF, ed.: Noninvasive diagnostic techniques in vascular disease, ed 3, St Louis, 1985, The CV Mosby Co.

111. Nielsen SL and Lassen NA: Finger systolic pressure in upper extremity testing for cold sensitivity (Raynaud's phenomenon). In Bernstein EF, ed.: Noninvasive diagnostic techniques in vascular disease, ed 3, St Louis, 1985, The CV Mosby Co.

112. Thulesius O: Problems in the evaluation of hand ischemia. In Bernstein EF, ed.: Noninvasive diagnostic techniques in vascular disease, ed 3, St Louis, 1985, The CV Mosby Co.

113. Dawson DL et al: The role of duplex scanning and arteriography before carotid endarterectomy: a prospective study, J Vasc Surg 18:673, 1993.

114. Roederer GO et al: Is siphon disease important in predicting outcome of carotid endarterectomy, Arch Surg 118:1177, 1983.

115. Kohler TR et al: Can duplex scanning replace arteriography for lower extremity arterial disease? Ann Vasc Surg 4:280, 1990.

116. Kimmey MB et al: Cross-sectional imagery method: a system to compare ultrasound, computed tomography and magnetic resonance with histologic findings, Invest Radiol 22:227, 1987.

117. Hale JD et al: MR imaging of blood vessels using three-dimensional reconstruction methodology, Radiology 157:727, 1985.

118. Herfkens RJ et al: Nuclear magnetic resonance imaging of the cardiovascular system: normal and pathologic findings, Radiology 147:749, 1983.

119. Shimizu K et al: Visualization of moving fluid: quantitative analysis of blood flow velocity using MR imaging, Radiology 159:195, 1986.

120. Barth K et al: Visualization and measurement of flow with magnetic resonance imaging, Biomed Tech 30:12, 1985.

CHAPTER FOUR

DIAGNOSTIC ANGIOGRAPHY

Bart Dolmatch
William J. Davros
Thomas M. Grist

The first angiogram was performed 100 years ago by injecting a radiopaque solution into the blood vessels of amputated extremities.[1] Since then there have been many advances in the application of angiographic technique to living humans. Refinements in radiopaque contrast materials, contrast delivery systems (including catheters, guidewires, and injectors), catheterization techniques, and imaging equipment allow safe and comfortable angiography from head to toe. But only in the past 20 years have technologic developments allowed us to broaden our concept of angiography beyond conventional "catheter and contrast" methods. These recent advances include the development of computed tomography (CT) in the 1970s, which marked the beginning of cross-sectional and multiplanar imaging. By the 1980s magnetic resonance imaging (MRI) techniques were being applied to image congenital great vessel anomalies and acquired disorders such as aortic aneurysms and dissections. Further advances in MRI led to magnetic resonance angiography (MRA) with an array of techniques to study both anatomy and blood flow in smaller arteries and veins. Developments in data storage and processing now allow computed tomographic angiography (CTA) and a burgeoning interest in three-dimensional (3D) angiographic renderings from both CTA and MRA.

It is not possible to draw a perfect representation of an artery or vein by any one technique alone. For example, catheter-based angiography, performed in a manner similar to that used in the 1950s, is the angiographic method commonly used for preoperative evaluation of an abdominal aortic aneurysm (AAA). If the clinical question concerns the size of the aneurysm, however, CT and MRI provide information about the extent of the aneurysm wall that is not available from catheter-based angiography. CT and MRI can assess the amount of mural thrombus and wall calcification. Angiographic images reconstructed from CT or MRI scans (CTA and MRA) give 3D displays of the AAA without arterial catheterization, potentially replacing catheter-based angiography altogether.

Because of the growing use of CTA and MRA in clinical practice, this chapter focuses on "conventional" catheter-based angiography, CTA, and MRA.

"CONVENTIONAL" CATHETER-BASED ANGIOGRAPHY: METHODS AND APPLICATIONS

Catheter-based angiography yields images of the vascular lumen. Any condition that requires luminal evaluation for diagnosis or characterization is best studied by this technique. Catheter-based angiography is of particular importance in the evaluation of atherosclerotic, thrombotic, and embolic occlusions; some congenital arterial and venous anomalies; many vasculitides; ischemia related to dissection or trauma; and deep vein thrombosis (DVT). It is also indispensable before most percutaneous and surgical vascular procedures related to renal, cerebrovascular, and lower-extremity atherosclerotic disease.

Catheter-based angiography combines three elements: radiopaque contrast material, delivery of a bolus of contrast material into the vascular system, and high-quality radiographic imaging during contrast administration.

Contrast Agents

Early contrast agents included iodinated oils, strontium bromide, sodium iodide, and organic iodides. These agents induced extreme pain during administration and often led to immediate or delayed toxic effects. Further work led to the development of triiodinated aromatic organic salts in the 1950s, including the meglumine and diatrizoate salts. These agents have a wide margin of safety but are not well tolerated in the arterial system because they produce sensations of heat, burning, and pain following injection. Nevertheless, they have achieved widespread use and provide excellent radiopacity.

In the 1970s research led to the discovery of new types of iodinated aromatic-acid salts. These new compounds, like the previous generation of contrast agents, incorporate covalently bound iodine into the structure of an organic

Table 4-1. Intravascular Contrast Agents Used for Angiography (Iodine Concentration Approximately 300 mg/ml for Each Agent)

Agent	Type of Agent	Osmolality mOsm/kg	Viscosity cP at 37° C
Diatrizoate	High-osmolar ionic	1340-1500*	2.3-6.1*
Iothalamate	High-osmolar ionic	1440-1700*	3.0-3.8*
Ioxaglate	Low-osmolar ionic	600	7.5
Iohexol	Low-osmolar nonionic	862	10.4
Iopamidol	Low-osmolar nonionic	796	9.4
Ioversol	Low-osmolar nonionic	716	6.0

(Modified from Cohan RH: Radiographic contrast media. In Kadir S, ed: Current practice of interventional radiology, Philadelphia, 1991, BC Decker with permission.)
*Value depends on specific preparation.

acid salt. Both the older triiodinated organic acid salts and the newer agents can be classified into one of three groups: high-osmolar ionics such as the diatrizoate and iothalamate salts (Conray and Renografin); low-osmolar nonionics including iohexol (Omnipaque), iopamidol (IsoVue), and ioversol (Optiray); low-osmolar ionics represented by ioxaglate (Hexabrix). Table 4-1 summarizes these agents and their physical properties, including osmolality and viscosity for agents approximately 60% by weight.

While the indications, risks, and benefits of these different intravascular contrast agents continue to be studied, it is clear that patients tolerate arterial injection of the lower-osmolar agents, both ionic and nonionic, better than the high-osmolar agents.[3] There is less burning and pain. Reduced pain also lessens patient movement, which usually produces better angiographic images. The low-osmolar agents generate a lower osmotic load (which may be important for those patients who are sensitive to intravascular volume increase, such as patients with congestive heart failure or patients who are hemodialysis dependent).

Compared with ionic contrast agents, nonionic agents offer a reduced risk of contrast-related anaphylactoid reactions such as urticaria, flushing, coughing, wheezing, dyspnea, facial edema, and sudden drop in blood pressure.[4] There is a threefold to eightfold reduction in the frequency of all contrast-related adverse reactions with the nonionic compounds.[2,4]

One adverse effect of contrast administration, renal toxicity, has not been appreciably reduced by use of the low-osmolality agents. Contrast-related nephrotoxicity, usually a self-limited problem, seems to occur equally with both the high- and low-osmolar agents when patients are well hydrated.[5,6] A prudent approach to avoid contrast-induced renal impairment has been summarized by Brezis

and Epstein.[7] They identify patients at risk for renal impairment before contrast administration, attempt to correct comorbid conditions (if possible), and assure appropriate hydration of the patient before the procedure. Then attempts are made to limit the amount of the intravascular contrast agent injected during the imaging study.

The selection of an appropriate contrast agent for angiography must be made based on many factors, and patient comfort and safety reflect only two of the issues. The cost of the low-osmolar agents is an important consideration, since they are currently 10 to 15 times that of the high-osmolar agents. This in part explains why the "safer" agents have not entirely replaced the high-osmolality ionics in daily practice.

There has been enthusiasm for the use of carbon dioxide gas as an intravascular contrast agent, particularly for study of abdominal aortic pathology, renal artery disease, and aortoiliac imaging[8-10] (Fig. 4-1, A and B). In addition, there are early indications that carbon dioxide gas may also provide an excellent agent for patients with arteriovenous grafts,[11] venous abnormalities,[12] and for placement of percutaneous intrahepatic portocaval shunts.[13] For patients with severe underlying renal insufficiency, labile intravascular volume status, or prior proven severe contrast reactions, carbon dioxide (CO_2) gas can produce images of diagnostic quality. Carbon dioxide gas causes no nephrotoxic effect,[14-17] is nonallergenic, and is well tolerated by patients with minimal discomfort. Eliminated by the lungs, CO_2 gas causes negligible change in the acid-base equilibrium and pH,[12] even when administered in large volumes (multiple 60-ml intravascular injections).

There are limitations to CO_2 as an intravascular contrast agent. Uneven intravascular distribution due to nondependent layering of gas may occur. Carbon dioxide must be injected by hand (since a suitable injector system has not been approved for use in the United States). Furthermore, CO_2 gas has not been proven safe in the ascending aorta or aortic arch. Animal work has shown multifocal cerebral infarction and disruption of the blood-brain barrier when CO_2 gas is injected into the cerebral vasculature.[18] Finally, for CO_2 gas to be used as a contrast agent, imaging must be performed with digital subtraction equipment. This, however, presents only a small barrier in most angiography suites, where digital subtraction imaging has become the standard of practice.

Perhaps the greatest hurdle for acceptance of carbon dioxide gas, aside from the lack of an injector system, is uncertainty regarding the ultimate profitability by the radiographic contrast industry. Quite simply, carbon dioxide gas is very inexpensive, costing only pennies for a typical angiographic study. A single small tank of carbon dioxide gas may last for years. Without a commercial proponent, carbon dioxide gas will probably never be marketed aggressively, and the necessary support equipment for carbon dioxide delivery may not be developed.

Contrast Agent Delivery: Catheterization

Transarterial catheter angiography is most often performed by puncture of the common femoral artery. This

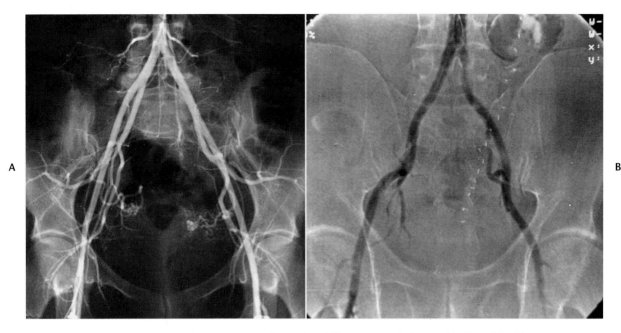

Fig. 4-1. A, Normal pelvic arteriogram obtained with film-screen technique and iodinated liquid contrast material. **B,** Carbon dioxide gas used as a contrast material. Digital subtraction pelvic arteriogram with computer overlap of bones and soft tissues.

technique, pioneered by Farinas[19] and improved by Seldinger,[20] has been refined with various needles and guidewires over the years. Simply stated, the common femoral artery is punctured to allow passage of a guidewire through the needle and into the common femoral artery, placing the wire tip into the aortoiliac circulation. Once the guidewire has been advanced sufficiently into the arterial system, the needle is removed, and a catheter is threaded over the guidewire and into the artery.

Improvements in catheter and guidewire technology have led to the development of new devices that permit selective catheterization of virtually any vessel from the common femoral approach. Catheter construction technology has produced a vast assortment of catheters differing in stiffness, shape, lumen size, and lubricity. Most catheters for selective contrast injection are preshaped and retain their shape even after multiple selective catheterizations. There have been many advances toward miniaturizing the outer diameter of newer catheters. Small high-flow catheters, with outer diameters ranging from 4 to 6 F (1.3 to 2.0 mm outer diameter; 1 F = 0.33 mm)[21] can handle contrast injection rates for virtually any angiographic study.

Advances in guidewire technology have led to the development of atraumatic "torque-controlled" wires. These devices, the products of combined metal alloy and plastic/polymer technology, come in differing degrees of stiffness, flexibility, and memory for their original or assumed shapes. The use of these new guidewires facilitates proper positioning of the angiographic catheter, and thereby reduces the length of time for intravascular catheter manipulation.

Once the catheter tip is seated at its desired location, a small test injection of contrast material is given to confirm that the catheter tip is positioned appropriately without

the possibility of migration during contrast injection. Then the catheter hub is connected to a contrast delivery system. This may be as simple as a syringe of contrast material that is hand injected or as complex as a mechanical injector that is integrated with the imaging equipment. As contrast material is injected, sequential images are obtained. After contrast injection, the catheter may be repositioned in other vessels for further angiography, or removed, with hemostasis being achieved at the puncture site by gentle pressure.

The incidence of common femoral artery puncture site complications, including transfusion-requiring hematoma (Fig. 4-2, *A*), pseudoaneurysm (Fig. 4-2, *B*), arteriovenous fistula (Fig. 4-2, *C*), arterial dissection, and puncture site thrombosis is 0.37% to 0.57%.[22-26] Recent work suggests that many postangiographic groin complications can be lessened by scrupulous technique. Altin et al[27] report that most postangiographic pseudoaneurysms and arteriovenous fistulas are related to femoral punctures at or below the femoral bifurcation. By assuring puncture into the common femoral artery, most pseudoaneurysms and arteriovenous fistulas can be avoided. Many pseudoaneurysms are now treated by ultrasound-guided compression, with thrombosis of the lumen of the pseudoaneurysm, as originally described by Fellmeth et al.[28] This noninvasive technique has largely replaced surgical treatment of groin pseudoaneurysms.

Other angiographic complications include distal thrombotic embolization, 0.10%,[22] and stroke during retrograde catheterization of the ascending aorta, 0.02% to 0.12%.[23-26,29] Femoral artery catheterization has an angiography-related mortality rate of 0.03% to 0.19%.[22-26]

Cholesterol embolization, a rare complication of arterial catheterization (particularly catheterization of the aorta), is believed to be associated with disruption of

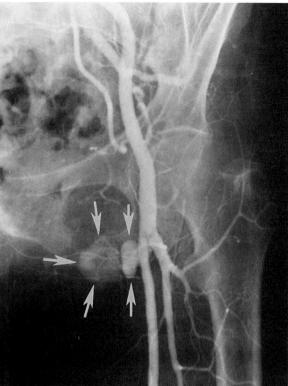

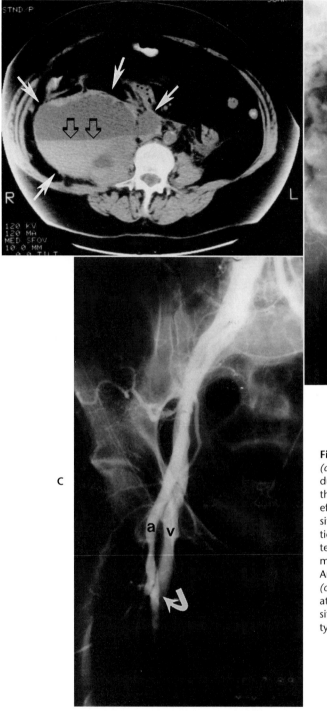

Fig. 4-2. **A,** Large bilobed right retroperitoneal hematoma *(arrows)* seen by CT. There is a fluid-fluid level *(open arrows)* due to layering of blood cells at the dependent portion of the hematoma and a serum supernatant ("hematocrit effect"). **B,** Pseudoaneurysm at a left femoral artery puncture site *(arrows).* The location is at the femoral artery bifurcation, well below the recommended site for safe femoral artery puncture (overlying the femoral head). This is typical for most puncture-related pseudoaneurysms at the groin. **C,** Arteriovenous fistula at a right femoral artery puncture site *(curved arrow).* The artery *(a)* and vein *(v)* communicate at the puncture site, which is well below the recommended site for safe femoral artery puncture. As in **(B)** this location is typical for most puncture-related AV fistulas at the groin.

cholesterol-rich aortic plaque. The embolic cholesterol crystals cause a dramatic (and often immediate) mottled blue skin discoloration (livedo reticularis) as well as agitation, hypertension, renal failure, stroke, and often death.[30,31] Although the direct embolic effects are certainly responsible for many of the clinical findings, a secondary autoimmune response may also be involved, characterized by early eosinophilia and prolonged erythrocyte sedimentation rate.[32]

Imaging Technology

For many years angiography has been accomplished using mechanical rapid film changers and film-screen radiographic technique. Although this method provides angiographic films with exceptional spatial resolution, there are a number of inherent problems and limitations. The radiation dose per image is high, and initial miscalculation of radiographic technique often necessitates repeated exposures of the same image. To set an appropriate

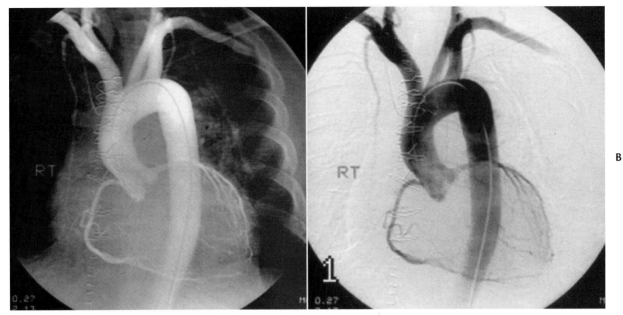

Fig. 4-3. A, Digital image (DI) of the thoracic aorta. The coronary arteries, aortic root, great vessels, and descending thoracic aorta are contrast filled. The cardiac silhouette, ribs, and sternal wires are seen as well. **B,** Digital subtraction angiogram (DSA). The same imaging data are used as for **(A);** however, all non–contrast-enhanced structures have been subtracted from the image by the computer. Only the vascular structures appear. The image may be reviewed as black-on-white or white-on-black (not shown).

radiographic technique, a "scout" film, which confirms the selection of appropriate positioning and technical settings for the ensuing angiogram, is required. Overall, this type of angiography is time-consuming and costly. It generates a series of angiographic images of high spatial resolution but often mediocre contrast resolution.

Digital angiography, a computerized method for acquiring angiographic images, has largely replaced film-screen angiographic studies. Rather than the image being captured on a silver-based film, the virtual radiographic image is converted to a light image by phosphors within an "image intensifier," and then transferred by a television-like camera system to the cathode-ray tube monitor. The digital angiographic image is displayed on the monitor almost immediately following image acquisition and can be electronically enhanced for improved contrast resolution. This often allows the use of smaller amounts of intravascular contrast agents for each study. The technical settings for obtaining optimal images are computer derived at the beginning of the angiographic run, avoiding the need for scout films. Because accurate technique is electronically adjusted, repetition of the injection or imaging sequence is rarely required. Radiation dose for a digital image is less than for a comparable film-screen image.[33] Finally, images can be acquired at a very rapid rate (7.5 to 30 frames per second), and only those images that provide useful information are ultimately saved on film. Hard-copy images are produced on a sheet of transparent photographic film, often using laser imaging techniques that preserve the resolution achieved by the imaging system.

There are two types of digital angiography: digital imaging (DI) and digital subtraction angiography (DSA). The first method, DI, simply records digital images. Bones, soft tissues, radiographic contrast agents, and gas all appear on the same image (Fig. 4-3, *A*). The advantage of DI is that any motion during the filming sequence (patient motion, cardiac or respiratory motion, or bowel gas movement) does not degrade the image. The disadvantage is that full-strength contrast, similar to conventional filming technique, is necessary to provide adequate contrast resolution.

DSA uses a technique where the system's computer electronically subtracts early images from later images in the same angiographic filming sequence (Fig. 4-3, *B*). Those structures that do not change during contrast injection are canceled out on the DSA image. In this way bone, calcifications, soft tissues, and air "disappear" from the final image, and only the injected contrast is seen. Compared with film-screen angiography and DI, DSA offers a marked improvement in contrast resolution. DSA, however, is limited by any form of movement, including overlying bowel gas movement and patient motion.

A digitally acquired angiogram can be archived on electronic storage media (magnetic tape, magnetic discs, or optical storage devices), whereas conventional film angiograms are bulky and require film storage libraries. In theory retrieval of digitally stored angiographic studies will be faster, easier, and less expensive than retrieval of stored radiographic films. It is hoped that future developments will foster electronic image transfer through computer networks. In the futuristic world of electronic imaging and image storage, conventional film-screen angiographic studies may become obsolete, and perhaps even hard-copy film images of digital studies will become unnecessary. Transmission of electronically stored images will allow simultaneous review of angiographic studies at different locations within the hospital or at off-site locations, without the need for conventional hard-copy films.

The only limitations of digital angiography are initial equipment costs compared with film-screen angiography and reduced spatial resolution (although systems can routinely resolve vessels that are 1.0 mm diameter or smaller).[34] Only when the highest spatial resolution is needed should conventional film angiography be considered a better choice than digital techniques.

ARTERIOGRAPHY

Although catheter-based arteriography can be performed in a similar manner for all patients undergoing the same type of examination, in reality the same type of study is almost never standardized. Factors relating to a patient's arterial anatomy and blood flow, as well as a directed diagnostic approach, require the angiographer to customize the arteriogram to take full advantage of a wide assortment of techniques. For example, carotid arteriography in a patient having transient ischemic attacks can be performed by nonselective aortic arch contrast injection, with oblique projections of the great vessels to show the carotid and vertebral arteries. But if the patient has poor cardiac output, carotid and vertebral artery tortuosity, or densely calcified carotid plaques, selective carotid artery catheterization may be necessary to obtain acceptable images. Decisions related to selective catheterization technique, catheter and guidewire selection, volume and rate of contrast injection, filming sequence, filming projections, and ultimate determination of study completion must be made from experience. Even with the finest equipment, the diagnostic quality of an arteriogram is dependent on many factors including the real-time decision-making process of the angiographer.

Beyond good equipment and an experienced angiographer, every study represents the result of an angiographic team. This team consists of the radiographic technologist, nurse, darkroom technician, receptionist, quality assurance unit, and trainees, as well as the staff angiographer. Without the strengths of this team, safe, complete, and accurate arteriography is not possible.

Ascending and Arch Aortogram

Historically used to evaluate aneurysms and dissections, catheter-based aortography has been widely replaced by transesophageal echo, CT, MRI, and MRA. Ascending and arch aortography is used today primarily for evaluation of stenoses or occlusions of the great vessels and for the evaluation of thoracic aortic transsection due to deceleration injury.

Most often accomplished by common femoral puncture technique, the tip of a high-flow multi-sidehole pigtail catheter is positioned at the aortic root. Typically two views of the arch are obtained, with one being the left anterior oblique (LAO) projection. The second view is

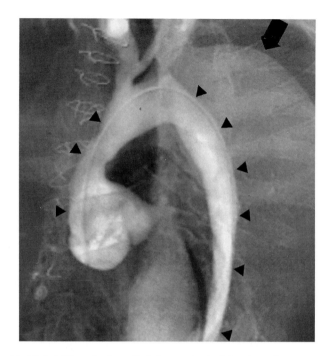

Fig. 4-4. LAO projection, digitally acquired, of the thoracic aorta. There is a dissection with aneurysmal dilatation of the entire thoracic aorta *(arrow)*. The dissection flap *(arrowheads)* separates the true lumen (contrast filled) from the thrombosed false lumen, which is seen to the left lateral aspect of the descending aorta as a broad soft tissue density that parallels the dissection flap.

usually a lateral or anterior projection. Contrast material is injected at a rate of 25 to 35 ml/sec for 2 seconds, and images are obtained at three frames per second or faster. During filming, the patient is asked to hold his breath. Although cardiac motion may give a small degree of artifact on one or two images, it rarely causes a problem for interpretation.

Fig. 4-4 shows LAO projection of the aortic arch in a patient who presented with an acute aortic dissection. Fig. 4-5, *A* shows a lateral arch aortogram in a patient who had previous coronary artery bypass grafting and has developed a false aneurysm at the proximal anastomosis of one of the vein grafts (which is now occluded). The LAO view (Fig. 4-5, *B*) was inadequate in showing the pseudoaneurysm, which is seen as a faint double density projected over the aortic contrast column. The false aneurysm is readily identified on a contrast CT image (Fig. 4-5, *C*).

Atherosclerotic occlusion of the left subclavian artery seen in Fig. 4-6, *A* has led to subclavian steal, with retrograde flow through the left vertebral artery to fill the distal left subclavian artery (Fig. 4-6, *B*). This type of occlusive lesion is best depicted by catheter-based arteriography, although it may be suspected from MRA or Doppler studies.

Carotid Arteriography

While there has been extensive investigation into noninvasive methods such as duplex Doppler, MRA, and CTA to detect and quantitate carotid artery stenoses, the gold standard remains carotid arteriography. Carotid artery

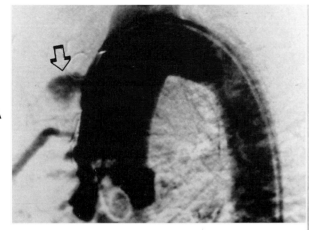

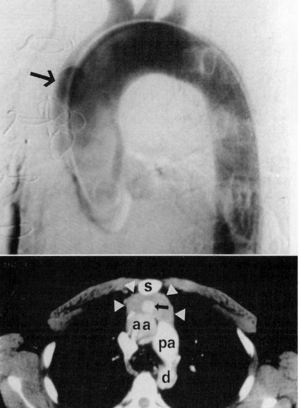

Fig. 4-5. **A,** Lateral arch aortogram shows a pseudo-aneurysm *(open arrow)* at the proximal anastomosis of a thrombosed coronary artery bypass graft. **B,** LAO arch aortogram in the same patient. The double density of the false aneurysm *(arrow)* is difficult to see in this projection. **C,** CT scan at the level of the pseudoaneurysm. The lumen of the pseudoaneurysm *(single black arrow)* is much smaller than its actual size, which includes the thrombosed lumen *(white arrowheads).* Note the relationship of this pseudoaneurysm to the sternum *(s),* which makes access via a median sternotomy hazardous. This relationship was not appreciated from the arteriogram. (*pa,* Pulmonary artery; *aa,* ascending aorta; *d,* descending aorta.)

Fig. 4-6. **A,** Film-screen arch aortogram in a patient with subclavian steal syndrome. Early image shows left subclavian artery occlusion *(arrowhead).* **B,** Late film shows retrograde flow in the left vertebral artery *(arrows),* reconstituting the left subclavian artery.

assessment is often possible from aortic arch injection; however, selective catheterization gives a much more accurate assessment of stenosis and can provide information regarding intracranial collateral flow from the vertebrobasilar system and the contralateral carotid circulation, which is not obtained from aortic contrast injection.

Selective carotid catheterization is performed with any one of a constellation of preshaped catheters, including the hockey-stick varieties, Simmons shapes, and "headhunter" designs. Catheter shaping with steam or air heat, still performed by some angiographers, is becoming less relevant in practice and retains importance mostly as a historical note.

Contrast injection during carotid arteriography is highly variable, and the selection of injection rate and total volume is based on catheter stability, blood flow during test injection of contrast material, size of the carotid artery, and type of imaging system: film-screen versus digital acquisition. Typically a rate of 3 to 10 ml/sec for a total volume of 5 to 14 ml is selected, with filming of two to four frames per second for the arterial phase and a slower frame rate into the venous phase of the study. At least two views are mandatory, typically lateral and anteroposterior, although oblique views are often needed to maximally visualize an internal carotid stenosis. The lateral projection, or a lateral oblique view, is usually best in showing proximal internal carotid stenosis as well as the carotid "siphon." The projection that reveals the "greatest" degree of stenosis is used to calculate percent diameter stenosis. The North American Symptomatic Carotid Endarterectomy Trial (NASCET) method of calculating carotid artery stenosis[35] compares the stenotic segment with the "normal" vessel beyond the stenosis. The anteroposterior view allows further assessment of the intracranial circulation and collateral flow pathways.

A technique similar to that described for carotid arteriography is used for cerebral angiography. If the carotid bifurcation is relatively free from occlusive disease, selective internal and external carotid artery catheterization is possible. Beyond this, microcatheters can now be placed into the intracranial arteries for cerebral arteriography as well as interventions such as thrombolysis and balloon angioplasty.

Flow rates and filming sequences for intracranial arteriography are highly variable. If the study is performed for evaluation of an intracranial arteriovenous malformation, larger volumes and ultrafast imaging sequences may be needed. However, for a patient with occlusive intracranial disease, very small volumes of contrast material and slow filming may suffice.

Abdominal Aortography: Renal, Mesenteric, and Aortoiliac Arteriography

Common indications for abdominal aortography include evaluation of occlusive diseases of the renal and mesenteric arteries, occlusive aortoiliac disease, and AAAs. Nonselective abdominal aortic catheterization is accomplished by placing the tip of a straight or pigtail multisidehole catheter at the level of the visceral arteries, usually corresponding to the position of the twelfth thoracic or first lumbar vertebral bodies. Contrast material is injected

at a rate of 15 to 30 ml/sec for a total volume of 30 to 60 ml. Large contrast volumes are necessary for evaluation of AAAs, whereas smaller volumes are adequate when occlusive disease is present. Filming sequences usually involve two to three images per second for aortic imaging and three images per second or faster when renal or visceral arteries are being evaluated.

Anteroposterior and lateral views provide most of the important information when the abdominal aorta and mesenteric vessels are being studied. Proximal renal artery stenoses may require frontal obliques: left or right anterior obliques, often with angulation of the imaging system in a cranial or caudal direction.

In Fig. 4-7, A and B an anteroposterior abdominal aortogram and the corresponding coronal MRI, respectively, are shown. In Fig. 4-7, C and D the lateral aortogram and MRI are shown. There is an AAA, and the features of importance regarding evaluation of this AAA are seen on both studies: patency of the proximal renal arteries and location of the proximal and distal aneurysm neck. There are, however, strengths and weaknesses of each modality. The aortogram can discern iliac artery stenoses, whereas the MRI shows mural thrombus lining the aneurysm.

As one of the correctable causes of hypertension, renal arterial stenosis can be detected and quantified by catheter-based arteriography. Unlike the multitude of noninvasive tests for renovascular hypertension and renal artery stenosis, catheter-based arteriography has an exceptionally high accuracy for renal artery occlusive disease and permits concurrent treatment with angioplasty and stenting techniques. Carbon dioxide arteriography is helpful in assessing renal patency when there is underlying impairment of renal function (Fig. 4-8, A and B).

Mesenteric ischemia on the basis of proximal mesenteric stenoses and occlusion is an uncommon but correctable condition. Lateral aortography is particularly helpful, as the mesenteric vessels arise from the anterior aortic wall (Fig. 4-9). The anteroposterior projection typically shows delayed filling of the mesenteric arteries via collateral pathways. In order for proximal mesenteric occlusive disease to cause ischemia, at least two of the three mesenteric vessels must be compromised. When the proximal mesenteric vessels are found to be patent, selective catheterization of the superior mesenteric artery may be helpful in elucidating branch vessel occlusion or embolic disease.

Aortoiliac occlusive disease, which can be studied by MRA, is probably better diagnosed by catheter-based arteriography, which allows the angiographer an opportunity to measure pressure gradients across stenoses of uncertain importance during the study. This can provide important physiologic data not possible by MRA techniques. Furthermore, stenoses and occlusions can be both diagnosed and treated (angioplasty with or without stenting) during the study.

Extremity Arteriography

Indications for arteriographic study of the arms and legs include exertional and resting ischemia due to atherosclerosis, thrombosis, embolus, and vasculitis. Additionally, peripheral aneurysms, vascular tumors, trauma-related

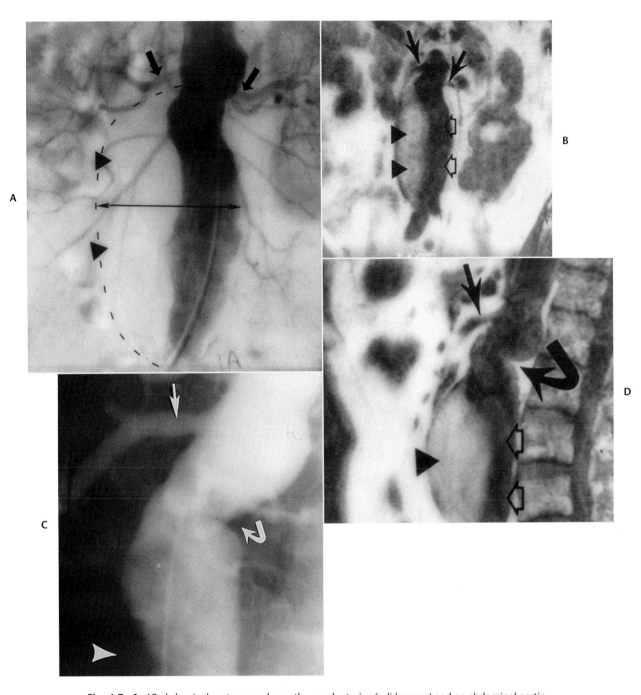

Fig. 4-7. A, AP abdominal aortogram shows the renal arteries *(solid arrows)* and an abdominal aortic aneurysm *(dashed line and horizontal double-headed arrow).* Only the lumen of the aneurysm fills with contrast; the thrombosed portion of the lumen is not seen by catheter-based arteriography. **B,** Coronal MRI of the aneurysm seen in **(A).** Without contrast, the aneurysm lumen *(open arrows),* thrombosed lumen *(arrowheads),* and renal arteries *(arrows)* are easily seen. **C,** Lateral catheter-based abdominal aortogram, shows the superior mesenteric artery *(arrow),* aneurysm neck *(curved arrow),* and thrombus at the anterior aspect of the aneurysm *(arrowhead).* **D,** Lateral MRI of the aneurysm seen in **(C).** The same features are seen. *(From Lindsay J, Jr: Diseases of the aorta, Baltimore, 1994, Williams & Wilkins with permission.)*

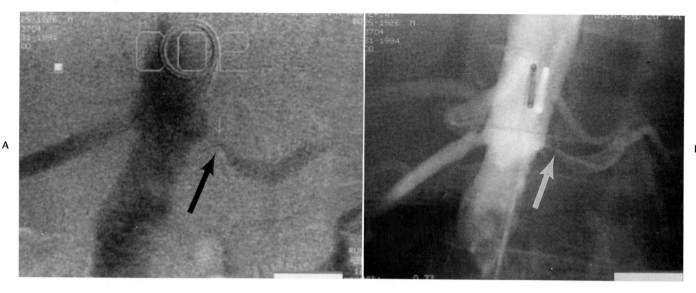

Fig. 4-8. **A,** Carbon dioxide (CO_2) aortogram shows a left renal artery stenosis *(arrow).* **B,** Catheter-based aortogram corresponding to the CO_2 images in **(A).** The left renal artery stenosis creates a jet of contrast *(arrow).*

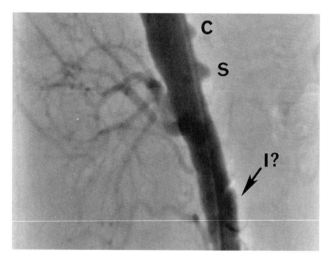

Fig. 4-9. Lateral abdominal aortogram of a patient with mesenteric ischemia presenting as postprandial abdominal angina. The celiac trunk *(c)* and superior mesenteric artery *(s)* are occluded at their origins. The inferior mesenteric artery *(I)* is occluded, and its origin is not evident.

injury, and evaluation of arterial anatomy before catheter-based or surgical intervention often necessitates peripheral arteriography.

Debate regarding the "better" site of femoral catheterization for leg arteriography will probably never be resolved. Some angiographers prefer to puncture the common femoral artery on the same side as the affected leg, and others insist on a contralateral approach. Rather than discuss the perceived merits of each approach, it should be recognized that both approaches are relatively safe, and there appears to be no correct solution.

The initial approach for peripheral arteriography is usually aortic contrast injection with filming over the area of interest. As the study progresses from the proximal to distal circulation, there is usually a decrease in the radiodensity of the contrast. When stenoses or occlusions intervene, the contrast density in the distal circulation may be inadequate for imaging, and selective catheterization may be required.

Contrast injection for peripheral arteriography of the legs with nonselective aortic injection starts with catheter positioning at the infrarenal aorta. If film-screen stepping-top technique is used, a single contrast injection is followed by stepwise movement of the angiography table. The contrast bolus is "followed" from the aorta to the feet, obtaining images along the way. Contrast material is injected at 7 to 9 ml/sec for a total volume of 70 to 120 ml. Since the stepping table moves in a preprogrammed manner, the volume and duration of contrast injection is often based on guesswork, and the quality of the final angiogram is dependent on luck as well as experience.

With digital acquisition, much of the guesswork can be eliminated. The study is performed with similar catheter position, but smaller contrast injections are given with stationary imaging over one arterial segment. For instance, the imaging equipment can be positioned over the aortoiliac circulation while contrast material is injected at a rate of 8 to 10 ml/sec for 2 to 3 seconds (total volume of 16 to 30 ml). Then the equipment is positioned over the femoral arteries for a similar injection and sequence. This is repeated until arteriography of the pedal vessels is completed. Usually five to six positions are required for a full study, using approximately 80 to 180 ml of contrast material. Some contrast saving is afforded by the high-contrast resolution of DSA, which can provide images using diluted contrast.

Recent advances have coupled the stepping table concept with digital angiographic techniques. The peripheral leg arteriogram in Fig. 4-10 was obtained by acquiring a digital images series without contrast material, then injecting contrast and allowing the mechanized imaging equip-

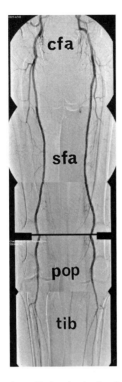

Fig. 4-10. DSA of the legs. Technologic developments of digital angiography equipment now permit their application in situations where film-screen techniques were used. With one injection of contrast material, the entire circulation of both legs has been recorded in this digitally acquired image. (*cfa,* Common femoral arteries; *sfa,* superficial femoral arteries; *pop,* popliteal arteries; *tib,* tibial arteries.)

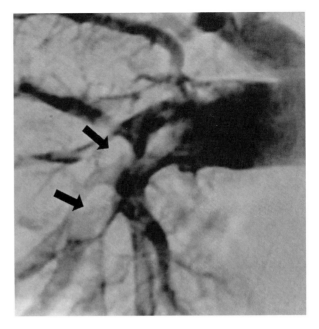

Fig. 4-11. DSA of the right pulmonary artery. Pulmonary emboli *(arrows)* are seen as filling defects in the contrast column.

ment to "follow" the contrast bolus. Although the final result appears similar to that obtained with a stepping table and film-screen technique, the process by which the images are obtained is completely different. The contrast bolus is actually monitored during the filming sequence, thereby eliminating the guesswork inherent in the stepping-table/film-screen technique. This new technique promises to save on time, film, film processing, radiation, and contrast material, and takes full advantage of the strengths of digital angiography.

Pulmonary Angiography

The overwhelming goal of pulmonary angiography is to detect pulmonary emboli and measure pressures within the pulmonary artery and right side of the heart. To do this, the femoral or jugular veins are punctured to allow placement of a high-flow, multi-sidehole catheter such as a pigtail or Grollman catheter. The catheter tip is positioned in the main pulmonary artery or the right or left pulmonary artery. Contrast material is injected at 25 to 35 ml/sec for a total of 40 to 60 ml, and images are obtained at three frames per second or faster. As with any form of right heart catheterization, catheter-induced irritation of the cardiac conduction pathways within the right ventricle can generate atrial and ventricular arrhythmias and induce a right-sided bundle branch block. One contraindication to pulmonary angiography is a left-sided bundle branch block, since a catheter-induced right-sided bundle branch

block will yield complete heart block. The patient with a left-sided bundle branch block should have placement of a temporary pacemaker before pulmonary angiography.

The cornerstone of diagnosing pulmonary embolus by angiographic technique is the "filling defect." Essentially, contrast material flows around the embolus, showing the embolus as a "defect" in the contrast-filled pulmonary artery (Fig. 4-11). There has been recent interest in digital pulmonary angiography, which can markedly reduce the length of the study. When respiratory movement degrades the DSA, conversion of the image to DI permits interpretation, although contrast resolution is reduced.

Venography

Duplex Doppler and compression ultrasound interrogation of the deep venous system has replaced contrast venography in all but a few indications. Sonographic techniques are the first line of diagnostic study for DVT. When the sonographic study is nondiagnostic, if DVT of the tibial veins is in question, or when the sonographic result is normal but the clinical suspicion for DVT is high, contrast venography may help.

The venographic approach has changed little over the past few decades. For lower-extremity venography, a small intravenous line is started in a pedal vein, preferably at the lateral dorsal aspect of the foot. Contrast material is injected by hand, and images of the tibial veins, popliteal vein, femoral veins, and iliac veins is obtained, with an attempt to see contrast entering the inferior vena cava. Clot is detected as a filling defect within the contrast column, as seen in Fig. 4-12. Chronic or recanalized DVT appears as strands or webs within the veins, often poorly defined because the contrast material is flowing through multiple small parallel channels within fibrotic old thrombus. When there is complete nonfilling of the deep venous

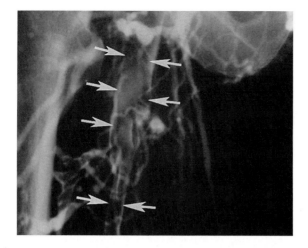

Fig. 4-12. Film-screen right leg venogram. There is extensive deep vein thrombus formation in the femoral venous system *(arrows)* seen as a filling defect within the contrast column.

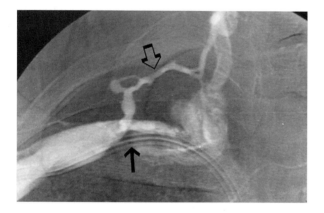

Fig. 4-13. Digitally acquired right subclavian venogram. A double-lumen dialysis catheter has been placed via the right subclavian vein. Thrombus formation on the catheter *(solid arrow)* causes subclavian vein stenosis, with collateral flow *(open arrow)* into the jugular vein.

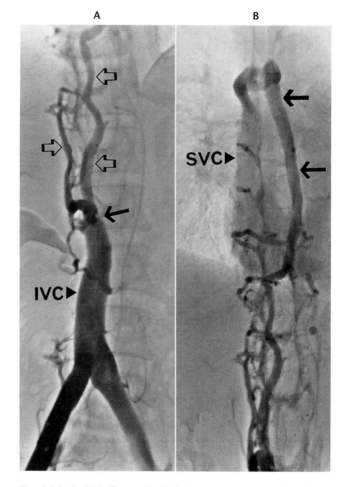

Fig. 4-14. A, Digitally acquired inferior vena cavogram. The inferior vena cava *(IVC)* is occluded *(solid arrow)* due to extension of tumor thrombus from a left renal cell carcinoma. Retroperitoneal collaterals *(open arrows)* divert venous flow into the azygos/hemiazygos venous system. **B,** Flow continues into the azygos vein *(arrows)*, with return to the right atrium via the superior vena cava *(SVC)*.

system, it is presumed that there is extensive DVT, although this may be either acute or chronic.

Upper-extremity contrast venography is particularly helpful when there is concern regarding the subclavian and brachiocephalic veins. Because of their location behind the clavicle, these venous structures cannot be studied reliably by Doppler or other ultrasound techniques. Even with contrast venography, however, differing degrees of subclavian vein stenosis may be difficult to quantitate, since flow from the internal jugular vein, which is not opacified, may mix with the contrast-mixed subclavian blood and give the appearance of a subclavian vein stenosis. Fortunately there are other venographic findings, such as the formation of collaterals, that can confirm the presence of a physiologically important venous stenosis (Fig. 4-13).

Caval Venography

Contrast venography of the superior and inferior vena cava remains an important test for caval patency. A tumor may invade, cause compression, or propagate within the cava. Radiation to the mediastinum can constrict the superior vena cava, and indwelling venous catheters may lead to caval thrombosis. Contrast venography is performed from any peripheral venous access but typically requires the placement of a multi-sidehole catheter into the central venous system. Contrast injection, 10 to 25 ml/sec for 20 to 50 ml, is followed by film-screen or digital angiographic technique at one to three images per second.

In Fig. 4-14, *A* and *B* a left renal cell carcinoma has propagated into the inferior vena cava. The segment of inferior vena cava below the level of the renal veins is patent. Blood flow enters the azygos system, and returns to the right side of the heart via the superior vena cava.

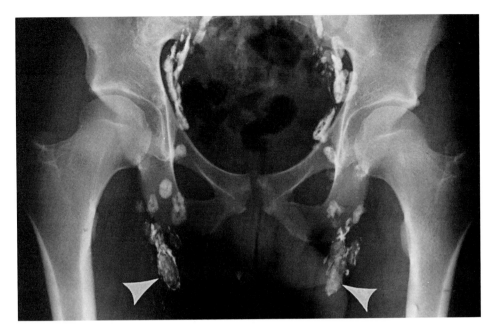

Fig. 4-15. At 24 hours, contrast material within the lymphatics has cleared. Nodal architecture is now appreciated, as contrast remains in the lymph nodes. The inguinal lymph nodes are enlarged but otherwise normal *(arrowheads)*.

Lymphangiography

There has been little development in lymphangiography during the past 30 years, despite it remaining the only direct imaging test for evaluating the lymphatic system. The technique most widely used for pelvic and abdominal lymphangiography calls for intradermal injection of a blue indicator dye between the toes. This dye is drained by the lymphatic system, coloring the lymph blue. Subsequent cutdown at the dorsum of the foot or ankle allows identification of a blue-stained lymphatic vessel, which is then cannulated with a 27- to 30-gauge needle. Either Ethiodol or Lipiodol (oily iodine-containing contrast agents) is slowly injected, typically with a small mechanical pump. At the conclusion of the procedure, the needle is removed, the cutdown closed, and radiographs of the abdomen and pelvis are obtained. The patient is instructed to return the following day for a series of abdominal and pelvic radiographs. The oily contrast material is sequestered within the lymphatics and lymph nodes along the draining pathways (Fig. 4-15).

Enlarged lymph nodes and abnormal contrast-filled lymph nodes are the cornerstones of diagnosing nodal abnormalities. Metastatic disease to the lymph nodes or granulomas appear as filling defects within the contrast-filled node.

Another application of lymphangiography is in the evaluation of a lymphatic leak. For instance, lymphangiography may diagnose the site of lymphatic injury in the patient with postoperative chylothorax.

Lymphangiography is time-consuming and uncomfortable for the patient. CT and MRI have largely replaced the need for this technique, although there are rare circumstances where it is necessary for accurate diagnosis. In some cases abnormal lymph nodes may not be enlarged, but lymphangiography may show architectural nodal abnormality that would otherwise require excisional nodal biopsy for diagnosis.

COMPUTED TOMOGRAPHIC ANGIOGRAPHY

Spiral Computed Tomographic Imaging

Spiral CT scanning involves moving a patient through the CT gantry at a constant velocity while simultaneously rotating the x-ray tube at a constant velocity around the patient. The combination of linear motion of the patient and circular motion of the x-ray tube combine to form a helical or spiral x-ray path about the patient. During the time the patient is being transported through the plane of the gantry, x-ray data are being collected. This data stream is continuous; it has no interruptions at slice interfaces as did the data stream from conventional CT scanners. Data from a spiral acquisition can be reconstructed into slices. If the distance between slices is less than the collimation of section thickness, overlapping slices are created without additional radiation. Spiral CT scans done with overlapping images lend themselves to multiplanar reformations, various two-dimensional (2D) projection renderings, and 3D displays.

CTA is dependent on proper contrast medium delivery. The delivery is itself dependent on the body part being imaged, injection site, injection rate, iodine concentration, and amount of contrast material used. For CTA of the head and neck, the goal is maximal opacification of the arteries while the veins are free of contrast medium. To accomplish this, the delay time (time between the onset of the injection and onset of image acquisition) is typically between 20 and 25 seconds, injecting at the antecubital vein. Contrast material is delivered at a rate of 2 ml/sec for a total volume of 75 to 100 ml. The patient is instructed to breathe quietly and to not move or swallow. Scanning for intracranial arterial lesions is most often started at the foramen magnum, proceeding to the midskull with collimation of 1 to 2 mm. Scanning the neck for carotid artery lesions is most often done by imaging from the C6 vertebral body to the skull base. Collimation of 3 mm is ideal.

CTA of the thorax typically calls for a delay time of 20 to 25 seconds. The injection is delivered via power injector at a rate of 2 to 4 ml/sec for a total volume of 100 to 150 ml. Breath-holding for up to 30 seconds is ideal, but if this is not possible, quiet breathing without movement or swallowing will suffice. Scanning in the thorax is most often done starting above the apices of the lungs, obtaining images to the lung bases. Collimation of 5 to 7 mm is typical.

In the abdomen the delay time is longer than it is for head, neck, and thoracic CTA. The delay time for abdominal CTA is between 50 and 70 seconds, depending on cardiac output. The injection delivered via power injector at a rate of 2 to 4 ml/sec may be as much as 120 to 150 ml total contrast volume. Again, breath-holding for up to 30 seconds is ideal. If this is not possible, then quiet breathing instructions are given. For extended scanning, clustered spiral scanning acquisitions separated with 5 seconds for a breath are often acceptable. Scanning in the abdomen is most often done from the dome of the liver to the iliac crest with collimation of 5 to 7 mm.

Intracranial Circulation

CTA of intracranial vasculature is advancing as a viable alternative to conventional angiography (Fig. 4-16, *A* and *B*). In a paper presented by Vieco, a series of patients with acute subarachnoid hemorrhage were imaged using CTA and DSA. Both modalities were assessed for number of segments of the circle of Willis visualized and the presence or absence of aneurysms. CTA and DSA were in agreement for nearly all of the segments of the cerebral circulation at the circle of Willis.[36]

CTA of the intracranial circulation is proving to be a valuable tool for evaluating other lesions of the circle of Willis, such as arterial stenoses.[37] Intracranial arteriovenous malformations can also be appreciated. Nevertheless, the role of CTA in relation to other imaging techniques remains to be better defined.

Carotid Bifurcation

CTA of the carotid bifurcation was first demonstrated in 1982 by Riles et al.[38] The theory behind using spiral CT to investigate the carotid bifurcation is to scan fast enough to capture the vessel while the iodinated contrast medium is at or near its maximum concentration but before venous return through jugular veins occurs. It is hoped that spiral CT of the carotid bifurcation may reduce the number of cases requiring traditional catheter-based angiography, providing accurate anatomic data (Fig. 4-17) with less risk and lower cost. A compilation of results of CTA compared with other modalities suggest that CTA of the carotid bifurcation is about 90% accurate in assessing severe stenosis.[37]

In a review of patients by Dillon et al,[39] 50 patients underwent spiral CT and conventional angiography. There was an 82% correlation between CTA and conventional angiography; 14 of 17 severe stenoses (greater than 90%

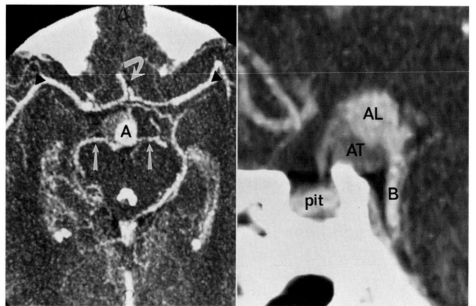

Fig. 4-16. **A,** CTA of a basilar tip cerebral aneurysm showing the relationship between the aneurysm and the cerebral arteries. (*A,* aneurysm; *white arrows,* posterior cerebral arteries; *white curved arrow,* anterior cerebral arteries; *black arrowheads,* middle cerebral arteries.) **B,** Midline sagittal CTA of the same basilar tip aneurysm as in **(A).** The pituitary gland *(pit)* and the basilar artery *(B)* are anatomic reference points. The aneurysm is partially thrombosed *(AT)* but has a patent lumen *(AL).* *(Used courtesy of Pedro T. Vieco, MD, University of Vermont, Burlington.)*

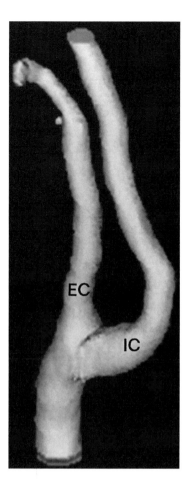

Fig. 4-17. Surface-shaded CTA of the normal carotid artery bifurcation in lateral projection. The internal carotid artery *(IC)* courses posteriorly, then cephalad, and the external carotid artery *(EC)* continues cephalad. *(From Zeman RK et al: Helical/spiral CT: a practical approach, New York, 1995, McGraw-Hill with permission.)*

diameter reduction) were correctly identified using CTA.

Thorax

CTA of the thorax can be broken down into two broad types of studies. The first involves imaging of the aortic arch and the great vessels.[40] Variants of the aortic arch, including double aortic arch, right arch, aortic coarctation, and pseudocoarctation can be imaged. Aneurysms and stenoses of the great vessels and aberrant branching patterns of the subclavian arteries are also visualized using CTA (Fig. 4-18, *A* and *B*). Aortic dissection[41] and aneurysms are easily imaged by CTA as well.

Another application of thoracic CTA involves imaging of the pulmonary circulation. The ability of spiral CTA to detect pulmonary artery emboli in the main pulmonary arteries as well as in second- and third-order branches has been studied.[42] Goodman et al[43] have demonstrated that CTA has an 86% sensitivity and 92% specificity to central vessel emboli and a 63% sensitivity and 89% specificity when segmental branches were included. Reliable evaluation of pulmonary vascular anatomy has recently been demonstrated.[44] Analysis of 28 pulmonary arteriovenous malformations (PAVMs), 25 simple and 3 complex, was provided by 3D reconstruction of spiral CT data. When

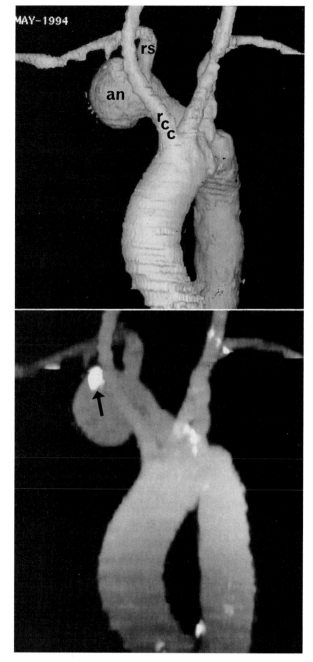

Fig. 4-18. A, Surface-shaded CTA of the aortic arch showing the right common carotid artery *(rcc)* and aberrant origin of the right subclavian artery *(rs)* with an aneurysm *(an)*. The projection is anteroposterior, and this surface-shaded display shows the relationship of the great vessels to the aneurysm. **B,** The corresponding "maximum intensity projection" CTA, which is less useful for determining the anatomic relationship of the great vessels but gives useful information regarding the aneurysm. Arrow indicates calcification in the aneurysm wall. *(From Zeman RK et al: Helical/spiral CT: a practical approach, New York, 1995, McGraw-Hill with permission.)*

combined with axial CT imaging, CTA provides an even more accurate evaluation of PAVMs.[45]

Abdomen

Helical scanning, because of its speed, is well suited for angiographic imaging of the abdominal vasculature. This

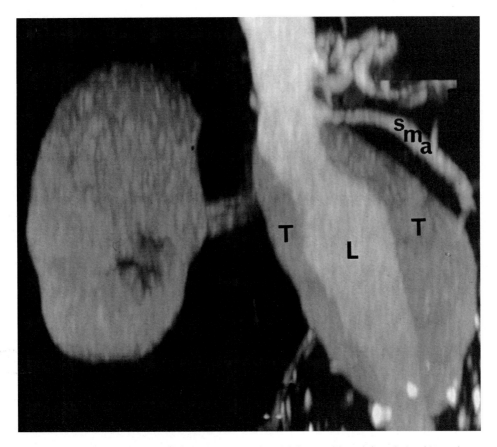

Fig. 4-19. CTA of an AAA in lateral projection. Thrombus *(T)*, lumen *(L)*, and the relationship to the superior mesenteric artery *(sma)* are seen on this "maximum intensity projection" CTA.

includes evaluation of the abdominal aorta; iliac arteries; renal arteries; hepatic, splenic, and superior mesenteric arteries; celiac axis; and portal vein. Vascular pathology such as thrombosis, stenosis, tumor encasement, aneurysm, and dissection can be imaged with CTA.

The abdominal aorta is relatively simple to assess using helical CTA. One of the more frequent examinations of the abdominal aorta is characterization of AAAs, including an assessment of diameter, length, lumen, mural thrombus, and involvement of other arteries such as the mesenteric renal and iliac arteries (Fig. 4-19). Zeman et al[46] describes a technique whereby collimation is changed during a single CT prescription for the purpose of tailoring the image acquisition to the anatomy. Scanning is done from cranial to caudal direction with 3-mm collimation, permitting accurate imaging of the aorta from the celiac axis to a level just beyond the renal arteries. Below this point the collimation is opened to 7 mm and imaging continues through the aneurysm to the iliac bifurcation. Images are then reconstructed into 3D renderings.[47]

Renal artery stenosis has been demonstrated using spiral CT.[48] Renal artery CTA is done with iodinated contrast media and a typical injection-to-scan delay of 40 seconds. Images are reconstructed with an image-to-image spacing of 1.5 mm or less if high-quality 3D modeling is desired.

Rubin et al[49] showed CTA of the renal arteries to have a 92% sensitivity and 83% specificity for the detection of renal artery stenosis.[49] However, the chance for misdiagnosing the degree of stenosis was high. Five of seven stenoses (90% diameter reduction) appeared occluded, and 9 of 17 moderate stenoses (50% to 69% diameter reduction) were misdiagnosed as hemodynamically significant (70% or greater diameter reduction).

Because of its ability to provide images of both luminal and mural anatomy, CTA will probably become more important in the evaluation of aneurysms throughout the body. For example, the common iliac artery aneurysm in Fig. 4-20 is located adjacent to the iliac artery bifurcation and within an extremely tortuous iliac artery circulation. These features can limit catheter-based angiography and MRA. CTA, however, provides a clear representation of the aneurysm and all related arteries.

Other areas where CTA is being explored for its usefulness are in the diagnosis of portal vein thrombosis, extent of renal vein involvement in renal cell carcinoma, vascular encasement by pancreatic carcinoma, and in the detection and pattern recognition of aberrant arterial branching of the celiac axis and superior mesenteric artery for presurgical planning. CTA is relatively new and exciting. But, as evident from this section, its application in the evaluation of vascular disorders must be more precisely defined.

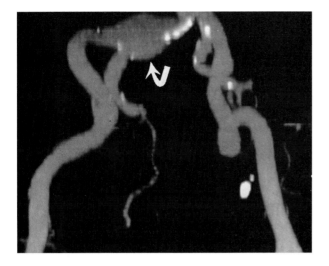

Fig. 4-20. Common iliac artery aneurysm *(curved arrow)* at the iliac bifurcation seen in the left anterior oblique projection. The iliac circulation is very tortuous. *(Used courtesy of Philip Costello, MD, Deaconess Hospital, Boston, MA.)*

MAGNETIC RESONANCE ANGIOGRAPHY

In 1985 Weeden et al showed that flowing blood could be imaged by MRI techniques.[50] Since then there has been a flood of investigation into the application of magnetic resonance techniques for imaging arteries and veins throughout the body.

MRA is based on MRI. Any description of advances in MRA require some familiarity with the physical concepts that allow images of human anatomy and physiology based on the magnetic properties of blood and adjacent tissues. Most of the imaging data provided by MRI are derived from the magnetic properties of protons in human tissues and the influence on these protons by their immediate chemical environment. When these protons are excited by a pulse of radiofrequency energy, they subsequently "relax" by emitting a radiofrequency signal. This signal can be recorded and reconstructed into an image that represents proton density and/or emitted energy. Many parameters influence the quantity and rate of energy emission that excited protons emit, but of particular importance in vascular imaging is the rate of flow of protons within blood through the signal-receiving field. In general, there are two ways in which MRI techniques are used to provide magnetic resonance angiograms: time-of-flight (TOF) and phase-contrast (PC) imaging, which are both discussed in the following material. For the reader who wishes to pursue an in-depth review of MRI and MRA physics, there are many insightful reviews in recent texts and review articles.[51,52] The intricacies of MRI and MRA physics, however, are not presented here.

Magnetic Resonance Angiographic Techniques: General Considerations

TOF imaging relies on the flow of fresh, fully magnetized protons into the imaging section. These protons provide high signal intensity necessary to image flow within the vessels. Simultaneously the background signal is suppressed by the rapid, repeated application of radiofrequency pulses. PC techniques, on the other hand, rely on phase shifts that are induced by user-prescribed magnetic field gradients. PC imaging techniques are analogous to Doppler ultrasound studies, in which blood flow is discriminated by phase shifts. In PC imaging it is necessary to select the peak velocity that is accurately encoded, also known as the velocity-encoding value (VENC). Typical VENCs used for the aorta are 100 to 200 cm/sec, whereas branch vessels may require a VENC of 30 to 40 cm/sec for optimal imaging.

TOF or PC angiographic images may be prepared by obtaining data from consecutive thin sections (2D acquisition) or by acquisition of a single large volume of information with subsequent division of the volume into multiple thin sections (3D acquisition). When overlapping MRA images are used to reconstitute a single rendering of the vessel, a technique called maximum image projection (MIP) is used.

The strengths of TOF are faster imaging and better spatial resolution per unit imaging time compared with PC. On the other hand, PC techniques allow visualization of smaller vessels and can be used to image vessels with slower flow because it offers better background suppression compared with TOF.

Regardless of whether TOF or PC is used, it is important to recognize that MRA is remarkably different from catheter-based angiography and CTA. Aside from obviating the need for invasive catheterization and contrast agent administration, MRA provides images based on the physiology of flowing blood. Catheter-based angiography and CTA rely on the anatomic features of the contrast-filled vessel lumen. By imaging blood flow rather than luminal anatomy, MRA may overlook or overaccentuate anatomic features of a blood vessel, depending on local flow characteristics.

For instance, the normal common carotid bulb is greater in diameter than the adjacent common carotid artery or the internal carotid artery. This area of dilation is consistently demonstrated in the nonatherosclerotic carotid circulation by catheter-based angiography. But when MRA images of the carotid bifurcation are obtained, the eddy-type vortex flow within the carotid bulb can show reduced or even absent forward flow, simulating an area of plaque with or without stenosis. This phenomenon has been recognized by duplex Doppler, which also images blood flow.

Laminar blood flow is most reliably imaged by MRA. As just discussed, eddy or vortex flow can simulate areas of disease. Turbulent flow can also lead to MRA vascular images that do not accurately depict vascular anatomy. Other conditions that lead to inaccurate MRA representation of vascular anatomy include blood flow above or below certain thresholds, small turbulent volumes of blood that enter the imaging plane (e.g., flow through high-grade stenoses), and blood flow not in alignment with the imaging plane. Yet with all of these caveats there are growing applications of MRA, and many investigators remain hopeful that MRA may replace catheter-based angiography in certain instances.

Carotid Magnetic Resonance Angiography

For the past decade there has been hope that MRA will replace catheter-based angiography in the evaluation of occlusive disease of the extracranial carotid artery. If MRA proves successful, its use will obviate the need for catheterization and contrast agent injection. The goal will be to eliminate groin complications, stroke, and adverse contrast effects while providing images that are sufficient to accurately assess carotid artery stenosis and occlusion. Additionally, MRA can provide information pertaining to the brain, such as prior stroke or nonvascular causes for the patient's presentation, all during one visit to the magnetic resonance scanner.

There are many reports of "successful" carotid imaging using MRA. Virtually all of these reports provide the reader with angiographic images of the carotid artery, as shown in Fig. 4-21, *A* and *B*. But despite many different approaches to carotid MRA, no single technique seems to consistently provide images with the anatomic precision of catheter-based angiography. At present, MRA is a good screening test for extracranial carotid artery disease but too unreliable for defining the degree of stenosis.[53] The shortcoming of MRA lies in its overestimation of stenosis. For carotid evaluation it is essential that the degree of stenosis be accurately determined so that a decision can be made regarding the appropriateness of medical or surgical therapy. Carotid MRA images, however, can be confusing for anyone except those who have had extensive experience in MRA interpretation. High-grade stenoses typically appear as complete occlusions on MRA images, and moderate stenoses may be difficult to quantitate.

Although MRA alone may not provide accurate information for quantifying occlusive disease of the carotid arteries, some workers believe that a combined approach using both MRA and duplex Doppler provides sufficient diagnostic accuracy for guiding further treatment.[54] Others believe that this combined approach still falls short of catheter-based angiography.[55] When procedural costs and risks are evaluated, the combined MRA/duplex Doppler approach seems safe and cost-effective. However, when broader issues of patient outcome and global costs of care are considered, there are no data to suggest that catheter-based angiography should be replaced by MRA with or without duplex Doppler studies at this time.

Thoracic and Abdominal Magnetic Resonance Angiography

Despite impressive advances in MRA of the head and neck, the role of MRA in the chest and abdomen has lagged behind. This delay in the diffusion of MRA technology is because of a number of factors including respiratory and bowel motion, lower signal-to-noise ratio available from the body coil compared with the head coil, and the relative abundance of fat-creating artifacts on the maximum-intensity pixel projection algorithms. An equally important problem is the pulsatile nature of aortic and pulmonary flow, which tends to create artifacts in the MRA sequences. Recently, however, technologic developments have led to widespread interest in MRA for the study of the thoracic and abdominal aorta, pulmonary arteries, renal arteries, and mesenteric circulation. There is great promise for the application of new pulse sequences designed to detect stenoses, occlusions, aneurysms, and thrombotic/embolic processes as discussed in the following material.

There are a growing number of applications of MRA in the chest. Thoracic aortic pathology such as dissection and aneurysm can be imaged by both MRI and MRA, and the images can often replace catheter-based arteriography. Thoracic aortic dissection is particularly well demonstrated (see Chapter 20). Differential flow velocities in the

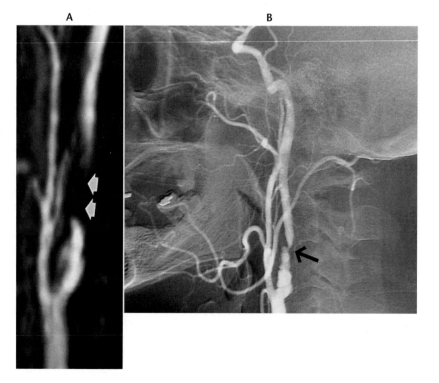

A   B

Fig. 4-21. A, MRA of a high-grade internal carotid artery stenosis. Predetermined MRA parameters may not detect fast flow across a tight stenosis, and the resulting signal void can be misinterpreted as showing total occlusion *(double arrows).* **B,** The corresponding arteriogram confirms a high-grade stenosis *(arrow)* rather than total occlusion.

true and false lumen of dissections can be detected, and slow flow can usually be distinguished from thrombus.[56,57]

Preliminary studies[58] indicate that MRA of the pulmonary arterial circulation may demonstrate pulmonary embolic disease. However, these preliminary studies also suggest that although the sensitivity for detecting embolic disease may be high, the specificity of the MRA study is low because of artifacts associated with slow blood flow. These slow-flow artifacts are most frequently seen in patients with significant pulmonary arterial hypertension. There-

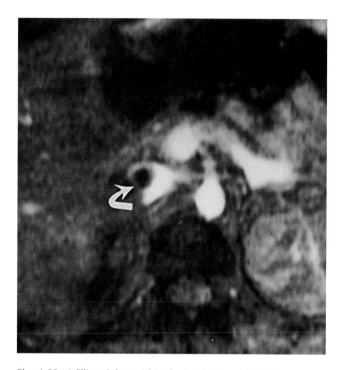

Fig. 4-22. A filling defect within the bright signal of inferior vena caval flow is indicative of caval thrombus *(curved arrow)* on this axial MR image.

fore the pulmonary MRA technique, if it is shown to be of value, will likely have the greatest impact when combined with MRV studies of the deep venous system (Fig. 4-22). Since neither conventional venography nor pulmonary angiography alone detects all patients with venous thromboembolic disease who require therapy, a technique that may be used to identify clots in the deep venous system and the pulmonary arterial system may be particularly useful.

One of the more exciting recent developments in MRA is the prospect of coronary artery MRA. In a preliminary report Manning and Edelman[59] showed the potential of a breath-held 2D TOF sequence for demonstrating coronary artery stenoses exceeding 50% in diameter. The technique is in the early stages of development at several institutions, and further clinical trials are necessary before the technique is accepted.

Magnetic Resonance Angiography of the Abdomen

The abdominal aorta is relatively simple to study with MRA techniques. Arlart et al[60] studied 36 patients with a variety of abdominal aortic diseases, including atherosclerotic occlusive disease, aneurysms, dissection, and renal artery stenosis. There was good correlation between MRA and DSA or CT in all cases. One drawback was encountered in AAAs where slow or turbulent flow caused signal loss and unsatisfactory spatial resolution. This limitation is shown in Fig. 4-23, *A* and *B*.

Although MRA may correlate with CT and angiography, the question remains as to its application in both the acute and chronic setting. For instance, when a patient presents with acute aortic occlusion, dissection, or aneurysm rupture, the role of MRA can be questioned, since MRA may not be available on an emergency basis, the unstable patient may not be able to be safely placed in the magnet, and the final images may not be of adequate resolution for operative decision making. Chronic processes, such

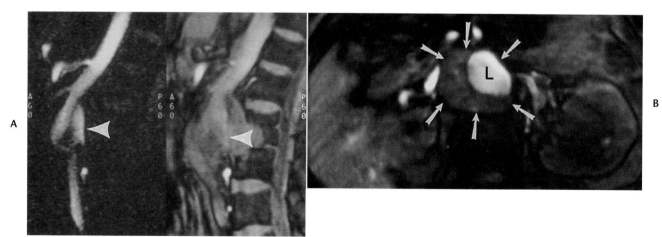

Fig. 4-23. A, Sagittal MRA of an AAA *(arrowheads),* with PC image on the left and a technique that shows MRI and MRA features on the right. Because of turbulent flow, neither image accurately depicts the luminal anatomy of the aneurysm. Images were obtained during one phase of the cardiac cycle (which was divided into 16 phases). This type of cardiac gating can reduce the artifact produced by pulsatile flow during the cardiac cycle. **B,** Axial MRI of the same AAA as in **(A).** With this technique, the lumen *(L)* and thrombus *(arrows)* are accurately displayed. *(From Grist TM: Magnetic resonance angiography of the aorta and renal arteries, MRI Clin North Am 1:255, 1993 with permission.)*

as aneurysms, may be easily evaluated by ultrasound, whereas angiography is often necessary for patients with occlusive disease and visceral involvement from dissection. The ultimate utility of MRA for abdominal aortic diseases, both acute and chronic, awaits comparative studies of patients randomized to different modalities with assessment of both image correlation and clinical outcome.

Evaluation of proximal renal artery stenosis in patients with azotemic renovascular disease is a reasonable expectation from the use of renal MRA. In young patients referred for evaluation of possible renovascular hypertension, however, MRA is of uncertain value since disease involving the segmental renal arteries is a potentially important radiographic finding that may not be detected. Although recent advances in MRA imaging of the more distal renal arteries may provide an important method for detecting segmental renal artery disease, these techniques await further clinical evaluation.

Problems are encountered in evaluation of the main renal arteries due to overlap from renal veins, the inferior vena cava, and the adrenal-gonadal vasculature. Finally, the inherent vessel tortuosity and complex flow patterns, as well as widely disparate flow velocities in the aorta and renal arteries, create problems in imaging the renal vessels with MRA. A report of 37 patients by Kim et al[61] demonstrated an overall sensitivity of 100% and specificity of 94% for detecting stenoses greater than 50% in diameter. They used coronal and axial breath-held gradient-echo images (TOF technique). As Kim et al point out, the spatial resolution of the technique was adequate only to evaluate the proximal renal arteries. The excellent results may thus at least be partly explained by the proximal location of the stenoses, which made them amenable to diagnosis with their technique. No branch vessel lesions, fibromuscular dysplasia, or lesions in accessory renal arteries were detected.

Debatin et al[62] compared the diagnostic accuracy of MRA with that of conventional arteriography to visualize the renal arteries and aid in the detection of renovascular disease. Thirty-three MRA studies, consisting of axial 2D PC, coronal 2D PC, and coronal 2D TOF acquisition, were obtained within 48 hours of conventional angiography. Evaluation was limited to the proximal 35 mm of each renal artery. Renal artery visualization and detection of renovascular disease were more complete with coronal PC (80% sensitivity, 91% specificity) than with the TOF images (53% sensitivity, 97% specificity). Combined axial and coronal PC images permitted visualization of the proximal 35 mm of all dominant renal arteries and detection of 13 of 15 stenoses (87% sensitivity, 97% specificity). The PC sequences were found to have a higher sensitivity than coronal breath-held TOF sequences in this study (sensitivity 87% vs. 53%).

An alternative protocol uses a combination of 3D PC, 2D TOF, and cardiac-gated cine 2D PC acquisitions to image the renal arteries. This technique was found to have a sensitivity of 86% and a specificity of 95% for detecting renal artery stenosis in a prospective comparison with conventional angiography.[63] Patients should be well hydrated, and baseline renal function is assessed by serum creatinine determination. The results of recent serum creatinine measurement allow estimation of the expected flow velocities in the renal arteries; a normal serum creatinine level implies normal renal blood flow, whereas an elevated serum creatinine level implies a reduced renal blood flow. In patients with reduced renal blood flow, a lower VENC (10 to 20 cm/sec) during the PC imaging sequences is frequently used.

In the absence of intravenous contrast medium, 3D TOF imaging strategies are not routinely used for examination of the abdominal aorta or renal arteries. These sequences require a very high rate of inflow of unsaturated spins to obtain adequate contrast between vascular structures and stationary structures. This condition is not easily satisfied in the abdominal aorta, where the rapid inflow is also required over a large imaging volume. However, Prince et al[64] have advocated a technique that uses a 3D TOF acquisition, in conjunction with an intravenous injection of gadolinium-DTPA (diethylenetriamine pentaacetic acid) for imaging the abdominal aorta and renal arteries. The administration of a contrast agent in this protocol allows imaging of the abdominal aorta in patients with poor cardiac output and evaluation of the renal arteries in patients with significant renal disease. Gadolinium-DTPA is administered with the use of an intravenous infusion during the 3-minute acquisition.

Localizer images of the kidneys are evaluated to determine if a reduction in renal parenchymal mass is present, a finding often associated with a significant long-standing renal artery stenosis. The presence of a renal artery stenosis is detected by a luminal narrowing identified within the vessel as well as by the presence of signal loss in the vessel from complex flow (Fig. 4-24, *A* and *B*). Since the stenotic renal artery segments frequently give rise to complex flow, which causes artifacts, Debatin et al[62] described a useful grading system that correlates with the severity of stenosis. A mild stenosis is associated with a luminal narrowing without evidence of signal loss. A moderate stenosis (50% to 75% in diameter) is associated with a luminal narrowing and incomplete signal loss or a focal signal loss within the renal artery of less than 5 mm in length. A severe stenotic segment is typically seen as a complete signal void longer than 5 mm, with reconstitution of flow distally. This grading scale is useful for evaluating the presence and severity of a renal artery stenosis. Caution should be exercised in patients with renovascular hypertension who recently began therapy with angiotensin converting enzyme inhibitors, since the sudden drop in blood pressure may cause a reduction in the flow disturbance at the site of the stenosis, therefore causing less signal loss.

MRA has been used to demonstrate celiac and superior mesenteric artery stenoses, using a combination of axial and sagittal 2D TOF acquisitions and 3D PC sequences. This work, however, is preliminary and will require further validation.

In addition to anatomic images, Li et al[65] have obtained preliminary flow measurements from patients with mesenteric arterial stenoses. They noted a blunted flow augmentation response after oral administration of Ensure in patients with mesenteric arterial stenosis, whereas normal patients showed augmentation of mesenteric blood flow

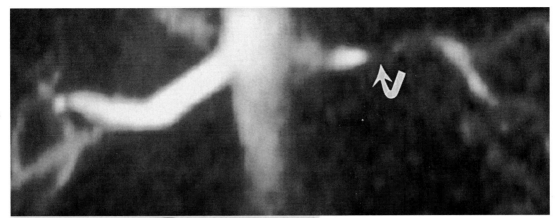

A

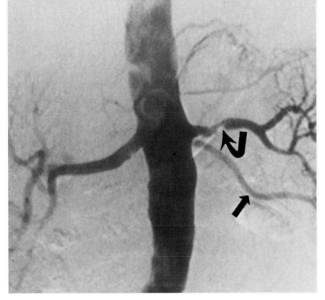

B

Fig. 4-24. A, Coronal MRA that demonstrates renal artery stenosis *(curved arrow).* **B,** Catheter-based aortogram for renal artery evaluation, corresponding to the same patient as **(A).** The left renal artery stenosis is apparent *(curved arrow).* An accessory lower pole left renal artery *(straight arrow)* was seen on this angiogram but not in the MRA images. This type of exclusion from the MRA projection represents one of the potential pitfalls of MRA renderings. *(From Grist TM: Magnetic resonance angiography of the aorta and renal arteries, MRI Clin North Am 1:265, 1993.)*

after feeding. This preliminary work was based on only a few patients.

Magnetic Resonance Angiography of the Lower-Extremity Circulation

Although there has been great enthusiasm for MRA of the peripheral run-off vessels from the iliac arteries to the tibial arteries, the clinical application of MRA techniques has met with only modest success. Precise definition of occlusive disease requires high spatial resolution—particularly when the degree of stenosis becomes important. Additionally, there is a level of comfort with the appearance of arterial anatomy seen on conventional film-screen or digital arteriograms. MRA images are less appealing to the vascular surgeon and vascular interventionalist, even though they may contain more information than contrast arteriograms.

In the iliac artery circulation, tortuosity and nonlaminar flow patterns can lead to studies that are false-positive for stenoses. This overestimation of iliac artery stenoses has been noted by several authors[66,67] who feel that inflow iliac artery stenoses detected by MRA should be viewed with caution and confirmed with other studies.

The infrainguinal circulation can be reliably imaged by

MRA (Fig. 4-25, *A* and *B*), but spatial resolution does not yet approach arteriography. Nevertheless, with the current techniques resolution of 1.25 mm is possible.[68] In a comparison between MRA and contrast arteriography, there was 100% agreement for significant occlusive disease in the infrainguinal circulation. Whether the images prove adequate for revascularization, however, remains to be seen. This is because the diagnosis of an occlusive segment (stenosis or total occlusion) is only the first step in surgical revascularization. Before surgery there must be identification of adequate target vessels for bypass graft anastomosis. This is especially important in the tibial artery circulation. As Owen et al[69] have shown, MRA may be more sensitive for distal tibial artery segments that are patent, compared with contrast arteriography, but the usefulness of this information for directing the surgeon to vascular segments that are suitable for bypass remains to be proved.

Finally, recent modifications of MRA technique for arterial studies of the lower extremities have decreased the time required for imaging. Douek et al[70] have described "fast MRA" using a technique that combines intravenous administration of gadolinium. With this contrast agent in the vascular system and modified imaging parameters, the aorta, iliac arteries, and arteries of the legs were imaged in

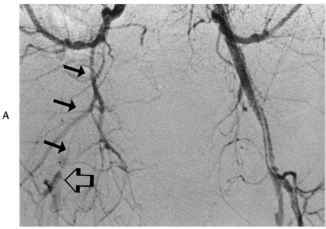

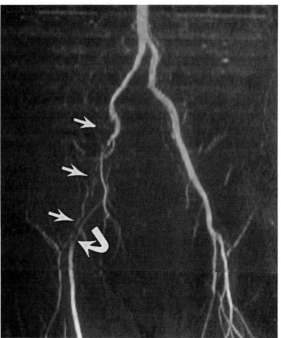

Fig. 4-25. A, DSA of right external iliac artery occlusion *(solid arrows),* with collateral reconstitution of the distal common femoral artery *(open arrow).* **B,** Corresponding 2D TOF MRA. The external iliac artery occlusion is noted *(straight arrows)* and the distal common femoral artery reconstitution *(curved arrow)* mirrors the DSA image.

less than 2 minutes. Their MRA results compared favorably with catheter-based angiography in 10 healthy volunteers and 20 patients with a variety of vascular disorders.

THORACIC VENOUS CIRCULATION

Indications

Magnetic resonance venography (MRV) is useful in evaluating thoracic venous abnormalities. The multiplanar acquisition capability of MRV is an important advantage relative to existing techniques such as conventional venography or CT angiography. Additionally, MRV is not limited by the acoustic window of duplex Doppler ultrasound, which limits evaluation of the superior vena cava. One disadvantage of MRV is image degradation by respiratory motion.

Technique

Breath-held 2D TOF acquisition constitutes the most useful technique. Unlike this imaging approach in the abdomen, however, images are acquired in the axial plane (for the superior vena cava) and the sagittal plane (for the subclavian veins). These techniques have generally demonstrated good accuracy for detecting venous thromboembolic disease in the thorax.[71]

ABDOMINAL MAGNETIC RESONANCE VENOGRAPHY

Indications for abdominal venography using MRV include suspected inferior vena cava or renal vein thromboembolic disease, bland thrombosis, and neoplastic thrombosis. In addition, MRV has been advocated to evaluate the portal venous circulation, particularly in patients with

either portal venous hypertension or for vascular imaging before liver transplantation.

Technique

Two-dimensional TOF MRA examinations constitute the workhorse of MRV. The 2D technique can be performed while the patient holds her breath at inspiration or at expiration, and therefore respiratory-related motion artifacts are minimized. Usually multiple coronal sections are acquired with an overlap of 20% to 30% to facilitate viewing of the portal venous system at multiple angles.

PC techniques also have been advocated for evaluating the venous system. PC images provide information regarding the speed and direction of blood flow and can be used for anatomic imaging as well as flow measurement. The PC studies may be performed with either an ungated or gated 2D acquisition. The ungated studies require less time and can be performed in a single breath-hold. However, the cardiac-gated cine examinations also provide qualitative information regarding the nature of the blood flow patterns.

Interpretation/Results

Venous thrombosis can be demonstrated with high accuracy using MRV. Since blood clots contain hemosiderin, thrombosis manifests as a very low signal void within the abdominal veins on gradient-recalled echo (GRE) images. Flowing blood, which appears very bright on GRE images, provides excellent contrast between normal blood flow and venous thrombosis. Several prospective trials have demonstrated the high accuracy of MRV for detecting venous thrombosis, with a sensitivity and specificity exceeding 95%.[72]

In addition, MRV has been used to demonstrate venous collateral pathways in patients with portal venous hypertension.[73] In this subject population MRV has been demonstrated to have a high accuracy for identifying the nature of collateral vessels, the level and length of occlusions, and the patency of portosystemic shunts.

SUMMARY

Recently developed MRA techniques currently provide useful information regarding arterial and venous abnormalities within the chest, abdomen, cerebrovascular, and extremity circulation. With further improvements in technique, MRA in the body is expected to provide extensive information regarding vascular pathology without the need for iodinated contrast agents or intravascular catheters. Further work is needed to evaluate the role of MRA with respect to other noninvasive imaging techniques.

REFERENCES

1. Haschek E and Lindenthal OT: A contribution to the practical use of the photography according to Roentgen, Wien Klin Wochenschr 9:63, 1896.
2. Cohan RH: Radiographic contrast media. In Kadir S, ed: Current practice of interventional radiology, Philadelphia, 1991, BC Decker.
3. The Society for Cardiac Angiography and Interventions: Guidelines for performance of peripheral percutaneous transluminal angioplasty, Cathet Cardiovasc Diagn 21:128, 1990.
4. Katayama H et al: Adverse reactions to ionic and nonionic contrast media, Radiology 175:621, 1990.
5. Schwab SJ et al: Contrast nephrotoxicity: a randomized controlled trial of a non-ionic and an ionic radiographic contrast agent, N Engl J Med 320:149, 1989.
6. Campbell RJ et al: A comparative study of the nephrotoxicity of iohexol, iopamidol, and ioxaglate in peripheral angiography, J Can Assoc Radiol 41:133, 1990.
7. Brezis M and Epstein FH: A closer look at radiocontrast-induced nephropathy, N Engl J Med 320:179, 1989.
8. Hawkins IF: Carbon dioxide digital subtraction arteriography, AJR 139:19, 1982.
9. Miller FJ et al: Clinical intra-arterial digital subtraction imaging, Radiology 148:273, 1983.
10. Weaver FA et al: Clinical applications of carbon dioxide/digital subtraction arteriography, J Vasc Surg 13:266, 1991.
11. Ehrman KO et al: Comparison of diagnostic accuracy with carbon dioxide versus iodinated contrast material in the imaging of hemodialysis access fistulas, J Vasc Interv Radiol 5:771, 1994.
12. Kerns SR and Hawkins IF Jr: Carbon dioxide digital subtraction angiography: expanding applications and technical evolution, AJR 164:735, 1995.
13. Rees CR et al: Use of carbon dioxide as a contrast medium for transjugular intrahepatic portosystemic shunt procedures, J Vasc Interv Radiol 5:383, 1994.
14. Seeger JM et al: Carbon dioxide gas as an arterial contrast agent, Ann Surg 217:688, 1993.
15. Miller FJ et al: Clinical intra-arterial digital subtraction imaging, Radiology 148:273, 1983.
16. Weaver FA et al: Clinical applications of carbon dioxide/digital subtraction arteriography, J Vasc Surg 13:266, 1991.
17. Harward TRS et al: Follow-up evaluation after renal artery bypass surgery with use of carbon dioxide arteriography and color-flow duplex scanning, J Vasc Surg 18:23, 1993.
18. Coffey R et al: The cerebrovascular effects of intra-arterial CO_2 in quantities required for diagnostic imaging, Radiology 151:405, 1984.
19. Farinas PL: A new technique for the arteriographic examination of the abdominal aorta and its branches, AJR 46:641, 1941.
20. Seldinger SI: Catheter replacement of the needle in percutaneous arteriography. A new technique, Acta Radiol 39:368, 1953.
21. Cope C: Minipuncture angiography, Radiol Clin North Am 24:359, 1986.
22. Hessel SJ: Complications of angiography and other catheter procedures. In Abrams HL, ed: Abrams angiography ed 3, Boston, 1983, Little, Brown.
23. Adams DF and Abrams HL: Complications of coronary arteriography: a follow-up report, Cardiovasc Radiol 2:89, 1979.
24. Davis K et al: Complications of coronary arteriography from the collaborative study of coronary artery surgery (CASS), Circulation 59:1105, 1979.
25. Kennedy JW: Complications associated with cardiac catheterization and angiography (from the Registry Committee of the Society for Cardiac Angiography), Cathet Cardiovasc Diagn 8:5, 1982.
26. Morton BC and Beanlands DS: Complications of cardiac catheterization: one centre's experience, Can Med Assoc J 131:889, 1984.
27. Altin RS, Flicker S, and Naidech HJ: Pseudoaneurysm and arteriovenous fistula after femoral artery catheterization: association with low femoral punctures, AJR 152:629, 1989.
28. Fellmeth BD et al: Postangiographic femoral artery injuries: nonsurgical repair with US-guided compression, Radiology 178:671, 1991.
29. Hansing CE: The risk and cost of coronary angiography: II. The risk of coronary angiography in Washington State, JAMA 242:735, 1979.
30. Colt HG et al: Cholesterol emboli after cardiac catheterization, Medicine (Baltimore) 67:389, 1988.
31. Palmer FJ and Warren BA: Multiple cholesterol emboli syndrome complicating angiographic techniques, Clin Radiol 39:519, 1988.
32. Rosman HS et al: Cholesterol embolization: clinical findings and implications, J Am Coll Cardiol 15:1296, 1990.
33. Detmer DE, Fryback D, and Strother CM: Cost effectiveness of digital subtraction arteriography. In Mistretta CA et al, eds: Digital subtraction arteriography: an application of computerized fluoroscopy, Chicago, 1982, Year Book Medical Publishers.
34. Kruger RA: Basic physics of computerized fluoroscopy difference imaging. In Mistretta CA et al, eds: Digital subtraction arteriography: an application of computerized fluoroscopy, Chicago, 1982, Year Book Medical Publishers.
35. Fox AJ: How to measure carotid stenosis, Radiology 186:316, 1993.
36. Vieco PT, Gross CE, and Shuman WP: Acute subarachnoid hemorrhage: detection of aneurysms of the circle of Willis with CT angiography and DSA, Paper presented at the ARRS 1994 meeting, New Orleans.
37. Vieco P: Helical/spiral CT: a practical approach, New York, 1995, McGraw-Hill.
38. Riles TS et al: The totally occluded carotid artery: preliminary observations using rapid sequential computerized tomographic scanning, Arch Surg 117:1185, 1982.
39. Dillon EH et al: CT angiography, AJR 160:1273, 1993.
40. Rosniak VH, Olson MC, and Demos TC: Aortic motion artifact simulating dissection on CT scans: elimination with reconstructive segmented images, AJR 161:557, 1993.
41. Costello P et al: Assessment of the thoracic aorta by spiral CT, AJR 158:1127, 1992.
42. Remy-Jardin M et al: Central pulmonary thromboembolism: diagnosis with spiral CT with the single-breath-hold

technique—comparison with pulmonary angiography, Radiology 185:381, 1992.

43. Goodman LR et al: Detection of pulmonary embolism in patients with unresolved clinical and scintigraphic diagnosis: helical CT versus angiography, AJR 164:1369, 1995.

44. White RI and Pollak JS: Pulmonary arteriovenous malformations: diagnosis with three-dimensional helical CT—a breakthrough without contrast media, Radiology 191:613, 1994.

45. Remy J et al: Angioarchitecture of pulmonary arteriovenous malformations: clinical utility of three-dimensional helical CT, Radiology 191:657, 1994.

46. Zeman RK et al: Abdominal aortic aneurysms: findings on three-dimensional display of helical CT data, AJR 164:917, 1995.

47. Zeman RK et al: Diagnosis of aortic dissection: value of helical CT with multiplanar reformation and three dimensional rendering, AJR 164:1375, 1995.

48. Galanski M et al: Renal arterial stenoses: spiral CT angiography, Radiology 189:185, 1993.

49. Rubin GD et al: Spiral CT of renal artery stenosis: comparison of three-dimensional rendering techniques, Radiology 190:181, 1994.

50. Wedeen V, Meuli R, Edelman R et al: Projective imaging of pulsatile flow with magnetic resonance, Science 230:946, 1985.

51. Hendrick RE: Basic physics of MR imaging: an introduction, Radiographics 14:829, 1994.

52. Edelman R: Basic principles of magnetic resonance angiography, Cardiovasc Intervent Radiol 15:3, 1992.

53. Atlas SW: MR angiography in neurologic disease, Radiology 193:1, 1994.

54. Polak JF et al: Carotid endarterectomy: preoperative evaluation of candidates with combined Doppler sonography and MR angiography. Work in progress, Radiology 186:333, 1993.

55. Masaryk TJ and Obuchowski NA: Noninvasive carotid imaging: caveat emptor, Radiology 186:325, 1993.

56. von Schulthess GK and Augustiny N: Calculation of T2 values versus phase imaging for the distinction between flow and thrombus in MR imaging, Radiology 164:549, 1987.

57. Chang JM et al: MR measurement of blood flow in the true and false channel in chronic aortic dissection, J Comput Assist Tomogr 15:418, 1991.

58. Grist T et al: Pulmonary angiography with MRA: preliminary clinical experience, Radiology 189:523, 1993.

59. Manning WJ, Li W, and Edelman RR: A preliminary report comparing magnetic resonance coronary angiography with conventional contrast angiography, N Engl J Med 328:828, 1993.

60. Arlart IP, Guhl L, and Edelman RR: Magnetic resonance angiography of the abdominal aorta, Cardiovasc Intervent Radiol 15:43, 1992.

61. Kim D et al: Abdominal aorta and renal artery stenosis: evaluation with MR angiography, Radiology 174:727, 1990.

62. Debatin J et al: Imaging of the renal arteries: value of MR angiography, AJR 157:981, 1991.

63. Grist T et al: Prospective evaluation of renal MR angiography: comparison with conventional angiography in 35 patients, Radiology 189:190, 1993.

64. Prince M et al: Dynamic gadolinium-enhanced three-dimensional abdominal MR arteriography, J MRI 3:877, 1993.

65. Li K et al: Phase contrast cine MRI for the diagnosis of mesenteric ischemia, Magn Reson Med 2:3109, 1992.

66. Mulligan SA et al: Peripheral arterial occlusive disease: prospective comparison of MR angiography and color duplex US with conventional angiography, Radiology 178:695, 1991.

67. Yucel EK et al: Atherosclerotic occlusive disease of the lower extremity: prospective evaluation with two-dimensional time-of-flight MR angiography, Radiology 187:637, 1993.

68. Cambria PR et al: The potential for lower extremity revascularization without contrast arteriography: experience with magnetic resonance angiography, J Vasc Surg 17:1050, 1993.

69. Owen RS et al: Magnetic resonance imaging of angiographically occult runoff vessels in peripheral arterial occlusive disease, N Engl J Med 326:1577, 1992.

70. Douek PC et al: Fast MR angiography of the aortoiliac arteries and arteries of the lower extremity: value of bolus-enhanced, whole-volume subtraction technique, AJR 165:431, 1995.

71. Evans A et al: Detection of deep venous thrombosis: prospective comparison of MR imaging with contrast venography, AJR 161:131, 1993.

72. Finn J et al: Imaging of the portal venous system in patients with cirrhosis: MR angiography vs duplex Doppler sonography, AJR 161:989, 1993.

73. Hansen M, Spritzer C, and Sostman H: Assessing the patency of mediastinal and thoracic inlet veins: value of MR imaging, AJR 155:1177, 1991.

CHAPTER FIVE

HEMOSTASIS AND THROMBOSIS

John R. Bartholomew
Kandice Kottke-Marchant

Hemostasis, the process by which a hemostatic plug is formed, is a normal physiologic response that prevents exsanguination after injury. Thrombosis, however, is a pathologic response to hemostasis at an abnormal time and location that may result in major morbidity and mortality. Thrombus formation may lead to ischemic injury as a result of decreased blood flow to the target organ, or the thrombus may become dislodged and embolize. Arterial thrombosis may result in stroke, myocardial infarction, or the loss of a limb, whereas venous thrombosis often presents as pulmonary embolism or deep vein thrombosis. For most of this century, research and interests have largely concentrated on bleeding disorders. Over the past few decades, however, congenital abnormalities of hemostasis have been identified that place patients at increased risk for thrombosis. These disorders are commonly referred to as *primary hypercoagulable states,* or *thrombophilias,* and have stimulated much interest and research (see box on this page). In addition, clinicians have long recognized that certain predisposing risk factors including malignancy, surgery, or trauma place individuals at an increased risk for thrombosis. These disorders are often referred to as *secondary hypercoagulable states* (see box, p. 90).

HISTORICAL BACKGROUND

In 1905 Morawitz[1] theorized that four factors were responsible for blood hemostasis. These factors included prothrombin, calcium ions, fibrinogen, and thromboplastin. His theory of hemostasis, also known as the *classical theory of coagulation,* or what we now refer to as the *extrinsic pathway,* remained the principal concept of hemostasis for most of this century. In 1964 the cascade, or waterfall, hypothesis was proposed by MacFarlane[2] and Davies and Ratnoff[3] independently. This idea, referred to as the *intrinsic pathway,* viewed hemostasis as a proteolytic cascade in which coagulation factors (normally existing as inert

precursors) are transformed into active enzymes in a step-by-step fashion. Recent research has led to new insights into the coagulation pathway, including a reassessment of the original role for factor XI in the intrinsic pathway and elucidation of the role of tissue factor path-

PRIMARY HYPERCOAGULABLE DISORDERS

Abnormalities of Natural Anticoagulants
Antithrombin III deficiency

Antithrombin III dysfunction

Protein C deficiency

Protein C dysfunction

Resistance to activated protein C

Protein S deficiency

Protein S dysfunction

Heparin cofactor II deficiency

Heparin cofactor II dysfunction

Disorders of Fibrinolysis
Plasminogen deficiency

Plasminogen dysfunction

t-PA deficiency

Plasminogen activator inhibitor-1

Lipoprotein(a)

Dysfibrinogenemia

Other disorders
Homocystinuria

Factor XII deficiency

Histidine-rich glycoprotein

SECONDARY HYPERCOAGULABLE STATES

Myeloproliferative disorders

Heparin-induced thrombocytopenia

Antiphospholipid antibody syndrome

Oral contraceptives/pregnancy

Nephrotic syndrome

Immobilization

Surgery

Trauma

Malignancy

Hyperlipidemias

Diabetes mellitus

Paroxysmal nocturnal hemoglobinuria

Elevated fibrinogen

Smoking

Implantation of artificial devices (catheters, pacemakers)

Disseminated intravascular coagulation

Vasculitis

Obesity

way inhibitor (TFPI).[4] Once the coagulation pathway is initiated, limitation of hemostasis to the sites of blood vessel injury is very important. Without control mechanisms, thrombin formation would go unchallenged, leading to thrombosis. Morawitz recognized this concept, and used the term "the progressive antithrombin activity" to describe the ability of human plasma to slowly neutralize thrombin and thus limit this potential. In 1954 Seegers et al[5] renamed this antithrombin III (ATIII) and recognized that a deficiency of this protein could lead to thrombosis. In 1965 Egeberg[6] reported the first patient with ATIII deficiency and thrombosis. Many other natural anticoagulants have since been identified. In 1960 protein C was discovered by Mammen, Thomas, and Seegers,[7] although it was originally called autoprothrombin II-A. Stenflo[8] later rediscovered this protein, but it was not until 1981 when the first case of a patient with protein C deficiency involving recurrent thrombophlebitis was described by Griffin et al.[9] Since these discoveries, protein S deficiency, and disorders of the fibrinolytic system have also been identified as causes of thrombophilia. More recently, resistance to activated protein C (APC) has been described.[10]

In this chapter we review the basic principles of hemostasis and discuss some of the hypercoagulable states that lead to the thrombosis problems seen in clinical practices.

PATHOGENESIS

The hemostatic system maintains a precarious balance between thrombosis and hemorrhage. Hemostasis is a complex mechanism that involves the blood vessels, plate-

lets, and coagulation proteins, as well as naturally occurring anticoagulants and platelet inhibitors (Fig. 5-1). The blood vessels and platelets are responsible for primary hemostasis, and the coagulation proteins are responsible for secondary hemostasis. Both primary and secondary hemostasis prevent bleeding, whereas the naturally occurring anticoagulants and platelet inhibitors are generally responsible for the prevention of thrombosis, and the fibrinolytic system regulates the extent of thrombosis when it occurs. An imbalance of the hemostatic system can lead to either thrombosis or hemorrhage (Fig. 5-2).

Primary Hemostasis

BLOOD VESSELS. Blood vessels participate in primary hemostasis through two mechanisms: vasoconstriction and endothelial function. Vasoconstriction may play an immediate, albeit temporary, role in hemostasis associated with injury of small vessels. It may be more important in arteries than in veins, because of the more substantial arterial muscular coat.[11] Vasoconstriction is thought to be initiated by vasoactive substances such as serotonin and thromboxane A_2 released from platelets during platelet activation, as well as endothelin released from the endothelial cells themselves.[12,13]

Endothelial cells actively participate in normal thromboresistance and are thought to be the primary factor responsible for maintaining blood in a fluid state in the vasculature. The nonthrombogenic properties of endothelial cells are maintained by production of prostacyclin, a potent antiplatelet agent, as well as by binding of the anticoagulant ATIII to heparan sulfate moieties on the endothelial surface and by the production of tissue plasminogen activator (t-PA), a potent activator of fibrinolysis.[14] Thrombomodulin, an integral endothelial cell membrane glycoprotein, binds and inhibits thrombin as it is generated during coagulation. The thrombin-thrombomodulin complex then activates protein C, which degrades coagulation factors Va and VIIIa, thereby further decreasing thrombin generation.[15] When injured, endothelial cells can rapidly develop prothrombotic properties due to expression of tissue factor (TF) activity, secretion of von Willebrand's factor (vWF), reduction of thrombomodulin activity, and development of phospholipid-based binding sites for coagulation complexes. In addition to mechanical injury, the prothrombotic function of endothelial cells is also stimulated by bacterial endotoxin, cytokines such as interleukin-1, and tumor necrosis factor and thrombin itself.[16,17] The hemostatic properties of endothelial cells vary with respect to location in the vascular tree. We are only just beginning to appreciate the role this functional variability may have in the pathogenesis and localization of vascular thrombosis.

PLATELETS. *Platelets* are nonnucleated cells, produced in the bone marrow from megakaryocytes, that play a major role in hemostasis. Platelets promote hemostasis by four mechanisms: (1) adhering to sites of vascular injury, (2) releasing procoagulant compounds from their alpha and dense granules, (3) aggregating together to form a hemostatic platelet plug, and (4) providing a procoagulant surface for activated coagulation protein complexes on their phospholipid membranes.

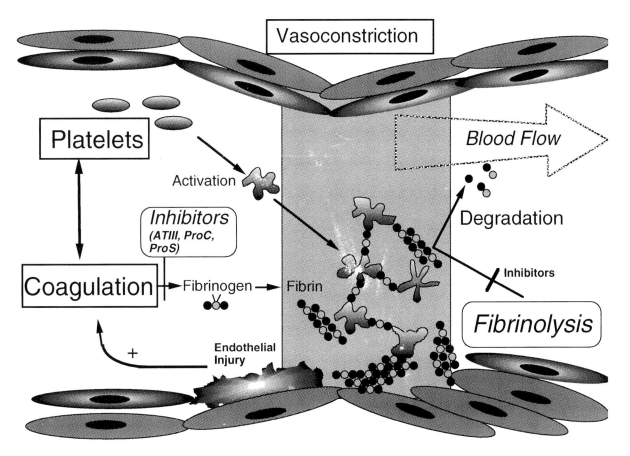

Fig. 5-1. Hemostasis is a normal physiologic response to form a fibrin-platelet thrombus after vessel injury. Hemostasis consists of prothrombotic primary responses (vasoconstriction, endothelial function, and platelet activation) as well as secondary responses (coagulation activation with fibrin formation). These are balanced by factors that have an anticoagulant effect (dilution of activated factors by blood flow and coagulation inhibitors such as antithrombin III, proteins C and S) and those that actively work to degrade the thrombus (fibrinolysis).

Platelet adhesion is the initial step in platelet plug formation. Platelets contain numerous adhesive glycoproteins on the outer surface of their plasma membrane. The ligands for these glycoproteins range from collagen to vWF and fibronectin. Interaction between the platelet-surface glycoproteins and their ligands mediates adhesion of platelets to both injured endothelial cells and exposed subendothelial matrix. After adhering to the subendothelium, platelets undergo a shape change with the development of pseudopods, and initiate a secretory release reaction whereby products from the alpha granules (platelet factor 4, β-thromboglobulin, thrombospondin, platelet-derived growth factor, fibrinogen, vWF) and dense granules (adenosine diphosphate [ADP] and serotonin) are released into the surrounding milieu.[18] The release of ADP from the dense granules initiates the process of aggregation, whereby platelet glycoprotein IIb-IIIa on one platelet is bound to adjacent platelets via a central fibrinogen molecule following a shape change of the glycoprotein IIb/IIIa molecule.[19] In addition to ADP, other agonists such as epinephrine, thrombin, collagen, and platelet-activating factor can initiate platelet aggregation by interaction with membrane receptors. Activated platelets also play a procoagulant role, with platelet phospholipids providing a

binding site for coagulation complexes that activate both factor X and prothrombin.[20]

Secondary Hemostasis
COAGULATION PROTEINS. Although vasoconstriction, endothelial cell function, and platelet plug formation play an important role in early hemostasis, the formation of a cross-linked fibrin clot by the coagulation cascade is essential for adequate hemostasis. Blood coagulation is a cascade-type process that involves multiple enzymes and cofactors, with the culmination being the conversion of fibrinogen to fibrin, and ultimately cross-linking of the fibrin clot into an insoluble network.

Blood coagulation traditionally has been thought to consist of four key reactions: (1) initiation, (2) activation of factor X, (3) formation of thrombin, and (4) formation of a fibrin clot. Coagulation is initiated via two mechanisms: (1) surface activation via the contact activation system (intrinsic pathway) and (2) extrinsic pathway activation from tissue injury and liberation of tissue thromboplastin (TF).[11]

A revised view of the coagulation process has been suggested because the older explanation did not adequately explain why patients with factor VIII or IX

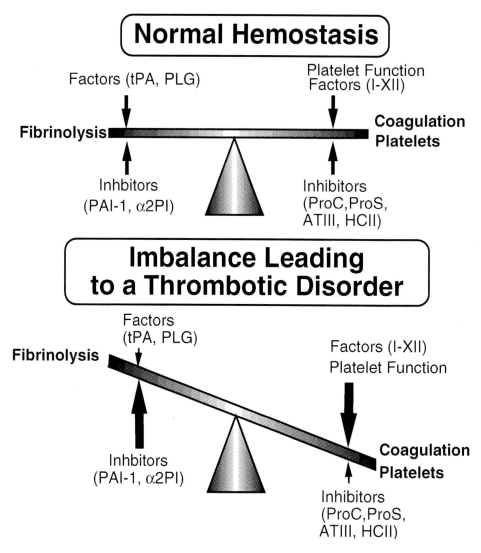

Fig. 5-2. *(Top)* For normal hemostasis there is a balance between activating and inhibiting factors for the coagulation and fibrinolytic systems. For the coagulation cascade the procoagulant factors (fibrinogen, prothrombin, etc.) are balanced by the inhibitors antithrombin III (ATIII), protein C (proC), protein S (proS), and heparin cofactor II (HCII). The profibrinolytic factors (plasminogen [PLG], tissue plasminogen activator [t-PA]) are balanced by the inhibitors (α_2-plasmin inhibitor [α_2PI]), and plasminogen activator inhibitor-1 (PAI-1). *(Bottom)* Imbalances leading to thrombosis are most often due to increased coagulation or decreased fibrinolytic function. Increased coagulation is most often due to deficiencies of the natural anticoagulants but may also be due to increased coagulation factor levels. Decreased fibrinolysis is most often due to decreased plasminogen, but increased levels of the inhibitors, especially PAI-1, have also been implicated.

deficiencies bleed, and those with factor XII and prekallikrein deficiencies do not.[21,22] Tissue factor released from injured cells complexes with factor VII to form the TF–factor VIIa–lipid complex that can activate not only factor X but also factor IX. This results in the production of thrombin with fibrin formation. However, thrombin can also activate factor XI.[23] The activated factor XI results in additional activation of factor IX.[22] A regulator of the activation of the coagulation cascade by this mechanism is TFPI, formerly called lipoprotein-associated coagulation inhibitor or extrinsic pathway inhibitor.[24] TFPI inhibits the factor VIIa–TF–factor Xa complex, thus preventing further factor Xa production by factor VIIa–TF.[24] The only remaining path for production of more factor IXa is then

from activation of factor XI or IX. This revised concept of the hemostasis pathway accounts for the importance of factors IX and VIII for adequate hemostasis, provides a role for factor XI in hemostasis and explains the lack of a bleeding diathesis in factor XII or prekallikrein deficiencies.[23,24] Fibrinogen is a large plasma protein (molecular weight 340,000) composed of two pairs of three polypeptide chains (A-α, B-β, and γ). The two pairs of polypeptide chains are linked by disulfide bonds near their N-terminal ends. The conversion of fibrinogen to fibrin involves cleavage of fibrinopeptides A and B from the A-α and B-β N-terminal regions by thrombin to form fibrin monomer, noncovalent aggregation, or polymerization of fibrin monomers via a half-staggered end-to-end and side-to-side association, and cross-linking of the γ chains by factor XIIIa to form insoluble fibrin.[25] The released fibrinopeptides can be assayed. Elevations in the level of these peptides have been used as sensitive indicators of fibrin formation.

Regulation of Hemostasis

Hemostasis is regulated by naturally occurring inhibitors of both platelets and the coagulation cascade, as well as by the fibrinolytic system, which degrades the fibrin clot, and by blood flow, which helps to dilute the activated coagulation factors as they form. Imbalances in these regulatory systems may predispose to thrombosis.

NATURAL ANTICOAGULANTS. Several proteins act to inhibit the coagulation cascade directly. ATIII inhibits thrombin and other activated coagulation proteins (VIIa, Xa, IXa, XIa, kallikrein, and plasmin) by forming a stable 1:1 complex with these enzymes.[26] These stable complexes can be assayed and serve as markers of coagulation activation. Heparin greatly accelerates this reaction by causing a conformational change in ATIII. The in vivo factor responsible for accelerating this reaction is heparan sulfate, located on the luminal surface of endothelial cells. A large proportion of ATIII is bound to luminal heparan sulfate, resulting in a pool of active inhibitor awaiting intravascular thrombin formation. Another inhibitor similar to ATIII is heparin cofactor II (HCII). However, HCII only inhibits thrombin, and its activity is accelerated by dermatan sulfate in addition to heparin. Patients with homozygous or heterozygous ATIII deficiency are predisposed to thrombosis, especially venous thrombosis. Although families with congenital HCII deficiency are known, there is not a clear association between HCII deficiency and thrombosis. Other plasma inhibitors of coagulation include α_2-macroglobulin, α_1-antitrypsin, and TFPI. As the extrinsic or TF pathway is thought to be the predominant physiologic pathway for coagulation activation, deficiencies of TFPI should be associated with thrombosis. However, no individual with TFPI deficiency has yet been identified.[24] Patients with abetalipoproteinemia have very low TFPI levels because of the absence of low-density lipoprotein (LDL), a carrier for TFPI, but do not have a tendency for thrombosis.[24] This suggests that plasma may not be the primary reservoir for TFPI.

Another unique thrombin inhibitory mechanism is provided by thrombomodulin, protein C, and protein S. Thrombomodulin is an intrinsic membrane glycoprotein found on endothelial cells, which forms a 1:1 molecular complex with thrombin.[27] Thrombomodulin alters the substrate specificity of thrombin from fibrinogen to protein C by binding to the anion-binding exosite of thrombin, turning it from a potent procoagulant molecule to an anticoagulant.[28] APC, produced by the thrombomodulin-thrombin complex, joins protein S in a complex on the phospholipid surface of platelets or endothelial cells and acts to selectively degrade factors Va and VIIIa[27] (Fig. 5-3). It also has profibrinolytic activity through inhibition of plasminogen activator inhibitor-1 (PAI-1). APC is inactivated by α_1-antitrypsin and protein C inhibitor. Deficiencies of protein C and protein S also predispose to thrombosis. No cases of thrombomodulin deficiency are

known, but this could also theoretically lead to thrombosis.

FIBRINOLYTIC SYSTEM. The *fibrinolytic system* is a series of proteins that, analogous to the coagulation system, is activated in a cascadelike fashion and results in the degradation of cross-linked fibrin (Fig. 5-4). *Plasmin* is the enzyme of the fibrinolytic cascade that degrades fibrin. Plasminogen is converted to plasmin by a group of enzymes known as *plasminogen activators*. These can be divided into two groups: intrinsic activators (factor XII, prekallikrein, high-molecular-weight kininogen, and prourokinase) and extrinsic activators (t-PA, urokinase, streptokinase).[29] Conversion of plasminogen to plasmin by plasminogen activators is thought to take place on the surface of the endothelial cells by binding to specific receptors.[30] As with the coagulation cascade, there are specific inhibitors of the fibrinolytic cascade. α_2-plasmin inhibitor is a rapidly acting inhibitor of plasmin, and PAI-1 is an inhibitor of the plasminogen activators t-PA and urokinase. Fibrinolytic disorders leading to thrombosis include deficiency of plasminogen, dysfunctional plasminogen, and defective t-PA release from endothelium. Elevated levels of PAI-1, the inhibitor of t-PA, have also been associated with thrombosis and are seen in patients with venous thrombosis, stroke, and myocardial infarction.[31,32]

CLINICAL PRESENTATION

In evaluating a patient for the cause of thrombosis, it is practical to use the classification listed in the boxes on pp. 89 and 90. The known primary hypercoagulable states, or thrombophilias, are generally congenital (autosomal dominant), and thrombosis usually involves the venous system. Secondary hypercoagulable states are usually acquired and are seen in a number of different clinical settings. A family history of thrombosis, thromboembolic event at an early age, unusual site for thrombosis (mesenteric vein, sagittal vein, hepatic vein), resistance to anticoagulation therapy, or a history of recurrence should lead the clinician to suspect a primary disorder. In addition, unexplained neonatal thrombosis, arterial thrombosis before age 30, and skin necrosis that develops while the patient is receiving warfarin should be investigated further (see the box on p. 96).

Secondary hypercoagulable states are often associated with acute or systemic illnesses. A history of recent surgery, pregnancy, recurrent miscarriage, trauma, or oral contraceptive use are important in identifying these patients (see the box on p. 96).

The incidence of primary hypercoagulable states is unknown. In one study involving 277 consecutive outpatients with venographically documented acute deep vein thrombosis, Heijboer et al[33] identified only 23 patients (8.3%) with a congenital hypercoagulable disorder. Malm et al[34] found a hereditary defect in only 5% of 439 individuals evaluated with thromboembolic disease despite 40% of these patients having a family history of thrombosis. Pabringer et al[35] studied 680 consecutive patients with a history of venous thrombosis, and at least one family member having the same clinical picture, and noted a prevalence of 7.1% for primary hypercoagulable

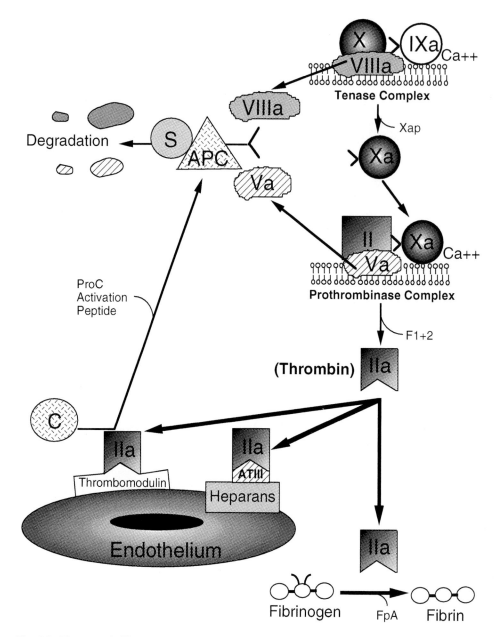

Fig. 5-3. The control of hemostasis. Coagulation activation at the common pathway begins with the formation of the tenase complex (factors IXa, VIIIa, X, phospholipid, and Ca^{++}), resulting in the activation of factor Xa and the release of a factor X activation peptide (Xap). Factor Xa then binds to phospholipid surfaces along with other coagulation factors (factor Va, Ca^{++}, and factor II-prothrombin) to form the prothrombinase complex. This results in the release of active thrombin (IIa) along with its cleavage product (F1+2). Thrombin then cleaves fibrinopeptide A (FpA) from fibrinogen, with the formation of fibrin, which polymerizes and is cross-linked. Regulation of this procoagulant process includes antithrombin III (ATIII), which is normally bound to heparan sulfate on endothelial surfaces, but readily binds activated thrombin, forming inactive thrombin–ATIII complexes. Thrombin also binds to an integral endothelial membrane protein, thrombomodulin, after which thrombin's substrate specificity is changed from fibrinogen to protein C (C). The thrombin-thrombomodulin complex activates protein C (APC) with liberation of a protein C activation peptide. APC complexes with its cofactor, protein S (S) and is responsible for the proteolytic degradation of factors Va and VIIIa to inactive products.

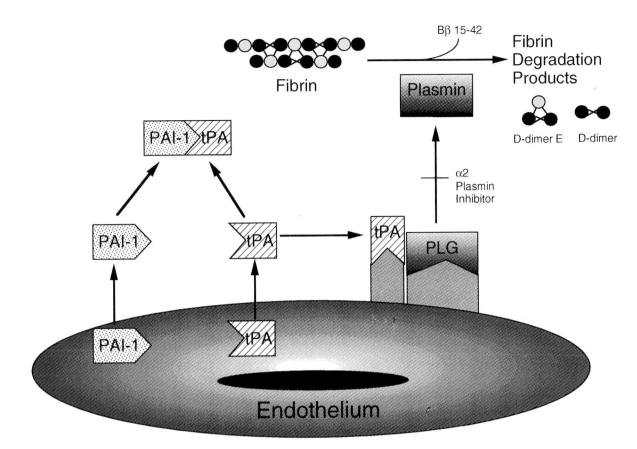

Fig. 5-4. The fibrinolytic system. The fibrinolytic system regulates hemostasis by the degradation of fibrin thrombi. The activity of the fibrinolytic system is centered on the endothelial cell, as several fibrinolytic proteins (tissue plasminogen activator [t-PA]), plasminogen activator inhibitor-1 (PAI-1), are produced by the endothelium and the endothelium has receptors on which the activation of plasmin by t-PA occurs. Plasmin activation can also occur on the fibrin thrombus, as both t-PA and plasminogen are able to bind directly to fibrin. Plasmin proteolytically degrades fibrin into multiple degradation products. One degradation product that is specific for the degradation of cross-linked fibrin is the D-dimer, which is the degradation product of adjacent cross-linked γ chains.

disorders. Bauer[36] has noted that hereditary defects can be detected in approximately 15% of patients presenting with venous thrombosis under the age of 45. These low reported prevalences of familial thrombophilia may be more reflective of our lack of knowledge of causes of these disorders than a true low prevalence. This is highlighted by recent reports that resistance to APC has been reported in as many as 64% of previously undiagnosed thrombophilia cases.[37]

The incidence of thrombosis may be higher in the secondary hypercoagulable states. For example, postoperative venous thrombosis occurs in approximately 70% of elderly patients with hip fractures and in up to 30% of general surgical patients. The overall incidence of thrombosis in cancer patients is about 5% to 15% and is even higher in patients with certain adenocarcinomas of the pancreas, stomach, lung or colon.[38]

Primary Hypercoagulable States

PROTEIN C. *Protein C* is a vitamin K–dependent glycoprotein that, in the presence of cofactor protein S, selectively inactivates factors Va and VIIIa and enhances fibrinolysis. Protein C is synthesized in the liver and has a

molecular weight of 56,000 Da. It is inherited in an autosomal dominant pattern, and patients with thrombosis have been recognized in both the heterozygous and homozygous states. In the heterozygous state venous thrombosis usually occurs before the age of 30, and the levels of protein C are 30% to 60% of normal. In the homozygous state thrombosis presents in infancy.

Two types of congenital protein C deficiency have been recognized. Most common is a true deficiency (type I) in which the plasma concentration of protein C is reduced using both functional and immunologic assays. Type I protein C deficiency is usually due to gene deletions or large gene defects. Type II protein C deficiency is characterized by a reduction in functional levels, although normal levels of protein C antigen are present. Type II protein C deficiency is most often due to point mutations leading to production of a dysfunctional protein. Patients with both types of protein C deficiency experience venous thromboembolic events.

Recurrent venous thrombosis at an early age, a family history of thrombosis, skin necrosis with the use of oral anticoagulants, and thromboembolic events occurring

FEATURES SUGGESTING A HYPERCOAGULABLE STATE

Primary Hypercoagulable State
Family history of thrombosis

Thromboembolism at an early age

Unusual site for thrombosis

Resistance to anticoagulation

Recurrent thromboembolic events

Neonatal thrombosis

Arterial thrombosis before age 30

Skin necrosis while receiving warfarin

Secondary Hypercoagulable State
Acute or systemic illness

Sepsis

Pregnancy or oral contraceptives

Recurrent miscarriages

Surgery and postoperative states

Trauma

Stroke

Myocardial infarction

Heparin

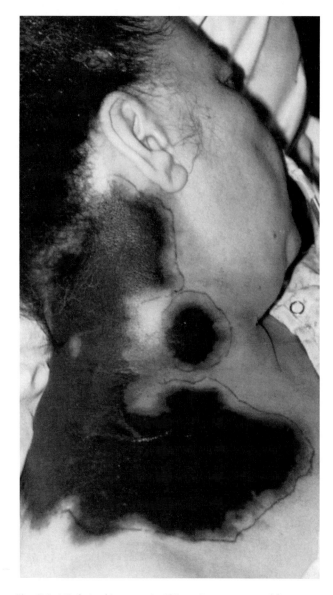

Fig. 5-5. Warfarin skin necrosis. This patient was treated for acute deep vein thrombosis. She developed cutaneous purpura and soft tissue necrosis while receiving warfarin therapy.

during infancy (purpura fulminans) are some of the manifestations of protein C deficiency. Superficial thrombophlebitis, deep vein thrombosis, pulmonary embolism, mesenteric vein thrombosis, and cerebral vein thrombosis have also been described. Arterial events are uncommon. Normal protein C levels are lower in infants and children compared with adults, so the diagnosis of protein C deficiency must be made with caution in this population.[39] Protein C levels may not reach adult levels until the child is 16 years of age.[40]

Acquired forms of protein C deficiency occur and may be seen in disseminated intravascular coagulation, warfarin therapy, liver disease, postoperative states, infection, malignancy, and adult respiratory distress syndrome. In the acquired form the other natural anticoagulants are often decreased.

Warfarin skin necrosis is reported to occur in less than 1% of patients receiving oral anticoagulant therapy[41] (Fig. 5-5). It generally is seen as a sudden, localized, painful skin lesion characterized by an initial erythematous or hemorrhagic appearance. This later develops into gangrenous necrosis. Warfarin skin necrosis usually develops between days 3 and 6 of therapy, appears more often in women, and is found more commonly in areas of increased subcutaneous fat, including the breasts, buttocks, and thighs.

Purpura fulminans is a devastating syndrome seen in infancy, often within hours of birth. Massive thrombosis of skin veins and capillaries leading to necrosis of the skin, sepsis, and death is seen.[42] Clinically the infant appears with ecchymoses about the head, extremities, and trunk.

Increased levels of protein C can sometimes be seen during an acute-phase response and are of doubtful significance. There has been no correlation between elevation of protein C and bleeding disorders.

RESISTANCE TO ACTIVATED PROTEIN C. Resistance to APC has only recently been described. In 1993 Dahlback et al[10] reported a familial thrombotic disorder characterized by a poor anticoagulant response to APC. Studies to date suggest that this defect is an autosomal dominant trait. The prevalence of this defect is reported to vary between 21% and 64% of patients presenting with venous thrombosis, whereas the prevalence of APC resistance in healthy control subjects has been noted to be 5%.[43-45] APC is a major risk factor for venous thrombosis, but it is not known if it is also a risk factor for arterial thrombosis.[43] In some studies patients with APC resistance tend to have a shorter activated partial thromboplastin time (APTT). An association between postoperative thrombosis and a short APTT has been previously noted.[46]

Dahlback et al developed an assay in which the addition of APC to plasma from a thrombotic patient does not result in prolongation of the APTT as expected. Dahlback proposed that degradation of factors VIIIa and Va by APC requires a previously unrecognized cofactor. This defect was later shown in the majority of patients to be due to a point mutation in factor V (factor V Leiden), which renders the mutant factor V resistant to degradation by APC.[47] Thus a molecular defect in factor V in the protein C pathway reduces APC anticoagulant activity.

PROTEIN S. Protein S deficiency is an autosomal dominant inherited disorder associated with venous thromboembolism and arterial thrombosis. Protein S was first discovered in 1977, although at that time it was given no function.[48] In 1980 Walker[49] proposed a role for protein S in expressing the anticoagulant activity of protein C. We now understand that protein S is a vitamin K–dependent plasma protein that inhibits thrombosis by serving as a cofactor for APC. It is required for both inactivation of factors Va and VIIIa and stimulation of fibrinolysis by protein C. It has a molecular weight of 69,000 Da and is synthesized in the liver and endothelial cells. Protein S is present in plasma in both a free and bound form. Free protein S is the active form and serves as a cofactor for protein C. The bound form is associated with a regulatory protein of the complement system, the C4b binding protein, and is inactive.

In 1984 Comp et al[50] reported two siblings who had recurrent venous thrombosis and lacked functional protein S activity. Since that time numerous reports have linked protein S deficiency to thrombosis. Superficial thrombophlebitis, deep vein thrombosis, mesenteric or cerebral vein thrombosis, and pulmonary embolism have been described. Stillbirth, purpura fulminans in homozygous deficient patients, and skin necrosis have also been reported.[41] More recently reports have linked stroke (Fig. 5-6) and arterial occlusive disease to protein S deficiency.[51-53] Protein S deficiency was associated with cerebrovascular accidents in 21 of 103 patients in one study, and in another series of 37 consecutive patients under the age of 45 presenting with arterial occlusive disease, 3 had protein S deficiency.[51,53] Despite these reports there is some question whether protein S is involved in acute arterial events. In a study of hereditary protein S deficiency from the Netherlands, none of the 12 families, of which 71 members were found to be heterozygous for protein S, had evidence of arterial disease before the age of 50.[54] Free protein S deficiency was also not considered to be a major risk factor for ischemic stroke in 94 hospitalized patients.[52]

Comp et al[55] have classified protein S deficiency into types I and II. Type I deficiency is associated with markedly decreased free levels of protein S and normal or mildly reduced total protein S antigen. Type II is characterized by greatly reduced total protein S antigen and free protein S levels. Both forms are associated with thrombosis. Not all families with protein S deficiencies have thrombosis problems. There are heterozygous patients and families who do not have an increased predisposition to thrombosis.

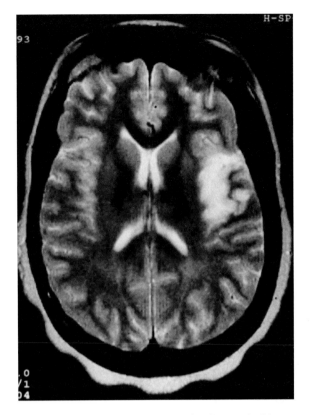

Fig. 5-6. A magnetic resonance imaging (MRI) scan of a 34-year-old patient demonstrates a stroke. This patient had laboratory evidence for protein S deficiency.

Low free protein S levels are not an uncommon finding.[52] Acquired protein S deficiency can be seen in liver disease, disseminated intravascular coagulation, pregnancy, and in patients using oral contraceptives. It has also been reported in patients with acute respiratory distress syndrome, acquired immunodeficiency syndrome, inflammatory bowel disease, warfarin therapy, nephrotic syndrome, renal failure, systemic lupus erythematosus, postmyocardial infarction, certain infections, diabetes mellitus, and in patients with anticardiolipin antibodies and malignancy.[56] In most patients with acquired protein S deficiency, the defect is not an isolated one. For example, patients receiving warfarin therapy will have low levels of protein C and S, as well as decreases in factors II, VII, IX, and X. Newborn infants are also reported to have low levels of protein S for at least the first month of life. Caution should be taken in classifying any acutely ill patient as protein S deficient. Because C4b binding protein is an acute-phase reactant, a decrease in free protein S levels can be expected in this setting because of a shift of protein S from the free to the bound form. This may help to explain why patients become hypercoagulable when acutely ill.[57]

ANTITHROMBIN III. ATIII deficiency is inherited in an autosomal dominant manner, with a reported prevalence of 1/2000 to 1/5000 in the general population. Heterozygotes have levels between 20% and 70% of normal plasma ATIII levels.[58,59] Both sexes are affected equally. ATIII is a glycoprotein synthesized in the liver and endothelial cells. It functions as a cofactor that dramatically enhances the anticoagulant properties of heparin and

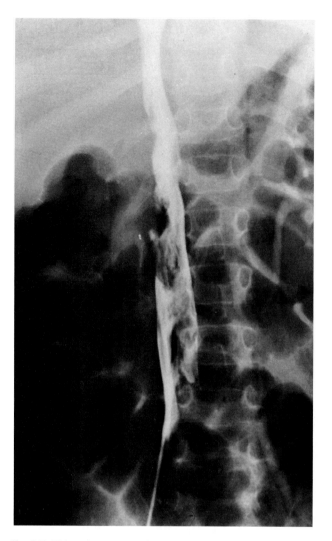

Fig. 5-7. This venacavogram demonstrates a thrombus in this patient with hereditary antithrombin III deficiency.

also exerts inhibitory activity against the serine proteases, factors IIa, IXa, Xa, XIa, and XIIa.

Many classifications for ATIII deficiency have been described. Type I, or the true deficiency, is characterized by a pure quantitative defect. Type II is a qualitative defect giving rise to normal levels of a dysfunctional protein. Type III is both a quantitative and qualitative defect. Because not all types of ATIII deficiency have a decreased antigenic level, it is best to screen for ATIII abnormalities using a functional assay, as this will detect type I, II, and III abnormalities. In ATIII deficiency most patients have their first thrombotic event during the second or third decade of life. Patients may experience deep vein thrombosis, pulmonary embolism, thrombosis at unusual sites including cerebral veins, mesenteric veins, portal or renal veins, inferior vena cava, retinal veins, and superficial thrombophlebitis (Fig. 5-7). Arterial thrombosis can also occur. Precipitating factors for thrombosis include pregnancy, surgery, the use of oral contraceptives, and trauma. Heparin resistance has been reported but is usually seen in patients with severe deficiencies. The diagnosis of ATIII deficiency can generally be excluded if the levels at the time of presentation of the acute thrombotic event are normal.

An acquired form of ATIII deficiency may be seen in patients with acute thrombosis, nephrotic syndrome, severe liver disease, disseminated intravascular coagulation, L-asparaginase therapy, or in patients using oral contraceptives. Lower ATIII levels can be seen during an acute thrombotic event or in patients receiving heparin.

HEPARIN COFACTOR II. Like ATIII, HCII is a serine protease inhibitor initially described in 1974. It is synthesized in the liver and differs from ATIII in that it inhibits only thrombin. Deficiencies of HCII are inherited in an autosomal dominant fashion. Heterozygotes have been reported in whom venous thromboembolism was seen.[59,60] However, family studies have often failed to document thrombosis in other affected family members, and the link between HCII deficiency and thrombosis has not been firmly established. Acquired HCII deficiencies may be seen in liver disease, disseminated intravascular coagulation, and preeclampsia. Unlike ATIII, HCII levels are not usually decreased during venous thrombotic events.[61]

DISORDERS OF THE FIBRINOLYTIC SYSTEM. The *fibrinolytic system* comprises the inactive zymogen plasminogen, active enzyme plasmin, plasminogen activators (both endogenous and exogenous), and plasminogen activator inhibitors. Excessive activation of the fibrinolytic system may result in bleeding, whereas decreased fibrinolytic activity may lead to thrombosis. Congenital and acquired disorders of the fibrinolytic system are well described.[62,63] Plasminogen abnormalities have been reported that include both true deficiency and dysfunctional plasminogen molecules (dysplasminogenemias). Type I plasminogen deficiencies are true deficiencies and are due to decreased synthesis of the protein. Both functional and immunologic plasminogen assays will be decreased in type I disorders. Type II plasminogen deficiencies include the dysfunctional proteins and are usually caused by a point mutation in the plasminogen molecule.[64] Laboratory studies will reveal functional activity decreased more than immunologic activity, which may be normal. In addition to hereditary deficiencies, plasminogen may be decreased in liver disease, disseminated intravascular coagulation, and during thrombolytic therapy.[65,66]

Very rare cases of congenital t-PA deficiency have been described and are not considered a major contributor to causes of the hypercoagulable state. However, abnormalities in t-PA release by endothelium may be more common and may account for a large number of cases of thrombotic tendencies. In a study of 120 patients with deep vein thrombosis and no known reason for a hypercoagulable state, 37% were poor responders to a venous occlusion test (VOT) and found to have defective t-PA release or elevated PAI-1 levels.[67,68] The VOT, like many tests of the fibrinolytic system, is cumbersome to perform and not available at all laboratories. This may be a reason why these deficiencies are not reported more often. Abnormal balance of t-PA and PAI-1 levels has been reported in survivors of myocardial infarction, patients with malignancy, in the postoperative state, in patients with liver failure, and during extracorporeal circulation.[69,70] It is unclear whether this abnormally high PAI-1 and/or defective t-PA release is a cause of thrombotic events or merely an epiphenomenon or part of the acute-phase reaction.

LIPOPROTEIN(a). Lipoprotein(a), or Lp(a), is an apolipoprotein associated with LDL. The molecular structure of Lp(a) is heterogeneous, but it is very similar to that of plasminogen in that it has multiple and variable repeats of kringle 4 and a nonfunctional protease domain.[71,72] Lp(a) may have a role in thrombotic disorders, as it can inhibit plasminogen or plasmin binding to t-PA on fibrin thrombi or endothelial cell surfaces leading to decreased fibrinolysis.[73] Elevated Lp(a) levels have been strongly associated with atherosclerosis and vascular disease and secondarily associated with thrombosis.[74]

DYSFIBRINOGENEMIA. Most disorders of fibrinogen, such as hypofibrinogenemias or many of the dysfibrinogenemias, result in a bleeding diathesis. However, several abnormal fibrinogens have been studied, where the affected kindreds display thrombotic tendencies. For full function, fibrinogen must be cleaved by thrombin, polymerized into fibrin polymers, cross-linked by factor XIIIa, allow the fibrinolytic factors to bind to it, and be degraded by plasmin. It is not surprising that a thrombotic tendency could arise if abnormal fibrinogen were either rapidly clotted by thrombin or resistant to plasmin degradation. Abnormal fibrinogens Dusard and Chapel Hill III are thrombin-clottable but cannot be degraded by plasmin.[75] They also display decreased plasminogen binding. Other types of dysfibrinogenemia associated with thrombosis have been shown to be rapidly clottable by thrombin, have increased function for platelet aggregation, or have defective binding to plasminogen or t-PA.[76] Patients with dysfibrinogenemias with thrombotic tendencies often have both arterial and venous thrombosis. Laboratory evaluation of dysfibrinogenemias will often show prolonged prothrombin time (PT) with normal or only slightly prolonged APTT, decreased clottable fibrinogen, normal or elevated immunologic fibrinogen, long thrombin time, and prolonged reptilase time. Dysfibrinogenemia can be acquired with liver disease, but the dysfunction is usually due to abnormal glycosylation and is not often associated with a thrombotic tendency.

HOMOCYSTINURIA. The genetic disease *homocystinuria,* caused by a defect and/or deficiency of cystathionine β-synthase, is inherited as an autosomal recessive trait and has been associated with vascular disease and thrombosis.[77] These patients have elevated blood levels of homocysteine, methionine and their metabolic products, with lower than normal cysteine levels. The major clinical manifestations of this disorder are dislocation of the optic lens (ectopia lentis), mental retardation, and osteoporosis. The most life-threatening clinical manifestations of homocystinuria are accelerated atherosclerosis and associated thromboembolic events in both arterial and venous systems. Stenotic vascular lesions consisting of concentric intimal proliferation, similar to changes observed in saphenous vein graft atherosclerosis, are seen diffusely in patients with homocystinuria and have been reported to involve coronary arteries, abdominal aorta and iliac arteries, as well as smaller arteries and arterioles. Arterial and venous thrombosis in coronary and cerebral circulations,

either superimposed on proliferative vascular lesions or de novo, may cause sudden death or severe morbidity.[78] An acute major vascular event is the cause of death in 70% of homocystinurics who die before the age of 30.[77]

Thrombosis and vascular disease are seen not only in homozygous homocystinurics but also in those with heterozygous cystathionine β-synthase defects and in patients with elevated homocysteine levels due to other causes. In a recent study of 185 patients with venous thrombosis, 25% were found to have elevated homocysteine levels.[79] Elevated plasma homocysteine levels, not related to nutritional vitamin B_{12} or folate deficiencies, have been observed in 17% of patients being evaluated for a hypercoagulable state in which no other causes for increased thrombosis could be found.[80] Further studies investigating the relationship of plasma homocysteine levels to premature vascular disease have found hyperhomocystinemia to be an independent risk factor for peripheral arterial occlusive disease, arteriosclerotic cerebrovascular disease, coronary artery disease, and aortoiliac disease.[81-83] The mechanism of these pathologic changes is not well understood but is thought to be caused by alteration of endothelial coagulant function by homocysteine.

Other Primary Hypercoagulable Disorders

HISTIDINE-RICH GLYCOPROTEIN. Histidine-rich glycoprotein (HRG) is a single-chain glycoprotein that may be involved in the fibrinolytic system and has been reported to be associated with thrombotic disease.[84,85] Whether this is a causal relationship remains to be established.

FACTOR XII DEFICIENCY (HAGEMAN FACTOR). Congenital factor XII deficiency has been reported to be a risk factor for the development of arterial and venous thromboembolism. It is inherited in an autosomal recessive manner and patients present with a markedly prolonged APTT in the homozygous state and a moderately prolonged APTT in the heterozygous state. Although generally regarded as a rare disorder, a recent paper suggested that the incidence is between 1.5% and 3% in the general population.[86] In other articles a high prevalence approaching 20% was noted in patients with factor XII deficiency and recurrent arterial thromboembolism and myocardial infarction.[87] In the same series an 8% prevalence was noted among patients with recurrent venous thromboembolism.[87]

Secondary Hypercoagulable States

ANTIPHOSPHOLIPID-ANTIBODY SYNDROME. The antiphospholipid-antibody syndrome is one of the most common causes of acquired or secondary hypercoagulable states. In a study of 499 healthy blood donors, the prevalence of the lupus anticoagulant was 4%, whereas anticardiolipin antibodies were noted to be 5%.[88] It is recognized clinically by thrombosis, thrombocytopenia, or fetal demise. Unlike disorders of the coagulation and fibrinolytic system mentioned earlier that predispose more to venous thrombosis, the antiphospholipid-antibody syndrome can lead to both venous and arterial thrombosis. The antiphospholipid-antibody syndrome consists of either anticardiolipin antibodies, lupus anticoagulant, or the biologic false-positive test for syphilis. Lupus anticoagulants are often identified during routine laboratory evaluation by the presence of a prolonged APTT and rarely a prolonged PT. The APTT may be normal, however, and is therefore not a reliable screening test. In patients in whom lupus anticoagulant is suspected, other tests including the dilute Russell's viper venom test, platelet neutralization procedure, tissue thromboplastin inhibition test, kaolin clotting time, or hexagonal-phase phospholipid neutralization procedure may be used to confirm the diagnosis. Most authors recommend a combination of any two of the preceding tests to confirm lupus anticoagulant.

Anticardiolipin antibodies have no activity in the clotting-based assays and therefore do not prolong the PT or APTT. They are demonstrated by the use of an enzyme-linked immunosorbent assay for the detection of immunoglobulin—IgG, IgA, or IgM—idiotypes.

Because lupus anticoagulant and anticardiolipin antibodies are different types of antibodies, some patients demonstrate both of these in their plasma, whereas others demonstrate only one of them.

Clinically patients with the antiphospholipid-antibody syndrome present with deep vein thrombosis, renal or hepatic vein thrombosis, or pulmonary embolism. Arterial events often involve the cerebral vessels and heart, presenting as transient ischemic attacks, cerebrovascular accidents, multiinfarct dementia, migraine headaches, myocardial infarction, intracardiac thrombus, cardiomyopathy, or valvular heart lesions. Cutaneous manifestations are a prominent feature as well. Livedo reticularis, thrombophlebitis, skin ulcerations, nodules, splinter hemorrhages, and gangrene are all reported (Fig. 5-8). Obstetric complications include recurrent miscarriages, intrauterine growth retardation, and deep vein thrombosis. Other reported manifestations include thrombocytopenia, chorea, pulmonary hypertension, Budd-Chiari syndrome, renal vein thrombosis, Addison's disease, and avascular necrosis.

Several recent articles have stressed the importance of the antiphospholipid-antibody syndrome in the vascular patient. Taylor et al[89] found positive antiphospholipid antibodies in 60 of 234 consecutive vascular surgery patients. These patients, more often female, were much more likely to have lower-extremity bypass failure. In their series of 1,078 patients, Shortell et al[90] found 19 patients with the antiphospholipid-antibody syndrome. They noted a failure of vascular reconstructions, an increase in upper-extremity involvement including digital ulcers and pain, severe claudication, and the blue toe syndrome. They recommended suspecting the antiphospholipid-antibody syndrome in young female nonsmokers presenting with vascular disease.[90]

More recently Asherson and Cervera[91] have attempted to classify this syndrome into primary, secondary, or catastrophic antiphospholipid-antibody syndromes. The primary antiphospholipid-antibody syndrome is seen most often. These patients do not have an underlying primary connective tissue disorder or other well-defined disease, generally have a low or negative titer antinuclear antibody, and may develop a vasculitic skin rash.[91] The secondary antiphospholipid-antibody syndrome is associated with underlying connective tissue disorders including systemic lupus erythematosus, rheumatoid arthritis, and scleroderma. It is also seen with medications including the phenothiazines, procainamide, hydralazine, quinidine, sulfonamides, and with certain infections and hematologic or malignant disorders. The catastrophic antiphospholipid-antibody syndrome is rarely seen but can be

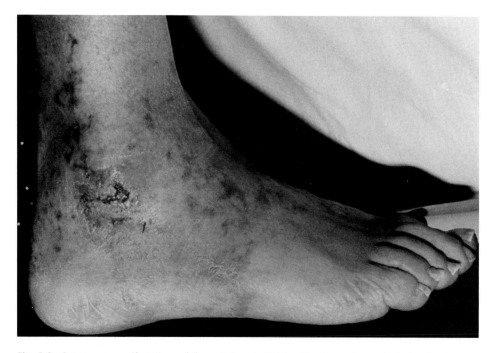

Fig. 5-8. Cutaneous manifestations of the antiphospholipid-antibody syndrome. Note the livedo reticularis and ischemic ulcerations.

devastating, generally involving multiple target organs and often resulting in death. There must be histopathologic evidence of multiple large- and small-vessel occlusions and serologic confirmation of antiphospholipid antibodies for this form to be present.[91]

HEPARIN-INDUCED THROMBOCYTOPENIA AND THROMBOSIS. Thrombocytopenia has been reported in association with heparin therapy in animals and humans since the early 1940s.[92,93] In 1958 Weismann and Tobin[94] described 10 patients with arterial and venous thromboembolic events occurring during heparin therapy, although no mention of thrombocytopenia was made. Since then, many reports have linked heparin and thrombocytopenia with thrombosis. Heparin-induced thrombocytopenia (HIT) with thrombosis, also referred to as the "white clot syndrome," is a well-known complication of therapy that can lead to myocardial infarction, stroke, arterial thrombosis with possible limb loss, or recurrent venous thromboembolic events. The incidence of HIT is reported to be between 5% and 10% of all patients receiving heparin. The incidence of thrombosis, however, occurs in less than 1% to 2%.[95-98]

There is more than one form of HIT. A mild and transient form, referred to as type I, occurs up to 3 to 4 days following initiation of heparin. The thrombocytopenia that develops seldom drops below 100,000/mm³ and it resolves despite continuing heparin. Thrombosis does not occur with this form.[99] It is thought to be an idiopathic reaction to heparin. Type II, a more severe form, typically occurs 5 to 14 days after heparin exposure and is associated with thrombosis.[100,101] Type II HIT has been shown to be caused by an antibody directed against a complex of heparin and platelet factor 4, the Fc portion of which binds to the platelet's Fc receptors, triggering platelet aggregation.[102] HIT has also been reported in patients receiving heparin flushes, on low-dose subcutaneous heparin, and with heparin-coated catheters.[103,104]

Heparin-induced thrombosis has been reported in patients with normal platelet counts and in those patients who have a decline in their platelet count but are not thrombocytopenic.[105-107] Thrombotic complications are much more frequent than the hemorrhagic manifestations of thrombocytopenia. The thrombosis occurs predominately on the arterial side of the circulation, is usually clinically distinct from the original event, may develop at multiple sites, and may continue until the heparin is discontinued. Arterial occlusions, ischemic strokes, and myocardial infarctions have all been reported. Skin necrosis, which may be at the site of subcutaneous heparin injections, has also been noted. Venous thrombotic events including pulmonary embolism, phlegmasia cerulea dolens (venous gangrene), and sagittal sinus thrombosis have also been described.[108-110]

In studies on the outcome in patients with HIT and thrombosis syndrome, deaths have been reported in 29% of patients, and limb amputation (Fig. 5-9) is reported as high as 21%.[97]

The diagnosis of HIT and thrombosis is primarily clinical. It should be suspected with any new or recurrent thromboembolic event that occurs despite adequate heparin therapy. It should also be suspected when there is

heparin resistance or an inability to maintain an adequate level of anticoagulation. Chong[101] has recommended that the diagnosis of HIT be based on these criteria: (1) occurrence of thrombocytopenia during heparin administration, (2) exclusion of other causes of thrombocytopenia, (3) resolution of thrombocytopenia when heparin is discontinued, and (4) demonstration in vitro of a heparin-dependent platelet antibody.

MALIGNANCY. Well over a century ago Trousseau recognized a relationship between malignancies and thromboembolic disorders. This syndrome, which still bears his name, is characterized by recurrent migratory superficial thrombophlebitis and arterial thrombosis.[111] The cancer is often an adenocarcinoma of the lung, pancreas, stomach, colon, gallbladder, or ovaries. The

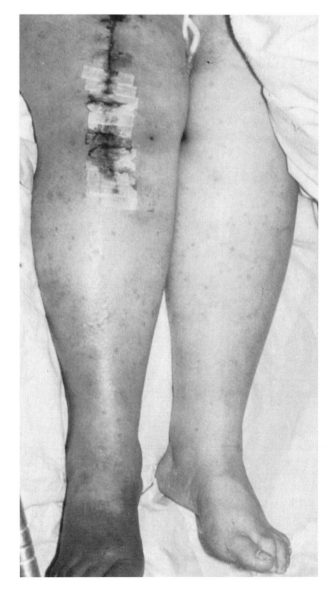

Fig. 5-9. Heparin-induced thrombocytopenia and thrombosis. This patient underwent a total knee replacement and postoperatively developed acute deep vein thrombosis. While receiving heparin, she developed an acute arterial occlusion, thrombocytopenia, and a positive heparin-associated antibody test.

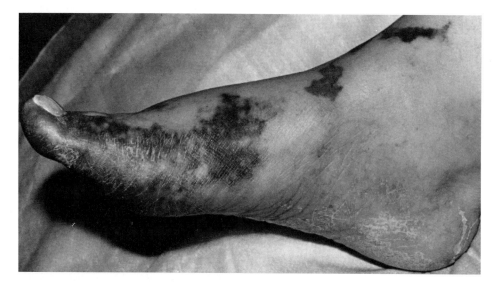

Fig. 5-10. Malignancy and thrombosis. This patient had adenocarcinoma of the lung and developed phlegmasia cerulea dolens (venous gangrene).

superficial thrombophlebitis or thromboembolic event may antedate the clinical diagnosis by months or years. Stroke, myocardial infarction, loss of an arm or leg due to arterial occlusion, and phlegmasia cerulea dolens (Fig. 5-10) may be other clinical manifestations. Patients may also present with nonbacterial thrombotic endocarditis. Bleeding is a less commonly recognized complication of this syndrome. In patients afflicted with Trousseau's syndrome, the coagulation and fibrinolytic systems are generally abnormal. The PT and APTT are usually prolonged, hypofibrinogenemia may be present, and an elevation in the D-dimer or fibrin degradation products can be expected. Microangiopathic hemolytic anemia is not uncommon, and review of the peripheral smear in this setting is an important key to the diagnosis. The etiology of thromboembolism in this syndrome remains unexplained.

Because many patients present with no identifiable precipitating factors for a venous thromboembolic event, cancer is always a concern. A thorough evaluation of all patients presenting as such can be expensive. In a recent review of 250 consecutive patients with no known cancer and a first episode of deep vein thrombosis, 7.6% were found to have a malignancy within a 2-year follow-up.[112] This compared with only 1.9% of those individuals with an identifiable precipitating factor.[112] The authors recommended a workup consisting of a complete history and physical examination, routine blood counts, chemistries, chest radiography, and erythrocyte sedimentation rate. More exhaustive testing was dependent on the initial screening. In another study by Gore et al,[113] the incidence of cancer within 2 years following the diagnosis of pulmonary embolism was 14.7%. Current recommendations for the workup of a single unexplained deep vein thrombosis should include a complete history and physical examination, complete blood cell count with a chemistry profile, screening mammography in women, prostate-specific an-

tigen in men, and testing for fecal occult blood. If the patient has a recurrent thromboembolic event, further testing including computed tomography of the chest, abdomen, and pelvis, and endoscopy and colonoscopy should be considered.

MYELOPROLIFERATIVE DISORDERS. The myeloproliferative disorders, including polycythemia vera, chronic myelogenous leukemia, essential thrombocythemia, myelofibrosis and myeloid metaplasia have all been associated with both bleeding and thrombotic problems.[114] Patients with polycythemia vera are most prone to thrombosis, although bleeding can also occur. The types of thrombosis seen include deep vein thrombosis, pulmonary embolism, cerebrovascular accidents, myocardial infarction, and peripheral arterial occlusion. These patients may have unusual thrombotic events, such as hepatic vein thrombosis (Budd-Chiari syndrome), microvascular thrombosis resulting in digital ischemia and cerebral ischemia.[114] The pathophysiology of thrombosis in the polycythemia vera patient may be due in part to the increased blood viscosity.

Thrombocytosis is often seen in the myeloproliferative disorders (Fig. 5-11). There is no clear relationship between the platelet count, however, and the degree of hemorrhage or thrombosis. Numerous studies have looked at platelet dysfunction in patients with myeloproliferative disorders.[114,115] A selective defect in epinephrine-induced platelet aggregation is often observed. Other abnormalities reported include platelet hyperaggregability, acquired storage pool disorders, abnormalities of prostaglandin D_2 receptors and Fc receptors, and defective arachidonic acid release and metabolism.[114-116] Abnormalities of tests such as epinephrine aggregation, spontaneous aggregation, circulating platelet aggregates, and the bleeding time may help to diagnose a myeloproliferative disorder, but they will not help predict whether the patient is at risk of bleeding or thrombosis.[114,115]

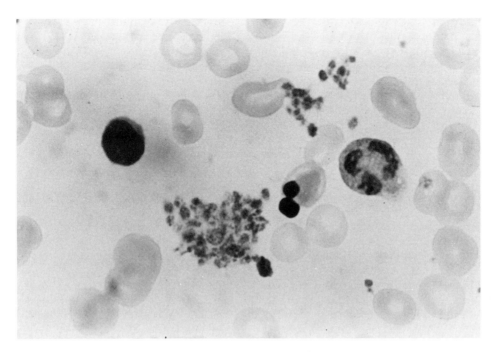

Fig. 5-11. This is a blood smear of a patient with well over a million platelets and a diagnosis of essential thrombocytosis.

DIAGNOSIS

The diagnosis of a hypercoagulable state requires a thorough history and physical examination. Particular attention should be paid to features suggesting a primary or secondary hypercoagulable state as listed in the box on p. 96.

The diagnosis of hypercoagulability relies heavily on the laboratory to aid the clinician. Routine coagulation studies should be performed including a complete blood cell count with peripheral blood smear, urinalysis, PT, APTT, fibrinogen, and chemistry profile. These studies may be more helpful in excluding secondary disorders—for example, thrombotic thrombocytopenia purpura, disseminated intravascular coagulation, abnormal hemoglobins, whereas the myeloproliferative disorders may be identified by a review of the peripheral blood smear. Thrombocytopenia may suggest paroxysmal nocturnal hemoglobinuria or HIT, whereas a prolonged APTT is suggestive of the lupus anticoagulant. More sophisticated laboratory testing is required to identify the primary disorders. These laboratory tests are not routinely available at all institutions. At our institution the hypercoagulation profile includes PT, APTT, circulating anticoagulant, fibrinogen, plasminogen, antithrombin III, proteins C and S, activated protein C resistance, dilute Russell's viper venom test, reptilase time, HCII, homocysteine, and anticardiolipin antibodies. A heparin aggregation test is ordered separately. Care should be used in interpreting results of these tests in the setting of an acute thrombotic event or in a patient receiving warfarin (Coumadin), heparin, or one of the thrombolytic agents. It cannot be assumed that the protein deficiency antedates the current thrombotic event; it may instead be a consequence of the initiating event or underlying illness. It also must not be overlooked that hypercoagulable disorders can be acquired in the setting of liver disease, nephrotic syndrome, in patients using certain medications, or in disseminated intravascular coagulation.

Limited testing may be helpful. For example, in patients with severe toxic hepatitis, nephrotic syndrome, or acute fatty liver of pregnancy, an ATIII test is recommended. In the setting of warfarin skin necrosis or purpura fulminans, protein C or S levels may be all that are necessary. With a history of unexplained arterial thrombosis, a lupus anticoagulant, anticardiolipin antibodies, or homocysteine level should be ordered. Although the hypercoagulation profile is commonly performed while the patient is hospitalized, it is best to perform it after the acute event has completely resolved and preferably once the patient is no longer receiving anticoagulation therapy. At times this will be impossible since the patient may require lifelong oral anticoagulation therapy. In this setting performing studies on immediate family members is recommended, especially when evaluation for protein C or S deficiency is desired. Another alternative is to perform certain studies including proteins C and S before oral anticoagulants are given. In addition, an ATIII level can be drawn once the patient is receiving warfarin.

An area of great laboratory interest is the development of a blood test that can identify the individual at increased risk for thrombosis, also referred to as the *prethrombotic state*. Prothrombin fragment 1+2, protein C activation peptide, fibrinopeptide A, D-dimer, thrombin-ATIII complex, and factor X activation peptide are some of the tests that have been studied. The aim of these laboratory tests is to assist the clinician in the diagnosis of venous or arterial thromboembolism, in the evaluation of high-risk individuals, and for monitoring patients at increased risk for thrombosis during exposure to stressful situations.

Plasma D-dimer has been used in a number of studies to diagnose venous thromboembolism. Goldhaber et al[117] analyzed D-dimer levels in 173 patients who underwent pulmonary angiography for suspected pulmonary embolism. Only 3 of 35 persons with abnormal angiograms had D-dimer levels under 500 ng/ml, and they concluded that a low D-dimer level may be helpful in excluding the diagnosis of pulmonary embolism. Yudelman et al[118] noted 89% of symptomatic patients with a positive lung scan or venogram had elevated levels of fibrinopeptide A. Bauer and Rosenberg[119,120] found that elevated levels of prothrombin fragment 1+2 and fibrinopeptide A were found in many individuals not receiving anticoagulation therapy who had congenital deficiencies of ATIII or protein C. Manucci et al,[121] however, found that only about one fourth of their patients with inherited syndromes had elevated levels of these two tests. Many of these sensitive markers for coagulation activation are difficult to obtain on a routine basis as results are extraordinarily sensitive to venipuncture technique and sample handling. It is not yet clear that the use of these markers can reliably document a prethrombotic state or predict a thrombotic event. The currently available tests may be able to indicate the presence of coagulation activation but are unable to indicate the cause of the thrombotic process. Further refinement is needed. However, these tests, or newer ones yet to be developed, may provide an important role in the diagnosis and treatment of hypercoagulable states.

TREATMENT

Once a primary disorder is found, lifelong anticoagulation therapy may be warranted if the patient has had an unexplained thrombotic event. If the setting of thrombosis occurs with identifiable risk factors present, treatment should be individualized. Family members should be tested as these individuals are more likely to suffer a thrombotic event in the setting of pregnancy, surgery, or trauma. By carefully identifying these patients and their family members at risk, appropriate prophylaxis and treatment will help to eliminate potentiating life-threatening thromboembolic disorders. In addition, the history of thromboembolism in other afflicted family members may give one a sense of how severely the family is affected. Commercial products for ATIII deficiency in the form of a concentrate are now available, and protein C and S concentrates may be available in the near future.

Pregnancy poses a special problem. Most agree that if an individual with a hereditary deficiency has had a thrombotic event during a previous pregnancy, anticoagulation therapy is necessary during the next pregnancy. In addition, anticoagulation therapy is probably indicated throughout the pregnancy in those individuals with a known hereditary deficiency but without a previous thrombotic episode. This may be more valid in persons with ATIII deficiency as opposed to those with protein C or

S deficiency. Warfarin is contraindicated, and heparin should be used in this setting.

Little information is available regarding therapy in asymptomatic individuals with a hereditary protein deficiency and no history of thrombotic events. In a study of 67 members of the ATIII Hamilton family, only 6 of 31 family members (19.4%) with true protein deficiency had one or more thrombotic events.[122] In five of these six subjects, the initial episode occurred in association with well-known established risk factors for thrombosis including recent surgery, pregnancy, the postpartum state, trauma, and the use of oral contraceptives. No nondeficient family member had a thrombotic event. Demers et al[122] concluded that lifelong anticoagulation therapy was not warranted in asymptomatic carriers, but that prophylaxis should be instituted in those afflicted individuals during periods of high risk for thrombosis. In a review of mortality in hereditary ATIII deficiency covering 171 individuals from 1830 to 1989, Rosendaal et al[123] concluded that lifelong treatment in symptom-free ATIII-deficient individuals was unlikely to improve survival. They also noted that there was no excess mortality in women aged 20 to 40 years, the time at which there is risk of thrombosis during pregnancy or the postpartum state.[123]

In the secondary disorders there is the potential to decrease the thrombotic tendency by treating or limiting the underlying inciting factors. For example, phlebotomy in patients with polycythemia vera or the use of chemotherapy in patients with essential thrombocythemia may help reduce the incidence of thrombosis. Monitoring platelet counts in persons receiving heparin and discontinuing this medication as soon as possible will help eliminate HIT and thrombosis syndrome. Cautious initiation of warfarin in individuals suspected of protein C or S deficiency, and overlapping this medication with heparin, may help reduce warfarin skin necrosis.

In the antiphospholipid-antibody syndrome, maintaining the international normalized ratio at or above 3 may be advisable.[124,125] The addition of low-dose aspirin (75 mg/day) is also more effective in preventing recurrence of thrombosis.[125]

Prophylaxis should be given to all patients with known primary and secondary hypercoagulable disorders on entering the hospital. Numerous agents are now available to help prevent thrombosis including low-molecular-weight heparin, unfractionated heparin, and warfarin, in addition to ambulation and the use of intermittent compression stockings.

In summary, patients and family members must be considered individually regarding treatment with either short-term or lifelong anticoagulation therapy. This decision must be based on the events leading to the thrombosis, the individual's compliance, the ability to monitor treatment, and the risk of hemorrhage and other complications from anticoagulation therapy.

REFERENCES

1. Morawitz P: Die chemie der blutgerinnung, Ergeb Physiol 4:207, 1905.

2. Macfarlane RG: An enzyme cascade in the blood clotting mechanism, and its function as a biochemical amplifier, Nature 202:498, 1964.
3. Davies EW and Ratnoff OD: Waterfall sequence for intrinsic blood clotting, Science 145:1310, 1964.
4. Rapaport SI and Rao LVM: Initiation and regulation of tissue factor-dependent blood coagulation, Arterioscler Throm 12:1111, 1992.
5. Seegers WH, Johnson JF, and Fall C: An antithrombin reaction related to prothrombin activation, Am J Physiol 176:97, 1954.
6. Egeberg O: Inherited antithrombin deficiency causing thrombophilia, Thromb Diath Haemorrh 13:516, 1965.
7. Mammen EF, Thomas WR, and Seegers WH: Activation of purified prothrombin to auto-prothrombin II (platelet cofactor II) or autoprothrombin II-A, Thromb Diath Haemorrh 5:218, 1960.
8. Stenflo J: A new vitamin K dependent protein: purification from bovine plasma and preliminary characterization, J Biol Chem 251:355, 1976.
9. Griffin JH, Evatt B, and Zimmerman TS: Deficiency of protein C in congenital thrombotic disease, J Clin Invest 68:1370, 1981.
10. Dahlback B, Carlsson M, and Svensson PJ: Familial thrombophilia due to a previously unrecognized mechanism characterized by poor anticoagulant response to activated protein C: prediction of a cofactor to activated protein C, Proc Natl Acad Sci USA 90:1004, 1993.
11. Saito H: Normal hemostatic mechanisms. In Ratnoff OD and Forbes CD, eds.: Disorders of hemostasis, ed 2, Philadelphia, 1991, WB Saunders.
12. Brenner BM, Troy JL, and Ballermann BJ: Endothelium-dependent vascular responses: mediators and mechanisms, J Clin Invest 84:1373, 1989.
13. Yanagisawa M et al: A novel potent vasoconstrictor peptide produced by vascular endothelial cells, Nature 332:411, 1988.
14. Jaffe EA: Cell biology of endothelial cells, Hum Pathol 18:234, 1987.
15. Esmon NL and Esmon CT: Protein C and the endothelium, Semin Thromb Hemost 14:210, 1988.
16. Bevilacqua MP et al: Interleukin-1 (IL-1) activation of vascular endothelium: effects on procoagulant activity and leukocyte adhesion, Am J Pathol 121:394, 1985.
17. Nawroth PP and Stern DM: Modulation of endothelial cell hemostatic properties by tumor necrosis factor, J Exp Med 163:740, 1986.
18. Holt JC and Niewiarowski S: Biochemistry of (alpha) granule proteins, Semin Hematol 22:151, 1985.
19. Kieffer N and Phillips DR: Platelet membrane glycoproteins: functions in cellular interaction, Annu Rev Cell Biol 6:329, 1990.
20. Walsh PN: Platelet-coagulant protein interaction. In Colman RW et al, eds.: Hemostasis and thrombosis: basic principles and clinical practice, ed 3, Philadelphia, 1994, JB Lippincott.
21. Mann KG, Krishnaswamy S, and Lawson JH: Surface-dependent hemostasis, Semin Hematol 29:213, 1992.
22. Nemerson Y: The tissue factor pathway of blood coagulation, Semin Hematol 29:170, 1992.
23. Gailani D and Broze GJ: Factor XI activation in a revised model of blood coagulation, Science 253:909, 1991.
24. Broze GJ: The role of tissue factor pathway inhibitor in a revised coagulation cascade, Semin Hematol 29:159, 1992.
25. Walz DA et al: Proteolytic specificity of thrombin, Thromb Res 4:713, 1974.
26. Rosenberg RB and Rosenberg JS: Natural anticoagulant mechanisms, J Clin Invest 74:1, 1984.
27. Esmon CT: The protein C anticoagulant pathway, Arterioscler Thromb 12:135, 1992.
28. Esmon CT: Molecular events that control the protein C anticoagulant pathway, Thromb Haemost 70:29, 1993.
29. Francis CW and Marder VJ: Physiologic regulation and pathologic disorders of fibrinolysis, Hum Pathol 18:263, 1987.
30. Hajjar KA and Nachman RL: Endothelial cell-mediated conversion of glu-plasminogen to lys-plasminogen. Further evidence for assembly of the fibrinolytic system on the endothelial surface, J Clin Invest 82:1769, 1988.
31. Jorgenson M and Bonnevie-Niesen V: Increased concentration of fast-acting plasminogen activator in plasma associated with familial venous thrombosis, Br J Haematol 65:175, 1987.
32. Engesser L et al: Elevated plasminogen activator inhibitor (PAI), a cause of thrombophilia? Thromb Haemost 62:673, 1989.
33. Heijboer H, Brandjes DP, and Buller HR: Deficiencies of coagulation-inhibiting and fibrinolytic proteins in outpatients with deep-vein thrombosis, N Engl J Med 323:1512, 1990.
34. Malm J et al: Thromboembolic disease—critical evaluation of laboratory investigation, Thromb Haemost 68:7 1992.
35. Pabringer I et al: Hereditary deficiencies of antithrombin III, protein C and protein S: Prevalence in patients with a history of venous thrombosis and criteria for rational patient screening, Blood Coag Fibrinolysis 3:547, 1992.
36. Bauer KA: Pathobiology of the hypercoagulable state: clinical features, laboratory evaluation and management. In: Hoffman R et al, eds.: Hematology: basic principles and clinical practice, New York, 1991, Churchill Livingstone.
37. Griffin JH et al: Anticoagulant protein C pathway defective in majority of thrombophilic patients, Blood 82:1989, 1993.
38. Schafer AI: The hypercoagulable states, Ann Intern Med 102:814, 1985.
39. Andrew M et al: Development of the human coagulation system in the full term infant, Blood 79:165, 1987.
40. Andrew M et al: Maturation of the hemostatic system during childhood, Blood 80:1998, 1992.
41. Cole MS, Minifee PK, and Wolma FJ: Coumarin necrosis—a review of the literature, Surgery 103:271, 1988.
42. Rick ME: Protein C and protein S, JAMA 263:701, 1990.
43. Svensson PJ and Dahlback D: Resistance to activated protein C as a basis for venous thrombosis, N Engl J Med 330:517, 1994.
44. Koster T et al: Venous thrombosis due to poor anticoagulant response to activated protein C: Leiden thrombophilia study, Lancet 342:1503, 1993.
45. Bauer KA: Hypercoagulability: A new cofactor in the protein C anticoagulant pathway, N Engl J Med 330:566, 1994.
46. Gallus AS, Hirsh J, and Gent M: Relevance of preoperative and postoperative blood tests to postoperative leg-vein thrombosis, Lancet 2:805, 1973.
47. Bertina RM et al: Mutation in blood coagulation factor V associated with resistance to activated protein C, Nature 369:64, 1994.
48. DiScipio RG et al: A comparison of human prothrombin, factor IX, factor X and protein S, Biochemistry 16:698, 1977.
49. Walker FJ: Regulation of activated protein C by a new protein, J Biol Chem 255:5521, 1980.

50. Comp PC et al: Familial protein S deficiency is associated with recurrent thrombosis, J Clin Invest 74:2082, 1984.
51. Sacco RL et al: Free protein S deficiency: a possible association with cerebrovascular occlusion, Stroke 20:1657, 1989.
52. Mayer SA, Sacco RL, and Hurlet-Jensen A: Free protein S deficiency in acute ischemic stroke, Stroke 24:224, 1993.
53. Allaart CF, Aronson DC, and Ruys TH: Hereditary protein S deficiency in young adults with arterial occlusive disease, Thromb Haemost 64:206, 1990.
54. Engesser L et al: Hereditary protein S deficiency: clinical manifestations, Ann Intern Med 106:677, 1987.
55. Comp PC et al: An abnormal plasma distribution of protein S occurs in functional protein S deficiency, Blood 67:504, 1985.
56. Forastiero RR et al: Differences in protein S and C4b-binding protein levels in different groups of patients with antiphospholipid antibodies, Blood Coagul Fibrinolysis 5:609, 1994.
57. D'Angelo A, Vigano-D'Angelo S, and Esmon CT: Acquired deficiencies of protein S, J Clin Invest 81:1445, 1988.
58. Nachman RL and Silverstein R: Hypercoagulable states, Ann Intern Med 119:819, 1993.
59. Tollefsen DM: Laboratory diagnosis of antithrombin III and heparin cofactor II deficiency, Semin Thromb Hemost 16:162, 1990.
60. Sie P et al: Constitutional heparin cofactor II deficiency associated with recurrent thrombosis, Lancet 2:414, 1984.
61. Toulon P, Vitoux JF, and Capron L: Heparin cofactor II in patients with deep venous thrombosis under heparin and oral anticoagulant therapy, Thromb Res 49:479, 1988.
62. Aoki N et al: Abnormal plasminogen. A hereditary molecular abnormality found in a patient with recurrent thrombosis, J Clin Invest 61:1186, 1978.
63. Hach-Wunderle V et al: Congenital deficiency of plasminogen and its relationship to venous thrombosis, Thromb Haemost 59:277, 1988.
64. Ichinose A et al: Two types of abnormal genes for plasminogen in families with a predisposition for thrombosis, Proc Natl Acad Sci USA 88:115, 1991.
65. Bick RL and Ucar K: Hypercoagulability and thrombosis, Hematol Oncol Clin North Am 6:1421, 1992.
66. McGann MA and Triplett DA: Laboratory evaluation of the fibrinolytic system, Lab Med 14:18, 1983.
67. Juhan VI, Valadier J, and Alessi MC: Deficient t-PA release and elevated PA inhibitor levels in patients with spontaneous or recurrent deep vein thrombosis, Thromb Haemost 57:67, 1987.
68. Petaja J: Fibrinolytic response to venous occlusion for 10 and 20 minutes in healthy subjects and in patients with deep vein thrombosis, Thromb Res 56:251, 1989.
69. Hamsten A et al: Increased plasma levels of a rapid inhibitor of tissue plasminogen activator in young survivors of myocardial infarction, New Engl J Med 313:1557, 1985.
70. Kruithof EKO, Gudinchet A, and Bachmann F: Plasminogen activator inhibitor 1 and plasminogen activator inhibitor 2 in various disease states, Thromb Haemost 59:7, 1988.
71. MBewu AD and Durrington PN: Lipoprotein(a): structure, properties and possible involvement in thrombogenesis and atherogenesis, Atherosclerosis 85:1, 1990.
72. Miles LA and Plow EF: Lp(a)A: an interloper into the fibrinolytic system, Thromb Haemost 63:331, 1990.
73. Hajjar KA et al: Lipoprotein(a) modulation of endothelial cell surface fibrinolysis and its potential role in atherosclerosis, Nature 339:303, 1989.
74. Genest J Jr et al: Prevalence of lipoprotein(a) (Lp(a)) excess in coronary artery disease, Am J Cardiol 67:1039, 1991.
75. Carrell N et al: Hereditary dysfibrinogenemia in a patient with thrombotic disease, Blood 62:439, 1983.
76. McDonagh J, Carrell N, and Lee MH: Dysfibrinogenemia and other disorders of fibrinogen structure and function. In Colman RW et al, eds.: Hemostasis and thrombosis: basic principles and clinical practices, ed 3, Philadelphia, 1994, JB Lippincott.
77. Mudd S, Levy HL, and Skovby F: Disorders of transsulfuration. In Scriver CR et al, eds.: The metabolic basis of inherited disease, ed 6, New York, 1989, McGraw-Hill.
78. Zimmerman R et al: Vascular thromboses and homocystinuria, AJR Am J Roentgenol 148:953, 1987.
79. denHeyer M et al: Is hyperhomocysteinaemia a risk factor for recurrent venous thrombosis? Lancet 354:882, 1995.
80. Kottke-Marchant K, Jacobsen D, and Green R: Elevated homocysteine levels in patients evaluated for a hypercoagulable state, Blood 78(suppl):214a, 1991.
81. Brattstrom L, Israelsson L, and Hultberg B: Plasma homocysteine and methionine tolerance in early-onset vascular disease, Haemostasis 19(suppl 1):35, 1989.
82. Brattstrom LE, Hardebo JE, and Hultberg BL: Moderate homocysteinemia—a possible risk factor for arteriosclerotic cerebrovascular disease, Stroke 15:1012, 1984.
83. Malinow MR et al: Prevalence of hyperhomocysteinemia in patients with peripheral arterial occlusive disease, Circulation 79:1180, 1989.
84. Engesser L et al: Familial elevation of plasma histidine-rich glycoprotein in a family with thrombophilia, Br J Haematol 67:355, 1987.
85. Shigekiyo T, Ohshima T, and Oka H: Congenital histidine rich glycoprotein deficiency, Thromb Haemost 70:2, 1993.
86. Halbmayer W-M et al: The prevalence of factor XII deficiency in 103 orally anticoagulated outpatients suffering from recurrent venous and/or arterial thromboembolism, Thromb Haemost 68:285, 1992.
87. Mannhalter C et al: Factor XII activity and antigen concentration in patients suffering from recurrent thrombosis, Fibrinolysis 1:259, 1987.
88. Shi W et al: Prevalence of lupus anticoagulant and anticardiolipin antibodies in a healthy population, Aust NZJ Med 20:231, 1990.
89. Taylor LM, Chitwood RW, and Dalman RL: Antiphospholipid antibodies in vascular surgery patients, Ann Surg 220:544, 1994.
90. Shortell CK, Ouriel K, and Green RM: Vascular disease in the antiphospholipid syndrome. A comparison with the patient population with atherosclerosis, J Vasc Surg 15:158, 1992.
91. Asherson RA and Cervera R: Antiphospholipid syndrome, J Invest Dermatol 100:21S, 1993.
92. Fidlar E and Jaques LB: The effect of commercial heparin on the platelet count, J Lab Clin Med 33:1410, 1948.
93. Copley AL and Robb TP: Studies on platelets: effect of heparin in vivo on platelet count in mice and dogs, Am J Clin Pathol 12:563, 1942.
94. Weismann RE and Tobin RW: Arterial embolism occurring during systemic heparin therapy, Arch Surg 76:219, 1958.
95. Ansell JE et al: Heparin-induced thrombocytopenia. What is its real frequency? Chest 88:878, 1985.
96. Bell WR and Royall RM: Heparin-associated thrombocytopenia: a comparison of three heparin preparations, N Engl J Med 303:902, 1980.
97. King DJ and Kelton JG: Heparin-associated thrombocytopenia, Ann Intern Med 100:535, 1984.
98. Becker PS and Miller VT: Heparin-induced thrombocytopenia, Stroke 20:1449, 1989.
99. Miller ML: Heparin-induced thrombocytopenia, Cleve Clin J Med 56:483, 1989.

100. Bell WR: Heparin-associated thrombocytopenia and thrombosis, J Lab Clin Med 111:600, 1988.
101. Chong BH: Heparin-induced thrombocytopenia, Aust NZJ Med 22:145, 1992.
102. Kelton JG et al: Heparin-induced thrombocytopenia: laboratory studies, Blood 72:925, 1988.
103. Johnson RA, Lazarus KH, and Henry DH: Heparin-induced thrombocytopenia. A prospective study, Am J Hematol 17:349, 1984.
104. Laster J and Silver D: Heparin-coated catheters and heparin-induced thrombocytopenia, J Vasc Surg 7:667, 1988.
105. Phelan BK: Heparin associated thrombosis without thrombocytopenia, Ann Intern Med, 99:637, 1983.
106. Lassepas MR et al: Heparin-induced thrombocytopenia in patients with cerebrovascular ischemic disease, Neurology 34:736, 1984.
107. Trono DP et al: Thrombocytopenia and heparin-associated thrombosis, Ann Intern Med 100:464, 1984.
108. Stanton PE et al: White clot syndrome, South Med J 81:616, 1988.
109. Sobel M, Adelman B, and Szentpetery S: Surgical management of heparin-associated thrombocytopenia, J Vasc Surg 8:395, 1988.
110. Warkentin TE and Kelton JG: Heparin and platelets, Hematol Oncol Clin North Am 4:243, 1990.
111. Sack GH, Levin J, and Bell WR: Trousseau's syndrome and other manifestations of chronic disseminated coagulopathy in patients with neoplasms: clinical pathophysiologic, and therapeutic features, Medicine 56:1, 1977.
112. Prandoni P et al: Deep-vein thrombosis and the incidence of subsequent symptomatic cancer, N Engl J Med 327:1128, 1992.
113. Gore JM et al: Occult cancer in patients with acute pulmonary embolism, Ann Intern Med 96:556, 1982.
114. Schafer AI: Bleeding and thrombosis in the myeloproliferative disorders, Blood 64:1, 1984.
115. Balduini CL et al: Platelet aggregation in platelet-rich plasma and whole blood in 120 patients with myeloproliferative disorders, Am J Clin Pathol 95:82, 1991.
116. Wehmeier A et al: Circulating activated platelets in myeloproliferative disorders, Thromb Res 61:271, 1991.
117. Goldhaber SZ et al: Quantitative plasma D-dimer levels among patients undergoing pulmonary angiography for suspected pulmonary embolism, JAMA 23:2819, 1993.
118. Yudelman IM, Nossel HL, and Kaplan KL: Plasma fibrinopeptide A levels in symptomatic venous thromboembolism, Blood 51:1189, 1978.
119. Bauer KA and Rosenberg RD: The pathophysiology of the prethrombotic state in humans, Blood 70:343, 1987.
120. Bauer KA: Laboratory markers of coagulation activation, Arch Pathol Lab Med 117:71, 1993.
121. Mannucci PM et al: Markers of procoagulant imbalance in patients with inherited thrombophilic syndromes, Thromb Haemost 67:200, 1992.
122. Demers C et al: Thrombosis in antithrombin-III deficient persons, Ann Intern Med 116:754, 1992.
123. Rosendaal FR et al: Mortality in hereditary antithrombin-III deficiency, Lancet 337:260, 1991.
124. Rosove MH, Petronella MC, and Brewer RN: Antiphospholipid thrombosis: clinical course after the first thrombotic event in 70 patients, Ann Intern Med 117:303, 1992.
125. Khamashta MA et al: The management of thrombosis in the antiphospholipid-antibody syndrome, N Engl J Med 332:993, 1995.

ANTICOAGULANTS AND ANTITHROMBOTIC AGENTS

K a n d i c e   K o t t k e - M a r c h a n t
J o h n   R .   B a r t h o l o m e w

A number of new drugs have been introduced during the past decade as anticoagulants and antithrombotic agents for the treatment of vascular disease. Although most of these agents remain investigational, low-molecular-weight heparin (enoxaparin) and ticlopidine (Ticlid) have been approved by the Food and Drug Administration (FDA) for the prevention of venous thrombosis and stroke. In addition, many of these new agents have been used for the compassionate treatment of heparin-induced thrombocytopenia and thrombosis. Others have been under investigation as adjunctive therapy in the prevention of restenosis following coronary angioplasty and stent placement and in the treatment of acute deep venous thrombosis, unstable angina, and ischemic stroke.

A number of changes have also occurred in the dosing and monitoring of the standard anticoagulants heparin and warfarin. The international normalized ratio (INR) is the method now recommended to monitor warfarin therapy, and a number of nomograms have been proposed to aid in the dosage of heparin. This decade promises to continue to be exciting for the physician treating vascular diseases with these newer agents, many of which are discussed in this chapter.

WARFARIN (COUMADIN)

The most common oral anticoagulants are derivatives of 4-hydroxycoumulants that inhibit hepatic vitamin K epoxide reductase and thus interfere with the posttranslational modification of the vitamin-K–dependent coagulation factors (II, VII, IX, X, protein C, and protein S). The most common 4-hydroxycoumarin anticoagulant used in the United States is warfarin (Coumadin). Warfarin stands for Wisconsin Alumni Research Foundation, the patent holder. The major indications for warfarin therapy are for long-term prophylaxis and treatment of thrombosis, especially deep vein thrombosis, pulmonary embolism, stroke, problems with mechanical heart valves, and atrial fibrillation. For the vitamin K–dependent coagulation factors to be fully functional, they must undergo conversion of glutamic acid residues to γ-carboxyglutamyl residues by the vitamin K carboxylase/epoxidase enzyme (Fig. 6-1, A). These additional carboxyl groups allow the factors to interact with both calcium and phospholipids. Vitamin K is a cofactor for the carboxylase enzyme and is converted from the hydroquinone form to the epoxide form. The epoxide form is then recycled to the hydroquinone form by vitamin K epoxide reductase and vitamin K reductase. Warfarin is an inhibitor of both of these enzymes and exerts its anticoagulant effect by trapping vitamin K in the nonactive epoxide form, thus leading to a decrease in the formation of γ-carboxyglutamyl residues on the vitamin K–dependent factors and a decrease in their function[1] (Fig. 6-1, A). Because warfarin interferes with protein synthesis, it is not a direct anticoagulant, and full anticoagulant effect takes several days to develop.

The prothrombin time (PT), one of the most commonly performed coagulation tests, measures the function of factor VII and the common pathway factors X, V, II, and fibrinogen. The PT has been widely used to monitor anticoagulant therapy with warfarin, as it is sensitive to the deficiency of three of the four vitamin K–dependent coagulation factors (VII, X, and II). The PT is performed using many different instruments and thromboplastin reagents (e.g., crude extracts of rabbit brain, human brain), and results of the PT may vary considerably from laboratory to laboratory. The variability is in large part due to the differing sensitivity of the types of thromboplastin to the levels of the vitamin K–dependent coagulation factors.[2] This variability makes it very difficult to monitor oral

Mechanism of Warfarin Anticoagulation

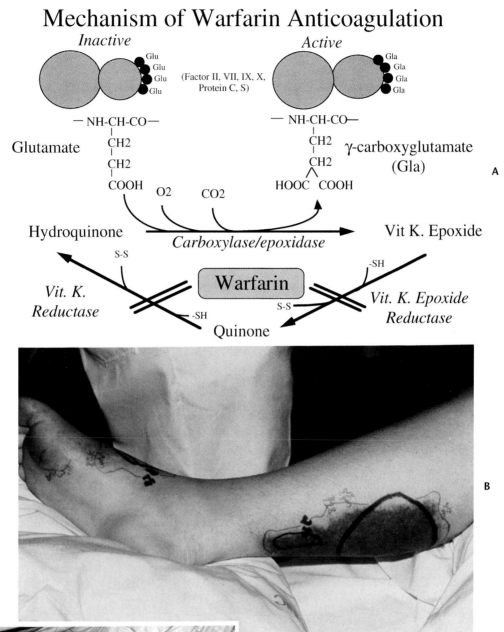

Inactive

Glu
Glu
Glu
Glu

(Factor II, VII, IX, X,
Protein C, S)

Active

Gla
Gla
Gla
Gla

A

Glutamate

— NH-CH-CO—
CH2
CH2
COOH

O_2 CO_2

— NH-CH-CO—
CH2
CH2
HOOC COOH

γ-carboxyglutamate
(Gla)

Hydroquinone

S-S

Carboxylase/epoxidase

Vit K. Epoxide

*Vit. K.
Reductase*

-SH

Warfarin

S-S

-SH

*Vit. K. Epoxide
Reductase*

Quinone

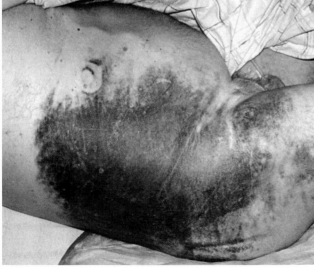

B

C

Fig. 6-1. A, Vitamin K is a cofactor for the vitamin K carboxylase/epoxidase enzyme in the formation of γ-carboxyglutamyl (Gla) residues in the vitamin K–dependent proteins (factors II, VII, IX, X, proteins C and S). This enzyme catalyzes the carboxylation of glutamic acid residues to Gla residues, usually clustered in a single domain of the proteins. Only proteins with Gla residues have coagulant activity. In the carboxylase/epoxidase reaction, vitamin K is changed from the hydroquinone to epoxide form. To regain cofactor activity, the vitamin K epoxide must be recycled to the hydroquinone form by the vitamin K epoxide reductase and vitamin K reductase enzymes. Warfarin's action as an anticoagulant stems from its inhibition of the two vitamin K recycling enzymes, thus preventing the reformation of vitamin K hydroquinone. **B,** Warfarin skin necrosis. This patient was treated for an acute deep vein thrombosis. She developed cutaneous purpura and soft tissue necrosis while receiving warfarin therapy. **C,** Hemorrhage while receiving heparin therapy. This patient was receiving a standard intravenous dose of heparin with the APTT measured within the standard range. The patient was elderly and had anemia and mild liver disease—all reported to increase the risk for bleeding.

anticoagulant therapy in patients who may have their PT monitored by different laboratories and also may lead to overanticoagulation in patients who are monitored using insensitive PT reagents.

The importance of the variability in the sensitivity of PT reagents to levels of vitamin K–dependent coagulation factors was highlighted by studies in the early 1980s that found that the dosage of warfarin was higher in the United States than in Europe, where the more sensitive human brain thromboplastin was used, and that there was a higher incidence of anticoagulant-related bleeding complications in the United States.[3] To address this problem, the INR—a method of standardizing the PT—was adopted by the World Health Organization (WHO).[1] The formula for the calculation of the INR is as follows:

$$INR = (PT_{patient}/PT_{normal})^{ISI} = (PT\ ratio)^{ISI}$$

The international sensitivity index (ISI) is a mathematic comparison of a particular thromboplastin to the primary WHO standard (assigned an ISI of 1.0).[1] Reagents with a low ISI have a greater sensitivity to deficiencies of extrinsic and common pathway factors. Each thromboplastin reagent is calibrated against the WHO primary thromboplastin standard, allowing the sensitivity of various thromboplastins to be determined relative to one another.[1,4] The use of the INR in PT testing allows for reporting of a standardized PT, so that the level of anticoagulation can be followed accurately.[5]

Although useful for standardizing PT testing, significant problems still exist with the INR. Lack of widespread reporting of the INR has been a problem, but a recent College of American Pathologists survey found that 91.8% of laboratories are now reporting the INR in one form or another.[6] The most common reporting format is to report both PT (in seconds) and INR. Additionally, due to the exponential dependence of the INR on the ISI, there is still a variability in the INR with reagents that vary widely in their ISI.[7] In the United States the most commonly used reagents have an ISI of approximately 2.7 but vary from 1 to 3. New reagents based on recombinant tissue factor show promise in terms of low ISI, standardization, lack of lot-to-lot variability, and sensitivity.[8,9] The recommended ranges for the INR during Coumadin therapy, as established by the National Heart, Lung, and Blood Institute are listed in Table 6-1.

A number of advantages are associated with the use of the INR for monitoring oral anticoagulant therapy. The INR allows physicians to make a direct comparison between PT results irrespective of the reagent sensitivities or site of test performance. Widespread implementation of the INR would enable physicians to more safely use PT information from different laboratories and to avoid overanticoagulation.[10] Standardization of the PT would result in the development of better treatment regimens by allowing research centers in this country and abroad to compare their data in a sound scientific fashion.

One of the major attractions of warfarin is that it can be administered both orally as well as intravenously. Current recommendations are to initiate treatment with a dose of between 5 and 10 mg on the first and second days, followed by adjusted doses dependent on the individual patient's

Table 6-1. Recommended INR Ranges

Situation	INR
Prevention of venous thrombosis	2-3
Treatment of venous thrombosis	2-3
Treatment of PE, TIA, A Fib	2-3
Prevention of recurrent DVT	2-3
Treatment post-MI	
Prevention of stroke	2-3
Reduced recurrence/mortality	3-4.5
Prevention of embolism	
Mechanical heart valves	2.5-3.5
Tissue heart valves	2-3

(From Hirsh et al: Oral anticoagulants: mechanism of action, clinical effectiveness, and optimal therapeutic range, Chest 102:312S, 1992.)
PE, Pulmonary embolism; *TIA,* transient ischemic attack; *A Fib,* atrial fibrillation; *MI,* myocardial infarction; *DVT,* deep vein thrombosis.

INR. For most acute thrombotic events, heparin should overlap with warfarin for 4 to 5 days. This is to ensure depletion of all the vitamin K–dependent factors. Occasionally one will observe an apparent "therapeutic" INR earlier in the course of treatment. This actually reflects rapid depletion of factor VII activity before the other vitamin K–dependent factors are consumed. Such patients are still not adequately anticoagulated until the levels of the remainder of the vitamin K–dependent factors are decreased.

A number of factors influence the dosage of warfarin. A genetically determined hereditary (autosomal dominant) resistance to the anticoagulant effects of warfarin has been reported.[11] Disorders that interfere with the availability, absorption, or utilization of vitamin K such as malnutrition, gastrointestinal disorders, sprue, cystic fibrosis, antibiotics that alter intestinal bacterial flora, biliary obstruction, or liver disease all increase the sensitivity to warfarin. Hypermetabolic states, excessive intake of alcohol, and congestive heart failure may also increase susceptibility to this anticoagulant. Concomitant administration of many other drugs may either potentiate or decrease the patient's response to warfarin. A partial list of these drugs is presented in the box on p. 111. The PT of patients receiving oral anticoagulants and any of these drugs must be monitored frequently. The simultaneous administration of other drugs may necessitate frequent alterations in the dose of the anticoagulant, either to maintain therapeutic effectiveness or to prevent potential bleeding disasters. The most common untoward reaction to warfarin is hemorrhage. The risk of major bleeding has been reported to vary from 0% to 19% of patients.[12] Risk factors that have predicted major bleeding in outpatients receiving warfarin include age over 65 years, history of stroke or gastrointestinal bleeding, a serious comorbid condition (myocardial infarction, renal insufficiency, liver disease, severe anemia), and atrial fibrillation.[12] Others have suggested that an increased risk for bleeding occurs with an elevated INR (greater than 4.5), during the first 3 months of warfarin therapy, and with an unstable INR due to medication

SOME DRUGS THAT AFFECT THE RESPONSE TO COUMARIN-INDANEDIONE ANTICOAGULANTS

Drugs that may potentiate anticoagulant effects
Pyrazolane compounds
- Phenylbutazone (Butazolidin)
- Oxyphenbutazone (Tandearil)

Antihyperlipidemic agents
- Clofibrate (Atromid-S)
- Dextrothyroxine (Choloxin)

Anabolic steroids
- Methandrostenolene (Dianabol)
- Norethandrolone (Nilevar)
- Oxymetholone (Adroyd)
- Nandrolone decanoate (Deca-Durabolin)

Muscle relaxants
- Phenyramidol (Analexin)

Salicylates—in large doses

Quinine, quinidine, cimetidine, amiodarone

Sulfonamides and antibiotics (moxalactam)

Disulfiram (Antabuse), mineral oil, glucagon

Drugs that may decrease anticoagulant effects
Sedatives and hypnotics
- Barbiturates
- Glutethimide (Doriden)
- Ethchlorvynol (Placidyl)

Griseofulvin (Fulvicin, Grifulvin, Grisactin)

Rifampin (Rimactane)

Mercurial diuretics and some thiazides

Multivitamins containing vitamin K

Tranquilizers
- Meprobamate (Miltown, Equanil)
- Haloperidol (Haldol)

Drugs that do not alter anticoagulant effects
Diazepam (Valium)

Chloridazepoxide (Librium)

Chlorothiazide (Diuril) in standard doses

Flurazepam (Dalmane)

Tolmetin (Tolectin)

Medication inactivated by warfarin
Cyclosporine

compliance, diet, use of other drugs, or presence of other illnesses.[13] In this study advanced age was not a significant factor as reported in other studies, whereas in a recent review an associated malignancy was the most important factor in predicting bleeding.[14]

Other adverse reactions to warfarin are rare but include skin necrosis and atheromatous embolization. Warfarin skin necrosis is reported to occur in less than 1% of patients receiving this medication. It is initially brought to the attention of the physician because of sudden, localized, painful skin lesions characterized by an erythematous or hemorrhagic appearance (Fig. 6-1, B). Lesions usually develop between the third and sixth day of therapy, appear more often in women, and are found more commonly in areas of increased subcutaneous fat including the breasts, buttocks, thighs, and calves. The cause of this entity is not clear, although some patients have been observed to have decreased levels of protein C and less commonly, protein S.[15,16] Treatment is aimed at recognizing and discontinuing warfarin immediately. Anticoagulation therapy with another agent is then recommended, although there have been reports that warfarin can be cautiously reintroduced at a later date if needed.[17]

The association of purple toes and warfarin is well described.[18] Initially thought to be an idiosyncratic reaction, it is now believed to be caused by cholesterol crystals (atheroemboli) that break loose from ulcerated atherosclerotic plaques and migrate distally. A number of other precipitating conditions can lead to atheromatous embolization including surgery, arteriography, thrombolytic therapy, and trauma. If atheromatous embolization is suspected, warfarin should be discontinued if possible. The source and cause of the embolization event should be sought.

Warfarin is contraindicated during pregnancy. It crosses the placenta and produces a characteristic embryopathy that may include nasal hypoplasia, stippled epiphyses, central nervous system abnormalities, and fetal bleeding. In this setting the use of heparin is recommended. Other side effects of warfarin include nausea, vomiting, diarrhea, and alopecia. Although unpleasant, they are not life-threatening and most patients adjust to them.

The anticoagulant effects of warfarin can be reversed by the administration of vitamin K_1, which can be administered intravenously, subcutaneously, or orally. The dose of vitamin K_1 depends on the amount and time of the last dose and the urgency of the situation. In patients with life-threatening hemorrhage, fresh frozen plasma should be given for an immediate reversal, and the intravenous route of vitamin K_1 is recommended. No more than 5 mg/min should be given in this manner as hypotension and anaphylaxis have been reported. Even given intravenously, the therapeutic effect of vitamin K_1 takes from 4 to 12 hours for complete reversal. Smaller doses can be administered subcutaneously if the indication for reversal is not life-threatening. As little as 1 mg can lower a markedly elevated INR without completely reversing the effects of warfarin.

HEPARIN

Heparin is an anticoagulant that has been used for over half a century. Heparin is a mucopolysaccharide consisting of unbranched chains of alternating sulfated hexosamine and uronic acid residues. When synthesized by cells,

The Mechanism of Heparin Anticoagulation

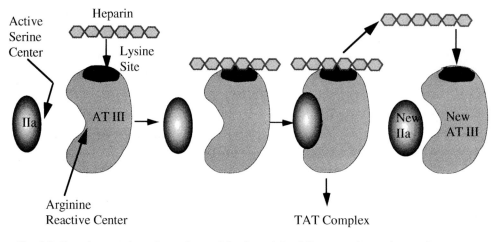

Fig. 6-2. Heparin exerts its anticoagulant activity through its ability to accelerate the reaction between antithrombin III (ATIII) and serine proteases: thrombin (IIa), IXa, Xa, XIa, XIIa. Once a thrombin-ATIII (TAT) complex has been formed, the heparin dissociates from the complex and binds to a new ATIII molecule.

heparin is attached to a backbone polypeptide by linkage sugars.[19] Heparin is most commonly derived from porcine intestinal mucosa but has also been obtained from bovine lung. In processing heparin for anticoagulant use, the mucopolysaccharide chains are cleaved from the peptide backbone, resulting in chains of 5,000 to 30,000 molecular weight. The anticoagulant activity of heparin has been localized to a unique pentasaccharide sequence, the third residue of which contains a 3-0-sulfated glucosamine that is required for binding to antithrombin III (ATIII).[20] Approximately 30% of most unfractionated heparin contains the active pentasaccharide sequence. Heparin's anticoagulant activity is due to the binding of the pentasaccharide sequence to a lysine-binding site in ATIII, thus imparting a conformational change in ATIII. This accelerates the binding of the arginine reactive center of ATIII to activated serine proteases over 2,000-fold, with the formation of inactive ATIII-protease complexes[21] (Fig. 6-2). Once binding of ATIII to the protease takes place, the heparin molecule dissociates and binds to a new ATIII molecule. The ATIII-protease (thrombin-antithrombin or TAT) complexes are removed by the reticuloendothelial system. This mechanism of action explains why heparin imparts anticoagulant activity quickly once infused intravenously and also explains why levels of ATIII often decrease during heparin therapy. The anticoagulant activity of heparin is also mediated by heparin cofactor II. Unlike ATIII, heparin cofactor II inhibits only thrombin and can accept either heparin or dermatan sulfate as cofactors.[22]

Unfractionated heparin inhibits thrombin through the activity of ATIII, but also inhibits multiple other serine proteases such as factors Xa, IXa, XIa, and XIIa.[23] Although unfractionated heparin inhibits multiple serine proteases, the mechanism of inhibition varies slightly for thrombin compared with other factors. For heparin to inhibit the

activity of thrombin, there is a requirement of at least 18 monosaccharide units, with the formation of a ternary complex between heparin, ATIII, and thrombin[24] (Fig. 6-3). The inhibition of factor Xa requires only the pentasaccharide sequence of heparin to bind to ATIII.[23] Direct binding of factor Xa to the heparin species is not needed. This difference in molecular weight requirements for heparin activity forms the basis for the specific anti–factor Xa activity of low-molecular-weight species of heparin, which is discussed later. When given intravenously, unfractionated heparin has a bioavailability of 30% and a half-life of 1 to 3 hours, with elimination by reticuloendothelial and renal routes.[23]

Monitoring of low-dose heparin administered subcutaneously for prophylactic use is not usually considered necessary, but high-dose intravenous therapy carries a substantial risk of hemorrhage and monitoring is recommended. There is no direct assay for heparin, as it acts as a cofactor in the inhibition of serine proteases by ATIII. Heparin's anticoagulant activity can be monitored by following its effects on coagulation assays, notably the activated partial thromboplastin time (APTT), activated clotting time (ACT), and thrombin time (TT).[25] Heparin can also be assayed by chromogenic substrate assays where the ability of heparin to inhibit the activity of either thrombin or factor Xa is measured. The sensitivity of the assays is anti-Xa(anti-IIa)> TT > APTT > ACT > PT. The PT is for the most part insensitive to the effect of heparin in the therapeutic range.

The most commonly used assay to monitor heparin therapy is the APTT, with an elevation of 1.5 to 2.5 times normal as the usual target range. This corresponds to a heparin activity of approximately 0.2 to 0.5 U/ml. Unfortunately the APTT is not the ideal test to monitor heparin therapy as the heparin sensitivity of the reagents varies

Mechanism of Interaction Between ATIII, Thrombin and fXa

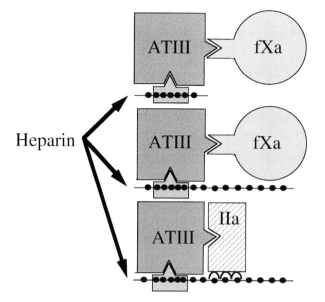

Fig. 6-3. The ability of heparin to facilitate the inhibition of coagulation factors by antithrombin III *(ATIII)* demonstrates a dependence on the size of the heparin chains. For heparin to inhibit thrombin *(IIa)*, heparin must contain at least 18 monosaccharide units, with the formation of a ternary complex between ATIII, heparin, and IIa. For inhibition of factor Xa, direct binding of heparin to factor Xa is not necessary, and the pentasaccharide sequence of heparin is sufficient to accelerate the reaction. This molecular weight dependence has important implications in the laboratory monitoring of heparin and low-molecular-weight heparin. As low-molecular-weight heparin inhibits only factor Xa, it can be monitored only by factor Xa inhibition assays. The APTT and ACT are relatively unaffected by low-molecular-weight heparin.

considerably.[26] For this reason, all laboratories should establish the heparin dose response of their APTT reagent. An in vivo dose response should be performed using samples from patients receiving intravenous heparin. Simple in vitro spiking of plasma with heparin often leads to much higher APTT values than similar levels of heparin in vivo. A standardization methodology analogous to the INR would be useful for monitoring heparin therapy with the APTT, but no such methodology has been widely adopted.

The APTT is not specific for the effect of heparin, and the APTT value is sensitive to abnormalities of the intrinsic pathway factors (XII, XI, IX, VIII) and common pathway factors (X, V, II, fibrinogen). Patients with congenital abnormalities of factor XI or XII may have very elevated baseline APTT values (e.g., 80 to 150 seconds), making heparin therapy difficult to follow with the APTT. Likewise, patients with the lupus anticoagulant, who often have thrombosis and require heparin therapy, will have an elevated baseline APTT. In these types of patients, heparin therapy can most accurately be followed by the chromogenic factor Xa inhibition assay.[27] Problems with the Xa inhibition assay include its increased cost in comparison to the APTT and the lack of a rapid turnaround time in many laboratories. Patients with increased levels of factor VIII may have a short baseline APTT. Heparin therapy in these patients often leads to a modest increase in APTT. Attempting to attain a 1.5-fold to 2.5-fold increase in the APTT in these patients may lead to overanticoagulation.[23] A heparin monitoring strategy is outlined in Fig. 6-4. Due to the prevalence of heparin-associated thrombocytopenia with attendant thrombosis, monitoring of the platelet count before and during heparin therapy is recommended.

In some patients administration of full-dose heparin fails to produce the desired 1.5-fold to 2.5-fold increase in the APTT. Apparent resistance to heparin's anticoagulant effect can be due to multiple factors. The most common causes of apparent heparin resistance are administration errors—that is, the patient is not receiving heparin because of a pharmacy error or a malfunctioning intravenous infusion. Another cause of heparin resistance is due to a deficiency of one of the heparin cofactors, ATIII, or heparin cofactor II. Patients with ATIII deficiency may display heparin resistance when their ATIII level is less than 50%.[28] However, ATIII levels must be interpreted with caution in patients receiving heparin therapy, as ATIII levels are known to decrease during the course of therapy. Increased levels of heparin-binding proteins such as platelet factor 4, histidine-rich glycoprotein, or vitronectin can also result in heparin resistance.[29] Apparent heparin resistance may also be caused by increased levels of factor VIII, which give rise to low basal APTT values. To investigate the cause of apparent in vitro heparin resistance where the patient's APTT is less than 1.5 times control despite adequate heparin dosage, it is recommended to assay the heparin levels using a chromogenic factor Xa inhibition assay. If the heparin level is greater than 0.2 U/ml, the cause of the heparin resistance may be due to ATIII deficiency or elevated factor VIII levels. If the heparin level is less than 0.2 U/ml, administration errors should be investigated. Furthermore, in vitro addition of heparin to the patient's plasma (in vitro dose-response curve) can be used to detect an inhibitor to heparin, such as elevated platelet factor 4 or an antibody.

Heparin may be given intravenously (continuously or intermittently) or subcutaneously. It is best administered through an intravenous infusion using a constant infusion pump. Subcutaneous administration may cause erratic absorption, is uncomfortable, and is a less desirable route

Monitoring Heparin Therapy

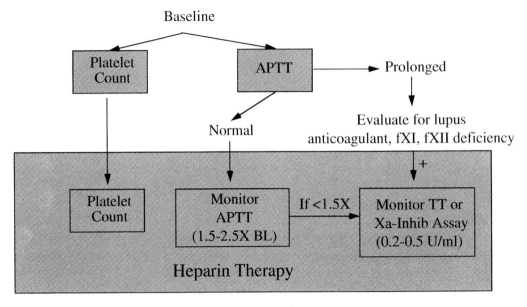

Fig. 6-4. Flow diagram for monitoring heparin therapy. Before initiating heparin therapy, measurement of the APTT may help to identify a lupus anticoagulant, or factor XI or XII deficiency. These result in an elevated APTT, making the thrombin time or Xa inhibition assay the best way to monitor heparin therapy in patients with these abnormalities. The target range for intravenous heparin therapy is an elevation of the APTT to 1.5 to 2.5 times the baseline. If the APTT fails to elevate more than the 1.5-fold increase, heparin resistance should be evaluated by performing the Xa inhibition assay. If the heparin level is greater than 0.2 U/ml, the cause of the heparin resistance may be due to antithrombin III deficiency or elevated factor VIII levels. If the heparin level is under 0.2 U/ml, administration errors or heparin inhibitors should be investigated.

in the inpatient setting. It may be necessary to prescribe subcutaneous heparin therapy for individuals refractory to oral warfarin, those with Trousseau's syndrome, warfarin skin necrosis, pregnant patients, or those in whom intravenous access is not available.

A loading dose between 5,000 and 10,000 U given slowly over 10 to 15 minutes is a standard dose for initiating intravenous heparin. This has been followed traditionally by a continuous infusion of 1,000 U/hr with adjustments made according to the APTT. Over the past few years several workers have devised nomograms for the initial dosing and adjustment of heparin. Recommendations have included a dose of 80 U/kg body weight bolus followed by 18 U/kg/hr continuous infusion or a bolus dose of 5,000 U of heparin followed by 1,280 U/hr.[30,31] Both of these nomograms recommended frequent monitoring of the APTT with adjustments made as needed. The advantage of the nomogram is the more rapid achievement of a therapeutic APTT, thus decreasing the incidence of recurrent thrombosis and bleeding events.

When the subcutaneous route is used, the approximated dosage and schedule is 10,000 to 25,000 U every 12 hours. The APTT should be measured at 6-hour intervals to ensure adequate anticoagulation, and the targeted APTT should be 1.5 to 2.5 times control. Some experts recommend checking an APTT 1 hour before the next dose to be certain the patient is adequately protected for the entire 12-hour period.

Hemorrhage is the most commonly encountered complication of treatment with heparin (Fig. 6-1, *C*). The incidence of serious hemorrhage is low and may be proportionate to the intensity of the regimen used. Fatalities have been reported, and moderate hemorrhage such as hematuria, ecchymosis, hematoma, epistaxis, and melena occurs in 10% to 33% of patients.[32-35]

Patients receiving heparin therapy should be examined daily to detect abnormal bleeding. Invasive procedures including arterial punctures, lumbar punctures, thoracentesis, paracentesis, and intramuscular injections should not be performed while the patient is receiving heparin.

Reactions to heparin other than hemorrhage are rare. Hypersensitivity and anaphylactoid reactions have ranged from mild fever, urticaria, rhinitis, and conjunctivitis to sudden severe hypertension, respiratory distress, and chest pain. Heparin skin necrosis has also been reported and may occur at the site of the subcutaneous injection. Hyperkalemia, hypoaldosteronism, elevation in transaminases, and transient alopecia have also been reported. The syndrome of heparin-induced thrombocytopenia and thrombosis can be devastating. Complications include acute limb ischemia and death. The overall incidence of thrombocytopenia is reported to vary between 2.4% to 15.6%.[23] Heparin-associated thrombosis is much less common and occurs in less than 1% of patients. A more detailed description of this entity is discussed in Chapter 5.

Osteoporosis has been reported in patients who receive

heparin for extended periods (more than 9 months).[36] It appears most related to the dose and duration of therapy. Vertebral fractures of the thoracic and lumbar spine are the most frequently seen complications. This complication is most likely seen in the pregnant patient receiving heparin during her entire pregnancy, or in patients with Trousseau's syndrome who have failed oral anticoagulation therapy and receive chronic heparin therapy. Protamine sulfate can reverse the anticoagulant effect of heparin. The dose depends on the amount of heparin present and the time and route of the last dose. The recommended dose is 1.0 mg for every 100 U of heparin present in the body. It should be administered slowly, intravenously, and at a rate not greater than 5 mg/min. No single injection of protamine should exceed 50 mg. The antiheparin effect lasts approximately 2 hours. An APTT should be checked approximately 15 minutes after the administration of protamine sulfate and before the next dose is given. Some heparin effect may reappear after a single dose of protamine sulfate, especially if a large dose of heparin was administered subcutaneously shortly before the injection of protamine. Transfusions of blood, plasma, or other blood products are not antidotes against heparin, although they are of value in replacement therapy after hemorrhage.

LOW-MOLECULAR-WEIGHT HEPARIN

Low-molecular-weight heparin is produced from unfractionated heparin by enzymatic or chemical degradation to produce mucopolysaccharide species with molecular weights in the range of 4000 to 6500.[37] Low-molecular-weight heparin contains the active pentasaccharide group in lower proportion than standard heparin (10% vs. 30%).[37] Because of its smaller size, low-molecular-weight heparin has a reduced ability to catalyze the inhibition of thrombin but maintains full inhibitory activity against factor Xa (Fig. 6-3). Low-molecular-weight heparin has been used for several years in Europe with considerable success. It is desirable because it produces less risk of bleeding complications at comparable anticoagulant effect compared with unfractionated heparin and has increased bioavailability and a longer half-life.[38] It also appears to have a reduced risk for development of heparin-associated thrombocytopenia and thrombosis compared with unfractionated heparin.[39] Drawbacks include its higher cost and limited availability in the United States (only enoxaparin has received FDA approval).

For prophylaxis and treatment of venous thrombosis, monitoring of low-molecular-weight heparin appears unnecessary.[40] However, in patients at special risk for hemorrhagic complications or in those applications using higher-dose therapy, monitoring may be desirable. In these instances the only assay suitable for monitoring low-molecular-weight heparin is the factor Xa inhibition assay, due to the lack of thrombin inhibition by the low-molecular-weight species.[41] The APTT and ACT are virtually unresponsive to low-molecular-weight heparin levels up to 2.0 U/ml.

Clinical use of the low-molecular-weight heparins has been primarily for prophylaxis of thrombosis, but it may also be useful for treatment of acute deep venous throm-

bosis and pulmonary embolism.[37] There is a reported lower incidence of recurrent venous thromboembolism, a decrease in bleeding, and even lower mortality.[42-46] The use of low-molecular-weight heparin is now well established in the prophylaxis of both knee and hip surgery and abdominal surgery. These are the only approved applications in the United States.

Low-molecular-weight heparin has been successfully used to treat patients with acute ischemic stroke, to prevent deep vein thrombosis in patients with spinal cord injury, and to replace heparin in cardiopulmonary bypass in those patients with heparin-associated thrombocytopenia.[47-49] Very little data are available concerning the intravenous use of the low-molecular-weight heparins. In those studies noted, however, it appears to be as effective and safe as regular heparin.[50-52] The standard dose for prophylaxis in hip and knee surgery is 30 mg administered subcutaneously every 12 hours. The first dose is generally given 12 to 24 hours following surgery. In the treatment of deep vein thrombosis and pulmonary embolism, a dose of 1 mg/kg by subcutaneous injection every 12 hours has been recommended.[42]

OTHER LOW-MOLECULAR-WEIGHT HEPARINS: HEPARINOIDS

The low-molecular-weight heparinoid, Danaparoid (Org 10172; Organon International BV, Oss, The Netherlands), is an antithrombotic agent available in the United States for compassionate use. It has a mean molecular weight of 5500 Da and is obtained from hog intestinal mucosa. It is a mixture of heparan sulfate, dermatan sulfate, and chondroitin sulfate. These three components help to determine the antithrombotic activity of the drug.[53] This low-molecular-weight heparinoid is a more selective inhibitor of factor Xa compared with either heparin or the low-molecular-weight heparins.[53] It also appears to have little cross-reactivity to heparin-induced platelet antibodies and therefore has been advocated as an alternative therapeutic agent in this setting.[54-56] Danaparoid has been used in the treatment of venous thromboembolism and resulted in significant reduction in both the recurrence and extension of thrombosis when compared with standard unfractionated heparin[53] and has a similar incidence of major and minor bleeding. Other potential uses include prophylaxis in hip fracture surgery, hip replacement surgery, in patients with nonhemorrhagic stroke, during hemodialysis, and in disseminated intravascular coagulation (DIC).[53,57]

ANTIPLATELET AGENTS

The strategy for inhibition of platelet function employed clinically has been to inhibit the thromboxane synthase pathway (aspirin, sulfinpyrazone), to increase intracytoplasmic cyclic adenosine monophosphate (cyclic AMP) levels (dipyridamole, prostaglandin I_2), or to interfere with the platelet membrane (ticlopidine). Antiplatelet agents have been found to be useful in the prevention of myocardial infarction and can be a beneficial adjunct to anticoagulant therapy in some clinical settings.

Inhibitors of Platelet Function

ASPIRIN AND SULFINPYRAZONE. Acetylsalicylic acid, or aspirin, is an inhibitor of prostaglandin synthesis.[58] It blocks production of the end product of platelet prostaglandin synthesis, thromboxane A_2, by irreversible acetylation of the cyclooxygenase enzyme[59,60] (Fig. 6-5). Aspirin thus inhibits platelet function for the entire platelet life span, approximately 7 to 10 days.[61,62] Endothelial cells also have a prostaglandin synthesis pathway, with the end product being prostaglandin I_2 (prostacyclin) instead of thromboxane A_2. Endothelial cell cyclooxygenase was initially thought to be less sensitive to aspirin,[62] but further studies have shown that platelet and endothelial forms of cyclooxygenase have equivalent sensitivities to aspirin.[63] It is now thought that equivalent doses of aspirin have a greater effect on platelets than endothelial cells primarily because the endothelial cell is able to produce more cyclooxygenase enzyme, whereas anucleate platelets cannot.[59] Aspirin prolongs the bleeding time and is able to inhibit in vitro platelet aggregation to adenosine diphosphate (ADP), epinephrine, and collagen. Aspirin does not inhibit platelet adhesion or release, so the aggregation tracing with aspirin will show a primary wave of aggregation followed by disaggregation and lack of a secondary wave of aggregation.[60,62,64,65] Aspirin is also able to completely inhibit aggregation due to arachidonic acid. Unresponsiveness to arachidonic acid during in vitro aggregation is highly indicative of aspirin ingestion.

A number of clinical applications are now recommended for the use of aspirin.[66] These include the prevention of myocardial infarction in asymptomatic men and women over the age of 50, in patients with unstable and stable angina, in the setting of acute myocardial infarction, transient ischemic attacks, thrombotic stroke, and in patients with peripheral arterial disease.[66] Aspirin may improve the results of percutaneous transluminal angioplasty and has been reported to be of benefit in lower-extremity bypass.[67-69] The recommended dose of aspirin suggested varies from as low as 60 mg/day to as high as 975 mg/day. Aspirin is also indicated in patients with atrial fibrillation who are unable to take warfarin. Aspirin has become the most widely used drug ever developed. Despite this, it must be remembered that aspirin has side effects and fatalities secondary to hemorrhage have been reported.[70] Other more common adverse reactions include heartburn or stomach pain, nausea, vomiting, constipation, and bloody stools. In a multicentered, prospective, cooperative study to compare endarterectomy plus aspirin to aspirin therapy alone for the treatment of asymptomatic carotid stenosis, fully 16% of patients were taken off aspirin because of adverse reactions, and 51% were converted to an enteric-coated product, and 27% were on a reduced dosage of aspirin at the time the trial ended.[71]

Sulfinpyrazone is a competitive inhibitor of cyclooxygenase whose mechanism of antithrombotic action is unknown.[62] Like aspirin, it inhibits in vitro platelet aggregation, but it additionally inhibits platelet adhesion.[65]

Sulfinpyrazone has been used in patients after myocardial infarction, aortocoronary bypass surgery, unstable angina, and stroke. In randomized trials evaluating sulfin-

Drugs That Interfere with Prostaglandin Synthesis

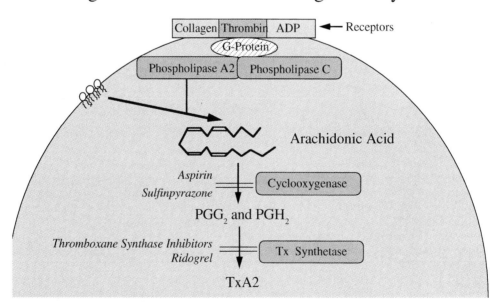

Fig. 6-5. One class of antiplatelet drugs acts to inhibit prostaglandin synthesis. Binding of agonists to membrane receptors results in the liberation of arachidonic acid from the phospholipid membrane by phospholipase A_2. Cyclooxygenase catalyzes the formation of the cyclic endoperoxides prostaglandin *(PGG$_2$)* and prostaglandin H_2 *(PGH$_2$)*. Thromboxane A_2 is next formed by thromboxane synthase. Aspirin acetylates cyclooxygenase, permanently blocking the function of the enzyme. Sulfinpyrazone also inhibits cyclooxygenase. Ridogrel is a new thromboxane synthase inhibitor that also blocks the thromboxane A_2 receptor.

pyrazone versus placebo and aspirin, more cerebrovascular events were noted with sulfinpyrazone than either aspirin or placebo.[72] Side effects include precipitation of uric acid stones and exacerbation of peptic ulcer.

DIPYRIDAMOLE AND PROSTAGLANDIN I₂ (PROSTACYCLIN). Cyclic AMP inhibits calcium uptake by the dense tubular system and also inhibits phosphoinositol 4,5-bisphosphate (PIP₂) hydrolysis to inositol 1,4,5-triphosphate (IP3).[73] IP3 is responsible for stimulating release of calcium from the dense tubular system, thus leading to platelet activation (Fig. 6-6). Classes of drugs have been developed that raise intracytoplasmic cyclic AMP levels, thus leading to inhibition of platelet activation. The two most widely used drugs in this class are dipyridamole and prostaglandin I₂ (prostacyclin) (Fig. 6-7). Prostacylin stimulates adenylate cyclase through activation of a G protein (Gs), leading to increased cyclic AMP levels.[74] Prostacyclin is a potent, short-acting inhibitor of platelet aggregation, platelet adhesion, and platelet release.[62] Iloprost, a stable analog of prostacylin (ZK36374; Schering AG, Berlin, Germany), has similar effects on platelet function.[75] Iloprost has been used in patients with peripheral vascular disease, thromboangiitis obliterans (Buerger's disease), Raynaud's phenomenon, and systemic sclerosis.[76,77] In addition, iloprost has been used in conjunction with heparin therapy in patients requiring cardiopulmonary bypass and in carotid endarterectomy in the setting of heparin-induced thrombocytopenia.[78,79] There are a few reports of increased platelet aggregability after iloprost therapy, giving rise to rebound hyperreactivity.[80] Iloprost also has several undesirable side effects including headache, nausea, vomiting, and hypotension.

At the time of this publication iloprost is not readily available for use in the United States.

Dipyridamole prevents the breakdown of cyclic AMP to 5'AMP by inhibiting phosphodiesterase and may also stimulate adenylate cyclase[81] (Fig. 6-7). At therapeutic plasma levels, dipyridamole has only limited effects on in vitro platelet function.[82] The only currently FDA-approved application for this agent is in the prevention of thromboembolism in patients with prosthetic heart valves. It is still commonly used, however, by many primary care physicians in the setting of transient ischemic attacks, stroke, peripheral vascular disease, and coronary artery disease even though it has no proven advantage over aspirin. Of ongoing interest, however, is the potential role dipyridamole may play in the prevention of homocysteine-induced atherosclerosis and in the prevention of atherogenesis.[83]

Other Platelet Inhibitors

TICLOPIDINE (TICLID). Ticlopidine and its analog clopidogrel are thienopyridine derivatives that are potent inhibitors of platelet aggregation.[84] Ticlopidine's mechanism of antithrombotic action is unknown, but it is a potent inhibitor of ADP-induced aggregation of human platelets.[85] It also inhibits low-dose aggregation by other agonists such as collagen, arachidonic acid, thromboxane A₂, thrombin, and platelet activating factor.[85] Although platelet aggregation may be inhibited as soon as 2 hours after a dose of ticlopidine, maximal anticoagulant effect takes up to 3 to 5 days to achieve, and the antiplatelet effect is seen for up to 10 days after drug withdrawal, suggesting that ticlopidine irreversibly affects platelet function.[84]

Mechanism of Platelet Release

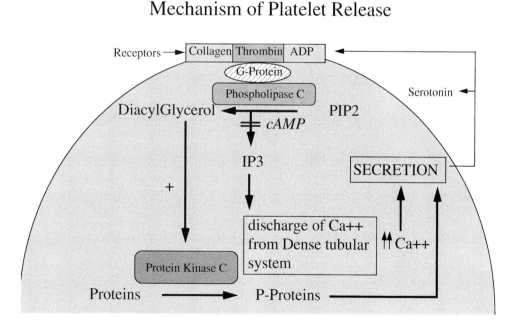

Fig. 6-6. Platelet secretion is stimulated by liberation of calcium from the dense tubular system. Cyclic adenosine monophosphate *(cAMP)* inhibits the conversion of phosphoinositol 4,5-bisphosphate *(PIP₂)* to inositol 1,4,5-triphosphate *(IP3)*. IP3 is responsible for stimulating release of calcium from the dense tubular system. Drugs that elevate cAMP levels would be expected to inhibit platelet release.

Drugs That Raise Platelet cAMP Levels

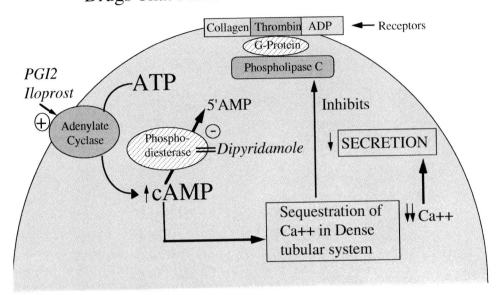

Fig. 6-7. Elevation of cyclic adenosine monophosphate *(cAMP)* levels prevents release of calcium from the dense tubular system and decreases platelet secretion. Drugs that elevate cAMP levels include prostaglandin I$_2$ *(PGI$_2$)* and its analog iloprost, which act by stimulating adenylate cyclase, thus resulting in the breakdown of adenosine triphosphate *(ATP)* to cAMP. Dipyridamole maintains elevated cAMP levels by inhibiting phosphodiesterase and preventing the breakdown of cAMP to 5'AMP.

Ticlopidine has a more profound effect on the bleeding time than aspirin[86] and may also reduce fibrinogen levels[87] and decrease platelet adhesiveness.[88] Ticlopidine and clopidogrel may inhibit the ADP-induced binding of fibrinogen to platelet glycoprotein IIb/IIIa, but it appears that they do not directly modify the structure of glycoprotein IIb/IIIa.[89] Other studies suggest that these drugs may not affect either ADP binding to platelet receptors or inhibit fibrinogen binding to glycoprotein IIb/IIIa, but rather inhibit a step in signal transduction between the two events.[90]

Ticlopidine is now approved for the use in patients with cerebrovascular disease, in patients with an allergy to aspirin or aspirin intolerance, and in patients who develop recurrent thromboembolism despite aspirin therapy.[66] In the largest trial of the drug for the prevention of stroke, it was found to be more effective than aspirin.[91] It has also been used successfully in decreasing the rate of vascular death and myocardial infarction in patients with unstable angina, to maintain graft patency after coronary artery bypass surgery, to prevent ischemic ulcers in patients with arterial occlusive disease, and shows promise in slowing the progression of diabetic microangiopathy.[91,92] A decrease in fibrinogen by as much as 10% to 25% has also been observed, and in one study this decrease was associated with clinical improvement and decreases in whole blood and plasma viscosities.[93] The recommended dose is 250 mg twice daily. A number of adverse reactions have been noted with this agent including diarrhea, nausea, vomiting, abdominal cramps, rash, increase in the serum cholesterol level, and neutropenia. The neutropenia is usually reversible. A baseline blood cell count is therefore recommended at initiation of therapy and then every 2 weeks for the first 3 months of treatment. Several cases of a fatal syndrome resembling thrombotic thrombocytopenia purpura have also been reported.

NEWER ANTITHROMBOTIC AGENTS

There is intense interest in the scientific and pharmaceutical communities for developing new antithrombotic agents. The search for these agents has been boosted from studies of snakes and blood-feeding animals, as many of these animals have developed elaborate mechanisms to prevent the clotting of blood.[94,95] Some of the strategies for development of new antithrombotic drugs target thrombin inactivation, prevention of thrombin generation, fibrinogen degradation, inhibition of endothelial thrombogenicity, or inhibition of platelet function. These are summarized in the box on p. 119.

Thrombin Inhibitors

HIRUDINS. Hirudin was one of the first antithrombotic agents ever discovered, when Haycraft described the antithrombotic properties of saliva from the medicinal leech *Hirudo medicinalis* in 1884.[96] Hirudin, now available in recombinant form, is a peptide of 65 amino acids that is an extremely specific thrombin inhibitor.[97] Structurally hirudin consists of a compact NH$_2$-terminal end with three intrachain disulfide bonds and a long peptide COOH-terminal end.[98] Thrombin is a serine protease, which, in addition to its active catalytic site, has an anion binding

NEWER STRATEGIES FOR THE DEVELOPMENT OF ANTITHROMBOTIC DRUGS

Target	*Approaches*
Thrombin inactivation	Hirudin and analogs
	Argatroban and P-PACK
	Thrombin receptor peptide antagonist
	Nucleotide-based thrombin inhibitors
Factors that inhibit thrombin formation	Tick anticoagulant peptide
	Antistasin
	Inactivated factor X
	Inactivated factor VIIa and blockade of tissue factor
Factors that degrade fibrinogen	Ancrod
Recombinant endogenous anticoagulants	Tissue factor pathway inhibitor
	Antithrombin III
	Activated protein C
	Thrombomodulin
Agents that block fibrinogen binding to platelet glycoprotein IIb/IIIa	Monoclonal antibodies against glycoprotein IIb/IIIa
	Peptide-based inhibitors mimicking RGD sequence of fibrinogen
Agents that block von Willebrand's binding to platelet glycoprotein Ib/IX	Fragments of von Willebrand's factor
New thromboxane receptor antagonists	Compounds that block binding of thromboxane A_2 to the platelet receptor
Combined inhibition of thromboxane synthase plus thromboxane receptor antagonism	Ridogrel
Agents that decrease vascular wall thrombogenicity	Dietary omega-3 fatty acids
	Agents acting directly on endothelium

exosite that is the binding site for fibrinogen. Binding of fibrinogen to the exosite helps to increase the specificity of thrombin for fibrinogen.[99] Hirudin is a direct inhibitor of thrombin and does not require ATIII for activity. The N-terminal portion of hirudin binds to the catalytic site of thrombin, the C-terminal portion of hirudin binds to the anion binding exosite,[98-100] and other portions of the molecule bind in multiple sites to other regions of thrombin. Other hirudin-like compounds have been developed. Hirugen is a synthetic hirudin derivative that is a peptide containing the 12 C-terminal amino acids of hirudin (aa 53 through 64).[101] Like the C-terminal portion of hirudin, hirugen binds to the anion binding exosite of thrombin and prevents thrombin binding to fibrinogen. Because it lacks the ability to inhibit the catalytic site of thrombin, hirugen is a less effective antithrombotic agent than hirudin.[102] Hirulog is a synthetic eicosapeptide that contains the N-terminal peptide D-Phe-Pro-Arg connected to hirugen through a polyglycine linker.[100] The N-terminal peptide of hirulog binds to the catalytic site of thrombin, and the hirugen portion of the molecule binds to the anion binding exosite. Thus hirulog retains the specific thrombin inhibitory properties of hirudin.

Hirudin is the most potent and specific thrombin inhibitor known due to its multifocal and specific binding to thrombin. Unlike heparin, hirudin is able to inhibit thrombin that is bound to fibrin or extracellular matrix.[103] Hirudin is not susceptible to inhibition by plasma proteins such as platelet factor 4 and histidine-rich glycoprotein like heparin. It also has a rapid half-life of approximately 36 minutes.[104] Thus hirudin is theoretically a more potent antithrombotic agent than heparin, and clinical trials of hirudin during angioplasty and in prevention and treatment of deep venous thrombosis have so far borne this out.[104-107] Large-scale clinical trials are now under way to study the antithrombotic properties of hirudin. One of these trials, the Global Use of Strategies to Open Occluded Arteries (GUSTO-IIb) is an ongoing study of 12,000 patients to compare the effect of hirudin versus heparin in the therapy of coronary thrombosis, which was completed in early 1996; however, the data will not be available until late 1996. These studies should provide important information in determining the antithrombotic efficacy of this new class of drug. Other potential uses for hirudin include the treatment of patients with heparin-induced thrombocytopenia and thrombosis, patients with

ATIII deficiency states, as an adjunct to thrombolytic therapy, renal dialysis patients, and as an effective surface coating for biomedical devices including tubings, catheters, dialysis membranes, and blood oxygenators.

In patients receiving intravenous heparin therapy, monitoring of anticoagulant effect is necessary due to the variable biologic responses of the drug. The hirudins display more consistent and reproducible anticoagulant properties than heparin[104-106] and may not require as much dose adjustment or monitoring as heparin. Hirudin has similar effects to heparin on many routine coagulation assays. At 2.5 μg/ml, hirudin has a greater effect on the thrombin time but a similar effect on the APTT, ACT and the anti-IIa amidolytic assay.[108] Like heparin, the PT is relatively insensitive to hirudin.[108] However, the usefulness of monitoring hirudin therapy with the APTT has not been confirmed, as the APTT may be insensitive to both low and high concentrations of hirudin.[108] There are specific immunologic assays being developed for hirudin, but these assays would determine plasma level of hirudin and not its anticoagulant effect.

One concern with the use of hirudin is lack of a specific antidote as seen with heparin and its antidote protamine sulfate. To date in most studies, bleeding has not been a major problem, probably because of hirudin's short half-life.

ARGATROBAN, P-PACK, AND EFEGATRAN. Argatroban and P-PACK (D-phenylalanyl-L-prolyl-L-arginyl chloromethylketone) are synthetic inhibitors of thrombin that, like hirudin, are not dependent on ATIII for their inhibitory activity. P-PACK is a tripeptide that mimics a portion of the structure of fibrinopeptide A, the peptide released from the alpha chain of fibrinogen by thrombin. It inhibits thrombin by binding to the active catalytic site of thrombin and is irreversible because it alkylates the active site histidine residue.[109] P-PACK has been shown to be effective in preventing thrombosis and reducing arterial reocclusion in animal models.[110] Argatroban, an arginine derivative, is also a specific thrombin inhibitor, but it is a competitive antagonist that binds to an apolar site adjacent to the catalytic site of thrombin.[111] Clinical trials using Novastan, a brand of argatroban (Texas Biotechnology Corporation, Houston, Tex.), as an alternative to heparin in patients with heparin-associated thrombocytopenia are under way. Argatroban has also been used in patients following cardiac surgery, in unstable angina, as an adjunct to thrombolysis, in the setting of chronic arterial occlusive disease, in hemodialysis, and in the treatment of DIC.[112] In patients treated for unstable angina, a recurrence of the angina was noted in 21% of patients in one study.[113]

Efegatran (D-methyl-phenylalanyl-prolyl-arginal) inhibits the same site on thrombin as argatroban, but is a slowly reversible inhibitor and has been shown to be effective in blocking the ex vivo generation of both thrombin and factor Xa.[114] It produces a dose-dependent anticoagulant effect on intravenous infusion. It has a short half-life, allowing for quick recovery of coagulation function, and no rebound phenomenon has yet been observed. It is being developed as an anticoagulant for prevention

and treatment of both arterial and venous thromboembolic disorders.

THROMBIN RECEPTOR PEPTIDE ANTAGONISTS. Thrombin is a physiologically important activator of platelets. The platelet thrombin receptor is activated by thrombin by a unique mechanism. Thrombin cleaves an N-terminal peptide from the receptor. The new N-terminal peptide activates the receptor as a tethered ligand and another portion of the receptor is a thrombin-binding site.[115] Peptides have been developed that inhibit thrombin activation of the thrombin receptor by mimicking the N-terminal domain or inhibiting thrombin binding to the receptor.[116,117]

NUCLEOTIDE-BASED THROMBIN INHIBITORS (APTAMERS). A novel class of thrombin inhibitors has been recently described that consists of single-stranded deoxynucleotides that bind to immobilized thrombin.[118] One thrombin aptamer, a synthetic oligonucleotide with a sequence of GGTTGGTGTGGTTGG, has been reported to display potent antithrombin activity in in vitro clotting assays.[118] It has also been reported to bind to clot-bound thrombin and to reduce arterial platelet thrombus formation[119] and thrombus formation in extracorporeal circuits.[120] Another thrombin aptamer has been reported to interact with thrombin's anion binding exosite and is able to compete with natural substrates, such as fibrinogen and platelet thrombin receptors.[121,122] Defibrotide, a polydeoxyribonucleotide agent with a polydisperse molecular weight range from 2,000 to 30,000 dal, functions as an antithrombotic agent, most likely by a direct antithrombin action.[123] It has also been reported that defibrotide may modulate endothelial cell function to increase cyclic AMP levels and increase tissue factor pathway inhibitor (TFPI) release.[121]

Factors that Inhibit Thrombin Formation

TICK ANTICOAGULANT PEPTIDE AND ANTISTASIN. Tick anticoagulant peptide (TAP) is a 60 amino acid polypeptide originally isolated from the soft tick *Ornithodoros moubata* and is now available in a recombinant form (rTAP).[124,125] rTAP acts as a reversible, competitive inhibitor of factor Xa. It is thought to inhibit factor Xa in a fashion analogous to the inhibition of thrombin by hirudin, requiring binding to the active site of factor Xa as well as an exosite.[126] Unlike ATIII, TAP is able to inhibit factor Xa even when the factor is bound to the prothrombinase complex, making TAP a potentially powerful antithrombotic agent. Several animal studies of arterial thrombosis have shown TAP to be an effective antithrombotic agent.[127,128]

Antistasin is a long-acting polypeptide inhibitor of activated factor Xa that has been isolated from the salivary gland of the leech, *Haementuria officinalis*.[129] It has been shown to enhance thrombolytic reperfusion and prevent reocclusion in an animal model of coronary thrombosis.[130] In a baboon model of vascular graft thrombosis, recombinant antistasin prevented platelet and fibrin deposition onto the graft surface.[131] It also caused a marked increase in APTT without affecting the bleeding time.[131]

INACTIVATED FACTOR X AND INHIBITORS OF PROTHROMBINASE COMPLEX FORMATION. Mutant forms of factor X have been developed that are catalytically inactive due to point mutations in the catalytic region of the protein.[132] This inactivated factor X is able to inhibit assembly of the prothrombinase complex and may prevent formation of thrombin.[133,134] It has been shown to be effective at inhibition of both arterial and venous thrombosis in animal models.[133,134] Inhibition of tenase complex formation has also been targeted as a possible antithrombotic approach by development of monoclonal antibodies that inhibit tissue factor[135] or by the production of an activated factor VII rendered non-catalytic by reacting with Glu-Gly-Arg chloromethylketone.[136]

Factors That Degrade Fibrinogen

ANCROD. A number of different snake venoms are able to degrade fibrinogen including ancrod, batroxobin, and crotalase.[116] Ancrod, extracted from the Malayan pit viper *(Akistrodon rhodostoma),* has been used clinically, mostly to treat venous thrombosis.[137] Ancrod cleaves fibrinopeptide A from fibrinogen and produces a fibrin that is very sensitive to fibrinolysis.[138] As ancrod does not activate factor XIII, the fibrin formed is un–cross-linked and soluble. Administration of ancrod results in a rapid decrease in plasma fibrinogen values with concomitant increases in fibrin(ogen) degradation products and decreases in plasminogen values.[139] Much of the use of ancrod has been anecdotal,[116] but recently ancrod has been suggested as a useful alternative to heparin in patients with heparin-associated thrombocytopenia[140] and in vascular surgery.[141]

Recombinant Endogenous Anticoagulants

TISSUE FACTOR PATHWAY INHIBITOR. Tissue factor (TF), released from injured cells, complexes with factor VII to form a TF/factor VIIa/lipid complex that can activate not only factor X but also factor IX. This results in production of thrombin with fibrin formation. A regulator of the activation of the coagulation cascade by this mechanism is TFPI, formerly called lipoprotein-associated coagulation inhibitor or extrinsic pathway inhibitor.[142] TFPI inhibits the factor VIIa/TF/factor Xa complex, thus preventing further factor Xa production by factor VIIa/TF.[142] Recombinant TFPI is available and has been shown to be comparable to low-molecular-weight heparin in inhibiting venous thrombosis.[143] It has also been shown to prevent reocclusion after tissue plasminogen activator (t-PA)–induced reperfusion in a canine femoral artery thrombosis model.[144]

ANTITHROMBIN III. ATIII is a rapid-acting inhibitor of thrombin and other serine proteases in the coagulation cascade. Recombinant ATIII is available clinically, but the primary indication for its use has been replacement therapy in patients with congenital deficiencies of antithrombin III.[145] Theoretically infusion of ATIII should neutralize thrombin and other active serine proteases, even in the absence of heparin, and make ATIII useful as an antithrombotic agent. Decreases in plasma ATIII levels are common in DIC and have been associated with a poor prognosis in this disorder.[146] Clinical trials of ATIII infusion in patients with sepsis have shown a decrease in the duration of DIC in treated patients.[146-148] Although a trend toward decreased mortality with ATIII infusion in DIC has been seen,[147] further definitive studies will be needed to address the efficacy of ATIII infusion in this clinical situation.

ACTIVATED PROTEIN C. Activated protein C, produced by the thrombomodulin-thrombin complex, is a potent natural anticoagulant that degrades coagulation factors Va and VIIIa.[149] Activated protein C has been studied as a potential antithrombotic agent and has been shown to prevent arterial reocclusion after thrombolysis in a canine coronary occlusion model.[150] Activated protein C has also been shown to be effective in preventing DIC in baboons infused with lethal concentrations of *Escherichia coli.*[151] α_1-Antitrypsin is an abundant inhibitor of activated protein C and could limit the effectiveness of administered activated protein C. A chimeric human/bovine protein C has been shown to be resistant to inhibition by α_1-antitrypsin, which could prolong the functionally useful half-life of infused activated protein C.[152] However, a relatively high prevalence of congenital resistance to activated protein C has been described recently in patients with thrombosis and is due to a mutation of factor V, called factor V Leiden.[153] A prevalence of resistance to activated protein C as high as 30% to 40% of patients with thrombophilia may limit the potential usefulness of activated protein C as an antithrombotic agent.

THROMBOMODULIN. Thrombomodulin is an intrinsic endothelial cell–based glycoprotein that binds to thrombin, and converts thrombin's substrate specificity from fibrinogen to protein C, thus resulting in activation of protein C.[149] Activated protein C proteolytically degrades factors Va and VIIIa, thus acting as a potent anticoagulant. Soluble thrombomodulin would be an attractive antithrombotic agent compared with simple thrombin inhibitors, as it would be able to both inhibit thrombin and stimulate production of activated protein C. Recombinant human thrombomodulin (rhTM) has been produced[154] and has been shown to prolong the thrombin time, PT, and APTT. In an animal model of DIC, rhTM has been shown to inhibit coagulation in vivo, independent of plasma ATIII levels.[155]

NEW ANTIPLATELET AGENTS

Glycoprotein IIb/IIIa Antagonists

The obligatory final step in platelet aggregation is the bivalent binding of fibrinogen to functional glycoprotein IIb/IIIa molecules (αIIb/β3 integrin) on adjacent platelets.[156] Glycoprotein IIb/IIIa binds many adhesive ligands, including fibrinogen, von Willebrand's factor (vWF), fibronectin, vitronectin, and thrombospondin, but fibrinogen appears to be the principal ligand at low shear rates, most likely due to the high plasma concentration of fibrinogen.[157] Fibrinogen contains two binding sites for glycoprotein IIb/IIIa, a unique domain and a domain shared with other adhesive proteins. The shared domain

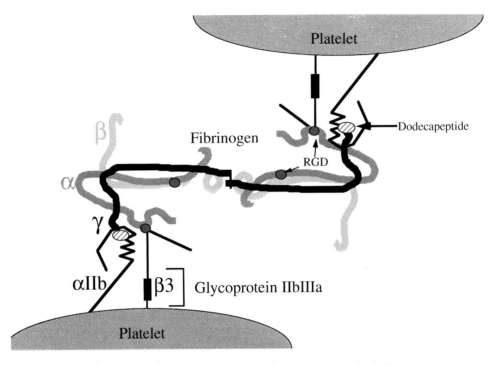

Fig. 6-8. The final step in platelet aggregation is the bridging of glycoprotein IIb/IIIa (integrin αIIb/β3) by fibrinogen. This entails binding of an arginine-glycine-asparagine *(RGD)* peptide sequence from the alpha chain of fibrinogen to the β3 integrin subunit as well as binding of the C-terminal dodecapeptide of the gamma chain of fibrinogen to the alpha IIb subunit of glycoprotein IIb/IIIa integrin. This binding site has become a target for development of a new class of antiplatelet drugs that block the binding of fibrinogen to glycoprotein PIIb/IIIa.

consists of an Arg-Gly-Asp (RGD) sequence, which is found in two locations in each of the alpha chains of fibrinogen (aa 95 through 97 and aa 572 through 574).[156,158] The adhesion domain unique to fibrinogen is a dodecapeptide at the C-terminal portion of each gamma chain, which does not contain the RGD sequence.[156,158] See Fig. 6-8.

Blockade of the binding between glycoprotein IIb/IIIa and fibrinogen has become a prime target for the development of new antithrombotic agents, due to its nature as an obligatory step in platelet aggregation. Three different categories of inhibitory compounds have been studied: (1) monoclonal antibodies against glycoprotein IIb/IIIa, (2) naturally occurring peptides that bind to glycoprotein IIb/IIIa (disintegrins), and (3) synthetic peptides based on the RGD sequence that bind to glycoprotein IIb/IIIa.[157,159] Murine monoclonal antibodies to human glycoprotein IIb/IIIa have been developed, and a chimeric antibody called c7E3 (abciximab or ReoPro) containing a murine F(ab')₂ fragment and a human Fc fragment has recently been approved by the FDA for clinical use.[157,160,161] In a large-scale clinical study (EPIC—evaluation of c7E₃ in preventing ischemic complications), c7E3 was found to reduce acute coronary complications when used during angioplasty in conjunction with heparin, although abnormal bleeding was a problem.[162] Antithrombotic doses of c7E3 were associated with markedly prolonged bleeding times and nearly complete inhibition of ADP-induced aggregation.[162]

Naturally occurring peptides that block the binding of fibrinogen to glycoprotein IIb/IIIa have been found in the venom of several types of snakes and include trigramin, echistatin, bitistatin 3, applagin, albolabrin, barbourin, elegantin, flavoridin, and kistrin.[163] The inhibitory activity of all of these compounds is due to an RGD group, held in an appropriate structural conformation by a disulfide loop.[164] In animal models the disintegrins have been shown to inhibit ADP-induced platelet aggregation in a dose-dependent manner and to prevent in vivo thrombus formation.[163,165,166] These compounds are unlikely to reach wide clinical use, however, because of problems with antigenicity and the development of thrombocytopenia during drug infusion in animal models.

Many synthetic compounds that block the binding of fibrinogen to glycoprotein IIb/IIIa have been developed, most based on the RGD binding sequence.[157,159] Cyclic compounds have been shown to be more resistant to enzymatic breakdown and can be designed with the RGD sequence held in a structural conformation suitable for binding to glycoprotein IIb/IIIa, which increases drug potency over linear forms.[167] Some of the compounds under investigation include MK-852 (Merck) and Integrelin (Cor Therapeutics).[168] Integrelin, a cyclic heptapeptide inhibitor based on a modified lysine-glycine-asparagine KGD sequence to improve the binding specificity to glycoprotein IIb/IIIa, has already undergone extensive clinical evaluation.[169] Clinical trials of Integrelin during coronary intervention (Impact trial) have shown Integrelin to be effective in inhibiting ADP-induced aggregation[169,170] but with a greater risk of bleeding compared with standard therapy. Synthetic peptide derivatives and nonpeptide inhibitors of fibrinogen binding to glycoprotein IIb/IIIa are being developed, as they may be more resistant to degradation and have a longer half-life than cyclic peptide compounds. An example of a peptide derivative compound is lamifiban (44-9883, Roche) and a nonpeptide-based compound is tirofiban (MK-383, Merck).[171] Clinical trials to test the efficacy of these nonpeptide compounds during angioplasty are under way.[172,173] Orally active glycoprotein IIb/IIIa inhibitors have been developed and have been designed as either a pro-drug or an orally active compound.[157] One such agent that has undergone limited clinical testing is xemilofiban (SC-54684A, Searle).[174]

Glycoprotein Ib/IX Antagonists

Platelet adhesion to subendothelium involves multiple components of the subendothelium, predominantly collagen and vWF, but other factors such as fibronectin, laminin, vitronectin, and thrombospondin may also be involved.[175] The binding between subendothelial vWF and the platelet surface glycoprotein Ib/IX is the primary mediator of platelet adhesion.[176] At high shear rates, the vWF/glycoprotein Ib/IX interaction is still important, but binding of vWF to glycoprotein IIb/IIIa through the RGD sequence in vWF also becomes important.[177,178] Binding sites on vWF for glycoprotein Ib/IX has been elucidated in the region containing domains A1, A2, and A3 and spanning amino acids 338 through 728.[179] There is an RGDS (Arg-Gly-Asp-Ser) sequence located at amino acids 1744 through 1747, which has been identified as the binding site for platelet glycoprotein IIb/IIIa and the αIIb/β3 integrin.[179] Because vWF interaction with platelets is an important step in platelet adhesion, the blockade of this binding has become a target for development of new antithrombotic drugs.

Strategies for inhibiting the binding of vWF to glycoprotein Ib/IX include (1) use of monoclonal antibodies against glycoprotein Ib/IX, (2) use of recombinant von Willebrand's peptide fragments, and (3) use of monoclonal antibodies to vWF or other substances that bind to vWF and block its interaction with glycoprotein Ib/IX. Monoclonal antibodies to glycoprotein Ib/IX have shown antithrombotic effects in experimental animal models, but thrombocytopenia has been an observed side effect.[180] Fragments of the A1 and A2 domain of von Willebrand's block ristocetin-induced platelet aggregation. One such fragment, comprising amino acids 445 through 733, has been shown to decrease in vitro platelet adhesion to collagen and extracellular matrix under flow conditions.[181,182] Unfractionated heparin may, however, bind to this fragment of vWF and counteract its inhibitory effect.[181] Antibodies against vWF have also shown antithrombotic effects in animal models.[183] Aurin tricarboxylic acid, a triphenylmethyl compound that inhibits the binding of glycoprotein Ib/IX to high-molecular-weight multimers of vWF inhibits ristocetin-induced platelet aggregation and shear-induced platelet aggregation.[184]

Thromboxane Receptor Antagonists

Thromboxane A_2 is an important modulator of platelet activation. Strategies have been developed for diminishing thromboxane A_2 function, either by inhibiting thromboxane synthase or blocking the platelet thromboxane A_2 receptor.[185,186] Animal studies have shown thromboxane A_2 receptor antagonists, such as vapiprost, to have antithrombotic properties greater than ticlopidine.[187] Ridogrel (Janssen) (R68070) combines both thromboxane A_2 receptor blockade with inhibition of thromboxane synthase[188] and has been shown to reduce ongoing in vivo platelet activation in patients with peripheral arterial disease in a small study.[189] Other platelet receptors have also been targeted for development of antagonists, including the serotonin receptor[190] and the platelet activating factor receptor.[191]

REFERENCES

1. Hirsh J et al: Oral anticoagulants: mechanism of action, clinical effectiveness, and optimal therapeutic range, Chest 102:312S, 1992.
2. Moriary HT, Lam-Po-Tang PR, and Anastas N: Comparison of thromboplastins using the ISI and INR system, Pathology 22:71, 1990.
3. Hull R et al: Different intensities of oral anticoagulant therapy in the treatment of proximal-vein thrombosis, N Engl J Med 307:1676, 1982.
4. Poller L and Hirsh J: Special report: a simple system for the derivation of international normalized ratios for the reporting of prothrombin time results with North American thromboplastin reagents, Am J Clin Pathol 92:124, 1989.
5. The International Committee on Thrombosis and Haemostasis, The International Committee for Standardization in Hematology: Prothrombin time standardization: report of the expert panel on oral anticoagulant control, Thromb Haemost 42:1073, 1979.
6. Meier FA and Schifman RB: The INR and monitoring of oral anticoagulation. In Data analysis and critique Q probes, Northfield, Ill, 1992, College of American Pathologists.
7. Taberner DA et al: Effect of international sensitivity index (ISI) of thromboplastins on precision of international normalized ratios (INR), J Clin Pathol 42:92, 1989.
8. Bader R et al: Multicentric evaluation of a new PT reagent based on recombinant human tissue factor and synthetic phospholipids, Thromb Haemost 71:292, 1994.
9. Hawkins PL et al: Prothrombin time reagents from recombinant human tissue factor produced in E. coli, Thromb Haemost 65:1215, 1991.
10. Bussey HI, Force RW, and Bianco TM: Reliance on prothrombin time ratios causes significant errors in anticoagulation therapy, Arch Intern Med 152:278, 1992.
11. Alving BM, Strickler MP, and Knight RD: Hereditary warfarin resistance, Arch Intern Med 145:499, 1985.
12. Landefeld CS and Goldman L: Major bleeding in outpatients treated with warfarin: incidence and prediction by factors known at the start of outpatient therapy, Am J Med 87:144, 1989.
13. Fihn SD et al: Risk factors for complications of chronic anticoagulation. A multicenter study, Ann Intern Med 118:511, 1993.
14. Gitter MJ et al: Bleeding and thromboembolism during anticoagulant therapy: a population based study in Rochester, Minnesota, Mayo Clin Proc 70:725, 1995.
15. Cole MS, Minifee PK, and Wolma FJ: Coumarin necrosis—a review of the literature, Surgery 103:271, 1988.
16. McGehee WG et al: Coumarin necrosis associated with hereditary protein C deficiency, Ann Intern Med 100:59, 1984.

17. Zauber NP and Stark MW: Successful warfarin anticoagulation despite protein C deficiency and a history of warfarin necrosis, Ann Intern Med 104:659, 1986.
18. Feder W and Auerback R: "Purple toes," an uncommon sequela of oral coumarin therapy, Ann Intern Med 55:911, 1961.
19. Lindahl U: Biosynthesis of heparin and related polysaccharides. In Lane DA and Lindahl U, eds: Heparin. Clinical and biological properties, clinical application, Boca Raton, Fla, 1989, CRC Press.
20. Thunberg L, Backstrom G, and Lindahl U: Further characterization of the antithrombin-binding sequence in heparin, Carbohydrate Res 100:393, 1982.
21. Bjork I, Olson ST, and Shore JD: Molecular mechanisms of the accelerating effect of heparin on the reactions between antithrombin and clotting proteinases. In Lane DA and Lindahl U, eds: Heparin. Clinical and biological properties, clinical application, Boca Raton, Fla, 1989, CRC Press.
22. Yamagishi R et al: Purification and biological property of heparin cofactor II; activation of heparin cofactor II and antithrombin III by dextran sulfate and various glycosaminoglycans, Thromb Res 36:633, 1984.
23. Hirsh J: Heparin. N Engl J Med 324:1565, 1991.
24. Danielsson A and Bjork I: Binding to antithrombin of heparin fractions with different molecular weights, Biochem J 193:427, 1981.
25. Barrowcliffe TW: Heparin assays and standardization. In Land DA and Lindahl U, eds: Heparin, London, 1989, Edward Arnold.
26. Brandt JT and Triplett DA: Laboratory monitoring of heparin. Effect of reagents and instruments on the activated partial thromboplastin time, Am J Clin Pathol 76:530, 1981.
27. Colvin BT: The British Society for Haematology guidelines on the use and monitoring of heparin 1992: second revision, J Clin Pathol 46:97, 1993.
28. Nielsen LE et al: Extensive thrombus formation with heparin resistance during extracorporeal circulation. A new presentation of familial antithrombin III deficiency, Arch Intern Med 147:149, 1987.
29. Young E et al: Heparin binding to plasma proteins, an important mechanism for heparin resistance, Thromb Haemost 67:639, 1992.
30. Raschke RA et al: The weight-base heparin dosing nomogram compared with a standard care nomogram, Ann Intern Med 119:874, 1993.
31. Cruickshank MK et al: A standard heparin nomogram for the management of heparin therapy, Arch Intern Med 151:333, 1991.
32. Pitney WR, Pettit JE, and Armstrong L: Control of heparin therapy, Br Med J 4:139, 1970.
33. Coon WW and Willis PW: Hemorrhagic complications of anticoagulation therapy, Arch Intern Med 133:386, 1974.
34. Glazier RL and Crowell EB: Randomized prospective trial of continuous vs. intermittent heparin therapy, JAMA 236:1365, 1976.
35. Levine MN, Raskob G, and Hirsh J: Hemorrhagic complications of long-term anticoagulation therapy, Chest 89:16S, 1986.
36. De Swiet M et al: Prolonged heparin therapy in pregnancy causes bone demineralization, Br J Obstet Gynaecol 90:1129, 1983.
37. Hirsh J and Levine MN: Low molecular weight heparin, Blood 79:1, 1992.
38. Carter CJ et al: The relationship between the hemorrhagic and antithrombotic properties of low molecular weight heparins and heparin, Blood 59:1239, 1982.

39. Warkentin TE et al: Heparin-induced thrombocytopenia in patients treated with low-molecular-weight heparin or unfractionated heparin, N Engl J Med 332:1330, 1995.
40. Boneu B: Low molecular weight heparin therapy: is monitoring needed? Thromb Haemost 72:330, 1994.
41. Harenberg J et al: Anti-factor Xa determination in blood: a new method for controlling heparin therapy, Semin Thromb Hemostas 19(suppl 1):79, 1993.
42. Simonneau G et al: Subcutaneous low-molecular-weight heparin compared with continuous intravenous unfractionated heparin in the treatment of proximal deep vein thrombosis, Arch Intern Med 153:1541, 1993.
43. Leizorovicz A et al: Comparison of efficacy and safety of low molecular weight heparins and unfractionated heparin in initial treatment of deep venous thrombosis: a meta analysis, Br Med J 309:299, 1994.
44. Thery C et al: Randomized trial of subcutaneous low-molecular-weight heparin CY216 (Fraxiparine) compared with intravenous unfractionated heparin in the curative treatment of submassive pulmonary embolism, Circulation 85:1380, 1992.
45. Prandoni P et al: Comparison of subcutaneous low-molecular-weight heparin with intravenous standard heparin in proximal deep-vein thrombosis, Lancet 339:441, 1992.
46. Lensing AWA et al: Treatment of deep venous thrombosis with low-molecular-weight heparin, Arch Intern Med 155:601, 1995.
47. Robitaille D et al: Cardiopulmonary bypass with a low-molecular-weight heparin fraction (enoxaparin) in a patient with a history of heparin-associated thrombocytopenia, J Thoracic Cardiovasc Surg 103:597, 1992.
48. Kay R, Wong KS, and Woo J: Pilot study of low-molecular-weight heparin in the treatment of acute ischemic stroke, Stroke 25:684, 1994.
49. Green D et al: Prevention of thromboembolism after spinal cord injury using low molecular weight heparin, Ann Intern Med 113:571, 1990.
50. Kroneman H et al: Pharmacokinetics of low-molecular-weight heparin and unfractionated heparin during elective aortobifemoral bypass grafting, J Vasc Surg 14:208, 1991.
51. Nurmohamed MT et al: Long term efficacy and safety of a low molecular weight heparin in chronic hemodialysis patients. A comparison with standard heparin, ASAIO Tran 37:M459, 1991.
52. Wilson NV et al: Intraoperative antithrombotic therapy with low molecular weight heparin in aortic surgery. How should heparin be administered? Eur J Vasc Surg 5:565, 1995.
53. de Valk HW et al: Comparing subcutaneous Danaparoid with intravenous unfractionated heparin for the treatment of venous thromboembolism, Ann Intern Med 123:1, 1995.
54. Ortel TL et al: Parenteral anticoagulation with the heparinoid Lomoparan (Org 10172) in patients with heparin induced thrombocytopenia and thrombosis, Thromb Hemostasis 67:292, 1992.
55. Doherty DC et al: "Heparin-free" cardiopulmonary bypass: first reported use of heparinoid (Org 10172) to provide anticoagulation for cardiopulmonary bypass, Anesthesiology 73:562, 1990.
56. Rowlings PA et al: The use of a low molecular weight heparinoid (Org 10172) for extracorporeal procedures in patients with heparin dependent thrombocytopenia and thrombosis, Aust N Z J Med 21:52, 1991.
57. Turpie AGG et al: A low-molecular-weight heparinoid compared with unfractionated heparin in the prevention

of deep vein thrombosis in patients with acute ischemic stroke, Ann Intern Med 117:353, 1992.

58. Vane JR: Inhibition of prostaglandin synthesis as a mechanism of action for aspirin-like drugs, Nature New Biol 231:232, 1971.

59. Roth GJ, Stanford N, and Majerus PW: Acetylation of prostaglandin synthase by aspirin, Proc Natl Acad Sci U S A 72:3073, 1975.

60. Tschopp TB: Aspirin inhibits platelet aggregation, but not adhesion to collagen fibrils: assessment of platelet adhesion and deposited platelet mass by morphometry and ^{51}Cr-labeling, Thromb Res 11:619, 1977.

61. Roth GJ and Calverely DC: Aspirin, platelets and thrombosis: theory and practice, Blood 83:885, 1994.

62. Stein B and Fuster V: Clinical pharmacology of platelet inhibitors. In Fuster V and Verstraete M, eds: Thrombosis in cardiovascular disorders, Philadelphia, 1992, WB Saunders.

63. Kyrle PA et al: Inhibition of prostacyclin and thromboxane A generation by low-dose aspirin at the site of plug formation in man in vivo, Circulation 75:1025, 1987.

64. Zucker MD and Peter J: Inhibition of adenosine diphosphate–induced secondary aggregation and other platelet functions by acetylsalicylic acid ingestion, Proc Soc Exp Biol Med 127:547, 1968.

65. Baumgartner HR: Effect of acetylsalicylic acid, sulfinpyrazone and dipyridamole on platelet adhesion and aggregation in flowing native and anticoagulated blood, Haemostasis 8:340, 1979.

66. Becker RC and Ansell J: Antithrombotic therapy, Arch Intern Med 155:149, 1995.

67. Clyne CAC et al: Random control trial of a short course of aspirin and dipyridamole for femorodistal grafts, Br J Surg 74:246, 1987.

68. Barnathan ES et al: Aspirin and dipyridamole in the prevention of acute coronary thrombosis, complicating coronary angioplasty, Circulation 76:125, 1987.

69. Schwartz L et al: Aspirin and dipyridamole in the prevention of restenosis after percutaneous transluminal angioplasty, N Engl J Med 318:1714, 1988.

70. Lekstrom JA and Bell WR: Aspirin in the prevention of thrombosis, Medicine 70:161, 1991.

71. Krupski WC et al: Adverse effects of aspirin in the treatment of asymptomatic carotid artery stenosis, J Vasc Surg 16:588, 1992.

72. Easton JD: Antiplatelet therapy in the prevention of stroke, Drugs 42(suppl 5):39, 1991.

73. Hawinger J, Brass LF, and Salzman EW: Signal transduction and intracellular regulatory processes in platelets. In Colman RW et al, eds: Hemostasis and thrombosis: basic principles and clinical practice, ed 3, Philadelphia, 1994, JB Lippincott.

74. Kerins DM, Murray R, and FitzGerald GA: Prostacyclin and prostaglandin E$_1$: molecular mechanisms and therapeutic utility. In Coller BS, ed: Progress in hemostasis and thrombosis, Philadelphia, 1991, WB Saunders.

75. Grant SM and Goa KL: Iloprost, a review of its pharmacodynamic and pharmacokinetic properties, and therapeutic potential in peripheral vascular disease, myocardial ischaemia and extracorporeal circulation procedures, Drugs 43:889, 1992.

76. Rademaker EDC et al: Comparison of intravenous infusions of iloprost and oral nifedipine in treatment of Raynaud's phenomenon in patients with systemic sclerosis: a double blind randomized study, Br Med J 298:561, 1989.

77. Fiessinger JN and Schafer M: Trial of iloprost versus aspirin treatment for critical limb ischaemia of thromboangiitis obliterans, Lancet 335:555, 1990.

78. Kappa JR et al: Carotid endarterectomy in patients with heparin-induced platelet activation: comparative efficacy of aspirin and iloprost (ZK36374), J Vasc Surg 5:693, 1987.

79. Kraenzler EJ and Starr NJ: Heparin-associated thrombocytopenia: management of patients for open heart surgery. Case reports describing the use of iloprost, Anesthesiology 69:964, 1988.

80. Kovacs IR, Mayou SC, and Kirby JD: Infusion of a stable prostacyclin analogue, iloprost, to patients with peripheral vascular disease: lack of antiplatelet effect, but risk of thromboembolism, Am J Med 90:41, 1991.

81. FitzGerald GA: Dipyridamole, N Engl J Med 316:1247, 1987.

82. George JN and Shattil SJ: The clinical importance of acquired abnormalities of platelet function, N Engl J Med 324:27, 1991.

83. Green D and Miller V: The role of dipyridamole in the therapy of vascular disease, Geriatrics 48:46, 1993.

84. McTavish D, Faulds D, and Goa KL: Ticlopidine, an updated review of its pharmacology and therapeutic use in platelet-dependent disorders, Drugs 40:238, 1990.

85. Defreyn G et al: Pharmacology of ticlopidine: a review, Semin Thromb Hemost 15:159, 1989.

86. Ellis DJ et al: The effects of ticlopidine hydrochloride on bleeding time and platelet function in man, Thromb Haemost 46:1973, 1981 (abstract).

87. Randi ML et al: Decrease of fibrinogen in patients with peripheral atherosclerotic disease by ticlopidine, Arzneimittelforschung 41:414, 1991.

88. Freund M et al: Experimental thrombosis on a collagen coated arterial shunt in rats: a pharmacological model to study antithrombotic agents inhibiting thrombin formation and platelet deposition, Thromb Haemost 69:515, 1993.

89. Gachet C et al: The thienopyridine PCR 4099 selectively inhibits ADP-induced platelet aggregation and fibrinogen binding without modifying the membrane glycoprotein IIb-IIIa complex in rat and in man, Biochem Pharmacol 40:229, 1990.

90. Hardisty RM, Powling MJ, and Nokes TJ: The action of ticlopidine on human platelets. Studies on aggregation, secretion, calcium mobilization and membrane glycoproteins, Thromb Haemost 64:150, 1990.

91. Flores-Runk P and Raasch RH: Ticlopidine and antiplatelet therapy, Ann Pharmacother 27:1090, 1993.

92. Ito MK, Smith AR, and Lee ML: Ticlopidine: a new platelet aggregation inhibitor, Clin Pharm 11:603, 1992.

93. Mazoyer E et al: How does ticlopidine treatment lower plasma fibrinogen? Thromb Res 75:361, 1994.

94. Bang NU: Leeches, snakes, ticks and vampire bats in today's cardiovascular drug development, Circulation 84:436, 1991.

95. Markwardt F: Inventory of coagulation inhibitors from animals feeding on blood. A report prepared on behalf of the scientific and standardization committee's registry of exogenous hemostatic factors, Thromb Haemost 72:477, 1994.

96. Haycraft JB: On the action of a secretion from the medicinal leech on the coagulation of blood, Proc R Soc 36:478, 1884.

97. Talbot M: Biology of recombinant hirudin (CGP 39393): a new prospect in the treatment of thrombosis, Semin Thromb Hemost 15:293, 1989.

98. Rydel TJ, Ravichandran KG, and Tulinsky A: The structure of a complex of recombinant hirudin and human alpha-thrombin, Science 249:277, 1990.

99. Stubbs MT and Bode W: A player of many parts: the spotlight falls on thrombin's structure, Thromb Res 69:58, 1993.

100. Maraganore JM: Thrombin, thrombin inhibitors, and the arterial thrombotic process, Thromb Haemost 70:208, 1993.

101. Skrzypczak-Jankun E et al: Structure of the hirugen and hirulog-1 complexes of alpha-thrombin, J Mol Biol 221:1379, 1991.

102. Kelly AB et al: Antithrombotic effects of synthetic peptides targeting different functional domains of thrombin, Proc Natl Acad Sci U S A 89:6040, 1992.

103. Weitz JI et al: Clot-bound thrombin is protected from inhibition by heparin–antithrombin III, but is susceptible to inactivation by antithrombin III–independent inhibitors, J Clin Invest 86:385, 1990.

104. Fox I et al: Anticoagulant activity of hirulog, a direct thrombin inhibitor, in humans, Thromb Haemostas 69:157, 1993.

105. Ginsberg JS et al: A phase II study of hirulog in the prevention of venous thrombosis after major hip or knee surgery, Circulation 86:409, 1992.

106. Topol EJ et al: Recombinant hirudin for unstable angina pectoris: a multicenter, randomized angiographic trial, Circulation 89:1557, 1994.

107. Parent F et al: Treatment of severe venous thromboembolism with intravenous hirudin (HBW 023): an open pilot study, Thromb Hemostas 70:386, 1993.

108. Walenga JM et al: Comparative studies on various assays for the laboratory evaluation of r-hirudin, Semin Thromb Hemost 17:103, 1991.

109. Powers JC and Kam CM: Synthetic substrates and inhibitors of thrombin. In Berliner LJ, ed: Thrombin: structure and function, New York, 1992, Plenum Press.

110. Harker L: Interruption of acute platelet-dependent thrombosis by the synthetic antithrombin D-phenylalanyl-L-propyl-arginyl chloromethylketone, Proc Natl Acad Sci U S A 85:3184, 1988.

111. Okamoto S, Hijikata A, and Kikumoto R: A potent inhibition of thrombin by the newly synthesized arginine derivative no. 805. The importance of stereostructure of its hydrophobic carboxamide portion, Biochem Biophys Res Commun 101:440, 1981.

112. Matsuo T et al: Effect of synthetic thrombin inhibitor (MD805) as an alternative drug on heparin induced thrombocytopenia during hemodialysis, Thromb Res 52:165, 1988.

113. Gold HK et al: Evidence for a rebound coagulation phenomenon after cessation of a 4-hour infusion of a specific thrombin inhibitor in patients with unstable angina pectoris, J Am Coll Cardiol 21:1039, 1993.

114. Callas DD, Hoppensteadt D, and Fareed J: Comparative studies on the anticoagulant and protease generation inhibitor actions of newly developed site-directed thrombin inhibitor drugs Efegatran, Argatroban, hirulog and hirudin, Semin Thromb Hemost 21:177, 1995.

115. Vu T-KH et al: Domains specifying thrombin-receptor interaction, Nature 353:674, 1991.

116. Harker LA, Maraganore JM, and Hirsh J: Novel antithrombotic agents. In Colman RW et al, eds: Hemostasis and thrombosis: basic principles and clinical practice, ed 3, Philadelphia, 1994, JB Lippincott.

117. Carney DH et al: Enhancement of incisional wound healing and neovascularization in normal rats by thrombin and synthetic thrombin receptor-activating peptides, J Clin Invest 89:1469, 1992.

118. Bock LC et al: Selection of single-stranded DNA molecules that bind and inhibit human thrombin, Nature 355:564, 1992.

119. Li WX et al: A novel nucleotide-based thrombin inhibitor inhibits clot-bound thrombin and reduces arterial platelet thrombus formation, Blood 83:677, 1994.

120. Griffin LC et al: In vivo anticoagulant properties of a novel nucleotide-based thrombin inhibitor and demonstration of regional anticoagulation in extracorporeal circuits, Blood 81:3271, 1993.

121. Fareed J et al: Recent developments in antithrombotic agents, Exp Opin Invest Drugs 4:389, 1995.

122. Paborsky LR et al: The single-stranded DNA aptamer binding-site of human thrombin, J Biol Chem 268:20808, 1993.

123. Bracht F and Schror K: Isolation and identification of aptamers from defibrotide that act as thrombin antagonists in vitro, Biochem Biophys Res Com 200:933, 1994.

124. Waxman L et al: Tick anticoagulant peptide is a novel inhibitor of blood coagulation factor Xa, Science 248:593, 1990.

125. Vlasuk GP: Structural and functional characterization of tick anticoagulant peptide (TAP): a potent and selective inhibitor of blood coagulation factor Xa, Thromb Haemost 70:212, 1993.

126. Jordan SP et al: Reaction pathway for inhibition of blood coagulation factor Xa by tick anticoagulant peptide, Biochemistry 31:5374, 1992.

127. Mellott MJ et al: Enhancement of recombinant tissue plasminogen activator-induced reperfusion by recombinant tick anticoagulant peptide, a selective factor Xa inhibitor, in a canine model of femoral arterial thrombosis, Fibrinolysis 17:195, 1993.

128. Nicolini FA et al: Superiority of selective factor Xa inhibition versus direct thrombin antagonism in facilitating rt-PA–induced thrombolysis in the canine model, Circulation 88(suppl I):545, 1993.

129. Dunwiddie C et al: Antistasin, a leech-derived inhibitor of factor Xa, J Biol Chem 264:16697, 1989.

130. Vlassuk G, Sitko G, and Shebuski R: Specific factor Xa inhibition enhances thrombolytic reperfusion and prevents acute reocclusion in the canine copper coil model of arterial thrombosis, Circulation 82(suppl III):603, 1990.

131. Schaffer LW et al: Anticoagulant efficacy of recombinant tick anticoagulant peptide, a potent inhibitor of coagulation factor Xa in a primate model of arterial thrombosis, Circulation 83:1741, 1991.

132. Sinha U et al: Expression, purification and characterization of inactive human coagulation factor Xa (Asn322Ala419), Protein Expr Purif 3:518, 1992.

133. Hollenbach S et al: A comparative study of prothrombinase and thrombin inhibitors in a novel rabbit model of non-occlusive deep vein thrombosis, Thromb Haemost 71:357, 1994.

134. Hollenbach S et al: Inhibition of arterial thrombosis by the prothrombinase complex inhibitor EGR-Xa, Blood 80:166a, 1992.

135. Jang IK et al: Antithrombotic effect of a monoclonal antibody against tissue factor in a rabbit model of platelet-mediated arterial thrombosis, Arterioscler Thromb 12:948, 1992.

136. Harker LA, Hanson SR, and Kelly AB: Antithrombotic benefits and hemorrhagic risks of direct thrombin antagonists, Thromb Haemost 74:464, 1995.

137. Voss D: Therapeutic defibrination: a new concept in anticoagulant therapy, Internist 9:389, 1968.

138. Carr M and Shen LLL: Physical studies of gels of fibrin and ancrod fibrin, Fed Proc 34:354, 1975.

139. Prentice CR et al: The fibrinolytic response to ancrod therapy: characterization of fibrinogen and fibrin degradation products, Br J Haematol 83:276, 1993.

140. Demers C et al: Rapid anticoagulation using ancrod for heparin-induced thrombocytopenia, Blood 78:2194, 1991.

141. Cole WE et al: Ancrod versus heparin for anticoagulation during vascular surgical procedures, J Vasc Surg 17:288, 1993.

142. Broze GJ: The role of tissue factor pathway inhibitor in a revised coagulation cascade, Semin Hematol 29:159, 1992.

143. Holst J et al: Antithrombotic effect of recombinant truncated tissue factor pathway inhibitor (TFPI1-161) in experimental venous thrombosis—a comparison with low molecular weight heparin, Thromb Haemost 71:214, 1994.

144. Haskel EJ, Torr SR, and Day KC: Prevention of arterial reocclusion after thrombolysis with recombinant lipoprotein-associated coagulation inhibitor, Circulation 84:821, 1991.

145. Menache D: Antithrombin III concentrate, Hematol Oncol Clin North Am 6:1115, 1992.

146. Vinazzer HA: Antithrombin III in shock and disseminated intravascular coagulation, Clin Appl Thromb/Hemost 1:62, 1995.

147. Fourier F et al: Double-blind, placebo-controlled trial of antithrombin III concentrates in septic shock with disseminated intravascular coagulation, Chest 104:882, 1993.

148. Blauhut B et al: Substitution of ATIII in shock and DIC: a randomized study, Thromb Res 39:81, 1985.

149. Esmon CT: The roles of protein C and thrombomodulin in the regulation of blood coagulation, J Biol Chem 264: 4743, 1989.

150. Sakamoto T et al: Prevention of arterial reocclusion after thrombolysis with activated protein C. Comparison with heparin in a canine model of coronary artery thrombosis, Circulation 90:427, 1994.

151. Taylor FB, Chang A, and Esmon CT: Protein C prevents the coagulopathic and lethal effects of Escherichia coli infusion in the baboon, J Clin Invest 79:918, 1987.

152. Holly RD and Foster DC: Resistance to inhibition by alpha-1-antitrypsin and species specificity of a chimeric human/bovine protein C, Biochemistry 33:1876, 1994.

153. Dahlback B: Inherited resistance to activated protein C, a major cause of venous thrombosis, is due to a mutation in the factor V gene, Haemostasis 24:139, 1994.

154. Gomi K et al: Antithrombotic effect of recombinant human thrombomodulin on thrombin-induced thromboembolism in mice, Blood 75:1396, 1990.

155. Aoki Y et al: Effect of recombinant human soluble thrombomodulin (rhsTM) on a rat model of disseminated intravascular coagulation with decreased levels of plasma antithrombin III, Thromb Haemost 71:452, 1994.

156. Phillips DR et al: The platelet membrane glycoprotein IIb-IIIa complex, Blood 71:831, 1988.

157. Lefkovits J, Plow EF, and Topol EJ: Platelet glycoprotein IIb/IIIa receptors in cardiovascular medicine, N Engl J Med 332:1553, 1995.

158. Plow EF, D'Souza SE, and Ginsberg MH: Ligand binding to GPIIb-IIIa: a status report, Semin Thromb Hemost 18:324, 1992.

159. Harker LA, Hanson SR, and Kelly AB: Antithrombotic benefits and hemorrhagic risks of direct thrombin antagonists, Thromb Haemost 74:464, 1995.

160. Coller BS et al: A murine monoclonal antibody that completely blocks the binding of fibrinogen to platelets produces a thrombasthenic-like state in normal platelets and binds to glycoproteins IIB and/or IIIa, J Clin Invest 72:325, 1983.

161. Coller BS et al: Abolition of in vivo platelet thrombus formation in primates with monoclonal antibodies to the platelet GPIIb/IIIa receptor. Correlation with bleeding time, platelet aggregation, and blockade of GPIIb/IIIa receptors, Circulation 80:1766, 1989.

162. The EPIC Investigators: Use of a monoclonal antibody directed against the platelet glycoprotein IIb/IIIa receptor in high-risk coronary angioplasty, N Engl J Med 330:956, 1994.

163. Gould RJ et al: Disintegrins: a family of integrin inhibitor proteins from viper venoms, Proc Soc Exp Biol Med 195:168, 1990.

164. Huang TF et al: Trigramin: primary structure and its inhibition of von Willebrand factor binding to glycoprotein IIb/IIIa complex on human platelets, Biochemistry 28:661, 1989.

165. Shebuski RJ et al: Prevention of canine coronary artery thrombosis with echistatin, a potent inhibitor of platelet aggregation from the venom of the viper, Echis carinatus, Thromb Haemost 64:576, 1990.

166. Musial J et al: Inhibition of platelet adhesion to surfaces of extracorporeal circuits by disintegrins. RGD-containing peptides from viper venoms, Circulation 82:261, 1990.

167. Barker PL et al: Cyclic RGD peptide analogues as antiplatelet antithrombotics, J Med Chem 35:2040, 1992.

168. Kottke-Marchant K et al: Inhibition of platelet aggregation with an infusion of MK-852 in patients with stable coronary artery disease, Blood 80(suppl 1):63a, 1992.

169. Tcheng JE et al: Multicenter, randomized, double-blind, placebo-controlled trial of the platelet integrin glycoprotein IIb/IIIa blocker Integrelin in elective coronary intervention, Circulation 91:2151, 1995.

170. Schulman SP et al: Integrelin in unstable angina: a double-blind randomized trial, Circulation 88:1608, 1993.

171. Jones CR et al: Ro 44-9833: a novel non-peptide GPIIb/IIIa antagonist in man, Thromb Haemost 69:560, 1993.

172. Kereiakes D et al: A dosing study in high-risk PTCA of MK-383, a platelet IIb/IIIa antagonist, Circulation 90:I-21, 1994.

173. Theroux P et al: A randomized double-blind controlled trial with the non-peptidic platelet GP IIb/IIIa antagonist RO 44-9883 in unstable angina, Circulation 90:I-232, 1994.

174. Cox D et al: The pharmacology of integrins, Med Res Rev 14:195, 1994.

175. Kieffer N and Phillips DR: Platelet membrane glycoproteins: functions in cellular interactions, Annu Rev Cell Biol 6:329, 1990.

176. Weiss HJ, Turitto VT, and Baumgartner HR: Effect of shear rate on platelet interaction with subendothelium in citrated and native blood. Shear rate dependent decrease of adhesion in von Willebrand's disease and the Bernard-Soulier syndrome, J Lab Clin Med 92:750, 1978.

177. Weiss HJ et al: Fibrinogen-independent platelet adhesion and thrombus formation on subendothelium mediated by glycoprotein IIb/IIIa complex at high shear rate, J Clin Invest 83:288, 1989.

178. Peterson DM et al: Shear-induced platelet aggregation requires von Willebrand factor and platelet membrane glycoproteins Ib and IIb-IIIa, Blood 69:625, 1987.

179. Ruggeri ZM and Ware J: The structure and function of von Willebrand factor, Thromb Haemost 67:594, 1992.

180. Miller JL, Thiam-Cisse M, and Drouet LO: Reduction in

thrombus formation by PG-1 F(ab')$_2$, an anti–guinea pig platelet glycoprotein Ib monoclonal antibody, Arterioscler Thromb 11:1231, 1991.

181. Alevriadou BR et al: Real-time analysis of shear-dependent thrombus formation and its blockade by inhibitors of von Willebrand factor binding to platelets, Blood 81:1263, 1993.

182. Dardik R et al: Platelet aggregation on extracellular matrix: effect of a recombinant GPIb-binding fragment of von Willebrand factor, Thromb Haemost 70:522, 1993.

183. Bellinger DA et al: Prevention of occlusive coronary artery thrombosis by a murine monoclonal antibody to porcine vWF, Proc Natl Acad Sci U S A 84:8100, 1987.

184. Phillips MD et al: Aurin tricarboxylic acid: a novel inhibitor of the association of von Willebrand factor and platelets, Blood 72:1898, 1988.

185. Smith BJ: Pharmacology of thromboxane synthetase inhibitors, Fed Proc 46:139, 1987.

186. Kotze HF et al: In vivo inhibition of acute platelet-dependent thrombosis in a baboon model by BAY U3405, a thromboxane A$_2$-receptor antagonist, Thromb Haemost 70:672, 1993.

187. Takiguchi Y, Wada K, and Nakashima M: Comparison of the inhibitor effect of the TXA$_2$ receptor antagonist, Vapiprost, and other antiplatelet drugs on arterial thrombosis in rats: Possible role of TXA$_2$, Thromb Haemost 68:460, 1992.

188. De Clerck F et al: R68070: Thromboxane A$_2$ synthetase inhibition and thromboxane A$_2$/prostaglandin endoperoxide receptor blockade combined in one molecule. II. Pharmacological effects in vivo and ex vivo, Thromb Haemost 61:43, 1989.

189. Hoet B et al: Ridogrel, a combined thromboxane synthase inhibitor and receptor blocker, decreases elevated plasma β-thromboglobulin levels in patients with documented peripheral arterial disease, Thromb Haemost 64:87, 1990.

190. Herbert JM et al: Potentiating effect of clopidogrel and SR 46349, a novel 5HT$_2$ antagonist, on streptokinase-induced thrombolysis in the rabbit, Thromb Haemost 69:268, 1993.

191. Herbert JM et al: Biochemical and pharmacological activities of SR 27417, a highly potent, long acting platelet activating factor receptor antagonist, J Pharmacol Exp Ther 259:44, 1991.

CHAPTER SEVEN

THROMBOLYTIC THERAPY

Anthony J. Comerota

Thrombolytic therapy is an important part of the care of patients with peripheral vascular disease, including patients with venous thromboembolism, arterial and bypass graft thrombosis, arterial embolism, thrombosed dialysis access grafts, and stroke. Less frequently patients with mesenteric ischemic (arterial and venous origin) renal artery occlusion and portal vein thrombosis have also been treated successfully with plasminogen activators.

Keys to successful therapy are proper patient selection, familiarity with the underlying disease, an understanding of the plasminogen-plasmin system, and knowledge of the available plasminogen activators. This chapter gives an overview of the fibrinolytic system and the available plasminogen activators, and concludes with a brief review of the indications for clinical use in patients with peripheral vascular disease.

Under physiologic conditions the body maintains an equilibrium between the coagulation and the fibrinolytic systems.[1] Complex interrelationships exist in which fibrin formation stimulates physiologic fibrinolysis. Since 1950 physicians have recognized that pharmacologic stimulation of the patient's fibrinolytic system could be therapeutically effective.[2]

Physicians involved in the management of patients with thromboembolic disorders of the arterial and venous systems should understand the interactions of the coagulation and fibrinolytic systems and the pharmacologic applications of plasminogen activation.

FIBRINOLYTIC SYSTEM

The primary purpose of the fibrinolytic system in humans is the physiologic dissolution of thrombi. Fibrinolysis is initiated by plasminogen activators, which activate the zymogen plasminogen to plasmin (Fig. 7-1), the key enzyme in this system, which is responsible for clot and thrombus dissolution. At least two distinct physiologic plasminogen activators have been identified: tissue-type

Supported in part by NIH Grant K 07 HL02658.

plasminogen activator (t-PA) and urokinase-type plasminogen activator (u-PA).

At least two physiologic pathways activate plasminogen to plasmin. Intrinsic activators consist of components normally found in the blood and include proteins of the contact phase of blood coagulation such as factor XII, and kallikrein, which can interact and generate plasmin at least in vitro. The physiologic relevance of these mechanisms is presently uncertain. Extrinsic activators arise from cells and tissues including vascular endothelial cells and neoplastic cells and are the main physiologic activators. These include t-PA and u-PA. The amount of plasmin generated by these pathways is the principal mechanism that the body calls on to dissolve intravascular thrombi; however, the rate at which this occurs may be too slow in many clinical situations. The overall goal of pharmacologic manipulation of the fibrinolytic system is to supply sufficient quantities of exogenous plasminogen activators in a well-controlled manner to induce rapid lysis of intravascular thrombi and restore blood flow, thereby minimizing the consequences of compromised perfusion. This topic has been addressed in several excellent reviews.[3,4]

Plasminogen

Plasminogen is synthesized in the liver and found in human plasma and serum in an average concentration of 21 mg/dl. It is a single-chain polypeptide with a molecular weight of 92,000 Da containing 790 amino acids with 24 disulfide bonds.[5,6] In addition there are five homologous triple-loop structures known as "kringles." Activators convert plasminogen to the two-chain plasmin molecule by cleavage of a single peptide bond (arginine 560–valine 561 bond), which splits the molecule into the heavy chain and light chain. The amino terminal 76 residues of native plasminogen (Glu-plasminogen) constitutes the activation peptide, which is released by plasmin, producing a smaller molecule containing an amino terminal lysine called Lys-plasminogen.[7] Lys-plasminogen has a much higher affinity for binding to fibrin both in purified systems and in plasma and also has greater reactivity with

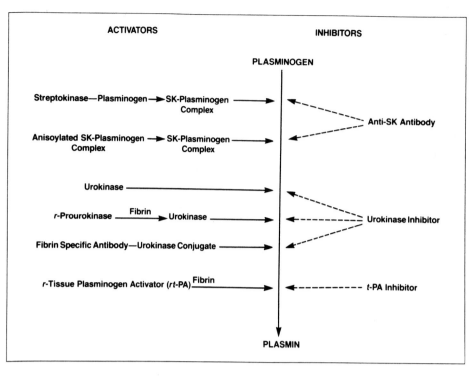

Fig. 7-1. Pathways of plasminogen activation to plasmin demonstrates the interaction of plasminogen activators as well as inhibitors of plasminogen activation. *(From Rubin RN: Streptokinase. In Comerota AJ, ed: Thrombolytic therapy for peripheral vascular disease, Philadelphia, 1995, JB Lippincott. Reproduced with permission.)*

plasminogen activators.[8] Plasminogen binding sites are present on fibrin molecules, are exposed by proteolysis, and have a particular affinity for Lys-plasminogen.[9] Therefore the formation of Lys-plasminogen accelerates and improves the efficiency of plasmin formation with subsequent fibrin dissolution. The heavy-chain portion of the molecule contains the kringles, which contribute to fibrin binding and interaction with plasminogen activators.[6,10]

Plasmin

Plasmin is a serine protease composed of two polypeptide chains linked by disulfide bonds. The light chain contains the enzyme's catalytic site.[11] Because plasminogen (Lys-plasminogen) is usually bound to fibrin, it can be converted by plasminogen activators to plasmin at the localized site of fibrin deposition, which is the primary focus of fibrinolytic activity.[12] Any plasminogen activation that occurs in the surrounding fluid phase is promptly neutralized by α_2-antiplasmin. Thus physiologic thrombolysis is a well-controlled and localized process (Fig. 7-2). Plasmin cleaves protein and peptide molecules at arginyl-lysyl bonds. In addition to fibrin and fibrinogen, plasmin hydrolyzes the coagulation factors V and VIII, components of serum complement, adrenocorticotropic hormone (ACTH), growth hormone, and glucagon. Plasmin also cleaves the activation peptide from plasminogen, which serves to further accelerate plasmin formation from Lys-plasminogen as part of a positive-feedback system.

Inhibitors

Plasmin's wide-ranging activity can have a profound effect on a large number of plasma proteins. Human

plasma contains inhibitors designed to regulate the activity of proteolytic enzymes.[13-15] α_2-plasmin inhibitor is the principal physiologic plasmin inhibitor. It is fast-acting and has the strongest affinity for plasmin, creating inactive plasmin-plasmin inhibitor complexes.[16] It is present in plasma in concentrations of 1 μM. A much slower-acting inhibitor, α_2-macroglobulin, exists in a concentration of approximately 3 μM.[16] The primary function of α_2-macroglobulin is to bind plasmin after α_2-plasmin inhibitor is depleted. Although the plasmin–α_2-macroglobulin complexes are active, they are rapidly removed from the circulation. Other plasmin inhibitors include α_1-antitrypsin, antithrombin III, and C1 esterase inhibitor—but they have a minimal physiologic effect in the blood. Plasminogen activator inhibitors are also important in the control of fibrinolysis. Inhibitors of t-PA and u-PA have been identified in human plasma[17] and derived from human platelets.[18] Other inhibitors have been obtained from cultured endothelial cells, from human umbilical vein, hepatoma cells, placenta, monocytes, and human fibroblasts.

Breakdown Products of Fibrinolysis

Under physiologic conditions the action of plasmin is limited to the site of fibrin deposition.[19] Circulating inhibitors bind to plasmin, forming inactive complexes, thus preventing breakdown of fibrinogen, clotting factors, and other circulating proteins. With the exogenous administration of plasminogen activators, or under certain pathologic conditions, plasmin levels exceed the inhibitor's capacity, resulting in a systemic plasminemia with breakdown of plasma proteins, especially fibrinogen. The

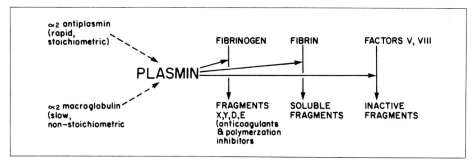

Fig. 7-2. Basic physiology of fibrinolysis. *(From Rubin RN: Streptokinase. In Comerota AJ, ed: Thrombolytic therapy for peripheral vascular disease, Philadelphia, 1995, JB Lippincott. Reproduced with permission.)*

action of plasmin on fibrinogen results in the segmental formation of several peptides including fragment X ($M_r = 250,000$ Da), which is degraded to yield fragments Y ($M_r = 150,000$), and D ($M_r = 100,000$). Fragment Y is degraded to yield fragments D and E ($M_r = 50,000$).[19,20]

Plasmin's action on non–cross-linked fibrin is identical to that on fibrinogen in the rate of breakdown and the end products except that B-β_{15-42} peptide rather than B-β_{1-42} is produced on cleavage of the B-β chain of fibrin. These peptides have been used to assess specific breakdown of fibrinogen versus fibrin by plasmin. Mature fibrin contains factor XIIIa–induced intramolecular bonds, causing a slower degradation by plasmin as well as different end products. D-Dimer is a unique derivative of the proteolysis of cross-linked moieties from adjacent fibrin monomers, which have been covalently bound by factor XIIIa.[21,22]

Plasminogen Activators

Since 1950 physicians have used plasminogen activators to dissolve fibrin in an attempt to improve patients' clinical outcome.[2] These activators have evolved from relatively impure and highly antigenic substances to pure, less antigenic and increasingly fibrin-specific agents. The ongoing improvement of these fibrinolytic agents, in addition to our increasing knowledge of the coagulation and fibrinolytic systems, will allow safer and more effective use of these agents.

The plasminogen activators currently in clinical use include streptokinase (SK), urokinase (UK) recombinant tissue plasminogen activator (rt-PA), prourokinase (proUK; also termed single-chain UK plasminogen activator [SCUPA]), and acyl-plasminogen SK activator complex (APSAC).

STREPTOKINASE. SK was first discovered in 1933 by Tillett and Garner[23] and was the first thrombolytic agent approved for clinical use. SK is a nonenzyme protein containing 415 amino acids with a molecular weight of 437,000, produced by group C β-hemolytic streptococci.[24] SK by itself is incapable of directly converting plasminogen to plasmin and therefore is not an enzyme. It indirectly activates plasminogen by forming a 1:1 complex with human plasminogen. This complex undergoes a conformational change to expose an active site on the plasminogen molecule. The plasminogen-SK complex is then capable of activating other plasminogen molecules to plasmin. An SK-plasmin complex also forms that is further capable of catalyzing plasminogen to plasmin. The various

cleavage products are SK fragments ranging in molecular weight from 10,000 to 40,000 Da, all of which are able to complex to plasminogen. These fragments have from 50% to 60% of the antigenic potential of the parent molecule. SK is highly antigenic and has the potential to cause allergic reactions. Patients with recent exposure to streptococci, or those recently treated with SK, have a high level of circulating antistreptococcal antibodies capable of neutralizing SK. Therefore patients who are resistant to SK therapy at standard doses may respond to higher doses. In vivo the activator complex formed by SK has a half-life of approximately 23 minutes.[25] In vitro testing is available to determine the SK dose needed for systemic fibrinogenolysis, although 95% of patients will be effectively treated by the standard recommended doses (bolus of 250,000 IU followed by 100,000 IU/hr infused intravenously).

SK has various systemic effects on the plasma coagulation and fibrinolytic systems and on platelets. Circulating levels of plasminogen and fibrinogen are markedly decreased during SK therapy. Systemic fibrinogenolysis results in increased plasma fibrinogen-split products; plasmin activity also causes a reduction of clotting factors V and VIII. These reductions alter normal hemostasis, which contributes to the increased hemorrhagic complications. Concomitantly there is a decrease in plasma plasminogen and plasma α_2-plasmin inhibitor. In addition there is evidence that platelets are also altered.[26] These effects are noted without exception with all of the thrombolytic agents, although SK appears to have a more pronounced effect than rt-PA. The major disadvantage of SK is its bacterial origin and antigenicity, which results in antibody formation in all patients, precluding reuse of SK within at least 6 months.

UROKINASE. UK was first isolated by MacFarlane and Pilling[27] in 1946 and Williams[28] in 1951. UK is a double-chain trypsinlike protease with a molecular weight of 54,000 to 57,000 Da. It was observed early on by several investigators that UK could exist in several molecular weights of approximately 22,000, 33,000 and 54,000 Da. The lower-molecular-weight molecules are fragments of the larger ones. The complete primary amino acid sequence of UK has been characterized.[29] Plasmin and kallikrein cleave proUK at position 156, which then produces UK in its two-chain form. The two chains are held together by a disulfide bond, which is important for the fibrinolytic activity of UK.

The preparations of UK used therapeutically are either extracted from human urine (as in the past) or are isolated from cultures of human fetal kidney cells (currently). UK can also be produced by recombinant genetic engineering in *Escherichia coli*. The problem in the production of UK from urine is the need for large quantities to produce adequate amounts of enzyme. Fifteen hundred liters of urine are required for the production of enough enzyme to treat one patient. The tissue culture techniques demonstrated by Bernik and Kwaan[30] indicated that improved production of UK could be achieved, and that the best fibrinolytic activity was seen in cultures from cells taken from 26- to 32-week fetuses. Recombinant DNA technology is now being used to produce recombinant-UK, which appears to have a similar clinical profile in terms of efficacy and safety to tissue culture UK.

UK converts the inactive forms of plasminogen to plasmin, with greater affinity for the fibrin-bound Lys-plasminogen. The conversion is due to the cleavage of a single Arg-560–Val bond. Activation of the fibrin-bound plasminogen allows fibrinolysis to occur in a relatively inhibitor-free environment, since there are no competing substrates for fibrin-bound plasmin. UK is rapidly cleared by the liver with about 3% to 5% cleared by the kidneys. It has a short half-life of about 16 minutes, which might be prolonged in patients with liver disease.

Although UK induces systemic fibrinogenolysis, it is not as intense as with SK. Because of the increased production costs of UK, the price of the drug is five to eight times that of SK for the treatment of an individual patient.

TISSUE PLASMINOGEN ACTIVATOR. The development of relatively fibrin-specific plasminogen activators was made possible once physiologic t-PA was extracted from human vascular endothelium,[31] and it was shown that the endothelial extract induced highly specific clot lysis when compared with the activity of SK or UK.[32] t-PA is a single-chain polypeptide serine protease with a molecular weight of approximately 68,000. The principal site of in vivo synthesis is the endothelial cell. It was initially purified from culture fluid of Bowes melanoma cells and other mammalian tissues but is now synthesized by recombinant DNA techniques.[33]

t-PA exists as a single chain that is rapidly converted to a double-chain form by enzymatic cleavage of the peptide bond Arg-275–Ile-276. In the absence of fibrin, t-PA is relatively inactive, but in the presence of fibrin, there is a 500-fold to 1000-fold increase of plasminogen activation.[34] This is due to an increased affinity of fibrin-bound t-PA for plasminogen. The high affinity of t-PA for plasminogen in the presence of fibrin allows activation of plasminogen on the clot, thus sparing plasma plasminogen. The half-life of t-PA is approximately 2 to 6 minutes due to binding by the rapid t-PA inhibitors and clearance by the liver. t-PA exists in plasma in both a free state and complexed with plasma serine protease inhibitors.

Although preliminary studies suggested that t-PA is fibrin specific and capable of inducing thrombolysis without causing systemic lytic effects,[35-37] overwhelming evidence from large trials indicate that therapeutic doses of rt-PA also induce systemic fibrinogenolysis, albeit less intense than with SK.[38,39] The first human application of

t-PA from melanoma cells was in a renal transplant recipient who suffered an iliofemoral venous thrombosis.[40] Extensive experience in acute myocardial infarction and pulmonary embolism indicate rt-PA is a highly effective thrombolytic agent.[41-44]

Although it was originally anticipated that the in vitro fibrin selectivity of rt-PA would result in fewer bleeding complications, this has not been borne out in clinical trials. The main reason is the inability of all of the potent thrombolytic agents to discriminate between thrombi responsible for hemostasis at sites of vascular breach and pathologic thrombi for which it is being administered to dissolve.

PROUROKINASE. A single-chain precursor to high-molecular-weight UK, proUK was isolated from urine in 1979.[45]

ProUK has been identified in human plasma, cultures of endothelial cells, explants of fetal organs, and various malignant cell lines.[46] This proenzyme is derived from human urine or genetically manipulated *E. coli* and has a molecular weight of approximately 54 kd.

ProUK is converted to high-molecular-weight UK by hydrolysis of the lysine 158–isoleucine 159 peptide bond. ProUK is not very effective as a plasminogen activator; however, this cleavage converts proUK into its two-chain structure and increases its activity 500-fold to 1000-fold.[41] ProUK differs from UK in several characteristics, mainly its higher fibrin affinity, lower specific activity, and its stability in plasma. Fibrin specificity of proUK does not depend on actual fibrin binding like t-PA, thus the mechanism of clot lysis is different between the two.[46] The half-life of proUK is approximately 7 minutes.

Studies with proUK in rabbits, dogs, and baboons demonstrated fibrin-selective clot lysis without fibrinogenolytic effects or hemorrhagic complications.[47] ProUK testing in dogs also revealed that although proUK had superior fibrin specificity, it was equal to UK in efficacy.[48]

The initial clinical application in humans was for acute myocardial infarction. A small pilot study followed by a multicenter study of acute myocardial infarction demonstrated a 60% reperfusion rate in patients with proven coronary artery thrombosis. Fifty mg of proUK was used with a mean time to lysis of approximately 55 minutes. Increasing the dose to 70 to 80 mg increased reperfusion to almost 70%; however, time to lysis was prolonged and several patients developed systemic fibrinogenolysis.[46] No hemorrhagic effects were noted. Additional studies combining UK and proUK as well as t-PA and proUK demonstrated a synergistic response between these agents because of complementary mechanisms of action.[49]

ACYLATED PLASMINOGEN-STREPTOKINASE ACTIVATOR COMPLEX. SK has significant fibrinogenolytic effects reflecting the wide-ranging proteolysis resulting from its use. In an effort to create a more efficient SK molecule with greater fibrin specificity, its molecular structure was modified. The addition of an acyl group accomplished the goal of improving fibrin specificity. Furthermore, the acyl group blocked the binding site of antistreptococcal antibodies, thereby eliminating its inactivation in plasma by the circulating inhibitors.[50,51]

The acylated SK molecule therefore is essentially inert

regarding the activation of plasminogen to plasmin in vitro. On the other hand, the acylation has little, if any, effect on the binding of the plasminogen-SK complex to fibrin. Since the fibrin binding site and the functionally active catalytic site are spacially separate, this compound retains its ability to bind to fibrin despite its lack of enzymatic activity when freely circulating. Activation then occurs via hydrolysis in which the compound deacylates to give free activator complex and anisic acid in equal concentrations. Since the majority of the deacylation occurs after fibrin binding, the result is improved concentration of the activator complex bound to fibrin and a relatively little amount of free activator complex circulating systemically. The deacylation half-life in plasma is approximately 90 to 105 minutes.[25] Since deacylation governs plasma clearance, the compound has a true half-life of approximately 90 to 105 minutes, with fibrinolytic activity persisting for 4 to 6 hours.

In trials of acyl-SK in rabbits and guinea pigs, this compound had higher thrombolytic activity compared with an equal amount of nonacylated SK complex and did not cause systemic fibrinogenolysis. A comparison of SK with acylated SK in a dog model of jugular venous thrombosis and pulmonary embolism demonstrated a minimal lytic response with SK; however, thrombolysis was radiographically complete with acylated SK. There was, however, significant fibrinogenolysis with a decrease in the circulating fibrinogen levels to approximately 50%.

Studies in human volunteers demonstrated the relative potency of APSAC and confirmed its potential to break down fibrinogen and deplete α_2-antiplasmin.[52,53] A 5-mg dose of APSAC is equivalent to 178,000 IU of SK.

Human trials in acute myocardial infarction show good recanalization rates (approximately 70%); however, these studies demonstrated a higher systemic fibrinogenolytic effect than was anticipated from the original animal data. Half the treated patients demonstrated fibrinogen levels of 30% or less. Decreases in plasminogen levels and α_2-plasmin inhibitor were likewise observed.[25]

The primary advantages of acylated SK are the prolonged half-life and the convenience of bolus administration.

CLINICAL APPLICATION OF THROMBOLYTIC AGENTS

Plasminogen activators have been used for patients suffering thrombotic and embolic problems, both on the arterial and venous side of the circulations (see box, this page). The clinical problems encompass many and diverse specialties that have an interest in the care of patients with thromboembolic disorders. During the past decade data have emerged demonstrating both acute and long-term benefits to patients treated for myocardial infarction, pulmonary embolism, venous thrombosis, arterial and graft occlusion, and stroke. This chapter presents short summaries of these applications.

The major concern with the use of all thrombolytic agents is hemorrhage. Although most hemorrhagic complications occur at sites of vascular invasion (current or recent), intracranial bleeding is the most devastating and

CLINICAL APPLICATIONS OF THROMBOLYTIC AGENTS

Myocardial infarction
- Reduction in mortality
- Improvement of ventricular function
- Slightly increased early mortality

Pulmonary embolism
- Rapid improvement of cardiopulmonary hemodynamics
- Improvement of long-term cardiopulmonary hemodynamics
- Reduction in mortality with "massive pulmonary embolism"

Acute deep vein thrombosis
- Improvement of patency of deep venous system
- Reduction of postthrombotic symptoms
- Preservation of long-term venous function

Axillo-subclavian vein thrombosis

Acute arterial and graft occlusion
- Graft salvage
- Reduction in major amputation
- Survival benefit (?)

Intraoperative intraarterial thrombolysis
- Bolus dose safe
- Isolated limb perfusion safe and effective

Other applications
- Thrombosed hemodialysis access grafts
- Mesenteric embolism/thrombosis
- Budd-Chiari syndrome
- Acute renal artery or renal vein thromboembolic occlusion
- Acute thrombosis of portosystemic shunts
- Thrombosis of central catheters

feared. Hemorrhagic complications have diminished with experience; however, hemorrhage continues to represent a source of morbidity and is the main reason why many patients are not offered lytic therapy. It is difficult to adequately place bleeding complications into a generic perspective since the risks versus benefits of treatment vary by indication. The reader is referred to the specific references by indication to appropriately estimate the risks of bleeding complication for a particular clinical problem.

Myocardial Infarction

Although the treatment of myocardial infarction is not considered part of peripheral vascular disease, lytic therapy has had such a profound impact on the care of these patients, it deserves several comments.

The medical community has witnessed a marked improvement in the treatment of myocardial infarction during the past 15 years. Mortality rates have decreased by 30% in patients who are eligible for myocardial reperfusion compared with conventional therapy.

Appreciating that coronary artery thrombosis is the underlying pathophysiology of acute myocardial infarction,[54] treatment aimed at eliminating the thrombotic occlusion and correcting underlying coronary artery disease has resulted in preserving myocardium, preserving ventricular function, and reducing mortality.[55] Due to the considerable interest in this area, more patients have been studied in prospective randomized trials of fibrinolytic therapy for the treatment of myocardial infarction than any other disease entity. Measured benefits of thrombolysis include reduction in mortality, improved left ventricular function, and improved patency of the infarct-related coronary artery.

There is a slight but apparent increased initial risk to patients treated with lytic therapy, demonstrated by a higher "early" mortality. Accepting this increased risk is due to cerebral hemorrhage, myocardial rupture, reperfusion arrhythmias, and other unexplained factors.[56] Accepting this increase in early risk appears more than justified considering the significantly reduced late mortality of patients treated with lytic therapy compared with controls. Many studies have demonstrated improved left ventricular function as a result of thrombolysis.[57] Although it might be intuitive that coronary artery patency would be improved following thrombolysis, this has been objectively confirmed,[58,59] with smaller infarct size associated with improved reperfusion.[60] A large recent trial demonstrated that 30-day mortality was related to coronary artery patency, and that accelerated thrombolysis was beneficial.[61]

Current efforts are directed at further improving outcomes by more rapid thrombolysis to obtain earlier reperfusion, and preserving patency of the infarct-related coronary artery with the use of newer antithrombotic agents.

Pulmonary Embolism

The benefit of thrombolytic therapy for the treatment of patients with pulmonary embolism was initially clarified by the National Institutes of Health (NIH)-sponsored trials,[62,63] which showed that SK and UK restored pulmonary perfusion that was demonstrated angiographically, and reduced pulmonary artery pressure and right ventricular end-diastolic pressure compared with standard heparin anticoagulation therapy. There was an increased risk of bleeding complications in the lytic group; however, this was attributed to the frequent invasive diagnostic testing and monitoring required as part of the protocols. Patients treated with heparin also had a substantially higher rate of bleeding than commonly observed.

A frequent criticism of lytic therapy for pulmonary embolism is that prior trials failed to show a mortality benefit from thrombolysis. However, prior trials were not designed to show a mortality benefit. Since this was not a primary or secondary end point, one cannot expect meaningful data in this regard. Furthermore, if patients entered into prior trials were not likely to die of their pulmonary embolism (PE), failure to show a reduction in mortality with lytic therapy is not a reasonable criticism. Therefore other measurable parameters should be evaluated.

Thirty-day and one-year follow-up physiologic studies of oxygen-diffusing capacity and pulmonary capillary blood volume showed significant improvement in patients treated with lytic therapy.[64] Although these results may not appear as "clinically relevant," since this testing is not part of the routine evaluation of patients with pulmonary or cardiopulmonary disease, these measurements do evaluate the functional unit of the lung.

Seven years following randomization into the prospective NIH trials, 21 patients were restudied with right-sided heart catheterization.[65] Patients initially randomized to receive thrombolysis for their acute PE had significantly lower pulmonary vascular resistance at rest and after exercise. There was also a trend toward better cardiopulmonary function at a clinical level in those whose PEs were lysed.

The recently performed PIOPED study[66] (Prospective Investigation of Pulmonary Embolism Diagnosis) reported the 1-year follow-up of 399 patients diagnosed with pulmonary emboli. Although reporting only a 2.5% early mortality in these patients with pulmonary emboli, there was progressive and significant mortality in all patients followed for up to 1 year. Patients treated with anticoagulation therapy alone had a 19% 1-year mortality compared with 9% for patients treated with lytic therapy. Although treatment was not randomized, these observations suggest that thrombolytic therapy for acute PE would improve long-term prognosis.

More contemporary clinical trials evaluating lytic therapy for PE uniformly demonstrated hemodynamic and angiographic improvement in patients treated with lytic agents.[44,67-75] High-dose early administration of rt-PA restored perfusion and lysed pulmonary emboli more rapidly compared with standard-dose UK, but by 6 hours lysis appeared equivalent. However, high doses of UK infused early demonstrated equivalence with rt-PA in terms of early and late lysis.[74]

Interestingly, right ventricular function also improved in patients with moderate to severe pulmonary embolism treated with lytic therapy.[44,75] A multicenter trial randomized 101 patients to either 100 mg of rt-PA over 2 hours followed by heparin or heparin alone. This was the largest randomized trial for PE since the NIH-sponsored trials. Results demonstrated marked improvement in right ventricular function and pulmonary perfusion compared with heparin alone.[75]

Current data support the use of thrombolytic therapy for acute PE; however, some physicians believe that the added risk and cost of thrombolytic agents outweigh their benefits. A trial currently under way is designed to answer the important question of whether lytic therapy for acute PE actually saves lives and/or reduces recurrent pulmonary emboli compared with conventional anticoagulation therapy.

Acute Deep Vein Thrombosis

The routine treatment for acute deep vein thrombosis (DVT) remains intravenous anticoagulation with heparin followed by oral anticoagulation with a warfarin compound. Such treatment effectively reduces the risk of pulmonary embolism; however, it does little to eliminate the clot in the deep venous system. Some patients may physiologically lyse their clot over time with minimal long-term symptoms. Others, however, have less effective physiologic lysis and have more severe postthrombotic symptoms. Physicians experiencing this inconsistent outcome believe that many patients do well with anticoagulation therapy and consider those with the postthrombotic syndrome to be the result of the adverse consequences of the disease and not a result of inadequate treatment for the acute DVT.

Natural history studies have demonstrated that the combination of obstruction and valvular incompetence produced the highest ambulatory venous pressures and the most severe postthrombotic syndrome.[76,77] As might be anticipated, rapid lysis of venous clot preserves valvular function; however, the concept of "rapid lysis" has recently changed.[78] Investigators have demonstrated that thrombosed vein segments undergoing "physiologic lysis" within 60 to 90 days of thrombosis have a significantly better chance of preserving valve function than those segments with delayed or no lysis.[79]

Pooled data from 13 studies that treated patients with either thrombolytic therapy or standard anticoagulation therapy after making the diagnosis with ascending phlebography and evaluating the outcome of therapy with repeat phlebography demonstrated significantly improved return of patency to the deep venous system in patients treated with thrombolytic therapy.[80] Results of thrombolysis have demonstrated improved symptomatic outcome in patients treated with lytic therapy[81,82] and improved long-term venous function in patients enjoying successful lysis.[83]

In light of these data, it appears reasonable to use plasminogen activators to accelerate lysis of acute DVT.

Lytic therapy has been used in patients with the most severe manifestations of acute DVT—namely, those patients with iliofemoral DVT, many of whom present with phlegmasia cerulea dolens. Failure is common with systemic delivery, since extensive venous thrombosis is the rule in these patients. Investigators have found improved outcome with direct intrathrombus infusion.[84-86] A strategy designed to eliminate thrombus in the iliofemoral venous system, restore unobstructed venous drainage into the vena cava, and prevent rethrombosis has yielded gratifying results.[84]

Axillo-Subclavian Vein Thrombosis

Treatment of acute primary axillo-subclavian vein thrombosis has evolved over the past several years. This has been spearheaded by Machleder.[87] Ineffective treatment of axillo-subclavian vein thrombosis is associated with prolonged disability in 25% to 74% of patients.[87-91]

Coupling catheter-directed thrombolysis with removal of extrinsic compression by first rib resection and correcting any residual intrinsic vein lesion, the long-term disability rate has been reduced to approximately 12%.[87] Interestingly, when bilateral phlebography was performed, a contralateral venous deformity at the thoracic

outlet was observed in 65% of the patients. This deformity is thought to represent a precursor to the acute thrombotic event.

Catheter-directed thrombolysis has also been used for treatment of secondary axillo-subclavian vein thrombosis.[92] Patients may present with the superior vena caval syndrome as a result of secondary subclavian vein thrombosis. Restoring patency in these patients will relieve acute symptoms, reduce the incidence of pulmonary embolism, restore patency to important veins required for venous access, and reduce chronic morbidity.

Acute Arterial and Graft Occlusion

Catheter-directed thrombolysis has become an established technique in most centers for the treatment of acute arterial and graft occlusion.[93] Refinements continue to be made in patient selection as well as the mechanics of drug delivery.

Direct delivery of plasminogen activators into the thrombus has demonstrated significant advantage in patients with peripheral arterial and graft occlusion. The most pertinent current question is which patient should be treated with thrombolysis and which patient should be treated surgically?

Most clinicians have appreciated that passage of a guidewire into and through the occlusion and proper embedding of the catheter into the occlusion are good prognostic indicators of success. Following successful lysis, it is imperative that the underlying cause of thrombosis be identified and corrected. Frequently arteriograms may not demonstrate an underlying lesion due to overlap of contrast material, particularly at anastomotic sites. If a patient has an underlying hypercoagulable disorder, this must be identified and treated.

Lower-extremity bypass graft occlusion is a common problem requiring catheter-directed thrombolysis. It has been noted that thrombosed suprainguinal bypass grafts enjoy a somewhat higher success rate from catheter-directed thrombolysis than occluded infrainguinal bypass grafts.[94,95]

When treating infrainguinal occluded bypass grafts, prosthetic grafts appear to have a higher initial success rate compared with autogenous vein grafts. However, due to an accelerated early failure rate of recanalized prosthetic grafts, recanalized saphenous vein grafts enjoy a better long-term patency rate.[96] As previously mentioned, the identification and correction of an underlying lesion is critical to long-term success. Grafts that have their underlying lesion corrected have significantly longer secondary patency than grafts without the lesion corrected, or without a lesion identified.

Two prospective randomized trials comparing catheter-directed thrombolysis with surgical revascularization have been completed. A single-center trial randomized 114 patients presenting with acute limb ischemia of less than 7 days duration to either catheter-directed UK or operative revascularization.[97] Angiographically successful thrombolysis was achieved in 70% of the patients randomized to the thrombolytic arm. An identifiable defect responsible for arterial bypass graft occlusion was found in only 37% of the patients. Primary amputation, overall major amputation, and in-hospital mortality were no different between the two treatment arms. Major bleeding was more common in the thrombolysis patients compared with those randomized to surgery (9% vs. 2%, $P = 0.09$). Interestingly, at 1 year, amputation-free survival was 75% in patients randomized to thrombolysis compared with 52% in patients randomized to surgery ($P = 0.03$). This difference was due mainly to the reduced mortality in the thrombolysis group, which was 16% as compared with 42% in the surgical group ($P = 0.02$). There was no difference in major amputation between the two groups.

Whether this mortality benefit is real or chance observation limited to this study remains to be proven. Interestingly a different prospective randomized trial (blinded and placebo controlled) of intraoperative UK infusion demonstrated a significant mortality benefit in patients receiving UK compared with those who received placebo.[98] This incidental but intriguing observation from these two prospective randomized studies justifies a prospective clinical trial designed to evaluate whether a survival benefit is possible as a result of thrombolysis in patients with advanced arterial occlusive disease.

The largest prospective randomized study to date, evaluating the role of catheter-directed thrombolysis was the STILE study (Surgery vs. Thrombolysis for the Ischemic Lower Extremity).[99] This trial evaluated patients with nonembolic lower-extremity ischemia who had progressive symptoms within 6 months of randomization. It was designed as an "all-inclusive" study in patients with nonembolic limb ischemia requiring intervention. After arteriography patients were randomized to either catheter-directed thrombolysis or surgical revascularization. If randomized to thrombolysis, patients were further randomized to either rt-PA or UK. After 393 patients were randomized, the study was terminated since a statistical end point was reached.

Catheter placement was not possible in 28% randomized to lysis (40% with graft occlusion and 21% with native arterial occlusion). Although significant differences were observed between the surgical and thrombolysis groups, results with rt-PA and UK were similar. When a plasminogen activator was infused, lysis was more successful for restoring patency to bypass grafts compared with native arteries (81% vs. 69%, $P =$ NS) and reduced the need for or magnitude of a subsequent surgical procedure ($P < 0.001$).

Overall conclusions indicated that patients were more effectively treated with operative revascularization compared with catheter-directed thrombolysis. However, when outcome was stratified by duration of ischemia, patients presenting with acute limb ischemia (14 days or less) enjoyed significantly lower amputation rates with catheter-directed thrombolysis than with surgical revascularization. On the other hand, in patients with more chronic ischemia (more than 14 days), operative revascularization had significantly less ongoing/recurrent ischemia (20% vs. 58%, $P < 0.001$) and showed a trend toward a reduction in major amputation.

Six-month follow-up was reported for the major end points of death and amputation. Interestingly there was no overall difference comparing the two treatment groups. However, when treatment strategies were stratified by duration of ischemia, once again differences were observed. Patients treated for acute limb ischemia (14 days or less) had significantly better amputation-free survival with catheter-directed thrombolysis, due to a significant reduction in major amputation. Operative revascularization was more effective in patients with chronic limb ischemia.

On the basis of these results, it appears that a treatment strategy that combines catheter-directed thrombolysis for patients with acute limb ischemia and operative revascularization for patients with chronic ischemia will offer the best overall results.

INTRAOPERATIVE, INTRAARTERIAL THROMBOLYTIC THERAPY

Animal laboratory experiments confirmed that following acute limb ischemia, arterial thrombosis occurred after 6 hours of inflow occlusion.[100] This extensive degree of thrombosis indicated that simple mechanical thrombectomy would not restore perfusion to the nutrient vessel from the main arteries.

An additional study demonstrated that thrombolysis following the best attempts at balloon catheter thromboembolectomy produced significantly improved angiographic results and a marked trend toward improved blood flow compared with control limbs.[101] Other animal studies have demonstrated that UK infusion aged more ischemic muscle compared with a control group.[102] Therefore experimental animal models confirmed the clinical observations that balloon catheter thromboembolectomy frequently left residual thrombus. Experimental data demonstrated that arteriolar perfusion could be restored, tissue salvaged, and reperfusion injury reduced with the judicious use of intraoperative, intraarterial infusion of lytic agents.[103]

Clinical trials have demonstrated that residual thrombi following balloon catheter thromboembolectomy can be effectively treated with intraoperative, intraarterial thrombolytic therapy.[104-106] An additional clinical benefit from intraoperative thrombolysis was that subsequent balloon catheter thromboembolectomy was more effective as a result of plasminogen activator infusion.[107,108]

A prospective, randomized, blinded, and placebo-controlled trial of intraoperative UK infusion was performed in patients undergoing lower-extremity revascularization procedures for severe limb ischemia.[98] Three doses of UK were used: 125,000, 250,000, and 500,000 IU, which were infused into the distal arterial circulation as a bolus at the time of the distal anastomosis. Analysis of plasma samples indicated a stepwise reduction in systemic plasminogen by dose, which reached statistical significance at the UK 500,000-IU level. Interestingly there was no significant fall in fibrinogen for any dose of UK infused. Fibrin degradation products increased with UK 500 and UK 250; and D-dimer increased significantly with all UK doses. There was no increase in bleeding complications in patients treated with UK compared with controls. An interesting but incidental observation was that patients receiving UK had a significantly lower mortality compared with placebo ($P = 0.034$).

Intraoperative infusion of thrombolytic agents apparently are of benefit in patients undergoing thromboembolectomy for acute (or chronic) arterial or graft occlusion. Whether the infused agent is enough to make a difference in an individual patient is a judgment to be made by the attending surgeon. The prospective randomized trial indicates that doses up to 500,000 units of UK given as a bolus are safe, and that fibrin will be broken down. Therefore both experimentally and clinically, intraoperative, intraarterial thrombolysis has been shown to be effective and can be used safely.

The technique of isolated limb perfusion of UK or rt-PA can be used in particularly difficult situations in which patients cannot be exposed to any potential of systemic fibrinolysis, and patients whose residual thrombus burden requires a high dose and sustained exposure to plasminogen activators to achieve adequate lysis.[105] This can be accomplished by applying a tourniquet to the proximal limb and inflating to above systolic pressure after exsanguinating the venous blood. Catheters are placed into the artery(ies) containing thrombus and the regional vein is drained by direct cannulation. The arterial catheter(s) is (are) infused with high-dose plasminogen activator, taking maximal advantage of tourniquet time (1 to 1½ hours). The venous effluent is collected and discarded. The limb is then flushed with heparinized saline solution, and the arteriotomy and venotomy closed. This is a valuable technique when dealing with small-vessel and multidistal vessel thrombi in patients not likely to respond to bolus dose intraoperative, intraarterial infusion and in patients in whom it is desirable to avoid systemic thrombolysis.

Acute Stroke

The resolution of stroke following the dissolution of cerebral emboli was observed over 35 years ago.[109] This area has had increased interest during the past 15 years. Selected patients have had remarkable recovery from profound neurologic deficits when acutely treated with thrombolytic agents for cerebral thrombotic/embolic events.

Intracerebral arterial occlusion occurs as a result of (1) in situ thrombosis on underlying atheromatous lesions, (2) cardiac source emboli, (3) emboli from a proximal artery that is diseased, and (4) intrinsic hemostatic abnormalities. The etiology of the neurologic deficit and the location of the occluded vessel may be important factors in the outcome of treatment.

An excellent, recently published review of thrombolytic therapy for stroke[110] addresses the issues of what is known about the natural history, diagnostic studies, review of previous trials, and ongoing trials.

As with most other acutely occluded vessels, regional/local delivery of plasminogen activators is associated with the greatest chance of success. For intracranial carotid territory occlusions, success rates of catheter-directed thrombolysis vary between 46% to 90%.[110-112] There is a relationship between the degree of recanalization and infarct size. However, there is a relatively high failure rate of proximal internal carotid artery occlusions. This failure of recanalization is likely due to the extensive atherosclerosis at the carotid bifurcation. Once occlusion occurs, the residual lumen that has thrombosed is minute and nearly impossible to cannulate.

Hemorrhagic infarction following treatment occurs in 18% to 20% of patients and appears independent of recanalization and resolves in the majority of patients.

Catheter-directed thrombolysis has demonstrated markedly improved outcomes in patients with vertebrobasilar thrombotic occlusion causing cerebellar and/or brainstem ischemia compared with conventional antithrombotic therapy.[113,114]

Although there is little information available regarding systemic lytic therapy for vertebrobasilar strokes, systemic lytic therapy has been studied in patients with carotid territory occlusion. Recanalization rates of 35% to 59% have been observed, with clinical outcome being related to recanalization. Patients receiving higher doses of lytic therapy appear to have higher rates of recanalization, which are uniformly better than placebo-treated patients.[115]

Hemorrhagic complications are always of paramount concern in patients treated with lytic therapy, especially in patients treated for stroke. The incidence of parenchymal hematoma appears to be 9% to 11% in patients treated with intraarterial lytic therapy, whereas the incidence of parenchymal hemorrhage appears less with systemic lytic therapy. It appears that there is no relationship between intracranial hemorrhage and recanalization of the occluded artery; however, the incidence of serious hemorrhagic complications with lytic therapy increases significantly with time from stroke onset to lytic therapy, with 6 hours emerging as a critical time interval. Although most hemorrhages occur within the ischemic area, there does not appear to be a relationship between the volume of the infarct size and the severity of hemorrhage.

A number of prospective randomized clinical trials are currently under way that will provide important information on clinical outcome of acute stroke treated with thrombolytic therapy.

Other Clinical Applications

There are a variety of additional clinical applications in which plasminogen activators are used to treat acute arterial, bypass graft, and venous occlusions. Patients with acute failure of their hemodialysis access grafts can have function restored after a relatively short course of catheter-directed thrombolysis. Patients with acute mesenteric ischemia due to embolic and thrombotic occlusion as well as mesenteric venous thrombosis have been selectively treated with thrombolytic agents. This requires good judgment with ongoing and intensive observation. However, in many of these patients their prognosis with conventional therapy is so poor that thrombolysis can be considered for potentially improving their outcome.

Acute occlusion of the renal arteries and veins, occluded central catheters, dural sinus thrombosis, retinal vein thrombosis, portal vein thrombosis, Budd-Chiari syndrome, and thrombosis of portosystemic shunts (both intrahepatic and extrahepatic) are but a few of the additional areas where lytic agents have been used. In most such cases the prognosis with conventional therapy is considered poor, and the anticipated risk of bleeding complications with lytic therapy was thought to be modest. In each instance physicians must be prepared to identify and correct the underlying cause of the thrombotic or embolic occlusion.

The use of thrombolytic agents for patients with thrombotic and embolic occlusions often reflects a degree of sophistication in the art and science of caring for these patients. During the past 15 years data have emerged demonstrating that risks can be reduced, and acute and long-term benefits can be offered to many of these patients.

REFERENCES

1. Astrup T: The haemostatic balance, Thromb Diath Haemorrh 2:347, 1958.
2. Sherry S: The origin of thrombolytic therapy, J Am Coll Cardiol 14:1085, 1989.
3. Marder VJ and Sherry S: Thrombolytic therapy, N Engl J Med 318:1512, 1988.
4. Marder VJ, Butler FO, and Barlow GH: Antifibrinolytic therapy. In Colman RW et al, eds: Hemostasis and thrombosis: basic principles and clinical practice, ed 2, Philadelphia, 1987, JB Lippincott.
5. Sottrup-Jensen L et al: The primary structure of human plasminogen: isolation of two lysine-binding fragments and one "mini" plasminogen (MW, 38,000) by elastase-catalyzed specific limited proteolysis. In Davidson JF et al, eds: Progress in chemical fibrinolysis and thrombolysis, vol 3, New York, 1978, Raven Press.
6. Dayhoff MO: Atlas of protein sequence and structure, vol 5 1978, suppl 3. Silver Spring, Maryland. National Biomedical Research Foundation.
7. Walther PJ et al: Activation of human plasminogen by urokinase: partial characterization of a preactivation peptide, J Biol Chem 249:1173, 1974.
8. Wallen P and Winman B: Characterization of human plasminogen II. Separation and partial characterization of different forms of human plasminogen, Biochem Biophys Acta 257:122, 1972.
9. Varadi A and Patthy L: Location of plasminogen-binding sites in human fibrin(ogen), Biochemistry 22:2440, 1983.
10. Markus G, DePasquale JL, and Wissler FC: Quantitative determination of the binding of epsilon-aminocaproic acid to native plasminogen, J Biol Chem 253:727, 1978.
11. Robbins KC et al: The peptide chains of human plasmin: mechanism of activation of human plasminogen to plasmin, J Biol Chem 242:2333, 1967.
12. Alkjaersig N, Fletcher AP, and Sherry S: The mechanism of clot dissolution by plasmin, J Clin Invest 38:1086, 1959.
13. Mullertz S: Natural inhibitors of fibrinolysis. In Davidson JF et al, eds: Progress in chemical fibrinolysis and thrombolysis, vol 3, New York, 1978, Raven Press.
14. Aoki N: Natural inhibitors of fibrinolysis, Prog Cardiovasc Res 21:267, 1979.
15. Wiman B: Human alpha-2-antiplasmin, Methods Enzymol 80:395, 1981.
16. Mullertz S and Clemmensen I: The primary inhibitor of plasmin in human plasma, Biochem J 159:545, 1976.
17. Thorsen S and Philips M: Isolation of tissue-type plasminogen activator-inhibitor complexes from human plasma: evidence for a rapid plasminogen activator inhibitor, Biochem Biophys Acta 802:111, 1984.
18. Erickson LA, Ginsberg MH, and Loskutoff DF: Detection and partial characterization of an inhibitor of plasminogen activator in human platelets, J Clin Invest 74:1465, 1984.
19. Francis CW and Marder VJ: Concepts of clot lysis, Annu Rev Med 37:187, 1986.
20. Budzynski AZ, Marder VJ, and Shainoff JR: Structure of plasmic degradation products of human fibrinogen: fibrinopeptide and poly-peptide chain analysis, J Biol Chem 249:2294, 1974.
21. Francis CW, Marder VJ, and Martin SE: Plasmic degradation of cross-linked fibrin. I. Structural analysis of the particulate clot and identification of new macromolecular soluble complexes, Blood 56:456, 1980.
22. Kopec M et al: Studies on "Double D" fragment from stabilized bovine fibrin, Thromb Res 2:283, 1973.
23. Tillett WS and Garner RL: The fibrinolytic activity of hemolytic streptococci, J Exp Med 58:485, 1933.
24. Kwaan HC: Hematologic aspects of thrombolytic therapy. In Comerota AJ, ed: Thrombolytic therapy, Orlando, 1988, Grune & Stratton.
25. Sherry S: Pharmacology of anistreplase, Clin Cardiol 5:3, 1990.
26. Coller B: Platelets and thrombolytic therapy, N Engl J Med 322:33, 1990.
27. MacFarlane RG and Pilling J: Fibrinolytic activity of normal urine, Nature 159:779, 1947.
28. Williams JRB: The fibrinolytic activity of urine, Br J Exp Pathol 32:520, 1951.
29. Grunzler WA et al: The primary structure of high molecular mass urokinase from human urine: the complete amino acid sequence of the A chain, Hoppe Seylers Z Physiol Chem 363:1155, 1982.
30. Bernik MB and Kwaan HC: Origin of fibrinolytic activity in cultures of human kidney, J Lab Clin Med 70P:650, 1967.
31. Aoki N and von Kaulla K: The extraction of vascular plasminogen activator from human cadavers: some of its properties, Am J Clin Pathol 5:171, 1971.
32. Gurewich V, Hyde E, and Lipinski B: The resistance of fibrinogen and soluble fibrin monomer in blood to degradation by a potent plasminogen activator derived from cadaver limbs, Blood 46:555, 1975.
33. Penneca D et al: Cloning and expression of human tissue plasminogen activator DNA in E coli, Nature 301:214, 1983.
34. Hoylaerts M et al: Kinetics of the activation of plasminogen by human tissue plasminogen activator: role of fibrin, J Biol Chem 257:2912, 1982.
35. Collen D, Stassen AJ, and Verstraete M: Thrombolysis with human extrinsic (tissue-type) plasminogen activator in rabbits with experimental jugular vein thrombosis, J Clin Invest 71:368, 1983.
36. Van de Werf F et al: Coronary thrombolysis with tissue-type plasminogen activator in patients with evolving myocardial infarction, N Engl J Med 310:609, 1984.
37. Korninger C et al: Thrombolysis with human extrinsic (tissue-type) plasminogen activator in dogs with femoral vein thrombosis, J Clin Invest 69:573, 1982.
38. Rao AK et al: Thrombolysis in myocardial infarction (TIMI) trial, phase I: hemorrhagic manifestations and changes in plasma fibrinogen and the fibrinolytic system in patients treated with recombinant tissue plasminogen activator and streptokinase, J Am Coll Cardiol 11:1, 1988.
39. Mueller HS, Rao AK, and Forman SA: Thrombolysis in myocardial infarction (TIMI): comparative studies of coronary reperfusion and systemic fibrinogenolysis with two forms of recombinant tissue-type plasminogen activator, J Am Coll Cardiol 10:479, 1987.
40. Weimer W et al: Specific lysis of an iliofemoral thrombus by administration of extrinsic (tissue-type) plasminogen activator, Lancet 2:1018, 1981.

41. The TIMI Study Group: The thrombolysis in myocardial infarction (TIMI) trial: phase I findings, N Engl J Med 312:932, 1985.

42. Verstraete M et al: Randomized trial of intravenous recombinant tissue-type plasminogen activator versus intravenous streptokinase in acute myocardial infarction: report from the European Cooperative Study Group for Recombinant Tissue-Type Plasminogen Activator, Lancet 1:842, 1985.

43. Goldhaber SZ: Thrombolytic therapy for pulmonary embolism, Semin Vasc Surg 5:89, 1992.

44. Come PC et al: Early reversal of right ventricular dysfunction in patients with acute pulmonary embolism after treatment with intravenous tissue plasminogen activator, J Am Coll Cardiol 10:971, 1987.

45. Husain SS, Lipinski B, and Gurewich V: Isolation of plasminogen activators useful as therapeutic and diagnostic agents (single-chain, high-fibrin affinity urokinase) US patent no. 4 381 346 (filed November 13, 1979, issued April 1983).

46. Gurewich V: Tissue plasminogen activator and prourokinase. In Comerota AJ, ed: Thrombolytic therapy, Orlando, 1988, Grune & Stratton.

47. Gurewich V et al: Effective and fibrin-specific clot lysis by a symogen precursor form of urokinase (prourokinase): a study in vitro and in two animal species, J Clin Invest 73:1731, 1984.

48. Collen D et al: Coronary thrombolysis in dogs with intravenously administered human prourokinase, Circulation 72:384, 1985.

49. Gurewich V and Pannell R: A comparative study of the efficacy and specificity of tissue plasminogen activator and prourokinase: demonstration of synergism and of different thresholds of nonselectivity, Thromb Res 44:217, 1986.

50. Smith R et al: Fibrinolysis with acylenzymes: a new approach to thrombolytic therapy, Nature 290:505, 1982.

51. Matsuo O, Collen D, and Verstraete M: On the fibrinolytic and thrombolytic properties of active-site p-anisoylated streptokinase-plasminogen complex (BRL 26921), Thromb Res 24:347, 1981.

52. Marder VJ, Francis CW, and Norry EC: Dose-ranging study of acylated streptokinase-plasminogen complex (BRL-26921), Thromb Haemost 50:321, 1983.

53. Marder VJ et al: Rapid lysis of coronary artery thrombi with anisoylated plasminogen streptokinase activator complex, Ann Intern Med 104:304, 1986.

54. DeWood M et al: Prevalence of total coronary occlusion during the early hours of transmural myocardial infarction, N Engl J Med 303:897, 1980.

55. Pietrolungo JF and Topol EJ: Thrombolytic therapy for acute myocardial infarction. In Comerota AJ, ed: Thrombolytic therapy for peripheral vascular disease, Philadelphia, 1995, JB Lippincott.

56. Baigent C for the Fibrinolytic Therapy Trialists' Collaboration CTS: Late benefit and early hazard associated with fibrinolytic therapy for acute myocardial infarction: results from six large randomized controlled trials, Circulation 86:1643, 1992.

57. Cairns JA, Fuster V, and Kennedy JW: Coronary thrombolysis, Chest 102(suppl):4825, 1992.

58. Lincoff AM et al: Is a coronary artery with TIMI grade 2 flow "patent"? Outcome in the Thrombolysis and Angioplasty in Myocardial Infarction Trial, Circulation 86(suppl):I-268, 1992 (abstract).

59. Voght A et al: 90-minute patency and optimal reperfusion of infarct-related coronary arteries, Circulation 86(suppl I):I-268, 1992 (abstract).

60. Anderson JL et al: Multicenter patency trial of intravenous anistreplase compared with streptokinase in acute myocardial infarction: the TEAM-2 Study investigators, Circulation 83:126, 1991.

61. The GUSTO Investigators: The international randomized trial comparing four thrombolytic strategies for acute myocardial infarction, N Engl J Med 329:673, 1993.

62. The Urokinase Pulmonary Embolism Trial. A national cooperative study, Circulation 47:II-1, 1973.

63. Urokinase-Streptokinase Pulmonary Embolism Trial—Phase 2 results. A cooperative study, JAMA 229:1606, 1974.

64. Sharma GVRK, Burleson VA, and Sasahara A: Effect of thrombolytic therapy on pulmonary capillary blood volume in patients with pulmonary embolism, N Engl J Med 303:842, 1980.

65. Sharma GVRK et al: Long-term hemodynamic benefit of thrombolytic therapy in pulmonary embolic disease, J Am Coll Cardiol 15(suppl):65A, 1990 (abstract).

66. PIOPED investigators value of ventilation-perfusion scan in acute pulmonary embolism. Results of the prospective investigation of pulmonary embolism, diagnosis (PIOPED), JAMA 263:2753, 1990.

67. Dalla-Volta S et al: PAIMS 2:alteplase combined with heparin versus heparin in the treatment of acute pulmonary embolism. Plasminogen Activator Italian Multicenter Study 2, J Am Coll Cardiol 20:520, 1992.

68. Meyer G et al on behalf of the European Cooperative Study Group for Pulmonary Embolism: Effects of intravenous urokinase versus alteplase on total pulmonary resistance in acute massive pulmonary embolism: a European multicenter double-blind trial, J Am Coll Cardiol 19:239, 1992.

69. Goldhaber SZ et al: Acute pulmonary embolism treated with tissue plasminogen activator, Lancet 2:886, 1986.

70. Goldhaber SZ et al: Perspectives on treatment of acute pulmonary embolism with tissue plasminogen activator, Semin Thromb Hemost 13:221, 1987.

71. Goldhaber SZ et al on behalf of the participating investigators: Thrombolytic therapy of acute pulmonary embolism: current status and future potential, J Am Coll Cardiol 10:96B, 1987.

72. Parker JA et al on behalf of the participating investigators: Early improvement in pulmonary perfusion after rt-PA therapy for acute embolism: segmental perfusion scan analysis, Radiology 166:441, 1988.

73. Goldhaber SZ et al: A randomized, controlled trial of recombinant tissue plasminogen activator versus urokinase in the treatment of acute pulmonary embolism, Lancet 2:293, 1988.

74. Goldhaber SZ et al: Recombinant tissue-type plasminogen activator versus a novel dosing regimen of urokinase in acute pulmonary embolism: a randomized, controlled multicenter trial, J Am Coll Cardiol 20:24, 1992.

75. Goldhaber SZ et al: Alteplase versus heparin in acute pulmonary embolism: randomized trial assessing right ventricular function and pulmonary perfusion, Lancet 341:507, 1993.

76. Shull KC et al: Significance of popliteal reflux in relation to ambulatory venous pressure and ulceration, Arch Surg 114:1304, 1979.

77. Johnson BF et al: Relationship between changes in the deep venous system and the development of the post-thrombotic syndrome after an acute episode of lower limb deep vein thrombosis: a one to six year follow-up, J Vasc Surg 21:307, 1995.

78. Killewich LA et al: Spontaneous lysis of deep vein thrombi: rate and outcome, J Vasc Surg 9:89, 1989.

79. Meissner MH et al: Deep venous insufficiency: the relationship between lysis and subsequent reflux, J Vasc Surg 18:596, 1993.

80. Comerota AJ: Thrombolytic therapy for acute DVT. In Comerota AJ, ed: Thrombolytic therapy for peripheral vascular disease, Philadelphia, 1995, JB Lippincott.

81. Elliot MS et al: A comparative randomized trial of heparin versus streptokinase in the treatment of acute proximal venous thrombosis: an interim report of a prospective trial, Br J Surg 66:838, 1979.

82. Arnesen H, Hoiseth A, and Ly B: Streptokinase or heparin in the treatment of deep vein thrombosis: follow-up results of a prospective study, Acta Med Scand 211:65, 1982.

83. Jeffrey P, Immelman E, and Amoore J: Treatment of deep vein thrombosis with heparin or streptokinase: long-term venous function assessment (abstract N. S20.3). In Proceedings of the Second International Vascular Symposium, 1989.

84. Comerota AJ et al: A strategy of aggressive regional therapy for acute iliofemoral venous thrombosis with contemporary venous thrombectomy or catheter directed thrombolysis, J Vasc Surg 20:244-S4, 1994.

85. Molina JE, Junter D, and Yedlicka JW: Thrombolytic therapy for iliofemoral venous thrombosis, Vasc Surg 26:630, 1992.

86. Semba CP and Dake MD: Iliofemoral deep venous thrombosis: aggressive therapy with catheter directed thrombolysis, Radiology 191:487, 1994.

87. Machleder HI: Evolution of a new treatment strategy for Paget-Schroetter syndrome: spontaneous thrombosis of the axillary-subclavian vein, J Vasc Surg 17:305, 1992.

88. Donayre CE et al: Pathogenesis determines late morbidity of axillosubclavian vein thrombosis, Am J Surg 152:179, 1986.

89. Gloviczki P, Kazmier FJ, and Hollier LH: Axillary-subclavian venous occlusion: the morbidity of a nonlethal disease, J Vasc Surg 4:333, 1986.

90. Tilney NL, Griffiths HJG, and Edwards EL: Natural history of major venous thrombosis of the upper extremity, Arch Surg 101:792, 1970.

91. Linblad B et al: Venous Hemodynamics of the upper extremity after subclavian vein thrombosis, Vasa 19:218, 1990.

92. Druy EM: Thrombolytic therapy for secondary axillosubclavian vein thrombosis. In Comerota AJ, ed: Thrombolytic therapy for peripheral vascular disease, Philadelphia, 1995, JB Lippincott.

93. Comerota AJ: Overview of catheter directed thrombolytic therapy for arterial and graft occlusion. In Comerota AJ, ed: Thrombolytic therapy for peripheral vascular disease, Philadelphia, 1995, JB Lippincott.

94. Durham JD et al: Regional infusion of urokinase into occluded lower-extremity bypass grafts: long-term clinical results, Radiology 172:83, 1989.

95. Gardiner GA Jr et al: Salvage of occluded arterial bypass grafts by means of thrombolysis, J Vasc Surg 9:426, 1989.

96. Gardiner GA Jr and Geoffrey A: Regional thrombolysis for failed lower extremity arterial bypass grafts. In Comerota AJ, ed: Thrombolytic therapy in peripheral vascular disease, Philadelphia, 1995, JB Lippincott.

97. Ouriel K et al: A comparison of thrombolytic therapy with operative revascularization in the initial treatment of acute peripheral arterial ischemia, J Vasc Surg 19:1021, 1994.

98. Comerota AJ et al: A prospective, randomized, blinded and placebo-controlled trial of intraoperative urokinase infusion during lower extremity revascularization: regional and systemic effects, Ann Surg 218:534, 1993.

99. The STILE Investigators: Results of a prospective trial of surgery vs thrombolysis for the ischemic lower extremity: the STILE trial, Ann Surg 220:251, 1994.

100. Dunnant JR and Edwards WS: Small vessel occlusion in the extremity after periods of arterial obstruction: an experimental study, Surgery 75:240, 1973.

101. Quinones-Baldrich WJ et al: Intraoperative fibrinolytic therapy: experimental evaluation, J Vasc Surg 4:229, 1986.

102. Belkin M, Valeri R, and Hobson RW: Intraarterial urokinase increases skeletal muscle viability after acute ischemia, J Vasc Surg 9:161, 1989.

103. Comerota AJ and Rao AK: Intraoperative, intra-arterial thrombolytic therapy. In Comerota AJ, ed: Thrombolytic therapy in peripheral vascular disease, Philadelphia, 1995, JB Lippincott.

104. Quinones-Baldrich WJ, Zierler RE, and Hiatt JC: Intraoperative fibrinolytic therapy: an adjunct to catheter thromboembolectomy, J Vasc Surg 2:319, 1985.

105. Parent NE et al: Fibrinolytic treatment of residual thrombus after catheter embolectomy for severe lower limb ischemia, J Vasc Surg 9:153, 1989.

106. Comerota AJ, White JV, and Grosh JD: Intraoperative, intra-arterial thrombolytic therapy for salvage of limbs in patients with distal arterial thrombosis, Surg Gynecol Obstet 169:283, 1989.

107. Norem RF, Short DH, and Kerstein MD: Role of intraoperative fibrinolytic therapy in acute arterial occlusion, Surg Gynecol Obstet 167:87, 1988.

108. Garcia R et al: Intraoperative, intra-arterial urokinase infusion as an adjunct to fogarty catheter embolectomy in acute arterial occlusion, Surg Gynecol Obstet 171:201, 1990.

109. Clarke RL and Cliffton EE: The treatment of cerebrovascular thrombosis and embolism with fibrinolytic agents, Am J Cardiol 30:546, 1960.

110. del Zoppo GJ and Otis SM: Thrombolytic therapy for acute stroke. In Comerota AJ, ed: Thrombolytic therapy for peripheral vascular disease, Philadelphia, 1995, JB Lippincott.

111. del Zoppo GJ et al: Local intra-arterial fibrinolytic therapy in acute carotid territory stroke: a pilot study, Stroke 19:307, 1988.

112. Mori E et al: Intracarotid urokinase with thromboembolic occlusion of the middle cerebral artery, Stroke 19:802, 1088.

113. Hacke W et al: Intra-arterial thrombolytic therapy improves outcome in patients with acute vertebrobasilar occlusive disease, Stroke 19:1216, 1988.

114. Matsumoto K and Satoh K: Topical intra-arterial urokinase infusion for acute stroke. In Hacke W, del Zoppo GJ, and Hirschberg M, eds: Thrombolytic therapy in acute ischemic stroke, Heidelberg, 1991, Springer-Verlag.

115. Mori E et al: Intravenous recombinant tissue plasminogen activator in acute carotid artery territory stroke, Neurology 42:976, 1992.

ARTERIAL DISEASES

CHAPTER EIGHT

PATHOGENESIS OF ATHEROSCLEROSIS

Paul E. DiCorleto
Henry F. Hoff
L. Allen Ehrhart
Richard E. Morton
Guy M. Chisolm, III

CHARACTERISTICS OF ATHEROSCLEROTIC DISEASE IN HUMANS

Atherosclerosis is a disease with both degenerative and regenerative characteristics that initially affects the tunica intima of major arteries in humans. In general, atherosclerosis leads to luminal narrowing of the affected artery and ischemia of the end organ. Atherosclerosis can lead to sufficient narrowing of the lumen at the iliac bifurcation and origins of the iliac arteries to induce ischemia of the lower limbs. Extensive atherosclerosis in the aorta that has progressed to involve the tunica media can result in dissecting aneurysms. In muscular arteries such as the coronary or cranial arteries, stenosis due to atherosclerosis can result in myocardial infarction or cerebral infarction (stroke), respectively. Available information on the evolution of the atherosclerotic plaque has been recently reviewed by an expert panel and has led to a proposed classification system for lesions,[1] which is summarized briefly in the following material.

The intima of an artery extends from the media to the endothelium and is composed of an internal elastic lamina and an acellular layer rich in connective tissue, especially proteoglycans. Intimal thickening, either focal or diffuse, occurs throughout the aortic, coronary, and carotid arteries in adult humans as an apparent response to regional differences in blood flow and wall tension. Adaptive intimal thickening first develops during fetal life, steadily increasing during puberty. This intimal thickening is self-limited in growth and is considered a physiologic rather than pathologic event, since it can be present without any development of atherosclerosis. However, advanced and clinically relevant atherosclerotic lesions consistently develop at anatomic sites that exhibit intimal thickening.

The initial atherosclerotic lesion (type I), which occurs in the absence of tissue damage, is visible only microscopically or by chemical analysis and consists of intimal accumulation of lipoproteins and some lipid-laden macrophages. This lesion develops into the fatty-streak lesion (type II). When sufficiently large, these lesions can be observed grossly as yellow elevations of the intimal surface. In the thoracic aorta they can be seen as yellow stripes running parallel to the vessel axis adjacent to the branches of the intercostal arteries (Fig. 8-1). Smaller fatty streaks can be seen grossly only following staining of the artery with lipid stains. Microscopically, cross sections of fatty streaks are characterized by an abundance of cells filled with vacuoles that contain predominantly cholesteryl esters (Fig. 8-2). These cells have been termed *foam cells* because of their foamy appearance under the microscope. Foam cells are usually observed in the intima close to the lumen immediately underlying the endothelium. Fatty streaks initially appear in the first decade of life in the aorta, in the second decade in coronary arteries, and in the third decade in cerebral arteries. These lesions are either progression prone (type IIa) when they are colocalized with adaptive intimal thickening or they are progression resistant (type IIb) and potentially quite reversible.

The type IIb lesion may progress to a preatheromic lesion (type III), which is characterized by microscopically visible tissue damage and increased quantities of extracellular lipid. These lesions are clinically silent, whereas the atheroma (type IV) found principally in individuals beyond the third decade of life may be either silent or overt.

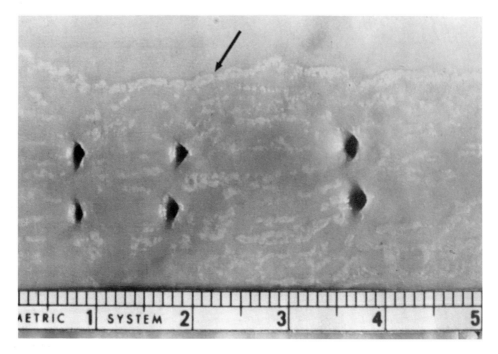

Fig. 8-1. Gross specimen of a human thoracic aorta shows raised fatty streaks (*arrow*) running parallel to orifices of the intercostal arteries.

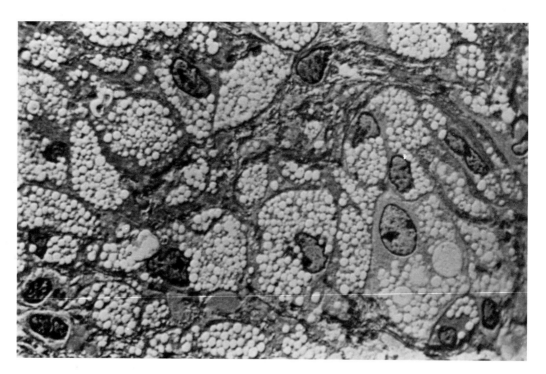

Fig. 8-2. Light micrograph of a cross section of a fatty streak from a human cerebral artery illustrates a close packing of round foam cells. Interference contrast microscopy was employed.

This lesion exhibits extensive structural damage to the intima. The next more advanced form of atherosclerotic lesion is the fibroatheroma (type V), which appears grossly as a raised, pearly white region of varied size (Fig. 8-3). Fibroatheromas are usually composed of two distinct parts.

One is a large region referred to as the necrotic core, which is frequently but not exclusively at the base of the lesion near the internal elastic lamina (Fig. 8-4). The core is composed of abundant extracellular lipid and extensive cell debris (Fig. 8-5). The second region is the fibrotic cap,

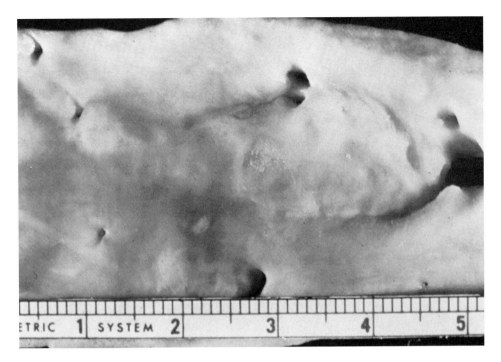

Fig. 8-3. Gross specimen of a fibrous plaque shows a slightly raised, pearly white lesion.

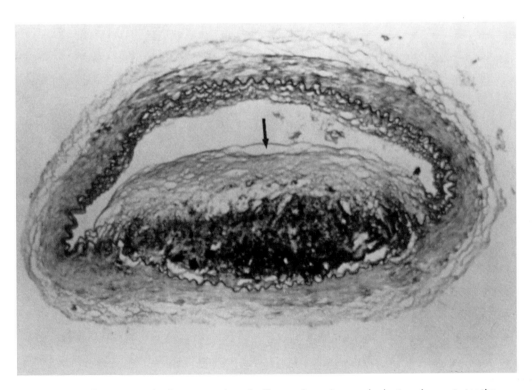

Fig. 8-4. Light micrograph of a cross section of a fibrous plaque in a cerebral artery demonstrates the eccentric location of the lesion and how the lesion compromises the lumen of the vessel. The lesion is composed of a necrotic core filled with lipid (*stained black*) and a fibrous cap (*arrow*).

which often comprises the largest portion of the atherosclerotic lesion (Fig. 8-6). The cap consists of numerous connective tissue components, especially collagen, surrounding smooth muscle cells. When these cells are present in abundance, this part of the lesion is referred to as a fibromuscular cap, whereas when few cells are present the term *fibrous* or *fibrotic cap* is usually used. The term *atherosclerosis* reflects the two major components of the

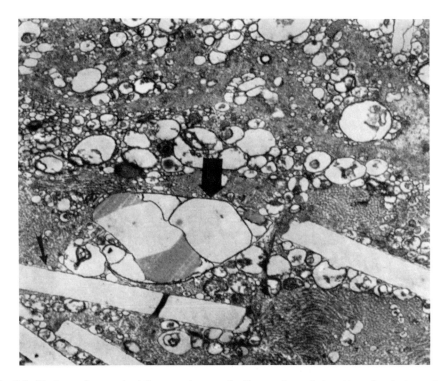

Fig. 8-5. Electron micrograph of the necrotic core of a fibrous plaque lesion. Note the cholesterol crystals (*small arrow*) and the extracellular lipid droplets (*large arrow*) embedded in a matrix of collagen.

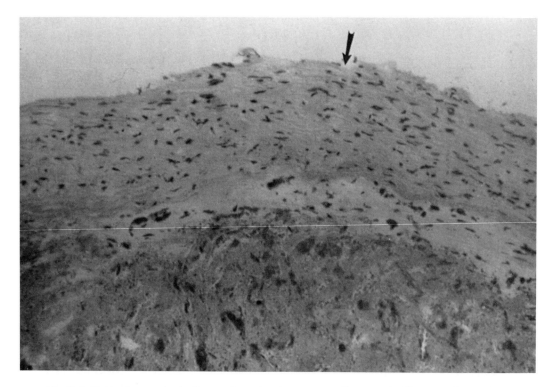

Fig. 8-6. Light micrograph of a fibrous plaque in a human aorta illustrates the fibromuscular cap (*arrow*) filled with smooth muscle cells (*nuclei are stained black*). Beneath the cap is the necrotic core, which is stained positive for lipid.

atherosclerotic lesion—that is, *athero* from the Greek word for gruel, corresponding to the necrotic debris at the base of the plaque, and *sclerosis* from the Greek word for hard, corresponding to the fibrotic cap.

In coronary arteries fibroatheromas may begin to appear as early as the second decade of life although the fourth decade and beyond is much more common. Numerous studies have indicated an association between the surface area occupied by fibroatheromas in the coronary arteries and subsequent myocardial infarction several decades later. No such association exists between fatty streaks and clinical manifestations. Indeed, fatty streaks present in children at several anatomic sites, such as the aortic arch and thoracic aorta, may disappear later in life. However, in the coronary and cranial arteries the early fatty streaks and the late fibrous plaques occur at similar anatomic sites. In addition, there are lesions that appear to represent transitions between these two types of lesions. These findings strongly suggest that fatty streaks are precursors of fibroatheromas.

The term *complicated lesion* (type VI) is used to identify a wide variety of advanced atherosclerotic lesions that exhibit characteristics not consistently found in the classic fibroatheroma. One form of complicated lesion, for example, is the ulcerated lesion (type VIa), which appears grossly as an open wound with an uneven surface more darkly colored than the surrounding intimal surface (Fig. 8-7). This lesion is believed to be formed by the erosion or fissure of the fibrous cap (Fig. 8-8), allowing direct interaction between the lipid and cell debris of the necrotic core and blood. This usually occurs when the cap above a large necrotic core filled with cholesterol crystals is very thin

(Fig. 8-9). Because of the thrombogenic nature of many of the plaque components in the core, such an event leads to mural thrombus formation. If this event occurs in a lesion that has already led to severe narrowing of the lumen, thrombus formation can completely occlude the vessel, resulting in myocardial infarction when occurring in the coronary circulation or stroke when occurring in the extraintracranial circulation. Recent studies using angioscopy have demonstrated a direct association between the appearance of such ulcerated lesions in coronary arteries and the clinical symptoms of unstable angina.[2] It is believed that rupture of the fibrous cap occurs at specific sites when the size of the necrotic core greatly exceeds that of the fibrous cap; lumen pressure then breaks the thin and fragile cap.

Another occasional feature of complicated lesions is the invasion of networks of capillaries, derived from both the vasa vasorum of the adventitia and new capillary sprouts originating from the lumen (Fig. 8-10). Hemorrhage occurring in the necrotic core due to the rupture of capillaries is frequently observed in ulcerated lesions. Such hemorrhagic lesions are classified as type VIb and those that exhibit thrombotic deposition as type VIc.

One of the most common characteristics of advanced, complicated lesions is the appearance of calcium in the form of apatite crystals in atherosclerotic lesions (Fig. 8-11), giving such lesions their characteristic brittleness. The phrase commonly used by the lay public, "hardening of the arteries," describes this calcific lesion (type VII). Any advanced lesion type that is composed predominantly of connective tissue (collagen) is referred to as a fibrotic lesion (type VIII).

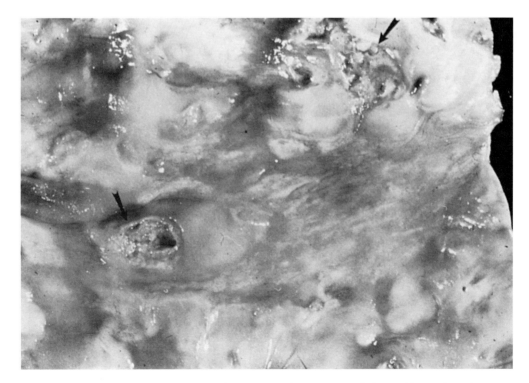

Fig. 8-7. Gross specimen of a human abdominal aorta illustrates several ulcerated lesions (*arrow*).

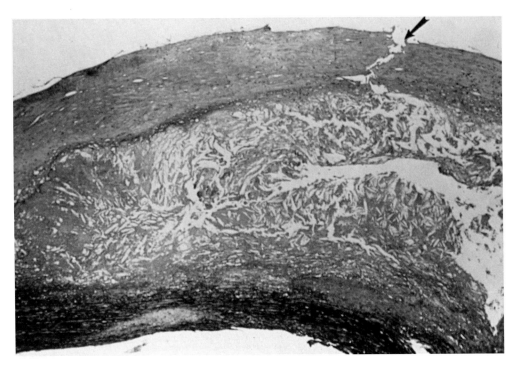

Fig. 8-8. Light microscopy of a cross section of a human aortic plaque illustrates a crack in the fibrous cap (*arrow*).

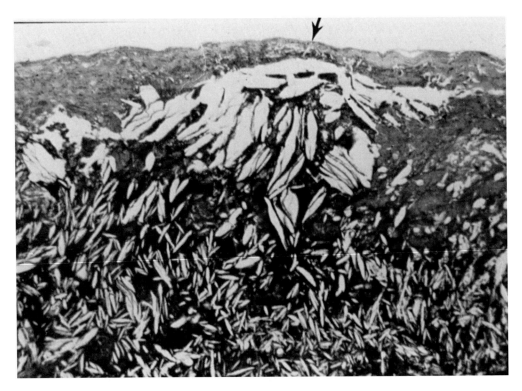

Fig. 8-9. Light microscopy of a cross section of a human aortic fibrous plaque shows how thin the fibrous cap can be at specific sites (*arrow*). Such areas are prone to rupture.

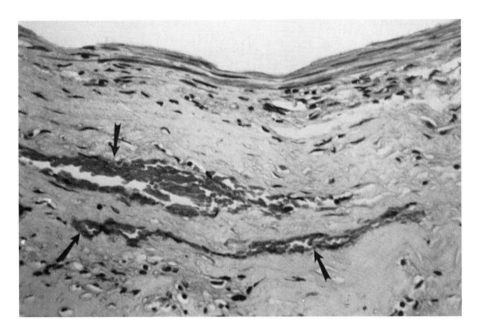

Fig. 8-10. Light micrograph of a cross section of a complicated lesion shows several capillaries filled with red blood cells (*arrow*).

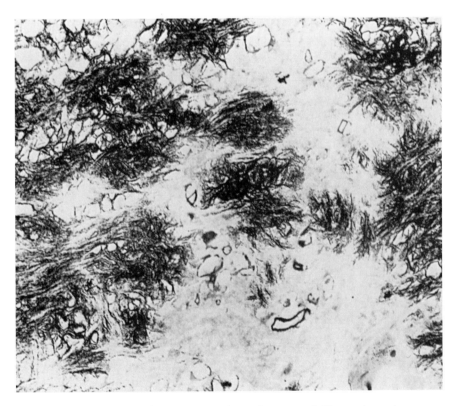

Fig. 8-11. Electron micrograph of a necrotic core from a human aortic fibrous plaque shows an area of calcification. Spicules of calcium apatite crystals (*dark structures*) can be seen throughout this area.

THEORIES OF ATHEROGENESIS

Historical Perspective

Even several decades ago descriptive pathology and animal experimentation allowed researchers to propose the sequence of events that occurs during the development of the atherosclerotic lesion. It was established early, for example, that the fatty-streak lesion is characterized by the accumulation of lipids,[3] primarily cholesterol in its esterified form.[4,5] Moreover, the smaller (and presumably newer) the lesion, the greater the fraction of lipid that is intracellular. Since both fatty streaks and fibrous plaques are characterized by the presence of cholesterol, primarily intracellular in fatty streaks and extracellular in fibrous plaques, it is understandable that much research has focused on how and why cholesterol accumulates. Virchow's early theory of atherogenesis[6] included the infiltration of lipids from the plasma into artery walls. Further refinements of the lipid hypothesis have been made over the years.[7,8] It is now believed that the primary source of lesion cholesterol is plasma low-density lipoprotein (LDL) that preferentially accumulates in the arterial intima. This accumulation may be the result of one or more of the following: (1) alterations in the permeability of the arterial intima to LDL, (2) increases in interstitial space in the intima, (3) poorer metabolism of LDL by vascular cells, (4) impeded transport of LDL from the intima to the media, (5) increased plasma LDL concentrations, or (6) specific binding of LDL to connective tissue components in the arterial intima. These factors are discussed in more detail in later sections. Studies of human arteries and studies of animals placed on high-cholesterol diets have clearly established that the LDLs accumulate to substantial levels in the tunica intima, even before lesions develop.[9,10] In fact, the primary site of such accumulation is the acellular zone close to the lumen within the thickened intima.[10] The wealth of studies in humans and experimental animal models demonstrating a direct association between diets rich in cholesterol and/or saturated fats, elevations in plasma LDL levels, and accelerated atherosclerosis, have established high plasma cholesterol and specifically elevated plasma LDL concentration to be a major risk factor for atherosclerosis and its clinical sequelae, myocardial infarction and stroke.

Response-to-Injury Theory

During the past two decades much has been learned about how cells respond to various stimuli. In particular a plethora of factors secreted by cells (cytokines) that dramatically affect the function of neighboring cells have been identified. This has led to a refinement of the earlier "nonspecific mesenchymal" theory to one in which specific factors are proposed to be responsible for the wound-healing reactions. In the early 1970s Ross and Glomset[11] proposed the response-to-injury theory of atherogenesis. Originally they proposed that different forms of injury (physical or chemical) induced frank denudation of the endothelial lining, leading to platelet adherence to the denuded areas of the arterial intima. Subsequent release of a growth factor, termed *platelet-derived growth factor (PDGF)*, triggered the movement of smooth muscle cells from the media to the intima and their subsequent proliferation. This theory may be correct in specific situations in which the endothelium has been mechanically removed, such as in balloon catheter injuries (experimental or during percutaneous transluminal coronary or peripheral artery angioplasty), or it may apply in later stages of lesion development. However, during the early stages of atherosclerosis, endothelial denudation is considered a rare event. More recent versions of the response-to-injury hypothesis have stressed the role of paracrine or local cell-derived factors provoked by vascular injury in the development of the atherosclerotic plaque,[12,13] as discussed in detail in later sections.

Hemodynamic Theory

Fatty streaks and fibrous plaques develop at specific anatomic sites of the vasculature. Likewise, the binding of blood monocytes to endothelium and the accumulation of LDL in the thickened intima of normal arteries are found to be focal. A theory of atherogenesis that attempts to explain the focal nature of the atherosclerotic process is the "hemodynamic theory" proposed in the 1950s by several investigators. It was theorized that hydrostatic and shear forces were primarily responsible for lesion development. The fact that atherosclerosis is accelerated in hypertension suggests a role for increased hydrostatic pressure in vascular disease. In addition, altered and/or fluctuating shear, including both turbulent flow and relatively stagnant flow, was shown to be present at anatomic sites where lesions preferentially develop such as at arterial branching sites. The association between altered shear forces and preferential lesion development is widely accepted as important in understanding lesion development. It is still not known how altered shear actually affects atherogenesis. Hemodynamics may change endothelial permeability to LDL or induce endothelial binding sites for monocyte adhesion, or it may alter other vascular processes.[14]

Lipoprotein Oxidation Theory

A relatively new theory of atherogenesis has emerged since the late 1970s that implicates lipoprotein oxidation as a precursor to and/or a causative agent in both lesion initiation and progression. The theory was proposed from the observations that (1) LDL following its oxidation injures vascular smooth muscle and endothelial cells in culture[15] and (2) endothelial and smooth muscle cells grown in culture are capable of oxidizing LDL, transforming it into both a ligand for scavenger receptor uptake by macrophages as well as a cytotoxin.[16,17] Macrophage scavenger receptors were identified and characterized by their recognition of chemically modified forms of LDL, such as acetylated LDL.[18] Uptake resulting from scavenger receptor binding of modified forms of LDL may result in unregulated uptake of the lipoprotein and storage of excess cholesterol in esterified form, a lipid engorgement resembling the foam cell formation of early fatty-streak lesions.

Oxidized LDL, unlike native LDL, changes cell function in vitro in ways that correspond to known features of atherosclerosis. For example, the cell functions suggestive of lesion formation, including endothelial cell injury, endothelial cell binding of monocytes, chemoattraction of monocytes, engorgement of lipoprotein lipid by mono-cyte-derived macrophages, stimulation of smooth muscle cell migration and proliferation, inhibition of endothelial wound healing, and expression of procoagulant agents are not readily induced in cell culture by native LDL; however, each of these processes can be induced by exposure of vascular cells to oxidized LDL.[19-22] Oxidized LDL injures cells, including endothelial cells, perhaps due to the potent cytotoxins formed during LDL oxidation, including 4-hydroxynonenal, lysophospholipids, and several oxyste-rols.[23] Oxidized LDL is a monocyte chemoattractant and promotes monocyte chemoattractant protein-1 (MCP-1) production and the expression of monocyte binding pro-teins on endothelial cells. HDL has been shown to be capable of inhibiting some of the effects of oxidized LDL. Cells present in vascular sites predisposed to lesion forma-tion, including smooth muscle cells, endothelial cells, stimulated monocytes and macrophages have all been shown to be capable of oxidizing LDL.[24-26]

The tenets of a theory of atherosclerosis invoking the above biologic activities that have been identified in cultured cells could begin with high plasma levels of LDL, leading to higher entry of LDL into the arterial intima and increased residence time particularly where the intima is thickened.[24] Next, oxidation by intimal endothelial cells, smooth muscle cells, or monocytes could begin the patho-logic process. Once oxidized the LDL may cause endothe-lial cell injury and dysfunction and may induce the endothelium to produce chemoattractants, procoagu-lants, and monocyte adhesion proteins (see next section). With invasion by monocytes comes the increased prob-ability that these free radical–producing cells will oxidize further the intimal pool of LDL. Macrophages express multiple receptors that recognize oxidized but not native LDL, including both class A type I and type II scavenger receptors, the class B scavenger receptors, SR-BI and CD36, and a subclass of macrophage Fc receptors.[19,22] Other means of macrophage recognition and uptake of oxidized LDL include ingestion via Fc receptor recognition of oxidized LDL bound to antibodies that recognize it; such antibodies have been identified in normal human plasma.[20] In addition, aggregates of oxidized LDL, known to form in vitro, may be ingested by phagocytosis. The effects of oxidized LDL on cytokine and growth factor production by various vascular cells could shift the balance of influences on smooth muscle cell behavior toward favoring migration and proliferation. The injury caused by oxidized LDL may enhance cell debris characteristic of late-stage lesions.[23] Oxidized LDL inhibits endothelium-dependent relaxation and enhances production of proco-agulants, which may enhance atherogenic processes.[19,23]

Supporting the lipoprotein oxidation theory of athero-sclerosis are data indicating that oxidized LDL is present in vascular lesions of animals and humans. Many properties of LDL isolated from lesions are similar to those of LDL oxidized in vitro, and antibodies that recognize oxidized but not native LDL bind lesion sites.[21,27] An array of antioxidants, including vitamin E, probucol, butylated hydroxytoluene, diphenylphenylenediamine, and β-caro-tene have been shown to limit atherosclerosis progression or symptoms in animals and humans.[19,28,29] Although

these data are consistent with the hypothesis that lipopro-tein oxidation plays a role in atherosclerosis, the agents mentioned above all exert side effects other than antioxi-dant activities, and since other studies using antioxidants have not inhibited atherosclerosis,[22,28] these data must be interpreted cautiously.

SEQUENCE OF EVENTS IN THE DEVELOPMENT OF THE ATHEROSCLEROTIC PLAQUE

Endothelial Cell Activation and the Initiation of Atherogenesis

The response-to-injury hypotheses has influenced the recent thoughts and experimental directions of vascular cell biologists and pathologists interested in atherogenesis. In the original model[12] described previously, the sole "function" of the endothelial cell in the disease process was its susceptibility to injury, leading to cell death and sloughing. Investigations by many laboratories during the past decade have failed to produce evidence that frank denudation of endothelium occurs as an early event in atherogenesis. Only in advanced atherosclerotic plaques have regions of vessel wall lacking intact endothelium been identified morphologically. The presence of an intact endothelium over lesion-prone areas of artery suggests the possibility of an active role for the endothelial cell in atherogenesis. Injury to the endothelium may shorten endothelial cell lifetime and cause increased endothelial cell turnover in specific regions of the artery. This may, in turn, lead to the expression of genes that are suppressed under physiologic rather than pathologic conditions. Spe-cific endothelial cell functions that may be directly rel-evant to atherosclerosis and its clinical sequelae include the expression of leukocyte binding sites on the endothe-lial cell surface; the altered production of paracrine growth factors, chemoattractants, and vasoreactive molecules; the ability to oxidize LDL and to respond to oxidized lipids and lipoproteins; the ability to express procoagulant rather than anticoagulant activities; and alterations in plasma component levels within the vessel wall through changes in permeability function (for recent review, see DiCorleto and Soyombo).[30]

An important question that remains unanswered is the source of injury (i.e., causative factor) that leads to altered endothelial cell gene expression during atherogenesis. Multiple candidates for the atherogenic agent have been proposed; however, rigorous identification of the mol-ecule(s) responsible for the initial changes in endothelial cell function that potentially lead to vascular disease has not been achieved. Candidates include chemical toxicity (cholesterol or its oxidized derivatives or homocysteine); immunologic injury (immune complexes); viral infection; and indirect mediators, such as tumor necrosis factor or thrombin, which are generated in the vessel wall in response to one of the preceding stimuli. In animal models a single intervention, such as high dietary cholesterol, generates a predictable atherosclerotic response in specific regions of the vasculature, but whether this is caused directly by an increased plasma cholesterol level or by a secondary initiating factor remains unknown. It has been proposed recently that the many putative injury agents may act through a common transcriptional factor(s), nuclear factor–kappa B (NF-κB), which is responsible for the inappropriate gene expression by endothelial cells.[31] Multiple other injury-induced signaling pathways may also be involved, as has been recently reviewed.[32,33]

A healthy physiologic endothelium presents a non-thrombogenic surface to blood cells; however, multiple pathways may be induced in activated endothelial cells that render these cells thrombogenic. The anticoagulant properties of the endothelium include the production of prostaglandin derivatives and other lipids that inhibit platelet aggregation and the elaboration of antithrombotic proteoglycans and proteins, such as thrombomodulin. Mechanisms by which the procoagulant state develops in large-vessel endothelial cells have been studied principally in vitro.[34] Activated endothelial cells express tissue factor, which initiates blood coagulation via the extrinsic pathway. Tissue factor activity has been shown to be induced in endothelial cells in response to various agonists such as endotoxin, interleukin-1 (IL-1), tumor necrosis factor, thrombin, and altered flow conditions. The tissue factor expressed by cultured endothelial cells in response to IL-1β has been found to be localized principally to the luminal or apical surface of the cell.[35]

In both native and activated states, the endothelium participates actively in the process of fibrinolysis as it relates to both clot dissolution and tissue repair.[36] Activated endothelial cells can inhibit fibrin degradation by reducing the expression of plasminogen activators while increasing expression of plasminogen activator inhibitor-1 (PAI-1). Oxidized lipoproteins, as well as native lipoproteins, were shown recently to cause increased synthesis of PAI-1 by cultured human endothelial cells.[37] Multiple proteases, including cathepsin-G, play a role in the fibrinolytic system by regulating the release of PAI-1 as well as plasminogen activator from the endothelial cell surface.[38] Finally, a link exists between vasoreactivity and the fibrinolytic activity of endothelial cells since endothelin (see the following material) has been found to augment release of both tissue plasminogen activator and PAI-1 from cultured endothelial cells.[39]

The ability of blood vessels to contract in response to humoral as well as paracrine vasoactive substances is affected by the diseased state of the vessel under study.[32,40] Understanding the regulation of endothelial cell production of vasoreactive molecules is therefore of direct relevance to clinical situations and end points, such as occlusion of blood flow. A key paracrine modulator of vascular reactivity is endothelin-1, a highly potent vasoconstrictive agent, which has been recently shown to be regulated both by oxidized lipoproteins and by shear stress.[41-43] Endothelin-1 is secreted by endothelial cells into the basolateral compartment,[44] and its secretion is suppressed by lysophosphatidylcholine (lysoPC), a major component of oxidized LDL.[41] Other modulators of endothelin-1 production by vascular endothelial cells include gamma interferon (IFN-γ), IL-1β, and thrombin.

The endothelium also controls vascular tone, depending on the physiologic state of the blood vessel, by secreting vasorelaxants such as nitric oxide. Multiple studies have examined the interrelationships between endothelium-dependent relaxation and hypercholesterolemia both in vitro and in vivo.[45-47] All of the studies, including those in humans, have demonstrated an inverse relationship between atherosclerotic plaque development and vasorelaxation. In an ex vivo rabbit model of hypercholesterolemia, increased neutrophil adherence to coronary artery endothelium was found to be caused by a reduction in nitric oxide release in the hypercholesterolemic state.[46] Hypoxia also causes abnormal contractile responses in the atherosclerotic rabbit aorta, potentially through reduced nitric oxide and cyclic guanosine monophosphate production.[48] In the same rabbit model, L-arginine administration, which would provide increased substrate for nitric oxide synthase, overcame the proatherogenic effects of hypercholesterolemia, further implicating nitric oxide production as an antiatherosclerotic event.[49] In humans impaired endothelium-dependent vasodilatation of forearm resistance vessels has been shown in hypercholesterolemic patients.[45] Also, patients with coronary risk factors and proximal atherosclerotic lesions were demonstrated to exhibit impaired responsiveness of their coronary vessels to acetylcholine.[50] These studies were further reinforced by those in hypercholesterolemic patients in which cholesterol-lowering therapy improved coronary endothelium-dependent relaxation.[51]

Two functional classes of compounds, antiinflammatory agents and antioxidants, have been tested in vitro for their ability to prevent endothelial cell activation in the presence of stimulators, such as cytokines. The antiinflammatory agent 3-deazaadenosine was found to inhibit thrombin-induced expression of PDGF and leukocyte adhesion molecules in cultured endothelial cells.[52] Multiple animal studies using various vascular disease models has led to much excitement regarding the possible antiatherosclerotic properties of antioxidants such as vitamin E (α-tocopherol) or probucol. The beneficial effects of these agents may be because of their ability to inhibit the generation of oxidized LDL—a putative triggering molecule in the atherosclerotic process. Recent results from several investigators point to a novel alternative mechanism of action of antioxidants—that is, through the scavenging of intracellular reactive oxygen intermediates that serve as second messengers in cytokine-induced gene activation in endothelial cells.[53-57] Vitamin E has also been demonstrated to enhance prostacyclin production by cultured endothelial cells,[58] suggesting a third mechanism by which this antioxidant may alter the progression of atherosclerosis.

Adhesion of Monocytes to the Endothelium

The past decade has been a very active period for the study of the molecular interactions between blood-borne leukocytes and the endothelium. This process is of great interest to atherosclerosis researchers because of the well-recognized involvement of both monocytes and T lymphocytes in the developing lesion. The monocyte-derived macrophage has been implicated in multiple aspects of atherosclerotic plaque development.[59] These cells contribute to the formation of fatty-streak lesions by ingesting massive amounts of lipid and thus developing into foam cells. They also produce growth factors for vascular smooth muscle cells, generate cytotoxic factors for neighboring cells, and emigrate as foam cells from the vessel wall, leading to physical damage to the endothelium.

The first step in monocyte recruitment into the subendothelial space is the attachment of this blood-borne cell to the endothelium. The focal adherence of mononuclear cells to lesion-prone regions of large vessels is one of the earliest, readily detectable events that occurs in experimentally induced atherosclerosis in various animal models. Topics that are currently under investigation in multiple laboratories include the nature of the underlying mechanisms regulating the expression of leukocyte adhesion proteins on the endothelial cell surface following cellular activation, the mechanism underlying the induction of adhesion by hypercholesterolemia, the specificity of this monocyte adhesion with little if any involvement of neutrophils, and finally the reason why monocytes adhere only to specific regions of the vasculature. A now well-accepted model to describe the process of leukocyte attachment to the endothelium and subsequent diapedesis involves the sequential involvement of various adhesion molecules and chemokines.[60,61] Both cell types play an active role in the process, which includes an initial rolling or tethering event (selectins), a signaling process (chemokines), and a strong attachment step (the immunoglobulin family members). In vivo data supporting this model have been limited to the microvasculature, and leukocyte adhesion to large vessels that develop atherosclerosis may not occur in the same way.

Many recent studies have implicated lipoproteins and their components in inducing leukocyte adhesion to endothelial cells. Minimally modified (oxidized) LDL, but not native LDL, has been shown to specifically increase monocyte adhesion to cultured endothelial cells.[62] Very low density lipoprotein (VLDL) that has been hydrolyzed by lipoprotein lipase was also found to induce increased monocyte adhesion to cultured aortic endothelial cells.[63] The underlying mechanism of action of lipoproteins and the specific components responsible for the effects of oxidized LDL and hydrolyzed VLDL on endothelial cells remain unknown. One advance in this direction has been recently provided by Kume et al,[64] who observed that lysophosphatidylcholine, a major component of oxidized LDL, increased mononuclear cell adhesion to cultured human and rabbit arterial endothelial cells. This lipid was found to induce the adhesion molecules VCAM-1 (vascular cell adhesion molecule-1) and ICAM-1 (intercellular adhesion molecule-1), but not E-selectin, on the endothelial cell surface, thus distinguishing this stimulus from many other agonists of leukocyte adhesion.

The specific leukocyte adhesion molecules responsible for monocyte adhesion in the absence of neutrophil adhesion in models of atherogenesis remain to be defined. Characteristics of the known endothelial cell/leukocyte adhesion molecules have been recently reviewed in detail.[59,65] The primary candidate to date for the "atherogenic" leukocyte adhesion molecule is VCAM-1.[66] The kinetics of expression of this cytokine-inducible leukocyte adhesion molecule are consistent with its involvement in monocyte adhesion to rabbit aorta following the feeding of a high-cholesterol diet.[67] Other adhesion molecules for which some evidence exists, albeit mostly in vitro, for their involvement in monocyte adhesion include E-selectin, ICAM-1, and P-selection.[59]

Lipoprotein Involvement in Atherogenesis

Much of the research pertaining to atherosclerosis and much of the focus in the treatment of atherosclerotic patients is related to the known link between the development of the disease and the plasma concentration of cholesterol or certain lipoproteins.[68-74] Total plasma cholesterol is correlated closely enough to coronary disease in humans that epidemiologic studies predict a monotonic increase in risk of coronary events with increases in total plasma cholesterol above about 170 to 200 mg/dl. This is an oversimplification, since the LDL cholesterol level is a very strong predictor of atherosclerosis, whereas the HDL cholesterol level is an inverse correlate of the disease. The roles the lipoproteins are believed to play in vascular diseases are related to their composition and their effects on cells and tissues,[75] which are reviewed briefly in the following material.

The major classes of plasma lipoproteins are chylomicrons, VLDL, LDL, intermediate-density lipoprotein (IDL), and HDL. The chylomicrons are produced in gut epithelial cells and traverse the mesenteric lymph to the thoracic duct where they enter the bloodstream. The chylomicron core consists chiefly of triglycerides and secondarily cholesteryl esters, which are synthesized by the epithelium from dietary fatty acids and cholesterol. Once in the bloodstream, chylomicrons are referred to as chylomicron remnants, since their catabolism begins immediately by the action of endothelium-associated lipoprotein lipase that breaks down the triglycerides. The liberated fatty acids are resynthesized to triglycerides in adipose cells for storage. The remnant is ultimately removed from the bloodstream via specific receptors on hepatic cells. In normal humans chylomicrons are cleared from the bloodstream within several hours after a fatty meal and are not appreciably present in the plasma after 12 hours of fasting.

VLDL is synthesized by the liver, and its principal function is the transport of cholesterol and triglycerides from liver to other tissues, including adipose tissue. Although smaller than chylomicrons, VLDL has similar composition with a predominance of triglyceride; it is also substrate for lipoprotein lipase. LDL is smaller than VLDL and has less triglyceride; LDL can be considered the final metabolic breakdown product of the VLDL remnant. In normal humans LDL carries most of the cholesterol present in fasting plasma. About 70% of LDL cholesterol is carried in esterified form; the balance is free cholesterol. About 21% of the mass of this lipoprotein particle is a single protein, called apolipoprotein B-100.

HDL is a smaller molecular complex and has the highest proportion of protein composing its mass. The protein component is a composite of several apolipoproteins, the most important of which are apolipoproteins A-1 (apoA-1) and A-2 (apoA-2). The various apolipoproteins of HDL influence specific metabolic activities, for example, apoA-2 plays a regulatory role in the action of hepatic lipase. HDL is believed to function in "reverse cholesterol transport," with the movement of cholesterol from peripheral tissues to liver. Consistent with such a beneficial role are epidemiologic data that show a correlation between less risk of atherosclerosis and the concentration of HDL cholesterol in plasma. HDL apolipoproteins are synthesized in liver as well as gut epithelium, and HDL is ultimately removed from the circulation by the liver.

Animal studies of dietary-induced elevations in lipoproteins that lead to the development of atherosclerosis, epidemiologic data in humans linking lipoproteins and disease, and studies showing atherosclerosis regression in both humans and primates following chronic, substantial reductions in plasma cholesterol, have led to the conclusion that lipoproteins can cause atherosclerosis. The identification of the mechanism(s) by which LDL or related lipoproteins can induce the documented cellular events that take place in the disease is the subject of the theories mentioned previously. Native or "normal" LDL does not lead to foam cell formation when it is incubated with macrophages or vascular smooth muscle cells in cell culture, but these two cell types are known to be the precursors of intimal foam cells in vivo.

Typically when animals are fed cholesterol, a distinct lipoprotein particle appears in plasma in concentrations related to the amount of cholesterol (and other fats) substituted in the diet. This lipoprotein is unlike the normally occurring lipoproteins and has been named β-VLDL, since upon electrophoresis of plasma proteins this particle migrates in the beta band along with LDL, yet it co-isolates with VLDL in the ultracentrifuge separation of plasma lipoproteins. β-VLDL can lead to cholesteryl ester accumulation in macrophages and is therefore considered to be an atherogenic particle; however, it is present in human plasma only in rare circumstances (type III hypercholesterolemia), and its presence certainly cannot explain the widespread incidence of this disease in humans in Western cultures.

It has been proposed that atherosclerosis is worsened by adverse interactions between arterial cells and lipoproteins following oxidative modification of the lipoprotein (see lipoprotein oxidation theory, earlier). However, other forms of lipoprotein modification have also been proposed. The pathologic lipoprotein may be synthesized in a modified form, as suggested by the demonstration that an LDL-related lipoprotein called lipoprotein(a), or Lp(a), exists in human plasma and its concentration, in general, correlates, with atherosclerosis risk.[76]

In 1973 Drs. Michael S. Brown and Joseph L. Goldstein discovered the cellular receptor for LDL. Their work, which led to their receiving the 1985 Nobel Prize in Medicine and Physiology, characterized the cellular pathway by which LDL can regulate cellular cholesterol metabolism via this receptor.[77] Increased cellular cholesterol due to the entry of LDL via its cellular receptor leads to the inhibition of cellular synthesis of cholesterol. In addition, the synthesis of the receptor is downregulated. The importance of these discoveries is far-reaching. Genetic defects in the receptor can result in the impaired removal of chylomicrons, VLDL, and LDL from plasma, allowing LDL cholesterol levels to increase. Their work led to therapeutic lowering of plasma cholesterol levels via suppression of 3-hydroxy-3-methylglutaryl coenzyme A (HMG CoA) reductase, the rate-limiting enzymatic step in cellular synthesis of cholesterol. This work revealed an important mechanism by which LDL can reach high plasma concentrations but did not explain how high LDL levels lead to atherosclerosis.

In recent decades numerous studies of the pathology of arterial lesions of humans and of experimental animals have revealed that apolipoprotein B accumulates in very high concentrations in the interstitial spaces. The interstitial fluid and lymphatic concentrations of plasma proteins are generally estimated at 10% to 30% of their plasma concentrations; however, estimates of LDL concentrations in lesions rival or exceed those of plasma.[9,10] The localization of LDL as demonstrated by immunofluorescence studies is primarily in the intima among foam cells in fatty-streak lesions (Fig. 8-12), at the intima-media border in transitional lesions—that is, those believed to represent the transition from fatty streaks to fibrous plaques (Fig. 8-13), and in the necrotic core of advanced fibrous plaques (Fig. 8-14). Studies in experimental animals suggest that excessive intimal lipoprotein accumulation is the earliest detectable change in a vascular site predisposed to lesion formation.

The interstitial intimal accumulation of plasma lipoproteins is the result of numerous processes, any of which may play a controlling role. Among these are (1) the ability of the endothelium to regulate the traffic of these large plasma molecules; (2) the sieving properties of the internal elastic lamina, which separates the intimal, or disease-prone, part of the arterial wall from the media, which becomes involved in the later stages of the disease; (3) the capabilities for degradation of the lipoprotein by smooth muscle cells that may be residing in the intima; and (4) the capacity for binding of lipoprotein by extracellular connective tissue components.

LDL can bind certain connective tissue substances. Large proteoglycans of the interstitial space as well as their glycosaminoglycan subunits have been shown to co-localize with LDL in the grossly normal intima and in fatty streaks (Figs. 8-15 and 8-16). They have also been shown to bind LDL in vitro under conditions believed to pertain in vivo. In addition, both collagen and elastin have been shown to bind LDL and certain lipids carried by LDL. Thus sequestration of certain lipoproteins by connective tissue may be an important contributor to the extracellular lipid accumulation of arterial lesions. In addition, certain of the complexes formed between lipoproteins and connective tissue proteins may be taken up by macrophages and contribute to foam cell formation.

Another variant of LDL known to occur in humans that has been studied intensely recently for its relationship to atherosclerosis and related disorders is Lp(a). Lp(a) is a macromolecular complex made up of one LDL particle associated with apolipoprotein(a), a protein of highly variable molecular weight, which is structurally homologous to plasminogen. Plasminogen is a naturally occurring serine protease that is a component of the fibrinolytic system. Plasma levels of Lp(a) are highly heritable, and a number of studies have linked plasma levels of Lp(a) to premature coronary disease in humans. Coupled with high plasma LDL concentrations, plasma Lp(a) levels have been shown by many to correlate with increased atherosclerosis

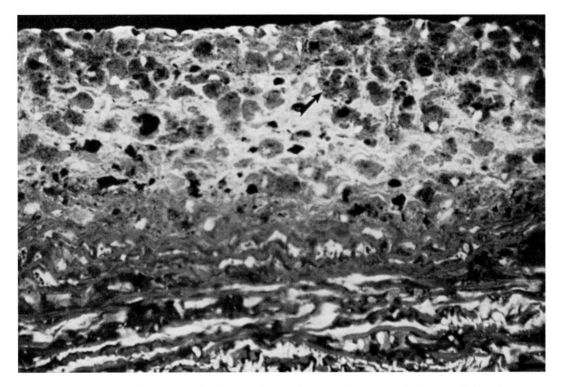

Fig. 8-12. Immunofluorescence localization of LDL (*white*) in a cross section of a fatty streak from the aorta of a hypercholesterolemic swine. LDL can be seen in the spaces between foam cells (*arrow*). Darkfield microscopy has been employed.

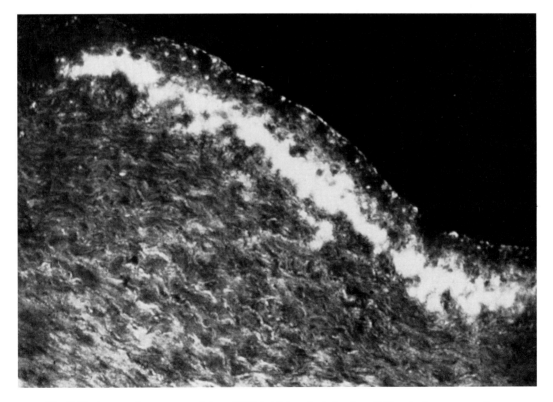

Fig. 8-13. Immunofluorescent staining of LDL (*white*) at the intimal-medial border in a cross section of a coronary artery lesion from a hypercholesterolemic swine.

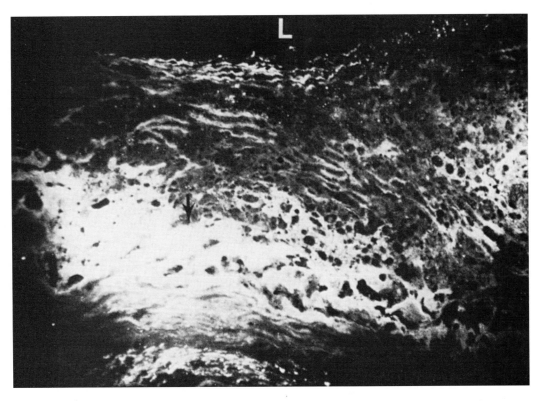

Fig. 8-14. Immunofluorescence localization of LDL (*white*) primarily in the necrotic core (*arrow*), but focally in the fibrotic cap, of a fibrous plaque in a human coronary artery (*L,* lumen).

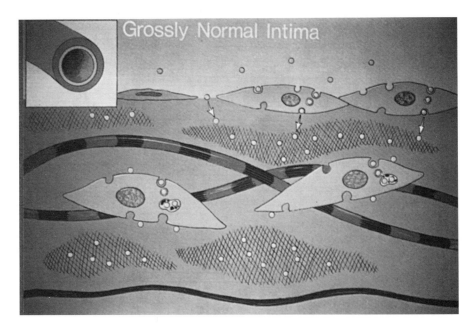

Fig. 8-15. Schematic representation of the deposition of LDL (spheres) in the grossly normal intima because of trapping by glycosaminoglycans in intima proteoglycans (*cross-hatched area*).

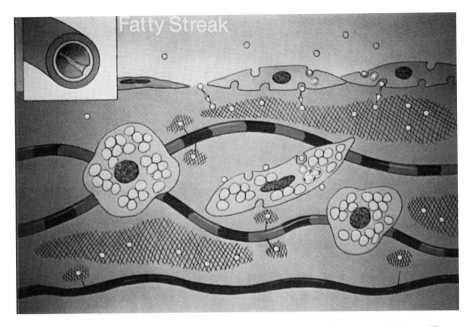

Fig. 8-16. Schematic representation of the deposition of LDL (*spheres*) in fatty-streak lesions. The lipid-laden cells (foam cells) are formed by the uptake of LDL accumulating in the extracellular space bound to proteoglycans (*cross-hatched section*).

risk above that predicted by high LDL alone; however, not all studies find Lp(a) to be an independent risk factor. There is speculation that Lp(a) and the genetic aberration contributing to its production can hasten the development of arterial lesions. The mechanism by which this modified lipoprotein may be involved in the disease is not known. Theories being pursued relate its putative atherogenicity to its tendency to self-aggregate and to bind proteoglycans better than LDL, its ability to interact with plasminogen receptors, its effects on smooth muscle proliferation, and its potential role in provoking an autoimmune response.[78]

That lipoproteins can play a causal role in atherosclerosis is no longer considered in doubt by the vast majority of physicians and scientists worldwide. The mechanisms by which lipoproteins interact with cells to injure them or disturb their metabolism, and thereby lead to fatty-streak formation and other complications, are incompletely understood. Research focusing on the interactions between vascular cells and lipoproteins suggests that certain steps in the mechanisms of these interactions offer opportunities to intervene in the processes that lead to vascular pathology.

Evolution of the Fatty-Streak Lesion—Foam Cell Development

Accumulated intimal lipoproteins and monocytes that have entered the intima to become macrophages clearly lead to foam cell formation.[59] The mechanisms by which this happens are currently under intense investigation (see theories, earlier). Fig. 8-17 illustrates the myriad of cholesterol-rich substrates that have been shown to induce lipid loading of macrophages in cell culture. Some of these substrates may also be responsible for foam cell formation

from smooth muscle cells (Fig. 8-18). As observed by electron microscopy, lipid-laden cells in lesions contain a heterogeneous array of inclusions believed to represent internalized lipoproteins at various stages of processing (Fig. 8-19).

LDL has been shown to form soluble and insoluble complexes with proteoglycans extracted from human aortic intima, in both grossly normal sites and atherosclerotic lesions.[14] Such complexes are avidly taken up by macrophages in culture. The mechanism of macrophage uptake of these insoluble complexes appears to be the same as for aggregated LDL following oxidation (i.e., by phagocytosis). The previously mentioned lipoprotein, Lp(a), also accumulates in human atherosclerotic lesions. It, too, forms insoluble complexes in vitro with arterial proteoglycans, and these complexes are avidly phagocytosed by macrophages in culture. This may explain why Lp(a) is considered an independent risk factor for atherosclerosis.

Two major forms of cholesterol are found in the extracellular space of atherosclerotic lesions in addition to that still residing on lipoproteins. One is the cholesteryl ester–rich droplets believed to be derived from lysed foam cells. These are rich in cholesteryl oleate, presumably resulting from cellular reesterification of ingested lipoprotein cholesterol. The other is a particle rich in both free cholesterol and cholesteryl linoleate believed to be derived directly from LDL without any intracellular processing. Recent data suggest that both types of particles can be internalized by macrophages, again contributing to the lipid loading of these cells. Uptake of dead cell debris (e.g., cell membranes) by macrophages may also contribute. These latter mechanisms may play a greater role in the transition of fatty streaks to more advanced atherosclerotic lesions.

Although most foam cells in early fatty-streak lesions

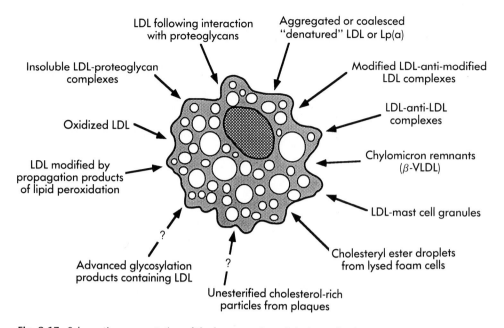

Insoluble LDL-proteoglycan complexes

LDL following interaction with proteoglycans

Aggregated or coalesced "denatured" LDL or Lp(a)

Modified LDL-anti-modified LDL complexes

Oxidized LDL

LDL-anti-LDL complexes

LDL modified by propagation products of lipid peroxidation

Chylomicron remnants (β-VLDL)

LDL-mast cell granules

Advanced glycosylation products containing LDL

Cholesteryl ester droplets from lysed foam cells

Unesterified cholesterol-rich particles from plaques

Fig. 8-17. Schematic representation of the large number of cholesterol-rich substrates that can be taken up by tissue macrophages leading to the formation of foam cells.

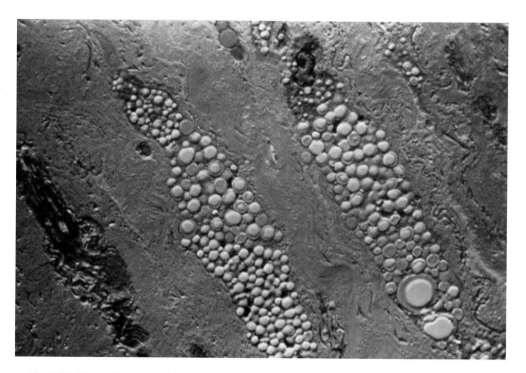

Fig. 8-18. Light micrograph of the cross section of a fatty streak in a human cerebral artery illustrates two spindle-shaped, lipid-laden foam cells, believed to be derived from smooth muscle cells. Interference contrast microscopy.

are presumed to represent monocyte-macrophages, in somewhat more advanced lesions, vascular smooth muscle cells also become foam cells (Fig. 8-18). The mechanisms by which smooth muscle cells become lipid laden are unclear. Smooth muscle cells under certain circumstances can express scavenger receptors, inviting speculation of a common mechanism with macrophages. However, it has also been demonstrated that smooth muscle cells in culture avidly take up lipid droplets derived from lysed, lipid-laden macrophages, suggesting that phagocytosis of cell debris by smooth muscle cells may be a mechanism by which smooth muscle cells become foam cells.[79]

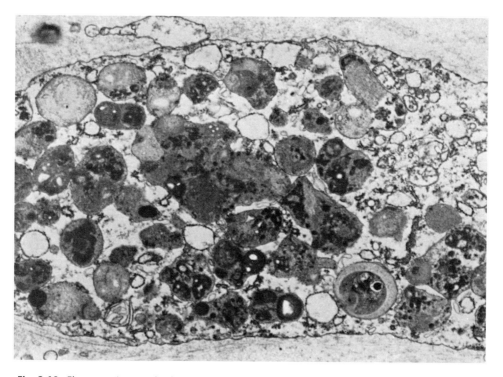

Fig. 8-19. Electron micrograph of a foam cell shows numerous lipid inclusions of different densities.

Intimal Hyperplasia of Smooth Muscle Cells

Smooth muscle cells are not homogeneously distributed through the distinct layers of the normal and atherosclerotic artery. In the normal artery smooth muscle cells are absent in the outermost, adventitial layer (containing primarily fibroblasts and connective tissue), but are the major cellular component of the medial layer of the normal artery. Their relative abundance in the media does not significantly change during development. Only a few smooth muscle cells are present in the intimal layer of the infant artery, but a gradual accumulation of intimal cells occurs during normal development. In the diseased artery smooth muscle cells are a significant component of the early fatty-streak lesion (although perhaps secondary to macrophages), but they are the predominant cellular component of the fibrotic plaque (Fig. 8-6).

Growth factors (or mitogens) are hormonelike proteins that bind to specific receptors on target cells, initiating a cascade of events that results in cell replication. Cultured smooth muscle cells possess receptors for, and are stimulated to divide by, PDGF. In addition, PDGF can act as a chemoattractant for smooth muscle cells, and a scenario can easily be imagined in which arterial cells situated near the lumen of the vessel secrete growth factors into the subendothelial space, thereby stimulating both migration of smooth muscle cells into the intima and proliferation of intimal cells. During the last decade attention has focused both on the function of PDGF, as well as possible sources of PDGF, in the artery wall. Much of our understanding of the regulation of production of PDGF from vascular cells is derived from in vitro studies. Endothelial cells were the first vascular cell (other than the platelet) shown to secrete PDGF.[80] Endothelial cells cultured from all major vessels,

and from all species examined to date, secrete PDGF into their medium. The regulation of production of PDGF by endothelial cells and evidence correlating PDGF expression by endothelial cells with dysfunction and vascular disease has been reviewed.[81] Recent studies have suggested novel ways in which PDGF production may be regulated within endothelial cells. Increasing the osmolarity or the glucose concentration of endothelial cell culture media caused a significant increase in the amount of PDGF produced by the cells.[82] These results may have relevance to the well-established association of atherosclerosis with diabetes. Other modulators of PDGF production that have been recently discovered include interleukin-6,[83] hydrogen peroxide,[84] and low-molecular-weight fibrinogen degradation products.[85] The most efficacious inducer of PDGF production by endothelial cells remains the coagulation system protease α-thrombin, which acts both transcriptionally and posttranslationally to cause release of PDGF.[86] Of great interest is the recent finding that the promoter of the PDGF B chain gene contains an element that confers shear stress responsiveness to this gene.[87] This observation, as well as previous studies reporting modulation of PDGF production by mechanical/physical activation, form a potential mechanistic link between regions of altered shear stress and susceptibility to atherosclerotic plaque development. The preceding studies highlight the multitude of factors that may modulate the level of growth factors produced by the endothelium under various pathophysiologic conditions.

The endothelium is also known to produce other growth factors in addition to PDGF, for example, insulin-like growth factor-1 (IGF-1), which can act to modulate gene expression and augment proliferation of neighboring smooth muscle cells.[88,89] Basic fibroblast growth factor, a ubiquitous mitogen, also exhibits regulated expression by the endothelium, as does the pluripotent growth factor/growth inhibitor, transforming growth factor-β (TGF-β). Endothelial cells respond to TGF-β as a growth inhibitor, and a recent report has suggested that this protein may also alter the differentiated state of endothelium, causing expression of genes by endothelial cells in culture previously thought to be smooth muscle cell specific.[90]

Evidence that endothelial cells are involved in smooth muscle cell proliferation in vivo is largely circumstantial. Intimal proliferation takes place even in the presence of an intact endothelium, suggesting that exogenous factors such as platelet products may not be required. Furthermore, intimal hyperplasia in many circumstances correlates with regions of endothelialization, for example, at the anastomoses of synthetic vascular grafts.

Vascular cells other than endothelial cells may also synthesize and secrete growth factors into the arterial wall. Several laboratories have shown that human peripheral blood monocytes, activated in vitro by bacterial lipopolysaccharide or by immune complexes, secrete PDGF. In addition, smooth muscle cells themselves, under certain circumstances, secrete growth factors. Smooth muscle cells cultured from the aorta of rat pups secrete significantly more PDGF than smooth muscle cells isolated from adult rats, suggesting that a normal function of PDGF may be related to blood vessel development. Cultured smooth muscle cells derived from the intima of mechanically injured rat arteries also produce more PDGF than medial smooth muscle cells from uninjured arteries. This concept is supported by a study reported by Wilcox et al[91] in which the method of in situ hybridization histochemistry is used to determine the in vivo location and identity of cells in atherosclerotic lesions expressing the genes for the A chain and B chain of PDGF. Endothelial cells and intimal smooth muscle cells express both gene transcripts, but medial smooth muscle cells and macrophages show little of either. These results suggest that smooth muscle cell-derived growth factors may stimulate their own growth in an autocrine fashion, similar to the mechanism postulated for the uncontrolled cell proliferation of certain tumors.

Certainly other factors besides PDGF contribute to the proliferation of arterial smooth muscle cells. Other growth factors may be involved, including fibroblast growth factors, transforming growth factors, heparin-binding epidermal growth factor, IGFs, and macrophage-derived cytokines. The physical structure and chemical composition of the extracellular matrix is known to regulate smooth muscle cell growth in vitro and is likely to play a key role in the vessel wall as well. Finally, the lipids present in the extracellular environment are likely to influence smooth muscle cell function and growth rate.

Synthesis and Composition of the Extracellular Matrix in Atherosclerotic Lesion Formation

One of the hallmarks of atherosclerosis is the gradual accumulation of an elaborate extracellular matrix in the arterial intima. This material, consisting mainly of collagen, glycoproteins, and proteoglycans, is synthesized by cells residing in the thickened intimal layer of the atherosclerotic vessel. Although the accumulation of collagen is generally regarded as a later event in the pathogenesis of atherosclerosis, usually associated with the development of the fibrous plaque, the synthesis and deposition of excessive collagen and other matrix components begins earlier.

Arteries of newborns are composed of an intima, which consists of a monolayer of endothelial cells covering an internal elastic lamina; a medial layer, in which the only cell is the smooth muscle cell; and the adventitia, in which fibroblasts are the predominant cell. As discussed in the preceding section, intimal thickening is an early event in atherosclerosis characterized by the proliferation of smooth muscle cells that have migrated from the media. These cells continue to proliferate as the lesion grows, but it is not certain that continued proliferation is a prerequisite for excessive matrix accumulation. In fact, a dissociation between active proliferation of smooth muscle cells and excessive production of extracellular matrix has been observed. Clowes et al[92] subjected rat carotid arteries to abrasive endothelial denudation by balloon catheter. Platelet deposition occurred within minutes of endothelial cell removal and stabilized within 24 hours, after which smooth muscle cells started to synthesize DNA as regeneration of the endothelium began. Migration of the proliferating, medial smooth muscle cells into the intima began at 4 days, and proliferation continued in the intima. The mass of smooth muscle cells increased to a maximum at 4 weeks. Intimal thickening, however, continued for another 8 to 12 weeks. The increase in thickness and mass of the intima during this time was due completely to additional accumulation of extracellular matrix synthesized by resident smooth muscle cells that were no longer proliferating. The chain of events seen in this experimental model may be relevant to the pathogenesis of restenosis, which follows percutaneous transluminal coronary angioplasty. Restenosis is frequently accompanied by additional intimal hyperplasia, hypertrophy, and deposition of extracellular matrix components, resulting in fibrotic and complicated lesions that are even more occlusive than those seen before angioplasty. It thus appears that regardless of whether the artery is in the early or later stages of atherosclerotic lesion formation, the predominant cell, if not the only cell, responsible for synthesis of extracellular collagen and other glycoproteins is the smooth muscle cell.

Although smooth muscle cells are thought responsible for the bulk of extracellular matrix production in the atherosclerotic intima, these cells are probably not the same as smooth muscle cells of the normal media. It has been proposed that there are two different phenotypes of arterial smooth muscle cells.[93] Medial smooth muscle cells are characterized as being in the "contractile" state and are filled with myofilaments. These cells are responsible for the normal contraction of arterial tissue and produce only a maintenance level of connective tissue components. The other phenotype is represented by smooth muscle cells that have been induced to migrate into the intima where they proliferate and exist in a "synthetic" state. These cells synthesize large amounts of extracellular matrix and contain increased levels of cytoplasmic rough endoplasmic reticulum, Golgi apparatus, and free ribosomes with very few filament bundles. Thus cells in atherosclerotic lesions that are producing excessive quantities of matrix most likely originated as medial smooth muscle cells but may no longer have all the characteristics of normal smooth muscle cells.

Other cellular components of human atherosclerotic plaques are macrophages and lymphocytes, but it is unlikely that they contribute significantly to the matrix components known to accumulate in developing lesions. The presence of various leukocytes in different types of lesions, however, suggests a strong potential for these cells to influence the composition of arterial matrix molecules by several mechanisms. Production of a variety of cytokines and other mediators of the inflammatory process, together with the secretion of matrix proteases, could profoundly affect the synthesis and accumulation of matrix components by resident smooth muscle cells.

Monocyte-derived macrophages have been shown to be present in fatty streak or fibrofatty lesions, as well as in advanced or complicated plaques.[94,95] Human arterial tissue taken from aortic, carotid, and femoral vessels showed two types of plaques beyond the fatty-streak stage, both of which contained extracellular connective tissue. The first type consisted of an elevated fibrous plaque without a necrotic core. The second was composed of a fibrous cap surrounding an atheromatous core. The fibrous plaque and the fibrous cap both contained collagen and elastin. In the lipid core of the complicated lesion, 60% of the cells were monocyte-derived macrophages, whereas in the overlying fibrous cap they represented 24% of the total cells.

The presence of macrophages in lesions suggests that atherosclerosis can be considered to be an inflammatory response. In most tissues inflammation is often accompanied by proliferation of fibroblasts, which is then followed by deposition of collagen and other extracellular matrix components. This sequence of events is analogous to the proliferation and subsequent matrix deposition in atherosclerotic arteries. In addition to smooth muscle cells and macrophages, T lymphocytes were found to account for nearly 20% of the cells in fibrous caps.[95] The presence of T cells together with activated macrophages in lesions also suggests the possibility of a cell-mediated, delayed-type hypersensitivity form of immune response.[96] Activated T cells produce a variety of proteins including IFN-γ, which is known to inhibit smooth muscle cell proliferation. This cytokine also inhibits collagen synthesis at the transcriptional level and may be responsible for reducing the elastin content of the tissue by increasing elastase activity. Smooth muscle cells, macrophages, and lymphocytes together produce a variety of growth factors, cytokines, and matrix protein hydrolytic enzymes. The coexistence of these cells in varying proportions in different types of lesions emphasizes the potential for regulation of extracellular matrix synthesis and remodeling as atherosclerotic plaques progress.

The macromolecular composition of the extracellular matrix of normal arteries and of atherosclerotic arteries consists of the fibrous proteins, collagen and elastin, together with other glycoproteins and various glycosaminoglycans and proteoglycans. During development of

atherosclerosis compositional changes occur in the absolute and relative concentrations of several of these macromolecules, and they may have profound influences on the structure and metabolism of the arterial wall. Some of the known alterations in the synthesis, degradation, and accumulation of these components are discussed in the following material.

Proteoglycans are composed of glycosaminoglycans or polymers of amino sugars, previously referred to as *mucopolysaccharides,* which are linked to specific core proteins. One of the major types of proteoglycans in the arterial wall is the chondroitin sulfate/dermatan sulfate (CS/DS) proteoglycan. This proteoglycan is increased with the progression of atherosclerosis.[97] CS/DS proteoglycan is reported to associate with collagen and to sequester apolipoprotein B–containing lipoproteins, which would contribute to the trapping and deposition of LDL cholesterol in the intima[97] (see Figs. 8-15 and 8-16).

The major structural components of all blood vessels are collagen and elastin. Collagen fibrils are the structures that provide the tensile strength throughout the entire cardiovascular system. Regulation of arterial smooth muscle cell collagen production is not well understood. Studies in which collagen synthesis was determined in isolated atherosclerotic arteries or in vivo concluded that one of the mechanisms responsible for the increased arterial collagen in atherosclerosis was an increase in the rate at which arterial collagen was synthesized.[98,99] This increase was significantly greater than that seen for noncollagen protein synthesis and was specific for arterial tissue. Whether a change in rates of arterial collagen degradation also accompanies the onset of atherosclerosis is not known.

These and other investigations established that arterial smooth muscle cells exhibit increased rates of collagen synthesis in response to changes taking place even in the relatively early stages of atherosclerosis in which lesion formation has not progressed beyond the fatty-streak stage. Types I and III collagen account for approximately 90% of all blood vessel collagen with less than 10% contributed by type V collagen and much smaller quantities of types IV, VI, and VIII.[100] Changes in the distribution or proportions of the various types of collagen that occur in atherosclerosis have been difficult to assess, but the relative percentages of types I and III in intimal plaques do not seem to differ significantly from that of the unaffected medial layer.

Elastin is the other major fibrous protein component of blood vessels. In the aortic arch and thoracic aorta elastin is present in larger quantities than collagen. In the abdominal aorta and in smaller blood vessels collagen becomes the predominant fibrous structural protein. Although elastin is seen in developing plaques in humans and in experimental atherosclerosis, it does not accumulate as collagen does. It is interesting that elastin synthesis appears to be increased in arteries of atherosclerotic rabbits to the same extent as collagen synthesis, when measured in isolated segments of thoracic aorta.[98] Increased production of elastin in the arterial intima thus appears to be offset by increased degradation. Elastin concentration does not increase, and many of the elastin fibers in lesions are fragmented.

Degradation of matrix proteins plays a major role in

atherosclerotic lesion formation and plaque rupture. In his extensive review Falk[101] concludes that the evolution of coronary atherosclerotic lesions is associated with frequent plaque ruptures accompanied by thrombosis, and that this process is probably the most important mechanism responsible for rapid plaque progression leading to acute coronary ischemic episodes. Lesions that rupture typically exhibit a fragmented internal elastic membrane beneath a lipid core and a thinning and weakening of the fibrous cap. The proteolytic enzymes responsible for these degradative events are synthesized by resident smooth muscle cells or by inflammatory cells, predominantly macrophages. Several matrix metalloproteinases (MMPs) secreted by smooth muscle cells have been identified including a 72-kDa MMP and a 92-kDa MMP, both of which are classified as gelatinases capable of hydrolyzing several types of collagen as well as elastin and other matrix proteins.[102] The 92-kDa enzyme, also known as gelatinase B and MMP-9, is produced by THP-1 cells, a human monocyte-macrophage cell, which when incubated with arterial segments, degraded elastin in the tissue.[103] Synthesis and degradation of matrix macromolecules in the vessel wall are thus key factors in vascular smooth muscle cell proliferation, lesion progression, and in atherosclerotic plaque rupture.

REGRESSION OF ATHEROSCLEROTIC LESIONS

The regression of atherosclerotic lesions ideally reflects a return of the vascular wall to the prelesion or normal state. However, in practice this ideal is rarely observed. The extent to which regression occurs has been documented in a number of animal models and in humans.[104-112] Regression in humans is discussed in detail in Chapter 9. Animal models of atherosclerosis have been invaluable in understanding the mechanisms of lesion development; however, these models rarely adequately replicate the severe lesions that typify advanced human atherosclerosis. This perhaps reflects the fact that human atherosclerotic lesions evolve slowly over decades, whereas animal models of this disease are developed in months to several years and are usually elicited by excessive elevations in blood cholesterol. Nevertheless, experimental models of atherosclerosis in rabbits, swine, and nonhuman primates do replicate many of the morphologic features of human atherosclerotic lesions, thus permitting a study of their potential for regression and the mechanisms involved.

Collectively the data obtained from regression studies in animal models have identified several important properties of the regression process.[106-112] Notably, regression is a common feature of lesions in both peripheral artery and coronary artery beds. Within these lesions most of the morphologic and biochemical alterations noted in atherosclerotic lesions are reversible. This includes the normalization of vascular wall cholesterol content by the removal or resolution of intracellular and extracellular lipid deposits, a reduction in smooth muscle cell number, the loss of necrotic material, and the repair of endothelial cell damage. Important exceptions to this trend are the connective tissue, particularly collagen, and calcium components of the atherosclerotic lesion, which usually increase during regression. Consistent with these conclusions, the extent to which lesion regression occurs is directly dependent on the severity of the initial lesion. Uncomplicated fatty-streak lesions induced by cholesterol feeding may completely regress when the induction stimulus is removed and the animals are returned to a normal diet. More complicated lesions, such as fibrofatty lesions, diminish markedly but never reach the prelesion state even after an extended regression period. Advanced, humanlike lesions regress only partially, often resulting in a highly fibrous, calcified lesion that is only slightly smaller in size than the original.

The cellular and biochemical mechanisms responsible for regression are poorly understood. The primary initial step in the regression of all lesions appears to be the loss of cholesteryl esters, resulting in a marked reduction in the number of foam cells. Evidence exists to support at least three mechanisms of foam cell regression: (1) cell death; (2) the egress of lipid-laden macrophages from the lesion into the circulation where they are cleared; and (3) cholesterol removal from intact foam cells, which is subsequently cleared from the extracellular space by effective cholesterol acceptors such as HDL. This latter process, referred to as *reverse cholesterol transport,* may explain why elevations in plasma HDL levels are correlated with enhanced lesion regression.[105,111] Secondary to foam cell loss, a reduction in smooth muscle cell number appears related to a normalization of cell division rates,[107] and the resolution of the necrotic debris of the lesion suggests that cell death stops and that adequate scavenger mechanisms exist to resolve large amounts of material when the input side of the equation is terminated. The mechanisms underlying the enhanced collagen production during the regression of fibrous lesions are unclear; however, it appears that this induction is dependent on the initial stimulation of collagen synthesis in the developing lesion.[110] The increase in fibrous lesion collagen content during regression is problematic in the return of vasodilation capacity. In some instances vessel stiffness decreases to near normal levels upon regression,[54] and in other studies the increased fibrosis prevents the regression of vasodilation capacity even when luminal diameter markedly improves.[112]

Thus, based on animal studies, it is understandable why the complicated lesions of advanced human atherosclerosis are slow to regress and require aggressive lipid-lowering therapy. The fact that the most easily resolved component of lesions, foam cells, represents a relatively small part of the advanced lesion, coupled with the propensity for collagen to accumulate in the resolving lesion, appears to impair effective lesion regression. These findings underscore the importance of reducing recognized risk factors for atherosclerotic lesion development in asymptomatic individuals.

REFERENCES

1. Stary HC: The evolution of human atherosclerotic lesions, Philadelphia, 1993, Merck & Co.
2. Falk E: Unstable angina with fatal outcome: dynamic coronary thrombosis leading to infarction and/or sudden death, Circulation 71:699, 1985.
3. McGill HC Jr: Fatty streaks in the coronary arteries and aorta, Lab Invest 28:560, 1968.

4. Adams CWM: Vascular histochemistry, Chicago, 1967, Year Book Medical Publishers.

5. St Clair RW: Pathogenesis of the atherosclerotic lesion; current concepts of cellular and biochemical events. In Recent advances in arterial disease: atherosclerosis, hypertension, and vasospasms, New York, 1986, Alan R Liss.

6. Virchow R: Gesammte Abhandlung zu wissenschafltiche, Medizin 550:458, 1856.

7. Page IH: Atherosclerosis: an introduction, Circulation 10:1, 1954.

8. Gofman JW and Young W: The filtration concept of atherosclerosis and serum lipids in the diagnosis of atherosclerosis. In Sandler M and Bourne GH, eds.: Atherosclerosis and its origins, New York, 1963, Academic Press.

9. Smith EB and Slater RS: Relationship between low density lipoproteins in aortic intima and serum lipid levels, Lancet 1:463, 1972.

10. Hoff HF, Gaubatz JW, and Gotto AM: ApoB concentration in the normal human aorta, Biochem Biophys Res Commun 85:1424, 1979.

11. Ross R and Glomset JA: The pathogenesis of atherosclerosis, N Engl J Med 295:369, 1976.

12. Ross R: The pathogenesis of atherosclerosis—an update, N Engl J Med 314:488, 1986.

13. Ross R: The pathogenesis of atherosclerosis: a perspective for the 1990s, Nature 362:801, 1993.

14. Davies PF et al: Influence of hemodynamic forces on vascular endothelial function, J Clin Invest 73:1121, 1984.

15. Hessler JR, Robertson AL Jr, and Chisolm GM: LDL-induced cytotoxicity and its inhibition by HDL in human vascular smooth muscle and endothelial cells in culture, Atherosclerosis 32:213, 1979.

16. Morel DW, DiCorleto PE, and Chisolm GE: Endothelial and smooth muscle cells alter low density lipoprotein in vitro by free radical oxidation, Arteriosclerosis 4:357, 1984.

17. Steinbrecher UP et al: Modification of low density lipoprotein by endothelial cells involves lipid peroxidation and degradation of low density lipoprotein phospholipids, Proc Natl Acad Sci USA 81:3883, 1984.

18. Brown MS and Goldstein JL: Lipoprotein metabolism in the macrophage: implications for cholesterol deposition in atherosclerosis, Ann Rev Biochem 52:223, 1983.

19. Penn MS and Chisolm GM: Oxidized lipoproteins, altered cell function and atherosclerosis, Atherosclerosis 108 (suppl):S21, 1994.

20. Parathasarathy S, Steinberg D, and Witztum JL: The role of oxidized low-density lipoproteins in the pathogenesis of atherosclerosis, Annu Rev Med 43:219, 1992.

21. Haberland ME and Steinbrecher UP: Modified low-density lipoproteins: diversity and biological relevance in atherogenesis, Monogr Hum Genet 14:35, 1992.

22. Chisolm GM and Penn MS: Oxidized lipoproteins and atherosclerosis. In Fuster V, Ross R, and Topol E, eds.: Atherosclerosis and coronary disease, New York, 1995, Raven Press.

23. Chisolm GM: Cytotoxicity of oxidized lipoproteins, Curr Opin Lipidol 2:311, 1991.

24. Chisolm GM: Oxidized lipoproteins. In Kreisberg RA and Segrest J, eds.: Plasma lipoproteins and coronary artery disease, Boston, 1992, Blackwell Scientific Publications.

25. Steinbrecher UP, Zhang H, and Lougheed M: Role of oxidatively modified LDL in atherosclerosis, Free Rad Biol Med 9:155, 1990.

26. Steinberg D et al: Beyond cholesterol. Modifications of low density cholesterol that increase its atherogenicity, N Engl J Med 320:915, 1989.

27. Yla-Herttuala S et al: Lipoproteins in normal and atherosclerotic aorta, Eur Heart J 11:88, 1990.

28. Chisolm GM: Antioxidants and atherosclerosis: a current assessment, Clin Cardiol 14:I-25, 1991.

29. Steinberg D and Workshop Participants: Antioxidants in the prevention of human atherosclerosis: summary of the proceedings of a National Heart, Lung, and Blood Institute workshop: September 5-6, 1991, Bethesda, Maryland, Circulation 85:2337, 1992.

30. DiCorleto PE and Soyombo AA: The role of the endothelium in atherogenesis, Curr Opin Lipidol 4:364, 1993.

31. Collins T: Endothelial nuclear factor-kappa B and the initiation of the atherosclerotic lesion, Lab Invest 68:499, 1993.

32. Luscher TF et al: Endothelial dysfunction in coronary artery disease, Annu Rev Med 44:395, 1993.

33. Gerritsen ME and Bloor CM: Endothelial cell gene expression in response to injury, FASEB J 7:523, 1993.

34. Antonov AS et al: Prothrombotic phenotype diversity of human aortic endothelial cells in culture, Thromb Res 67:135, 1992.

35. Narahara N et al: Polar expression of tissue factor in human umbilical vein endothelial cells, Arterioscler Thromb 14:1815, 1994.

36. Van Hinsbergh VWM: Impact of endothelial activation on fibrinolysis and local proteolysis in tissue repair, Ann NY Acad Sci 667:151, 1992.

37. Tremoli E et al: Increased synthesis of plasminogen activator inhibitor-1 by cultured human endothelial cells exposed to native and modified LDL: an LDL receptor-independent phenomenon, Arterioscler Thromb 13:338, 1993.

38. Pintucci G et al: A polymorphonuclear cell protease, affects the fibrinolytic system by releasing PAI-1 from endothelial cells and platelets, Ann N Y Acad Sci 667:286, 1992.

39. Yamamoto C et al: Effect of endothelin on the release of tissue plasminogen activator and plasminogen activator inhibitor-1 from cultured human endothelial cells and interaction with thrombin, Thromb Res 67:619, 1992.

40. Kisanuki A et al: Contribution of the endothelium to intimal thickening in normocholesterolemic and hypercholesterolemic rabbits, Arterioscler Thromb 2:1198, 1992.

41. Jougasaki M et al: Suppression of endothelin-1 secretion by lysophosphatidylcholine in oxidized low density lipoprotein in cultured vascular endothelial cells, Circ Res 71:614, 1992.

42. Boulager CM et al: Oxidized low density lipoproteins induce messenger RNA expression and release of endothelin from human and porcine endothelium, Circ Res 70:1191, 1992.

43. Kuchan MI and Frangos JA: Shear stress regulates endothelin-1 release via protein kinase C and cGMP in cultured endothelial cells, Am J Physiol 264:H150, 1993.

44. Wagner OF et al: Polar secretion of endothelin-1 by cultured endothelial cells, J Biol Chem 267:16066, 1992.

45. Chowienczyk PJ et al: Impaired endothelium-dependent vasodilation of forearm resistance vessels in hypercholesterolaemia, Lancet 340:1430, 1992.

46. Lefer AM and Ma X: Decreased basal nitric oxide release in hypercholesterolemia increases neutrophil adherence to rabbit coronary artery endothelium, Arterioscler Thromb 13:771, 1993.

47. Galle J et al: Cyclosporine and oxidized lipoproteins affect vascular reactivity: influence of the endothelium, Hypertension 21:315, 1993.

48. Simonet S et al: Hypoxia causes an abnormal contractile response in the atherosclerotic rabbit aorta: implication of

reduced nitric oxide and cGMP production, Circ Res 72:616, 1993.

49. Cooke JP et al: Antiatherogenic effects of L-arginine in the hypercholesterolemic rabbit, J Clin Invest 90:1168, 1992.

50. Egashira K et al: Impaired coronary blood flow response to acetylcholine in patients with coronary risk factors and proximal atherosclerotic lesions, J Clin Invest 91:29, 1993.

51. Leung W-H, Lau C-P, and Wong C-K: Beneficial effect of cholesterol-lowering therapy on coronary endothelium-dependent relaxation in hypercholesterolaemic patients, Lancet 341:1496, 1993.

52. Shankar R, de la Motte Ca, and DiCorleto PE: 3-Deaza-adenosine inhibits thrombin-stimulated platelet-derived growth factor production and endothelial-leukocyte adhesion molecule-1–mediated monocytic cell adhesion in human aortic endothelial cells, J Biol Chem 267:9376, 1992.

53. Faruqi R, de la Motte CA, and DiCorleto PE: α-Tocopherol inhibits agonist-induced monocytic cell adhesion to cultured human endothelial cells, J Clin Invest 91:592, 1994.

54. Schreck R and Baeuerle PA: A role for oxygen radicals as second messengers, Trends Cell Biol 1:39, 1991.

55. Marui N et al: Vascular cell adhesion molecule-1 (VCAM-1) gene transcription and expression are regulated through an antioxidant-sensitive mechanism in human vascular endothelial cells, J Clin Invest 92:1866, 1993.

56. Yang J et al: Regulation of adhesion molecule expression in Kaposi's sarcoma cells, J Immunol 152:361, 1994.

57. Schreck R, Rieber P, and Baeuerle PA: Reactive oxygen intermediates as apparently widely used messengers in the activation of the NF-κB transcription factor and HIV-1, EMBO J 10:2247, 1991.

58. Kunisaki M et al: Vitamin E binds to specific binding sites and enhances prostacyclin production by cultured aortic endothelial cells, Thromb Haemost 68:744, 1992.

59. Faruqi RM and DiCorleto PE: Mechanisms of monocyte recruitment and accumulation, Br Heart J 69:S19, 1993.

60. Springer TA: Traffic signals for lymphocyte recirculation and leukocyte emigration: the multistep paradigm, Cell 76:301, 1994.

61. Butcher EC: Leukocyte-endothelial cell recognition: three (or more) steps to specificity and diversity, Cell 67:1033, 1991.

62. Berliner JA et al: Minimally modified low density lipoprotein stimulates monocyte endothelial interactions, J Clin Invest 85:1260, 1990.

63. Saxena U et al: Lipoprotein lipase-mediated lipolysis of very low density lipoproteins increases monocyte adhesion to aortic endothelial cells, Biochem Biophys Res Commun 189:1653, 1992.

64. Kume N, Cybulsky MI, and Gimbrone MA Jr: Lysophosphatidylcholine, a component of atherogenic lipoproteins, induces mononuclear leukocyte adhesion molecules in cultured human and rabbit arterial endothelial cells, J Clin Invest 90:1138, 1992.

65. Bevilacqua MP: Endothelial-leukocyte adhesion molecules, Annu Rev Immunol 11:767, 1993.

66. Cybulsky MI and Gimbrone MA Jr: Endothelial expression of a mononuclear leukocyte adhesion molecule during atherogenesis, Science 251:788, 1991.

67. Li H et al: An atherogenic diet rapidly induces VCAM-1, a cytokine-regulatable mononuclear leukocyte adhesion molecule, in rabbit aortic endothelium, Arterioscler Thromb 13:197, 1993.

68. The Lipid Research Clinics Program: The lipid research clinics coronary prevention trial results. I. Reduction in incidence of coronary heart disease, JAMA 251:351, 1984.

69. The Lipid Research Clinics Program: The lipid research clinics coronary primary prevention trial results. II. The relationship of reduction in incidence of coronary heart disease to cholesterol lowering, JAMA 251:365, 1984.

70. Castelli WP et al: Incidence of coronary heart disease and lipoprotein cholesterol levels: the Framingham Study, JAMA 256:2835, 1986.

71. Multiple Risk Factor Intervention Trial Research Group: Multiple Risk Factor Intervention Trial: risk factor changes and mortality results, JAMA 248:1465, 1982.

72. Report of the National Cholesterol Education Program Expert Panel on detection, evaluation, and treatment of high blood cholesterol in adults, Arch Intern Med 148:36, 1988.

73. Stamler J, Wentworth D, and Neaton JD: Is relationship between serum cholesterol and risk of premature death from coronary heart disease continuous and graded? Findings in 365,222 primary screenees of the Multiple Risk Factor Intervention Trial (MRFIT), JAMA 256:2823, 1986.

74. Schaefer DJ and Levy RI: Pathogenesis and management of lipoprotein disorders, N Engl J Med 312:1300, 1985.

75. Mahley RW et al: Plasma lipoproteins: apolipoprotein structure and function, J Lipid Res 25:1277, 1984.

76. Utermann G: The mysteries of lipoprotein(a), Science 246:904, 1989.

77. Brown MS and Goldstein JL: A receptor-mediated pathway for cholesterol homeostasis, Science 232:34, 1986.

78. Dahlen GH: Lp(a) lipoprotein in cardiovascular disease, Atherosclerosis 108:111, 1994.

79. Wolfbauer G et al: Development of the smooth muscle foam cell: uptake of macrophage lipid inclusions, Proc Natl Acad Sci USA 83:7760, 1986.

80. DiCorleto PE and Bowen-Pope DF: Cultured endothelial cells produce a platelet-derived growth factor-like protein, Proc Natl Acad Sci USA 80:1919, 1983.

81. DiCorleto PE and Fox PL: Growth factor production by endothelial cells. In Ryan U, ed.: Endothelial cells, vol II, Boca Raton, 1988, CRC Press.

82. Mizutani M et al: High glucose and hyperosmolarity increase platelet-derived growth factor mRNA levels in cultured human vascular endothelial cells, Biochem Biophys Res Commun 187:664, 1992.

83. Calderon TM et al: Interleukin-6 modulates c-sis gene expression in cultured human endothelial cells, Cell Immunol 143:118, 1992.

84. Montisano DF, Mann T, and Spragg RG: H_2O_2 increases expression of pulmonary artery endothelial cell platelet-derived growth factor mRNA, J Appl Physiol 73:2255, 1992.

85. Lorenzet R et al: Low molecular weight fibrinogen degradation products stimulate the release of growth factors from endothelial cells, Thromb Haemost 68:357, 1992.

86. Soyombo AA and DiCorleto PE: Stable expression of human platelet-derived growth factor B chain by bovine aortic endothelial cells: cell-association and selective proteolytic cleavage by thrombin, J Biol Chem 269:17734, 1994.

87. Resnick N et al: Platelet-derived growth factor B chain promoter contains a cis-acting fluid shear-stress-responsive element, Proc Natl Acad Sci USA 90:4591, 1993.

88. Taylor WR, Nerem RM, and Alexander RW: Polarized secretion of IGF-I and IGF-I binding protein activity by cultured aortic endothelial cells, J Cell Physiol 154:139, 1993.

89. Gajdusek CM, Luo Z, and Mayberg MR: Sequestration and secretion of insulin-like growth factor-I by bovine aortic endothelial cells, J Cell Physiol 154:192, 1993.

90. Arciniegas E et al: Transforming growth factor beta-1 promotes the differentiation of endothelial cells into smooth muscle-like cells, J Cell Sci 103:521, 1992.

91. Wilcox JN et al: Platelet-derived growth factor mRNA detection in human atherosclerotic plaques by in situ hybridization, J Clin Invest 82:1134, 1988.

92. Clowes AW et al: Regulation of smooth muscle cell growth in injured artery, J Cardiovasc Pharmacol 14(suppl 6):S12, 1989.

93. Campbell GR and Campbell JH: Smooth muscle phenotypic changes in arterial wall homeostasis: implications for the pathogenesis of atherosclerosis, Exp Mol Pathol 42:139, 1985.

94. Gown AM, Tsukada T, and Ross R: Human atherosclerosis. II. Immunocytochemical analysis of the cellular composition of human atherosclerotic lesions, Am J Pathol 125:191, 1986.

95. Hansson GK et al: Immune mechanisms in atherosclerosis, Arteriosclerosis 9:567, 1989.

96. Munro JM and Cotran RS: The pathogenesis of atherosclerosis: atherogenesis and inflammation, Lab Invest 58:249, 1988.

97. Berenson GS et al: Carbohydrate-protein macromolecules and arterial wall integrity—a role in atherosclerosis, Exp Mol Path 4:267, 1984.

98. Ehrhart LA and Holderbaum D: Aortic collagen, elastin and non-fibrous protein synthesis in rabbits fed cholesterol and peanut oil, Atherosclerosis 37:423, 1980.

99. Opsahl WP, DeLuca DJ, and Ehrhart LA: Accelerated rates of collagen synthesis in atherosclerotic arteries quantified in vivo, Arteriosclerosis 7:470, 1986.

100. Mayne R: Collagenous proteins of blood vessels, Arteriosclerosis 6:585, 1986.

101. Falk E: Why do plaques rupture? Circulation 86(suppl III):III-30, 1992.

102. Newby AC, Southgate KM, and Davies M: Extracellular matrix degrading metalloproteinases in the pathogenesis of atherosclerosis, Basic Res Cardiol 89(suppl 1):59, 1994.

103. Katsuda S et al: Matrix metalloproteinase-9 (92 kd gelatinase/type IV collagenase equals gelatinase B) can degrade arterial elastin, Am J Pathol 145:1208, 1994.

104. Blankenhorn DH: Regression of atherosclerosis: dietary and pharmacologic approach, Can J Cardiol 5:206, 1989.

105. Brown BG et al: Lipid lowering and plaque regression: new insights into prevention of plaque disruption and clinical events in coronary disease, Circulation 87:1781, 1993.

106. St Clair RW: Atherosclerosis regression in animal models: current concepts of cellular and biochemical mechanisms, Prog Cardiovasc Dis 26:109, 1983.

107. Kim DN et al: The "turning off" of excessive cell replicative activity in advanced atherosclerotic lesions of swine by a regression diet, Atherosclerosis 71:131, 1988.

108. Hollander W et al: Changes in the connective tissue proteins, glycosaminoglycans and calcium in the arteries of the cynomolgus monkey during atherosclerotic induction and regression, Atherosclerosis 51:89, 1984.

109. Strong JP et al: Long-term induction and regression of diet-induced atherosclerotic lesions in rhesus monkeys. I. Morphological and chemical evidence for regression of lesions in the aorta and carotid and peripheral arteries, Arterioscler Thromb 14:958, 1994.

110. Langner RO and Bement CL: Lesion regression and protein synthesis in rabbits after removal of dietary cholesterol, Atherosclerosis 5:74, 1985.

111. Badimon JJ, Fuster V, Badimon J: Role of high density lipoproteins in the regression of atherosclerosis, Circulation 83(suppl III):III-86, 1992.

112. Armstrong ML et al: Hemodynamic sequelae of regression of experimental atherosclerosis, J Clin Invest 71:104, 1983.

CHAPTER NINE

DIAGNOSIS AND TREATMENT OF LIPID DISTURBANCES

Jeffrey W. Olin

Michael D. Cressman

Byron J. Hoogwerf

Cheryl E. Weinstein

In the last three decades results of several epidemiologic studies have been published and have confirmed the observation that increased serum total cholesterol (TC) or low-density lipoprotein cholesterol (LDL-C) levels and decreased high-density lipoprotein cholesterol (HDL-C) levels are strongly associated with the development of complications resulting from atherosclerotic vascular disease. In addition, controlled clinical trials have demonstrated that lowering serum cholesterol levels decreases the risk of developing coronary heart disease (CHD) (i.e., primary prevention). There are now several randomized, controlled clinical trials that present convincing evidence that aggressive lowering of LDL-C and/or raising of HDL-C can result in regression of atherosclerosis and fewer cardiovascular events in subjects with CHD (i.e., secondary prevention). Because of the interest in the role of lipoproteins in the pathogenesis of atherosclerosis, this chapter discusses the epidemiologic evidence linking blood lipids to atherosclerotic vascular disease, evidence that cholesterol-lowering therapy decreases cardiovascular morbidity and mortality rates, and the role that lipids play in the progression and regression of atherosclerosis. This discussion is followed by reviews of lipoprotein metabolism and clinical aspects of various lipid and lipoprotein disorders, including the treatment of these conditions.

ROLE OF BLOOD LIPIDS IN PATHOGENESIS OF ATHEROSCLEROTIC VASCULAR DISEASE

The Framingham Study was one of the first epidemiologic studies demonstrating a strong association between TC levels and the development of cardiovascular disease.[1]

The 8-year probability of developing CHD was directly related to the level of TC even when the TC values were still within the "normal" range. The Framingham data also showed that CHD risk at any cholesterol level was highly dependent on the presence or absence of other cardiovascular risk factors (glucose intolerance, hypertension, cigarette smoking, electrocardiographic [ECG] evidence of left ventricular hypertrophy). The risk was substantially increased in patients with multiple risk factors. In 4374 Framingham participants less than 50 years old, Anderson, Castelli, and Levy[2] noted that for each 10-mg/dl increment in TC there was a 9% increase in cardiovascular mortality.

In the Multiple Risk Factor Intervention Trial (MRFIT), 6-year follow-up data were obtained from more than 350,000 middle-aged men who had no history of atherosclerotic coronary artery disease.[3] There was a strong correlation between the TC level at screening and the 6-year CHD death rates (Table 9-1). This relationship was continuous and graded. In agreement with the Framingham Study, cigarette smoking and/or increased blood pressure substantially increased the CHD mortality rate at any given TC level. The relationship between TC level and stroke mortality rate was also examined during the 6-year MRFIT follow-up.[4] A significant positive correlation ($P = 0.007$) between nonhemorrhagic stroke and TC level was found using a proportional hazards regression analysis controlling for age, cigarette smoking, diastolic blood pressure, and race or ethnic group. Tell, Crouse, and Furberg[5] reported that a positive relationship between elevated blood lipid and lipoprotein levels and clinical evidence of cerebrovascular atherosclerosis was apparent in 23 of 26 studies reviewed. An association between increased TC levels and decreased HDL-C levels and the

Table 9-1. MRFIT: 6-Year Coronary Mortality Rate

Quintile	Serum Cholesterol (mg/dl [mmol/L])	CHD Mortality		
		Number of Deaths	Rate per 1000	Relative Risk
1	≤181 (≤4.68)	196	3.2	1.0
2	182-202 (4.71-5.22)	288	4.2	1.29
3	203-220 (5.25-5.69)	395	5.6	1.73
4	221-224 (5.72-6.31)	533	7.1	2.21
5	≥245 (≥6.34)	846	11.1	3.42

(From Stamler J, Wentworth D, and Neaton JD: Is the relationship between the serum cholesterol and risk of premature death from coronary heart disease continuous and graded? Findings in 356,222 primary screenees of the Multiple Risk Factor Intervention Trial (MRFIT), JAMA 256:2833, 1986. Copyright 1986, American Medical Association.)

development of peripheral arterial atherosclerotic disease was also noted in the Lipid Research Clinics Program Prevalence Study.[6]

Although most of the early epidemiological studies focused on the relationship between TC and the risk of atherosclerosis, it has become apparent that separation of cholesterol-containing lipoproteins into different lipoprotein fractions improves the predictive power of this risk assessment. For example, LDL-C levels have been shown superior to TC levels in predicting CHD risk.[7] A very strong inverse relationship between HDL-C levels and CHD risk has also been reported.[8,9] The risk is particularly great when HDL-C levels are below 35 mg/dl.

In the Framingham Study (after 12 years of follow-up) myocardial infarction occurred in six times as many patients in the lowest quartile of HDL-C distribution (HDL-C less than 46 mg/dl) compared with those in the highest HDL-C quartile (HDL-C 67 mg/dl or greater).[10] For this reason, screening with TC levels may be inadequate in predicting cardiovascular risk since some high-risk individuals with normal TC levels may have low HDL-C levels and escape detection.[11] Although reduction of TC and LDL-C have been shown to decrease CHD risk (see the following material), no trials have adequately shown that raising HDL-C levels decreases CHD risk in patients with TC levels below 200 mg/dl.[12] However, the magnitude of risk reduction in gemfibrozil-treated patients in the Helsinki Heart Study[13] was greater than the risk reduction observed in the cholestyramine-treated participants of the Lipid Research Clinics Coronary Primary Prevention Trial (LRC-CPPT)[14,15] even though gemfibrozil and cholestyramine produced similar effects on LDL-C levels. Since the study groups were similar, this difference may be due to the 10% increase in HDL-C levels that occurred in patients treated with gemfibrozil in the Helsinki Heart Study. No change in HDL-C levels was noted in the cholestyramine-treated group of the LRC-CPPT.

There is conflicting information regarding the association between elevated cholesterol levels and CHD morbidity and mortality in the elderly population.[16-18] Benfante and Reed[16] studied 1480 men aged 65 to 74 years and demonstrated that elevated cholesterol was an indepen-

dent risk factor for the development of CHD (relative risk, 1.64). However, Krumholz et al[17] recently failed to show a correlation between elevated levels of TC and LDL-C or low HDL-C and CHD or all-cause mortality in persons older than 70 years. In a recent editorial Hulley and Newman[18] suggested that the absolute risk attributable to high blood cholesterol (in CHD deaths per thousand people) may be greater in the patient 70 years of age or older compared with those 60 years of age or younger even though the relative risk is smaller. They estimate that true relative risk for those in their sixties and seventies may be as high as 1.6 in men and 1.3 in women. Unfortunately the cholesterol reduction in the Seniors Program Trial has been canceled because of a lack of funding. Perhaps the recently initiated Antihypertensive, Lipid Lowering to Prevent Heart Attack Trial (ALLHAT) will provide an answer to two important questions: Is elevated cholesterol a risk for CHD in the elderly? and Does lowering TC and LDL-C decrease CHD and all-cause mortality in the elderly? Until these important questions are answered, we will continue to treat the elderly patient who has atherosclerosis aggressively with life-style modification and lipid-lowering pharmacologic therapy. Perhaps a less aggressive approach should be taken with the elderly patient who does not have atherosclerosis (i.e. primary prevention).

Plasma Triglycerides and Cardiovascular Disease

Whether triglycerides are an independent risk factor for cardiovascular disease is a matter of continued controversy. Elevated serum triglycerides have been shown to correlate with the risk of developing CHD using univariate analysis, but when multivariate analysis is used to take into consideration other risk factors, most of this correlation is lost.[19] It is difficult to determine the importance of triglycerides alone because of the complicated interplay between elevated triglycerides, low HDL-C and small dense LDL particles (LDL subclass phenotype B). These small dense LDL particles are associated with elevated plasma triglycerides and are particularly atherogenic.[20-22] Elevated triglycerides may be a stronger risk factor for CHD in women than in men.[22] Although triglycerides are usually measured in the fasting state, some investigators have suggested that it may be important to study triglyceride metabolism in the postprandial state rather than the fasting state. Using multivariate analysis, Patsch et al[23] showed that a single postprandial triglyceride level 6 to 8 hours after a meal was an accurate predictor of the risk for developing CHD.

A subgroup analysis from the Helsinki Heart Study[24] demonstrated that the relative risk for the development of CHD was 3.8 for subjects with an LDL/HDL ratio greater than 5 and triglycerides greater than 200 mg/dl compared with subjects with an LDL/HDL ratio of 5 or less and triglycerides greater than 200 mg/dl. In subjects with triglycerides greater than 200 mg/dl and an LDL/HDL ratio greater than 5 treated with gemfibrozil, there was a 71% lower incidence of CHD events than in subjects in the placebo subgroup. Grundy and Vega[25] have summarized the various views of the relationship of hypertriglyceridemia to CHD.

EVIDENCE THAT CHOLESTEROL-LOWERING THERAPY REDUCES CARDIOVASCULAR RISK

A number of well-controlled clinical trials have been designed to determine the effects of lipid-lowering therapy on cardiovascular morbidity and mortality. Only the most important studies are discussed in the following material.

Primary Prevention Trials*
LIPID RESEARCH CLINICS CORONARY PRIMARY PREVENTION TRIAL. The LRC-CPPT was a randomized, placebo-controlled double-blind multicenter trial designed to test the effectiveness of cholesterol-lowering therapy in reducing the risk of developing CHD.[14,15,16] Enrolled in this study were 3806 middle-aged men (35 to 59 years at entry) with plasma cholesterol levels of 265 mg/dl or higher and LDL-C levels of 190 mg/dl or higher. Participants had no clinical evidence of atherosclerotic heart disease at entry. All participants were advised to follow a cholesterol-lowering diet and were randomly assigned to treatment with a placebo (*n* = 1900) or the bile acid binding resin cholestyramine (*n* = 1906) at a dose of 24 g/day. Patients were followed 7 to 10 years (mean, 7.4 years). Definite CHD death plus definite nonfatal myocardial infarction were the primary end points. There was a 19% reduction in these primary end points in the cholestyramine group versus the placebo group (*P* < 0.05) (Fig. 9-1). CHD death and nonfatal myocardial infarction were reduced by 24% and 19%, respectively, in the cholestyramine versus placebo groups. There were also a 25% reduction in the development of positive exercise tests, a 20% reduction in angina pectoris, a 21% reduction in coronary artery bypass surgery, and a 15% reduction in intermittent claudication in the group receiving cholestyr-

---

*The West of Scotland Coronary Prevention Study (New Engl J Med 333:1301, 1995) was recently published demonstrating that pravastatin reduced coronary heart events by 31% (*P* < 0.001) and death by any cause by 22% (*P* = 0.051) compared to placebo in men with no previous myocardial infarction.

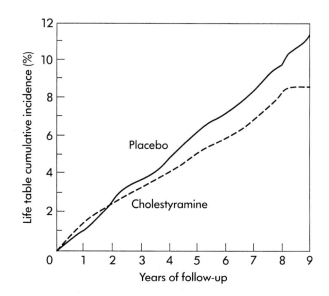

Fig. 9-1. Life-table cumulative incidence of primary end points in treatment groups computed by Kaplan-Meier method. *(From Lipid Research Clinics Program, JAMA 251:365, 1984.)*

amine compared with the group receiving a placebo. All-cause mortality, however, was no different in the two groups. The trial was not designed to show a difference in all-cause mortality, and the absence of a difference was due to an increased number of accidental and violent deaths in the cholestyramine group compared with the placebo group.

Not all participants in the trial took full doses of cholestyramine. Approximately 50% of the cholestyramine-treated patients ingested 20 to 24 g of cholestyramine per day; approximately 25% took 8 g or less. The relationship between the total dose of cholestyramine taken and the reduction in TC and LDL-C levels was significant. There was a significant relationship between the reduction in LDL-C and the reduction in CHD risk. For every 1% reduction in the TC level, there was a 2% reduction in CHD risk. Although there were no differences in mean HDL-C levels at baseline or after treatment in the cholestyramine group versus the placebo group, some patients did demonstrate an increase in HDL-C. In these patients there was a 5.5% decrease in CHD risk for each 1-mg/dl increment in HDL-C.[26]

HELSINKI HEART STUDY. The Helsinki Heart Study[13] was a randomized, double-blind, 5-year primary prevention trial comparing a placebo with the fibric acid derivative gemfibrozil (600 mg twice daily) in 4081 middle-aged men (40 to 55 years). In contrast to cholestyramine, which lowers only TC and LDL-C levels, gemfibrozil lowers TC, triglycerides, and LDL-C and very low density lipoprotein cholesterol (VLDL-C) levels. Gemfibrozil also increases HDL-C levels. There were similar changes in TC and LDL-C in the gemfibrozil-treated patients as in the cholestyramine-treated LRC-CPPT patients. In the Helsinki Heart Study gemfibrozil produced a 9% decrease in TC, an 8% decrease in LDL-C, and a 10% increase in HDL-C. Participants with the lowest HDL-C levels at entry had the greatest increase in HDL-C during gemfibrozil treatment. Triglyceride levels were reduced by approximately 35% in the gemfibrozil-treated group.

The life-table curves for primary end points in the Helsinki Heart Study were almost identical to those of the LRC-CPPT. There was a 34% reduction in the incidence of fatal and nonfatal myocardial infarction and cardiac death in the gemfibrozil-treated groups versus the placebo group. Nonfatal myocardial infarction was reduced by 37%, whereas CHD mortality was reduced by 26%. As in the LRC-CPPT the overall mortality rate was no different between the placebo group and the gemfibrozil group in the Helsinki Heart Study. An increased incidence of accidental and violent deaths occurred in gemfibrozil-treated patients versus placebo-treated patients in this trial. The relationship between serum cholesterol level and the risk of death from violence or accidents has been examined in a cohort of 1580 Finnish men, and no correlation was found.[27]

As previously stated, for every 1% reduction in TC or LDL-C levels, there was a 2% decrease in CHD risk in the LRC-CPPT. In the Helsinki Heart Study, for every 1% decrease in TC or LDL-C levels there was approximately a 3.8% reduction in fatal and nonfatal myocardial infarction and cardiac death in the gemfibrozil group. The more favorable effect of gemfibrozil compared with cholestyramine may be attributed to the rise in HDL-C levels observed in the gemfibrozil group. However, gemfibrozil also reduced triglyceride levels and may also have produced favorable effects on the composition of other atherogenic lipoproteins.

Secondary Prevention Trials

CORONARY DRUG PROJECT. The Coronary Drug Project (CDP)[28,29] assessed the effect of various drugs in 8341 men with a history of myocardial infarction. Although conjugated estrogens, clofibrate, or dextrothyroxine sodium showed no benefit compared with a placebo, patients treated with nicotinic acid demonstrated a reduced incidence of nonfatal myocardial infarction and an 11% decrease in all-cause mortality after 15 years of follow-up ($P = 0.0004$). Interestingly this favorable effect was not apparent after 6 years of follow-up when the formal CDP ended and drug therapy was discontinued. Although the exact cause of this late benefit of niacin is not clear, it has been suggested that the drug either prevented mild non–life-threatening myocardial infarction early or reduced progression of coronary atherosclerosis during the period of niacin administration. Theoretically these effects could reduce the rate of later ischemic complications. Although additional similar benefits may be seen in the LRC-CPPT and Helsinki Heart Study participants with a longer period of follow-up, the availability of new lipid-lowering agents to participants after those trials were completed, and a more aggressive approach to lipid management beginning in 1988, may dilute any long-term effect of the agents used during the trials in the treated subjects.

SCANDINAVIAN SIMVASTATIN SURVIVAL STUDY. More recently the Scandinavian Simvastatin Sur-

vival Study[30] has demonstrated that aggressive cholesterol lowering not only reduced the risk for CHD events but also reduced the risk for all-cause mortality. This was a randomized double-blind trial in 4444 patients in which simvastatin lowered the TC by 25%, LDL-C by 35%, and raised the HDL-C by 8%. At slightly more than 5 years of follow-up, the relative risk of death in the treated group was 0.79 (95% CI 0.58 to 0.85). Eight percent of patients in the treatment group died compared with twelve percent in the placebo group. Similarly, 28% of patients in the placebo group had CHD events compared with 19% in the simvastatin group. The effects of treatment on mortality and CHD events became evident only after more than 1 year of therapy. The study demonstrated a reduction of CHD events in women on simvastatin compared with those receiving a placebo, although all-cause mortality was not different in women. Analysis of participants greater than 60 years old also showed that simvastatin reduced CHD and mortality in this subgroup of patients.

Regression of Atherosclerosis

There have been numerous animal studies over the last 30 to 40 years demonstrating that regression of atherosclerosis is possible with a low-cholesterol, low–saturated-fat diet. Over the last 2 decades an enormous amount of literature has emerged demonstrating that regression of atherosclerosis is possible in humans. Most of the recently reported regression studies used quantitative angiography to measure progression and regression of coronary and peripheral atherosclerosis. The actual degree of regression measured by quantitative arteriography is quite small, suggesting that something other than changes in luminal diameter accounted for the marked reduction in atherosclerotic events that occurred in these trials. De Feyter et al[31] and Hong et al[32] have summarized the value, limitations, and implications of quantitative coronary angiography. Several recent reviews have summarized the results of the available randomized controlled clinical trials using coronary angiography to assess the role that aggressive lipid management plays in the progression and regression of atherosclerosis.[33-35] Brown et al[33] have summarized some of these results in Table 9-2.

Most of the regression studies used pharmacologic lipid-lowering therapy to achieve regression of atherosclerosis. However, in the Lifestyle Heart Trial, Ornish et al[39] used intensive life-style modification such as diet, exercise, and stress management as a means to lower lipid values and decrease CHD events. In the Program on Surgical Control of Hyperlipidemia (POSCH) Trial,[38] patients with a previous myocardial infarction were randomized to diet alone or to diet and partial ileal bypasses as a means of lowering cholesterol. There was a 35% reduction in the CHD event rate in the patients undergoing partial ileal bypass compared with the control group receiving diet alone. In addition, more regression occurred in the actively treated group. A detailed description of every regression study published to date is beyond the scope of this chapter. However, several studies are discussed in the following material.

The Cholesterol Lowering Atherosclerosis Study[37]

Table 9-2. Lipid Lowering and Plaque Regression (Results of 9 Arteriographic Trials)

| Study (Ref) | n | Control Regimen | Treatment Regimen | Treatment Response | | Years | Control Patients | | Treatment Patients | | % Event Reduction |
				LDL %	HDL %		Progression (%)	Regression (%)	Progression (%)	Regression (%)	
NHLBI[36]	143	Diet	D + R	−31	+8	5	49	7	32	7	33
CLAS I[37]	188	Diet	D + R + N	−43	+37	2	61	2	39	16	25
POSCH[38]	838	Diet	D + PIB + R	−42	+5	9.7	65	6	37	14	35
Lifestyle[39]	48	Usual	D + M + E	−37	−3	1	32	32	14	41	0 vs 1
FATS (N + C)[40]	146	Diet ± R	D + R + N	−32	+43	2.5	46	11	25	39	80
FATS (L + C)[40]			D + R + L	−46	+15	2.5	46	11	22	32	70
CLAS II[41]	138	Diet	D + R + N	−40	+37	4	83	6	30	18	43
UCSF-SCOR[42]	97	Usual	D + R + N + L	−39	+25	2	41	13	20	33	1 vs 0
STARS (D)[43]	90	Usual	D	−16	0	3	46	4	15	38	69
STARS (D + R)[43]			D + R	−36	−4	3	46	4	12	33	89
SCRIP[44-46]	300	Usual	D+(R/N/L/F) + BP + E	−215	+13	4	–	10	–	21	50
Heidelberg[47]	113	Usual	D + E	−8	+3	11	42	4	20	30	27
MARS[48]	270	Usual	D + L	−38	+10	2	65	11	47	23	–

(From Brown BG et al: Lipid lowering and plaque regression. New insights into prevention of plaque disruption and clinical events in coronary disease, Circulation 87:1781, 1993, with permission.)
D, diet; *R*, resin; *N*, niacin; *PIB*, partial ileal bypass; *L*, lovastatin; *F*, fibric acid derivatives; *M*, meditation; *E*, exercise; *BP*, blood pressure.

(CLAS) reported on 162 nonsmoking, highly compliant men aged 40 to 59 who had undergone previous coronary artery bypass surgery. Patients were randomized to receive a placebo or a combination of colestipol and nicotinic acid. Patients were studied angiographically at the initiation of the study and 2 years after treatment was initiated. There was a 26% reduction in TC, a 43% reduction in LDL-C, and a 37% increase in HDL-C in patients receiving active drug. There was less progression of atherosclerosis ($P < 0.03$) and more regression of atherosclerosis ($P < 0.03$) in the native coronary arteries of patients treated with colestipol and niacin compared with patients treated with placebo. In patients undergoing coronary artery bypass grafting, there were fewer new lesions and less progression of atherosclerosis in patients receiving active drug compared with placebo ($P < 0.03$). Regression of atherosclerosis at the end of 2 years occurred in 16.2% of patients treated with colestipol-niacin as compared with 2.4% of patients treated with placebo ($P < 0.002$). Of the original 162 subjects, 132 were treated for 4 years, and repeat coronary arteriography was performed at that time.[41] Again, there was significantly more regression and fewer new native coronary lesions in the actively treated group compared with those treated with placebo. Brown et al[40] used computer-assisted quantitative coronary angiography in 120 men with apolipoprotein B levels of 125 mg/dl or higher and a positive family history for CHD. All patients were instructed on a low-cholesterol, low–saturated-fat diet and were then randomized to one of three groups: placebo (with the addition of colestipol if needed) ($n = 46$), lovastatin and colestipol ($n = 38$), or niacin and colestipol ($n = 36$). LDL-C was reduced by 7% in the placebo-colestipol group, 46% in the lovastatin-colestipol group, and 32% in the niacin-colestipol group. The HDL-C was increased 5% in the placebo-colestipol group, 15% in the lovastatin-colestipol group, and 43% in the niacin-colestipol group.

Apolipoprotein B decreased from 149 to 142 in the conventional therapy group, from 159 to 103 in the lovastatin-colestipol group, and from 155 to 111 in the niacin-colestipol group. Regression occurred much more commonly in the actively treated groups ($P < 0.005$) compared with the placebo group. In addition to arteriographic regression, cardiovascular events were fewer in both the lovastatin-colestipol group and the niacin-colestipol group ($P < 0.005$). The Monitored Atherosclerosis Regression Study[48] (MARS) compared the 3-hydroxy-3-methylglutaryl coenzyme A (HMG CoA) reductase inhibitor lovastatin to placebo. This is the only trial to prospectively evaluate coronary angiographic films by a computerized quantitative coronary angiographic system with automated edge detection algorithms as the primary end-point methodology and panel-based reading as a secondary end-point methodology. B-mode ultrasound measurements to the distal carotid artery far wall intima-media thickness (IMT) was an additional end point. The MARS Trial was one of the few regression studies to include a large number of women. Subgroup analysis showed that the women had better lesion regression response to lipid-lowering therapy than men and estrogen replacement therapy enhanced the response to lipid-lowering therapy. These data are similar to the data reported in the UCSF-SCOR Study.[42] Blankenhorn and Hodis[49] performed a metaanalysis using the data from the NHLBI Type II,[36] CLAS,[37,41] POSCH,[38] UCSF-SCOR,[42] FATS,[40] St. Thomas Atherosclerosis Regression Study (STARS),[43] and the Lifestyle Heart Trial[39] evaluating the role of lipid-lowering therapy in regression of atherosclerosis and in secondary prevention of CHD. A summary of their findings is demonstrated in Figs. 9-2 and 9-3. In the actively treated group of patients ($n = 688$), the odds ratio of achieving regression of atherosclerosis was 2.0 and progression of atherosclerosis was 0.4 when compared with control subjects ($n = 593$). Further analysis was

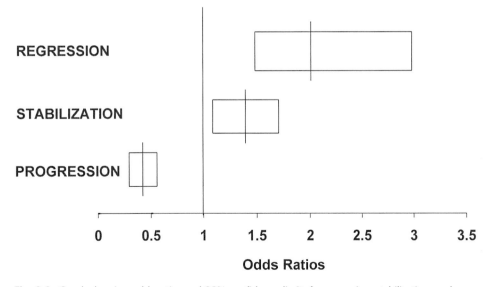

Fig. 9-2. Graph showing odds ratios and 95% confidence limits for regression, stabilization, and progression comparing 688 treated subjects with 593 control subjects with entrance and exit angiograms derived from seven coronary angiographic trials. *(From Blankenhorn DH and Hodis HN: Arterial imaging and atherosclerosis reversal, Arterioscler Thromb 12:177, 1994, with permission.)*

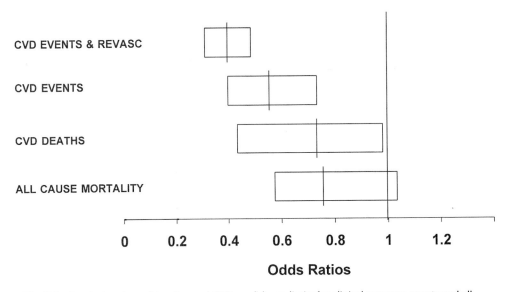

Fig. 9-3. Graph showing odds ratios and 95% confidence limits for clinical coronary events and all-cause mortality, comparing all 793 treated subjects with 708 control subjects from seven coronary angiographic trials. *(From Blankenhorn DH and Hodis HN: Arterial imaging and atherosclerosis reversal, Arterioscler Thromb 12:177, 1994, with permission.)*

conducted on 793 treated patients and 708 control patients. Cardiovascular disease events, revascularization, and deaths were significantly less in the treated group compared with the control patients. The odds ratio for all-cause mortality was reduced but fell short of the 95% confidence level for significance.

The exact mechanism by which regression occurs is unknown. Regression may actually mean a shrinkage of intimal plaque due to a reduction in the components of the plaque such as lipid components, macrophages, smooth muscle cells, and connective tissue. Certain components of the plaque such as calcification of fibrous tissue may make regression less likely.[50] Other mechanisms such as lysis of occlusive thrombi or mural thrombi, healing or remodeling of an acutely disruptive plaque, physiologic remodeling independent of plaque size, relaxation of arterial vasomotor tone (vasodilator or vasoconstrictor responses), and the role of the endothelium itself may be important.[50] Treasure et al[51] demonstrated in a randomized double-blind placebo-controlled trial that cholesterol-lowering therapy with lovastatin significantly improved endothelium-mediated responses in the coronary arteries in patients with atherosclerosis. Anderson et al[52] randomly assigned 49 patients with coronary artery disease to receive one of three treatments: American Heart Association step I diet (diet group, $n = 11$), lovastatin and cholestyramine (LDL-lowering group, $n = 21$), or lovastatin and probucol (LDL-lowering antioxidant group, $n = 17$). Endothelium-dependent coronary artery vasomotion in response to an intracoronary infusion of acetylcholine was assessed at baseline and after 1 year of therapy. The greatest improvement in vasoconstrictor response occurred in the LDL-lowering antioxidant group compared with diet ($P < 0.01$) with a lesser response in the LDL-lowering group compared with diet ($P = 0.08$). These investigators and others[53] suggest that the improvement in

endothelial function may at least in part account for the decreased cardiac event rate that occurs in patients treated with lipid-lowering therapy.

There has been an extensive amount of published data on the use of noninvasive imaging (B-mode ultrasound) of the carotid and other peripheral arteries to serve as a marker of underlying atherosclerosis and to assess whether regression of atherosclerosis has occurred. Population-based ultrasonography studying eastern Finnish men has demonstrated a strong association between IMT measured by B-mode ultrasound and cardiovascular disease.[54] Similar data is available in women.[55] The CLAS[56,57] has shown that over 48 months of follow-up, patients receiving placebo had an increase in intima-media wall thickness compared with a decrease in patients receiving active drug (Fig. 9-4). The IMT of the common carotid artery correlated with the quantitative computed angiographic measurement of carotid atherosclerosis with an r value of 0.702 ($P < 0.001$).

LIPOPROTEIN METABOLISM

Cholesterol and triglycerides are transported in the blood in complexes called lipoproteins. The plasma lipoproteins contain a core of water-insoluble lipids (cholesterol esters and triglycerides) surrounded by a coat containing a small amount of unesterified cholesterol, phospholipids, and specialized proteins referred to as apoproteins (apo).[58] Lipoproteins are mainly synthesized in intestinal cells and hepatocytes but are modified considerably in the circulation by lipolytic enzymes and transfer of several lipoprotein components between the various plasma lipoproteins. Thus they are extremely heterogeneous structures. Classically the plasma lipoproteins are separated into five major classes: (1) chylomicrons, (2) very low density lipoproteins (VLDLs), (3)

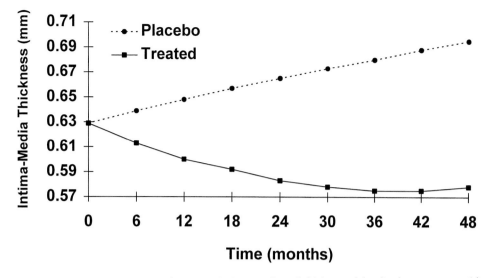

Fig. 9-4. Effect of lipid-lowering therapy on intima-media wall thickness of the distal common carotid artery in the Cholesterol Lowering Atherosclerosis Study. *(From Mack WJ et al: One-year reduction and longitudinal analysis of carotid intima-media thickness associated with colestipol-niacin therapy, Stroke 24:1779, 1993.)*

Table 9-3. Classification of Plasma Lipoproteins

Lipoprotein	Source	Major Density (g/ml)	Apoproteins	Lipids
Chylomicrons	Intestine	<1.006	B-48, E, C, A-I, A-II, A-IV	TG > C
VLDL	Liver	<1.006	B-100, E, C	TG > C
IDL	VLDL	1.006-1.019	B-100, E	TG = C
LDL	IDL	1.019-1.063	B-100	C > TG
HDL	Liver, intestine	1.063-1.21	A-I, A-II, C, E	C > TG

TG, Triglycerides; *C*, cholesterol.

intermediate-density lipoproteins (IDLs), (4) low-density lipoproteins (LDLs), and (5) high-density lipoproteins (HDLs). This separation is based on their flotation density *(d)*, which is determined by ultracentrifugation (Table 9-3). Clinically the dyslipoproteinemias are often classified on the basis of the concentration of these major lipoprotein classes. Alternatively a genotypic classification can be used if the disorder appears to have a genetic basis.[59]

Chylomicrons are large triglyceride-rich lipoproteins *(d < 1.006 g/ml)* that are synthesized in intestinal cells. Chylomicrons transport dietary fats through the lymphatics to the systemic circulation. Triglycerides are removed from chylomicrons by lipoprotein lipase, which is located on the luminal side of endothelial cells in adipose tissue and muscle (Fig. 9-5). Remnants of these particles are rapidly removed by the liver. In healthy individuals chylomicrons are no longer present in blood a few hours after a meal.

The liver secretes VLDLs *(d < 1.006 g/ml)* that are similar to chylomicrons but contain a large apoprotein called ApoB-100 (subsequently referred to as apoB). Each VLDL particle contains one apoB molecule, but the triglyceride

content of specific VLDLs varies widely. VLDLs are converted to VLDL remnants through lipoprotein lipase–stimulated removal of triglycerides from these particles. Some of these particles reside in the IDL range *(d, 1.006 to 1.019 g/ml)* and are removed by hepatic LDL receptors, which avidly bind the apoE on the IDL particle. Others are converted to LDLs *(d, 1.019 to 1.063 g/ml)*. However, the precise mechanisms responsible for conversion of IDLs to LDLs are not known.

LDLs, the major atherogenic lipoproteins, contain apoB as their sole apoprotein. In general, two thirds of the TC is carried in LDLs. Although factors regulating LDL synthetic rate are poorly understood, considerable progress in understanding LDL catabolism has been made in recent years. Goldstein and Brown[60] characterized an LDL receptor-mediated process (referred to as receptor-mediated endocytosis) that is tightly coupled to the regulation of intracellular cholesterol synthesis. It has become apparent that a complex interaction exists between LDL receptor-mediated removal of plasma LDL, recycling of LDL receptor protein into the cell membrane, synthesis of intracellular cholesterol, regulation of new LDL receptor synthesis,

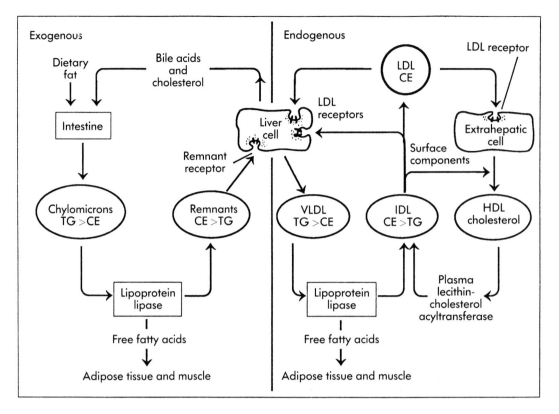

Fig. 9-5. Endogenous and exogenous metabolism of lipoproteins, emphasizing the importance of lipoprotein lipase in chylomicron and VLDL metabolism and of liver cell and extrahepatic cell specific receptors in LDL metabolism. *(From Goldstein JL and Brown MS: Familial hypercholesterolemia: a genetic receptor disease, Hosp Pract 20:35, 1985.)*

and conversion of intracellular cholesterol to bile acids. This interaction maintains the intracellular cholesterol concentration at a constant level. The number and activity of LDL receptors apparently is particularly important in regulating plasma LDL concentration.[61] The intestine and liver also synthesize HDLs that seem to be involved in "reverse cholesterol transport." Conceptually this is a process by which HDLs (d, 1.063 to 1.21 g/ml) transport cholesterol from extrahepatic tissues. HDLs exchange a variety of structural components (lipids and apoproteins) with other lipoproteins.[62] Certain HDLs may be removed by the liver, although the routes of HDL catabolism have not been completely characterized. Apoproteins A-1 and A-2 are the major HDL apoproteins.

PHENOTYPIC CLASSIFICATION OF THE DYSLIPOPROTEINEMIAS

Fredrickson, Levy, and Lees[63] developed a classification scheme based on the concentration of four of the major lipoprotein classes. The scheme does not include HDL-C. Although this phenotypic approach does not provide information about specific abnormalities of apoprotein structure, lipolytic enzyme function, or lipoprotein receptor activity, it is useful for the clinical classification of disorders of lipoprotein metabolism and is particularly helpful when drug treatment is considered. Several genetic syndromes (e.g., heterozygous familial hypercholesterol-

Table 9-4. Fredrickson Classification of Dyslipoproteinemias

Lipoprotein Phenotype	Elevated Lipoprotein Fraction	Frequency
I	Chylomicrons	Rare
IIa	LDL	Common
IIb	LDL and VLDL	Common
III	IDL	Rare
IV	VLDL	Common
V	Chylomicrons and VLDL	Uncommon

emia) have been identified, although laboratory techniques to confirm presumed genetic disorders are not always available.[64] For these reasons, we review the Fredrickson phenotypic classification initially and then discuss some of the familial dyslipoproteinemias associated with a high risk of atherosclerosis. There are five major Fredrickson phenotypic lipoprotein abnormalities (Table 9-4). The type I and type V hyperlipidemias are characterized by fasting chylomicronemia. In type I, the least common Fredrickson phenotype, concentrations of the other lipoproteins (VLDL, IDL, LDL) are usually decreased. The familial form generally is identified in the first decade of life and is due to a marked reduction in lipoprotein lipase activity.[65] Episodes of eruptive xanthomas and/or pancreatitis dominate the clinical picture. The risk of developing premature atherosclerosis is probably not increased. Affected individuals have fasting triglyceride levels of 1,500 mg/dl or higher, and triglyceride levels greater than 10,000 mg/dl are not unusual. Chilled plasma from type I patients contains a creamy layer above clear plasma. Treatment requires severe dietary fat restriction, although medium-chain triglycerides can be added to the diet since they are not transported in chylomicrons. This lipoprotein disorder is not amenable to lipid-lowering drug therapy.

In patients with type V hyperlipidemia there is fasting chylomicronemia with severe hypertriglyceridemia. Patients also have elevated VLDL levels.[66] With this disorder chilled plasma contains a creamy layer and a milky layer. Since VLDLs carry some cholesterol, fasting triglyceride and cholesterol levels are usually both increased. LDL and HDL levels are usually reduced. As is true in patients with type I hyperlipidemia, the clinical picture in patients with type V hyperlipidemia is dominated by eruptive xanthomas and pancreatitis. Carbohydrate intolerance, obesity, hyperuricemia, and excess alcohol intake are often present. Treatment consists of correction of these underlying medical conditions and institution of a low-fat, low-calorie diet. Administration of nicotinic acid and/or a fibric acid derivative is indicated if triglyceride levels are greater than 500 mg/dl despite these measures. The risk of atherosclerosis may be increased, although this increase may be caused by associated factors such as diabetes mellitus, hyperinsulinemia, obesity, low HDL-C, or small dense LDL particles.

Hypertriglyceridemia is also the predominant lipid abnormality in type IV hyperlipidemia. VLDL levels are increased, and LDL and HDL levels are generally below normal.[67] Fasting chylomicronemia is not present. TC levels may be low, normal, or increased. Type IV hyperlipidemia is quite common, particularly in patients with obesity, poorly controlled diabetes mellitus, excess alcohol intake, or chronic renal failure. High-carbohydrate diets and certain drugs such as the diuretics, β-blockers, estrogens, corticosteroids, or isotretinoin can cause or exacerbate hypertriglyceridemia. In addition, genetic forms of this phenotypic disorder have been identified. Treatment of patients with type IV hyperlipidemia begins with correction of associated conditions. A moderately low-fat diet, restricted in calories when appropriate, should be initiated. "Tight" control of blood sugar levels in patients with diabetes mellitus should be emphasized. The omega-3 fatty acids contained in fatty fish may reduce triglyceride levels, but many of the fish oil capsules contain a considerable amount of calories and cholesterol.[68] A paradoxic rise in LDL-C may occur. In addition, hyperglycemia has been noted in previously well-controlled diabetics who take large doses of fish oils. Nicotinic acid and the fibric acid derivatives are the most useful triglyceride-lowering drugs (see section, "Pharmacologic Treatment of Lipid Disorders"). The HMG CoA reductase inhibitors and probucol are relatively ineffective in treating type IV hyperlipidemia. The bile acid sequestrants may exacerbate preexisting hypertriglyceridemia.

Type III hyperlipidemia is an uncommon disorder caused by the presence of a structurally abnormal apoE that does not bind to the LDL receptor.[69] ApoE exists in three isoforms (apoE-2, apoE-3, apoE-4) and six genotypes (E-2/2, E-2/3, E-2/4, E-3/3, E-3/4, and E-4/4). The E-2/2 genotype is present in approximately 1% percent of the population and most commonly is associated with type III hyperlipidemia. Since the apoE-2 isoform does not bind to the LDL receptor, chylomicron remnants and IDLs can both accumulate in the circulation, particularly when obesity, diabetes mellitus, or hypothyroidism is present. In patients with type III hyperlipidemia the plasma cholesterol and triglyceride levels are elevated to a similar degree. Palmar and tuberous xanthomas may occur, and these patients have a significantly increased risk of atherosclerosis. Dietary treatment (saturated fat restriction, weight loss) may be quite effective. Nicotinic acid, fibric acid derivatives, and HMG CoA reductase inhibitors have been used with variable degrees of success.

Type II hyperlipidemias are characterized by either an isolated elevation of LDL (type IIa) or a combined increase in LDL and VLDL (type IIb). The current approach to reduce the incidence of atherosclerotic vascular disease depends primarily on the detection and treatment of patients with elevated LDL levels. Plasma LDL levels are under the influence of a variety of environmental and genetic factors. The high-saturated-fat diet habitually consumed in the United States is believed to contribute to the high prevalence of mild elevations of LDL-C seen in a subset of the population. In contrast, it has become apparent that genetic factors also play a major role in regulating plasma LDL levels. The most obvious example is the twofold to threefold elevation of LDL levels seen in patients with heterozygous familial hypercholesterolemia, a relatively common disease with an autosomal dominant mode of inheritance.[70] Several other genetic disorders such as the familial combined hyperlipidemia (FCHL) syndrome, the hyperapobetalipoproteinemia syndrome, and a syndrome characterized by elevated levels of lipoprotein(a) (Lp[a]), a plasminogen-like glycoprotein covalently bound to apoB in an LDL-like lipoprotein, have been described.[71] A spectrum of defects in the genetic control of lipoprotein synthesis, apoprotein structure, and LDL receptor defects have been characterized over the last several years.

GENETIC DYSLIPIDEMIAS ASSOCIATED WITH ATHEROSCLEROSIS

Familial Hypercholesterolemia

Familial hypercholesterolemia is the prototype of the genetic dyslipidemia that is due to a single gene defect that results in failure to produce functionally active cell-surface receptors that normally bind apoB in LDLs.[70] The heterozygous form of familial hypercholesterolemia is present in approximately 0.2% of the U.S. population. The disease is transmitted as an autosomal dominant trait. Individuals who inherit one normal and one abnormal gene (heterozygote) have only half the normal number of LDL receptors and a twofold to threefold increase in circulating LDL-C (usually 250 to 400 mg/dl) (Fig. 9-6). Tendon xanthomas and overt CHD are frequent in the third or fourth decade

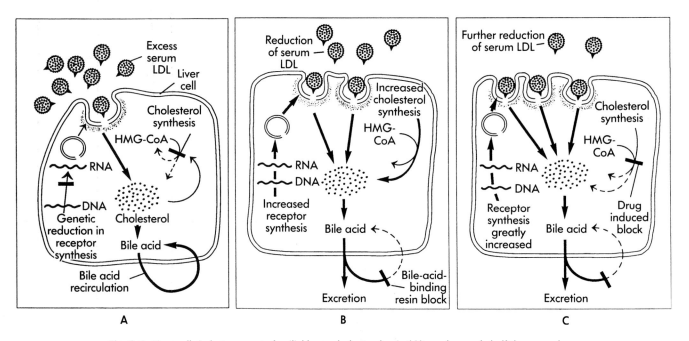

Fig. 9-6. Liver cells in heterozygote familial hypercholesterolemia **(A)** produce only half the normal number of LDL receptors. As a result, LDL accumulates in serum. Treatment with a resin that binds bile acids **(B)** reduces intracellular cholesterol slightly and thereby upregulates receptor synthesis and lowers serum LDL; however, the effect is partially offset by increased cholesterol synthesis. Addition of a drug that blocks this process **(C)** upregulates receptor formation still further and produces near-normal LDL serum levels. *(From Goldstein JL and Brown MS: Familial hypercholesterolemia: a genetic receptor disease, Hosp Pract 20:35, 1985.)*

of life. Patients with the rare homozygous form of the disease have no functioning LDL receptors and develop massive hypercholesterolemia, accelerated atherosclerosis, and death in the first to third decades. Five percent of patients with myocardial infarction below the age of 55 to 60 years have familial hypercholesterolemia.[72]

Although LDL receptor assays in fibroblasts and peripheral blood lymphocytes can be used to confirm the presence of the LDL receptor defect in patients with heterozygous familial hypercholesterolemia,[64] these tests are usually not necessary to establish the diagnosis since the patient often has the triad of (1) tendinous xanthomas, (2) LDL-C levels greater than 250 mg/dl, and (3) a family history of severe hypercholesterolemia and/or premature CHD in approximately 50% of the patient's first-degree relatives.

It is important to screen relatives of patients with familial hypercholesterolemia for lipid abnormalities. With affected adult relatives, teenagers' serum TC levels will nearly always exceed 250 mg/dl. The elevation in LDL-C is apparent at birth (and should be two to three times the level of a normal neonate). In adults adequate treatment often requires diet, a bile acid sequestrant, and an HMG CoA reductase inhibitor. Some patients require three or four drugs.

Familial Combined Hyperlipidemia

Goldstein et al[73] proposed this designation, FCHL, to characterize families exhibiting multiple lipoprotein phe-

notypes (IIa, IIb, IV, and occasionally V). These investigators originally suggested that an autosomal dominant mode of inheritance was present in this syndrome as it is in familial hypercholesterolemia. Unfortunately there is no unique marker for this syndrome, thus impairing the ability to determine its prevalence or mode of inheritance precisely. The diagnosis depends on finding elevated levels of cholesterol and triglycerides in affected patients and their first-degree relatives. Multiple lipoprotein phenotypes are often observed in a single patient. In addition to the abnormalities of lipoprotein concentration, the composition of lipoproteins is often abnormal, and there is an increased risk of premature CHD in these families.[74] Ten percent of patients less than 60 years old with myocardial infarction have FCHL. The LDL fraction often contains a wide range of LDL particle size and a high number of small dense LDL particles with a relative reduction in cholesterol. The concentration of apoB in whole plasma is often increased, but the LDL-C level may be normal. The situation is analogous to the hyperapobetalipoproteinemia syndrome described by Sniderman et al.[75] Perhaps these structural abnormalities contribute to the high risk of premature CHD noted in patients with this syndrome.

The nature of the metabolic defect(s) leading to FCHL is not clear. Several lines of evidence suggest that there is an increased hepatic apoB synthetic rate.[76] This could lead to simultaneous overproduction of LDL. However, the fractional catabolic rate of LDL tends to be high so that LDL levels, and particularly LDL-C levels, may not be increased.

Thus in patients with FCHL there apparently is overproduction of apoB-containing lipoproteins, many of which are small, dense, and highly atherogenic.

It seems prudent to recommend a diet moderately low in saturated fat and cholesterol and low in calories if the patient is obese. However, weight reduction may cause a paradoxic rise in LDL-C when triglycerides are reduced in patients with this syndrome. Nicotinic acid seems the most logical drug to use since it reduces synthesis of all of the apoB-containing lipoproteins, increases lipoprotein lipase activity, and raises HDL-C. Bile acid sequestrants or HMG CoA reductase inhibitors can be added to nicotinic acid if LDL-C levels remain high. The bile acid sequestrants or HMG CoA reductase inhibitors have been given in combination with gemfibrozil as well.[77]

Lipoprotein(a)

Lipoprotein(a), or Lp(a), is an atherogenic lipoprotein structurally related to LDL.[71] The lipid composition of Lp(a) and LDL is similar, and both of these cholesterol-rich lipoproteins contain apoB. The presence of a glycoprotein, apo(a), that is covalently bound to apoB in the Lp(a) accounts for the immunologic properties of Lp(a) and its higher density when compared with LDL. Apo(a) may be responsible for the markedly reduced binding of Lp(a) by the hepatic LDL receptor. Lp(a) apparently is synthesized by the liver, but its route of catabolism is not known.[78] Serum Lp(a) does not appear to interact with other lipoproteins, and Lp(a) levels do not correlate with other lipoprotein levels.

Lp(a) levels apparently are primarily under genetic control, with different Lp(a) glycoprotein phenotypes related to serum Lp(a) concentrations.[71] The Lp(a) glycoprotein phenotypes associated with the highest Lp(a) levels are relatively uncommon in the population, so that the frequency of distribution of Lp(a) levels is highly skewed, with higher frequencies of low Lp(a) values. This skewed distribution of Lp(a) levels has been observed in all white populations studied. Hoefler et al[79] found that approximately 15% of 1486 white men had Lp(a) levels greater than 25 mg/dl, which are associated with approximately a 2½ higher risk of myocardial infarction. Similar conclusions were reached by Kostner et al.[80] At this time few laboratories routinely measure serum Lp(a) levels, but there is interest in including this assay in patients with significant atherosclerosis and no apparent risk factors. Lp(a) levels are not affected by diet, and the only drugs known to reduce Lp(a) levels are neomycin, nicotinic acid,[81] and estrogen.[82]

Familial Hypoalphalipoproteinemia

Most of the current knowledge about the relationship between HDLs and atherosclerosis is derived from studies relying on measurement of cholesterol in HDLs (HDL-C). These studies have generally shown that patients with HDL-C in the lowest decile of the HDL-C distribution have a high risk of atherosclerosis. This correlates with an HDL-C level of approximately 35 mg/dl or less. A variety of factors such as physical activity, diet composition, triglyceride levels, estrogen levels, and smoking habits influences

HDL-C levels, but it appears that genetic factors play a major role in the etiology of low HDL levels in 50% of these individuals.[62] This syndrome seems to be inherited in an autosomal dominant mode and is characterized by premature atherosclerosis without corneal opacifications or xanthomas. Approximately one third of patients with premature CHD have this syndrome. There is no specific way to establish this genotypic diagnosis; the presence of HDL-C levels less than 35 mg/dl in a patient and in approximately 50% of his relatives is suggestive. This is particularly true if obesity, diabetes mellitus, or hypertriglyceridemia is not present.

Several rare genetic HDL deficiency states have been identified, including familial lecithin, cholesterol acyltransferase deficiency, fish eye disease, Tangier disease, and several syndromes caused by the presence of apoA-1 mutations. Corneal opacifications are often present in these uncommon disorders. A detailed discussion of these syndromes is beyond the scope of this text but may be found in the comprehensive review by Schaefer et al.[83]

EVALUATION OF THE PATIENT WITH HYPERLIPIDEMIA

The principal goals of the evaluation of the patient with a presumed or documented dyslipoproteinemia are to (1) confirm the presence of the lipoprotein disorder, (2) assess the patient's overall state of health, (3) evaluate and treat other cardiovascular risk factors, (4) detect the presence of atherosclerotic vascular disease, and (5) rule out secondary causes of dyslipoproteinemia. Detection of abnormalities in lipoprotein metabolism may result from cholesterol screening programs or during patient contact with a physician in the office setting.

SECONDARY DYSLIPIDEMIAS

In addition to the primary hyperlipidemias, many other factors and diseases can influence serum lipoprotein metabolism, producing a secondary dyslipoproteinemia.[84] The common causes of secondary dyslipoproteinemias are shown in the box on p. 178.

In the Lipid Research Clinics Prevalence Study, less than 10% of the dyslipoproteinemias could be attributed to other diseases on the basis of laboratory abnormalities.[85] However, if obesity, alcohol use, medications, or menopause are included, the prevalence of secondary forms is considerably higher. The importance of identifying secondary causes of dyslipoproteinemia is that alteration of the secondary factor may ameliorate the lipid disorder. In patients with primary lipid and lipoprotein abnormalities, secondary factors may exacerbate the lipid abnormalities.

Obesity is commonly associated with hypercholesterolemia, hypertriglyceridemia, and low HDL-C levels. Hypertriglyceridemia and low HDL-C are particularly common and, when detected, should prompt a careful assessment of glucose metabolism. Weight reduction may alleviate the lipid disorder, reduce fasting blood glucose levels, correct hyperinsulinemia, and decrease blood pressure. Of particular importance is upper-body (android)

CAUSES OF SECONDARY DYSLIPOPROTEINEMIA

Common

Obesity

Ethanol use

Diabetes mellitus

Hypothyroidism

Obstructive liver disease

Chronic renal failure

Nephrotic syndrome

Medication (β-blockers, diuretics, isotretinoin, etretinate, cyclosporine A, progesterones, estrogens, corticosteroids), amiodarone, anabolic steroids)

Menopause

Uncommon

Cushing's syndrome

Pancreatitis

Dysgammaglobulinemia

Glycogen storage disease

Acute intermittent porphyria

Acromegaly

obesity. It is associated with a waist-hip ratio greater than 0.85 and is associated with increased cardiovascular risk.[86,87] Alcohol consumption contributes to obesity and also may adversely affect lipoprotein metabolism, leading to elevations in triglycerides and VLDL levels even in the absence of obesity. Alcohol also may contribute to the development of hypertension and may worsen glucose tolerance.

The CHD mortality rate is two to four times higher in diabetics than in nondiabetics and is the main cause of death in patients with non–insulin-dependent diabetes mellitus (NIDDM) and insulin-dependent diabetes mellitus (IDDM). The relative risk of cardiovascular death in diabetic versus nondiabetic individuals was 2.1 for men and 4.9 for women in the Framingham Study.[88] Even mild abnormalities of glucose metabolism increased the risk of CHD mortality. Lipid disorders may contribute to the increased risk of atherosclerosis in diabetics. As noted previously, there is controversy regarding the role of high plasma triglyceride levels (the most common lipid abnormality in patients with diabetes) and CHD. The low HDL-C levels frequently observed in these patients may contribute to this risk. Alterations in metabolism of VLDLs and LDLs may cause certain lipoproteins to be particularly atherogenic. For example, hypertriglyceridemia may be a marker for the presence of increased levels of VLDL remnants or may be associated with small, dense LDLs. Massive hypertriglyceridemia and chylomicronemia with eruptive xanthomas, lipemia retinalis, and chronic abdominal pain or pancreatitis can occur in patients with poorly controlled

diabetes. In treating the dyslipidemia of diabetes, obese patients will benefit from weight reduction. Control of blood sugar with diet,[89] oral glucose-lowering agents and/or insulin often correct the underlying lipid disturbance.[90]

The fibric acid derivative gemfibrozil has been demonstrated to lower triglycerides more than 25% in diabetic patients with a corresponding increase in HDL-C of more than 10% after 12 weeks of therapy.[91] In the Helsinki Heart Study the percent reduction of triglycerides and percent increase in HDL-C were less in diabetic subjects than in nondiabetic subjects. Nevertheless, the incremental risk reduction for CHD death and myocardial infarction was greater in diabetic subjects than in the nondiabetic subjects.[13,92]

In patients with hypothyroidism TC, VLDL-C, and LDL-C may all be increased.[84,93,94] There are increased synthesis and decreased catabolism of LDL. The association of elevated cholesterol levels with hypothyroidism has been recognized for many years and was used as an aid to the diagnosis of hypothyroidism in the past. Patients with "subclinical hypothyroidism" (elevated thyroid-stimulating hormone levels with normal thyroxine levels) may also develop hypercholesterolemia.[94] Treatment of hypothyroidism with thyroid replacement usually improves or corrects the underlying lipid abnormality.

A variety of abnormalities of lipoprotein concentration and/or composition occurs in patients with chronic renal failure.[95,96] Hypertriglyceridemia and low HDL-C levels are the most frequently observed abnormalities. It is not certain if the abnormalities in lipoprotein metabolism contribute to the development of progression of atherosclerosis in these patients. Marked hypercholesterolemia frequently occurs in patients with nephrotic syndrome.[95] Overproduction of apoB-containing lipoproteins by the liver apparently is the major cause of these abnormalities. There is considerable controversy about the role of the dyslipoproteinemia of nephrotic syndrome in the development of atherosclerosis.

Certain drugs may adversely affect blood lipids and lipoproteins.[97,98] In some patients β-blockers (except those with both α- and β-blocking activity or those with intrinsic sympathomimetic activity)[99] and diuretics may increase triglycerides and decrease HDL-C.[98] Isotretinoin[100] and etretinate may cause marked hypertriglyceridemia and modest increases in TC and LDL-C. Amiodarone has been shown to increase TC and LDL-C.

Estrogens and progestins may have beneficial effects on some lipoprotein fractions and deleterious effects on others (see the following material).[101] Corticosteroids may also have an adverse effect on blood lipids. A detailed discussion of other causes of secondary hyperlipidemia is beyond the scope of this chapter.

The most useful laboratory tests that should be included in the evaluation of patients with hypercholesterolemia or other lipoprotein abnormalities include measurement of (1) fasting blood glucose, (2) thyroid-stimulating hormone, (3) alkaline phosphatase, (4) serum creatinine, (5) serum albumin, and (6) urinalysis. Most of the secondary dyslipoproteinemias will be detected with these relatively inexpensive tests.

EYE AND SKIN MANIFESTATIONS OF HYPERLIPIDEMIAS

During the physical examination several ocular and cutaneous abnormalities may suggest the presence of an abnormality of lipoprotein metabolism or suggest a specific genotypic or phenotypic dyslipidemic state. Xanthelasmas (yellow to gray plaques on the eyelids and periorbital skin) and corneal arcus (a light gray pigment deposition in the periphery of the cornea) are seen with increased frequency with aging and may be associated with presence of hypercholesterolemia. In the Lipid Research Clinics Program Prevalence Study xanthelasmas were noted in approximately 1% of the 8998 study participants, and corneal arcus was present in approximately 20%.[102] Corneal arcus was more common in blacks than whites and more prevalent in men than in women. The presence of xanthelasmas and corneal arcus was associated with an increased risk for developing ischemic heart disease, particularly in men less than 49 years of age, but it was not associated with manifestations of peripheral arterial disease. The clinical findings of xanthelasmas or corneal arcus, especially in younger patients, should serve as a reminder to assess lipid status and other cardiovascular risk factors.

Lipemia retinalis, which is a salmon or creamy coloration of the retinal blood vessels, occurs with marked elevation of triglycerides to greater than 2500 mg/dl. These patients usually have fasting hyperchylomicronemia and a phenotype V dyslipoproteinemia.

Cutaneous markers for lipoprotein disorders are associated with both primary and secondary lipid disorders.[103] Deposition of lipids, lipoproteins, and their remnants in tissues close to the surface of the body causes xanthomas of various types. Recognition of these physical findings should lead to a complete lipoprotein evaluation and may allow the physician to recognize specific disease states. The type of lesion frequently correlates with the types of lipid or lipoproteins that are elevated.

Tendon xanthomas are firm to hard subcutaneous nodules with normal-appearing overlying skin that can be moved over the nodules easily. These xanthomas are often noted as a swelling or prominence in the Achilles tendon or on the extensor tendons of the digits. Tendon xanthomas strongly suggest the presence of familial hypercholesterolemia. Two unusual disorders produce tendon xanthomas because of accumulation of other steroid molecules: (1) cerebrotendinous xanthomatosis is a disorder of bile acid metabolism, and (2) β-sitosterolemia is caused by accumulation of plant sterols. Both of these conditions are rare and are associated with an increased risk for the development of atherosclerosis.

Eruptive xanthomas are reddish-yellow, 1- to 4-mm dermal papules that are somewhat acneiform and develop rapidly in crops or showers. They tend to form on the extensor surface of the hands, arms, knees, and buttocks. They can also arise on the flexor creases, the face, or in areas of trauma. Acutely they may be quite pruritic and tender. Eruptive xanthomas usually occur in patients with hyperchylomicronemia from primary or secondary causes. They tend to resolve rapidly with treatment of the lipid disorder.

Tuberoeruptive and tuberous xanthomas appear on the elbows, knees, and buttocks, and less commonly in other areas. The tuberous form is nodular and noninflammatory. The tuberoeruptive xanthomas have an inflammatory component that begins as dermal papules. They are most commonly seen in association with familial dysbetalipoproteinemia (type III) or heterozygous familial hypercholesterolemia.

Planar xanthomas may be diffuse or well-circumscribed noninflammatory dermal macules or plaques. Intertriginous xanthomas are slightly raised yellow plaques with a cobblestone-like surface seen in the finger web spaces and sometimes in the axillary antecubital and popliteal fossae. They are pathognomonic for homozygous familial hypercholesterolemia.

Palmar crease xanthomas (xanthoma palmaris striatum) are identified as a yellow-to-orange discoloration in the creases of the palms and fingers that is very easily overlooked. They are pathognomonic of familial dysbetalipoproteinemia (type III).

SCREENING AND MANAGEMENT OF LIPID ABNORMALITIES

On the basis of the Framingham Study, MRFIT, and other[1-3] population-based epidemiologic studies, one may identify most patients at increased risk by measuring total serum cholesterol. In most people the major contributor to the total serum cholesterol value is LDL-C. Total concentrations of cholesterol in the blood are not markedly affected by ingestion of a meal. Therefore fasting is not required when TC levels are used as a screening tool. This observation and the low cost of total serum cholesterol measurements are major advantages, and for these reasons the first report of the expert panel on detection, evaluation, and treatment of high blood cholesterol in adults recommended screening individuals with TC alone.[104]

However, there are several major limitations of screening people using only a TC determination, including the following: (1) variability of cholesterol measurements; (2) failure to detect potentially significant dyslipidemias such as low HDL-C; (3) failure to discriminate high levels of HDL-C; and (4) variability of nonfasting cholesterol as a result of changes in chylomicrons or VLDL-C concentration. For these reasons the second Adult Treatment Panel (ATP II) recommended measuring TC and HDL-C as initial screening.[20]

The evidence that low HDL-C is associated with increased risk for atherosclerotic vascular disease is quite convincing,[8,10] and in fact there is suggestive evidence that raising HDL-C may reduce the risk for CHD events.[13,25] In 125 consecutive patients with lower-extremity arteriosclerosis obliterans at our institution, 48% of patients had low HDL-C, and 28% of the entire group had TC less than 200 mg/dl.[105]

Not all elevations of TC are associated with an increased risk of CHD. This is true for a subgroup of people with high HDL-C levels and includes many women—especially premenopausal women and postmenopausal women receiving estrogen therapy. According to Framingham data, a person with an LDL-C level of 100 mg/dl and an HDL-C level of 25 has a higher risk for the development of CHD (relative risk, 1.2) than a person with an LDL-C level of 220 and HDL-C level of 80 (relative risk, 0.3).[106] Frequently, undue anxiety is generated by the use of high TC levels alone, and such persons may initiate unnecessarily restrictive diets and inappropriate over-the-counter medications; in some cases physicians who treat on the basis of TC levels alone may initiate the use of lipid-lowering drugs.

The National Cholesterol Education Program (NCEP) expert panel on Detection, Evaluation and Treatment of High Blood Cholesterol in Adults (Adult Treatment Panel II)[20] is significantly different from the first adult panel in several respects: (1) There is increased emphasis on CHD risk status in guiding the type and intensity of treatment. Patients with coronary heart disease or atherosclerosis elsewhere are treated much more aggressively, whereas patients at low risk for coronary disease (primary prevention) are treated less aggressively. (2) High-risk postmenopausal women and high-risk elderly patients are candidates for cholesterol-lowering medications. (3) More attention is given to HDL-C as a CHD risk factor. (4) There is increased emphasis on physical activity and weight reduction in addition to dietary therapy. (5) There is reduced emphasis on treating young low-risk persons.

Risk status based on the presence of CHD and other risk factors is shown in Table 9-5. An algorithm for screening and managing adults without evidence of CHD or other significant risk factors (primary prevention) is shown in Fig. 9-7. Treatment decisions (whether dietary and/or drug therapy) should be based on the level of LDL-C as shown in Table 9-6. However, if the patient has evidence of underlying atherosclerosis, a more aggressive approach is war-

Table 9-5. Risk Status Based on Coronary Heart Disease Risk Factors Other Than LDL Cholesterol

Positive
  Age, years
    Men ≥45
    Women ≥55 or premature menopause without estrogen replacement therapy
  Family history of premature coronary heart disease
  Smoking
  Hypertension
  HDL cholesterol <35 mg/dl
  Diabetes mellitus
Negative
  HDL cholesterol ≥60 mg/dl

(From Expert Panel on Detection, Evaluation and Treatment of High Blood Cholesterol in Adults: NCEP guidelines II, JAMA 269:3015, 1993.)

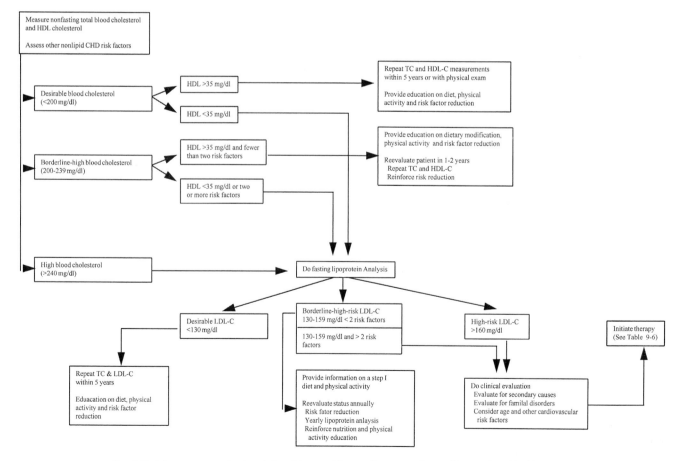

Fig. 9-7. Primary prevention in adults without evidence of coronary heart disease. *(Modified from NCEP Adult Treatment Panel II, JAMA 269:3015, 1993.)*

ranted. All such patients should have a complete lipid profile to include measurement of TC, triglycerides, HDL-C, and LDL-C. The goal LDL-C is less than 100 mg/dl for patients with coronary disease or atherosclerosis elsewhere. A useful algorithm from the National Cholesterol Education Program, Adult Treatment Panel II,[20] is shown in Fig. 9-8. A complete lipid profile should be obtained in all patients who are obese, have a strong family history for vascular disease and/or lipid disturbances, or have diabetes mellitus.

DIETARY TREATMENT OF LIPID DISTURBANCES

The initial steps to lower cholesterol involve dietary intervention. Useful dietary guidelines are outlined in the NCEP report.[20,104] For obese persons the first goal is to reduce calories to achieve desirable body weight. The next step is to reduce the total fat intake in the diet to 30% or less of the total calories. Since saturated fat contributes more substantially to elevations of LDL-C than polyunsaturated or monounsaturated fat, the total saturated fat intake should be reduced to 10% or less. Saturated fat intake should be reduced to less than 7% of total calories for persons whose cholesterol levels are not reduced to target levels with the 10% saturated fat ingestion level. The most common sources of saturated fat in the American diet are hamburger meat, other red meats, fried foods, and dairy products, including milk and cheese. Increasing the quantity of fish and poultry and changing the nature of dairy products to skim milk and nonfat cheese may help bring the diet into conformity with these recommendations for saturated fat intake. The third goal is to reduce the amount of cholesterol intake to less than 300 mg/day for a step I diet and less than 200 mg/day for a step II diet. This usually occurs if saturated fat intake is reduced. Common sources of cholesterol include egg yolks, organ meats, shell fish, and animal meats. Increasing dietary fiber, especially soluble fiber such as that found in oats, lentils, and beans has a beneficial effect on lipid levels. Additional dietary recommendations include the restriction of ethanol ingestion, especially in obese patients for whom it is a source of "empty" calories and in persons with elevated triglyceride levels.

Fast foods, snack foods, and restaurant dining account for a large amount of the increased fat intake in the United States. The commonly used vegetable oils in the fast food industry and in many snack foods include coconut oil, palm oil, and palm kernel oil. These oils contain a large amount of saturated fats. Their widespread use is the result of stability with storage and heating as well as general palatability. Furthermore, many restaurants use butters and sauces containing saturated fats to enhance the flavor of their meals. Persons on cholesterol-lowering diets must be instructed in these more subtle forms of fat intake in conjunction with overall proper nutrition instruction.

Table 9-6. Treatment Decisions Based on LDL Cholesterol Level

Patient Category	Initiation Level	LDL Goal
Dietary Therapy		
No CHD, <2 risk factors	≥160	<160
No CHD, >2 risk factors	≥130	<130
CHD	>100	≤100
Drug Therapy		
No CHD, <2 risk factors	≥190	<160
No CHD, >2 risk factors	≥160	<130
CHD	≥130	≤100

(From Expert Panel on Detection, Evaluation and Treatment of High Blood Cholesterol in Adults: NCEP guidelines II, JAMA 269:3015, 1993.)

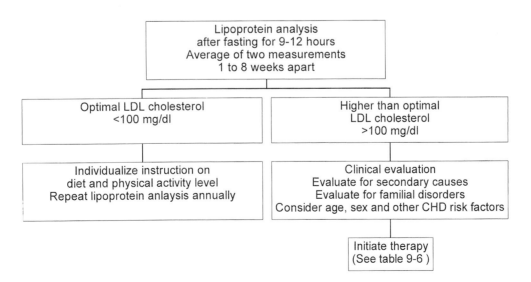

Fig. 9-8. Secondary prevention in adults with evidence of coronary heart disease or other vascular disease. *(From NCEP Adult Treatment Panel II, JAMA 23:3020, 1993.)*

Dietary counseling by a registered dietitian is recommended for all patients who do not have a satisfactory dietary response to physician counseling alone. Table 9-6 provides useful guidelines for dietary treatment based on LDL-C.

ROLE OF HORMONE REPLACEMENT THERAPY IN THE TREATMENT OF LIPID DISORDERS

The availability of information relating to the development and treatment of atherosclerosis in women has increased considerably over the last decade. Estrogen deficiency, attributable to surgical menopause or premature natural menopause, triples the incidence of CHD in women. Literature supports an expanding consensus that estrogen replacement therapy decreases the relative risk of CHD by 40% to 50% and decreases overall mortality by 30% (Table 9-7).[107-113] Postmenopausal estrogen replacement therapy for women with established CHD (i.e., secondary prevention) is more beneficial than it is in healthy women. In a cohort study of 1822 women, Sullivan et al[110] demonstrated a 4% 10-year mortality in estrogen-using women with angiographically documented severe coronary artery disease compared with a 35% 10-year mortality among nonusers. There was an 89% reduction in cardiovascular risk with the use of estrogens.

There is insufficient and contradictory observational evidence with respect to the effect of estrogen and estrogen-progestin replacement therapy on stroke incidence and mortality in postmenopausal women.

Reports of the increased incidence of adenocarcinoma of the endometrium with unopposed estrogen replacement therapy emerged in the early 1980s. Progestational agents have been added to estrogen replacement therapy in a variety of cyclic and continuous regimens for women who have a uterus. In a recent report 34% of women receiving unopposed estrogen therapy demonstrated adenomatous or atypical endometrial hyperplasia.[111] A preliminary report of a prospective cohort of 23,000 women in Sweden reported a relative risk of 0.69 for heart disease in users of estrogen alone and 0.53 in women receiving combined estrogen and progesterone (levonorgestrel).[112] The results of the Heart and Estrogen Replacement Study (HERS), a prospective secondary prevention trial of estrogen-progestin replacement therapy, and the Women's Health Initiative (WHI) are anxiously awaited to more clearly define the benefits and risks of the combination of estrogen-progestin therapy with respect to CHD and overall mortality.

The proposed mechanisms for the beneficial effects of estrogen replacement therapy with respect to decreasing cardiovascular risk include altering lipid levels,[114] which may account for 25% to 50% of the benefit, modulation of vascular tone by direct effects on the vascular endothelium,[115] decreasing stress-related vasoconstriction, and antioxidant properties of estrogen.

Most of the available information with respect to the alteration of lipid and lipoprotein levels in postmenopausal women deals with the effects of unopposed estrogen. Unopposed oral estrogen therapy in postmenopausal women increases HDL-C by 10% to 15% and decreases

Table 9-7. Prospective Studies of Postmenopausal Estrogen Use and Cardiovascular Disease

Study	Year	No. of Subjects	Age-Adjusted Relative Risk
Potocki	1971	158	0.31
Burch	1974	737	0.43
Hammond	1979	610	0.33
Nachtigall	1979	168	0.33
Lafferty	1985	124	0.17
Stampfer	1985	33,317	0.3
Wilson	1985	1,234	1.94
Bush	1987	2,270	0.34
Petitti	1987	6,093	0.9
Hunt	1987	4,544	0.48
Criqui	1988	1,868	0.75
Henderson	1988	8,807	0.47
Avila	1990	24,900	0.7
Sullivan	1990	2,268	0.16
Stampfer	1991	48,470	0.56

(From Kuhn FE and Rackley CE: Coronary artery disease in women. Risk factors, evaluation, treatment, and prevention, Arch Intern Med 153:2626, 1993.)

LDL-C by a similar percentage.[101,114] Transdermal estrogen replacement does not have a significant beneficial effect on HDL-C. Unopposed estrogen replacement therapy remains appropriate for women without a uterus. However, for women with a uterus, combination estrogen-progestin therapy is required to prevent a therapy-related increase in endometrial hyperplasia and carcinoma.

Information is beginning to emerge that addresses the differences in lipid and lipoprotein effects of various natural and synthetic estrogen compounds, delivery systems, in combination with natural and synthetic progestational agents with differing androgenicity. The first randomized multicentered double-blind, placebo-controlled trial of the effects of estrogen and estrogen-progestin replacement therapy in healthy postmenopausal women was recently reported.[111] Eight hundred and seventy-five postmenopausal women aged 45 to 64 years were randomized to placebo, conjugated equine estrogen 0.625 mg/day, conjugated equine estrogen 0.625 mg/day plus cyclic medroxyprogesterone acetate 10 mg/day for 12 days a month, conjugated equine estrogen 0.625 mg/day plus consecutive medroxyprogesterone acetate 2.5 mg/day, or conjugated equine estrogen 0.625 mg/day plus cyclic micronized progesterone 200 mg/day for 12 days a month. Trial end points were risk factors of cardiovascular disease, HDL-C, systolic blood pressure, serum insulin, and fibrinogen, rather than cardiovascular events. There was improvement in lipoprotein values and decreased fibrinogen without detectable effects on postchallenge insulin or blood pressure measurements.

The adult treatment guidelines of the National Cholesterol Education Program[20] (NCEP) advised consideration of estrogen replacement therapy for postmenopausal women with elevated cholesterol levels, particularly if they have coronary artery disease. Judelson[116] emphasized that the NCEP (ATP II) definition of a low HDL-C level at less than 35 mg/dl is appropriate for men but not for women, who frequently have HDL levels above 50 mg/dl. Women have a relative risk of developing CHD of 1.7 with an HDL-C less than 50 mg/dl compared with HDL-C over 50 mg/dl.

PHARMACOLOGIC TREATMENT OF LIPID DISORDERS

Pharmacologic therapy of patients with lipid abnormalities (Table 9-8) generally involves use of drugs that reduce LDL-C concentrations.[20] These drugs include the bile acid sequestrants, nicotinic acid, and the HMG CoA reductase inhibitors. Gemfibrozil and other fibric acid derivatives are primarily triglyceride-lowering agents that tend to increase HDL-C concentrations.[13] Nicotinic acid is the most potent HDL-C raising agent currently available and has been used in combination with one of the bile acid sequestrants in several studies that demonstrated reduced progression of atherosclerosis in patients with preexisting coronary artery disease.[37,40,56]

Bile acid binding resins include cholestyramine (Questran and Questran Light) and colestipol (Colestid). Their major effect is to lower LDL-C levels.[117,118] These agents bind bile acids in the gut and increase the ratio of intrahepatic conversion of cholesterol to bile acids. This results in increased hepatic LDL receptor activity.

Frequently encountered side effects of the bile acid binding resins are gastrointestinal in origin and include bloating, midepigastric pain, and constipation. These side effects reduce the degree of adherence to treatment with these agents. Serum triglyceride levels may increase during treatment with these agents, particularly in patients with mild increases in triglycerides.[119] In addition, the bile acid sequestrants bind several drugs in the gut and reduce absorption of these agents, which include warfarin (Coumadin), thyroid hormone, and the thiazide-type diuretics. There is also evidence that bile acid sequestrants delay absorption of β-blocking agents.

Cholestyramine and colestipol have been administered alone or in combination with nicotinic acid or an HMG CoA reductase inhibitor in clinical trials that showed a reduced CHD risk. When the bile acid resins are used with other agents, lower doses can be used and therefore compliance will be better.[120]

Cholestyramine and colestipol are available in 4- and 5-g packets, respectively, and in bulk containers that are used to dispense the once to twice daily doses of these agents. The dosage of cholestyramine ranges from 4 to 24 g/day; that of colestipol ranges from 5 to 30 g/day. Recently, colestipol was released as a caplet.

Nicotinic acid is a very effective drug for lowering VLDL-C and LDL-C levels and is the most potent HDL-C raising agent that is currently available. Although niacin frequently causes flushing, the severity of this adverse effect tends to diminish with time. In addition, use of aspirin and administration of nicotinic acid with food, and avoidance of ingestion of hot liquids, reduce the severity of flushing. Niacin (particularly the slow-release preparation)

can cause a chemical hepatitis, abdominal pain, or gastritis. Niacin can also induce insulin resistance and may raise blood glucose levels. However, significant blood glucose elevations are relatively uncommon during niacin treatment in nondiabetic patients. Nicotinic acid should not be used in patients with active peptic ulcer disease or recurrent episodes of gouty arthritis. Slow-release niacin preparations reduce the cutaneous side effects but appear to be associated with a higher risk of hepatitis when compared with crystalline niacin.[121,122] For these reasons, we generally advise use of a crystalline niacin preparation and suggest use of low-dose aspirin (if no contraindication to aspirin use exists) to reduce the severity of flushing. Patients should have liver function tests (alanine aminotransferase [ALT]) monitored at least as frequently as those patients receiving HMG CoA reductase inhibitors (see the following material). Patients are advised to begin therapy with 100-mg niacin doses administered with breakfast and dinner. Avoidance of hot beverages around the time of each niacin dose is advised. The daily dose of niacin should be slowly increased to the 1500 to 2000 mg/day range over approximately 3 to 4 weeks. Since niacin-induced side effects are clearly dose related, we tend to limit daily doses to the 2- to 3-g range and prefer addition of second lipid-altering agent if the response to niacin is inadequate. There are some patients, however, who require larger doses of niacin to get the desired lipid-lowering or HDL-C raising effect.

There are currently four *HMG CoA reductase inhibitors* that have been approved by the Food and Drug Administration for use in clinical practice; the availability of these agents has markedly increased the LDL-C lowering efficacy and reduced the side effect profile that was associated with use of the bile acid binding resins, nicotinic acid, or the fibric acid derivatives. These agents primarily reduce LDL-C concentrations but tend to reduce serum triglyceride and increase HDL-C levels to a lesser extent.[123] These effects occur through competitive inhibition of the enzyme HMG CoA reductase, which catalyzes the rate-limiting enzyme in endogenous cholesterol synthesis. This reduction in cholesterol synthesis causes a decrease in intracellular cholesterol stores and a corresponding increase in the hepatic LDL receptor activity (Fig. 9-6). This increases hepatic removal of LDL from the plasma. HMG CoA reductase inhibitors are generally well tolerated but can cause elevation of liver transaminase levels.[123-125] For this reason, patients taking an HMG CoA reductase inhibitor are advised to have liver enzymes (ALT) monitored every 6 weeks for the first 3 months, every 8 weeks for the remainder of the first year and periodically thereafter (i.e., every 4 to 6 months). Slight elevations in hepatic transaminase levels occur in approximately 3% of patients but are frequently transient and do not usually necessitate discontinuing these drugs. When the liver enzymes increase to greater than three times normal, the medication should be stopped.[126] Baseline and annual ophthalmologic examinations to check for cataracts were originally recommended for patients receiving an HMG CoA reductase inhibitor; however, there is no direct evidence that cataracts form in humans as a result of the HMG CoA reductase inhibitor treatment. Another side effect of HMG CoA

Table 9-8. Lipid-Lowering Drugs

Drug	Usual Dosage (Total/day)	Times (per day)	Mechanism of Action	Comments
Bile acid sequestrants*				
Cholestyramine	4-24 g	2-3	Increases clearance of cholesterol binding bile acids	Anticipated side effects Bloating Midepigastric fullness or pain Constipation (may be decreased by adding 3-4 g psyllium to each dose of resin) Tolerance increased by slow upward dose titration Colestipol also available in caplet form Possible binding of other agents including antihypertensive agents; in general, give other drugs at least 1 hr before or 4 hr after resin Avoid with serum triglyceride levels >400 mg/dl unless gemfibrozil or niacin is also given
Colestipol	5-30 g	2-3	Increases LDL receptor-mediated catabolism of LDL cholesterol	
Nicotinic acid	1000-4000 mg	2-3	Inhibits lipoprotein synthesis Inhibits apolipoprotein B synthesis	Anticipated side effects Flushing—especially with regular crystalline niacin preparations; usually diminished with time, administration with food, and/or addition of low-dose aspirin Gastrointestinal distress/dyspepsia—probably more common with slow-release preparations and may represent early symptoms of chemical hepatitis May cause itching, headache, insomnia, recurrence of gout, unmasking of glucose intolerance, or diabetes mellitus; may cause toxic amblyopia, acanthosis nigricans, dry skin, or myositis (particularly when combined with an HMG CoA reductase inhibitor)
HMG CoA reductase inhibitors				
Lovastatin	20-80 mg	1-2	Inhibits the rate-limiting enzyme in cholesterol synthesis	Capable of lowering LDL-C by 35%-45% in high percentage of patients Side effects infrequent, liver enzyme elevations frequently occur but are of questionable significance, liver function testing still recommended Mainly lowers LDL-C level; modest elevation of HDL-C level and reduction of serum triglyceride level also occur Does not cause cataracts; most feared side effect is myositis, which is rare except when used with niacin, gemfibrozil, cyclosporin, or possibly erythromycin Most cost-effective use may be in high-risk patients, addition of low-dose resin therapy may be particularly effective
Pravastatin	10-40 mg	1		
Simvastatin	10-40 mg	1	Increases LDL receptor-mediated catabolism of LDL cholesterol	
Fluvastatin	20-40 mg	1		
Gemfibrozil	1200 mg	2	Increases lipoprotein lipase activity	Most potent and consistently effective triglyceride-lowering agent, tends to increase HDL-C level and reduce LDL-C by 10%-20%; seems to be more effective in reducing primary CHD risk in hypertriglyceridemic patients with high LDL-C/HDL-C ratios than predicted by its LDL-C lowering effect

*May be given as a single dose at bedtime (1-2 scoops or packets). Daytime doses should be given before meals.

reductase inhibitor treatment is myositis. The risk for myositis apparently increases when these drugs are used in conjunction with cyclosporin A, erythromycin, nicotinic acid, or gemfibrozil. HMG CoA reductase inhibitors should usually be discontinued when patients are hospitalized before elective surgery because of concerns about potential increased risk of developing a drug-related myopathy in the perioperative period.

Gemfibrozil is the only *fibric acid derivative* that is frequently prescribed in the United States. Clofibrate has been available in the United States for many years but is currently used infrequently because of concerns about long-term toxicity that emerged from several previously conducted clinical trials. In contrast, gemfibrozil was shown to be effective in reducing CHD risk in men with no clinical evidence of CHD who participated in the Helsinki Heart Study.[13] The fibric acid derivatives have several effects on lipoprotein metabolism, including an increase in cholesterol secretion into the bile. This may account for the lithogenic effect of the fibric acid derivatives. These agents also stimulate lipoprotein lipase activity that increases the fractional catabolic rate of triglyceride-rich lipoproteins.[127,128] Gemfibrozil reduces serum triglyceride levels by approximately 40% in hypertriglyceridemic patients and has a variable effect on LDL-C concentrations. Although the LDL-C lowering effect of gemfibrozil tends to be greater in patients with phenotype IIa when compared with phenotype IIb dyslipidemic syndromes, a subset analysis of participants in the Helsinki Heart Study suggested that the CHD-reducing effect of gemfibrozil was actually greatest in participants who had serum triglyceride levels exceeding 200 mg/dl and LDL-C/HDL-C ratio above 5.0.[24] This subset of Helsinki Heart Study participants appeared to have a 70% reduction in CHD risk during gemfibrozil therapy when compared with placebo therapy.

Gastrointestinal symptoms occur in approximately 5% to 10% of gemfibrozil-treated patients but are generally more bothersome than serious. Gemfibrozil is available in 600-mg tablets; the usual dose is 600 mg twice daily. Since little monitoring of blood tests to detect systemic toxicity of gemfibrozil is required, the overall cost of reducing blood lipid levels during gemfibrozil treatment is not excessive.

Combinations of drugs may be particularly effective when the drugs work by different mechanisms of action and have major effects on different lipids and lipoproteins. For example, nicotinic acid and the bile acid binding resins were a very effective combination in a number of clinical trials. There are accumulating trials on the use of HMG CoA reductase inhibitors and bile acid binding resins, particularly for patients with familial heterozygote hypercholesterolemia.[126] Furthermore, many lipid experts find that using low doses of more than one agent frequently reduces the side effect profile and increases efficacy.[120] Hence there is a trend away from using full doses of a single medication before moving to another medication. Increasingly, it has become necessary to use a fibric acid derivative such as gemfibrozil and an HMG CoA reductase inhibitor together. The risk of myositis is increased with this combination. However, if the patient is educated about this possibility and followed frequently, this combination of drugs can be safely administered.

REFERENCES

1. Kannel WB, Castelli WP, and Gordon T: Cholesterol in the prediction of atherosclerotic disease. New perspectives based on the Framingham Study, Ann Intern Med 90:85, 1979.
2. Anderson KM, Castelli WP, and Levy D: Cholesterol and mortality—30 years of follow-up from the Framingham Study, JAMA 257:2176, 1987.
3. Stamler J, Wentworth D, and Neaton JD: Is the relationship between the serum cholesterol and risk of premature death from coronary heart disease continuous and graded? Findings in 356,222 primary screenees of the Multiple Risk Factor Intervention Trial (MRFIT), JAMA 256:2823, 1986.
4. Iso H et al: Serum cholesterol levels and 6 year mortality from stroke in 350,977 men screened for the Multiple Risk Factor Intervention Trial, N Engl J Med 320:904, 1989.
5. Tell GS, Crouse JR, and Furberg CD: Relation between blood lipids, lipoproteins and cerebrovascular atherosclerosis. A review, Stroke 19:423, 1988.
6. Pomrehn P et al: The association of dyslipoproteinemia with symptoms and signs of peripheral arterial disease. The Lipid Research Clinics Program Prevalence Study, Circulation 73(suppl I):I100, 1986.
7. Kannel WB, Gordon T, and Castelli WP: Role of lipids and lipoprotein fractions in assessing atherogenesis. The Framingham Study, Prog Lipid Res 20:339, 1981.
8. Gordon T et al: High density lipoprotein as a protective factor against coronary heart disease. The Framingham Study, Am J Med 62:707, 1977.
9. Castelli WB et al: The incidence of coronary heart disease and lipoprotein cholesterol levels: The Framingham Study, JAMA 256:2835, 1986.
10. Abbott RD et al: High density lipoprotein cholesterol, total cholesterol screening, and myocardial infarction. The Framingham Study, Arteriosclerosis 8:207, 1988.
11. Freedman DS et al: The relation of documented coronary artery disease to levels of total cholesterol and high-density lipoprotein cholesterol, Epidemiology 5:80, 1994.
12. Gordon DJ and Rifkind BM: High density lipoprotein— the clinical implications of recent studies, N Engl J Med 321:1311, 1989.
13. Frick MH et al: Helsinki Heart Study: Primary-Prevention Trial with gemfibrozil in middle aged men with dyslipidemia, N Engl J Med 317:1237, 1987.
14. Lipid Research Clinics Program: The Lipid Research Clinics Coronary Primary Prevention Trial results. I. Reduction in incidence of coronary heart disease, JAMA 251:351, 1984.
15. Lipid Research Clinics Program: The Lipid Research Clinics Coronary Primary Prevention Trial results. II. The relationship of reduction in incidence of coronary heart disease to cholesterol lowering, JAMA 251:365, 1984.
16. Benfante R and Reed D: Is elevated serum cholesterol level a risk factor for coronary heart disease in the elderly? JAMA 263:393, 1990.
17. Krumholz HM et al: Lack of association between cholesterol and coronary heart disease mortality and morbidity and in all-cause mortality in persons older than 70 years, JAMA 272:1334, 1994.
18. Hulley SB and Newman TB: Cholesterol in the elderly. Is it important? JAMA 272:1372, 1994.
19. Criqui MH et al: Plasma triglyceride level and mortality from coronary heart disease, N Engl J Med 328:1220, 1993.

20. Expert Panel on Detection, Evaluation and Treatment of High Blood Cholesterol in Adults: Summary of the second report on the National Cholesterol Education Program (NCEP). Expert panel on the detection, evaluation, and treatment of high blood cholesterol in adults (Adult Treatment Panel II), JAMA 269:3015, 1993.

21. Austin MA et al: Low-density lipoprotein subclass patterns and risk of myocardial infarction, JAMA 260:1917, 1988.

22. Austin MA and Hokanson JE: Epidemiology of triglycerides, small dense low-density lipoprotein, and lipoprotein a as risk factors for coronary heart disease, Med Clin North Am 78:99, 1994.

23. Patsch JR et al: Relation of triglyceride metabolism and coronary artery disease. Studies in the post-prandial state, Arterioscler Thromb 12:1336, 1992.

24. Manninen V et al: Joint effects of serum triglyceride and LDL cholesterol and HDL cholesterol concentrations on coronary heart disease risk factors in the Helsinki Heart Study. Implications for treatment, Circulation 85:37, 1992.

25. Grundy S and Vega GL: Two different views of the relationship of hypertriglyceridemia to coronary heart disease. Implications for treatment, Arch Intern Med 152:26, 1992.

26. Gordon DJ et al: High density lipoprotein cholesterol and coronary heart disease in hypercholesterolemic men: the Lipid Research Clinics Coronary Primary Prevention Trial, Circulation 74:1217, 1986.

27. Pekkanen J et al: Serum cholesterol and risk of accidental or violent death in a 25-year follow-up, Arch Intern Med 149:1589, 1989.

28. Levy RI et al: The influence of changes in lipid values induced by cholestyramine and diet on progression of coronary artery disease: results of the NHLBI Type II Coronary Intervention Study, Circulation 69:325, 1984.

29. Canner PL: Fifteen year mortality in coronary drug project patients: long-term benefit with niacin, J Am Coll Cardiol 8:1245, 1986.

30. Scandinavian Simvastatin Survival Study Group: Randomized trial of cholesterol lowering in 4444 patients with coronary heart disease: the Scandinavian Simvastatin Survival Study, Lancet 344:1383, 1994.

31. de Feyter PJ et al: Quantitative coronary angiography to measure progression and regression of coronary atherosclerosis. Value, limitations and implications for future clinical trials, Circulation 84:412, 1991.

32. Hong MK et al: Limitations of angiography for analyzing coronary atherosclerosis. Progression and regression, Ann Intern Med 121:348, 1994.

33. Brown BG et al: Lipid lowering and plaque regression. New insights into prevention of plaque disruption and clinical events in coronary disease, Circulation 87:1781, 1993.

34. Superko HR and Krauss RM: Coronary artery disease regression. Convincing evidence for the benefit of aggressive lipoprotein management, Circulation 90:1056, 1994.

35. Levine GN, Keaney JF, and Vita JA: Cholesterol reduction in cardiovascular disease. Clinical benefits and possible mechanisms, N Engl J Med 332:512, 1995.

36. Brensike JF et al: Effects of therapeutic cholestyramine on progression of coronary arteriosclerosis. Results of NHLBI Type II Coronary Intervention Study, Circulation 69:313, 1984.

37. Blankenhorn DH et al: Beneficial effects of combined colestipol-niacin therapy on coronary atherosclerosis and coronary venous bypass grafts, JAMA 257:3233, 1987.

38. Buchwald H et al: Effect of partial ileal bypass surgery on mortality and morbidity for coronary heart disease in patients with hypercholesterolemia. Report of the Program on Surgical Control of Hyperlipidemia (POSCH), N Engl J Med 323:946, 1990.

39. Ornish D, Brown SE, and Scherwitz LW: Can lifestyle changes reverse coronary artery disease? The Lifestyle Heart Trial, Lancet 336:129, 1990.

40. Brown BG et al: Regression of coronary artery disease as a result of intensive lipid-lowering therapy in men with high levels of apolipoprotein B, N Engl J Med 323:1289, 1990.

41. Cashin-Hemphill L et al: Beneficial effects of colestipol-niacin on coronary atherosclerosis. A four-year follow-up, JAMA 264:3103, 1990.

42. Kane JP et al: Regression of coronary atherosclerosis during treatment of familial hypercholesterolemia with combined drug regimens, JAMA 264:3007, 1990.

43. Watts GF et al: Effects of coronary artery disease on lipid-lowering diet or diet plus cholestyramine in the St. Thomas Atherosclerosis Regression Study (STARS), Lancet 339:563, 1992.

44. Alderman E et al: Beneficial angiographic and clinical response to multi-factor modification in the Stanford Coronary Risk Intervention Project (SCRIP), Circulation 84(suppl II):II-140, 1991 (abstract).

45. Haskell WL et al: The effects of the intensive multiple risk factor reduction on coronary atherosclerosis and clinical cardiac events: the Stanford Coronary Risk Intervention Project (SCRIP), Circulation 89:975, 1994.

46. Quinn TG et al: Development of new coronary atherosclerotic lesions during a 4-year multifactor risk reduction program: The Stanford Coronary Risk Intervention Project (SCRIP), J Am Coll Cardiol 24:900, 1994.

47. Schuler G et al: Regular physical exercise and low-fat diet: effects on progression of coronary artery disease, Circulation 86:1, 1992.

48. Blankenhorn DH et al: Coronary angiographic changes with the lovastatin study. The Monitored Atherosclerosis Regression Study (MARS): coronary angiographic changes with lovastatin therapy, Ann Intern Med 119:969, 1993.

49. Blankenhorn DH and Hodis HN: Arterial imaging and atherosclerosis reversal, Arterioscler Thromb 14:177, 1994.

50. Loscalzo J: Regression of coronary atherosclerosis, N Engl J Med 323:1337, 1990.

51. Treasure CB et al: Beneficial effects of cholesterol-lowering on the coronary endothelium in patients with coronary artery disease, N Engl J Med 332:481, 1995.

52. Anderson TJ et al: Effect of cholesterol-lowering and anti-oxidant therapy on endothelium—the dependent coronary vasomotion, N Engl J Med 332:488, 1995.

53. Benzuly KH et al: Functional improvement precedes structural regression of atherosclerosis, Circulation 89:1810, 1994.

54. Salonen R and Salonen JT: Determinants of carotid intima-media thickness: a population-based ultrasonography study in eastern Finnish men, J Intern Med 229:225, 1991.

55. Bonithon-Kopp C et al: Risk factors for early carotid atherosclerosis in middle-aged French women, Atheroscler Thromb 11:966, 1991.

56. Blankenhorn DH et al: Beneficial effects of colestipol-niacin therapy on the common carotid artery. Two- and four-year reduction in intima-media thickness measured by ultrasound, Circulation 88:20, 1993.

57. Mack WJ et al: One-year reduction and longitudinal analysis of carotid intima-media thickness associated with colestipol-niacin therapy, Stroke 24:1779, 1993.

58. Schaefer EJ and Levy RI: Pathogenesis and management of lipoprotein disorders, N Engl J Med 312:1300, 1985.

59. Goldstein JL and Brown MS: Familial hypercholesterolemia: a genetic receptor disease, Hosp Pract 20:35, 1985.
60. Goldstein JL and Brown MS: The LDL receptor locus and the genetics of familial hypercholesterolemia, Ann Rev Genet 13:259, 1979.
61. Slater HR et al: Contribution of the receptor pathway to low density lipoprotein catabolism in humans. New methods for quantitation, Arteriosclerosis 4:604, 1984.
62. Krauss RM: Regulation of high density lipoprotein levels, Med Clin North Am 66:403, 1982.
63. Fredrickson DS, Levy RI, and Lees RS: Fat transport in lipoproteins—an integral approach to mechanisms and disorders, N Engl J Med 276:32, 1967.
64. Cuthbert JA et al: Detection of familial hypercholesterolemia by assaying functional low-density-lipoprotein receptors on lymphocytes, N Engl J Med 314:879, 1986.
65. Glueck CJ, Levy RI, and Fredrickson DS: Norethindrone acetate, postheparin lipolytic activity, and plasma triglycerides in familial types I, III, IV and V hyperlipoproteinemia, Ann Intern Med 75:345, 1971.
66. Brunzell JD and Bierman EL: Chylomicronemia syndrome, Med Clin North Am 66:455, 1982.
67. Kissebah AH et al: The mechanism of action of clofibrate and tetranicotinoylfructose (Bradilan) on the kinetics of plasma free fatty acid and triglyceride transport in type IV and type V hypertriglyceridemia, Eur J Clin Invest 4:163, 1974.
68. Phillipson BE et al: The reduction of plasma lipids, lipoproteins and apoproteins in hypertriglyceridemic patients by dietary fish oils, N Engl J Med 312:1210, 1985.
69. Davignon J, Gregg RE, and Sing CF: Apolipoprotein E polymorphism and arteriosclerosis, Arteriosclerosis 8:1, 1988.
70. Goldstein JL and Brown MS: Hyperlipidemia in coronary heart disease: a biochemical genetic approach, J Lab Clin Med 108:174, 1986.
71. Utermann G et al: LP(a) glycoprotein phenotypes. Inheritance and relation to LP(a)-lipoprotein concentrations in plasma, J Clin Invest 80:458, 1987.
72. Hazzard WR et al: Hyperlipidemia in coronary heart disease. III. Evaluation of lipoprotein phenotypes of 156 genetically surveyed survivors of myocardial infarction, J Clin Invest 52:1569, 1973.
73. Goldstein JL et al: Hyperlipidemia in coronary heart disease. II. Genetic analysis of lipid levels in 176 families and delineation of a new inherited disorder, combined hyperlipidemia, J Clin Invest 52:1544, 1973.
74. Grundy SM, Chait A, and Brunzell JD: Familial combined hyperlipidemia workshop, Arteriosclerosis 7:203, 1987.
75. Sniderman AS et al: Association of coronary atherosclerosis with hyperapobetalipoproteinemia (increased protein but normal cholesterol levels in human plasma low density [beta] lipoproteins), Proc Natl Acad Sci USA 77:604, 1980.
76. Kissebah AH, Alfarsi S, and Evans DJ: Low density lipoprotein metabolism in familial combined hyperlipidemia. Mechanism of the multiple lipoprotein phenotypic expression, Arteriosclerosis 4:614, 1984.
77. East C, Bilheimer DW, and Grundy SM: Combination drug therapy for familial combined hyperlipidemia, Ann Intern Med 109:25, 1988.
78. Krempler S et al: Turnover of lipoprotein(a) in man, J Clin Invest 65:1483, 1980.
79. Hoefler G et al: Lipoprotein Lp(a). A risk factor for myocardial infarction, Arteriosclerosis 8:398, 1988.
80. Kostner GM et al: Lipoprotein Lp(a) and the risk for myocardial infarction, Atherosclerosis 38:51, 1981.
81. Gurakar A et al: Levels of lipoprotein Lp(a) decline with neomycin and niacin treatment, Atherosclerosis 57:293, 1985.
82. Soma MR et al: The lowering of lipoprotein[a] induced by estrogen plus progesterone replacement therapy in postmenopausal women, Arch Intern Med 153:1462, 1993
83. Schaefer EJ et al: Genetic high density lipoprotein deficiency states in atherosclerosis. In Angel A and Frolich J, eds: Lipoprotein deficiency syndromes, New York, 1986, Plenum Press.
84. LaRosa JC: Secondary hyperlipoproteinemia. In Rifkin BM and Levy RI, eds: Hyperlipidemia: prognosis and therapy, New York, 1977, Grune & Stratton.
85. Wallace RS: The Lipid Research Clinics Program Prevalence Study. Alterations in clinical chemistry levels associated with dyslipoproteinemias, Circulation 73(suppl I):I62, 1986.
86. Peiris AN et al: Adiposity, fat distribution and cardiovascular risk, Ann Intern Med 110:677, 1989.
87. Kaplan NM: The deadly quartet. Upper-body obesity, glucose intolerance, hypertriglyceridemia and hypertension, Arch Intern Med 149:1514, 1989.
88. Kannel WB and McGee DL: Diabetes and cardiovascular disease. The Framingham Study, JAMA 241:2035, 1979.
89. Frantz MJ et al: Nutrition principles for the management of diabetes and related conditions (review), Diabetes Care 17:490, 1994.
90. Dunn FL: Treatment of lipid disorders in diabetes mellitus, Med Clin North Am 72:1379, 1988.
91. Vinik A, Colwell JA, and the Hyperlipidemia in Diabetes Investigators: Effects of gemfibrozil on triglyceride levels in patients with NIDDM, Diabetes Care 16:37, 1993.
92. Koskinen P et al: Coronary heart disease incidence in NIDDM patients in the Helsinki Heart Study, Diabetes Care 15:820, 1992
93. O'Reilly DSTJ: Hypercholesterolaemia and thyroid hormone status, J Endocrinol 118:349, 1988.
94. Althans BU et al: LDL/HDL-changes in subclinical hypothyroidism: possible risk factors for coronary heart disease, Clin Endocrinol 28:157, 1988.
95. Wheeler DC, Varghese Z, and Moorhead JF: Hyperlipidemia in nephrotic syndrome, Am J Nephrol 9(suppl I):78, 1989.
96. Grundy SM: Management of hyperlipidemia of kidney disease, Kidney Int 37:847, 1990.
97. Henkin Y et al: Secondary dyslipidemia. Inadvertent effects of drugs in clinical practice, JAMA 267:961, 1992.
98. Kasiske BL et al: Effects of antihypertensive therapy on serum lipids, Ann Intern Med 122:133, 1995.
99. Disler LJ, Joffe BI, and Seftel HC: Massive hypertriglyceridemia associated with atenolol, Am J Med 85:586, 1988.
100. Bershad S et al: Changes in plasma lipids and lipoproteins during isotretinoin therapy for acne, N Engl J Med 313:981, 1985.
101. Hirvonen E, Malkonen M, and Manninen V: Effects of different progestogens on lipoproteins during post-menopausal replacement therapy, N Engl J Med 304:560, 1981.
102. Segal P et al: The association of dyslipoproteinemia with corneal arcus and xanthelasma. The Lipid Research Clinic Program Prevalence Study, Circulation 73(suppl I):I108, 1986.
103. Cruz PD, East C, and Bergstresser PR: Dermal, subcutaneous and tendon xanthomas: diagnostic markers for specific lipoprotein disorders, J Am Acad Dermatol 19:95, 1988.
104. The Expert Panel: Report of the National Cholesterol Education Program Expert Panel on Detection, Evaluation and

Treatment of High Blood Cholesterol in Adults, Arch Intern Med 148:36, 1988.

105. Olin JW et al: Lipoprotein abnormalities in patients with lower extremity arteriosclerosis obliterans, Cleve Clin J Med 59:491, 1992.

106. Kannel W: Lipids, diabetes, and coronary heart disease: insights from the Framingham Study, Am Heart J 110:1100, 1985.

107. Kuhn FE and Rackley CE: Coronary artery disease in women. Risk factors, evaluation, treatment and prevention, Arch Intern Med 153:2626, 1993.

108. Bush TC et al: Cardiovascular mortality and noncontraceptive use of estrogens in women: results from the Lipid Research Clinic Program Follow-Up Study, Circulation 75:1102, 1987.

109. Stampfer MJ et al: A prospective of post-menopausal estrogen therapy and coronary heart disease, N Engl J Med 313:1044, 1985.

110. Sullivan JM et al: Estrogen replacement and coronary artery disease. Effect on survival in post-menopausal women, Arch Intern Med 150:2557, 1990.

111. The Writing Group for the PEPI Trial: Effect of estrogen or estrogen/progestin regimens on heart disease risk factors in postmenopausal women—The Postmenopausal Estrogen/Progestin Interventions (PEPI) Trial, JAMA 273:199, 1995.

112. Persson et al: The effect on myocardial infarction (MI) risk of estrogens and estrogen-progestin combinations, Presented at the 6th International Congress on the Menopause, Bangkok, Thailand, 1990.

113. Barrett-Conner E and Bush TL: Estrogen and coronary artery disease in women, JAMA 265:1861, 1991.

114. La Rosa JC: Metabolic effects of estrogens and progestins, Fertil Steril 62(suppl 2):1405, 1994.

115. Lieberman EH et al: Estrogen improves endothelium-dependent, flow-mediated vasodilation in postmenopausal women, Ann Intern Med 121:936, 1994.

116. Judelson DR: Coronary heart disease in women: risk factors and prevention, JAMA 49:186, 1994.

117. Hoeg JM, Gregg RE, and Brewer HB Jr: An approach to the management of hypercholesterolemia, JAMA 255:512, 1986.

118. Heel RC et al: Colestipol: a review of its pharmacological properties and therapeutic efficacy in patients with hypercholesterolemia, Drugs 91:161, 1980.

119. Crouse JR: Hypertriglyceridemia: a contraindication to the use of bile acid binding resins, Am J Med 83:243, 1987.

120. Sprecher DL et al: Low-dose combined therapy with fluvastatin and cholestyramine in hyperlipidemic patients, Ann Intern Med 120:537, 1994.

121. Knopp RH et al: Contrasting effects of unmodified and time-release forms of niacin on lipoproteins and hyperlipidemic subjects: clues to mechanism of action, Metabolism 34:642, 1985.

122. Mullin GE, Greenson JK, and Mitchell MC: Fulminant hepatic failure after ingestion of sustained-release nicotinic acid, Ann Intern Med 111:253, 1989.

123. Illingworth DR, Tobert JA: A review of clinical trials comparing HMG–CoA reductase inhibitors, Clin Ther 16:366, 1994.

124. Shear CL et al: Expanded clinical evaluation of lovastatin (EXEL) study results: effect of patient characteristics on lovastatin-induced changes in plasma concentrations of lipids and lipoproteins, Circulation 85:1293, 1992.

125. Grundy SM: Drug therapy: HMG-CoA reductase inhibitors for the treatment of hypercholesterolemia, N Engl J Med 319:24, 1988.

126. Illingworth DR: Mevinolin (lovastatin) plus colestipol in therapy for severe heterozygous familial hypercholesterolemia: a multicenter trial, Ann Intern Med 104:598, 1984.

127. Samuel J: Effects of gemfibrozil on serum lipids, Am J Med 74(suppl 5A):23, 1983.

128. Grundy SM and Vega GL: Fibric acids: effects on lipids and lipoprotein metabolism, Am J Med 83(suppl 5B):9, 1987.

CHAPTER TEN

HYPERTENSION

Donald G. Vidt

Approximately 50 million individuals in the United States have arterial hypertension, which is defined as systolic blood pressure (SBP) of 140 mm Hg or greater and/or diastolic blood pressure (DBP) of 90 mm Hg or greater, and/or the taking of antihypertensive medication. Prevalence of hypertension increases with advancing age, and blacks are affected more than whites.[1,2] Hypertension is the most common public health problem in the United States today. It has been clearly demonstrated that cardiovascular risk increases progressively as SBP and DBP levels rise.[3] Although incremental risk is apparent in both men and women, the overall mortality experienced at any given range of blood pressure is lower among women than it is among men. The absolute cardiovascular risk of any given blood pressure level depends on the presence or absence of other associated cardiovascular risk factors.

PATHOGENESIS

Today it is recognized that 90% to 95% of all patients with hypertension have what is termed *essential or primary hypertension*—that is, the pathogenesis of the disease remains unclear. There has been an extraordinary development in the knowledge of regulatory mechanisms of blood pressure control, as well as numerous other factors that may contribute to our understanding of essential hypertension.[4] The role of heredity in the etiology of essential hypertension cannot be discounted. Population studies have clearly demonstrated the tendency for hypertension to aggregate within family groups; however, the manner in which heredity affects the numerous mechanisms involved in the control of blood pressure remains uncertain. More recently intensive investigation has focused on mechanisms of sodium and other cation transport, as well as the role of the central nervous system and the renin-angiotensin-aldosterone system in blood pressure control. In addition, distinct racial influences on the prevalence of hypertension have been well recognized, as well as the role of socioeconomic environment, obesity, physical inactivity, cigarette smoking, and alcohol consumption.

New drug development over the last several decades has certainly reflected the multiple mechanisms that influence blood pressure. The selection of drugs and regimens for controlling blood pressure continues to evolve. As new information becomes available, we can expect that future drug development will reflect evolving knowledge regarding mechanisms and other factors inherent in the onset and natural history of essential hypertension. Progressive renal failure as a consequence of untreated or inadequately treated malignant hypertension is well recognized. Although the incidence of malignant hypertension has decreased dramatically with new drug development and more aggressive treatment of hypertension, the incidence of progressive renal failure in young, predominantly black individuals with hypertension has certainly not declined.[5] There is a growing body of experimental and clinical data suggesting a cause-and-effect relationship for progressive renal failure in association with mild to moderate arterial hypertension.[6,7] These data suggest that more aggressive treatment and blood pressure control is indicated in patients with mild to moderate hypertension (now stage I or II). Yet there are no data from carefully controlled clinical trials to show that renal protection will result from more aggressive blood pressure control. Again, current and future studies with newer classes of antihypertensive agents to assess the potential for "renal protection" through effects on intrarenal hemodynamics may affect future treatment considerations.

CURRENT CLASSIFICATION

In recognizing the fact that the traditional classification of hypertension has failed to convey the impact of high blood pressure on the overall risks of cardiovascular disease (CVD), a new classification has emerged.[8] The traditional terms "mild hypertension" and "moderate hypertension" have been deleted because they fail to convey the major impact of high blood pressure on eventual risk. The new classification describes stages of blood pressure and recognizes that all stages of hypertension are associated with

Table 10-1. Classification of Blood Pressure for Adults 18 Years and Older*

Category	Blood Pressure (in mm Hg)	
	Systolic	Diastolic
Normal†	<130	<85
High normal	130-139	85-89
Hypertension**		
Stage I (mild)	140-159	90-99
Stage II (moderate)	160-179	100-109
Stage III (severe)	180-209	110-119
Stage IV (very severe)	≥210	≥120

Note: In addition to classifying stages of hypertension based on average blood pressure levels, the clinician should specify presence or absence of target-organ disease and additional risk factors. For example, a patient with diabetes and a blood pressure of 142/94 mm Hg plus left ventricular hypertrophy should be classified as "stage I hypertension with target-organ disease (left ventricular hypertrophy) and with another major risk factor (diabetes)." This specificity is important for risk classification and management.
*Not taking antihypertensive drugs and not acutely ill. When SBP and DBP fall into different categories, the higher category should be selected to classify the individual's blood pressure status. For instance, 160/92 mm Hg should be classified as stage II, and 180/120 mm Hg should be classified as stage IV. Isolated systolic hypertension (ISH) is defined as SBP ≥140 mm Hg and DBP <90 mm Hg and staged appropriately (e.g., 170/85 mm Hg is defined as stage II ISH).
†Optimal blood pressure with respect to cardiovascular risk is SBP <120 mm Hg and DBP <80 mm Hg. However, unusually low readings should be evaluated for clinical significance.
**Based on the average of two or more readings taken at each of two or more visits following an initial screening.
(From the fifth report of the Joint National Committee on Detection, Evaluation, and Treatment of High Blood Pressure [JNC-V], Arch Intern Med 153:154, 1993.)

Table 10-2. Manifestations of Target-Organ Disease

Organ System	Manifestations
Cardiac	Clinical, electrocardiographic, or radiologic evidence of coronary artery disease
	Left ventricular hypertrophy (LVH) or "strain" by electrocardiography or LVH by echocardiography
	Left ventricular dysfunction or cardiac failure
Cerebrovascular	Transient ischemic attack or stroke
Peripheral vascular	Absence of one or more major pulses in the extremities (except for dorsalis pedis) with or without intermittent claudication; aneurysm
Renal	Serum creatinine ≥130 μmol/L (1.5 mg/dl)
	Proteinuria (1+ or greater)
	Microalbuminuria
Retinopathy	Hemorrhages or exudates, with or without papilledema

(Adapted from the fifth report of the Joint National Committee on Detection, Evaluation, and Treatment of High Blood Pressure [JNC-V], Arch Intern Med 153:154, 1993.)

increased morbidity and mortality from CVD events (Table 10-1). The higher the blood pressure, the greater the risk. High blood pressure, stage I, previously termed "mild," is the most common form of hypertension in the adult population and is responsible for a large proportion of the excess morbidity, disability, and mortality attributable to hypertension.

This new classification also specifies the presence or absence of additional risk factors, together with surrogate target-organ end points. For example, other major cardiovascular risk factors such as dyslipidemia, cigarette smoking, diabetes mellitus, physical inactivity, and obesity should be identified. Detection and treatment of other major cardiovascular risk factors are critical to the successful management of persons with hypertension.[9,10]

The clinical manifestations of target-organ disease are also specified in the new classification system. The risks of CVD at any level of high blood pressure are increased severalfold for persons with target-organ disease, as described in Table 10-2. For example, a patient with diabetes and blood pressure of 142/94 mm Hg, plus left ventricular hypertrophy (LVH) should be classified as stage I hypertension with target-organ disease (LVH) and with another major risk factor (diabetes).

This degree of specificity in identifying other cardiovas-cular risk factors and/or surrogate end points is important for a more precise risk classification of the hypertensive patient. Expectations are that the increased specificity and sensitivity will benefit clinicians both in deciding to treat or not to treat and determining the aggressiveness of therapy warranted. In some situations this specificity of classification should also help in the appropriate selection of initial and subsequent antihypertensive therapy.

DIAGNOSIS

The recommendations of the Joint National Committee on Detection, Evaluation, and Treatment of High Blood Pressure (JNC-V) are useful for the practicing physician.[8] The diagnosis of hypertension in adults is confirmed when the average of two or more diastolic measurements on at least two office visits is 90 mm Hg or greater or when the average of multiple systolic measurements on two or more visits is 140 mm Hg or greater. Blood pressure confirmation on subsequent visits will help determine whether initial elevations remain high and therefore require further evaluation and therapy, or whether they have returned to normal and may therefore require only periodic remeasurement. The diagnosis of hypertension and treatment decisions must never be made on the basis of a single blood pressure reading. Blood pressure measurement techniques as outlined by the American Heart Association are recommended.[11]

EVALUATION OF THE HYPERTENSIVE PATIENT

With approximately 20% of the population at risk from hypertension and its complications, initial evaluation of the new hypertensive patient should be thorough but must also be cost-effective. The initial evaluation of patients with sustained hypertension should be designed to answer several questions:

1. Does the patient have primary or secondary hypertension?
2. Is target-organ involvement present?
3. Are cardiovascular risk factors other than hypertension present?

The medical history should include any family history of hypertension, premature CVD or mortality, diabetes, renal disease, or pheochromocytoma. If the patient has been previously diagnosed as hypertensive, the duration of disease should be established as well as prior antihypertensive therapy prescribed, response to therapy, and adverse effects of treatment. A careful history of both prescription and over-the-counter medications should be obtained for all patients since numerous agents may interact with antihypertensive drugs to raise blood pressure or block the effectiveness of antihypertensive medications. The presence or absence of other cardiovascular risk factors such as obesity, smoking, hyperlipidemia, and carbohydrate intolerance must be established. Psychosocial and environmental factors such as emotional stress, socioeconomic status, or specific cultural food practices that may have a bearing on blood pressure control and on subsequent compliance with medication regimens should be noted. In particular, an estimate of daily sodium intake and alcohol use should be established. The use of oral contraceptives in younger women and excessive alcohol intake in both men and women represent the two most common causes of reversible hypertension.

Symptoms of target-organ involvement may be revealed by obtaining a history of transient ischemic attack, stroke, myocardial infarction, angina pectoris, atherosclerotic heart disease, or lower-extremity arteriosclerosis obliterans. A change in the diurnal pattern of urine flow may be an early clue to concentrating defects secondary to hypertension-induced renal disease or other forms of renal parenchymal disease.

The physical examination should help verify the degree of target-organ involvement and may also provide additional clues to secondary causes of hypertension. Careful measurement of blood pressure, height, and weight, and a thorough funduscopic evaluation for evidence of arteriolar narrowing, arteriovenous compression, hemorrhages, exudates, or papilledema should be made. Auscultation and palpation of the neck should be performed for evidence of carotid bruits, distended neck veins, or an enlarged thyroid gland. Examination of the heart should establish size, rate, and rhythm, as well as the presence or absence of murmurs or gallop sounds. Careful auscultation of the lungs for rhonchi, rales, or wheezes will help establish the presence or absence of congestive heart failure or possibly chronic pulmonary disease. Examination of the abdomen should include both auscultation and palpation for evidence of bruits, enlarged kidneys, other abdominal masses, or dilation of the abdominal aorta. Examination of the extremities may reveal diminished or absent peripheral arterial pulses, bruits, or edema, and careful neurologic assessment will establish the presence of fixed neurologic deficits.

The history and physical examination should be complemented by a few carefully selected laboratory studies, preferably performed before initiating therapy.[8] The determination of a hemoglobin, hematocrit, urinalysis, serum potassium, serum creatinine, and an electrocardiogram will help determine the severity of vascular disease or the presence of target-organ involvement and may provide clues to secondary hypertension. The addition of a lipid profile, serum calcium, fasting blood sugar, and serum uric acid will help identify other cardiovascular risk factors. Many of these studies are easily obtainable as part of an automated blood chemistry profile. The decision to perform additional diagnostic studies should be determined by the presence or absence of clinical clues to secondary hypertension uncovered in the course of the history, physical examination, and screening studies. Clinical clues that may be helpful in identifying secondary and potentially reversible causes of hypertension are outlined in the box on p. 192. When the diagnosis of hypertension has been established, the process of patient education should be initiated. For subsequent therapy to be successful, patients must recognize that hypertension is a lifelong disease, that it is usually asymptomatic since the symptoms do not correlate with blood pressure levels, and that therapy will, in most instances, have to be maintained for life. Patients must recognize that effective therapy will control hypertension and that optimal control is usually compatible with an excellent long-term prognosis and quality of life. Adherence with a prescribed regimen is the key to successful therapy and will relate directly to the patient's willingness to comply with recommended medications and, when appropriate, to undertake selected behavioral modification.

LIFE-STYLE MODIFICATION

The benefits of therapy have been demonstrated in numerous clinical trials during the last 25 years. The decision to initiate therapy in the individual patient requires that both the severity of the hypertension and the presence or absence of other cardiovascular risk factors or disease conditions be considered. Life-style modification has received increasing attention in recent years as evidence has continued to mount regarding the effectiveness of selected nonpharmacologic measures in the control of blood pressure, particularly in patients with stage I hypertension. Selected life-style interventions can also be of adjunctive value in patients with more severe hypertension receiving pharmacologic therapy.

The use of nondrug therapies as initial treatment for most patients, at least for the first 3 to 6 months after recognition of their hypertension, has been widely advocated.[12,13] Effective life-style changes include appropriate reduction of calories, salt, alcohol, and fat consumption. In

CLINICAL CLUES FOR SECONDARY CAUSES OF HYPERTENSION

Renovascular Hypertension

Systolic-diastolic epigastric bruit

Accelerated or malignant hypertension

Unilateral small kidney discovered by an investigative study

Onset of hypertension before the age of 30 or after the age of 50

Refractory hypertension

Hypertension and unexplained impairment in renal function

Impairment in renal function in response to angiotensin-converting enzyme inhibitor

Evidence of extensive arteriosclerosis obliterans: carotid, coronary, peripheral

Coarctation of the Aorta

Absent or reduced pulses in the lower extremities

Palpable pulsations over intercostal arteries in the posterior thorax

Bruits over the intercostal arteries

Rib notching on chest x-ray

Absent aortic knob

Cushing's Syndrome

Recent change in physical appearance and weight gain

Extreme weakness with muscle wasting

Typical body habitus with moon facies, skin changes, and hirsutism

Glucose intolerance

Neutrophilia with relative lymphocytopenia

Pheochromocytoma

Symptomatic paroxysms of hypertension with headache, tachycardia, palpitations, tremor, and sweating

History of labile blood pressure

Substandard weight or recent weight loss

A pressor response to antihypertensive drugs or during induction of anesthesia

Refractory hypertension

Occasional occurrence with neurocutaneous syndromes

Unusual lability of blood pressure or orthostatic hypotension

Abnormal glucose tolerance

Primary Aldosteronism

Weakness, periodic paralysis, paresthesia, and tetany (rare)

Hypokalemia with inappropriate kaliuresis

Refractory hypertension

addition to these measures, avoidance of tobacco and participation in regular exercise need to be considered.

Sodium Restriction

Moderate dietary sodium restriction carries no risk for the hypertensive individual and may benefit selected patients by modest reductions in blood pressure. Almost half the patients who reduce their daily sodium intake into the range of 2 g of sodium or 5 to 6 g of salt will lower their blood pressure by about 5 mm Hg. In some stage I hypertensive patients this may be sufficient to normalize blood pressure without medication, whereas in others sodium restriction will enhance the antihypertensive efficacy of most antihypertensive medications.[14] Since a high proportion of daily sodium intake comes from prepared foods, merely undertaking a no-added-salt diet at the table or in food preparation may not be sufficient in many individuals. Thus appropriate counseling should include educational information regarding the labeling of processed foods and an increased awareness of the sodium content of frequently purchased foods.

The role of other agents such as potassium, calcium, and magnesium in the genesis of hypertension remains controversial. A modest beneficial effect on blood pressure has been noted after potassium supplementation in hypertensive patients who have been rendered hypokalemic from using diuretics; thus potassium supplements and prevention of hypokalemia in diuretic-treated patients may be beneficial.[15] Preliminary nutritional data have suggested that calcium intake is lower among hypertensive individuals than normotensive individuals, and that calcium supplementation may lower blood pressure in hypertensive patients.[16,17] Calcium supplements may be considered for patients in whom rigid restriction of dairy products has been undertaken for control of hyperlipidemia. Similarly, lower magnesium levels have been noted in hypertensive individuals.[18] Diuretic therapy may induce hypomagnesemia along with hypokalemia, and, if documented, supplementation may be considered in the diuretic-treated hypertensive patient.

Weight Reduction

The relationship between obesity and blood pressure has now been clearly established from numerous epidemiologic and intervention studies.[19,20] It is appropriate to recommend weight reduction for all obese hypertensive patients, with the goal of reducing body weight to within 15% of ideal weight. There is now evidence to suggest that upper body obesity correlates to hypertension, impaired glucose tolerance, and hypertriglyceridemia.[21] An increased coronary risk has also been associated with upper body obesity, thus suggesting that the risks related to obesity may not be a matter of weight alone, but also may be related to the distribution of that increased weight.[22] Although blood pressure reduction represents the primary benefit of weight reduction, favorable effects on plasma lipid abnormalities should also be considered. The high rate of recidivism following successful weight reduction is well recognized, stressing the importance of ongoing, long-term counseling and reassurance.

Restriction of Alcohol

Heavy alcohol consumption (more than 1 oz daily of ethanol) may elevate arterial pressure.[23] One oz of ethanol is contained in 2 oz of 100-proof whiskey, 8 oz of wine, or 24 oz of most beers. Hypertensive patients who drink should be encouraged to moderate their alcohol intake to comply with these limits.

Cessation of Smoking

Although there is little evidence to suggest that smoking is a risk factor for the development of hypertension, avoidance of tobacco products can considerably improve the overall cardiovascular health of the hypertensive patient. Smokers clearly increase their risks for cancer and chronic pulmonary disease, more than double their risk for coronary artery disease and sudden death, and increase their risk of stroke from twofold to tenfold.[24] Smokers may require higher dosages of a β-blocker to control blood pressure than nonsmokers. Avoidance of smoking should be strongly encouraged in hypertensive patients regardless of their age.

Exercise

A regular program of aerobic (isotonic) exercise facilitates cardiovascular conditioning, can aid the obese hypertensive individual in weight reduction, and may provide some benefit in reducing blood pressure.[25] Physical fitness is associated with lower all-cause mortality as well as cardiovascular and cancer mortality.[26] Additional benefits may be reflected in favorable changes in the lipid profile. A regular isotonic exercise program is strongly encouraged, whereas isometric exercise, such as that associated with weight lifting, should be discouraged because of exaggerated rises in systolic and diastolic blood pressure observed with this form of exercise.

Potassium Supplementation

Potassium supplementation may play a role in the prevention of high blood pressure but it is unlikely to be as important as reducing the amount of sodium intake. A number of clinical trials in hypertensive patients have suggested a blood pressure–lowering effect of potassium supplementation. A major cooperative research group trial, INTERSALT, identified an inverse relationship between blood pressures and measures of serum, urine, total body, and dietary intake of potassium.[27,28] Potassium supplementation in combination with other life-style modifications may provide an optimal strategy for the prevention of high blood pressure. Potassium supplementation may also play an important role in the prevention of hypertension among subgroups of the population, such as blacks, and others with a diet that is deficient in potassium intake.

Evidence is less convincing for other life-style interventions such as stress management, fish oils, fiber, and for alteration in macronutrient consumption.[29] It must be recognized, however, that in many instances, available data are insufficient to make a final judgment on the potential role of these factors in the control or primary prevention of hypertension.

CURRENTLY AVAILABLE ANTIHYPERTENSIVE AGENTS

Drug treatment of hypertension has changed significantly in the past decade. Many new classes of antihypertensive agents have been introduced for clinical use such as the α- and β-adrenergic blockers, the angiotensin-converting enzyme (ACE) inhibitors, and calcium channel blocking drugs. The effectiveness of these agents, their favorable adverse effect profiles, and the high degree of patient acceptance have led to their increasing popularity and changes in physician prescribing patterns. The primary attention of clinicians is no longer focused on the safety and efficacy issues of available drugs, since all approved agents share these characteristics. Attention is now focused on selection of agents for initial and subsequent therapy that control blood pressure and provide an optimal quality of life for the hypertensive patient, thus ensuring better patient adherence with long-term therapy. Another important trend in therapy has been the use of lower doses of individual agents, which is probably best demonstrated by the change in prescribing of thiazide diuretics.

The following section focuses on special characteristics, as well as potential advantages or disadvantages of different classes and selected agents. A review of the pharmacologic and metabolic properties of antihypertensive drugs is beyond the scope of this chapter but is available from other sources.[8,30-32] A complete listing of currently available drugs and recommended dosages is provided in Table 10-3.

Thiazide and Related Sulfonamide Diuretics

Diuretics have been the cornerstone of antihypertensive therapy since the introduction of the prototype agent chlorothiazide in 1958. These agents have been an integral part of every major clinical trial on hypertension during the past 25 years. Two important observations have significantly affected the use of diuretics in recent years and have led to a trend toward the use of lower doses of these agents. The first has been the clarification that therapeutic efficacy is obtained with once-a-day administration of doses ranging from 12.5 to 50 mg of hydrochlorothiazide or chlorthalidone in many patients (compared with doses of 50 to 100 mg, which were used previously). The second has been the accompanying observation that adverse effects such as hypokalemia and the risk of cardiac arrhythmias are less commonly observed with lower doses.

The major clinical trials, all of which included diuretics, demonstrated that optimal blood pressure control can drastically reduce cardiovascular morbidity and mortality, particularly the risk of stroke. A metaanalysis of 14 randomized treatment trials has indicated a 42% reduction in stroke from a 5 to 6 mm Hg lowering of DBP.[33] This reduction in stroke rate was highly consistent with long-term observational studies that predicted a 35% to 40% reduction with this blood pressure difference. The same long-term analyses predicted a 20% to 25% reduction in the rate of coronary heart disease. However, the observed reduction from the 14 pooled trial results was 14% over 4 to 6 years. The longitudinal observational trials to which these intervention results were compared extended for considerably longer periods.[34] It seems apparent that the

Table 10-3. Antihypertensive Agents (In all patients, life-style modifications should also be advised.)

Type of Drug	Usual Dosage Range (Total mg/day)*	Frequency (Per day)	Comments
Initial Antihypertensive Agents			
Diuretics			For thiazide and loop diuretics, lower doses and dietary counseling should be used to avoid metabolic changes.
Thiazides and Related Agents			
Bendroflumethiazide	2.5-5	1	More effective antihypertensive than loop diuretics except in patients with serum creatinine ≥221 μmol/L (2.5 mg/dl).
Benzthiazide	12.5-50	1	
Chlorothiazide	125-500	2	
Chlorthalidone	12.5-50	1	Hydrochlorothiazide or chlorthalidone is generally preferred; were used in most clinical trials.
Cyclothiazide	1.0-2	1	
Hydrochlorothiazide	12.5-50	1	
Hydroflumethiazide	12.5-50	1	
Indapamide	2.5-5	1	
Methyclothiazide	2.5-5	1	
Metolazone	0.5-5	1	
Polythiazide	1.0-4	1	
Quinethazone	25.0-100	1	
Trichlormethiazide	1.0-4	1	
Loop Diuretics			
Bumetanide	0.5-5	2	Higher doses of loop diuretics may be needed for patients with renal impairment or congestive heart failure.
Ethacrynic acid	25.0-100	2	
Furosemide	20.0-32.0	2	
Torsemide	5.0-200		Ethacrynic acid is the *only* alternative for patients with allergy to thiazide and sulfur-containing diuretics.
Potassium Sparing			
Amiloride	5-10	1 or 2	Weak diuretics.
Spironolactone	25-100	2 or 3	Used mainly in combination with other diuretics to avoid or reverse hypokalemia from other diuretics.
Triamterene	50-150	1 or 2	
			Avoid when serum creatinine ≥221 μmol/L (2.5 mg/dl).
			May cause hyperkalemia, and this may be exaggerated when combined with ACE inhibitors or potassium supplements.
Adrenergic Inhibitors			
β-Blockers			
Atenolol	25-100†	1	Selective agents will also inhibit β₂-receptors in higher doses (e.g., all may aggravate asthma.)
Betaxolol	5-40	1	
Bisoprolol	5-20	1	
Metoprolol	50-200	1 or 2	
Metoprolol (extended release)	50-200	1	
Nadolol	20-240†	1	
Propranolol	40-240	2	
Propranolol (long-acting)	60-240	1	
Timolol	20-40	2	
β-Blockers with Intrinsic Sympathomimetic Activity (ISA)			
Acebutolol	200-1200†	2	No clear advantage for agents with ISA except in those with bradycardia who must receive a β-blocker; they produce fewer or no metabolic side effects.
Carteolol	2.5-10†	1	
Penbutolol	20-80†	1	
Pindolol	10-60†	2	
α-β–Blocker			
Labetalol	200-1200	2	Possibly more effective in blacks than other β-blockers.
			May cause postural effects, and titration should be based on standing blood pressure.

Table 10-3. Antihypertensive Agents (In all patients, life-style modifications should also be advised.)—cont'd

Type of Drug	Usual Dosage Range (Total mg/day)*	Frequency (Per day)	Comments
α₁-Receptor Blockers			
Doxazosin	1.0-16	1	All may cause postural effects, and titration
Prazosin	1.0-20	2 or 3	should be based on standing blood pressure.
Terazosin	1.0-20	1	
ACE Inhibitors			
Benazepril	10.0-40†	1 or 2	Diuretic doses should be reduced or discon-
Captopril	12.5-150†	2	tinued prior to starting ACE inhibitors
Cilazapril	2.0-5.0	1 or 2	whenever possible to prevent excessive
Enalapril	2.5-40†	1 or 2	hypotension.
Fosinopril	10.0-40	1 or 2	Reduce dose of those drugs market "†" in
Lisinopril	5.0-40†	1 or 2	patients with serum creatinine ≥221 μmol/L
Perindopril	1.0-16†	1 or 2	(2.5 mg/dl)
Quinapril	5.0-80†	1 or 2	May cause hyperkalemia in patients with renal
Ramipril	1.25-20†	1 or 2	impairment or in those receiving potassium-
Spirapril	12.5-50†	1 or 2	sparing agents.
			Can cause acute renal failure in patients with severe bilateral renal artery stenosis or severe stenosis in an artery to a solitary kidney.
Calcium Antagonists			
Diltiazem	90-360	3	These agents also block the slow channels in
Diltiazem (sustained release)	120-360	2	the heart and may reduce sinus rate and
Diltiazem (extended release)	180-360	1	produce heart block.
Verapamil	80-480	2	
Verapamil (long acting)	120-480	1 or 2	
Dihydropyridines			
Amlodipine	2.5-10	1	Dihydropyridines are more potent peripheral
Felodipine	5-20	1	vasodilators than diltiazem and verapamil
Isradipine	2.5-10	2	and may cause more dizziness, headache,
Nicardipine	60-120	3	flushing, peripheral edema, and tachycardia.
Nifedipine	30-120	3	
Nifedipine (GITS)	30-90		
Supplemental Antihypertensive Agents			
Centrally acting α₂-Agonists			
Clonidine	0.1-1.2	2	Clonidine patch is replaced once a week.
Clonidine TTS (patch)‡	0.1-0.3	1 *weekly*	None of these agents should be withdrawn
Guanabenz	4-64	2	abruptly. Avoid in nonadherent patients.
Guanfacine	1-3	1	
Methyldopa	250-2000	2	
Peripheral-acting Adrenergic Antagonists			
Guanadrel	10-75	2	May cause serious orthostatic and exercise-
Guanethidine	10-100		induced hypotension.
Rauwolfia Alkaloids			
Rauwolfia root	50-200	1	
Reserpine	0.05-0.25	1	
Direct Vasodilators			
Hydralazine	50-200	2 to 4	Hydralazine is subject to phenotypically
Minoxidil	2.5-80	1 or 2	determined metabolism (acetylation). For both agents: should treat concomitantly with a diuretic and a β-blocker due to fluid retention and reflex tachycardia.

*The lower dose indicated is the preferred initial dose, and the higher dose is the maximum daily dose. Most agents require 2-4 weeks for complete efficacy, and more frequent dosage adjustments are not advised except for severe hypertension. The dosage range may differ slightly from the recommended dosage in *Physicians' Desk Reference* or package insert.
†Indicates drugs that are excreted by the kidney and require dosage reduction in the presence of renal impairment (serum creatinine ≥221 μmol/L [2.5 mg/dl]).
‡Weekly patch is 1, 2, 3 equivalent to 0.1-0.3 mg per day.

benefits of therapy in preventing stroke are seen early, whereas the multifactorial influences on significant coronary heart disease require considerably longer periods of therapy to show benefits.

Approximately 50% of mild to moderate hypertensive individuals will have a suitable blood pressure response to 12.5 to 50 mg of hydrochlorothiazide per day or its equivalent.[31] Thiazide diuretics are particularly effective in managing black individuals with hypertension, possibly because more blacks have a salt-sensitive, low-renin hypertension with a normal to modestly expanded plasma volume. Despite the fact that elderly individuals with hypertension tend to have a decreased plasma volume and a high peripheral resistance, diuretics are nevertheless effective as initial or subsequent therapy.

The Systolic Hypertension in the Elderly Program (SHEP) demonstrated a 36% reduction in fatal and nonfatal stroke, a 27% reduction in coronary heart disease incidence, and a 32% reduction in all major cardiovascular events.[35] The results were associated with a treatment regimen in which the primary agent was low-dose chlorthalidone.

The most common adverse effects associated with the thiazide or thiazide-like diuretics are volume depletion and electrolyte imbalance. Chronic administration predisposes patients to hypokalemia. It is apparent that the general trend toward lower doses of these agents has resulted in fewer problems with symptomatic hypokalemia. Hypomagnesemia, associated with weakness, tremors, and anorexia, can also be observed as a dose-related complication of thiazide therapy. Hyperuricemia is commonly associated with administration of these agents, but symptomatic gout seldom occurs unless the patient has a family or personal history of acute podagra. In the patient with a history of gout in whom thiazides are deemed necessary for control of hypertension, hyperuricemia can usually be controlled by the concomitant administration of allopurinol.

The major concern for the hypokalemic individual with hypertension relates to a possible increased risk for ventricular arrhythmias and sudden death in the setting of intrinsic cardiac disease or in the patient receiving a digitalis preparation.[36,37] Severe hypokalemia (less than 3 mEq/L) is less common with the use of low doses of diuretics. Probably the most effective way to prevent significant hypokalemia during thiazide therapy is to ensure that a patient adheres to a modest sodium-restricted diet. The use of potassium supplements, potassium-sparing diuretics, or ACE inhibitors also minimizes the risk of hypokalemia (less than 3.5 mEq/L).

Thiazide therapy has been associated with increases in plasma glucose and with the development of overt diabetes mellitus in selected patients. The mechanism of thiazide-induced impaired glucose tolerance probably relates to impaired insulin release and/or peripheral insulin resistance.[38] These changes may occur within weeks of initiation of diuretic therapy and are reversible upon discontinuation of these agents. The risk of impaired glucose tolerance appears to be enhanced by diuretic-induced hypokalemia.

In the management of the hypertensive diabetic with established nephropathy and edema, the use of a diuretic is often mandatory for adequate control of edema. Risk of deterioration in glycemic control associated with diuretic therapy is probably small if obesity and caloric intake can be carefully controlled. Prevention of hypokalemia and prudent use of recommended lower doses of diuretics can further reduce the risk of thiazide-induced hyperglycemia. Concurrent use of an ACE inhibitor will further blunt diuretic-induced hypokalemia.

Multiple observations have demonstrated elevations of total cholesterol, low-density lipoprotein (LDL) cholesterol, and triglycerides in association with thiazide diuretic therapy.[39,40] Careful adherence to a low-cholesterol diet during therapy has been shown to blunt the hyperlipidemic effects. These concerns will continue to influence the choice of initial therapy for many patients with mild to moderate hypertension.[41] It would seem prudent to avoid diuretics, at least as initial therapy, in patients with hypertension and hyperlipidemia, particularly those with LDL cholesterol levels greater than 160 mg/dl. In these high-risk patients, suitable initial alternative therapies are available that do not adversely affect the lipid profile. When diuretic therapy is indicated in the hypertensive, hyperlipidemic patient, concurrent treatment with a low-cholesterol diet, controlled caloric intake, liberal use of increased soluble dietary fiber, and the lowest effective diuretic dosage is recommended.

Loop Diuretics

The antihypertensive effects of loop diuretics are similar to those of the thiazide and thiazide-like agents. Unlike thiazides, the potency of loop diuretics can be increased by increasing the dose in stepwise fashion, and it is often possible to establish diuresis in patients who are otherwise refractory to thiazide diuretics. Loop diuretics may be preferable to thiazide diuretics in patients with refractory hypertension or congestive heart failure and in patients with impaired renal function (serum creatinine level greater than 2.5 mg/dl and glomerular filtration rate [GFR] less than 25 ml/min). Ethacrynic acid has never attained the popularity enjoyed by furosemide or bumetanide but may be a useful alternative for patients with known hypersensitivity to these agents.

A new loop diuretic, torsemide, is rapidly absorbed with high bioavailability of 80% following oral administration; and oral and intravenous forms are therapeutically equivalent (milligram for milligram).[42] Effects can be observed for 6 to 8 hours and approximately 20% of the dose is eliminated in the urine and the rest by hepatic cytochrome oxidation to inactive metabolites.[43]

Intravenous administration of loop diuretics may be preferred in patients with refractory edema and as concurrent therapy with other parenteral agents in the management of hypertensive urgencies or emergencies. Transient deafness has been reported with furosemide and ethacrynic acid and is most common with administration of high parenteral doses in patients with renal insufficiency. The ototoxic potential from bumetanide is significantly less than that observed with other loop diuretics.

Potassium-Sparing Diuretics

The potassium-sparing agents include spironolactone, triamterene, and amiloride. Unfortunately spironolactone and amiloride are less potent diuretic and antihypertensive agents than are the thiazides, and triamterene has no significant antihypertensive effects when used alone, making them inappropriate agents for initial therapy of patients with stage I or II hypertension.

Potassium-sparing agents reduce potassium losses secondary to other diuretics and in states of increased circulating aldosterone. They may potentiate the effectiveness of a thiazide or loop diuretic when used concurrently.

Hyperkalemia is the most common adverse effect of potassium-sparing agents, and severe renal insufficiency represents an absolute contraindication to their administration because of the danger of inducing hyperkalemia. Concurrent therapy with potassium-sparing agents, ACE inhibitors, and oral potassium supplements should be avoided because of the risk of hyperkalemia.

Adrenergic Blocking Agents

The antihypertensive effects of adrenergic blocking agents may be caused by prevention of sympathetic responses to changes in posture, exertion, and plasma volume deficits, or to suppression of renin secretion by selected sympathetic depressant drugs. Prevention of vasoconstriction in the arterial vascular bed results in a modest reduction in blood pressure. The normal baroreceptor influences mediated by sympathetic nerves are blunted under the influence of sympathetic depressant drugs. Cardiac contractility, heart rate, and cardiac output may be reduced, and decreased sympathetic activity in the veins results in increased venous capacitance, decreased cardiac output, and possibly postural hypotension. Subtle changes in renal plasma flow and GFR following reduction of blood pressure may lead to salt retention and increase in plasma volume, a consequence of therapy with most of the sympathetic depressant drugs.

β-Adrenergic Blocking Agents

Currently 11 β-adrenergic blockers have been approved for hypertension, and when used in appropriate doses, there is little evidence to suggest that any one has major advantages over the others in hypertension control. There are, however, differences in the clinical pharmacology of these agents that affect their use in associated diseases and may contribute to specific differences in the adverse effect profiles of these drugs. All β-blockers, including those with cardioselectivity and partial agonist activity, can induce bronchoconstriction in patients with poorly controlled asthma. These agents may aggravate heart failure in patients with preexistent cardiac disease. In insulin-dependent diabetics, who are prone to hypoglycemia, premonitory symptoms may be masked by β-blockade, and there is some evidence to suggest that prolonged therapy with propranolol may impair carbohydrate tolerance.[38] An area of current concern relates to the effects of some β-blockers on lipid metabolism.[44] Nonselective agents appear to increase plasma triglycerides as well as very low density lipoprotein (VLDL) cholesterol, and may decrease the high-density lipoprotein (HDL) cholesterol. The propensity for these adverse lipid changes is lessened in the presence of cardioselectivity or partial agonist activity.[45]

All β-blockers cross the blood-brain barrier to some degree, although higher central nervous system concentrations have been evidenced with the more lipophilic agents. As a result, symptoms of fatigue, depression, sleep disturbances, and occasional nightmares have been commonly observed with this class of agents. Clinical experience suggests that the hydrophilic β-blockers have less propensity for these central nervous system adverse effects. β-blockers should be used with caution in patients receiving digitalis glycosides, since excessive bradycardia has been reported in patients receiving both agents.

Some β-adrenergic blockers are less effective in lowering blood pressure in black individuals with hypertension, and side effect profiles may vary from agent to agent. The β-blockers are the only antihypertensive drugs shown to reduce the risk of ischemic heart disease, particularly as it relates to morbidity and mortality following an initial myocardial infarction. In general, immediate reductions in blood pressure are not expected with administration of a β-blocker. Continued therapy for several days to a week or longer is needed to appreciate the full pharmacologic effects of these agents.

The parenteral β_1 cardioselective β-blocker, esmolol, has demonstrated immediate antihypertensive effects. It is ultrashort acting and is used primarily for the control of supraventricular tachycardia, but it has been used successfully for the control of perioperative hypertension. After a loading dose of 500 µg/kg is administered over 1 minute, a maintenance infusion of 25 to 200 µg/kg/min is titrated by increments of 50 µg/kg/min at 5- to 10-minute intervals. Increments in dosage may be preceded by reboluses of 500 µg/kg.

Combined α- and β-Blocker

Labetalol differs from currently available β-adrenergic blocking agents in its ability to block both α- and β-adrenergic receptors. Systemic vascular resistance and arterial blood pressure are reduced, while heart rate is unchanged or slightly suppressed and cardiac output is generally unaffected. This hemodynamic profile is observed within minutes of an intravenous injection of labetalol, and changes persist during long-term oral administration. Labetalol also demonstrates mild intrinsic agonist activity for β_2-adrenergic receptors, an effect that may help explain its improved tolerance in patients with asthma or chronic obstructive pulmonary disease (COPD). Clinical studies have demonstrated labetalol to be more effective in black and elderly individuals than other β-blockers.

As with other β-adrenergic blockers, labetalol should be avoided or used with caution in patients with asthma, heart block greater than first-degree, severe sinus bradycardia, or decompensated congestive heart failure. The most common adverse effect observed with oral administration of labetalol is postural hypotension, a manifestation of the α-blocking properties of this agent.

The immediate effectiveness of labetalol by intravenous infusion or intermittent pulse administration has made labetalol the drug of choice for many clinicians in the initial management of hypertensive urgencies or emergencies, including pheochromocytoma.[46,47] The observation of peak antihypertensive effects within 90 to 120 minutes after oral administration has led to increasing usage in the initial management of severe hypertension or hypertensive urgencies.

Central Adrenergic Inhibitors

The four agents in this family of drugs—methyldopa, clonidine, guanabenz, and guanfacine—appear to exert their major effects on central nervous system vasomotor centers. These agents function primarily by decreasing sympathetic outflow from the central nervous system.

Dryness of the mouth and drowsiness occur frequently with these agents and are the most common adverse effects. No significant adverse effects have been reported on either carbohydrate metabolism or blood lipid concentrations. In fact, clinical trials have suggested that guanabenz may reduce total cholesterol and triglycerides. The decrease in cholesterol appears primarily because of a reduction in the LDL fraction. A pronounced withdrawal reaction may develop within 12 to 48 hours after sudden discontinuation of clonidine or guanabenz therapy. The withdrawal syndrome occurs most commonly in patients receiving larger doses of either agent and is associated with restlessness, irritability, tremors, tachycardia, abdominal pain, and marked rebound hypertension. The hypertension is associated with increased plasma and urinary catecholamines. Patients must be warned of the risk of this withdrawal syndrome, should they abruptly discontinue medication. A longer duration of action of guanfacine enables once-daily administration, whereas other agents in this class are administered twice daily.

Clonidine may be administered transdermally in an adherent skin patch that provides sufficient drug treatment for 7 days at a time. The transdermal preparation is available in sizes delivering the equivalent of 0.1, 0.2, or 0.3 mg of clonidine per day. Although the incidence of drowsiness and dry mouth appear less with the transdermal preparation, a major limitation in its usage has been the development of localized skin reactions with pruritus.[48] The central α-agonists are useful in treating a broad range of patients with hypertension, including those with renal insufficiency, asthma or COPD, and diabetes mellitus. The absence of adverse metabolic effects, particularly on plasma lipid profiles, provides a potential advantage in treating hypertensives at high risk for progression of atherosclerosis. Adverse effects can be minimized by concomitant administration of a small dose of a diuretic to enable smaller daily dosages of the agent of choice.

α-Adrenergic Blocking Agents

Two early α-adrenergic blockers, phentolamine and phenoxybenzamine, are currently reserved for the diagnosis and treatment of hypertensive states associated with high circulating levels of catecholamines. Intravenous administration of phentolamine is followed by a transient α-adrenergic blockade. Significant cardiac stimulation with tachycardia and occasional cardiac arrhythmias may be associated with its use. A transient and sometimes marked reduction in blood pressure will be observed in patients with high circulating levels of catecholamines from an actively secreting tumor or from rebound hypertension following abrupt discontinuation of clonidine or guanabenz.

Similarly, oral phenoxybenzamine is still used in the preoperative management of patients with pheochromocytoma. It is a short-acting agent, and its administration is also associated with profound postural hypotension and reflex tachycardia.

Three α_1-blockers—prazosin, terazosin, and doxazosin—are currently available and induce functional blockade of postsynaptic α_1-adrenergic receptors to reduce peripheral vascular resistance. They dilate both arterioles and veins, and unlike phentolamine and phenoxybenzamine, do not induce reflex tachycardia. The most common side effect of the α_1-blockers is postural hypotension, which can be minimized by initiating therapy with a low dosage and increasing it gradually. Terazosin and doxazosin differ from prazosin in having more predictable absorption and a longer duration of action that enables once-daily administration.

In selected hypertensive men with benign prostatic hypertrophy (BPH), α-adrenergic blockers can provide beneficial effects on the symptoms of BPH.[49] α_1-Adrenergic receptors are located in the bladder body, bladder base, prostate, and urethra. An α_1-blockade can relieve the dynamic obstructive component by inducing relaxation of the bladder outlet without impairing the contractile properties of the bladder body. α_1-Blockade is well suited for hypertensive patients with moderate symptoms of BPH but who are fully compensated with little or no residual urine and no significant obstruction.

All three agents can be administered to hypertensives with renal insufficiency without changing the dosage. Use of these agents in hypertensive patients with congestive heart failure has not been associated with any significant reduction in mortality. These agents have no detrimental effects on pulmonary function and can be useful in hypertensive patients with asthma. No adverse effects have been demonstrated in carbohydrate metabolism or in lipid levels. In fact, clinical studies have suggested a slight decrease in total cholesterol and a rise in the HDL cholesterol with long-term therapy, making the α-blockers suitable treatment choices for high-risk hypertensive patients with hyperlipidemia. Because of the propensity for postural hypotension following α_1-blockade, these agents must be used with caution in patients with autonomic impairment, including elderly individuals, in whom baroreceptor responses are often impaired.

Rauwolfia Alkaloids

The rauwolfia alkaloid compounds, including reserpine, were among the earliest available sympathetic inhibiting agents for treating hypertension. The use of reserpine has declined progressively over the last two decades with the emergence of many new classes of effective and better-tolerated agents.

The major limitations in the use of reserpine have been

its modest efficacy and significant adverse effect profile. The sedative and depressive effects of reserpine are subtle and have been mostly observed with dosages exceeding 0.25 mg daily. It is expected that the use of reserpine will continue to progressively decline.

Peripheral-Acting Adrenergic Antagonists

Guanethidine and guanadrel inhibit the function of postganglionic sympathetic neurons by accumulation and displacement of norepinephrine from neuronal storage granules. Blood pressure reduction is associated with a decrease in cardiac output, caused primarily by pooling of blood in capacitance vessels and decreased venous return to the heart. The use of these agents today is reserved for patients with severe or refractory hypertension in whom combinations of other, better-tolerated agents have been ineffective. The clinical pharmacology and problems experienced with guanethidine are similar to guanadrel, with one caveat. The major advantage of guanadrel over guanethidine is its shorter duration of action, an advantage that is most notable in the patient who develops incapacitating postural symptoms on guanethidine. The potential for drug interactions is the same as that observed with guanethidine. These compounds are infrequently required in the therapy of hypertension today since the vast majority of patients can be controlled with one or a combination of other agents that are far better tolerated.

Direct Vasodilating Agents

Since direct vasodilators reduce peripheral vascular resistance, the primary hemodynamic abnormality in essential hypertension, they should be preferred therapeutic agents. Unfortunately their effectiveness is limited by the responsiveness of homeostatic mechanisms, which tend to blunt the pharmacologic response to vasodilators (increased cardiac output, increased plasma renin activity, and increased plasma volume). Vasodilators have largely been relegated to use in combination with adrenergic blocking agents and diuretics.

HYDRALAZINE. Hydralazine lowers peripheral vascular resistance by a direct effect on arteriolar smooth muscle.[50] Reflex increases in heart rate and cardiac output accompany its use as monotherapy because it has little effect on venous capacitance; in patients with coronary artery disease, the increased cardiac work may precipitate anginal symptoms. Stimulation of the renin-angiotensin-aldosterone system contributes to sodium and water retention and expansion of plasma volume, which may lead to rapid pseudotolerance.

The major metabolism of hydralazine occurs in the liver by ring hydroxylation and subsequent conjugation. Most reported cases of hydralazine toxicity, including the development of antinuclear antibodies and rheumatoid arthritis–like symptoms, have probably occurred in slow acetylators.[51] Patients with renal failure acetylate hydralazine more slowly, and adjustment in dosage may be required because of slow acetylation and decreased renal clearance of the unchanged drug.

Hydralazine has been used parenterally to manage selected hypertensive emergencies. Although affording the convenience of either intramuscular or intravenous administration, it is not as consistently effective as newer vasodilating agents such as diazoxide or sodium nitroprusside. Hydralazine remains a favorite with some clinicians to manage eclampsia of pregnancy.

MINOXIDIL. Minoxidil is an extremely potent vasodilating agent with hemodynamic actions similar to those of hydralazine. Vasodilation is accompanied by reflex tachycardia, increased cardiac output, and a propensity for sodium and water retention. Minoxidil combined with a β-blocker to control reflex cardiac stimulation and a loop diuretic to control fluid retention is a potent combination in the management of severe or refractory hypertension.

Although the drug has a relatively short plasma half-life of approximately 4 hours, once-daily administration is effective in most patients. The most common adverse effects are those common to direct vasodilating agents, such as headache, tachycardia, palpitations, and aggravation of anginal symptoms. A common adverse effect of prolonged use, hirsutism, can be of considerable cosmetic concern to some patients. The use of topical minoxidil in the treatment of pattern baldness has not been associated with any adverse effects on blood pressure in hypertensive patients.

DIAZOXIDE. When administered intravenously, diazoxide is a potent arteriolar vasodilator with rapid onset of action. The maximum hypotensive effect is usually observed within 3 to 5 minutes following injection and may persist for variable periods of 1 to 12 hours or longer.[52] The rapid, dose-related reduction in blood pressure has been associated with impaired regional blood flow in patients with significant coronary or cerebrovascular disease. It is recommended that diazoxide be administered in repeated, small pulse doses of 50 to 75 mg, given at intervals of 5 to 15 minutes. With repeated pulse administration, a more gradual and controllable reduction in blood pressure can be obtained, thus minimizing the risk of cerebral or myocardial ischemia.[53] Concomitant administration of a β-adrenergic blocker is useful in patients with coronary artery disease to prevent reflex tachycardia, and concomitant administration of a loop diuretic is recommended to prevent sodium and water retention with repeated dosages.

Diazoxide induces hyperglycemia; occasionally adjustments in insulin dosage may be required in diabetic patients. The hypotensive effects of diazoxide may be exaggerated by concomitant administration of other antihypertensive agents, particularly other vasodilators, and by intravascular volume depletion. Since diazoxide displaces coumarin anticoagulants from their binding sites on serum albumin, reduction of the anticoagulant dose may be necessary in patients receiving both diazoxide and a coumarin derivative. Diazoxide should only be considered in the initial management of patients with severe hypertension or in hypertensive emergencies.

SODIUM NITROPRUSSIDE. This agent differs from other direct vasodilators in that both resistance and capacitance vessels are affected; thus decreases in both arterial pressure and central venous pressure accompany its use.[54] Because of its ability to improve left ventricular function without inducing reflex tachycardia, it has been a particularly useful agent in managing the hypertensive crisis associated with congestive heart failure or following acute myocardial infarction. The rate of reduction in blood pressure during intravenous administration of sodium nitroprusside depends on the rate of infusion. Its rapid onset of effect, and rapid disappearance following discontinuation, necessitate administration of a controlled infusion in an intensive care environment with constant nursing supervision. Nitroprusside is almost universally effective and will lower blood pressure when other potent antipressor agents have failed.

Sodium nitroprusside is rapidly metabolized to cyanogen and subsequently converted to thiocyanate, which is excreted by the kidneys. Acute toxicity is primarily related to excessive vasodilation and hypotension, and symptoms disappear promptly when the infusion is stopped or slowed. In patients with renal failure, excessive accumulation of thiocyanate may occur after several days of administration and may produce manifestations of toxicity ranging from weakness, nausea, and tinnitus, to overt psychosis. There is a small but significant risk of cyanide toxicity, which has been observed with prolonged use of nitroprusside in patients with refractory heart failure and poor tissue perfusion.[55] Rapid decomposition of nitroprusside on exposure to light necessitates the use of opaque wrappings during administration and periodic replacement with fresh solutions.

NITROGLYCERIN. Intravenous nitroglycerin shares several of the advantages of sodium nitroprusside, including its rapid onset and offset of action and the ability to titrate the drug to a desired goal blood pressure under close supervision. Unlike nitroprusside, nitroglycerin predominantly dilates venous capacitance vessels, but when large doses are administered, arteriolar dilation may also be observed. By reducing both left ventricular filling pressure and mean arterial pressure, end-diastolic volume and pressure and myocardial oxygen demand are reduced. Collateral coronary blood vessels are also dilated, and improved perfusion to ischemic areas and myocardium can be observed, as opposed to sodium nitroprusside, which decreases flow to ischemic myocardium. Thus nitroglycerin is efficacious in hypertensive patients with significant coronary artery disease and has proved particularly effective in the management of hypertensives following coronary artery bypass surgery.[56,57] It is also a treatment of choice in congestive heart failure when blood pressure before treatment is normal or only modestly elevated.

Nitroglycerin's ultrashort half-life, measured in minutes, requires close and constant supervision of continuous infusions. Headache, flushing, and dizziness may be observed during infusion, but can usually be minimized by starting with small initial infusion rates. Because of variable absorption by plastic containers and tubing, glass containers must be employed for dilution and storage, combined with nonabsorbing administration tubing. Nitroglycerin may be useful in managing hypertension with renal failure, since it lacks the risk of cyanide and/or thiocyanate toxicity.

Angiotensin-Converting Enzyme Inhibitors

Experience with ACE inhibitors has clearly demonstrated that blood pressure can be substantially reduced in a majority of patients by blockade of the renin-angiotensin-aldosterone system.[58,59] The major action of the ACE inhibitors resides in their ability to inhibit the conversion of angiotensin I to the potent vasoactive peptide, angiotensin II, thus inducing vasodilation and reduced peripheral vascular resistance. A secondary decrease in aldosterone secretion prevents sodium and water retention and adds to the usefulness of this class of agents as monotherapy in managing mild and moderate hypertension. Their combined vasodilator and natriuretic effects have led to their wide acceptance as primary agents in managing congestive heart failure with or without complicating hypertension. Vasodilation and reduced blood pressure are accomplished without reflex cardiac stimulation, possibly caused in part by the parasympathomimetic action of these agents. Other potential mechanisms of action may include accumulation, via ACE inhibition, of vasodilator bradykinins and prostaglandins, or possibly by interactions within the central nervous system, as well as the peripheral sympathetic nervous system to blunt baroceptor responsiveness. Emerging evidence suggests the existence of tissue-specific renin-angiotensin systems, including vascular endothelium. It is intriguing to consider the possibility that future developments may provide ACE inhibitors with different tissue-specific responses.[58]

ACE inhibitors are excreted wholly or in part by the kidney, and adjustments in dosage may be required in patients with renal insufficiency. These agents have no adverse effects on lipid metabolism, pulmonary function, or carbohydrate metabolism, and recent studies suggest that ACE inhibitors reduce proteinuria and have the potential for preservation of renal function in hypertensive diabetics with nephropathy.[60] ACE inhibitors have now been approved for afterload reduction in the management of congestive heart failure and decreased left ventricular function following a myocardial infarction.[61,62] Clinical experience suggests that ACE inhibitors, when used as monotherapy, are more effective in whites and younger individuals than they are in blacks or older individuals. When combined with a diuretic, additive effects are noted on BP, and the age and racial differences of effect are no longer apparent.

Several adverse effects occur with ACE inhibitors as a class that deserve attention. Potentially hazardous hypotension may follow the initial dose of an ACE inhibitor if administered to a patient who is volume depleted. It is appropriate to discontinue diuretics for several days before initiating ACE inhibitor therapy. If this is not practical, the first dose should be administered under close clinical surveillance. Sudden, severe hypotension and oliguric renal failure has been observed with ACE inhibitors administered to patients with bilateral high-grade renal artery stenosis or high-grade stenosis to a solitary functioning kidney.[63] The increasing prevalence of generalized arteriosclerotic occlusive disease, including renovascular disease or cholesterol emboli and azotemia, in older patients makes this a noteworthy caution when considering ACE inhibitors in this population.[64] Hyperkalemia is routinely observed with ACE inhibitors, and although these agents may blunt the tendency toward hypokalemia when used with diuretics, the clinician must be aware of a significant risk of hyperkalemia if potassium-sparing agents or potassium supplements are used concurrently. A dry, nonproductive cough is now clearly the most common adverse effect observed with ACE inhibitors, and, when searched for, may be observed in as many as 15% of patients.[65,66] Although the mechanism for cough is unclear, a possible pulmonary effect of accumulated bradykinin on J receptors and pulmonary C fibers is suspected.[67] While rarely observed, angioedema is a potentially life-threatening adverse effect. Adverse effects such as leukopenia, nephrotic-range proteinuria, dysgeusia, and skin rashes are rarely observed with current, therapeutic doses of captopril and have rarely been observed with subsequent generations of ACE inhibitors.

Calcium Channel Blockers

Although representing a chemically diverse group of compounds, calcium channel blockers all act by selective inhibition of calcium influx through cell membranes. Despite sharing the same pharmacologic mechanism of action at the cell level, clinical effects of subgroups of calcium channel blockers are quite different, particularly as they relate to the contractile process of the heart, vascular smooth muscle and skeletal muscle, and cardiac nodal conduction tissue.[68,69] These differences apparently relate to differences in relative specificity of different calcium channel blockers for effector tissues.

Extensive first-pass metabolism and short plasma half-lives once necessitated frequent doses to maintain an adequate clinical response. The availability of long-acting preparations of currently available agents, verapamil, diltiazem, and newer dihydropyridines, now enables once-daily or twice-daily administration in most patients.

Calcium channel blockers have no adverse effects on lipid metabolism or carbohydrate metabolism with prolonged use and can be safely administered to the asthmatic hypertensive patient. A natriuretic and diuretic effect observed with most calcium channel blockers may explain the lack of sodium and volume retention, which enables administration of these agents as monotherapy.

Clinical observations suggest that calcium channel blockers are particularly efficacious in older and black hypertensive patients, who share a tendency toward normal to low plasma renin activity. Use of calcium channel blockers need not be restricted to these groups since their efficacy in younger, white hypertensive patients has also been established. Nifedipine deserves special mention, since it has emerged as an agent of choice in the initial treatment of patients with hypertensive urgencies or emergencies.[70] The ease of administration sublingually or orally and a rapid dose response within 15 to 30 minutes have undoubtedly contributed to its popularity. However, a word of caution must be offered. In older patients with significant occlusive cerebral or coronary vascular disease, the uncontrolled, initial response to nifedipine may be accompanied by symptomatic cerebral or coronary ischemia.

Nicardipine is the first dihydropyridine calcium antagonist approved for short-term, intravenous treatment of hypertension, when oral therapy is not feasible or desirable.[71,72] It is a rapid-acting, systemic, and coronary artery vasodilator. Cardiac depression is minimal and atrial ventricular conduction defects, as seen occasionally with verapamil, have not been described. Onset of action is observed within 15 to 30 minutes of initiating an infusion. The effects of nicardipine correlate well with plasma concentrations, and like other calcium antagonists, nicardipine undergoes hepatic degradation with no active metabolites. Nicardipine can be titrated for rapid or gradual reduction of blood pressure levels. Effects last for 10 to 15 minutes after stopping the infusion. Nicardipine has proved to be particularly effective in the management of postoperative hypertension of multiple etiologies, and may provide a greater ease of titration than sodium nitroprusside.

The predominant vasodilator effects of the dihydropyridine derivatives may cause headache, reflex tachycardia, dizziness, and edema. The latter is caused by fluid redistribution, not retention. These symptoms are less common with newer dihydropyrides such as isradipine, felodipine, and amlodipine. Constipation is the most prominent side effect of negative inotropic agents such as verapamil and diltiazem. Diltiazem and verapamil should be used with caution in combination with β-blockers in patients with atrial ventricular conduction disturbances.

The efficacy of the calcium channel blockers, together with their high degree of patient acceptance, has contributed to their rapid increase in clinical use.[73] Experimental observations suggesting a potential antiatherogenic effect and an ability to mitigate renal ischemia, together with a host of other noncardiovascular effects, tend to enhance the future promise of this class of agents.

TREATMENT

The goal of treating patients with hypertension is to prevent morbidity and mortality associated with high blood pressure and to control blood pressure by the least intrusive means possible. This strategy can be accomplished by achieving and maintaining arterial pressure below 140 mm Hg systolic and 90 mm Hg diastolic, while controlling other cardiovascular risk factors.[74,75] Further reductions to levels of 130/85 mm Hg may be pursued with due regard for cardiovascular function, especially in older persons. How far the diastolic pressure should be reduced below 85 mm Hg remains uncertain.

Life-style modifications, including weight reduction, increased physical activity, and moderation of dietary sodium and alcohol intake are used as adjunctive or definitive therapy for hypertension. Properly used, life-style modification interventions offer the ability to improve the cardiovascular risk profile. Even when not adequate in themselves to control hypertension, they may still reduce the number and doses of antihypertensive medications required to manage the patient. Life-style modifications are particularly helpful in the large proportion of hypertensive patients who have additional risk factors for premature cardiovascular disease, such as dyslipidemia or diabetes. Cigarette smoking, although unrelated to hypertension, is a major risk factor for CVD, and avoidance of tobacco is essential.

If blood pressure remains at or above 140/90 mm Hg after 3 to 6 months, in patients with stage I and II hypertension, despite encouragement of life-style modifications, antihypertensive medications should be initiated.[8] Progression to pharmacologic therapy is particularly important in individuals with target-organ damage and/or other known cardiovascular risk factors.[76,77]

In the absence of target-organ damage, and other major risk factors, some clinicians may elect to continue life-style modifications and carefully monitor blood pressure for patients with stage I hypertension. If this course is selected, careful and frequent follow-up is critical since clinical trial data suggest that antihypertensive drug therapy is best initiated before the development of target-organ damage.

Initial therapy for stage I and stage II hypertension should be started with a single drug (monotherapy). Because diuretics and β-blockers have been shown to reduce cardiovascular morbidity and mortality in controlled clinical trials, these two classes of agents may be preferred for initial drug therapy if there are no contraindications to their administration in the individual patient, and in the absence of any special indications for initiating therapy with an alternative agent. The alternative drugs: calcium antagonists, ACE inhibitors, α_1-receptor blockers, and the α-β–blocker (labetalol) are equally effective in reducing blood pressure but unfortunately have not been used in long-term, controlled clinical trials to demonstrate their efficacy in reducing morbidity and mortality. There is indeed an urgent need to evaluate the effectiveness of these several classes of agents in reducing long-term cardiovascular morbidity and mortality.

The reappraisal of diuretics and β-blockers should not suggest that all patients should be started on one of these two classes of agents. As noted, individual patients may have relative contraindications to the use of a specific drug, and further there may be special indications for selecting a drug in any available class of agents.[8] Other factors must be considered in the selection of drugs including cost of medication, metabolic and/or subjective side effects, potential drug-drug interactions, and the presence of other concomitant illnesses that may be benefitted or aggravated by the selection of a given agent for initial therapy.

Figure 10-1 provides a simple treatment algorithm, as recommended by JNC-V. If after 1 to 3 months, response to initial therapy is inadequate, the patient is not experiencing significant side effects and adherence to therapy is adequate, several options for subsequent therapy should be considered: (1) increase the dose of the first dose to or toward maximum levels; (2) substitute an agent from another class; (3) add a second drug from another class.

Combining antihypertensive drugs with different modes of action will often allow smaller doses of drugs to be used to achieve control and minimize the potential for dose-dependent side effects. If a diuretic is not selected as the first drug, it will often be useful as a second-step agent because its addition usually enhances the effects of other agents. If addition of a second agent produces satisfactory blood pressure control, an attempt to withdraw the first agent may be considered, because monotherapy with virtually all agents provides blood pressure control for at least half of all patients.

For patients with stage III and IV hypertension, it may be necessary to add a second or third agent after a short interval if no control is achieved. In some patients it may be necessary to initiate treatment with more than one agent. Patients with average diastolic blood pressures of 120 mm Hg or greater require more immediate therapy, and if significant target-organ damage is present, may require hospitalization for further evaluation and aggressive treatment.

A Reasoned Approach to Treatment

As one reads or listens to the continuing debate regarding individualized step care versus tailored care, or discussions in defense of traditional versus alternative therapy, clinicians become aware that the differences expressed appear more semantic than real. In fact, educators in hypertension must bear the risk of providing a disservice for primary physicians by suggesting that these approaches to treatment really differ. The simple treatment algorithm provided in JNC-V was designed to provide the physician with a rational and practical stepwise guideline to the patient with hypertension. This treatment algorithm should in no way limit the clinician's versatility in selecting initial and subsequent agents based not only on special indications for a given drug but also on the basis of concomitant illnesses and/or conditions, adverse effects, and/or prior medication experiences with the patient and a given class of drugs. JNC-V exhaustively reviewed potential limitations for individual classes based on drug interactions, adverse effects, and/or special cautions to be considered. With this information base, each clinician should be able to make a selection based on appropriate information available regarding the patient and learned experience with each and every available antihypertensive agent.

There is sufficient evidence from comparative clinical trials to suggest that all of the currently available classes of antihypertensive agents are efficacious and will effect blood pressure control in about half of patients with stage I or II hypertension treated with initial therapy.[76-78] It is interesting that two drugs in combination, as long as they are not two drugs in the same class, will control blood pressure in 85% to 90% with stage I or II hypertension. Recognizing that we can control the vast number of patients with hypertension with available therapy, the issues come down to understanding the clinical pharmacology of individual agents to take advantage of selected clinical parameters that should enable skillful individualization or tailoring of treatment to the hypertensive patient.

Cost of Care

As we view cost-effectiveness, it is true that older agents are inexpensive by today's standards, which can be a major factor in a patient's long-term adherence to therapy. On the other hand, newer classes of agents have favorable adverse effect profiles, and may in fact provide a better

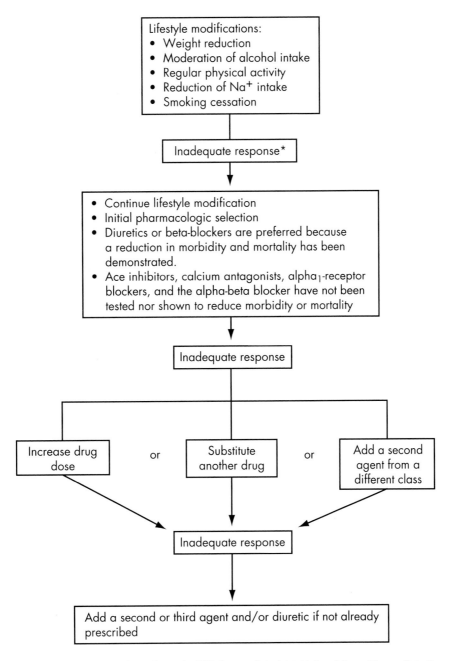

Fig. 10-1. Treatment algorithm. *(From the Fifth Report of the Joint National Committee on Detection, Evaluation and Treatment of High Blood Pressure [JNC-V], Arch Intern Med 153:154, 1993.)*

quality of life than that observed on some older therapies. The quality-of-life issue also represents an important factor from the standpoint of long-term adherence to therapy. The bottom line regarding cost-effectiveness is clearly the ability to maintain optimal adherence and ensure long-term control of blood pressure, to minimize morbid events and the extraordinary costs associated with these events.

It must be remembered that long-term therapy of hypertension represents a significant component of the nation's financial commitment to health.[79] Drug costs can amount to 70% to 80% of the total expenditure for treating hypertension. Thus for individual as well as societal reasons, minimizing costs must be an essential component of

the health care provider's responsibility. Keep in mind that the determination of cost in the care of the hypertensive patient includes not only the initial evaluation but also follow-up visits, drug costs, and confirmation strategies undertaken in the course of a patient's management.

When to Refer the Hypertensive Patient

Each physician's comfort level in managing the hypertensive patient will differ depending on individual training, areas of clinical interest, and expertise. Recommendations regarding detection and initial evaluation of hypertensive patients are applicable to most clinical practices regardless of the specialty interest of the physician.

Clinical situations that may warrant referral include but are not necessarily limited to the following:

1. *Initial evaluation provides clinical clues or findings consistent with a secondary form of hypertension.* How much of the evaluation will or should be done by the patient's primary physician (or case manager) will be determined by the individual physician's training, expertise, and clinical interest. Appropriate differential studies may be obtained before referral and/or the patient may be referred for completion of further studies. Clinical clues that should suggest the possibility of the more common secondary forms of hypertension have been reviewed earlier in this chapter.

2. *Intolerance to antihypertensive medications.* This intolerance may occur for a number of reasons. Intolerance may be due to the development of a side effect to a specific medication or through a drug-drug interaction with other medications in the patient's treatment regimen. Adverse effects may be associated with specific medications in the presence of other associated disease conditions in the hypertensive patient or may be due to the development of adverse effects associated with the metabolism or the excretion of the medication.

   Numerous drug-drug interactions have been reported, although not necessarily documented as to cause and effect, and have been cataloged in selected publications.[8,30]

3. *The patient with resistant hypertension.* Hypertension should be considered resistant if blood pressure in an adherent patient cannot be reduced to less than 140/90 mm Hg by an adequate and appropriate triple-drug regimen prescribed in near maximal doses, when the pretreatment blood pressure was less than 180/115 mm Hg. For patients with initial blood pressures greater than 180/115 mm Hg, resistance can be defined as blood pressure that cannot be controlled below 160/100 mm Hg with an appropriate three-drug regimen. It is also suggested that an adequate and appropriate regimen should include at least three different pharmacologic agents including a diuretic.[80,81] An algorithm for the evaluation of patients with possible resistant hypertension is included (Fig. 10-2).

4. *Hypertension in special populations and situations.* Finally, physicians may prefer to refer patients in special situations where the disease may be considered outside of their field of expertise. There are many hypertensives who have other significant concomitant illnesses that may serve as relative or absolute contraindications to the use of selected antihypertensive agents. Referral to a physician who is expert in hypertension and especially in the clinical pharmacology of the antihypertensive agents may be considered appropriate. Many physicians are not comfortable in managing hypertension during pregnancy and would prefer to leave treatment decisions to the patient's obstetrician. Particular challenges to the management of hypertension

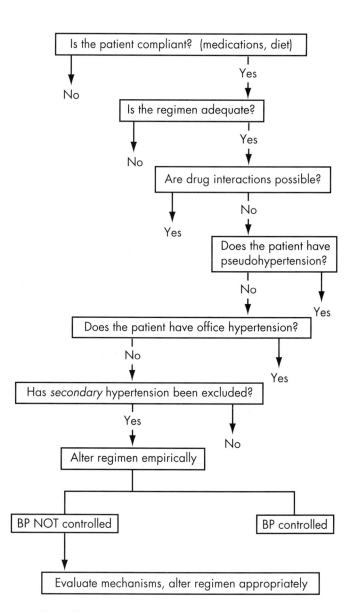

Fig. 10-2. Algorithm for the management of resistant hypertension.

are presented in patients with concomitant cerebrovascular disease or peripheral vascular insufficiency, progressive renal insufficiency, coronary artery disease, or congestive heart failure. Diabetic patients with advanced nephropathy may be better managed by a nephrologist in view of dosing limitations and potential adverse effects associated with therapy. Each physician's comfort level will determine how much of the evaluation and/or management of the hypertensive patient will be accomplished.

HYPERTENSIVE URGENCIES AND EMERGENCIES

Most hypertensive urgencies and emergencies arise as a result of poorly controlled chronic hypertension from primary or secondary causes. Increased awareness, widespread detection efforts, and more aggressive therapy of

Table 10-4. Drugs for the Management of Hypertensive Emergencies and Urgencies

Preparation	Dose	Reaction Time	Cautions
Vasodilators			
Sodium nitroprusside	0.3-10 µg/kg/min as IV infusion	Instantaneous	Nausea, vomiting, muscle twitching, thiocyanate intoxication, methemoglobinemia
Nitroglycerin	5-100 µg/min as IV infusion	2-5 min	Headache, tachycardia, vomiting, flushing, methemoglobinemia
Diazoxide	50-150 mg IV bolus, repeated, or 15-30 mg/min by IV infusion	1-2 min	Hypotension, tachycardia, aggravation of angina pectoris, hyperglycemia with repeated injections
Nifedipine	10-20 mg PO or SL (perforated capsules), repeat after 30 minutes	15-30 min	Rapid, uncontrolled reduction in blood pressure may precipitate congestive heart failure in patients with aortic stenosis
Nicardipine	10-15 mg/hr by IV infusion	5-15 min	Hypotension, tachycardia, nausea, and vomiting
Verapamil	5-10 mg IV bolus, or 3-25 mg/hr by IV infusion	1-5 min	Avoid in patients with cardiac conduction abnormalities, adverse interaction with other negative inotropes
Enalaprilat	0.625-1.25 mg q6h IV	15-60 min	Renal failure in patients with bilateral renal artery stenosis
Captopril	25-50 mg PO or SL, repeat as required	15-30 min	Hypotension, renal failure in bilateral renal artery stenosis, hypotension
Adrenergic Inhibitors			
Phentolamine	5-15 mg IV	1-2 min	Reflex tachycardia, occasional arrhythmias, abdominal cramping
Trimethaphan camsylate	1-4 mg/min as IV infusion	1-5 min	Paresis of bowel and bladder, orthostatic hypotension, blurred vision, dry mouth
Labetalol	20-80 mg IV bolus every 10 min; 2 mg/min IV infusion; 200-400 mg PO, repeat q2-3h	5-10 min 30 min-2 hr	Bronchoconstriction, heart block, orthostatic hypotension
Methyldopa HCl	250-500 mg IV infusion q6h	30-60 min	Drowsiness
Esmolol	500 µg/kg/bolus injection IV or 25-200 µg/kg/min by infusion	1-5 min	Avoid in patients with heart block, congestive heart failure, uncontrolled asthma
Clonidine	0.1-0.2 mg PO or SL, repeated qh as required	30-60 min	Hypotension, drowsiness, dry mouth

IV, Intravenous; *PO,* by mouth; *SL,* sublingual.
(Modified from the 1993 Fifth Report of the Joint National Committee on Detection, Evaluation and Treatment of High Blood Pressure (JNC-V), Arch Intern Med 153:154, 1993.)

mild and moderate hypertension have contributed to a progressive decline in the incidence of hypertensive urgencies and emergencies. A distinction between a hypertensive urgency and a true emergency can be helpful in determining the required expediency for therapy as well as the selection and route of administration of appropriate drugs.[82,83] A true hypertensive emergency represents a life-threatening condition in which blood pressure should be lowered to a safer level within minutes to 1 hour. Hypertensive urgencies are those situations in which the immediate risk to the integrity of the cardiovascular system is less, but prompt institution of drug therapy (usually oral) and reduction of blood pressure over several hours to 24 hours will be appropriate. Several agents have been successfully used by repeated administration or "loading dosages" to induce progressive but controlled reduction of blood pressure in hypertensive urgencies. These agents include clonidine, minoxidil, nifedipine, captopril, and more recently, labetalol. The rapid onset of effect, within 15 to 30 minutes, following administration of nifedipine has led to its becoming the most popular agent in this group.

Agents currently available for treatment of the hypertensive emergency or urgency are listed in Table 10-4. These agents generally fall into two classes, direct vasodilating drugs and those agents that act through inhibition at various sites in the sympathetic nervous system.

In managing the hypertensive emergency or urgency, prompt initiation of therapy should take precedence over time-consuming diagnostic procedures. The agent selected, and the method of administration, should enable a controlled reduction of blood pressure to a safer level, usually a diastolic pressure of 100 to 110 mm Hg. Additional diagnostic studies, if considered necessary, can be undertaken after blood pressure has been safely controlled. A thorough knowledge of the pharmacologic properties and proper indications of the currently available agents is essential for optimal management.

REFERENCES

1. Cornoni-Huntley J, LaCroix AZ, and Havlik RJ: Race and sex differentials in the impact of hypertension in the United States: the National Health and Nutrition Examination Survey I epidemiologic follow-up study, Arch Intern Med 149:780, 1989.
2. Ibrahim M et al: Hypertension prevalence and the status of awareness, treatment, and control in the United States: final report of the Subcommittee on Definition and Prevalence of the 1984 Joint National Committee, Hypertension 7:457, 1985.
3. Kannel WB: Role of blood pressure in cardiovascular morbidity and mortality, Prog Cardiovasc Dis 17:5, 1974.
4. Page IH: The mosaic theory. In Page IH: Hypertension mechanisms, New York, 1987, Grune & Stratton.
5. Eggers PW, Connerton R, and McMullan M: The Medicare experience with end-stage renal disease trends in incidence, prevalence, and survival, Health Care Financ Rev 5:69, 1984.
6. Hostetter TH, Rennke HG, and Brenner BM: The case of intrarenal hypertension in the initiation and progression of diabetic and other glomerulopathies, Am J Med 72:375, 1982.
7. Lindeman RD, Tobin JD, and Shock NW: Association between blood pressure and the rate of decline in renal function, Kidney Int 26:861, 1984.
8. The fifth report of the Joint National Committee on Detection, Evaluation, and Treatment of High Blood Pressure (JNC-V), Arch Intern Med 153:154, 1993.
9. Stamler J, Neaton JD, and Wentworth DN: Blood pressure (systolic and diastolic) and the risk of fatal coronary heart disease, Hypertension 13(suppl I):I-2, 1989.
10. Neaton JD and Wentworth D: Serum cholesterol, blood pressure, cigarette smoking and death from coronary heart disease, Arch Intern Med 152:56, 1992.
11. Frohlich ED et al: Recommendations for human blood pressure determination by sphygmomanometers: report of a special task force appointed by the Steering Committee, American Heart Association, Hypertension 11:209A, 1988.
12. Kaplan NM: Treatment of hypertension: nondrug therapy and the rationale for drug therapy. In Kaplan NM: Clinical hypertension, ed 4, Baltimore, 1986, Williams & Wilkins.
13. Nonpharmacologic approaches to the control of high blood pressure: final report of the Subcommittee on Non-Pharmacologic Therapy of the Joint National Committee on Detection, Evaluation, and Treatment of High Blood Pressure, Hypertension 8:444, 1986.
14. Erwteman TM et al: β blockade, diuretics, and salt restriction for the management of mild hypertension: a randomised double blind trial, Br Med J 289:406, 1984.
15. Kaplan NM et al: Potassium supplementation in hypertensive patients with diuretic-induced hypokalemia, N Engl J Med 312:746, 1985.
16. McCarron DA: Calcium, magnesium, and phosphorus balance in human and experimental hypertension, Hypertension 4(suppl III):III-27, 1982.
17. Resnick LM, Nicholson JP, and Laragh JH: Outpatient therapy of essential hypertension with dietary calcium supplementation, J Am Coll Cardiol 3:616, 1984 (abstract).
18. Resnick LM, Gupta RK, and Laragh JH: Intracellular free magnesium in erythrocytes of essential hypertension: relation to blood pressure and serum divalent cations, Proc Natl Acad Sci USA 81:6511, 1984.
19. Aristimuno GG et al: Influence of persistent obesity in children on cardiovascular risk factors: the Bogalusa heart study, Circulation 69:895, 1984.
20. Barrett-Connor E and Khaw KT: Is hypertension more benign when associated with obesity? Circulation 72:53, 1985.
21. Haffner SM et al: Do upper body and centralized adiposity measure different aspects of regional body fat distribution? Relationship to non-insulin-dependent diabetes mellitus, lipids, and lipoproteins, Diabetes 36:43, 1987.
22. Donahue RP et al: Central obesity and coronary heart disease in men, Lancet 1:821, 1987.
23. MacMahon SW and Norton RN: Alcohol and hypertension: implications for prevention and treatment, Ann Intern Med 105:124, 1986.
24. Dawber TR: The Framingham Study: the epidemiology of atherosclerotic disease, Cambridge, Mass, 1980, Harvard University Press.
25. Kaplan NM: Therapy for mild hypertension: toward a more balanced view, JAMA 249:365, 1983.
26. Blair SN et al: Physical fitness and all-cause mortality: a prospective study of healthy men and women, JAMA 262:2395, 1989.
27. Intersalt Cooperative Research Group: Intersalt: an international study of electrolyte excretion and blood pressure, results of 24 hours urinary sodium and potassium excretion, Br Med J 297:319, 1988.
28. Intersalt Cooperative Research Group: Sodium, potassium, body mass, alcohol and blood pressure: the Intersalt Study, J Hypertens 6(suppl 4):S594, 1988.
29. Working Group report on Primary Prevention of Hypertension, Arch Intern Med 153:186, 1993.
30. AMA Drug Evaluations, ed 5, Chicago, 1983, American Medical Association.
31. McMahon FG: In management of essential hypertension: the new low dose therapy, ed 2, Mount Kisco, NY, 1984, Futura Publishing Co.
32. Vidt DG: Antihypertensive agents. In Wang RIH, ed: Practical drug therapy, Milwaukee, 1987, Medstream Press.
33. Collins R et al: Blood pressure, stroke and coronary heart disease; Part 2. Short term reductions in blood pressure: overview of randomized drug trials in the epidemiologic context, Lancet 335:827, 1990.
34. MacMahon S et al: Blood pressure, stroke and coronary heart disease; Part 1. Prolonged observational studies corrected for the regression dilution bias, Lancet 335:765, 1990.

35. Systolic Hypertension in the Elderly Cooperative Research Group: Prevention of stroke by antihypertensive drug treatment in older persons with isolated systolic hypertension, JAMA 265:3255, 1991.
36. Holland OB, Nixon JV, and Kuhnert L: Diuretic-induced ventricular ectopic activity, Am J Med 70:762, 1981.
37. Hollifield JW and Slaton PE: Thiazide diuretics, hypokalemia, and cardiac arrhythmias, Acta Med Scand Suppl 647:67, 1981.
38. Houston MC: The effects of antihypertensive drugs on glucose intolerance in hypertensive nondiabetics and diabetics, Am Heart J 115:640, 1988.
39. Ames R: Effects of diuretic drugs on the lipid profile, Drugs 36(suppl 2):33, 1988.
40. Weidmann P and Gerber A: Effects of treatment with diuretics on serum lipoproteins, J Cardiovasc Pharmacol 6:S260, 1984.
41. Kaplan NM: Importance of coronary heart disease risk factors in the management of hypertension: an overview, Am J Med 86(suppl 1B):1, 1989.
42. Friedel HA and Buckley MM: Torsemide. A review of its pharmacological properties and therapeutic potential (review), Drugs 41:81, 1991.
43. Rudy DW et al: The pharmacodynamics of intravenous and oral torsemide in patients with chronic renal insufficiency, Clin Pharmcol Ther 56:29, 1994.
44. Pollare T et al: Sensitivity to insulin during treatment with atenolol and metoprolol: a randomised, double blind study of effects on carbohydrate and lipoprotein metabolism in hypertensive patients, Br Med J 298:1152, 1989.
45. Chait A: Effects of antihypertensive agents on serum lipids and lipoproteins, Am J Med 86(suppl 1B):5, 1989.
46. Dal Palu C et al: Intravenous labetalol in severe hypertension, Br J Clin Pharmacol 13(suppl 1):978, 1982.
47. Vidt DG: Intravenous labetalol in the emergency treatment of hypertension, J Clin Hypertens 2:179, 1985.
48. Chen S and Vidt DG: Patient acceptance of transdermal clonidine: a retrospective review of 25 patients, Cleve Clin J Med 56:21, 1989.
49. Kirby RS et al: Prazosin in the treatment of prostate obstruction: a placebo controlled study, Br J Urol 60:136, 1987.
50. Koch-Weser J: Hydralazine, N Engl J Med 295:320, 1976.
51. Perry HM Jr: Late toxicity to hydralazine resembling systemic lupus erythematosus or rheumatoid arthritis, Am J Med 54:58, 1973.
52. Miller WE et al: Management of severe hypertension with intravenous injections of diazoxide, Am J Cardiol 24:870, 1969.
53. Wilson DJ, Lewis RC, and Vidt DG: Control of severe hypertension with pulse diazoxide. In Vidt DG, ed: Cardiovascular Clinics, Philadelphia, 1982, FA Davis Co.
54. Cohn JN and Burke LP: Nitroprusside, Ann Intern Med 91:752, 1979.
55. Vesey CJ, Cole PV, and Simpson PJ: Cyanide and thiocyanate concentrations following sodium nitroprusside infusion in man, Br J Anaesth 48:651, 1976.
56. Cottrell JE and Turndorf H: Intravenous nitroglycerin, Am Heart J 96:550, 1978.
57. Flaherty JT et al: Comparison of intravenous nitroglycerin and sodium nitroprusside for treatment of acute hypertension after coronary artery bypass surgery, Circulation 65:1072, 1982.
58. Frohlich ED: Angiotensin converting enzyme inhibitors, Hypertension 13(suppl I):I-125, 1989.
59. Williams GH: Converting-enzyme inhibitors in the treatment of hypertension, N Engl J Med 319:1517, 1988.
60. Lewis EJ et al: The effect of angiotensin-converting-enzyme inhibition on diabetic nephropathy, New Engl J Med 329:1456, 1993.
61. The SOLVD Investigators: Effect of enalapril on survival in patients with reduced left ventricular ejection fractions and congestive heart failure, New Engl J Med 325:293, 1991.
62. Pfeffer MD et al: Effect of enalapril on mortality and morbidity in patients with left ventricular dysfunction after myocardial infarction. Results of the survival and ventricular enlargement trial, New Engl J Med 327:669, 1992.
63. Hricik DE et al: Captopril-induced functional renal insufficiency in patients with bilateral renal artery stenosis or renal artery stenosis in a solitary kidney, N Engl J Med 303:373, 1983.
64. Vidt DG et al: Atheroembolic renal disease: association with renal arterial stenosis, Cleve Clin J Med 56:407, 1988.
65. Coulter DM and Edwards IR: Cough associated with captopril and enalapril, Br Med J 294:1521, 1987.
66. Hood S, Nichollas MG, and Gilchrist NL: Cough with angiotensin converting enzyme inhibitors, N Z Med J 100:6, 1987.
67. Martinez EJ and Seleznick MJ: Respiratory tract side effects of angiotensin converting enzyme inhibitors: current knowledge, Southern Med J 84:1343, 1991.
68. Braunwald E: Mechanism of action of calcium-channel-blocking agents, N Engl J Med 307:1618, 1982.
69. Kates RE: Calcium antagonists: pharmacokinetic properties, Drugs 25:113, 1983.
70. Bertel O et al: Nifedipine in hypertensive emergencies, Br Med J 286:19, 1983.
71. IV Nicardipine Study Group: Efficacy and safety of intravenous nicardipine in the control of post operative hypertension, Chest 99:393, 1991.
72. Clifton GG and Wallin JD: Intravenous nicardipine: an effective new agent for the treatment of severe hypertension, Angiology 41:1005, 1990.
73. Kaplan NM: Calcium entry blockers in the treatment of hypertension: current status and future prospects, JAMA 262:817, 1989.
74. MacMahon SW et al: The effects of drug treatment for hypertension on morbidity and mortality from cardiovascular disease: a review of randomized controlled trials, Prog Cardiovasc Dis 24(suppl 1):99, 1986.
75. Strasser T and Genten D, eds: Mild hypertension: from drug trials to practice, New York, 1987, Raven Press.
76. Alderman MH: Mild hypertension: new light on an old clinical controversy, Am J Med 69:653, 1980.
77. Swales JD et al: Treating mild hypertension: agreement from the large trials. Report of the British Hypertension Society working party, Br Med J 298:694, 1989.
78. Reid JL: First-line and combination treatment for hypertension, Am J Med 86(suppl 4A):2, 1989.
79. Shulman NB et al: Financial cost as an obstacle to hypertension therapy, Am J Public Health 76:1105, 1986.
80. Gifford RW Jr and Tarazi RC: Resistant hypertension: diagnosis and management, Ann Intern Med 88:661, 1978.
81. Vidt DG: The patient with resistant hypertension: cations, volume and renal factors, Hypertension 11(suppl II):II-76, 1988.
82. Garcia JY and Vidt DG: Current management of hypertensive emergencies, Drugs 34:263, 1987.
83. Vidt DG and Gifford RW Jr: A compendium of the treatment of hypertensive emergencies, Cleve Clin Q 51:421, 1984.

CHAPTER ELEVEN

ATHEROSCLEROSIS OF THE AORTA AND LOWER-EXTREMITY ARTERIES

Leonard P. Krajewski
Jeffrey W. Olin

HISTORICAL PERSPECTIVES

Arteriosclerosis obliterans (ASO) affecting the lower extremities may involve the abdominal aorta and/or its major branches to both lower extremities. Atherosclerosis of the lower extremities occurs in various "patterns of disease."[1] These patterns may affect local segments of the arterial anatomy, or they may occur in combinations of multiple segments.[2] Recognition of the pattern of disease is extremely useful for a plan of management, whether that involves medical treatment, endovascular therapy, or surgical reconstruction. The modern era of direct arterial repair of lower-extremity occlusive vascular disease began in the early 1950s. The pioneering experiments in 1906 by Carrel and Guthrie[3,4] using vascular suture demonstrated that direct arterial reconstruction was technically feasible. During the first half of this century the techniques of arteriography, blood transfusion, anesthetic management, anticoagulation, and antibiotics were developed and led to the ability to perform successful vascular reconstruction.[5] Before the early 1950s arterial grafting with venous replacements was occasionally reported. However, it was not until 1949 that Kunlin[6] reported a successful femoropopliteal bypass using reversed greater saphenous vein. In 1950 Oudot[7] replaced the aortoiliac bifurcation with an arterial homograft.

These two landmark reports initiated a new era of arterial reconstruction for lower-extremity occlusive disease. Before this time lumbar sympathectomy and arteriectomy, as advocated by Leriche, were the only other recognized methods of surgical treatment. The technique of thromboendarterectomy had been introduced in 1947 when Jao Cid Dos Santos and his father Reynaldo[8] extended their interest in arterial embolectomy to perform "desobliteration" of the iliofemoral and subclavian-axillary segments. Endarterectomy was soon extended to the abdominal aorta and other peripheral arteries.[9] In the early 1950s the techniques of endarterectomy and vein bypass caught on rapidly and were used at a number of medical centers in the United States. Within a few years fabric prostheses were created and used successfully as arterial replacements.[10] Extensive endarterectomy gradually fell into disfavor compared with either venous bypass grafts for femoropopliteal disease or dacron prostheses for aortoiliac-femoral reconstructions. During the 1950s and into the 1960s most lower-extremity bypass reconstructions were performed to the above-knee popliteal artery and less commonly to the below-knee popliteal artery. A few reports of bypasses to tibial vessels were published in the early-to-mid 1960s, but it was not until the 1970s that larger series with acceptable results were reported.[11-13]

Interest in the use of the saphenous vein in a "non-reversed" position for lower-extremity bypass reconstruction spread gradually.[14] However, this method proved to be very tedious and time-consuming because of the difficulty of reliable valve disruption. After Leather, Powers, and Karmody[15] reintroduced the "in situ" method for saphenous vein bypass in 1979, widespread interest in more distal tibial bypass occurred. In the United States Leather et al developed new techniques and instrumentation that made valve disruption easier and more reproducible. Since then, the in situ method has become the preferred technique for infrapopliteal bypass by many surgeons when the ipsilateral saphenous vein is available, whereas prosthetic replacement grafts remain the preferred method for aortoiliac-femoral reconstructions.

INCIDENCE AND PREVALENCE

Data from the Framingham Study[16] have reported an annual age-adjusted incidence of intermittent claudication of 0.3% in men and 0.1% in women. McDaniel and Cronenwett[17] reviewed available literature and determined that approximately 1.8% of patients under 60 years of age, 3.7% of those 60 to 70 years, and 5.2% over 70 years had intermittent claudication. The Framingham Study examined 1813 men and 2504 women with 34-year follow-up data and demonstrated that if diabetes mellitus was present, the incidence of claudication was increased twofold to threefold.[18] This study also showed that in those who developed diabetes and intermittent claudication there was an especially high risk of associated cardiovascular events. In patients under 40 years old, aortoiliac occlusive disease is the most common site of atherosclerosis, whereas in those over 40, femoropopliteal disease accounts for 65% of the patients with claudication.[17] When lower-extremity atherosclerosis does become symptomatic in patients under 50 years old, it generally follows a particularly virulent course.[19] Virtually all patients are heavy cigarette smokers, and the ratio of men to women is approximately equal.

The incidence of asymptomatic arterial disease is much higher than the numbers just cited.[20,21] Data from the Systolic Hypertension in the Elderly Study[20] showed that the ankle/brachial [systolic blood pressure] index (ABI) was 0.9 or less in 25.5% of the 1537 participants. In an ancillary study to the Multicenter Study of Osteoporotic Fractures,[21] the ABI was 0.9 or less in 5.5% of 1492 women entered into this study. As is discussed later, a decreased ABI directly correlates with increased cardiovascular mortality.

RISK FACTORS AND ATHEROSCLEROSIS

The etiology and pathogenesis of atherosclerosis is a subject of intense research (see Chapter 8). The cellular and biochemical events leading to the development of an atherosclerotic plaque are probably similar whether the plaque occurs in the coronary arteries or in the peripheral arterial circulation.

Traditional risk factors such as age and sex, presence of hypertension, diabetes, elevated total and low-density lipoprotein (LDL) cholesterol, decreased high-density lipoprotein (HDL) cholesterol, elevated plasma triglycerides, smoking, obesity, sedentary life-style, family history of vascular disease, and genetic factors are as important in patients with peripheral atherosclerosis as in those with coronary disease. More recently recognized risk factors such as increased levels of lipoprotein(a), increased plasma homocysteine, elevated anticardiolipin antibodies, and altered platelet function may also be important in the pathogenesis of atherosclerosis. These risk factors are discussed in detail in Chapters 8, 9, and 10.

Diabetes mellitus remains a particularly important risk factor in the development of lower-extremity ASO. The Framingham Study[18,22] demonstrated that any degree of impaired glucose tolerance was associated with an increased risk of ASO. Glycosuria increased the relative risk of ASO to 3.5% among men and 8.6% among women. In the Framingham Study[18] the 2-year incidence of intermittent claudication for nondiabetic men was 8.8 per 1000 compared with a rate of 22.9 per 1000 for diabetic men. The rate for nondiabetic women was 5.1 per 1000 compared with 17.3 per 1000 for diabetic women. These differences are highly statistically significant. If diabetes mellitus, impaired glucose tolerance, or glycosuria is present, the incidence of ASO is equal in men and women. The severity and extent of disease are often greater in individuals who have diabetes mellitus compared with those without diabetes. Patients with diabetes mellitus have a higher incidence of tibial peroneal disease, a similar incidence of femoropopliteal disease, and a lower incidence of aortoiliac disease than their nondiabetic counterparts.

In the Framingham Study[22] hypertension imposed a threefold increased risk of intermittent claudication during a follow-up of 26 years. No reports have been published on the effect of antihypertensive treatment on the course of clinically evident lower-extremity occlusive disease. Nevertheless, control of hypertension is considered an important factor in lowering overall cardiovascular risk.

In 1990 it was estimated that approximately 400,000 deaths (19% of total deaths) were directly attributable to tobacco use in the United States.[23] In 1990 46.3 million adults (25.7% of the population) were smokers.[24] Many investigators have suggested that smoking is the single most important risk factor for ASO of the aorta and lower-extremity arteries.[25-28] In the Framingham Study[22] cigarette smoking doubled the risk of lower-extremity ASO for both men and women. There was a dose-related response between the number of cigarettes smoked and the rate of intermittent claudication for all age groups.

Cigarette smoking is also strongly associated with advanced lower-extremity ASO in patients under 50 years of age. Jonason and Ringquist[29] found that in patients who quit smoking after they developed intermittent claudication, none progressed to rest pain. Sixteen percent of patients who continued to smoke developed rest pain. Patients who stopped smoking had fewer amputations, fewer myocardial infarctions, less rest pain, and lived twice as long as those who continued to smoke. Cigarette smoking is probably the most important factor related to the acceleration and progression of peripheral atherosclerotic arterial disease. In addition, smoking after vascular reconstructive surgery significantly decreases the patency rate of prosthetic bypass grafts and autologous saphenous vein bypass grafts.[30-32]

Although the risk of cardiac death from cigarette smoking seems to be related to the number of cigarettes smoked in a dose-response fashion, abstinence from smoking may reduce the risk of death from coronary artery disease by 50% after 2 years of cessation with a further reduction of risk to nonsmokers after 20 years of cessation.[33] Excluding patients with diabetes, nonsmokers comprise only 1% of all patients with intermittent claudication.[34] The risk of claudication is nine times greater for smokers than for nonsmokers.[35] There have been increasing reports suggesting that environmental tobacco smoke (passive smoking) is an important cause of ischemic heart disease and may also play a role in ASO of the lower extremities as well.[36] In addition, the Atherosclerosis Risk and Community Study[37] has demonstrated that patients exposed to environmental tobacco smoke had greater intima-media wall thickness on carotid ultrasound compared with those patients who were not exposed.

There are many mechanisms by which cigarette smoking causes atherosclerosis.[23] Perhaps one of the most important is that cigarette smoke directly damages the endothelium, causing structural damage and endothelial dysfunction. Smoking increases peripheral vascular resistance, platelet aggregation, plasma viscosity, carbon monoxide levels, fibrinogen levels, and thrombotic tendencies. Cigarette smoking directly stimulates the sympathetic nervous system, therefore increasing heart rate, blood pressure, stroke volume, and cardiac output.[28] There are marked regional disturbances in blood flow that have been demonstrated with cigarette smoking.

The habit of cigarette smoking has recently been accepted as a recognized medical disorder described as tobacco dependency disorder (TDD). It is defined by Pollin[38] as the "inability to discontinue smoking despite awareness of its medical consequences." It is difficult to persuade smokers who have ASO to give up their smoking habit. Physicians should strongly recommend the cessation of smoking to all of their patients, not only those with clinically significant vascular disease.

The role that lipids play in the progression and regression of peripheral arterial disease are discussed in detail in Chapter 9. It should also be mentioned that elevated levels of lipoprotein(a)[39] and elevated plasma homocysteine[40] may be important independent risk factors for the development of intermittent claudication and lower-extremity atherosclerosis.

The relation between hemostatic factors and atherosclerosis has recently been of interest. Thrombosis in a region of severe ASO is the final event that may precipitate more severe symptoms or signs such as ischemic rest pain, focal gangrene, or ischemic ulceration. Abnormalities of regulating proteins, circulating lupuslike anticoagulant, and altered platelet reactivity have been identified in patients with peripheral ASO.[41] When present, these blood coagulation abnormalities may lead to early failure of arterial

reconstruction. Hemorrheologic factors such as increases in blood viscosity, elevated hematocrit, and elevated fibrinogen levels may also influence the success of reconstruction.[42]

NATURAL HISTORY OF PERIPHERAL VASCULAR DISEASE

Limb-Related Complications

It is important to recognize that many patients with ASO of the lower extremities remain asymptomatic.[20,21] Patients who have disease to a single segment (i.e., superficial femoral artery) often have adequate collaterals, and their limb is not jeopardized.[43]

Most individuals require tandem lesions and/or multisegment disease to experience severe limb-threatening ischemia. Table 11-1 demonstrates the late incidence of amputation, severe ischemia, or operation in patients with lower-extremity claudication.

Virtually all studies involving large numbers of patients have shown that progression to severe ischemia or amputation is unusual in patients with intermittent claudication. Many studies support a rate of progression of approximately 1.4%/yr. Jonason and Ringqvist[46] have studied 224 nondiabetic patients and 47 diabetic patients and followed them over 6 years. Gangrene occurred in 31% of diabetics as opposed to only 5% of patients without diabetes ($P < 0.001$) and rest pain and/or gangrene occurred in 40% of patients with diabetes mellitus and only in 18% of those without ($P < 0.001$). These investigators[47] also evaluated the effects that smoking had on the eventual development of ischemic rest pain. In the 304 patients who continued to smoke, rest pain occurred in 16% of patients after 7 years of follow-up, whereas in the 39 patients who were able to stop smoking, none developed rest pain ($P < 0.05$). In a retrospective study, Cox et al[48] reported that in 377 patients (520 limbs) with superficial femoral artery disease, the risk for patients requiring surgery or endovascular treatment was 11% at 5 years and 14% at 10 years, again illustrating

Table 11-1. Late Incidence of Amputation, Severe Ischemia, and/or Operation in Patients with Lower-Extremity Claudication

Series	No.	Follow-up Years	Severe Ischemia and/or Operation		Amputation	
			No.	%	No.	%
Juergens et al[44] 1960	336	5	NA		10	3
Humphries et al[45] 1963	1552*	4 (mean)	356	23	105	7
Stable claudication	661*		171	26	53	8
Progressive claudication	891*		185	21	52	6
McDaniel and Cronenwett[17] 1989†						
History and physical examination	2469	7	NA	19	NA	7
Vascular laboratory and/or angiography	1624	5	NA	27	NA	4

(From Hertzer NR: The natural history of peripheral vascular disease. Implications for its management, Circulation 83 (suppl I):I-12, 1991.)
NA, data not available.
*Limbs.
†Collected series (weighted means).

that a conservative approach to the treatment of intermittent claudication is warranted in most patients.

Long-Term Survival

Intermittent claudication is a marker for atherosclerosis elsewhere. As previously mentioned, decreases in ABI correlate with long-term cardiovascular mortality.[20,21] Population-based studies and follow-up studies of surgically treated patients indicate that for those individuals with lower-extremity occlusive vascular disease, the mortality rate at 5 years is approximately 30%, at 10 years 50%, and at 15 years 70% to 75%.[49] An overall 10-year decline in life expectancy occurs in patients with lower-extremity ASO.[49] Hertzer et al[50] have demonstrated that in patients with intermittent claudication shown to have no or mild coronary artery disease, the 5-year survival was 85%. In those patients with advanced but compensated coronary artery disease, the 5-year survival was 64%. In patients with severe coronary artery disease undergoing coronary artery bypass grafting, the 5-year survival was approximately 72%. In patients with severe coronary artery disease not undergoing bypass and in patients with severe inoperable coronary artery disease, the estimated 5-year survival using life-table analysis was 43% and 22%, respectively.

Criqui et al[51] performed a population-based study of 565 men and women for the presence of large-vessel peripheral arterial disease and identified 67 subjects with disease who were followed prospectively over 10 years; 61.8% of men and 33.3% of women with peripheral arterial disease died during the 10-year follow-up compared with 16.9% of men and 11.6% of women without evidence of peripheral arterial disease. The relative risk of dying among subjects with peripheral arterial disease compared with those without was 3.1 for deaths from all causes, 5.9 for all deaths from cardiovascular disease, and 6.6 for deaths from coronary heart disease.

These data illustrate that there are really two important aspects in the treatment of patients with intermittent claudication. The first involves management of leg symptoms and the second involves long-term survival. Factors that affect the natural history of peripheral arterial disease are discussed in the section under Medical Treatment.

PATHOPHYSIOLOGY

The pathology of atherosclerosis is discussed in detail in Chapter 8. Atherosclerotic plaque tends to occur on the posterior aspect of the lower-extremity arteries. As the plaque develops, it may involve the artery circumferentially in certain areas. Atherosclerosis is most often present at the origin of arteries or at sites of arterial bifurcation. Other areas of local involvement include the common femoral artery, distal superficial femoral artery at Hunter's canal, and the tibial-peroneal trunk. The superficial femoral artery itself is often diffusely involved with occlusive disease (Fig. 11-1). As the obstructing plaque accumulates, thrombus may be deposited on the obstructing lesion as well as on the adjacent arterial wall. Eventually the obstructing plaque may become unstable and may rupture, causing intraplaque hemorrhage or thrombose, thereby completely obstructing the artery.[52] As atherosclerosis

progresses, segmental occlusion of the arterial supply to the lower extremities develops, and nutritive blood flow to the extremities is impaired. Tissues distal to the obstruction experience ischemia, although the degree of ischemia depends on the location and extent of the occlusive process and the development of collateral channels. The most common symptom is intermittent claudication of the calf, which is most often related to occlusion of the superficial femoral artery. This process usually is initiated at Hunter's canal and gradually extends to involve occlusion of the entire superficial femoral artery. Blood flow to distal tissues is usually maintained through collateral channels. In most cases the process is so gradual that collateral pathways develop that adequately maintain viability of more distal tissue. If occlusion occurs more abruptly (i.e., emboli), the onset of acute symptoms may be more dramatic.

The collateral pathways that often develop to maintain distal circulation include the lumbar aortic branches or

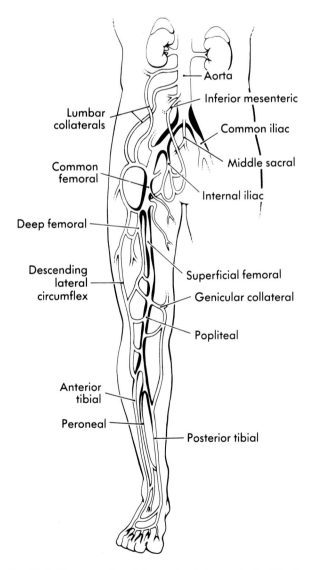

Fig. 11-1. Common sites of atherosclerosis *(shown in black)* in the aorta and lower extremities.

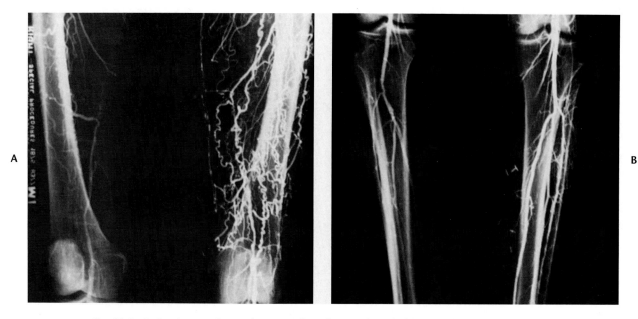

Fig. 11-2. A, Arteriogram shows adequate collateralization through the profunda femoris artery.
B, This artery supplies blood to the popliteal and tibioperoneal vessels where the superficial femoral
artery is occluded.

internal iliac system in relation to common iliac occlusion, the circumflex femoral vessels in relation to common femoral occlusion, and the profunda femoris system in relation to superficial femoral artery occlusion. The geniculate collaterals around the knee also perform a vital collateral function when occlusive disease more extensively involves both the superficial femoral and popliteal arteries (Fig. 11-1). The extent of development in these collateral beds may be quite dramatic when the occlusive process progresses slowly (Fig. 11-2). In fact, patients may be symptomatic only when walking long distances or when walking briskly.

The more severe manifestations of lower-extremity occlusive disease such as pain at rest, gangrene, or ischemic ulceration usually occur when the collateral pathways are inadequate to provide enough oxygen to maintain tissue viability. In these individuals the obstructive process usually involves multiple levels or compromise of the main trunk of the collateral bed. Collateral circulation in diabetic patients is often not as well developed as in nondiabetic patients. Occasionally, distal embolization or thrombosis in situ of the distal vascular bed may acutely compromise the viability of more distal ischemic tissues. Frequently some minor degree of external trauma will be an initiating factor for a more serious ischemic lesion. If arterial blood flow has been compromised sufficiently, even minor degrees of trauma may lead to the development of gangrene or ischemic ulceration.

CLINICAL MANIFESTATIONS

The symptoms of atherosclerotic occlusive disease of the lower extremities usually are of gradual onset. The individual may often be unaware of subtle symptoms. In fact, the extent of disease may be quite severe and involve multiple arterial segments before the patient becomes aware that a problem exists. Most often the symptoms are so insidious and gradual in their progress that they may be brought to medical attention only at a far advanced stage. Some evidence also suggests that milder symptoms may remain stable for many years. At times, however, acute occlusion (thrombosis in situ) superimposed on preexisting disease may make the problem acutely apparent.

Intermittent Claudication

The primary symptom of lower-extremity occlusive disease is intermittent claudication. Its onset is usually gradual and often unrecognized by many older adults who may attribute their symptoms to arthritis or simply to aging. Intermittent claudication is usually described as an aching sensation associated with walking. This discomfort occurs in a muscle group distal to an arterial obstruction. Most characteristically it occurs in the calf as a result of superficial femoral artery obstruction. The specific location of the obstruction is commonly at the adductor tendon (Hunter's canal) in the distal thigh. Intermittent claudication may also occur in the thigh, hip, and buttock if the obstruction involves the aortoiliac segment or internal iliac arteries. Intermittent claudication rarely may be felt in the foot alone. This most commonly occurs in patients with small-vessel occlusive disease such as thromboangiitis obliterans (Buerger's disease). If multilevel occlusive disease is present, the most distal muscle group is affected first, followed by more proximal muscle groups if the patient continues to walk. An exception to this general rule may occur in an individual who has mainly proximal occlusive disease that involves the common and internal iliac arteries. This individual may experience hip or buttock claudication only. The aching or cramplike sensation of intermittent claudication is progressive as the individual

Table 11-2. Differentiating True Claudication from Pseudoclaudication

	Intermittent Claudication	Pseudoclaudication
Character of discomfort	Cramping, tightness, tiredness	Same or tingling, weakness, clumsiness
Location of discomfort	Buttock, hip, thigh, calf, foot	Same
Exercise induced	Yes	Yes or no
Distance to claudication	Same each time	Variable
Occurs with standing	No	Yes
Relief	Stop walking	Often must sit or change body positions

exercises, but it diminishes rapidly with rest. Intermittent claudication is usually unilateral at its onset. It may appear as a bilateral symptom in those individuals who have occlusion of the distal abdominal aorta. More commonly, one leg is affected first, followed by the onset of similar symptoms in the opposite lower extremity.

Once intermittent claudication has been identified as a symptom of atherosclerotic occlusive disease, the patient may recognize that it has been present for years, in a lesser degree. If questioned carefully, the individual usually can identify the approximate time when the symptoms started. Most patients also can provide an accurate description of their walking distance before claudication occurs. The onset of symptoms usually occurs when the patient walks between one half and two city blocks at a normal pace on level ground. Walking up a grade or at increased speed brings on the discomfort more quickly. In most patients the symptoms are consistent and reproducible. In those who are poor observers, the treadmill exercise test is an excellent means of determining their functional disability. Some individuals describe the ability to "walk through" their symptoms. These individuals usually have a well-developed collateral circulation and will adjust their walking pace to compensate for the degree of arterial insufficiency. In addition, walking exercise will often result in "conditioning" of the affected muscle bed that permits the individual to walk demonstrably greater distances even though the segmental arterial pressures and pulse waveforms may not change appreciably on follow-up treadmill testing. True claudication must be differentiated from pseudoclaudication (neurogenic claudication) caused by lumbar canal stenosis or disk disease.[53,54] This differentiation can usually be made on the basis of the patient's history and physical examination (Table 11-2). Since many patients with pseudoclaudication have concomitant ASO, lower-extremity pulses may be diminished or absent. The patient's history is quite important in determining which disease is actually responsible for the symptoms. There are three major clinical features in patients with intermittent claudication.[45] Depending on variables such as the grade of the terrain and the pace of walking, intermittent claudication is reproducible with a consistent level of exercise from day to day. Second, it completely resolves within 2 to 3 minutes after exercise has been stopped unless the patient has walked to the point of severe leg pain in which an enormous amount of lactic acid has accumulated, and then it may take longer for the discomfort to go away. Last, discomfort occurs again at approximately the same distance once walking has been resumed.

Rest Pain

Progression to critical ischemia is evidenced by the onset of rest pain. Pain at rest characteristically occurs at night when the patient lies supine. Usually described as a dull aching sensation in the toes or forefoot, this sensation may awaken the patient from sleep. The patient may hang the foot over the side of the bed or get up and walk around for relief. As the symptom persists, the individual may start to sleep in a chair with the legs dependent. This often results in a moderate degree of lower-extremity edema. The affected foot usually demonstrates dependent rubor.[55] In patients who have rest pain, the degree of arterial insufficiency is severe and usually involves multiple arterial segments.

Ischemic Ulceration and Gangrene

If an individual is able to tolerate ischemic pain at rest, eventually ischemic necrosis between two toes ("kissing ulcer") may occur. Dry gangrene or ulcerations (Fig. 11-3) may also begin at the tips of the toes or over pressure points and is common after minor trauma such as nail trimming. By the time tissue necrosis occurs, the individual's ability to walk is usually severely limited.

Ischemic Neuropathy

If ischemia is severe and long-standing, an individual may develop pain along the distribution of a peripheral sensory nerve. This pain, referred to as *ischemic monomelic neuropathy*,[56] may occur in the absence of ulceration or gangrene and is often described as a sensation of numbness, deadness, or burning. Ischemic neuropathy may occur after acute arterial thrombosis and subsequent revascularization, particularly if the ischemia has been quite prolonged. This type of pain is very difficult to treat and may persist indefinitely in some individuals.

Disuse Atrophy

Patients with severe arterial insufficiency who are sedentary and nonambulatory may experience considerable loss of muscle mass in the lower extremity and foot. Occasionally their complaint of pain in the limb is out of proportion to the findings on segmental blood pressure measurements. These individuals may experience pain on simple palpation of the calf or thigh muscles, and os-

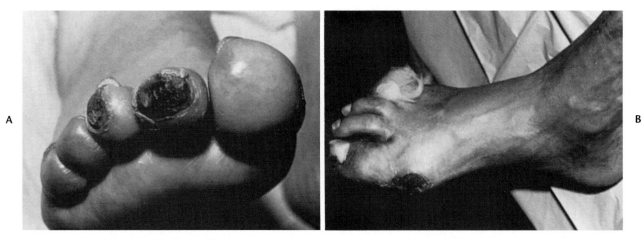

Fig. 11-3. Typical ischemic ulcer caused by arteriosclerosis obliterans. These ulcers occur distally **(A)** or over pressure points **(B)** where trauma is more likely. The base is dry and necrotic and does not contain healthy granulation tissue.

teoporosis may be demonstrated on plain x-ray films of the limb. This condition of disuse phenomenon, or reflex sympathetic dystrophy, is discussed in detail in Chapter 32. This condition may also cause problems for rehabilitation after lower-extremity arterial reconstruction. A supervised course of physical therapy may be needed to rehabilitate the postoperative patient when the disuse syndrome is present.

Other Sensory Disturbances

Many individuals with arterial insufficiency describe cold sensitivity of the feet, often stating that they have had cold feet for many years. Patients with diabetes mellitus may have a peripheral neuropathy in which they note burning or a sharp pain in the feet and toes. Some of the individuals may note the sensation of tightness and decreased mobility of the toes. These symptoms may occur even in the presence of adequate circulation. Diabetic patients with impaired sensation may develop traumatic ulceration over the plantar metatarsal heads, which are referred to as *neurotrophic ulcers* (see Chapter 40). Foot sepsis may occur if secondary infection supervenes. The infection may progress rapidly in the tissues, and the extent of infection may preclude salvage of an otherwise viable foot.

Muscular Weakness and Joint Stiffness

In situations of severe arterial insufficiency, muscle weakness inevitably occurs because of the limited degree of ambulation and associated atrophy. As previously noted, this condition may be associated with pain. Muscle pain may persist even after revascularization, and considerable rehabilitation may be required to restore muscle mass and normal function. In certain situations of acute and prolonged arterial insufficiency, entire muscle groups become infarcted following revascularization. This condition is most common in the anterior compartment syndrome. Urgent decompression of the swollen muscles (fasciotomy) is often necessary to preserve muscle viability.

Joint stiffness and flexion contractures at the hip and knee may occur as a result of chronic arterial insufficiency,

since many individuals will keep the hip and knee flexed in an effort to relieve pain. These contractures may be difficult to treat after successful revascularization or amputation. Physical therapy should be recommended to maintain joint mobility and muscle strength for individuals with severe arterial insufficiency.

PHYSICAL EXAMINATION

The combination of a careful history and physical examination should lead the experienced clinician to an accurate diagnosis of the anatomic location and severity of arterial occlusive disease. However, in patients with relatively mild occlusive disease, the physical diagnostic findings may be minimal. It is helpful to compare one lower extremity with the other, because one limb is usually affected more severely than the other. Simultaneous visual examination of both lower extremities will also allow the physician to evaluate the color and skin nutrition of both lower extremities. Physical findings such as gangrene, ulceration, edema, and atrophy will all be readily apparent. The skin should be examined for dryness and cracking. The distribution of hair growth is a poor indicator of arterial insufficiency since it may decrease normally with advancing age. When both legs and feet are examined and compared with each other, a temperature difference may often be evident. The limb with severely impaired circulation may feel cool, and often an obvious area of demarcation in temperature is present.

Palpation of the arterial pulses at the femoral, popliteal, posterior tibial, and dorsalis pedis areas is one of the most important clinical diagnostic maneuvers (see Chapter 2). A systematic approach should be used to examine the relative strength and quality of the arterial pulsation. Initial examination of the blood pressure in both upper extremities and the palpation of both radial pulses will generally provide a baseline evaluation for comparison with lower-extremity pulses. Lower-extremity pulsation should be compared in a stepwise fashion beginning with the femoral areas bilaterally. The popliteal, posterior tibial, and

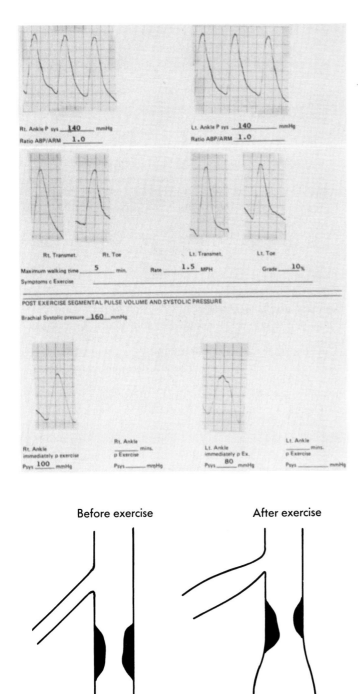

Fig. 11-4. Pulse-volume recordings and Doppler blood pressures were normal at rest. The ankle/arm blood pressure ratio was 1.0 bilaterally. The patient walked for 5 minutes on the treadmill and developed bilateral calf claudication. After excercise, the arm blood pressure increased to 160 mm Hg, and the ankle blood pressure decreased to 80 mm Hg on the left and to 100 mm Hg on the right, indicating the presence of underlying arterial occlusive disease.

Before exercise   **After exercise**

Fig. 11-5. At rest *(left)* there is an area of obstruction that is not severe enough to cause an abnormality in pressure distal to the obstruction. Therefore the pulses and blood pressure at rest are normal. Exercise increases the metabolic demand to the muscles. However, the obstruction only allows oxygen to be delivered at a fixed rate. In an attempt to compensate, more blood is shunted in the collateral vessels proximal to the obstruction. The vessels distal to the obstruction dilate so less blood is delivered to dilated segments of the distal vessels and the pressure decreases.

dorsalis pedis pulses of both limbs should be compared with each other, and both of these should be compared with the quality of the radial pulsation. The pulses should be graded as normal, diminished, or absent. Some individuals may have nonpalpable dorsalis pedis pulses with essentially normal lower-extremity arterial perfusion. This is most often the result of an anomaly of the below-knee arterial anatomy.[57] Patients with significant ASO may demonstrate pallor on elevation and rubor on dependency. Occasionally patients with typical complaints of intermittent claudication may have palpable pedal pulses at rest. A brief period of walking exercise and reexamination may be required to determine if the pulses disappear and if segmental blood pressure decreases with exercise (Figs. 11-4 and 11-5). A sensory examination is also very helpful. Diabetics particularly will demonstrate impaired sensation for vibration, pain, and light touch, even though they may not have severe arterial insufficiency. Also, individuals with ischemic neuropathy often have impaired sensation, and at times hyperesthesia is present.

LABORATORY STUDIES

During the past several decades the use of noninvasive methods of circulatory assessment has increased dramatically (see Chapter 3). Techniques range from simple measurement of the ankle/brachial index (ABI) to the use of magnetic resonance imaging (MRI) to measure arterial blood flow. Although the recording of ABI provides some information at the bedside, segmental Doppler systolic blood pressures and pulse waveform analysis by plethysmography provide more objective information about the level and severity of occlusive disease. Arteriography is the definitive examination when interventional or surgical treatment is being considered.

Doppler Ankle/Brachial Index

The simplest vascular laboratory test for lower extremity circulation is the ABI. The equipment is inexpensive and consists of an ordinary blood pressure cuff and a Doppler ultrasonic velocity detector. The blood pressure cuff is placed over both brachial areas and inflated above systolic pressure. Resumption of blood flow is detected with the Doppler probe over the brachial artery. If there is a discrepancy in the readings of the two arms, the higher of the two arm systolic blood pressures is used. Next the blood pressure cuff is moved to the ankle and inflated above systolic blood pressure. The Doppler detector is then placed alternately over the posterior tibial artery at the ankle and the dorsalis pedis artery. The ABI is obtained by dividing the ankle systolic blood pressure by the brachial systolic pressure.

Under most circumstances the ABI correlates quite well with functional symptoms.[58] In a normal individual at rest, the index will range from 0.9 to 1.3. Patients with intermittent claudication will have an index that generally ranges from 0.35 to 0.9. Patients experiencing ischemic rest pain will usually have an index of less than 0.4. Ischemic ulceration or impending gangrene is usually found when the index is below 0.25.

The ABI can also be used to identify individuals who have relatively normal pulses at rest but who complain of typical claudication symptoms. These individuals should be exercised and the ankle systolic pressure index measured following exercise (Fig. 11-4). If there is no significant drop in the ankle systolic pressure index following exercise, the cause of the symptoms is something other than ASO. Measurement of ABI can also be used as a convenient means of observing patients who have had bypass reconstructions. The level of improvement following the reconstruction can be compared with future measurements during follow-up visits. This method of surveillance may detect functional deterioration of the bypass before limb-threatening occlusion occurs.

Some investigators believe that the absolute systolic pressures may also provide information about the expectation of healing.[59] However, in our opinion, the absolute ankle pressure may be erroneous especially in diabetics with calcified, noncompressible arteries. In this situation pulse waveform analysis is needed to accurately evaluate the circulation.

Segmental Pressures

Segmental pressures can be measured by placing blood pressure cuffs at the high thigh, calf, and ankle level to determine the level of occlusive disease. This examination is usually performed in combination with segmental volume plethysmography or analysis of Doppler-derived pulse waveforms. Vascular stress testing with walking exercise or reactive hyperemia produces increased arterial

blood flow in an extremity and can be used to unmask subcritical stenoses or marginally significant stenotic lesions. Treadmill exercise provides a functional evaluation of the patient's symptoms. Standard stress measurements are used, such as walking at 2.0 mph on a 12% grade for 5 minutes. The time of onset of symptoms is recorded as well as the maximum walking time. Postexercise ankle pressures and recovery at 2 minutes after exercise are recorded (Fig. 11-4). Several investigators[60,61] have suggested that a progressive treadmill test is more reproducible than a single-stage treadmill test. In the single-stage treadmill test there is a fixed speed (2.0 mph) and grade (12%). The patients walk until they get claudication that forces them to stop or for 5 minutes, whichever occurs first. In the progressive or graded treadmill test there is a fixed speed (2.0 mph) but the grade increases over time to produce an increased work load. Hiatt et al[60] have stated that progressive treadmill testing is the best objective method of determining improvement in exercise capacity in patients undergoing clinical trials using an exercise program and/or medication.

Segmental Volume Plethysmography

Pulse waveform analysis can be performed with a system that incorporates mercury strain gauges or the pneumoplethysmograph (pulse-volume recorder, Life Sciences, Inc., Greenwich, Conn.). We prefer the pulse-volume recorder (PVR) as the method of evaluation along with segmental pressure measurements and treadmill walking exercise. The PVR waveforms can be analyzed by qualitative analysis of the waveform profile or PVR category criteria. A combination of segmental limb pressure measurements and PVR waveform analysis has been accurate to the 97th percentile in predicting the level and extent of occlusive disease.[62]

Transcutaneous Oxygen Measurement

This technique assesses tissue metabolism as a function of perfusion and is therefore thought by many to yield a more accurate evaluation of the degree of ischemia. Absolute values may be used (transcutaneous oxygen pressure [$tcPo_2$]) or a calf/brachial partial pressure of oxygen (Po_2) index can be calculated.[63] Studies have suggested that this method can be predictive of the success of ulcer healing or the ability to heal an amputation site.

Duplex Ultrasonography

Recently duplex ultrasonography has been extended to the evaluation of lower-extremity arterial occlusive disease. This method can assess both arterial anatomy and physiology. By spectral analysis it evaluates the hemodynamic effect of localized stenoses. Measurements of velocity profiles can be compared before and after endovascular procedures such as atherectomy and balloon dilation, or following bypass reconstructions. However, tibial vessels cannot yet be reliably evaluated with this technique. Duplex ultrasound has proved to be an extremely useful tool in following patients after undergoing lower-extremity arterial bypass operations. By periodically studying the patient with surveillance ultrasound examinations, one can accurately detect restenosis or a failing saphenous vein bypass graft. The underlying abnormality can then be corrected before thrombosis of the graft occurs.[64]

Magnetic Resonance Imaging

MRI has been receiving increasing attention for studying the peripheral circulation.[65,66] With MRI blood flow velocity can be estimated, and contrast agent administration is not needed to enhance the images obtained. Images can be obtained in transverse, sagittal, and coronal planes. Moreover, the technique has no known harmful effects. The patient under study is placed in a magnetic field and subjected to millisecond bursts of high-frequency energy that alters the alignment of nuclei in the magnetic field and thus creates a condition of "excitement." When bursts of radiofrequency energy stop, the nuclei "relax" and realign in the magnetic field. This relaxation is associated with the emission of radiofrequency energy that can be detected and analyzed by two-dimensional Fourier reconstruction to produce an image. Owen et al[67] prospectively used both conventional angiography and magnetic resonance angiography (MRA) in 23 patients (25 legs) with peripheral atherosclerosis who underwent lower-extremity revascularization. They showed that MRA detected all vessels identified by conventional angiography, whereas conventional angiography failed to detect 22% of run-off vessels identified by MRA. Other investigators have demonstrated similar results.[68] However, MRA continues to be plagued by overestimating the degree of stenosis that is present in some vascular beds.

Blood Chemistry Studies

Several chemistry studies should be considered for every patient undergoing evaluation of lower-extremity atherosclerosis. If a fasting blood glucose level is elevated, Hb A_{1c} should be measured to assess diabetic control. A complete lipid profile should also be obtained after a 12-hour fast (see Chapter 9). A complete blood cell count and a kidney and liver profile should be performed as well. Some individuals with ASO, particularly those who smoke, have a high hematocrit value, which may contribute to increased blood viscosity and possibly arterial thrombosis. Some evidence suggests that fibrinogen levels may also be significantly elevated in smokers who have vascular disease and that this elevation may be a contributing factor in thrombosis.[69]

Cardiac Testing

Long-term survival in patients with lower-extremity atherosclerosis is directly related to their underlying cardiac status.[70,71] All patients seen for initial evaluation should have a 12-lead electrocardiogram. Since a history of myocardial infarction or electrocardiographic evidence of myocardial infarction places the individual in a higher risk category for future cardiac events, this information is important for prognosis. If surgical reconstruction is being considered, cardiac stress testing is advisable. If the patient cannot exercise, a dobutamine echocardiogram, a dipyridamole thallium scan, or positron emission tomography may be performed. If the patient has clinical symptoms of angina pectoris or resting electrocardiographic evidence of ischemia, a cardiac catheterization may be indicated.

Plain X-ray Films

In the presence of digital gangrene or ischemic ulceration, plain x-ray films of the foot may help detect underlying osteomyelitis or deep soft tissue infection. Patients with diabetes and individuals with chronic renal failure may have severe diffuse calcification of the leg and foot arteries. Diabetics who have neurotrophic ulcers may have underlying osteomyelitis with relatively little external evidence of chronic infection. Thus the radiograph may help determine whether other conservative or more aggressive treatment is indicated, including the possibility of amputation as primary treatment for the involved digit.

Arteriography

With the advent of reliable noninvasive vascular laboratory testing, arteriography is no longer necessary unless endovascular or surgical treatment is being considered. Adequate information can be obtained from the patient's clinical history, physical diagnosis, and noninvasive testing to assess the level and extent of occlusive vascular disease. Clear guidelines have been developed to determine when more aggressive treatment is indicated. If endovascular or surgical treatment is being considered, complete arteriography of the abdominal aorta and run-off vessels in both lower extremities should be performed. Arteriography is performed using a transfemoral Seldinger catheter approach.[72] With the aid of fluoroscopic control, flexible guidewires, preformed catheters, and power injection of contrast material, detailed and complete studies can be obtained (Fig. 11-6). The development of equipment with moving tables and the use of digital subtraction techniques has increased the quality of radiographic studies while limiting the contrast load. (See Chapter 4.) Complete studies, including the pedal arch of the foot, should be obtained. Oblique views may also be needed to define certain areas such as the iliac or femoral bifurcation. Intraoperative arteriography still has an important role in distal lower-extremity bypass reconstruction.[73]

Diagnosis

To establish the diagnosis of atherosclerosis of the extremities, it is necessary to combine all of the information obtained by a careful clinical history, physical examination, and noninvasive vascular laboratory testing. Intermittent claudication is a classic symptom, and when clearly described by a reliable observer, it is strongly indicative of vascular disease. Associated risk factors such as hypertension, diabetes, and cigarette smoking are commonly present in patients with symptoms of intermittent claudication, ischemic rest pain, or digital gangrene. A clinician who is experienced in the evaluation of peripheral vascular disease will usually recognize when some aspect of the patient's history, physical examination, or laboratory findings do not fit the picture of peripheral arteriosclerosis obliterans. Several other vascular and nonvascular conditions may simulate symptoms of atherosclerosis. These differential diagnoses are discussed in detail in other chapters of this book and are summarized in the box on p. 220.

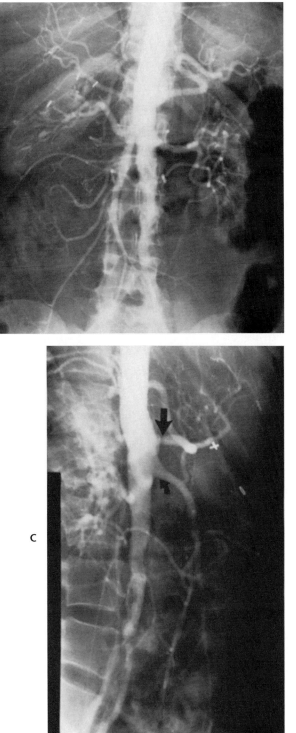

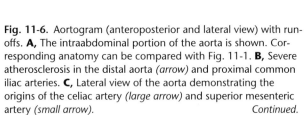

Fig. 11-6. Aortogram (anteroposterior and lateral view) with run-offs. **A,** The intraabdominal portion of the aorta is shown. Corresponding anatomy can be compared with Fig. 11-1. **B,** Severe atherosclerosis in the distal aorta *(arrow)* and proximal common iliac arteries. **C,** Lateral view of the aorta demonstrating the origins of the celiac artery *(large arrow)* and superior mesenteric artery *(small arrow).*   *Continued.*

MEDICAL TREATMENT

Medical management in patients with lower-extremity occlusive vascular disease is indicated for all patients with intermittent claudication. Some patients will undergo medical management alone, whereas others will undergo surgical treatment or endovascular therapy (percutaneous transluminal balloon angioplasty [PTA] and/or stent) in addition to medical management. Traditionally surgical therapy has been reserved for patients who develop limb-threatening ischemia with ischemic rest pain, tissue necrosis, or life-style-disabling claudication. With the advent of new nonsurgical techniques (PTA, stent), indications for intervention are changing. A therapeutic algorithm for treating patients with ASO is shown in Fig. 11-7 and the

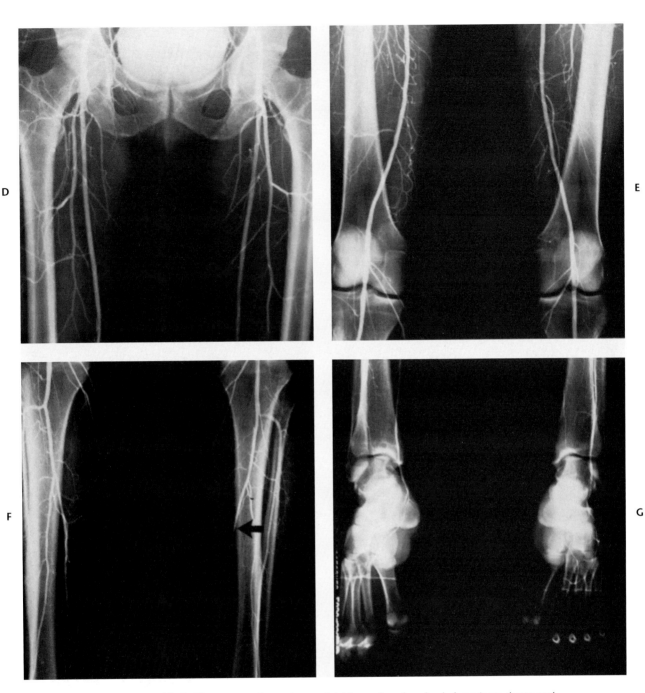

Fig. 11-6, cont'd. **D,** The common femoral, superficial femoral, and profunda femoris are shown and are normal. **E,** Normal superficial femoral and popliteal arteries. **F,** Tibial peroneal vessels are shown in this view. The posterior tibial artery in the left leg is occluded *(arrow)*. **G,** Anterior and posterior tibial arteries are patent into the right foot.

box on p. 220. The medical approach to treating patients with ASO is discussed in the following material.

Discontinue Cigarette Smoking

Since cigarette smoking is so highly correlated with the presence of ASO and its progression, the cessation of smoking is strongly recommended. It is the single most important measure that may prevent the progression of atherosclerosis. Patients who are able to stop smoking

successfully have been shown to improve their treadmill walking distance, compared with those who continued to smoke.[74] It has also been demonstrated that long-term graft patency in both the aortofemoral and femoral popliteal locations is adversely affected by continued cigarette smoking.[75,76] The evidence is conclusive that smoking cessation is associated with fewer adverse events related to lower-extremity atherosclerosis.[25] Progressive claudication, ischemic rest pain, and amputations are less

DIFFERENTIAL DIAGNOSIS IN PATIENTS WITH A HISTORY SUGGESTIVE OF INTERMITTENT CLAUDICATION

1. Atherosclerosis
2. Thromboangiitis obliterans (see Chapter 21)
3. Takayasu's arteritis (see Chapter 22)
4. Giant cell arteritis (see Chapter 22)
5. Arterial embolism (see Chapter 15)
6. Chronic pernio (see Chapter 35)
7. Popliteal artery entrapment syndrome (see Chapter 24)
8. Fibromuscular dysplasia (ssee Chapter 24)
9. Ergotamine use and abuse
10. Phlegmasia cerulea dolens (venous gangrene) (see Chapter 26)
11. Cystic adventitial disease of the popliteal artery (see Chapter 24)
12. Atheromatous emboli (see Chapter 14)
13. Lumbar canal stenosis and lumbar disk disease
14. Degenerative joint disease of the hip and back

TREATMENT OF PATIENTS WITH SEVERE ARTERIOSCLEROSIS OBLITERANS OF THE LOWER EXTREMITIES *(PREVENTION, FOOT CARE, AND PALLIATION)*

Put bed in a vascular position (reverse Trendelenburg) for patients with rest pain or ischemic ulcers that will not heal

Foot Care

  Daily inspection of the feet

  Careful trimming of the toenails

  Avoid trauma or injury to the feet

  Keep skin in good condition (i.e., use a lanolin-based cream 2 to 4 times per day)

  Treat underlying tinea infection

  Wear properly fitting soft shoes or orthotics

  Wear protective foam or wool boots, and use lamb's wool between the toes to prevent pressure (kissing) ulcers

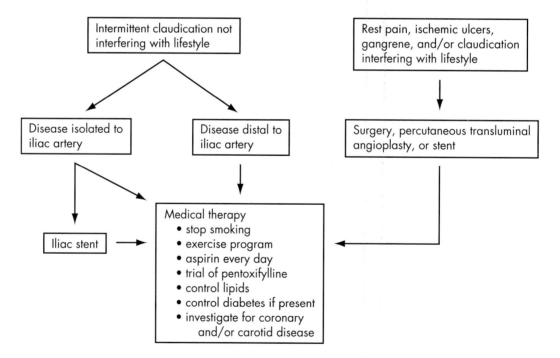

Fig. 11-7. Algorithm for treating patients with arteriosclerosis obliterans.

frequent in the individual who discontinues smoking cigarettes compared with those individuals who continue smoking. In addition, overall cardiovascular morbidity and mortality is improved. Every effort should be made to offer assistance to individual patients in their efforts to stop smoking completely. Numerous programs are available for guidance and assistance in stopping this addictive behavior.

Exercise Therapy

Besides discontinuing cigarette smoking, an exercise program is perhaps the most important aspect in the medical management of the patient with intermittent claudication. Skinner and Strandness[77] demonstrated that a physical training program of repeated walking exercise improved resting limb blood flow, reduced the onset of claudication symptoms, and increased maximal walking

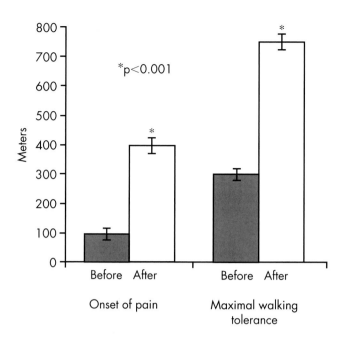

Fig. 11-8. Walking tolerance of patients with intermittent claudication (*n* = 129) before and after 4 to 6 months of physical training. (From Elkroth R et al: Physical training of patients with intermittent claudication: indications, methods, and results, Surgery 84:640, 1978.)

time. Elkroth et al[78] studied 148 patients who had intermittent claudication for more than 6 months. After a 4- to 6-month training period, walking distance increased in 88% of the patients and the average increase was a staggering 234%. Despite an improvement in walking distance, calf blood flow remained unchanged. After the training period more than 40% of the patients could walk 1000 m or more (Fig. 11-8). Hiatt et al[79] placed patients with intermittent claudication on an exercise conditioning program for 12 weeks and demonstrated that the treated subjects increased their peak walking time 123%, peak oxygen consumption 30%, and pain-free walking time 165%. All parameters were statistically significantly better than those in a control group. In this study maximum calf blood flow increased 38% (±45%) (*P* < 0.05), but this change was not correlated with an increase in peak walking time. There was a 26% decrease in resting short-chain acylcarnitine concentration, and this correlated strongly with peak walking time. Radack and Wyderski[25] and Hiatt and Regensteiner[80] have nicely summarized the available data on exercise rehabilitation in patients with peripheral arterial disease. Although most patients with intermittent claudication improve after an exercise program, the precise mechanism for this improvement is unknown. The possibilities include a training effect, increased collateral blood flow, improved hemorrheology, decreased whole blood and plasma viscosity, and/or an improved oxidative metabolism of skeletal muscle.[79]

It appears that a structured exercise program in a vascular rehabilitation center is superior to informally instructing the patient in the office. Williams et al[81] studied 45 patients who completed a vascular rehabilitation program. Thirty-eight patients (88%) had a docu-

mented increase in walking distance greater than 100% (range, 122% to 450%). Long-term follow-up was available in all patients. Thirty-eight patients (84%) maintained or improved walking distances for 2 years. Therefore after being instructed in a formalized setting, it appears that many patients will continue the exercise program long-term.

At the very least, if an exercise rehabilitation center is not available, the patient should be instructed to walk for 30 to 40 minutes 4 to 5 days weekly. We instruct the patient to walk at a pace fast enough to bring on the discomfort at approximately one block. The patient should then walk a little farther, stop, stand still, and wait until the discomfort disappears. He or she should then continue walking again and repeat this cycle for 30 to 40 minutes.

Pharmacologic Therapy

The three major goals of pharmacologic therapy in patients with atherosclerosis of the aorta and lower extremities are to:

1. Increase walking distance (functional improvement)
2. Decrease the need for surgical revascularization or endovascular therapy
3. Prevent the progression of atherosclerosis and reduce cardiac and cerebrovascular mortality and morbidity

Vasodilating drugs have been popular in the past, although no convincing studies support their use.[82] Despite this, physicians still prescribe this class of drug, and some investigators[83] believe that some drugs in this class (Naftidrofuryl, buflomedil) have a favorable effect on walking distance.

Most of the data regarding walking distance in patients with intermittent claudication involves the drug pentoxifylline (Trental). Pentoxifylline is currently the only hemorrheologically active pharmacologic agent approved by the Food and Drug Administration for the treatment of intermittent claudication.[25] Pentoxifylline improves red blood cell membrane flexibility, reduces hyperviscosity, platelet hyperactivity, and hypercoagulability. Nine of twelve randomized control trials concluded that pentoxifylline was significantly more effective than placebo regarding walking distance in patients with intermittent claudication.[25] Similarly, Cameron, Waller, and Ramsay[84] reviewed seven placebo-controlled trials of pentoxifylline and showed that there was an overall 65% increase in claudication distance in those patients on active drug versus placebo. However, these investigators noted a significant negative correlation between sample size and response (*r* = –0.79, *P* < 0.05). They suggested that this was related to bias of nonpublication of negative results. Duprez and Clement[85] further illustrated some of the problems with methodology in many of the studies involving pentoxifylline. They noted that in a total of 252 patients in seven placebo-controlled trials, the initial walking distance was 159 m and the average response was an increase in 44 m with placebo and 148 m with pentoxifylline. This represents an overall increase of approximately 65%. However, the sample size of these trials was small. If one includes only the two largest trials of pentoxifylline, the response is smaller.[86,87]

Table 11-3. Pentoxifylline in Arteriosclerosis Obliterans

	Initial Claudicating Distance (meters)		Actual Claudicating Distance (meters)	
	Pentoxifylline (*n* = 42)	Placebo (*n* = 40)	Pentoxifylline (*n* = 42)	Placebo (*n* = 40)
Baseline	111	117	172	181
Week 24	195	180	268	250
Increase (%)	59	36	38	25

(Modified from Porter JM et al: Pentoxifylline efficacy in the treatment of intermittent claudication: multicenter controlled double blind trial with objective assessment of chronic occlusive arterial disease patients, Am Heart J 104:66, 1982.)

A multicenter, prospective, randomized study performed in the United States has supported the use of pentoxifylline[86] (Table 11-3). There was a 19% increase in walking distance, but the clinical relevance of an increase such as this is uncertain. Despite the overall favorable statistical significance in many of the studies using pentoxifylline, many investigators continue to believe that the increase in walking distance attributable to pentoxifylline is unpredictable, is not clinically relevant when compared with a group of patients receiving placebo who also participate in a walking program, and may not be cost-effective.[25]

We currently favor a program that initially stresses the importance of discontinuation of cigarette smoking and participation in a regular walking program. If the patient does not get the desired response with these modalities of life-style modification, we will then give the patient a 2-month trial of pentoxifylline. Twenty percent of patients note a subjective improvement at a dose of 400 mg three times a day. The most common side effect of gastrointestinal intolerance can be avoided in most patients if the medication is taken with meals.

Antiplatelet agents have received increasing attention in the treatment of patients with ASO. In the Physicians Health Study, Goldhaber et al[88] performed a randomized double-blind placebo-controlled trial among 22,071 healthy U.S. male physicians aged 40 to 84 and followed them for a mean of 60.2 months. The relative risk of peripheral arterial surgery in the aspirin group (one 325-mg aspirin every other day) was 0.54 (95% confidence interval, 0.30 to 0.95, P = 0.03). In addition, it has been previously demonstrated that aspirin also decreases cardiovascular morbidity and mortality.

Ticlopidine is a thienopyridine derivative with a broad spectrum of platelet antiaggregating activity. It inhibits adenosine diphosphate (ADP)-induced platelet aggregation, reduces fibrinogen levels and blood viscosity in patients with peripheral arterial disease, and has been demonstrated to normalize platelet adhesiveness, erythrocyte deformability, and β-thromboglobulin release in diabetic patients. Ticlopidine inhibits the ADP-induced exposure of the fibrinogen-binding site of the glycoprotein IIb/IIIa complex.[89] Several studies have now demonstrated[90,91] that when ticlopidine was used in patients with intermittent claudication, sudden death, fatal or nonfatal myocardial infarction, fatal or nonfatal stroke, cardiovascular intervention and overall mortality were significantly diminished. In the Swedish Ticlopidine Multicenter Study 341 patients were randomized to placebo and 346 patients to ticlopidine 250 mg twice daily.[90] The mortality rate was 29.1% lower in the ticlopidine group compared with placebo (P = 0.015). Phagher[91] and the Swedish Ticlopidine Multicenter Study Group randomized 101 patients with intermittent claudication to ticlopidine 500 mg daily or placebo. After 5 years of treatment there were no significant increases in walking distance, leg blood flow variables, ABI, and probably no clinically relevant effects on slowing the progression of atherosclerosis. Despite these shortcomings, ticlopidine has a favorable effect on cardiovascular events and mortality in patients with intermittent claudication.

When physical training is coupled with pharmacologic therapy, the results are significantly better.[92,93] Scheffler et al[92] performed a randomized open study using intravenous prostaglandin E_1 (PGE$_1$), or pentoxifylline with a controlled vascular training program in patients with peripheral arterial occlusive disease, Fontaine stage IIB. The duration of therapy was 4 weeks. In all three groups there was a significant increase in walking distance. There was 119% increase in symptom-free walking distance in the exercise group only. The combination of pentoxifylline and exercise provided no additional increase in walking distance. However, administration of PGE$_1$ combined with exercise achieved a remarkable improvement of 604% (P < 0.05). Mannarino et al[93] studied the efficacy of physical training alone or combined with antiplatelet therapy (dipyridamole and aspirin) in 30 patients with stage II peripheral arterial occlusive disease. The maximum walking time improved significantly in all three groups. Both pain-free walking time and maximal walking time were significantly increased in patients receiving the combination of platelet inhibitors and exercise compared with either one alone.

Other pharmacologic agents such as ketanserin and L-carnitine have been investigated for their potential usefulness in the treatment of intermittent claudication, but thus far they have not been clearly demonstrated to be effective.[94,95] Intraarterial infusions of prostaglandin have been suggested to be beneficial in patients with advanced lower-extremity arterial insufficiency.[96,97] However, a multicenter randomized trial by Schuler et al[98] failed to demonstrate effectiveness when prostaglandin was administered intravenously. In another study Cronenwett et al[99] infused prostacyclin intravenously to treat ischemic ulcers and rest pain, but no objective improvement was noted. Thus the search continues for an effective pharmacologic agent to treat lower-extremity ASO.

Aggressive management of lipoprotein abnormalities should be undertaken as recommended in Chapter 9. Reasonable evidence now exists that regression of atherosclerosis may occur in some patients who follow a program of aggressive risk factor modification.[100,101]

Associated blood clotting disorders such as protein C, protein S, and antithrombin III deficiency have all been identified in more recent years.[102] Other blood clotting disorders have also been recognized such as hyperaggregable platelet dysfunction, lupus anticoagulant, and abnormal plasminogen activator inhibitor levels. Since heparin is so frequently used to treat acute lower-extremity ischemia, heparin-associated antibodies may also occur and promote thrombosis rather than the desired therapeutic effect of anticoagulation. When these conditions are identified as coexisting with peripheral atherosclerosis, the use of long-term anticoagulant therapy for patients with ASO may be considered. Although anticoagulant therapy has not demonstrated a significant improvement in either the amputation rate or long-term survival, recent reports have shown that it may improve the patency rate of infragenicular prosthetic bypass reconstructions.[103,104]

SURGICAL TREATMENT

Preoperative Considerations

Progression of intermittent claudication to severe disabling symptoms is an indication to proceed with surgical treatment of lower-extremity atherosclerosis. Limb-threatening symptoms such as ischemic ulceration or rest pain are more definitive symptoms for which surgical treatment may be recommended. The noninvasive vascular laboratory can be very helpful in confirming the degree of arterial impairment, which should correlate with the severity of symptoms. Once the history, physical examination, and objective assessment in the noninvasive laboratory confirm that an individual does have severe arterial insufficiency, an arteriogram should be obtained that will define the extent of occlusive disease and help determine the options for successful surgical intervention. When this information has been obtained and analyzed, a decision can be made regarding the surgical alternatives for treatment such as endovascular therapy (catheter-directed intervention), bypass reconstruction, or in rare instances primary amputation.

For a patient who demonstrates progressive or severely restrictive claudication symptoms, surgical treatment is usually considered elective. In this circumstance the patient and the immediate family should be informed completely about treatment alternatives including continued medical management, endovascular techniques, and vari-

ous options for bypass reconstruction. This will usually require some discussion regarding the advantages and disadvantages as well as the risks related to various treatment options. It also requires the use of clinical judgment based on the experience of the treating physician. For example, an elderly individual with a sedentary life-style and the recent onset of two- to three-block claudication may require only reassurance that the claudication symptoms are not limb-threatening and continued medical management should be pursued. On the other hand, if the individual is employed and supporting a family or retired and actively pursuing recreational interests, even relatively mild claudication symptoms may be intolerable. In these circumstances more aggressive treatment with endovascular therapy or bypass reconstruction may be considered. It is the obligation of the treating physician to provide the individual with the expected benefits to be derived with surgical intervention versus the potential risks involved with undertaking surgical treatment.

If patients elect to pursue surgical treatment, they may require more in-depth investigation of the medical risk. In patients with lower-extremity atherosclerosis, the most critical risk factor is the presence of coronary artery disease.[105] Patients under consideration for bypass reconstruction in the lower extremities who underwent coronary bypass grafting before vascular surgical reconstruction had a 30% higher 5-year survival rate than a comparable group who did not have myocardial revascularization in the presence of severe correctable coronary disease.[105] The assessment of coronary disease in vascular patients is discussed more completely in Chapter 13. If clinically significant coronary artery disease is present and it cannot be corrected, some alternative less stressful operative intervention may be considered such as axillofemoral or femorofemoral bypass reconstruction rather than an intraabdominal aortobifemoral procedure. Other medical risks also need to be evaluated such as the presence of chronic obstructive pulmonary disease, renal insufficiency, poorly controlled hypertension, and uncontrolled diabetes mellitus. Age alone is not a contraindication to surgical treatment.

The presence of rest pain or ischemic ulceration is a more compelling reason to recommend surgical treatment. In these circumstances the patient may be facing limb loss if the arterial perfusion to the extremity cannot be improved. Therefore a decision to pursue surgical treatment becomes a more urgent matter. The same process of evaluation as mentioned previously for intermittent claudication is necessary but may be more compressed in terms of time frame for evaluation. The individual with rest pain or ischemic ulceration will usually be a more challenging problem to manage due to multiple levels of involvement with the atherosclerotic process. The risks for failure of the reconstruction and possible amputation are greater in the individual with limb-threatening ischemia than they are in patients with intermittent claudication. These factors must also be made clear to the patient and family regarding the expectations of treatment.

The arteriogram will define the extent and severity of ASO. This study should include the entire abdominal aorta and the lower-extremity arteries throughout both limbs including the feet (Fig. 11-6). Lateral or oblique views of selected areas such as the iliac and femoral bifurcations may be necessary. The use of digital subtraction arteriography has generally supplanted the use of multiple sequential standard radiographs for the evaluation of lower-extremity ASO.[107] In more distal lower-extremity atherosclerosis, it is especially important to visualize whether the tibial vessels are in continuity with the vessels of the foot itself. Selective injections of contrast agent and delayed views may be necessary in some circumstances.

Preoperative Preparation

Once the preliminary preoperative studies have been performed and a decision has been made to proceed with surgical treatment, the patient should be prepared medically. A review of the patient's medications is important. If the individual has been under treatment with daily aspirin for its antiplatelet effect, this medication should be stopped at least 1 week before aortic reconstruction. Although aspirin does not cause a measurable effect on blood coagulation, many surgeons find increased bleeding and delayed clotting in retroperitoneal dissection. In addition, if the patient has been taking diuretics for antihypertensive management, the total body potassium may be depleted; these patients should receive replacement therapy to avoid cardiac complications. For individuals with known coronary artery disease, perioperative transcutaneous or intravenous nitrates may also be beneficial. Assessment of pulmonary function with screening spirometry and cessation of cigarette smoking, if only for a few days, may be extremely helpful in the mobilization of pulmonary secretions. Preoperative respiratory therapy with bronchodilators or steroids may be helpful for some individuals with severe chronic pulmonary disease. Adequate hydration is also important, particularly in patients who may have marginal renal function and have recently undergone arteriographic studies. In those who have known impairment of ventricular contractility, preoperative assessment in the intensive care unit with Swan-Ganz catheter placement and hemodynamic evaluation may be useful.

Prophylactic antibiotics are recommended by most vascular surgeons when the use of a prosthetic vascular conduit is anticipated. *Staphylococcus, Streptococcus,* and *Escherichia coli* are the most common organisms associated with perioperative wound infections and major complications of graft infection. Therefore most surgeons commonly employ a cephalosporin effective against these organisms.

Each hospital should also be aware of the most common flora present in its own operating rooms and intensive care units. Most institutions do surveillance testing with antibiotic sensitivities to the organism most commonly encountered in a particular environment. Ideally selection of antibiotic prophylaxis should be based on this information for individual institutions.

Most aortic reconstructions require transfusion of at least 2 or 3 U of blood during or immediately after the surgical procedure. Although the risk of hepatitis and acquired immunodeficiency syndrome is very low from the transfusion of anonymous donor-banked blood, some institutions have developed a program of predonation of autologous blood that will be used during major aortic reconstructive operations. Most surgeons also employ a blood recovery system and retransfuse autologous packed red blood cells during major aortic reconstructions.[108] Rarely is there sufficient blood loss during femoropopliteal reconstructions alone to require the use of autotransfusion devices. However, for reoperations, predonation of autologous blood is also a reasonable consideration.

Lumbar Sympathectomy

Surgical lumbar sympathectomy has been employed as treatment for lower-extremity occlusive disease since the concept was advocated by Leriche in 1913.[109] Diez[110] elaborated on the technique and included the use of ganglionectomy along with periarterial sympathectomy. In 1925 Adson and Brown[111] first used lumbar sympathectomy in the United States for the treatment of Raynaud's disease. For the next three decades sympathectomy was the only surgical alternative to amputation for the treatment of lower-extremity occlusive disease. Even after direct reconstructive procedures were introduced in the early 1950s, surgical sympathectomy was used either as sole treatment for patients with distal, tibial occlusive disease or as an adjunct for reconstructive procedures.

The effectiveness of sympathectomy has always been controversial. Although laboratory studies have demonstrated that sympathectomy can increase total limb blood flow in normal subjects, no convincing clinical studies have demonstrated improved limb blood flow in patients with arterial occlusive disease. Experimental studies by Rutherford and Valenta[112] and Cronenwett and Lindenauer[113] have shown that most of the increased blood flow following sympathectomy involves redistribution to the skin rather than to muscle. These studies support the impression that sympathectomy does not relieve symptoms of intermittent claudication or rest pain. However, sympathectomy may be useful in patients who have ischemic skin ulceration related to arterial insufficiency and local trauma. Clinical studies by Persson, Anderson, and Padberry[114] and Walker and Johnston[115] suggested that patients with ischemic rest pain or ulceration may be reasonable candidates for lumbar sympathectomy if they have an ABI of greater than 0.30, if the symptoms are limited to the forefoot, and if sensory neuropathy is absent. Yao and Bergan[116] reported in 1973 that more than 90% of patients who had an ABI lower than 0.35 failed to experience symptomatic relief from lumbar sympathectomy alone. Diabetic patients with sensory neuropathy are particularly unresponsive to the effects of lumbar sympathectomy for ischemic foot lesions.

The use of lumbar sympathectomy as an adjunct to surgical reconstruction has gradually declined among vascular surgeons. The resurgence of interest in the use of in situ or reversed saphenous vein bypass to distal tibial and pedal vessels in recent years has resulted in revascularization of many extremities that were previously considered "nonoperable." The success of these distal arterial reconstructions has consequently reduced the use of sympathectomy. Some surgeons continue to use lumbar sympathectomy in association with aortic reconstruction when there is evidence of digital ischemia from atheroembolization or in the presence of severe multilevel disease. However, no conclusive evidence supports the persistence of this practice.[117] Sympathectomy may be useful in the treatment of causalgia, thromboangiitis obliterans (Buerger's disease), frostbite, or digital ischemia if a trial of percutaneous lumbar sympathetic blocks demonstrates a positive response. Chemical sympathectomy with a phenol or alcohol injection has also been advocated by some,[118] and it may be as effective as surgical sympathectomy.

Aortoiliac-Femoral Reconstruction

Patients with the onset of calf claudication followed by thigh and hip claudication commonly have proximal disease involving the aortoiliac region. Patients with short-distance claudication, pain at rest, or ischemic necrosis of the feet will often have diffuse multisegment disease involving the aortoiliac region, femoropopliteal segment, as well as tibial occlusive disease. Isolated aortoiliac occlusive disease, when associated with impotence in men and with diminished femoral pulses, is often referred to as the *Leriche syndrome*. Although originally described by Leriche as complete aortic occlusion at the bifurcation of the abdominal aorta, this term has come to be applied loosely to patients who have stenotic lesions in the aortoiliac segment.

If atherosclerosis affects the patient at multiple segments, the proximal segments are treated initially if they are hemodynamically significant. Current methods of noninvasive testing that measure segmental pressures as well as intraarterial pressure measurements at the time of the arteriographic study may help define the significance of arteriographically demonstrated lesions.

The first aortic reconstructive operations performed in the early 1950s used cadaver homograft replacements.[7] Within a short time the technique of thromboendarterectomy was also applied to atherosclerotic lesions of the aortoiliac segment.[9] At the same time dacron fabric prostheses were constructed that were found to be adequate replacements for occluded vessels in the aortoiliac and femoral segments.[10] The use of homografts has been abandoned because of the deterioration of the conduit by aneurysm formation. However, thromboendarterectomy is still a useful technique for patients who have localized disease, particularly in younger individuals with disease confined to the aortic bifurcation.[119,120] Endovascular therapy using balloon dilatation and/or stent placement in the iliac segment for localized lesions has been employed effectively in recent years as an alternative to thromboendarterectomy or graft placement (see Chapter 12).

Prosthetic graft replacement has become the standard reconstructive method for most patients with aortoiliac and femoral occlusive disease, although there are still some controversial aspects. Controversies include the method of proximal anastomosis (i.e., end-to-end vs. end-to-side) and the type of prosthesis (i.e., knitted vs. woven dacron material and standard vs. velour construction). Polytetrafluoroethylene (PTFE) grafts are also favored by some surgeons over dacron grafts. Controversy also exists over whether the optimal approach to the aorta is a transabdominal midline incision or retroperitoneal exposure through the flank.[121] Most vascular surgeons continue to

use a transabdominal midline approach. Since different approaches may have specific benefits for selected patients, the vascular surgeon should be familiar with a wide variety of anatomic approaches and reconstructive techniques.

For aortofemoral reconstruction it is important to be aware of the blood supply to the left side of the colon.[122,123] The arteriogram will demonstrate whether the inferior mesenteric artery is occluded or patent and whether prominent collateral circulation exists between the inferior mesenteric bed and the superior mesenteric artery distribution. If an end-to-end proximal aortic to graft anastomosis is constructed, and there is significant external iliac occlusive disease, some alternative means may be needed to maintain perfusion to the internal iliac arteries or inferior mesenteric artery. This can be accomplished by reimplantation of the inferior mesenteric artery or branched prosthetic limbs to the internal iliac or common iliac arteries when the main reconstruction extends to the common femoral arteries bilaterally. Frequently, substantial disease is present in the common femoral arteries that may extend a short distance into the profunda femoris or superficial femoral origin. A localized femoral endarterectomy may be needed to ensure adequate outflow for the aortofemoral reconstruction. This procedure is even more important if combined segment disease is present with significant stenosis or segmental occlusions of the superficial femoral artery.[124]

Other alternatives exist for the treatment of aortoiliac occlusive disease. These include axillofemoral-femoral reconstruction or femoral-femoral bypass if unilateral iliac occlusive disease is present. In general, these alternative forms of reconstruction are used for the medically high-risk individual in cases where a transabdominal procedure would place the patient at substantial risk. They are particularly useful for patients who have nonreconstructible coronary disease or severe pulmonary disease. However, these extraanatomic bypasses are not as durable as an aortoiliac or aortofemoral reconstruction.[125]

Profunda Femoris Reconstruction

In 1961 Morris et al[126] as well as Leeds and Gilfillan[127] recognized the importance of the profunda femoris artery in lower-extremity collateral circulation. The concept of profunda femoris reconstruction was later emphasized by Martin, Bernhard, and others.[2,128,129] The profunda femoris or deep femoral artery serves as a bridge or a major collateral pathway between the aortofemoral segment and the femoropopliteal segment when the superficial femoral artery is occluded. Therefore the profunda femoris artery plays an important role in both "inflow" and "outflow" lower-extremity reconstructions. Maintenance of profunda femoris blood flow is always an objective of lower-extremity revascularization when the superficial femoral artery is occluded. In many situations the prosthetic graft may be extended down onto the profunda femoris for a short distance to provide unobstructed outflow. In femoropopliteal reconstruction it is important to assess whether a profundaplasty may be needed to maintain this collateral pathway. This adjunct to femoropopliteal reconstruction may help maintain limb viability if the femoropopliteal or tibial bypass subsequently becomes occluded.

For a time there was considerable interest in profunda reconstruction as an isolated procedure for limb salvage. However, further study has indicated that although profunda reconstruction alone may help relieve symptoms of intermittent claudication, it is often insufficient to heal ischemic necrosis of the foot or relieve rest pain when critical ischemia is present.[130] Therefore profunda reconstruction is most often an adjunct to either an inflow aortofemoral procedure or to outflow femoropopliteal reconstruction. At times if disease in the profunda femoris is quite extensive, a procedure referred to as "extended profundaplasty" may be required to preserve its function.[131,132] This condition is particularly common in patients with associated diabetes mellitus.

Profundaplasty alone, as an isolated procedure for limb salvage, should be considered in highly selected patients. Boren et al[130] have advocated the use of a profunda-popliteal collateral index as a means of providing an objective criterion for success. Limb salvage may be expected in 91% of limbs with an index of less than 0.19. Calculation of the index may be influenced by the presence of iliac inflow disease and should not be relied on as the only criterion for performing profundaplasty. Profundaplasty should also be considered for those patients who have "nonreconstructible" disease before a major amputation is undertaken, since the level of amputation may be reduced from above the knee to below the knee in some patients.[132]

Femoropopliteal and Femorotibial Reconstruction

The first successful surgical reconstructions for lower-extremity vascular disease were femoropopliteal bypass operations using a reversed greater saphenous vein. Early experience confirmed that the saphenous vein was a reliable conduit.[133] For the most part bypasses were performed to the above-knee or below-knee popliteal artery, whereas reversed vein bypass to tibial arteries were less commonly performed. In the United States it was not until 1979 that a large well-analyzed series of tibioperoneal bypasses was reported.[13] At the same time some surgeons believed that the use of the reversed saphenous vein had reached the limits of its effectiveness for surgical treatment of femoropopliteal disease.[134] Leather, Powers, and Karmody[15] reintroduced the use of the saphenous vein in situ as a conduit for femoropopliteal and tibial reconstruction. The resurgence of interest in this technique, as well as many of their adjuncts to the in situ technique, have helped spur the advancement of bypass reconstruction to more distal tibial vessels. During the 1980s the in situ method of saphenous vein bypass reconstruction has become a firmly established reconstructive technique. Although many surgeons believe that this method represents a distinct advancement in technique, others maintain that similar results can be obtained with reversed saphenous vein to tibial vessels.[135]

Several prosthetic conduits have been used for femoropopliteal reconstruction. These include dacron, bovine heterografts, umbilical vein, PTFE, and composites of dacron-PTFE. Unfortunately these prosthetic materials are unable to achieve the same primary patency rates as autogenous vein for bypass reconstructions to the above-knee popliteal, below-knee popliteal, or tibial arteries. The development of a suitable prosthetic conduit for small-caliber arteries has been elusive during the past two decades. Carefully analyzed studies demonstrate that PTFE has inferior patency rates compared with vein bypass at all levels. The primary patency drops off dramatically in bypasses to the below-knee popliteal artery or individual tibial vessels.[136] Attempts to coat the lumen of the PTFE bypass with endothelial cells have also been studied. To date none of these methods has substantially improved the patency of prosthetic material in distal bypass reconstructions. Other technical adjuncts such as vein patch at the distal anastomosis and local or distal arteriovenous fistulas have also been tried.[137-140] Extensive femoropopliteal thromboendarterectomy was also used for a time. These methods consisted of both closed and semi-open techniques with and without vein or dacron patch angioplasty.[141,142] However, the experience over time was that these reconstructed femoropopliteal arteries eventually reoccluded as a result of myointimal hyperplasia.

The indications for bypass reconstruction of the femoropopliteal and femoral tibial segments are generally more stringent than for aortofemoral reconstruction. Intermittent claudication is an acceptable indication if the patient's walking distance is extremely limited. Some differentiation is necessary about the extent of femoropopliteal disease and the available conduit. If an above-knee bypass can be performed with either the saphenous vein or a prosthetic conduit and distal run-off is unimpaired, the results of surgical treatment are quite acceptable—that is, 60% to 80% 5-year graft patency. However, when reconstruction requires bypass to the below-knee popliteal or individual tibial arteries, the results of prosthetic conduits may not be durable enough to justify reconstruction in the presence of intermittent claudication as the sole symptom. In patients with extensive lower-extremity occlusive disease, ischemic pain at rest or tissue necrosis that threatens limb viability are more acceptable indications for operation. Most centers have reserved distal tibial bypass reconstruction for patients with limb-threatening ischemia using venous conduits. The results of more recent reports indicate that bypass to individual tibial arteries is comparable to bypass to the below-knee popliteal artery if either an in situ or reversed saphenous vein graft is used when the vein conduit is 3 mm or larger in diameter.[143,144] The use of prosthetic conduits to tibial arteries has very poor 5-year patency (12% to 20%).[136,145]

Many subtle technical variations have been reported for femoropopliteal and femorotibial reconstruction. When a sufficient length of autogenous greater saphenous vein is unavailable, other sources of autogenous conduit have been suggested such as the lesser saphenous or cephalic veins and endarterectomized superficial femoral artery.[146-150] Other combinations of autogenous and prosthetic material have been recommended as have the use of sequential bypasses.[151] Alternative inflow sites such as the profunda femoris artery or distal superficial artery have been suggested when the length of vein is inadequate for distal bypass reconstruction. Another reported variation in technique is the use of short tibiotibial vein interposition bypasses.[152] Even bypasses to the dorsalis pedis artery have been reported to have very acceptable results for limb salvage.[153] These innovative techniques have resulted in successful bypass reconstructions to arteries previously considered nonreconstructible.

Most series report significant attrition of bypass patency during the first 1 to 2 years of follow-up study. Table 11-4 shows the results of reported series for femoropopliteal and femorotibial reconstructions. Some investigators have reported that if distal bypass reconstructions are observed carefully postoperatively, failing bypasses can be identified, and timely intervention may be able to salvage a failing bypass.[154,155] However, secondary reconstructions in the lower extremity are significantly less successful than primary reconstruction (50% patency at 1 year in most series). In more recent years noninvasive techniques provide a convenient method of objective follow-up. Rutherford et al[156] have recommended a standard scheme of reporting of lower-extremity bypass reconstruction so that series from different centers can be compared. Standardized reporting should lead to more accurate comparisons of surgical techniques and graft materials among published series. Continued refinements of surgical technique, graft materials, and objective means of assessment should lead to improvements and salvage of lower extremities with arterial insufficiency due to ASO.

Endovascular Therapy

From 1980 to 1990 the use of catheter-directed interventional techniques for lower-extremity ASO has become more widely used. The use of percutaneous catheter-directed techniques for the treatment of lower-extremity ASO was initially introduced by Dotter[157] in the 1960s. This approach used progressively increasing sizes of coaxially placed catheters to dilate an area of arterial stenosis. The next major advance occurred in 1974 when Gruntzig introduced a reliable polyvinylchloride balloon dilatation catheter.[158] These balloon catheters could be produced to provide a specified length and fixed diameter of dilatation. The catheters were constructed to expand to a predetermined size without any further enlargement. They were also capable of withstanding high inflation pressures, which provided a means to dilate (crack) rather rigid atherosclerotic plaques.

During the past decade a wide array of catheter-delivered devices have been used in the treatment of lower-extremity ASO. These devices have included hot-tipped laser probes for recanalization, directional atherectomy devices, as well as rotational atherectomy devices. Many of these technologies have met with limited success and some, such as the hot-tipped laser, have been abandoned. Another development during the 1980s has been the introduction of the balloon expandable stent by

Table 11-4. Published Results of Femoropopliteal and Femorotibial Bypass Grafts

Author	No. of Bypasses	Graft Material	Location Bypass	1-Year Patency (%)	1-Year Limb Salvage (%)	5-Year* Patency (%)	5-Year* Limb Salvage (%)
DeWeese and Rob[70] (1977)	113	Vein	Popliteal (above and below knee)	65		59	
Reichle et al[13] (1979)	474	Vein and dacron	Popliteal (above and below knee)		67.6		59.7
		Vein	Tibial-peroneal		53.9		46.9
Harris et al[148] (1984)	70	Vein	Popliteal and tibial-peroneal	85		68	85
Weaver et al[147] (1987)	29	Vein	Tibial-peroneal	72			
Veith et al[136] (1986)	522	Vein	Proximal popliteal	80		61	75
			Distal popliteal	84		76	76
			Tibial-peroneal	75		49	57
		PTFE	Proximal popliteal	80		38	70
			Distal popliteal	84		54	70
			Tibial-peroneal	56		12	61
Leather et al[146] (1988)	725	Vein (in situ)	Distal popliteal	90.8		78.5	
			Tibial-peroneal	91.7		74.3	
Taylor, Edwards, and Porter[143] (1990)	516	Vein	Proximal popliteal	86.6		76.6	
			Distal popliteal	92		80.2	90.2
			Tibial-peroneal	81.2		69.1	
Pomposelli et al[153] (1995)	384	Vein (in situ translocated reversed)	Dorsalis pedis	83†	94†	68	87

*Four-year patency/limb salvage data for Veith et al.[136]
†Estimated.

Palmaz.[159] The use of stents has allowed treatment of arterial stenoses that were resistant to balloon dilatation alone. Stents have proven to be very useful in treating patients with iliac artery stenosis. A variety of stent designs are currently undergoing evaluation. The technology for catheter-directed intervention has developed rapidly over the past several years and is still undergoing evaluation for effectiveness, durability, and freedom from long-term complications. In 1991 Parodi introduced the first clinical use of a stented abdominal aortic dacron graft placed from a femoral approach by a carrying catheter.[160] This technical capability may have significant long-range influence on the treatment of arterial aneurysms and lower-extremity ASO.

The technique of PTA by means of balloon dilatation has been the most widely employed and therefore the most widely studied interventional technique. Despite the fact that balloon angioplasty has been used for more than 20 years, there are relatively few large well-studied series from which to gather information on specific indications and outcomes. One thoroughly analyzed study by Johnston et al, has stratified the results of angioplasty for iliac and femoropopliteal lesions according to length.[161-163] This study demonstrated that common iliac lesions of limited length resulted in an 81.1% 1-year and 60% 5-year patency. However, when lesions were extensive, the long-term patency was less following balloon angioplasty. As a result of this and other studies, balloon angioplasty has been primarily used for localized iliac stenosis or occlusion.

Short stenoses in both the iliac and superficial femoral segments have the best reported results. If an artery has multiple areas of stenosis or diffuse disease, the durability of the technique diminishes significantly. Selection of patients for treatment should be dependent on the degree of symptomatology, noninvasive vascular studies demonstrating impaired segmental pressures or depressed waveforms consistent with the clinical symptoms, and finally an arteriographically documented lesion that is considered suitable for endovascular treatment. Success of balloon dilatation in the external iliac artery has also been reported to be inferior to treatment of common iliac stenosis. Success has been progressively inferior as the balloon dilatation is performed in more distal segments of the lower extremity such as the superficial femoral, popliteal, and tibial-peroneal arteries.

Complications of PTA include thrombosis, embolization, and bleeding from the catheter introduction site. Bleeding may be manifest as a hematoma, acute false aneurysm, or arteriovenous fistula. However, morbidity requiring surgical treatment has occurred in only approximately 5% of most reported series. Mortality is less than 1% in most series with cardiac complications being the primary cause of death. Balloon dilatation may result in plaque dissection at the site of the stenotic lesion. This dissection can result in early thrombosis or late restenosis due to intimal fibroplasia. Arterial rupture in the iliac and femoropopliteal areas or distal embolization are both rare complications of the treatment.

Occasionally, localized arterial segments are refractory to attempts at balloon dilatation due to either dense calcification or elastic recoil of the plaque and artery. To more effectively treat such patients with interventional techniques, endovascular stents have been developed and successfully used in the iliac and femoral segments. A number of different designs have been developed. The Palmaz stent is currently the only device approved by the Food and Drug Administration for use in the iliac segment. Early results suggest that in the high-flow iliac location placement of these stents can be very effective.

Other adjunctive measures have been helpful in the interventional treatment of atherosclerotic lesions. These include the use of intravascular ultrasound for precise placement of the stents and to assure complete expansion of the stent. In addition, the use of intraarterial thrombolytic therapy may help dissolve some of the accumulated thrombus or reopen short occlusions and thus reveal the precise contour of the underlying plaque. These lesions can then be treated more specifically with balloon angioplasty and/or stent placement after the occluding thrombus has been lysed. Streptokinase, urokinase, and tissue plasminogen activator have been the lytic agents used for this purpose. In the arterial system the agent is usually directly infused into the thrombus by a multiple-holed catheter. It appears that the selective use of thrombolytic therapy in both acute and chronic arterial thrombosis can be advantageous in defining more precisely the arterial plaque anatomy responsible for the occlusion. The obstructing lesion may then be treated with endovascular therapy or alternatively by endarterectomy or a bypass reconstruction. These issues of endovascular therapy and thrombolytic therapy are discussed in more detail in Chapters 7 and 12.

Amputation

Treatment of lower-extremity occlusive disease will inevitably require amputation for some patients. Fortunately the number is small compared with the number of patients who have symptomatic ASO. Lalka and Malone[164] stated that "the purpose of amputation surgery is to remove gangrenous, necrotic, or infected tissue; relieve pain; obtain primary healing of the most distal amputation possible; and achieve maximal rehabilitation after amputation. These goals can only be met by careful preoperative evaluation and aggressive preparation of patients for surgery." Amputation of a limb is an emotional issue for patients. Some individuals will go to great lengths to avoid major amputation, often enduring many attempts at revascularization or extended periods of intense pain in an effort to avoid an inevitable amputation. The physician should view amputation as an alternative treatment option for selected patients with the long-term goal of functional rehabilitation.

Amputations are characterized as primary or secondary, depending on whether they are undertaken as definitive surgical treatment for lower-extremity ischemia or whether they follow a previous attempt at revascularization. Primary amputation versus revascularization for patients with limb-threatening ischemia is a controversial issue. Methods to assess the possibility of limb salvage by revascularization as opposed to the need for definitive amputation include Doppler ankle systolic pressures, pulse-volume waveform measurements, skin temperature measurements, laser Doppler velocity measurements, xenon-133 skin blood flow measurements, fluorescein dye injections, and transcutaneous oxygen measurements. After analysis of these and other methods, the final decision to pursue primary amputation or revascularization depends on the surgeons's clinical judgment. The surgeon's decision also includes personal experience and subjective factors such as the patient's potential for rehabilitation and willingness to accept amputation as the recommended definitive treatment. Other issues in this decision-making process include the patient's general medical condition and history of myocardial infarction, previous stroke, chronic organic brain syndrome, and chronic renal insufficiency.

Secondary amputations are those that follow a previous vascular reconstructive procedure. The decision to perform a secondary amputation depends on the type and location of previous vascular reconstruction, the number of repeated attempts at maintaining bypass graft patency, the type of bypass employed in femoral distal reconstructions (e.g., vein or PTFE), and the presence of coexisting factors such as sepsis.

Amputation may be required for acute (as opposed to chronic) limb-threatening conditions. Acute or urgent amputations are often required for those patients who have such extensive tissue necrosis that salvage of a viable foot is not possible. Ischemia accompanied by extensive soft tissue infection with signs of systemic sepsis is another indication for urgent amputation, often found in patients with coexistent diabetes mellitus. Many surgeons prefer a guillotine amputation at the ankle level as an initial procedure to eliminate the source of sepsis rather than definitive below-knee amputation when extensive sepsis is present.[165] The patient can be treated for several days with antibiotics and surgical drainage to allow time for the infection to subside. Diabetes mellitus has been associated with more than 50% of major amputations in patients with lower-extremity occlusive disease.[166] Secondary amputation may also be considered for the patient who has intractable ischemic rest pain following occlusion of previous bypass reconstruction.

Minor amputations of individual toes, or transmetatarsal amputation, may be necessary in some individuals who undergo a reconstructive procedure. In general, revascularization will improve perfusion sufficiently to heal local amputation of toes or amputations in the midfoot region. If more than two digits are involved with fixed gangrenous changes that preclude conservative management, a full transmetatarsal amputation is usually preferable to individual toe amputation. Patients tolerate transmetatarsal amputation quite well without functional disability. They will often benefit from the use of a custom-fitted, toe-filling orthotic for the shoe.

Major amputation involves below-knee amputation through the midcalf or above-knee amputation in the distal thigh. Standard techniques have been described elsewhere in surgical texts. Although the Syme amputation technique (through the ankle) has been advocated by some as an acceptable alternative to below-knee amputation, in general we have found that this technique has very limited applicability. Because of recent advances in prosthetic

design and patient rehabilitation therapy, below-knee amputees should have excellent functional recovery.

Perioperative mortality from amputation ranges from 9% to 15%, depending on the patient's age and associated risk factors.[167] The same risk factors are present for patients who require amputation as for those who are candidates for lower-extremity revascularization. In general, the risk might be expected to be even higher because many of these individuals have advanced nonreconstructible occlusive disease. Survival of amputees has been reported to be approximately 30% at 5 years for major amputations.[168]

Rehabilitation therapy for patients who are able to retain the knee joint is so superior to above-knee amputation that a conservative approach should be used before a major amputation is undertaken. In some cases the level of amputation may be reduced by proximal revascularization.[169] For example, some patients may require only below-knee amputation if a reconstruction in the aortoiliac segment or above-knee femoropopliteal bypass is undertaken. In addition, profundoplasty alone may aid in maintaining a below-knee level of amputation in selected cases.

Amputations through the knee and hip joints do not usually offer any advantage over standard below-knee or above-knee amputations. Knee disarticulation is an alternative means of debridement when acute infection involves the leg above the ankle. Hip disarticulation is usually reserved for those individuals who have extensive ischemia that extends proximally in the thigh and precludes an above-knee amputation through the femur. Functional rehabilitation in patients with hip disarticulation is poor.

More than half of patients who undergo lower-extremity amputation have coexisting diabetes mellitus. Diabetics often develop a sensory neuropathy that leads to bony changes in the foot and to neurotrophic ulceration over bony prominences. These individuals may develop extensive foot sepsis with little awareness of pain or discomfort. If arterial circulation to the foot is preserved, their condition often responds dramatically to aggressive surgical drainage and antimicrobial therapy. Occasionally excision of an involved metatarsal head may be required to allow the foot ulcer to heal. If sepsis can be controlled locally, and if arterial perfusion is adequate, foot salvage is often possible.[170]

It is extremely important that amputees receive physical therapy or supervised rehabilitation. Some patients may require transfer to an inpatient rehabilitation facility if their progress during in-hospital convalescence is not adequate. Various prosthetic options are available. Prosthetics may be fitted immediately to allow the patient to begin walking soon after surgery. In some patients with vascular disease who have delayed wound healing, prosthetic fitting should be delayed for 2 to 3 months until the amputation site has healed completely. An experienced prosthetist is very important to help the patient achieve the proper fitting and adjustment of the artificial limb. A close working relationship between the physician, prosthetist, physical therapist, and patient is important for the best functional recovery of the patient with vascular disease who requires an amputation.

REFERENCES

1. Darling RC et al: Aortoiliac reconstruction, Surg Clin North Am 59:565, 1979.
2. Samson RH, Scher LA, and Veith FJ: Combined segment arterial disease, Surgery 97:385, 1985.
3. Carrel A and Guthrie CC: Results of biterminal transplantation of veins, Am J Med Sci 132:415, 1906.
4. Carrel A and Guthrie CC: Unilateral and biterminal venous transplantation, Surg Gynecol Obstet 2:266, 1906.
5. Dale WA: The beginnings of vascular surgery, Surgery 76:849, 1974.
6. Kunlin J: Le traitement de l'arterite obliterante par la greffe veneuse, Arch Mal Coeur 42:371, 1949.
7. Oudot J: La greffe vasculaire dans les thromboses du carrefour aortigue, Presse Med 59:234, 1951.
8. Dos Santos JC: Sur la desobstruction des thromboses arterielles anciennes, Mem Acad Chir 73:409, 1947.
9. Wylie EJ: Thromboendarterectomy for arteriosclerotic thrombosis of major arteries, Surgery 23:275, 1952.
10. Blakemore A and Voorhees AB: The use of tubes constructed from Vinyon-N cloth in bridging arterial defects: experimental and clinical, Ann Surg 140:324, 1954.
11. Imparato AM et al: The results of tibial artery reconstruction procedures, Surg Gynecol Obstet 138:33, 1974.
12. Maini BS and Mannick JA: Effect of arterial reconstruction on limb salvage: a ten year appraisal, Arch Surg 113:1297, 1978.
13. Reichle FA et al: Long-term results of 474 arterial reconstructions for severely ischemic limbs: a 14 year follow-up, Surgery 85:93, 1979.
14. Hall V: The great saphenous vein used in-situ as an arterial shunt after extirpation of the vein valves, Surgery 51:492, 1962.
15. Leather RP, Powers SR, and Karmody AM: A reappraisal of the in-situ saphenous vein arterial bypass and its use in limb salvage, Surgery 86:453, 1979.
16. Kannel WB and McGee DL: Diabetes and cardiovascular disease: the Framingham Study, JAMA 241:2035, 1979.
17. McDaniel MD and Cronenwett JL: Basic data related to the natural history of intermittent claudication, Ann Vasc Surg 3:273, 1989.
18. Brand FN, Abbott RD, and Kannel WB: Diabetes, intermittent claudication, and risk of cardiovascular disease. The Framingham Study, Diabetes 38:504, 1989.
19. McCready RA, Vincent AE, and Schwartz RW: Atherosclerosis in the young: a virulent disease, Surgery 96:863, 1984.
20. Newman AB et al: Morbidity and mortality in hypertensive adults with a low ankle/arm blood pressure index, JAMA 270:487, 1993.
21. Vogt MT et al: Decreased ankle/arm blood pressure index and mortality in elderly women, JAMA 270:465, 1993.
22. Kannel WB and McGee DL: Update on some epidemiologic features of intermittent claudication: the Framingham Study, J Am Geriatr Soc 33:13, 1985.
23. Bartecchi CE, MacKenzie TD, and Schrier RW: The human costs of tobacco use (first of two parts), N Engl J Med 330:907, 1994.
24. Cigarette smoking among adults—United States, 1991, MMWR Morb Mortal Wkly Rep 42:230, 1993.
25. Radack K and Wyderski RJ: Conservative management of intermittent claudication, Ann Intern Med 113:135, 1990.
26. Kannel WD and Shurtleff D: The Framingham Study. Cigarettes and the development of intermittent claudication, Geriatrics 28:61, 1973.
27. Krupski WC: The peripheral vascular consequences of smoking, Ann Vasc Surg 5:291, 1991.
28. Couch NP: On the arterial consequences of smoking, J Vasc Surg 3:807, 1986.
29. Jonason T and Ringquist I: Factors of prognostic importance for subsequent rest pain in patients with intermittent claudication, Acta Med Scand 218:27, 1985.
30. Myers KA et al: The effect of smoking on the late patency of arterial reconstruction in the legs, Br J Surg 65:267, 1978.
31. Greenhalgh RM et al: Smoking and arterial reconstruction, Br J Surg 68:605, 1981.
32. Herring M, Gardner A, and Glover J: Seeding human arterial prostheses with mechanically derived endothelium. The detrimental effect of smoking, J Vasc Surg 1:279, 1984.
33. Kannel WB: Update on the role of cigarette smoking in coronary heart disease, Am Heart J 101:319, 1981.
34. Thomas M: Smoking and vascular surgery, Br J Surg 68:601, 1981.
35. Hughson WG, Mann JI, and Garrod A: Intermittent claudication: prevalence and risk factors, Br Med J 1:1379, 1978.
36. Wells AJ: Passive smoking as a cause of heart disease, J Am Coll Cardiol 24:546, 1994.
37. Howard G et al: Active and passive smoking are associated with increased carotid wall thickness. The Atherosclerosis Risk and Community Study, Arch Intern Med 154:1277, 1994.
38. Pollin W: The role of the addictive process as a key step in causation of all tobacco related diseases, JAMA 252:2874, 1984.
39. Molgaard J et al: Significant association between low-molecular-weight apolipoprotein a isoforms and intermittent claudication, Arterioscler Thromb 12:895, 1990.
40. Molgaard J et al: Hyperhomocyst(e)inaemia: an independent risk factor for intermittent claudication, J Intern Med 231:273, 1992.
41. Eldrup-Jorgenson J et al: Hypercoagulable states and lower limb ischemia in young adults, J Vasc Surg 9:334, 1989.
42. Ciuffetti G et al: The hemorrheological role of cellular factors in peripheral vascular disease, Vasa 17:168, 1988.
43. Hertzer NR: The natural history of peripheral vascular disease. Implications for its management, Circulation 83(suppl I):I-12, 1991.
44. Jurgens JL, Barker NW, and Hines EA Jr: Arteriosclerosis obliterans: review of 520 cases with special reference to pathogenic and prognostic factors, Circulation 21:118, 1960.
45. Humphries AW et al: Evaluation of the natural history and results of treatment in occlusive arteriosclerosis involving the lower extremity in 1,850 patients. In Wesolowski SA and Dennis C, eds: Fundamentals of vascular grafting, New York, 1963, McGraw-Hill.
46. Jonason T and Ringqvist I: Diabetes mellitus and intermittent claudication. Relation between peripheral vascular complications and location of occlusive atherosclerosis in the legs, Acta Med Scand 218:217, 1985.
47. Jonason T and Bergstrom R: Cessation of smoking in patients with intermittent claudication: effects on the risk of peripheral vascular complications, myocardial infarction and mortality, Acta Med Scand 221:253, 1987.
48. Cox GS et al: Non-operative treatment of superficial femoral artery disease: long-term follow up, J Vasc Surg 17:172, 1993.
49. Coffman JD: Intermittent claudication: not so benign, Am Heart J 112:1127, 1986.
50. Hertzer NR et al: Late results of coronary bypass in patients with peripheral vascular disease: I. Five-year survival ac-

cording to age and clinical cardiac status, Cleve Clin Q 53:133, 1986.

51. Criqui MH et al: Mortality over a period of 10 years in patients with peripheral arterial disease, N Engl J Med 326:381, 1992.

52. Mecley M et al: Atherosclerotic plaque hemorrhage and rupture associated with crescendo claudication, Ann Intern Med 117:663, 1992.

53. Castronuevo JJ and Flanigan DP: Pseudoclaudication of neurospinal origin, Vasc Diag Ther 5:21, 1984.

54. Stephens MM, O'Connell D, and McManus F: Neurogenic claudication (spinal stenosis), Br Med J 77:235, 1984.

55. Kozol RA et al: Dependent rubor as a predictor of limb risk in patients with claudication, Arch Surg 119:932, 1984.

56. Wilbourn AJ et al: Ischemic monomelic neuropathy, Neurology 33:447, 1983.

57. Kim D, Orron DE, and Skillman JJ: Surgical significance of popliteal arterial variants and a unified angiographic classification, Ann Surg 210:776, 1989.

58. Yao JST: Hemodynamic studies in peripheral arterial disease, Br J Surg 57:761, 1970.

59. Hodgson KJ and Sumner DS: Noninvasive assessment of lower extremity arterial disease, Ann Vasc Surg 2:174, 1988.

60. Hiatt WR et al: Clinical trials for claudication. Assessment of exercise performance, functional status, and clinical endpoints, Circulation 92:614, 1995.

61. Gardner AW et al: Progressive vs. single-stage treadmill test for evaluation of claudication, Med Sci Sports Exer 23:402, 1991.

62. Rutherford RB, Lowenstein DH, and Klein MF: Combining segmental systolic pressures and plethysmography to diagnose arterial disease of the legs, Am J Surg 138:211, 1979.

63. Kram HB, Appel PL, and Shoemaker WC: Multisensor transcutaneous oximetric mapping to predict below knee amputation wound healing: use of a critical P_{O_2}, J Vasc Surg 9:796, 1989.

64. Bandyk DF: Essentials of graft surveillance, Semin Vasc Surg 6:92-102, 1993.

65. Rhodes RS and Cohen AM: Magnetic resonance imaging and spectroscopy in the study of cardiovascular disease, J Vasc Surg 2:354, 1985.

66. Mitchell DG and Carabasi A: Vascular applications of magnetic resonance imaging, Ann Vasc Surg 3:400, 1989.

67. Owen RS et al: Magnetic resonance imaging of angiographically occult runoff vessels in peripheral arterial occlusive disease, N Engl J Med 326:1577, 1992.

68. Cambria RP et al: The potential for lower extremity revascularization without contrast arteriography: experience with magnetic resonance angiography, J Vasc Surg 17:1050, 1993.

69. Dientfass L: Elevation of blood viscosity, aggregation of red cells, hematocrit values and fibrinogen levels in cigarette smokers, Med J Aust 1:617, 1975.

70. DeWeese JA and Rob CG: Autogenous venous grafts ten years later, Surgery 82:775, 1977.

71. Hertzer NR et al: Late results of coronary bypass in patients presenting with lower extremity ischemia: the Cleveland Clinic Study, Ann Vasc Surg 1:411, 1986.

72. Seldinger S: Catheter replacement of the needle in percutaneous arteriography, Acta Radiol 39:368, 1953.

73. Dardik I et al: Routine intraoperative angiography: an essential adjunct in vascular surgery, Arch Surg 110:184, 1975.

74. Quick CRG and Cotton LT: The measured effect of stopping smoking on claudication, Br J Surg 69(suppl):24, 1982.

75. Robicsek F et al: The effect of continued cigarette smoking on the patency of synthetic vascular grafts in Leriche syndrome, J Thorac Cardiovasc Surg 70:107, 1975.

76. Greenhalgh RM et al: Smoking and arterial reconstruction, Br J Surg 68:605, 1981.

77. Skinner JS and Strandness DE Jr: Exercise and intermittent claudication. II. Effect of physical training, Circulation 36:23, 1967.

78. Elkroth R et al: Physical training of patients with intermittent claudication: indications, methods, and results, Surgery 84:640, 1978.

79. Hiatt WR et al: Benefits of exercise conditioning for patients with peripheral arterial disease, Circulation 81:602, 1990.

80. Hiatt WR and Regensteiner JG: Exercise rehabilitation in the treatment of patients with peripheral arterial disease, J Vasc Med Biol 2:163, 1990.

81. Williams LR et al: Vascular rehabilitation: benefits of a structured exercise/risk modification program, J Vasc Surg 14:320, 1991.

82. Coffman JD: Vasodilator drugs in peripheral vascular disease, N Engl J Med 300:713, 1979.

83. DeFelice M, Gallo P, and Masotti G: Current therapy of peripheral obstructive arterial disease. The non-surgical approach, Angiology 41:1, 1990.

84. Cameron HA, Waller PC, and Ramsay LE: Drug treatment of intermittent claudication: a critical analysis of the methods and findings of published clinical trials, 1965-1985, Br J Clin Pharmacol 26:569, 1988.

85. Duprez D and Clement DL: Medical treatment of peripheral vascular disease: good or bad? Eur Heart J 13:49, 1992.

86. Porter J et al: Pentoxifylline efficacy in the treatment of intermittent claudication: multicenter controlled double blind trial with objective assessment of chronic occlusive arterial disease patients, Am Heart J 104:66, 1982.

87. Lindgard F et al: Conservative drug treatment in patients with moderately severe chronic occlusive peripheral arterial disease, Circulation 80:1549, 1989.

88. Goldhaber SZ et al: Low dose aspirin and subsequent peripheral arterial surgery in the Physicians Health Study, Lancet 340:143, 1992.

89. McTavish D, Fauds D, and Goa KL: Ticlopidine. An updated review of its pharmacology and therapeutic uses in platelet-dependent disorders, Drugs 40:238, 1990.

90. Ganzon L et al: Prevention of myocardial infarction and stroke in patients with intermittent claudication: effects of ticlopidine. Results from STIMS, the Swedish Ticlopidine Multicentre Study, J Intern Med 227:301, 1990.

91. Phagher B: On behalf of the STIMS Group. Long-term effects of ticlopidine on lower limb blood flow, ankle/brachial index and symptoms in peripheral arteriosclerosis. A double-blind study, Angiology 45:777, 1994.

92. Scheffler et al: Intensive vascular training in stage IIB of peripheral arterial occlusive disease. The additive effects of intravenous prostaglandin E_1 or intravenous pentoxyfilline during training, Circulation 90:818, 1994.

93. Mannarino E et al: Physical training and anti-platelet treatment in stage II peripheral arterial occlusive disease: alone or combined? Angiology 41:513, 1991.

94. Prevention of Atherosclerotic Complications with Ketanserin Trial Group: Prevention of atherosclerotic complications: controlled trial of ketanserin, Br Med J 298:424, 1989.

95. Brevetti G et al: Increases in walking distance in patients with peripheral vascular disease treated with L-carnitine: a double-blind, crossover study, Ther Prevent 77:767, 1988.

96. Carlson LA and Erikksson I: Femoral artery infusion of

prostaglandin E in severe peripheral vascular disease, Lancet 1:155, 1976.

97. Gruss JD et al: Conservative treatment of inoperable arterial occlusion of the lower extremities with intraarterial prostaglandin E_1, Br J Surg 69(suppl II):II-103, 1982.

98. Schuler JJ et al: The efficacy of prostaglandin E_1 (PGE_1), in the treatment of lower extremity ischemic ulcers secondary to peripheral vascular occlusive disease: results of a prospective, randomized, double-blind, multicenter clinical trial, J Vasc Surg 1:160, 1984.

99. Cronenwett JL et al: Prostacyclin treatment of ischemic ulcers and rest pain in unreconstructable peripheral arterial occlusive disease, Surgery 100:369, 1986.

100. Brown BG et al: Regression of coronary artery disease as a result of intensive lipid-lowering therapy in men with high levels of apolipo-protein B, N Engl J Med 323:1289, 1990.

101. Blankenhorn DH et al: Beneficial effects of combined colestipol-niacin therapy on coronary atherosclerosis and coronary venous bypass grafts, JAMA 257:3233, 1987.

102. Rick ME: Protein C and protein S: vitamin K dependent inhibitors of blood coagulation, JAMA 263:701, 1990.

103. Flinn WR et al: Improved long-term patency of infragenicular polytetrafluoroethylene bypass grafts, J Vasc Surg 7:685, 1988.

104. Baxter BR et al: Prospective assessment of antithrombotic therapy following primary below knee prosthetic bypass. Paper presented at the meeting of the Society for Vascular Surgery, Los Angeles, June 1990.

105. Hertzer NR: Fatal myocardial infarction following lower extremity revascularization, Ann Surg 193:492, 1981.

106. Hertzer NR et al: Late results of coronary bypass in patients with peripheral vascular disease. I. Five year survival according to age and clinical cardiac status, Cleve Clin Q 53:133, 1986.

107. Blakeman BM, Littody FN, and Baker WH: Intra-arterial digital subtraction angiography as a method to study peripheral vascular disease, J Vasc Surg 4:168, 1986.

108. O'Hara PJ et al: Intraoperative autotransfusion during abdominal aortic reconstruction, Am J Surg 145:214, 1983.

109. Ewing M: The history of lumbar sympathectomy, Surgery 70:791, 1971.

110. Diez J: Un neuro metodo de simpatectomia perferica para el tratamiento de affecionas trofilas y gangrenosas de las miembrios, Med Soc Cir Buenos Aires 8:10, 1924.

111. Adson AW and Brown CE: Treatment of Raynaud's disease by lumbar ramisection and ganglionectomy and perivascular sympathectomy neurectomy of the common iliacs, JAMA 84:1908, 1925.

112. Rutherford RB and Valenta J: Extremity blood flow and distribution: the effect of arterial occlusion, sympathectomy and exercise, Surgery 69:332, 1971.

113. Cronenwett JL and Lindenauer SM: Hemodynamic effects of sympathectomy in ischemic canine hind limbs, Surgery 87:417, 1980.

114. Persson AV, Anderson LA, and Padberry FT Jr: Selection of patients for lumbar sympathectomy, Surg Clin North Am 65:393, 1985.

115. Walker PM and Johnston KW: Predicting the success of sympathectomy: a retrospective study using discriminant function and multiple regression analysis, Surgery 87:216, 1980.

116. Yao JST and Bergan JJ: Predictability of vascular reactivity relative to sympathetic ablation, Arch Surg 107:767, 1973.

117. Satiani B et al: Prospective randomized study of concomitant lumbar sympathectomy with aortoiliac reconstruction, Am J Surg 143:755, 1982.

118. Walker PM et al: Phenol sympathectomy for vascular occlusive disease, Surg Gynecol Obstet 146:741, 1978.

119. Naylor AR, Ah-See AK, and Engeset J: Aortoiliac endarterectomy: an eleven year review, Br J Surg 77:190, 1990.

120. Costantino MJ, Smith RB III, and Perdue GD: Segmental aortic occlusion: an unusual lesion found in menopausal women, Surgery 114:318, 1979.

121. Sicard GA et al: Comparison between the transabdominal and retroperitoneal approach for reconstruction of the infrarenal aorta, J Vasc Surg 5:19, 1987.

122. Ernst CB: Prevention of intestinal ischemia following abdominal aortic reconstruction, Surgery 93:102, 1983.

123. Fisher DR Jr and Fry WJ: Collateral mesenteric circulation, Surg Gynecol Obstet 164:487, 1987.

124. Martinez BD, Hertzer NR, and Beven EG: Influence of distal arterial occlusive disease on prognosis following aorto-bi-femoral bypass, Surgery 88:795, 1980.

125. Rutherford RB, Patt A, and Pierce WH: Extra-anatomic bypass: a closer view, J Vasc Surg 5:437, 1987.

126. Morris GC Jr et al: Surgical importance of profunda femoris artery: analysis of 102 cases with combined aortoiliac and femoropopliteal occlusive disease treated by revascularization of the deep femoral artery, Arch Surg 82:52, 1961.

127. Leeds FH and Gilfillan RS: Revascularization of the ischemic limb: importance of the profunda femoris artery, Surgery 82:25, 1961.

128. Martin P, Renwick S, and Stephenson CL: On the surgery of the profunda femoris artery, Br J Surg 55:539, 1968.

129. Bernhard VM, Ray LI, and Militello JP: The role of angioplasty of the profunda femoris artery in revascularization of the ischemic limb, Surg Gynecol Obstet 142:840, 1976.

130. Boren CH et al: Profunda popliteal collateral index: a guide to successful profundaplasty, Arch Surg 115:1366, 1980.

131. David TE and Drezner AD: Extended profundaplasty for limb salvage, Surgery 84:758, 1978.

132. Edwards WH et al: Extended profundaplasty to minimize pelvic and distal tissue loss, Ann Surg 211:694, 1990.

133. Dale WA, DeWeese JA, and Scott JM: Autogenous venous shunt grafts, Surgery 46:145, 1959.

134. Szilagyi DE et al: Autogenous vein graft in femoropopliteal atherosclerosis: the limits of its effectiveness, Surgery 86:836, 1979.

135. Taylor LM Jr et al: Reversed vein bypass to infrapopliteal arteries: modern results are superior to or equivalent to insitu bypass for patency and vein utilization, Ann Surg 205:90, 1987.

136. Veith FJ et al: Six-year prospective multicenter randomized comparison of autologous saphenous vein and expanded polytetrafluoroethylene grafts in infrainguinal arterial reconstructions, J Vasc Surg 3:104, 1986.

137. Taylor RS, McFarland RJ, and Cox MI: An investigation into the causes of failure of PTFE grafts, Eur J Vasc Surg 1:335, 1987.

138. Tyrrell MR et al: Experimental evidence to support the use of interposition vein collars/patches on distal PTFE anastomoses, Eur J Vasc Surg 4:95, 1990.

139. Ibrahim IM et al: Adjunctive arteriovenous fistula with tibial and peroneal reconstruction for limb salvage, Am J Surg 140:246, 1980.

140. Paty PSK et al: Remote distal arteriovenous fistula to improve infrapopliteal bypass patency, J Vasc Surg 11:171, 1990.

141. Edwards WS: Composite reconstruction of the femoral ar-

tery with saphenous vein after endarterectomy, Surg Gynecol Obstet 111:651, 1960.

142. Sobel I et al: Gas endarterectomy, Surgery 59:517, 1961.

143. Taylor LM, Edwards JM, and Porter JM: Present status of reversed vein bypass grafting: five year results of a modern series, J Vasc Surg 11:193, 1990.

144. Donaldson MC, Mannick JA, and Whittemore AD: Femoral-distal bypass with the in-situ greater saphenous vein and long term results using the Mills valvulotome, Ann Surg 213:457, 1991.

145. Quinones-Baldrich WJ et al: Long term results of infrainguinal revascularization with polytetrafluoroethylene: a ten year experience, J Vasc Surg 16:209, 1992.

146. Leather RP et al: Resurrection of the in situ saphenous vein bypass, Ann Surg 208:435, 1988.

147. Weaver FA et al: The lesser saphenous vein: autogenous tissue for lower extremity revascularization, J Vasc Surg 5:687, 1987.

148. Harris RW et al: Successful long-term limb salvage using cephalic vein bypass grafts, Ann Surg 200:785, 1984.

149. Balshi JD et al: The use of arm veins for infrainguinal bypass in end-stage peripheral vascular disease, Arch Surg 124:1078, 1989.

150. Mukherjee D, Schickler WJ, and Inahara T: The superficial femoral artery as a conduit: an alternative to prosthetic material, J Vasc Surg 2:739, 1989.

151. DeLaurentis DA and Friedman P: Sequential femoropopliteal bypasses: another approach to the inadequate saphenous vein problem, Surgery 71:400, 1972.

152. Veith FJ et al: Tibiotibial vein bypass grafts: a new operation for limb salvage, J Vasc Surg 2:552, 1985.

153. Pomposelli FB et al: Dorsalis pedis arterial bypass and durable limb salvage for foot ischemia in patients with diabetes mellitus, J Vasc Surg 21:375, 1995.

154. Bandyk DF et al: Monitoring functional patency of in-situ saphenous vein bypasses: the impact of a surveillance protocol and elective revision, J Vasc Surg 11:207, 1990.

155. Green RM et al: Comparison of infrainguinal graft surveillance techniques, J Vasc Surg 11:207, 1990.

156. Rutherford RB et al: Suggested standards for reports dealing with lower extremity ischemia, J Vasc Surg 4:80, 1986.

157. Dotter CT and Judkins MP: Transluminal treatment of arteriosclerotic obstructions: description of a new technique and a preliminary report of its application, Circulation 30:654, 1964.

158. Gruntzig A and Hopff H: Percutaneous rekanlisation chronish arterieller verschlasse mit einem neuen dilationskatheter, Dtsch Med Wochenschr 99:2502, 1974.

159. Palmaz JC et al: Intraluminal stents in atherosclerotic iliac artery stenosis: preliminary report of a multicenter study, Radiology 168:727, 1988.

160. Parodi JC, Palmaz JC, and Barone HD: Transfemoral intraluminal graft implantation for abdominal aortic aneurysms, Ann Vasc Surg 5:491, 1991.

161. Johnston KW et al: Five year results of a prospective study of percutaneous transluminal angioplasty, Ann Surg 206:403, 1987.

162. Johnston KW: Femoral and popliteal arteries: reanalysis of results of balloon angioplasty, Radiology 183:767, 1992.

163. Johnston KW: Iliac arteries and reanalysis of balloon angioplasty, Radiology 186:207, 1993.

164. Lalka SG and Malone JM: Patient evaluation and preparation for amputation. In Rutherford RB, ed: Vascular surgery, ed 3, Philadelphia, 1989, WB Saunders.

165. McIntyre KE Jr et al: Guillotine amputation in the treatment of nonsalvageable lower extremity infections, Arch Surg 119:450, 1984.

166. Malone JM and Goldstone J: Lower extremity amputation. In Moore WS, ed: Vascular surgery: a comprehensive review, New York, 1986, Grune & Stratton.

167. Plecha FR et al: The early results of vascular surgery in patients 75 years of age and older: an analysis of 3259 cases, J Vasc Surg 2:769, 1985.

168. Couch NP et al: Natural history of the leg amputee, Am J Surg 133:469, 1977.

169. Johansen K et al: Improvement of amputation level by lower extremity revascularization, Surg Gynecol Obstet 153:707, 1981.

170. Martin JD et al: Radical treatment of mal perforans in diabetic patients with arterial insufficiency, J Vasc Surg 12:264, 1990.

CHAPTER TWELVE

ENDOVASCULAR TREATMENT OF PERIPHERAL VASCULAR DISEASE

J. Michael Bacharach
Timothy M. Sullivan

Charles T. Dotter's initial experience with transluminal dilatation and his report of treating ischemic extremities with this new technique in 1964 represents the beginning of a new era in the treatment of peripheral vascular disease.[1] Following Dotter's lead, numerous individuals including Porstmann, Wierney, Zeitler, van Andel, and Grüntzig contributed to the early development of endovascular techniques.[2-6] With time, percutaneous transluminal angioplasty (PTA) has evolved from a novelty to an important therapeutic modality in the treatment of peripheral vascular disease.

Modern endovascular therapy encompasses an array of mechanical techniques including balloon angioplasty, atherectomy, and a variety of endoluminal stents and stent grafts. Catheter-directed thrombolytic therapy has complemented these techniques and expanded their applicability. Pharmacologic therapies aimed at the cellular and subcellular levels may in the future dramatically alter the way in which peripheral vascular diseases are treated.

It is beyond the scope of this chapter to provide an in-depth review of all the currently available endovascular techniques. Rather, it provides an overview of endovascular therapies and some insight into what lies on the horizon.

PATIENT SELECTION

The traditional indications for lower-extremity revascularization (surgical and nonsurgical) have included limb-threatening arterial insufficiency such as rest pain and tissue loss (nonhealing ulcers or gangrene). Life-style or work-limiting claudication has been a sufficient, though less compelling, indication. As the results of percutaneous revascularization have improved, the indications for nonsurgical intervention have relaxed somewhat. Those patients who might not have otherwise been offered treatment (i.e., stable claudicators) are now considered acceptable candidates for endovascular intervention. Technologic developments and improved patient selection have produced significant improvements in procedural results, in both the short- and long-term. However, it is important to assess an individual's degree of disability, the likelihood of technical success, and the overall chance for clinical improvement before subjecting any patient to an interventional procedure.

Patients who have significant medical comorbidities that place them at increased risk for surgical revascularization may benefit from percutaneous revascularization. Many of these patients, however, have diffuse, multilevel occlusive disease and therefore may not be ideal candidates for percutaneous treatment alone. Before considering an endovascular procedure, it is imperative to consider what surgical options exist should the procedure fail, be partially successful, or result in a complication requiring urgent surgical repair. It is especially important to recognize that a combination of percutaneous and standard surgical techniques may be the best option for some patients. An example is the patient with both suprainguinal and infrainguinal disease who might avoid an aortic reconstruction by PTA and stenting of an iliac lesion to improve inflow, followed by a femoral-femoral or femoral-popliteal bypass to salvage a threatened lower extremity.

Another group of patients who lend themselves well to percutaneous intervention are those with life-style–limiting claudication whose disease is focal and limited to short segments of the arterial tree. Generally these lesions are easily and durably treated by endovascular therapy. Finally, there is a segment of patients with limb-threatening ischemia who have had multiple failed surgical revascularizations for femoral-popliteal and tibial disease in whom a suitable available conduit (i.e., autologous vein) is limited. These patients may be candidates for a percutaneous procedure. This challenging group of patients may require a variety of techniques such as catheter-directed thrombolytic therapy and mechanical intervention with balloon angioplasty, atherectomy, and/or stents.

The practitioner must weigh the risks and potential benefits for the individual patient before considering any type of therapy whether medical, surgical, or interventional. It is important to recognize that some of these techniques do have limitations in terms of initial technical success, durability, and risk.

TECHNICAL AND SAFETY CONSIDERATIONS

Physicians treating patients with vascular disease are well acquainted with the basic principles underlying the mechanism of balloon angioplasty. Many new devices use similar principles and technologies, or in the case of stents, augment balloon angioplasty by providing a structural framework to overcome elastic recoil and intimal dissection. Although the presumed mechanisms of transluminal catheter techniques are important, it is perhaps more helpful to the practitioner caring for vascular patients to have an understanding of the basic issues regarding safety and the incidence of complications with endovascular techniques. With this understanding, patient selection can be enhanced, and both physician and patient can have realistic expectations of technical success and associated procedural risks.

Endovascular intervention, by definition, requires vessel access remote from the site of proposed intervention either by cutdown or by percutaneous needle puncture. Devices such as catheters, guidewires, balloon catheters, and stents are manipulated and directed through the peripheral vasculature to the site of pathology. Mechanical device–related complications may occur at a number of locations: at the entry site adjacent to the target lesion or at points in between. Because of their inherent thrombogenicity, these devices may cause thrombotic complications as well.

COMPLICATIONS

The overall complication rate for endovascular intervention is higher than for diagnostic angiography alone. The spectrum of complications ranges from minor local complications requiring no therapy to those more severe requiring urgent surgical repair. Death as a result of endovascular therapy is rare. Published data from a number of series support a mortality of less than 0.5%. When death does occur, it is usually in patients who have significant comorbidities related to cerebrovascular or cardiovascular disease.

Access site complications clearly comprise the majority of those associated with endovascular therapy. Puncture site hematomas, arteriovenous (AV) fistulas, and pseudoaneurysms occur in 2% to 8% of cases.[7] Significant puncture site complications that require surgical repair generally occur in less than 1% of cases. In a study of the anatomic and clinical factors associated with complications of transfemoral arteriography, Lily et al reviewed 10,589

transfemoral arteriographic procedures over 4 years.[8] A total of 47 complications requiring surgical intervention were discovered, for an overall surgical repair rate of 0.44%. The total risk of puncture site–related complications in their large series was estimated at less than 1%. A recent evaluation of 381 patients who underwent percutaneous interventional procedures at the Cleveland Clinic revealed AV fistulas in 1.4%, pseudoaneurysms in 3.1%, and hematomas in 13.3%. Transfusions were required in 7.3% of all patients. Factors associated with bleeding and vascular complications were postprocedure anticoagulation, multiple procedures performed concurrently, female gender, and older age group.

An additional complication important to recognize is that of distal embolization. Although this complication tends to occur in less than 1% of cases, it can have important clinical consequences.

Complications at the Site of Intervention

The most common and serious complication at the site of peripheral intervention is acute occlusion, which is estimated to occur in 1% to 7% of cases. Thrombosis is generally the underlying etiology, although focal dissection with disruption of an intimal flap or local spasm can contribute. Systemic anticoagulation during angioplasty is an important adjunct in preventing focal thrombosis. This is particularly true when dealing with smaller arteries or in situations where there is low flow.

Subintimal dissection or perforation at a stenosis site can also occur. In most cases, especially in vessels below the inguinal ligament, there is no significant clinical consequence. With the development of improved steerable guidewires, and enhanced imaging capabilities including intravascular ultrasound (IVUS), many of these complications can be avoided.

PERCUTANEOUS TRANSLUMINAL ANGIOPLASTY

Background

It is only through morphologic and pathologic studies of treated arteries that the mechanisms of balloon angioplasty, atherectomy, and stent placement have been elucidated. Much of the data pertaining to peripheral angioplasty have been gleaned from the extensive experience gained in the cardiac interventional laboratory with work done on coronary arteries. Dotter and Judkins[1] initially proposed that the method of arterial luminal enlargement involved remodeling and redistribution of arteriosclerotic plaque. Grüntzig[9,10] in the late 1970s attributed the results of arterial dilatation to controlled injury to the artery, resulting in compression of the atheroma with intimal tearing and enlargement of the outer wall of the vessel. Restoration of adequate flow through the diseased arterial segment was believed to have a major role in the process. Lee et al[11] studied the effect of balloon dilatation on fresh human cadaver hearts. They found a number of histologic changes in coronary arteries after angioplasty, including endothelial disruption, disruption of the collagen and elastin within the tunica intima and tunica media, as well as disturbance of the smooth muscle within the media, stretching of the adventitia, and compression of atheroma with calcified plaques remaining intact. In addition, they noted that none of the intimal tears were severe and that the vessels showed no gross evidence of damage.

More recent studies, however, do not show any evidence of plaque compression as a mechanism of angioplasty.[12-17] These studies suggest that two other mechanisms are involved in the pathophysiology of PTA including desquamation of superficial plaque elements and splitting of the plaque with retraction of intimal flaps as healing occurs. Block et al[18] studied the histologic effects of angioplasty in normal canine coronary arteries, human coronary arteries (postmortem), and in an atherosclerotic rabbit coronary model. In the canine arteries PTA was histologically associated with a loss of endothelium and exposure of subendothelial connective tissue without evidence of intimal splitting. An adherent layer of platelets, fibrin, and red blood cells was found over the denuded portion of the vessel. Autopsy studies of human coronary arteries suggested that luminal enlargement was secondary to "splitting and disruption" of the plaque and media, without evidence of compression of the atherosclerotic plaque. Finally, in a model using an atherosclerotic rabbit aorta, similar findings were reported: loss of endothelial integrity with platelet/fibrin thrombus formation and splitting of the intima to the level of the internal elastic lamina. At 2 weeks the intimal splits were fibrotic, which appeared to cause retraction of the intimal flap and further enlargement of the lumen.

The effects of balloon angioplasty are also mediated by changes in the medial layer of the arterial wall. Castaneda-Zuniga et al[19] reiterated the findings that compression of atheroma was not part of the mechanism of balloon angioplasty. In experimental balloon angioplasty of human cadaver and animal arteries, they demonstrated widening of the artery due to compaction and stretching of elastic fibers, particularly smooth muscle cells. The muscle cell nuclei elongated, resulting in a characteristic corkscrew appearance. In some cases there was disruption of the media and healing by fibrous tissue. They postulate that during balloon angioplasty, the stretched media distends. As it is freed from the underlying intima and plaque, it distends further and can remain distended by blood pressure and "adapt" to circulatory needs. This mechanism is in contrast to that of directional atherectomy, in which the endothelial layer and variable thicknesses of atherosclerotic plaque and media are excised from the lumen of the diseased vessel.[20]

Results of Percutaneous Transluminal Angioplasty

Percutaneous transluminal angioplasty (PTA) has become an accepted and important modality in the treatment of patients with occlusive disease of the peripheral arteries. In recent years the enthusiasm for PTA has risen dramatically because of its less invasive nature and low complication rates when compared to standard surgical therapy. It is especially attractive in those patients with significant comorbid conditions, considered to be at high operative risk, and in those with relatively low levels of disease who would not otherwise be considered for surgery. In selected patients PTA may be the treatment of choice; overall success rates, however, are generally not as high as those of reconstructive surgery with the possible exception of iliac PTA and stenting. As such, it is important to identify which lesions are most amenable to angioplasty, which may be better treated with a traditional surgical approach, and which may be treated with a combination of modalities.

As with any invasive procedure, the risk-benefit ratio must be carefully examined before proceeding. Indications for lower-extremity PTA include those patients with life-style or work-limiting claudication who have failed a trial of conservative therapy (e.g., risk and life-style modification, exercise program) and those with more advanced degrees of ischemia (ischemic rest pain, tissue necrosis). All patients should be evaluated objectively with pulse-volume recording (PVR) and segmental limb pressures before and after the procedure. As vascular interventional procedures are generally performed with patients under local anesthesia with light sedation, few individuals are excluded on the basis of underlying comorbid medical conditions; in fact it is for those patients with severe cardiopulmonary disease (who are at high risk for surgery) that PTA is most attractive. Contraindications to PTA based on anatomic considerations are considered relative and must be weighed against the risk of other forms of therapy. Conditions that have an increased risk of complications with PTA include long-segment occlusions, extremely tortuous vessels, occlusions that contain thrombus, and stenoses adjacent to aneurysms. Patients with atheromatous embolization secondary to an ulcerated atherosclerotic lesion have not been considered for PTA in the past because of the perceived risk of further atheromatous embolization with intervention; recent experience suggests that many of these lesions can be successfully treated with PTA and stents.

Johnston et al[21] reported the results of a prospective series of 984 consecutive patients treated with PTA for peripheral arterial disease in 1987. Variables thought to be prognostically important were recorded and analyzed to assess which were most influential on long-term success. Success (or failure) was determined by a combination of clinical and vascular laboratory criteria. Variables predictive of success included (1) indication (claudication vs. limb salvage), (2) site of dilatation (common iliac vs. other), (3) severity of lesion (stenosis vs. occlusion), and (4) run-off (good vs. poor). For all cases the initial success rate was 88.6%; the success rate (*not* excluding initial failures) at 5 years was 48.2%. The predictive importance of these variables has been reiterated by other authors.[22-25]

In general, large, high-flow vessels in the proximal circulation with good run-off are well treated with PTA; as one travels more distally in the circulatory tree, the results become less durable.

The results of PTA for specific sites and their complications are represented graphically in Figs. 12-1 through 12-4.[21,23-27]

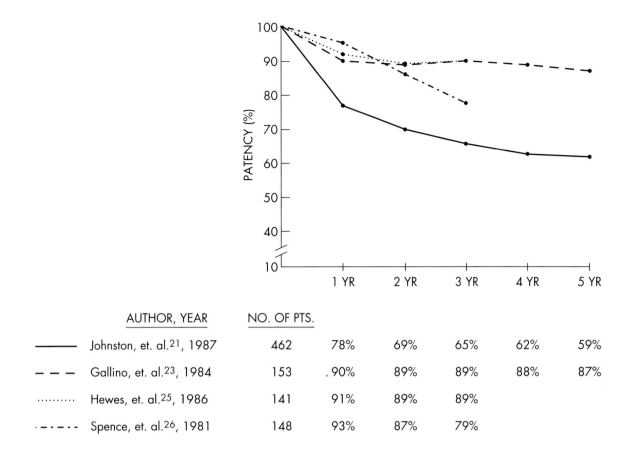

AUTHOR, YEAR	NO. OF PTS.					
Johnston, et. al.[21], 1987	462	78%	69%	65%	62%	59%
Gallino, et. al.[23], 1984	153	90%	89%	89%	88%	87%
Hewes, et. al.[25], 1986	141	91%	89%	89%		
Spence, et. al.[26], 1981	148	93%	87%	79%		

Three- and 5-year patency rates for four series of patients undergoing PTA for aortoiliac arteriosclerotic vascular disease.

Fig. 12-1. Results of aortoiliac PTA from four series reporting 3- and 5-year results. *(From Wilson SE, Sheppard B: Results of percutaneous transluminal angioplasty for peripheral vascular occlusive disease. In Porter JM, Taylor LM, eds: Basic data underlying clinical decision making in vascular surgery, St Louis, 1994, Quality Medical Publishing.)*

INTRAVASCULAR STENTS

Background

Despite reasonable success rates, problems remain with balloon angioplasty including abrupt closure, dissection, and difficulty in treating heavily calcified lesions or total occlusions. Intraluminal vascular stents are designed to improve upon the short- and long-term results of balloon angioplasty. The idea of an intraluminal stent was first proposed by Dotter in 1964.[1] He speculated that an endovascular splint could maintain vessel patency until endothelialization could take place. In 1969 he reported on the use of two types of intravascular stents used in canine femoral and popliteal arteries.[28] The first, an experimental tubular Silastic device, was prone to migrate and thrombose. Some success was achieved, however, with stainless steel wire coils, which were found to endothelialize over

time, promoting long-term patency. Stents may be effective in overcoming elastic recoil of the vessel wall, preventing or treating intimal dissections, and may more effectively treat calcified vessels or those with eccentric plaque. Put simply, they accomplish this by acting as a "scaffold," which tacks the damaged intima and media to the adventitia.

There are, in general, three types of intravascular stents. Thermal memory stents are composed of *nitinol*, an alloy of nickel and titanium. They change shape when exposed to a warm environment (e.g., blood) to adopt a configuration of predetermined shape. Spring-loaded (self-expanding) stents are generally composed of tempered stainless steel wire. They are preloaded into a sheath device and are deployed into the target vessel by removing the sheath. Their final diameter is determined by the residual elasticity of the stent and by the elastic recoil of the vessel wall. They

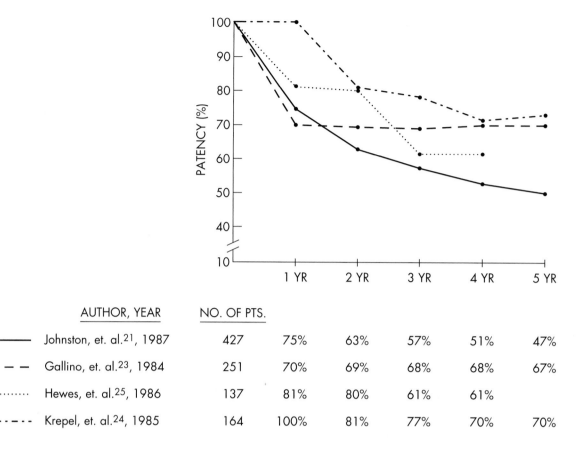

AUTHOR, YEAR	NO. OF PTS.					
——— Johnston, et. al.[21], 1987	427	75%	63%	57%	51%	47%
– – – Gallino, et. al.[23], 1984	251	70%	69%	68%	68%	67%
·········· Hewes, et. al.[25], 1986	137	81%	80%	61%	61%	
-·-·-·· Krepel, et. al.[24], 1985	164	100%	81%	77%	70%	70%

Four- and 5-year patency rates for four series of patients undergoing PTA for femoropopliteal arterio-sclerotic occlusive disease.

Fig. 12-2. Results of femoropopliteal PTA from four studies reporting 4- and 5-year results. *(From Wilson SE, Sheppard B: Results of percutaneous transluminal angioplasty for peripheral vascular occlusive disease. In Porter JM, Taylor LM, eds: Basic data underlying clinical decision making in vascular surgery, St Louis, 1994, Quality Medical Publishing.)*

Results of Infrapopliteal Angioplasty

	Data
Procedure	
Limbs/vessels at risk	126/161
Initial anatomic success (limbs)	119 (94)
Initial clinical results (limbs)	
No amputation	109 (86)
Healed amputation	13 (10.3)
Pre-PTA AAI (mean of 114 limbs)	0.27
Post-PTA AAI (mean of 114 limbs)	0.61
Follow-up	
AAI at 2 yr (mean of 37 limbs)	0.59
Pain-free limbs at 2 yr	32/37

Fig. 12-3. Results of infrapopliteal angioplasty. *(AAI, ankle arm index.) (From Becker GJ, Katzen BT, Dake MD: Noncoronary angioplasty,* Radiology *170:921, 1989.)*

may, however, be further expanded by balloon dilatation. Examples of self-expanding stents are the Gianturco stent and the Wallstent. Plastic or balloon-expandable stents are constructed of a malleable metal such as annealed stainless steel. They are expanded beyond their elastic limit by a coaxial balloon. The Palmaz-Schatz stent is an example.

Desirable characteristics of intravascular stents relate to their deliverability, versatility, and biocompatibility. Ease of deliverability is enhanced by a low profile permitting percutaneous access, longitudinal flexibility allowing the stent to be delivered around tortuous vessels, radiopacity for ease of visualization, reliable expansion, and stable apposition to the vessel wall once deployed. Versatility relates to a high expansion ratio and suitability for numerous vascular sites. Finally, a biocompatible stent is one that promotes rapid endothelialization and does not promote myointimal hyperplasia. A stable nonshifting, nonflexible scaffold is thought to promote the growth of intima; excessive wire thickness, an increased metal-to-free-space ratio, and unstable apposition of the stent to the vessel wall have been implicated in myointimal hyperplasia. Histo-

Complications of 4,662 PTAs (Peripheral and Renal)

Complication	Number (%)
Major	
Death	11 (0.23)
Limb/kidney loss	10 (0.21)
Arteriovenous fistula	4 (0.09)
Thrombus/embolism, any vessel	223 (4.8)
Arterial rupture/ perforation	12 (0.26)
Subtotal (major)	260 (5.57)
Minor	
Hematoma, false aneurysm, minor entry site injury	171 (3.7)
Transient ATN	<41 (<0.88)
Subtotal (minor)	<212 (<4.58)
Total	<472 (<10.1)
Subtotal requiring surgery or other treatment	117 (2.5)

Fig. 12-4. Complications of PTA. (*ATN,* acute tubular necrosis.) *(From Becker GJ, Katzen BT, Dake MD: Noncoronary angioplasty,* Radiology *170:921, 1989.)*

logic studies of the Palmaz-Schatz stent in canines have demonstrated that immediately after implantation, the stent is covered by fibrin and thrombus.[29] At 1 week the fibrin is colonized by immature endothelial cells. From 3 to 8 weeks myofibroblasts and proliferating fibroblasts dominate, followed by regression of matrix over the next 24 weeks. By 32 weeks the stent is covered by a thin neointima.

Clinical Applications of Intravascular Stents

AORTOILIAC. Percutaneous angioplasty of the aortoiliac arterial segment, especially the common iliac arteries, is one of the most common locations of PTA. The 2-year patency rates of common iliac angioplasty exceed 80% in most series. The 5-year rates are from 50% to 87%, with an average of about 72%.[21,27] Stents have been used in the aortoiliac segment in an attempt to improve on these already satisfactory results. In 1992 Palmaz et al[30] reported the results of a multicenter trial of intraluminal stenting of the iliac arteries using the Palmaz stent. The trial, begun in 1987, enrolled 486 patients who had a total of 587 procedures. Eighty-one patients had bilateral iliac stent placements. In follow-up (range, 1 to 48 months; mean, 13.3 months) sustained clinical benefit was obtained in 91% at 1 year, 84% at 2 years, and 67% at 43 months. Two hundred one patients had angiographic follow-up at an average of 8.7 months; the angiographic patency rate (defined as less than 50% stenosis) was 92%. The overall complication rate of 10% was primarily related to the arterial entry site and was not different between the centers involved. As with standard balloon angioplasty, diabetes and poor run-off had a significant negative effect on clinical outcome. These results are similar to other reported series using the Palmaz stent for iliac lesions.[31,32]

Similar results have been reported with the Wallstent, although the number of patients treated is significantly less than those reported with the Palmaz stent.[33,34] Richter et al[35] have reported on the results of a large, randomized, multicenter trial comparing the results of primary PTA alone versus PTA with primary Palmaz stenting for iliac lesions. The mean transstenotic pressure gradient before treatment was similar for the two groups, but the gradient after treatment was significantly less in the stent group (*P* < 0.001). The mean percent restenosis was 27% in the PTA group compared with 14% in the stent group at 24 months, although this difference did not reach statistical significance. Finally, 2% of the stent patients and 28% of the PTA patients required further intervention at 36 months. Others have reported small series of short-term results with PTA and primary stenting of the infrarenal abdominal aorta, with good results.[36-40] Based on these results many investigators recommend primary stenting for stenosis of the aortoiliac arterial segment.

INFRAINGUINAL VESSELS. The role of stents for stenosis or occlusion of infrainguinal blood vessels is less clear than it is for the aortoiliac segment. It is hoped that intravascular devices may improve the success of infrainguinal PTA, especially for long stenoses and occlusions, where the results are less than ideal. Do-dai-Do et al[41] studied the results of 26 patients with lesions of the femoropopliteal arteries treated with balloon angioplasty alone and compared them with 26 matched patients treated with balloon angioplasty and placement of a Wallstent. In the stent group 5 had early thrombosis requiring intervention; at 12 months 10 of the 26 had recurrent stenoses secondary to myointimal hyperplasia. The cumulative secondary patency rate in this group was 69% at 12 months. In comparison the primary PTA group had a 65% primary patency rate at 12 months. The authors concluded that this type of stent does not improve the patency rate of femoropopliteal lesions compared with PTA alone. They may, however, be useful secondarily after an unsuccessful PTA. Others have documented the presence of myointimal restenosis within the stent 3 to 6 months from the time of stent insertion.[42] In one study 8 of 40 patients (20%) developed recurrent lesions of 30% or greater. Using the Strecker stent Liermann et al[43] found a 62% patency rate in femoropopliteal occlusions and 84% in stenotic lesions at 19 months mean follow-up. Published data on the Palmaz stent in the femoral and popliteal vessels are unavailable; enrollment in the FAST (Femoral Artery Stent Trial) study has been terminated and follow-up data are being compiled. Palmaz stents have been used in the tibial vessels to improve the results of failed angioplasty. Anecdotal reports[44] are available, but no series have been published to date. Significant problems remain with the use of intravascular stents in the infrainguinal vessels, especially related to myointimal hyperplasia within the stented segment of vessel. There are no convincing data to support the use of stents as primary therapy in lesions of the femoropopliteal segment. However, stents may be useful in situations where the results of balloon angioplasty alone are unsatisfactory.

RENOVASCULAR DISEASE. Balloon angioplasty is currently the treatment of choice for renovascular disease in which the underlying etiology is fibromuscular dysplasia. It also can be quite beneficial in patients who have nonosteal atherosclerotic stenoses. The most significant problem associated with renal artery stenosis is atherosclerotic plaque that involves the renal ostium. This is, in essence, aortic plaque that extends into the origin of the renal artery and is generally refractory to angioplasty alone. Endoluminal stents have made a significant contribution to the treatment of osteal renal artery disease, and to calcific atherosclerotic disease that does not lend itself well to balloon angioplasty.

Patients most suited to renal revascularization are those who have renovascular hypertension that is not responsive to a good medical regimen. In addition, an increasing number of patients have either bilateral renal artery stenoses or renal artery stenosis to a solitary functioning kidney. This may lead to ischemic nephropathy and renal dysfunction. Many investigators believe that preservation of renal function can be achieved (surgical or endovascular therapy) in patients with severe bilateral disease (see Chapter 18).

Based on available natural history data[45,46] and the observed clinical benefit from surgical revascularization on both hypertension control and renal preservation, there is growing support for a more aggressive approach to the treatment of patients with atherosclerotic renal artery disease. Operative revascularization has demonstrated efficacy and durability, but the associated surgical morbidity and mortality is not inconsequential. This is especially true in high-risk patients who require combined aortic replacement and renal revascularization.[47] Percutaneous techniques may offer lower morbidity and mortality and a shorter hospital stay.

RENAL ARTERY STENTS. The development of endovascular stents has significantly improved the ability to revascularize renal arteries percutaneously. This is particularly true in patients with osteal disease and in those arteries with iatrogenic dissections from angioplasty.

The collective experience with endovascular stents using the Palmaz stent in renal arteries has demonstrated a patency rate of 60% to 90%. European trials with the Wallstent have demonstrated an average patency of approximately 80%. Results of renal artery stenting with these two types of stents is difficult to compare; Palmaz stents were generally used for osteal renal artery stenoses whereas less than half of those who received the Wallstent had osteal disease.

A preliminary study of 98 renal arteries in 77 patients performed at the Cleveland Clinic has been analyzed with respect to patency and clinical outcome. At 12 months of mean follow-up, the patency rate was 81%. Clinical improvement or stabilization of renal function at 12 months was 70% and improvement in blood pressure at 6 months was 66%.

These preliminary data would suggest that renal artery stents may have a significant role in the treatment of renovascular disease. Prospective trials of renal artery stenting compared with surgical revascularization and balloon angioplasty alone will be important in fully defining the role of endovascular stents in the treatment of renal artery disease.

BRACHIOCEPHALIC VESSELS. Symptomatic stenoses and occlusions of the branches of the aortic arch, including the innominate, left common carotid, and left subclavian arteries have been traditionally treated with direct reconstruction (bypass) from the ascending aorta or by extraanatomic bypass with satisfactory results. Endovascular treatment is particularly attractive in these lesions, which are not readily accessible without median sternotomy. Angioplasty alone for these vessels is associated with significant rates of restenosis. For example, restenosis of the subclavian artery following PTA range from 14% to 50% in long-term follow-up.[48-50] A total of 47 patients with stenosis or occlusion of the proximal innominate (6), left common carotid (7), and left subclavian (34) arteries were treated at the Cleveland Clinic with PTA and primary Palmaz stenting. Initial technical success was achieved in 96% of patients. The majority of the subclavian and innominate lesions were treated via a retrograde brachial approach. Of the subclavian and innominate arteries, 39 remain patent in short-term follow-up (range, 1 to 24 months; mean, 3 months). All left common carotid artery repairs were approached via direct retrograde common carotid puncture in the operating room, allowing distal control and prevention of embolization. Three of seven common carotid stents were placed in conjunction with carotid endarterectomy. Initial technical success was achieved in 100%, and in short-term follow-up none has restenosed or occluded. In the short-term this technique yields excellent results and avoids the need for extraanatomic grafting or direct surgical repair. It must be, however, compared with the results of standard surgical techniques over time.

CEREBROVASCULAR INTERVENTIONS. Considerable interest has been generated in the last several years with the use of PTA and primary stenting of stenotic lesions of the internal carotid artery. The North American Symptomatic Carotid Endarterectomy Trial (NASCET)[51] and recently published Asymptomatic Carotid Atherosclerosis Study (ACAS)[52] trials have identified carotid endarterectomy as the treatment of choice for high-grade symptomatic and asymptomatic lesions of the carotid bifurcation and proximal internal carotid artery. A report summarizing the results of carotid PTA for symptomatic cerebrovascular disease in 165 patients concluded that the initial technical success rate was 85% and the complication rate less than 4%.[27] Most of the studies cited offer little data regarding recurrence rates or follow-up, and therefore a valid comparison cannot be made to standard carotid endarterectomy. Similarly, complete data concerning the use of PTA in the vertebral arteries is scarce; as such no recommendations can be made regarding its proper role at this time. There are currently no published reports of the results of PTA and primary stenting of the extracranial carotid artery; anecdotal reports indicate that the procedures are technically feasible and are associated with a moderate risk of complications including stroke. The results of prospective, randomized trials comparing carotid stenting with that of standard bifurcation endarterectomy will be needed to determine the exact role of carotid artery stenting. To be considered a satisfactory form of therapy for patients with cerebrovascular disease, it must be cost-effective and achieve rates of initial technical success, stroke morbidity and mortality, and recurrence equal to or better than that of carotid endarterectomy.

OTHER APPLICATIONS. The proliferation of stents and other interventional devices has opened up a wide array of potential applications for intravascular therapy. A number of conditions that are presently, albeit infrequently, treated by interventional means may be of some interest to the practicing clinician. Among these is the superior vena cava syndrome, from both benign and malignant causes. Because of the fibrous, unyielding nature of these extravascular lesions, they are not readily or permanently well treated by PTA alone. Several reports in the literature have documented the efficacy of stents in large central veins with excellent symptom relief and secondary patency rates as high as 94%.[53-57] Stents clearly represent a significant advance in the treatment of patients with symptomatic lesions of the central veins, a condition with few other successful treatment options. Intravascular stents have also been used in the treatment of aortic dissection in conjunction with fenestration procedures,[58] in failing dialysis fistulas or grafts, and in the mesenteric circulation. They will obviously play an increasing role in the management of peripheral vascular disease as technology and designs improve, and as the problem of restenosis is solved.

The use of PTA with and without stents will likely continue to increase over time. This increase may be due to patient preference, cost savings per treatment relative to surgery (including hospital stay), and improved results of interventional therapies. Several studies have examined the cost issue, concluding that the cost of surgical revascularization is three to five times that of revascularization with PTA, although the additional cost of stents and other new technologies and of additional interventional procedures for recurrence may narrow that difference.[59-61]

Bernstein et al[62] examined changes in their practice with respect to peripheral intervention over three 1-year periods from 1987 to 1992. They found—based on an intention-to-treat analysis—the following: (1) the number of patients evaluated has steadily increased; (2) more patients are being treated with intervention as the initial treatment modality; (3) the results of interventional therapies have not improved significantly over the 5-year study; (4) the percentage of patients undergoing surgery has not changed nor have the excellent results of these surgical procedures; and (5) the number of operations for aortoiliac disease have declined, while the number of distal reconstructions have increased.

Examples of a number of endovascular techniques and their applications are depicted in Figs. 12-5 through 12-8.

ATHERECTOMY

Atherectomy is a technique that attempts to debulk atheroma, thereby mimicking surgical endarterectomy. There are two types of atherectomy devices currently available: rotational and directional. The Simpson directional atherectomy catheter was the first atherectomy catheter to be used in the treatment of peripheral arterial occlusive disease.[63] The directional atherectomy catheter consists of a rotating cutter that is connected to a motor drive unit. A cutting window is held in place against the atheroma by a low-pressure balloon located opposite the window. As the cutting blade is advanced, plaque is excised and collected in a chamber just beyond the cutting window. The rotational device uses a rapidly rotating cutting head to cut atheroma into microfragments.

The potential benefits of atherectomy over angioplasty are that the debulking of irregular calcified atheroma takes place and can reduce recoil. It may have advantages in treating very eccentric lesions or in postoperative bypass restenosis where stenotic lesions tend to be fibrotic and where recoil is often a problem.

The completeness of debulking with atherectomy, either directional or rotational, is often very difficult to measure. Angiography may underestimate the completeness of atherectomy. Intravascular ultrasound (IVUS) can help direct the debulking process and may assure a better luminal result and perhaps improved long-term patency. The relationship between the degree of lesion debulking and long-term patency is unclear.

There have been no randomized trials comparing balloon angioplasty with atherectomy in the peripheral circulation. In fact, the results of atherectomy have not proven superior to those achieved with angioplasty alone. The 2-year patency rates for directional atherectomy have ranged from 37% to 86%.[64-68] In some of these reports adjuvant balloon angioplasty was used.[69] Kim et al[64] did demonstrate 3-year patency rates of 80% to 85% by using aggressive atherectomy and IVUS guidance, leaving less than 30% residual plaque.

The Rotablator rotational atherectomy device has been proposed as particularly useful in unfavorable lesions and in the distal leg arteries. Henry et al observed a restenosis rate of 21% with the Rotablator in the infrapopliteal arteries.[70] The device may have specific usefulness in dealing with tibial arteries, particularly those that have eccentric lesions or diffuse calcification that does not lend itself well to balloon angioplasty. Another important application of atherectomy may be specifically in the area of bypass restenosis. Dolmatch et al[71] demonstrated excellent initial success rates using a directional atherectomy device for anastomotic restenosis in bypass grafts. The technical success rate was 92% with a graft patency of 88% at a mean follow-up of 14 months.

Although there may be advantages to atherectomy for specific lesion types, long-term results are unknown. In addition, cost and procedure time are higher than for balloon angioplasty alone. At the present time atherectomy is a device that has a somewhat limited role in the treatment of peripheral vascular disease.

THROMBOLYSIS

Significant progress has been made in the clinical application of thrombolytic therapy for peripheral arterial occlusive disease since McNichol[72] first attempted the direct local delivery of streptokinase 30 years ago. Catheter-directed intraarterial thrombolysis is now a well-

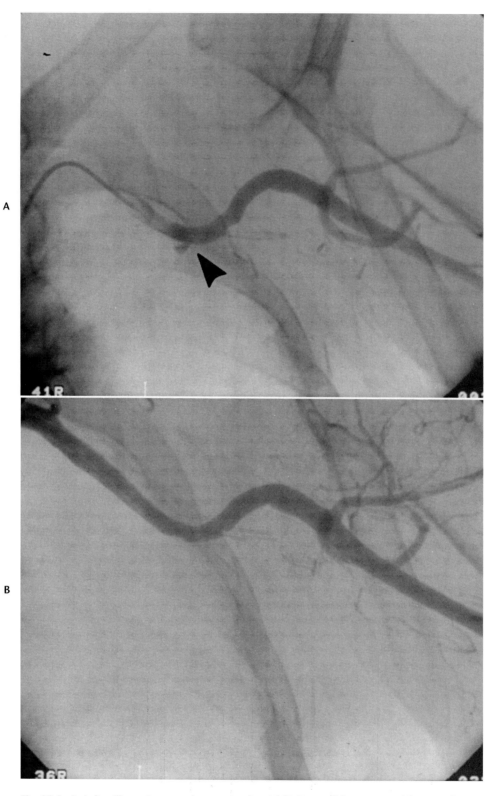

Fig. 12-5. A, Left axillary artery pseudoaneurysm *(arrow).* **B,** Successful treatment with covered stent utilizing vein.

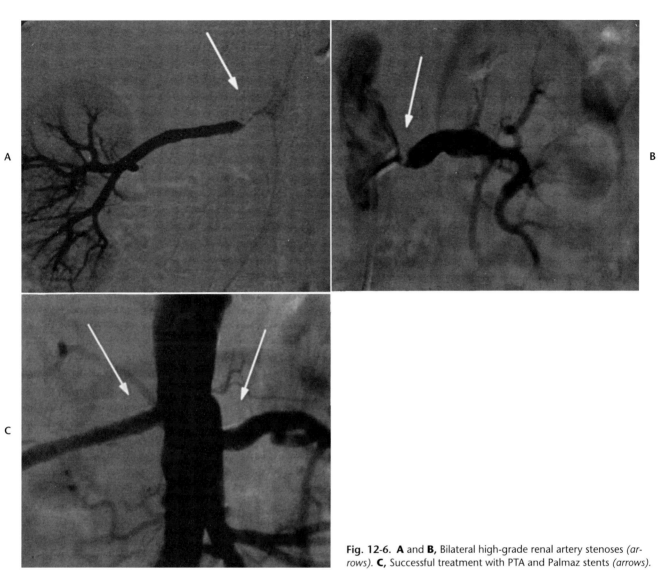

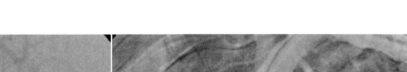

Fig. 12-6. **A** and **B,** Bilateral high-grade renal artery stenoses *(arrows).* **C,** Successful treatment with PTA and Palmaz stents *(arrows).*

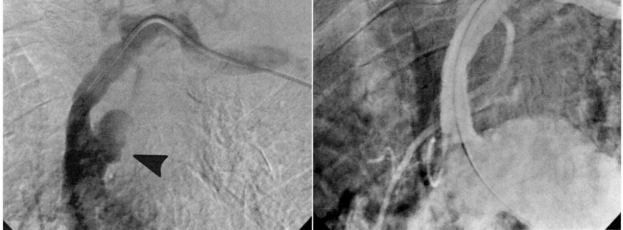

Fig. 12-7. **A,** Left subclavian artery aneurysm *(arrow).* **B,** Treated with PTFE-covered stent via left brachial cutdown.

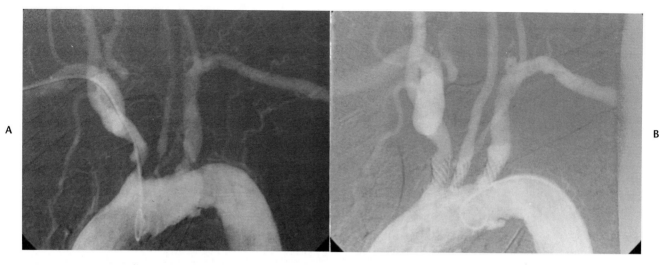

Fig. 12-8. **A,** Stenoses of the brachiocephalic arteries treated with intraluminal stents. **B,** Innominate and left subclavian stents placed via percutaneous right and left brachial punctures. Left common carotid stent placed via open common carotid approach.

established method for the treatment of arterial occlusive disease of both native arteries and bypass grafts in the peripheral circulation. A variety of techniques and infusion catheters have been developed and promoted. Although the designs differ, the general principle of seating the catheter into or through the thrombus to ensure efficient delivery of the thrombolytic agent is similar. Lysis occurs most effectively when the drug is delivered directly into the clot, resulting in high local concentrations of the lytic agent. Catheter-directed thrombolysis improves the likelihood of clot lysis and allows lysis to be achieved with a shorter duration infusion. As a result, clot lysis times of 24 to 72 hours can be shortened to 12 hours or less. Effective clot lysis has been achieved in as little as 4 to 8 hours, using intraarterial infusion of tissue plasminogen activator (t-PA).[73]

Long-term patency of both native arteries and bypass grafts is influenced by a variety of factors. The most important factor is the identification and correction of an underlying stenotic lesion that caused the initial thrombotic event. McNamara and Bamberger[74] demonstrated this convincingly on a group of patients treated for femoral-popliteal occlusions. In patients who had untreated residual stenosis in the reopened arterial segment, the 6-month patency was only 48%, compared with 77% of patients without residual stenosis. The influence of persistent hemodynamic lesions on bypass graft patency is even more dramatic. The same authors reported a 6-month patency rate of 80% for infrainguinal grafts that did not have persistent stenosis, and only 7% in bypass grafts with persistent lesions. Gardiner et al[75] reported a 1-year patency rate of 86% in bypass grafts that had a correctable lesion compared with 37% in lysed grafts with lesions that could not be corrected. Other factors that have played a role in outcome after thrombolytic therapy include initial degree of ischemia,[76] the anatomic location of the lesion, the duration of the occlusion, and the type of graft used (vein vs. prosthetic).[77-80]

The use of thrombolytic agents for the treatment of deep venous thrombosis remains controversial. The basis

for thrombolysis in the treatment of iliofemoral deep vein thrombosis is the preservation of venous valve function, which may help prevent postphlebitic syndrome and reduce venous insufficiency.[81,82] Although thrombolytic therapy has been demonstrated more effective than heparin alone in producing complete lysis of acute deep vein thrombosis, it has not been firmly established to reduce the frequency of the postphlebitic syndrome. Moreover, thrombolytic therapy has not been proven better than standard anticoagulation therapy in decreasing the incidence of pulmonary embolism and its associated mortality.[83]

Although it is our belief that thrombolytic therapy for patients with proximal deep venous thrombosis decreases the likelihood of developing the postphlebitic syndrome, this subject is controversial.[84] Large, prospectively randomized studies comparing heparin, urokinase, and t-PA need to be performed before it can be determined if thrombolytic therapy can lower the incidence of chronic venous insufficiency in patients with proximal venous thrombosis.

Phlegmasia cerulea dolens (venous gangrene) is a form of ileofemoral deep venous thrombosis that results in distal extremity ischemia. Thrombolysis and/or thrombectomy are the treatments of choice for this condition. Catheter-directed thrombolysis into the proximal iliac venous clot and/or direct infusion of the thrombolytic agent into the arterial segment have been successfully employed in this condition.

A detailed discussion of the role of thrombolytic therapy in the treatment of patients with peripheral arterial and venous diseases can be found in Chapter 7.

ENDOVASCULAR GRAFTING FOR THE TREATMENT OF ANEURYSMAL DISEASE

One of the most exciting areas of endovascular therapy involves the placement of endoluminal grafts for the treatment of abdominal aortic aneurysm (AAA). Rupture of AAA remains a significant problem; it is associated with a mortality rate approaching 75% and is the thirteenth leading cause of death in the United States. Standard treatment of AAA involves direct surgical replacement of the diseased (aneurysmal) vessel with a prosthetic conduit of dacron or polytetrafluoroethylene (PTFE). Elective repair of AAA can be performed with a mortality rate of less than 5% in most large medical centers;[85] the operative mortality rate for elective repair at the Cleveland Clinic Foundation is 1.86% (Department of Vascular Surgery Quality Assessment Registry, 1989 to 1995). Despite these excellent results, there is significant morbidity associated with operative repair. Other forms of treatment have been investigated in an attempt to improve these results. Parodi et al began to investigate the feasibility of placing a graft *within* the aneurysm via endovascular means in 1976, reporting on their first clinical series in 1991.[86,87] Their technique involves placing a thin-walled, crimped, knitted dacron graft into the aneurysm via a femoral artery cutdown. The graft is sutured to a Palmaz stent on either end, and the entire device is loaded into a sheath of 18 or 21 Fr. The graft is held in place by the stents, which are fixed to normal artery above and below the aneurysm. Their initial experience was with aortoaortic grafts; an additional number of patients have been treated with aortoiliac grafts in conjunction with occlusion of the contralateral common iliac artery and a femoral-femoral crossover graft. Parodi reported on his first 50 patients in 1995.[88] In this initial experience 40 of the 50 procedures were considered successful. Success was defined as complete exclusion of the aneurysm and restoration of normal blood flow. Complications (in 10 patients) included incomplete deployment of the stent with migration, visceral ischemia related to embolization, fatal atheromatous embolization, stent misplacement and proximal leaks (3 patients) and distal leaks (2 patients). There have been four early procedure-related deaths (8% operative mortality), one late procedural death, and four unrelated deaths in follow-up (range, 1 to 43 months; mean 17 months). Some form of secondary treatment has been required in 6 of the remaining 41 patients, including 2 open operations and 4 secondary endovascular procedures. Despite this favorable early experience, a number of problems limit the use of this particular procedure, including small-caliber iliac arteries, distal leak with a small distal "neck," stent migration, and microembolization with large, tortuous aneurysms. Parodi has now treated over 90 patients; most are treated with the aortoiliac endovascular graft at this time (personal communication, 1992).

Dake et al[89] have recently reported their experience with endovascular repair of descending thoracic aortic aneurysms. They treated 13 patients with atherosclerotic, anastomotic, and posttraumatic true and false aneurysms and aortic dissections of the thoracic aorta with custom-designed endoprostheses. The stent graft was successfully deployed in all patients; there were no deaths and no instances of paraplegia, stroke, or distal embolization. On average follow-up of 11.6 months, there are no perigraft leaks; one patient required surgical repair because of progressive enlargement of the native aorta. Other investigators have reported results with endoluminal grafts to treat aneurysms and injuries of the abdominal aorta and peripheral arteries with varying degrees of success and complication rates.[90-96] At the present time, it appears that a minority of patients will have anatomy suitable for endovascular repair of an AAA using the currently available devices. Yusuf et al[97] evaluated 29 patients for endoluminal graft repair with a bifurcated device and found suitable anatomy in only 5 (17%). With improvements in design and materials, and with continued experience with these evolving techniques, it is likely that an increasing number of aneurysms will be repaired with endoluminal grafts in the future, especially in those patients at high risk for standard open vascular surgical repair.

INTRAVASCULAR ULTRASOUND

Although contrast angiography has been the gold standard for evaluation of arterial pathology, it does not give an accurate three-dimensional picture of the lesions being studied. In fact, angiography does not directly visualize atherosclerotic plaque but rather the residual lumen of the diseased vessel, and as such tends to underestimate the degree of atherosclerosis present, even when taken in multiple projections. This shortcoming is enhanced when studying the results of peripheral vascular interventions.

Intravascular ultrasound (IVUS) has been developed in an attempt to better evaluate vascular morphology. Currently available IVUS catheters range from 2.25 MHz (for imaging large vascular structures such as the aorta) to higher-frequency catheters used to image the coronary arteries (20 to 40 MHz). The most commonly used devices consist of a rotating transducer enclosed within a plastic sheath to protect both the transducer and the vessel being studied. They are generally able to be passed over a guidewire to the site of interest within the vascular tree. IVUS demonstrates the vascular wall as a three-layered structure. The most centrally located layer is the intima, which is of varying thickness depending on the degree of intimal proliferation. The internal elastic membrane is highly echogenic, followed by the echolucent muscular media. The media is seen as a dark zone before the echogenic adventitia. Investigators have found a close correlation between the thickness of plaque on IVUS when compared with histologic sections.[98]

IVUS is ideal for assessing the results of interventional procedures including balloon angioplasty, stent and covered stent placement, and atherectomy. In the coronary circulation IVUS has been useful in determining the presence and type of dissection following PTA, including those types of dissection that may lead to higher rates of restenosis.[99] IVUS may be particularly useful in visualizing intravascular stent deployment. Full apposition of the stent to the vessel wall and full stent expansion may be important in preventing acute and subacute thrombosis, especially in the coronary arteries. Initial stent expansion in the coronaries may be inadequate in up to 70% of cases when examined by IVUS.[100] In the periphery, inadequate stent expansion may lead to early thrombosis or stent migration, and overexpansion may lead to perforation of the vessel or to excessive intimal hyperplasia.[101]

We studied a total of 101 consecutively placed stents in the iliac system in patients with symptomatic occlusive arterial disease of the aortoiliac system.[102] Twenty-five stents (24.7%) were either undersized or incompletely deployed despite normal completion arteriograms and

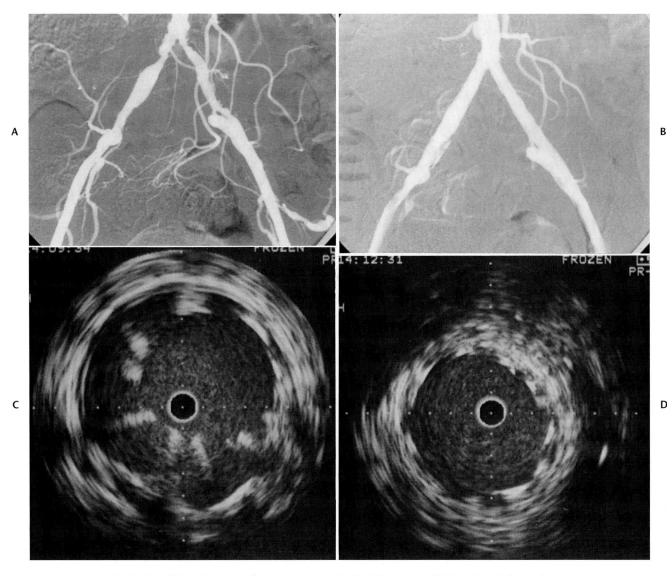

Fig. 12-9. **A,** Bilateral common iliac stenoses treated with Palmaz stents **(B).** Despite satisfactory hemodynamic and angiographic result, note the incomplete deployment of the right iliac **(C)** stent and complete apposition of the left iliac stent to the vessel wall **(D)** when examined with intravascular ultrasound.

normal transstent pressure measurements (Fig. 12-9). IVUS allowed correction of these deficiencies before termination of the interventional procedure. In summary, IVUS is useful in stent deployment to (1) assess the need for stenting, (2) measure arterial diameter proximal and distal to the lesion, (3) select an appropriate balloon and stent, and (4) assess stent position and degree of expansion.[103] In addition, IVUS will likely be invaluable in the deployment of stent grafts in the treatment of AAA.

FUTURE CONSIDERATIONS

As the development of devices, particularly endoluminal stents, has progressed, so have a variety of new applications. Alternatives in the treatment of cerebrovascular disease are now being pursued. Balloon angioplasty, and now endoluminal stents, are actively being tested in the cerebrovascular circulation, particularly for the treatment of carotid artery stenosis. Another area of interest is in the use of cerebral intraarterial thrombolysis. Preliminary data suggest some benefit in patients with evolving thromboembolic stroke.

One of the more exciting areas of future development in endovascular therapy is the intraarterial delivery of drugs or oligonuclear peptides that may provide for a significant reduction in intimal hyperplasia and restenosis. These drugs may be delivered to the target lesion via infusion catheters or via intraarterial stents to which the drug is bonded. As the field of molecular biology progresses, there will be further potential applications for transgenic therapy using molecular-derived growth factors (such as endothelial-derived growth factor) to stimulate angiogenesis, or oligonuclear peptides that can influence the cellular response to injury. Investigators are currently exploring transcatheter gene therapy for the promotion of angiogenesis, and human trials are under way. The area of cellular and molecular biology may well prove to be the most exciting and fruitful area of endovascular therapy.

REFERENCES

1. Dotter CT, Judkins MP: Transluminal treatment of arteriosclerotic obstruction: description of a new technique and a preliminary report of its application, Circulation 30:654, 1964.
2. Porstmann W, Wiermy L: Intravasale rekanalisation, inoperable arterieller obliterationer, Zentralbi Chir 92:1586, 1967.
3. Zeitler E, Muller R: Erste ergebnisse mit, der katheterrakanalisation nach dotter, be, Arterieller Verschivsskrankheit RaFa 111:345, 1969.
4. Van Andel GJ: Percutaneous transluminal angioplasty—The Dotter procedure, Amsterdam, 1976, Excerpta Medic.
5. Gruntzig A: Die perkutane rekanalisation chronischer arterielles verschlusse (Dotter - Prinzip), Miteinem Neven Doppellumigers Dilatjonskatheter Rofo (1):80, 86 1976.
6. Dotter CT: Transluminal angioplasty: a long view, Radiology 135:561, 1980.
7. Gardiner GA et al: Complications of transluminal angioplasty, Radiology 159:201, 1986.
8. Lilly MP et al: Anatomic and clinical factors associated with complications of transfemoral arteriography, Ann Vasc Surg 4:264, 1990.
9. Gruntzig A: Transluminal dilatation of coronary artery stenosis (letter), Lancet 1:263, 1978.
10. Gruntzig AR, Senning A, Siegenthaler WE: Nonoperative dilatation of coronary artery stenosis: percutaneous transluminal coronary angioplasty, N Engl J Med 301:61, 1979.
11. Lee G et al: Evaluation of transluminal angioplasty of chronic coronary artery stenosis. Value and limitations assessed in fresh human cadaver hearts, Circulation 61:77, 1980.
12. Mizuno K, Kurita A, Imazeki N: Pathologic findings after percutaneous transluminal angioplasty, Br Heart J 52:588, 1984.
13. Zarins CK et al: Arterial disruption and remodeling following balloon dilatation, Surgery 92:1086, 1982.
14. Soward AL, Essed CE, Serruys PW: Coronary arterial findings after accidental death immediately after successful percutaneous transluminal coronary angioplasty, Am J Cardiol 56:794, 1985.
15. Potkin BN, Roberts WC: Effects of percutaneous transluminal coronary angioplasty on atherosclerotic plaques and relation of plaque composition and arterial size and outcome, Am J Cardiol 62:41, 1988.
16. Fallon JT: Pathology of arterial lesions amenable to percutaneous transluminal angioplasty, AJR 135:913, 1980.
17. Faxon DP et al: Acute effects of transluminal angioplasty in three experimental models of atherosclerosis, Arteriosclerosis 2:125, 1982.
18. Block PC, Fallon JT, Elmer D: Experimental angioplasty: lesions from the laboratory, AJR 135:907, 1980.
19. Castaneda-Zuniga WR et al: The mechanism of balloon angioplasty, Radiology 135:565, 1980.
20. Johnson DE, Braden L, Simpson JB: Mechanism of directed transluminal atherectomy, Am J Cardiol 65:389, 1990.
21. Johnston KW et al: Five-year results of a prospective study of percutaneous transluminal angioplasty, Ann Surg 206:403, 1987.
22. Cambria RP et al: Percutaneous angioplasty for peripheral arterial occlusive disease: correlates of clinical success, Arch Surg 122:283, 1987.
23. Gallino A et al: Percutaneous transluminal angioplasty of the arteries of the lower limbs: a five-year follow up, Circulation 70:619, 1984.
24. Krepel VM et al: Percutaneous transluminal angioplasty of the femoropopliteal artery; initial and long-term results, Radiology 156:325, 1985.
25. Hewes RC et al: Long-term results of superficial femoral artery angioplasty, AJR 146:1025, 1986.
26. Spence RK et al: Long-term results of transluminal angioplasty of the iliac and femoral arteries, Arch Surg 116: 1377, 1981.
27. Becker GJ, Katzen BT, Dake MD: Noncoronary angioplasty, Radiology 170:921, 1989.
28. Dotter CT: Transluminally placed coil-spring endarterial tube grafts, long-term patency in canine popliteal artery, Invest Radiol 4:329, 1969.
29. Schatz RA et al: Balloon expandable intracoronary stents in the adult dog, Circulation 76:450, 1987.
30. Palmaz JC et al: Stenting of the iliac arteries with the Palmaz stent: experience from a multicenter trial, Cardiovasc Intervent Radiol 15:291, 1992.
31. Richter GM et al: First long-term results of a randomized multicenter trial: iliac balloon-expandable stent placement versus regular percutaneous transluminal angioplasty, Radiology 177:152, 1990 (abstract).
32. Henry M et al: Palmaz-Schatz stents in the treatment of peripheral vascular disases, J Am Coll Cardiol 17:302A, 1991 (abstract).
33. Vowerk D, Guenther RW: Mechanical revascularization of occluded iliac arteries with use of self-expandable endoprostheses, Radiology 175:411, 1990.
34. Zollikofer CL et al: Arterial stent placement with use of the Wallstent: midterm results of clinical experience, Radiology 179:449, 1991.
35. Richter GM et al: Initial long-term results of a randomized five-year study: iliac stent implantation versus PTA, Vasa 35(suppl):192, 1992.
36. Diethrich EB et al: Preliminary observations on the use of the Palmaz stent in the distal portion of the abdominal aorta, Am Heart J 125:490, 1993.
37. Williams JB et al: Balloon angioplasty with intraluminal stenting as the initial treatment modality in aortoiliac occlusive disease, Am J Surg 168:202, 1994.
38. Long AI et al: Infrarenal aortic stents: initial clinical experience and angiographic follow up, Cardiovasc Intervent Radiol 16:203, 1993.
39. El Ashmaoui A et al: Angioplasty of the terminal aorta: follow up of 20 patients treated by PTA or PTA with stents, Eur J Radiol 13:113, 1991.
40. Roeren T et al: Stent angioplasty of the infrarenal aorta and aortic bifurcation. Clinical and angiographical results of a prospective study, Radiology 34:504, 1994.
41. Do-Dai-Do et al: A comparison study of self-expandable stents vs. balloon angioplasty alone in femoropopliteal occlusions, Cardiovasc Intervent Radiol 15:306, 1992.
42. Rousseau H et al: Treatment of femoropopliteal stenoses by means of self-expandable endoprostheses: midterm results, Radiology 172:961, 1989.
43. Liermann D, Strecker EP, Peters J: The Strecker stent: indications and results in iliac and femoropopliteal arteries, Cardiovasc Intervent Radiol 15:298, 1992.
44. Dorros G, Hall P, Prince C: Successful limb salvage after recanalization of an occluded infrapopliteal artery utilizing a balloon expandable (Palmaz-Schatz) stent, Cathet Cardiovasc Diagn 28:83, 1993.

45. Schreiber MJ, Pohl MA, Novick AC: The natural history of atherosclerotic and fibrous renal artery disease, Urol Clin North Am 11:383, 1984.

46. Zierler RE et al: Natural history of atherosclerotic renal artery stenosis. A prospective study with duplex ultrasound, J Vasc Surg 19:250, 1994.

47. Hallett JW et al: Renovascular operations in patients with chronic renal insufficiency. Do the benefits justify the risks? J Vasc Surg 5:622, 1987.

48. Duber C et al: Percutaneous transluminal angioplasty for occlusion of the subclavian artery: short and long-term results, Cardiovasc Intervent Radiol 15:205, 1992.

49. Millaire A et al: Subclavian angioplasty: immediate and late results in 50 patients, Cathet Cardiovasc Diagn 29:8, 1993.

50. Mathias KD, Luth I, Haarmann P: Percutaneous transluminal angioplasty of proximal subclavian artery occlusions, Cardiovasc Intervent Radiol 16:214, 1993.

51. North American Symptomatic Carotid Endarterectomy Trial Collaborators: Beneficial effect of carotid endarterectomy in symptomatic patients with high-grade carotid stenosis, N Engl J Med 325:445, 1991.

52. Executive Committee for the Asymptomatic Carotid Atherosclerosis Study: Endarterectomy for asymptomatic carotid artery stenosis, JAMA 273:1421, 1995.

53. Elson JD et al: Vena caval and central venous stenoses: management with Palmaz balloon-expandable intraluminal stents, J Vasc Interv Radiol 2:215, 1991.

54. Rosenblum J et al: Intravascular stents in the management of acute superior vena cava obstruction of benign etiology, J Parenteral Enteral Nutr 18:362, 1994.

55. Solomon N, Wholey MH, Jarmolowski CR: Intravascular stents in the management of superior vena cava syndrome, Cathet Cardiovasc Diagn 21:245, 1991.

56. Khanna S et al: Superior vena cava stenosis associated with hemodialysis catheters, Am J Kidney Dis 21:278, 1993.

57. Dake MD, Semba CP, Wexler L: Venous stents: results in 125 cases, J Endovasc Surg 2:201, 1995 (abstract).

58. Walker PI et al: The use of endovascular techniques for the treatment of complications of aortic dissection, J Vasc Surg 18:1042, 1993.

59. Kinnison ML et al: Cost incentives for peripheral angioplasty, AJR 145:1241, 1985.

60. Jeans WD et al: A comparison of the costs of vascular surgery and balloon dilatation in lower limb ischaemic disease, Br J Radiol 59:453, 1986.

61. Wolf GL, McClean GK: Comparison of the cost of bypass surgery and transluminal angioplasty for peripheral vascular disease, Semin Intervent Radiol 1:237, 1984.

62. Bernstein EF et al: Changing pattern practice patterns in peripheral arterial disease, Ann Vasc Surg 8:186, 1994.

63. Simpson JB et al: Transluminal atherectomy. Initial clinical results in 27 patients, Circulation 74:203, 1986.

64. Kim DS: Peripheral directional atherectomy. Four year experience, Radiology 183:773, 1992.

65. Dorros G et al: Angiographic follow up and clinical outcome in 126 patients. After percutaneous directional atherectomy for occlusive peripheral vascular disease, Cathet Cardiovasc Diagn 22:79, 1991.

66. Graor RA, Whitlow P: Directional atherectomy for peripheral vascular disease: two year patency and factors influencing patency, J Am Coll Cardiol 17:106A, 1991.

67. Katzen BT et al: Long-term follow up of directional atherectomy in the femoral and popliteal arteries, J Vasc Intervent Radiol 3:30, 1992.

68. Von Polnitz A et al: Percutaneous peripheral atherectomy: angiographic and clinical follow up of 50 patients, J Am Coll Cardiol 15:682, 1990.

69. Dorros G, Lyer S, Zaitoun R: Acute angiographic and clinical outcome of high speed percutaneous rotational atherectomy (Rotablater), Cathet Cardiovasc Diagn 22:157, 1991.

70. Henry M et al: Percutaneous peripheral rotational ablation using the Rotablater: immediate and mid-term results, Int Angiol 12:231, 1993.

71. Dolmatch BL et al: Treatment of anastomotic bypass graft stenosis with directional atherectomy: Short-term and intermediate term results, J Vasc Interv Radiol 6:105, 1995.

72. McNichol GT et al: Treatment of peripheral arterial occlusion by streptokinase perfusion, BMJ 1:1508, 1963.

73. Graor RA et al: Thrombolysis with recombinant human tissue-type plasminogen activator in patients with peripheral artery and bypass graft occlusions, Circulation 74:15, 1986.

74. McNamara TO, Bamberger RA: Factor affecting initial and 6 month patency rates after intraarterial thrombolysis with high dose urokinase, Am J Surg 152:709, 1986.

75. Gardiner GA, Harrington DP, Kolton W: Salvage of occluded arterial bypass grafts by means of thrombolysis, J Vasc Surg 9:426, 1989.

76. McNamara TO, Bamberger RA, Merchant RF: Intraarterial urokinase as the initial therapy for acutely ischemic limbs, Circulation 1:1, 1991.

77. Durham JD, Geller SC, Abbott W: Regional infusion of urokinase into occluded lower extremity bypass grafts: long-term clinical results, Radiology 172:83, 1989.

78. Hess H, Mietasehk A, Bruckle R: Peripheral arterial occlusion: a 6 year experience with local low dose thrombolytic therapy, Radiology 163:753, 1987.

79. Sullivan KL et al: Efficacy of thrombolysis in infrainguinal bypass grafts, Circulation 83:99, 1991.

80. McNamara TG, Goodwin SC, Kandarper K: Complications of thrombolysis, Semin Intervent Radiol 11:134, 1994.

81. Marko A, Strandness D: The potential role of thrombolytic therapy in venous thrombosis, Arch Intern Med 152:1265, 1992.

82. Meissner MH et al: Deep venous insufficiency. The relationship between lysis and subsequent reflux, J Vasc Surg 18:596, 1993.

83. Duckert F: Treatment of deep venous thrombosis with streptokinase, Br Med J 1:479, 1975.

84. Ott P et al: Streptokinase therapy and the routine management of deep venous thrombosis in the lower extremities, Acta Med Scand 219:295, 1986.

85. Brown OW et al: Abdominal aortic aneurysm and coronary disease: a reassessment, Arch Surg 116:1484, 1981.

86. Laborde JC et al: Intraluminal bypass of abdominal aortic aneurysm: feasibility study, Radiology 184:185, 1992.

87. Parodi JC, Palmaz JC, Barone HD: Transfemoral intraluminal graft implantation for abdominal aortic aneurysm, Ann Vasc Surg 5:491, 1991.

88. Parodi JC: Endovascular repair of abdominal aortic aneurysms and other arterial lesions, J Vasc Surg 21:549, 1995.

89. Dake MD et al: Transluminal placement of endovascular stent-grafts for the treatment of descending thoracic aortic aneurysms, N Engl J Med 331:1729, 1994.

90. White GH et al: A new non-stented balloon-expandable graft for straight or bifurcated endoluminal bypass, J Endovasc Surg 1:16, 1994.

91. May J: Comparison of the Sydney and EVT prostheses for treatment of aneurysmal disease, J Endovasc Surg 2:122, 1995 (abstract).

92. Cragg AH: Development of the Cragg endoluminal graft to

treat peripheral occlusive and aneurysmal disease, J Endo-vasc Surg 2:123, 1995 (abstract).

93. Fogarty TJ: Thoracic aortic aneurysm: endovascular stent-graft repair, J Endovasc Surg 2:124, 1995 (abstract).

94. Marin ML et al: Transluminally placed endovascular stented graft repair for arterial trauma, J Vasc Surg 20:466, 1994.

95. Mialhe C: Clinical experience with the Stentor bifurcated device for treatment of abdominal aortic aneurysmal disease, J Endovasc Surg 2:125, 1995 (abstract).

96. Chuter TAM et al: Early clinical experience with bifurcated endovascular grafts for abdominal aortic aneurysm repair, J Endovasc Surg 2:126, 1995 (abstract).

97. Yusuf SW et al: Transfemoral endoluminal repair of abdominal aortic aneurysm with bifurcated graft, Lancet 344:650, 1994.

98. Tobis JM et al: Lessons from intravascular ultrasonography: observations during interventional angioplasty procedures, J Clin Ultrasound 21:589, 1993.

99. Honye J et al: Morphologic effects of coronary balloon angioplasty in vivo assessed by intravascular ultrasound imaging, Circulation 85:1012, 1992.

100. Fitzgerald PJ, Yock PG: Mechanisms and outcomes of angioplasty and atherectomy assessed by intravascular ultrasound imaging, J Clin Ultrasound 21:579, 1993.

101. Busquet J: The current role of vascular stents, Int Angiol 12:206, 1993.

102. Navarro F, Sullivan TM, Bacharach JM: The use of intravascular ultrasound to assess peripheral vascular intervention, Circulation 92(suppl):1, 1995.

103. Scoccianti M et al: Intravascular ultrasound guidance for peripheral vascular interventions, J Endovasc Surg 1:71, 1994.

CHAPTER THIRTEEN

ASSOCIATION OF CORONARY ARTERY DISEASE WITH PERIPHERAL VASCULAR DISEASE

J. Michael Bacharach
Thomas H. Marwick

Atherosclerosis is a systemic disease with the potential to affect multiple vascular beds. The specific association of coronary artery disease and peripheral vascular disease (PVD) is well established. The resultant comorbidity impacts on the perioperative risk associated with surgical revascularization and significantly affects overall survival.

One of the most challenging tasks that the vascular physician and surgeon faces is assessing risk and then adapting or modifying the management decisions to achieve appropriate risk-benefit and long-term outcomes. The development of new technologies to assess cardiac function and the presence of cardiac ischemia allows for improved stratification of risk. These new technologies, however, have also contributed to significant confusion as to how they should be applied to achieve the optimal clinical benefit in a cost-effective manner. A fundamental component of caring for patients with PVD is assessing their cardiovascular status, but the optimal way to do this remains uncertain. This chapter should provide some insight into the available technologies and how they can be selectively and judiciously applied.

PREVALENCE OF CORONARY ARTERY DISEASE IN THE PERIPHERAL VASCULAR DISEASE PATIENT

The reported prevalence of significant coronary artery disease in patients with PVD varies from 16% to 92%.[1-49] The variability can be explained by different methods of assessment and the type of patient studied. Patients undergoing coronary angiographic assessment have typically had higher reported prevalence of coronary artery disease than those patients who were assessed on the basis of clinical evidence of disease.[50]

In a comprehensive analysis by Hertzer,[51] the collective experience of approximately 50 series representing more than 10,000 patients was summarized. Clinical evidence of coronary disease was present in approximately 50% of patients with aortic aneurysms, carotid artery disease, or lower-extremity occlusive disease, ranging from 22% to 70% in individual series. Significant coronary artery disease was observed in approximately 60% of patients in the series where coronary angiography was performed.[51] Additional data from the Cleveland Clinic in a consecutive series of 1,000 patients undergoing coronary angiography demonstrated that even among patients without clinical indications of coronary disease significant coronary artery stenoses were observed in as high as 37% of patients.[22] This compared with observed significant stenoses as high as 78% in patients with clinical indications of coronary artery disease. In addition, multivessel disease was present in the majority of patients with significant angiographic findings.[22,52,53]

Patients stratified according to PVD location have also been shown to have different prevalences of associated coronary artery disease. Patients with abdominal aortic aneurysms have the highest rate of coronary artery disease compared with patients who have isolated PVD involving the carotid arteries or with lower-extremity occlusive disease.* It is important to recognize that irrespective of location, patients with PVD have significantly greater coronary artery disease compared with a normal age-matched population.

*References 13, 16, 17, 22, 23, 54.

IMPACT OF ASSOCIATED CORONARY ARTERY DISEASE ON SURVIVAL

The impact of comorbid coronary artery disease in patients with PVD is twofold. First, the prognosis for perioperative morbidity and mortality in the patient undergoing vascular reconstructive surgery is primarily determined by the presence and extent of associated coronary artery disease. The specific perioperative events include myocardial infarction, congestive heart failure, and arrhythmia. Cardiac etiology accounts for 40% to 60% of early deaths in patients undergoing vascular reconstructive surgery.[13,27,51,55-57] It is estimated that the perioperative mortality rate is approximately four times higher in patients with coronary artery disease compared with those without. Based on 29 reported series of more than 14,000 patients, those without overt evidence of coronary artery disease had an operative mortality of 1.3% compared with an operative mortality of 6.8% in patients with clinical evidence suggesting comorbid coronary artery disease.[50,51] In a population-based study from The Mayo Clinic analyzing elective abdominal aortic aneurysm repair, there was a marked difference in perioperative complications. Patients with overt coronary artery disease had a complication rate of 21% compared with only 7% in patients without overt cardiac disease.[56]

It is likely that the impact of associated cardiac disease on perioperative risk varies substantially with the type of vascular reconstruction. One cannot assign the same perioperative risk of an adverse outcome to carotid endarterectomy or to lower-extremity arterial reconstruction as one would to aortic aneurysm repair. This, however, does not negate the potential adverse effect of associated coronary artery disease on presumably less stressful surgical procedures such as carotid artery endarterectomy or femoropopliteal bypass. In a comparison of cardiac morbidity between aortic and infrainguinal operations, Krupski et al[58] observed a very similar incidence of postoperative cardiac events including nonfatal myocardial infarction, unstable angina, ventricular tachycardia, and congestive heart failure.

Late mortality is the second impact of cardiac disease on patients with PVD. Before the development of modern vascular reconstructive surgical techniques, Juergens, Barker, and Hines[1] at The Mayo Clinic reviewed and described the pathogenic and prognostic factors of a cohort of patients with PVD. From this early natural history study, it was observed that the majority of deaths were cardiac related (in this group of patients). Patients with aortoiliac disease had a worse survival rate than patients with infrainguinal disease. However, survival in both groups was much worse than age- and gender-matched controls. More recent studies have demonstrated 5-year mortality rates that are two to three times that of the general population in patients with symptomatic claudication.[59,60] Criqui, Coughlin, and Fronek[61] reported that the 10-year risk of death caused by cardiovascular disease was 10 to 15 times greater for patients with symptomatic or large-vessel peripheral artery disease compared to those without.

In patients who have undergone vascular surgery, there is a well-established decrease in survival in patients with evidence of cardiac disease. Crawford et al[17] collected extensive long-term survival data on patients who underwent aortic surgery for either aneurysms or occlusive disease. Actuarial survival rates at 5 years were 84% to 89% for patients without clinically indicated coronary artery disease and only 54% in patients with coronary disease. Hertzer et al[62,63] demonstrated very similar results in a series of patients treated at the Cleveland Clinic.

More recently a number of population-based studies have evaluated the influence of coronary artery disease on long-term survival in patients undergoing vascular surgery and have strikingly confirmed the adverse impact it has on long-term survival. Eight-year survival in patients following abdominal aneurysmectomy was 59% in patients without suspected or overt coronary disease. Multivariate analysis demonstrated a twofold increased risk of death and a fourfold increased risk of late cardiac events in patients with suspected but uncorrected coronary artery disease.[56] Farkouh et al[64] analyzed survival rates at 5 and 10 years in a population-based study of patients undergoing lower-extremity revascularization. Survival rate after operation at 5 and 10 years was 77% and 51%, respectively, in patients without overt coronary disease. This compared with survival of 54% and 24% at the same time intervals in patients with known coronary artery disease.

Based on the extensive data available, cardiac disease is the primary determinant of survival in patients with PVD. There is therefore strong support for the concept that the patient with PVD requires careful longitudinal observation independent of whether they require a vascular surgical procedure if optimal survival is to be achieved.

IMPACT OF MYOCARDIAL REVASCULARIZATION

The previous data demonstrate unequivocally the striking influence that cardiac disease has on both perioperative events and long-term survival. In assessing the benefits and indications of myocardial revascularization, it is important to recognize that the goal of reducing perioperative cardiac events and the goal of improving long-term survival need to be considered independently. From nonrandomized studies there are data suggesting that the risk of vascular surgery is low following prior coronary bypass surgery. Data from the Coronary Artery Surgery Study (CASS) demonstrated that the morbidity and mortality rates for noncardiac surgery in patients who had had prior coronary artery surgery were similar to those who had insignificant coronary artery disease based on angiography.[65-68] In a review of seven series of more than 1200 patients, the mean operative mortality for vascular surgical procedures was 1.5% in the cohort who had undergone prior coronary artery surgery. These results were quite similar to the rate of 1.3% observed in patients without evidence of coronary artery disease and were substantially lower than the 6.8% mortality rate observed in patients with uncorrected coronary artery disease.[51] There are also data supporting the survival benefit of coronary artery bypass surgery in patients with PVD. The European Coronary Surgery Study Group demonstrated an 8-year survival rate of 85% in patients who had PVD and were treated with coronary artery surgery, compared with 52% survival in the group randomized to medical therapy. In patients without PVD the survival rates between surgical and medical therapy were 90% and 81%, respectively.[69] In a review of later mortality in vascular patients according to associated coronary artery disease, Hertzer et al[63] summarized a large cumulative experience and found a mean 5-year mortality of 21% in patients with prior coronary artery bypass surgery, compared with 20% in patients with no coronary disease and 41% in patients with suspected coronary disease.

The Cleveland Clinic experience has clearly shown that in select patients with significant coronary artery disease there is an improved 5-year survival rate following vascular surgery in patients treated with coronary artery bypass.[52] Despite the demonstrated benefit of myocardial revascularization with coronary artery bypass, there are associated risks especially in the patient with PVD. With the recognition that associated coronary disease substantially impacts on management considerations for the patient with PVD, the second portion of this chapter concentrates on the goals of assessment and an approach to stratifying risk.

GOALS OF ASSESSMENT

Avoidance of Late Cardiac Mortality

As previously described, PVD and coronary heart disease often coexist. In this situation PVD may be the "index" illness that leads the patient to seek medical care. Many such patients are asymptomatic from the cardiac standpoint, often because their exercise capacity is compromised by claudication or prior stroke, and sometimes because their ischemia is "silent" (e.g., because of diabetes or medical therapy). In these circumstances prognostically important coronary disease may be unidentified.

The concern consequently arises that patients may either succumb to coronary disease or develop symptoms once their vascular disease is treated. Follow-up studies have demonstrated that in the absence of coronary intervention, the rate of significant cardiac events in patients after aortic aneurysm surgery is unacceptably high, ranging from 15% in patients without recognized coronary disease to 61% in patients with suspected or known (but uncorrected) disease.[56] In a follow-up study of 131 patients undergoing elective aortic aneurysm repair at The Mayo Clinic, Roger et al[56] also reported the estimated survival at 8 years to range from 59% to 34% in the same groups. The association of uncorrected coronary disease with a twofold increased risk of death and fourfold increased risk of cardiac events is a strong argument in favor of cardiac risk stratification at the time of presentation with vascular disease. If this evaluation is carried out before surgery, coronary intervention may forestall perioperative ischemia and cardiac events.

Avoidance of Perioperative Complications

FREQUENCY AND NATURE OF CARDIAC COMPLICATIONS. With improvements of surgical and anesthetic techniques, cardiac complications of surgery have become the major cause of mortality and morbidity following many operations. Patients with a history of cardiac disease have a 25% to 50% higher mortality rate than normal,[70] and in the setting of emergency surgery this risk increases between two and four times. The risk of cardiac complications is greater in vascular operations than other procedures of similar magnitude because of the hemodynamic stresses on the circulation, especially if the intervention involves aortic cross-clamping,[71] and the high prevalence of coexisting coronary disease in this group.

Perioperative cardiovascular complications of vascular surgery include cardiac death, myocardial infarction, myocardial ischemia, congestive heart failure, arrhythmias, and severe hypertension. Both major cardiac events—death and myocardial infarction—are rare. Myocardial infarction occurs perioperatively in 0.15% of patients without prior clinical evidence of heart disease but is reported in 3% to 18% of patients with prior infarction.[72] This complication has a high mortality since these patients are unsuitable for thrombolytic therapy, which has substantially reduced infarct mortality rate in other circumstances. Although infarction seems to be infrequently associated with intraoperative ischemia, it correlates quite strongly with postoperative ischemia.[73] Many non–Q wave infarctions occur within 24 hours of surgery, although the typical timing of myocardial infarction postoperatively is within 3 days. Two underlying processes are responsible for perioperative infarction. The first is the severity of the underlying coronary lesions and the second is coronary thrombosis. Although the former component is predictable by preoperative testing, the latter is difficult to predict and may occur with rupture of a minor plaque as well as in the context of a flow-limiting stenosis.

Despite myocardial ischemia, heart failure, hypertension, and arrhythmias being classified as "minor" events, which may not be included as end points in some prognostic studies, they may be responsible for increasing the duration of hospital stay. Nonetheless, a good argument can be made for using only death and myocardial infarction as serious events, as the others are often present to a variable degree preoperatively and usually respond well to treatment.

Despite the high prevalence of coronary disease in patients with vascular disease, perioperative cardiac events are relatively infrequent. In the absence of preoperative coronary intervention, the overall event rate in one series was 18%, although both the mortality and the frequency of nonfatal myocardial infarction were 1%.[73] This low frequency of major end points poses a statistical challenge for the use of preoperative testing to identify patients at risk of cardiac events. According to Bayes' theorem, the posttest probability of disease is most influenced by the results of testing if the patient is at intermediate (pretest) probability of disease (e.g., 20% to 80%). Fortunately the rationale of preoperative testing is not based purely on the reduction of operative risk but also on the reduction of subsequent cardiac events, which are more frequent.

CAUSES OF PERIOPERATIVE CARDIAC EVENTS. The causes of perioperative cardiac events include intraoperative and postoperative phenomena. Intraoperative cardiovascular stresses occur as a response to surgery and the direct and indirect effects of anesthetic agents (reduced myocardial contractility, tachycardia, or hypotension).

Hypotension may be caused by the vasodilator effects of anesthetics, intermittent positive-pressure ventilation, and hypovolemia, whereas hypertension may be induced by intubation. Patients may become hypoxemic because of anesthetic effects. Increased autonomic activity provoked by surgery may induce cardiovascular instability. Spinal and regional anesthetics are arguably "safer" for patients with cardiac disease,[74] but hypotension caused by vasodilation and increased autonomic activity resulting from inadequate pain relief may be potent contributors to cardiovascular complications. Indeed, the nature of the anesthetic is probably less important than careful monitoring and rapid response to the development of cardiovascular problems. In the postoperative period circulatory stress may be contributed to by hemorrhage, infection, and pain. Additionally the development of a hypercoagulable response to surgery over the subsequent few days may contribute to the development of coronary thrombosis and venous thromboembolic disease.

Although careful intraoperative and postoperative anesthetic care may avoid factors that initiate a cardiac event, the underlying substrate of many events is coronary artery disease. As coronary disease becomes increasingly prevalent with the aging of the surgical population, the preoperative assessment of cardiac risk is increasingly important.

CARDIAC RISK STRATIFICATION

Association of Clinical Features with Cardiac Events

The probability of coronary artery disease may be calculated on the basis of the clinical history, based specifically on the patient's age, gender, history of angina, infarction, diabetes, smoking, and hypertension.[75,76] The same factors—apart from gender, smoking, and hypertension—were found by Pryor et al[76] to predict subsequent cardiac events in patients undergoing vascular surgery. Similarly, Jamieson et al[20] reported previous vascular surgery, clinically evident coronary disease, and diabetes to predict late mortality; the presence of one and two factors being associated with a 20% and a 33% late mortality, respectively. In a study of 566 patients undergoing vascular surgery, Cooperman et al[77] showed mortality to be increased in the presence of prior myocardial infarction, heart failure, stroke, arrhythmias, and abnormal electrocardiogram (ECG), especially if more than one of these factors were present.

Clinical Approach to Risk Stratification

The history and physical examination (rather than routine noninvasive testing) are the cornerstones of preoperative risk assessment. The resting ECG and chest x-ray should be performed if there is any suspicion of cardiac disease. Further investigations should be undertaken in patients with intermediate or indeterminate pretest probability of developing complications.

The clinical history should focus on current cardiovascular symptoms and exercise capacity, together with the medical history. In relation to exercise capacity, if a patient is able to exercise within classes I or II (doing housework or

able to walk briskly for a couple of blocks), they are probably increasing the rate-pressure product to the level that would be expected during general anesthesia. If the patient's history seems unreliable in this context, a standard exercise test is a reasonable means of confirming exercise capacity. If the patient is unable to exercise, investigations examining myocardial function, perfusion, or both may be combined with a pharmacologic stress test. With respect to history, specific questions should be directed toward the presence and timing of previous angina and myocardial infarction, previous myocardial revascularization, coexisting valvular disease, congestive heart failure, arrhythmias, or the presence of a permanent pacemaker.

RECENT MYOCARDIAL INFARCTION. Twenty years ago patients undergoing general anesthesia within 3 months of infarction were found to have a 30% risk of reinfarction or cardiac death, which decreased to 15% between 3 and 6 months following infarction. However, with recent improvements in monitoring and treatment, these risks have fallen to between 0% and 6% in the first 3 months and less than 2% in the first 6 months.[78] Nonetheless, if the patient has had recent myocardial infarction and truly elective surgery is planned, the most prudent policy is to delay 6 months; conversely, surgery clearly must proceed irrespective of risk for emergent indications. The most difficult (and most frequent) decisions are required in postinfarction patients needing semielective surgery—for example, for cancer or painful and limiting arthritic problems. In these situations it is prudent to wait 4 to 6 weeks for the myocardial scar to heal and then assess risk on the basis of usual clinical indicators. Thus patients at highest risk are the elderly, those with postinfarction ischemia, severe left ventricular dysfunction, and extensive reversible perfusion defects; perioperative risk may be reduced in these patients by revascularization before the planned operation. However, in lower-risk patients without significant jeopardized tissue, surgery less than 6 months after infarction is likely to be safe.

CHRONIC STABLE ANGINA AND PAST MYOCARDIAL INFARCTION. Patients with chronic stable angina and previous infarction have known coronary disease and often engender concerns regarding the occurrence of new infarction under anesthesia. In these situations the extent as well as presence of ischemia is an important concern, and preoperative stress testing is often performed to further identify coronary risk.

PREVIOUS MYOCARDIAL REVASCULARIZATION. From a retrospective analysis of the CASS study,[68] it was found that the mortality rate of patients with significant coronary artery disease undergoing major operations without bypass surgery was 2.4% compared with 0.9% in patients with previous myocardial revascularization. However, the reduction of cardiovascular risk was greatest in those with impaired left ventricular function, congestive heart failure, the elderly, and diabetics. Noncardiac operations are safe following myocardial revascularization, although it is prudent to delay 1 month, particularly after open heart surgery, if possible.

VALVULAR HEART DISEASE. Patients with valvular heart disease are at increased risk of congestive heart failure, endocarditis, and embolization perioperatively and frequently do not tolerate tachycardia. Noncardiac surgery is contraindicated in the presence of severe aortic and mitral stenosis. If cardiac surgery is inappropriate, a balloon valvuloplasty may be a reasonable option to permit noncardiac surgery to proceed.[79] In addition to predicting perioperative risk, anticoagulant cover and endocarditis prophylaxis in valvular heart disease patients must be carefully planned.

CONGESTIVE HEART FAILURE. Patients with a history or clinical signs of congestive heart failure should be treated for this problem preoperatively. Surgery should be delayed for about a week to allow establishment of a steady state before noncardiac surgery. In patients older than 40 years, perioperative congestive heart failure occurs in about 2% of cases overall, including 6% of patients with controlled congestive heart failure, and in 16% of cases with poorly controlled congestive heart failure.[56]

OVERALL COMPUTATION OF CARDIAC RISK. The results of the clinical history, examination, and simple investigations have been combined into various risk indices for noncardiac surgery. Some caution needs to be applied to the application of general surgical risk indices such as the ASA criteria to the vascular surgery population, among whom coronary disease and its risks are a substantial concern. Similarly, although the Goldman et al score[80] has been shown to indicate perioperative risk in an initial series of 1000 unselected patients, it does not account for smoking and other coronary risk factors, remote myocardial infarction, and even mild angina, which have been shown to be important predictors of outcome in the vascular surgery group, as previously discussed. This index underestimates risk[81] in patients with a high-risk status on the basis of clinical factors or who is undergoing abdominal aortic aneurysm surgery. The modification of this score by Detsky et al[82] to include angina and a history of pulmonary edema may have rendered this score more attractive for patients with vascular disease. Nonetheless, in elderly patients with reduced exercise capacity, cardiac events have been documented in the absence of significant risk status on the Goldman et al score.[83] This is an important shortcoming in patients with vascular disease, among whom exercise capacity is often compromised.

In patients undergoing general anesthesia (but not necessarily for vascular surgery), Ashton et al[84] have reported on the complication rates associated with particular cardiac risk profiles in nearly 1500 patients. Among patients with *diagnosed* coronary disease (prior infarction, angina, or angiographically documented disease), the perioperative cardiac mortality was 2%, with myocardial infarction occurring in 4%. In those with *suspected* disease (atypical angina or diagnosed vascular disease), these events occurred in 0.4% and 0.8%, respectively. Finally, in patients at low risk (risk factors or age over 70 years), the cardiac mortality was 0.4%. This approach is similar to that developed by Eagle et al[85] specifically for use in patients with vascular disease. According to this profile, the clinical markers of cardiac risk include age over 70 years, diabetes, angina, and prior myocardial infarction. The cardiac event rate at vascular surgery is 5% in patients without these factors, 15% in the presence of one or two, and 50% in the setting of three or more factors.[85]

The accuracy of various risk factor scores for the prediction of perioperative cardiac events has been studied by Lette et al[86] in a group of 125 patients undergoing vascular surgery, 13 of whom suffered cardiac events.[86] The assignment of high or intermediate risk using the Goldman or ASA scores was associated with unacceptably low sensitivity. The Detsky, and particularly the Eagle, score had a greater sensitivity, but at the cost of low specificity. These results suggest that patients predicted by clinical scoring to be at intermediate risk should be stratified further with a functional test.

NONINVASIVE TESTING FOR CORONARY ARTERY DISEASE

A bewildering variety of diagnostic techniques may be used for the detection of coronary disease. These may be performed at rest or using exercise, pharmacologic, or other stressors. However, although exercise testing is an important means of diagnostic and prognostic evaluation in most patients with suspected coronary disease, the accuracy of all testing modalities (ECG, thallium, or echocardiography) is dependent on the performance of adequate stress, which is difficult in many patients with vascular disease.[87] Thus the major alternative functional studies for prediction of perioperative risk in patients with vascular disease are dipyridamole, adenosine, or dobutamine stresses in combination with myocardial perfusion imaging (thallium, [MIBI], or positron emission tomography [PET] studies) or stress echocardiography, and ambulatory ST-segment monitoring.

EXERCISE ELECTROCARDIOGRAM. In addition to the dependence of the exercise ECG on an adequate cardiac work load, the results of this test may be influenced by antihypertensive and antianginal therapies, digoxin, occult left ventricular hypertrophy, and hypokalemia secondary to diuretic use—all of which are common in patients with vascular disease. Nonetheless, Cutler et al[18] reported that no major perioperative events occurred in patients attaining greater than 75% of age-predicted maximal heart rate with a normal exercise ECG. In contrast, patients with an ischemic response had a 4% incidence of infarction, and those who had a positive test at a submaximal heart rate had a 26% incidence of infarction and a perioperative cardiac mortality of nearly 20%.

NUCLEAR VENTRICULOGRAPHY. Resting ejection fraction (EF) is an important prognostic determinant in most patients with cardiac diseases. Preexisting left ventricular dysfunction (often associated with prior infarction or congestive heart failure) is associated with cardiac events, and hence the specificity of this test is higher in patients with more severe left ventricular dysfunction (EF < 30% to 35%). However, this technique does not identify myocardial ischemia, so that in most studies it has been shown to be insensitive for the prediction of perioperative events in vascular surgery patients.[88,89]

STRESS MYOCARDIAL PERFUSION IMAGING. Exercise myocardial perfusion scintigraphy (most commonly using thallium-201 or technetium isonitrile com-

Table 13-1. Clinical Picture, Events, and Event Rates in Various Diagnostic Groups Using Dipyridamole Thallium Imaging for Perioperative Risk Stratification in Patients Undergoing Vascular Surgery

Author	n	Events	Events	Tl-isc	Tl-isc ER	Tl-scar ER	ER of nl
Boucher et al[92]	48	Death, MI, UAP	8 (17%)	16 (33%)	8 (50%)	0 (0%)	0 (0%)
Eagle et al[93]	111	Death, MI, UAP, CHF	18 (16%)	42 (38%)	16 (38%)	6 (18%)	–
Lette et al[94]	66	Death, MI	9 (14%)	27 (41%)	9 (43%)	0 (0%)	0 (0%)
Younis et al[44]	111	Death, MI	8 (7%)	50 (45%)	6 (12%)	2 (10%)	0 (0%)
Marwick and Underwood[95]	86	Death, MI, UAP	10 (12%)	9 (10%)	3 (16%)	(See isch)	7 (11%)
Mangano et al[96]	60	Death, MI, UAP, CHF	13 (22%)	22 (37%)	6 (27%)	4 (22%)	3 (15%)
Hendel et al[97]	327	Death, MI	294 (9%)	186 (57%)	26 (14%)	22 (12%)	1 (1%)
Cambria et al[98]	58	Death, MI	2 (3%)	26 (45%)	2 (15%)	–	–
Takase et al[99]*	53	Death, MI, UAP, CHF	13 (25%)	15 (28%)	8 (53%)	2 (33%)	3 (9%)
Younis et al[100]*	161	Death, MI, UAP, CHF	25 (15%)	50 (31%)	15 (30%)	5 (23%)	5 (6%)
Baron et al[101]	457	Death, MI, UAP, CHF, VT	86 (19%)	160 (35%)	31 (19%)	23 (24%)	32 (16%)

*Includes major nonvascular surgery.
Tl-isc, Ischemia at dipyridamole thallium imaging; *CHF,* congestive heart failure; *ER,* event rate (calculated in nonrevascularized patients); *MI,* myocardial infarction; *UAP,* unstable angina; *Tl-scar,* Thallium scar; *VT,* ventricular tachycardia.

pounds) is usually reported to have a sensitivity of greater than 90% for the detection of coronary artery disease.[90] The specificity of thallium single photon emission computed tomography (SPECT) has been reported to be in the 70% to 80% range; false positives may be caused by factors that are quite prevalent in the vascular surgery population, including soft tissue attenuation, left ventricular hypertrophy, and left-sided bundle branch block. Failure to exercise maximally compromises the sensitivity of this technique,[91] and in these circumstances dipyridamole stress testing is an acceptable alternative. Most of the literature on risk stratification for vascular patients using myocardial perfusion imaging has focused on dipyridamole stress. However, patients who are able to exercise maximally should do so, as exercise capacity is prognostically important and may facilitate decisions regarding myocardial revascularization.

A number of studies using either thallium or technetium-99m sestamibi in combination with planar and SPECT imaging have demonstrated that the absence of myocardial ischemia at myocardial perfusion imaging is predictive of a low risk of perioperative cardiac events, whereas its presence is somewhat correlated with events (Table 13-1). However, the clinical impact of perfusion scintigraphy continues to be debated, and several researchers have found this method of risk stratification to be ineffective. The reason for this inconsistency is unclear, but it may relate to population selection. The predictive value of these tests for major cardiac events is related to the pretest probability of these events; this relationship has become important as the incidence of serious perioperative cardiac events (death or myocardial infarction) has fallen. In our experience most events occurring in the absence of preoperative ischemia were myocardial infarctions, whereas the presence of inducible ischemia at preoperative evaluation was predictive of perioperative ischemia induced by the stresses of surgery. Although some perioperative myocardial infarctions originate as ischemic episodes, the occurrence of infarction reflects atherosclerotic

plaque rupture and perioperative disturbances of coagulation pathways, which may both contribute to coronary thrombosis. These phenomena cannot be predicted by preoperative perfusion imaging, so that some false-negative results are inevitable.

Resting defects do not predict postoperative cardiac events; previous studies suggesting a correlation between fixed thallium defects and postoperative events may be explained by the potential of severe ischemia masquerading as a fixed thallium defect. The presence of ischemia at perfusion imaging is predictive of subsequent events in only 30% to 50% of patients. One explanation is that the presence of a stress-induced perfusion defect infers the presence of coronary disease, but not all patients with coronary disease are necessarily at high risk. To focus on risk rather than diagnostic aspects, Lette et al[94] have suggested stratification based on the assessment of defect extent using semiquantitative evaluation of thallium scans. However, in our experience the incidence of major postoperative cardiac events remains very low, even in patients with a considerable ischemic burden. It is likely that surgical and anesthetic factors (e.g., hemodynamic monitoring, which may be modified in light of preoperative test results) may explain the poor positive predictive value of reversible perfusion defects.

PET differs from conventional SPECT imaging on the basis of higher energy emissions, greater count rates, and attenuation correction. All of these features favor the accuracy of PET over SPECT, but unfortunately the technique is expensive and not widely available. The sensitivity and specificity of PET for prediction of perioperative events in patients undergoing vascular surgery has recently been reported to be 79% and 76%, respectively.[102] The expense of the technique limits its application for this purpose, but its use may be justifiable for patients in whom imaging is challenging due to obesity and possibly prior myocardial infarction.

PHARMACOLOGIC STRESS ECHOCARDIOGRAPHY. The diagnosis of coronary artery disease using stress

Table 13-2. Studies of Pharmacologic Stress Echocardiography for Perioperative Risk Stratification in Patients Undergoing Vascular Surgery

Author	n	Events	Stress	Events		Sensitivity	Specificity
Tischler et al[104]	109	MI, UAP	DIPY	8	(7%)	88%	98%
Lane et al[105]	57	Death, MI, CABG	Db	4	(7%)	100%	56%
Lalka et al[106]	60	Death, MI, UAP, CABG	Db	10	(17%)	83%	58%
Davila-Roman et al[107]	91	MI, UAP, CABG	Db + atro	17	(19%)	100%	92%
Poldermans et al[108]	131	MI, UAP, CHF	Db + atro	15	(11%)	100%	83%

CABG, Coronary artery bypass grafting; *DIPY,* Dipyridamole; *Db,* Dobutamine; *atro,* Atropine.

echocardiography is based on the detection of stress-induced wall motion abnormalities in the setting of myocardial ischemia. In patients who cannot exercise, dobutamine stress testing is a feasible and accurate alternative, and the accuracy of this test is comparable to that of myocardial perfusion imaging using vasodilator or dobutamine stress.[103] The availability and relative inexpensiveness of stress ECG make this an attractive technique for risk stratification in vascular surgery patients, and preliminary data suggest that pharmacologic stress echocardiography is effective in this setting (Table 13-2).

Dobutamine stress echocardiography has been the most widely used form of this technique for perioperative risk stratification. The predictive value of a negative dobutamine echocardiogram in patients undergoing vascular surgery has been high, reflecting the high sensitivity of dobutamine echocardiography. Indeed, on multivariate testing, the presence of ischemia provoked by dobutamine echocardiography increases the risk of an event by over fortyfold.[108] Even in those patients with a positive test who have surgery canceled, there is a high prevalence of events at follow-up. The predictive value of a positive dobutamine ECG for perioperative cardiac events has been somewhat lower, consistent with the identification of milder coronary disease and correlating with the experience of dipyridamole thallium imaging.

Dipyridamole echocardiography has been used for risk stratification before vascular surgery. The need of dipyridamole to create coronary steal to induce ischemia usually requires the presence of severe or extensive stenoses—hence the technique is relatively insensitive to mild or single-vessel disease and is thereby less sensitive for the diagnosis of coronary disease than is perfusion scintigraphy. The high positive predictive value (78%) of this test reported by Tischler et al[104] in a group of 109 vascular surgery patients may reflect the relatively selective detection of multivessel disease—and therefore those patients who are more likely to develop complications from the stress and hemodynamic challenges of vascular surgery. In contrast, patients with single-vessel disease, who may not be detected with dipyridamole echocardiography, are less likely to suffer a major cardiac event at the time of surgery. Moreover, the lower sensitivity of dipyridamole echocardiography for milder coronary disease did not compromise its negative predictive value (99%).

PERFUSION SCINTIGRAPHY OR STRESS ECHOCARDIOGRAPHY. The various pharmacologic stress imaging combinations share a high negative predictive value for the identification of patients unlikely to suffer perioperative complications. Studies comparing the diagnostic accuracy of these tests have reported them to be comparable, with slightly higher sensitivities for perfusion imaging (but comparable sensitivities for multivessel disease) and somewhat higher specificities for stress echo. Few data exist comparing the prognostic capacity of stress echocardiography and stress perfusion imaging. In our experience the two have been comparable, with the predictive power of a positive stress ECG being greater, possibly reflecting its greater specificity. However, the number of patients with events is small, and a large comparative series is needed to establish the relative roles of these tests.

AMBULATORY ELECTROCARDIOGRAM MONITORING. Spontaneous (usually silent) episodes of ST depression during daily living activities may be recorded using ambulatory ECG monitoring. These may be used as a marker of ischemia in the same way as ST-segment changes during exercise testing. In the existing studies of this technique, the sensitivity of this test for prediction of perioperative events has been favorable,[38] but specificities of 53% to 63% have been recorded.[109,110] The place of this approach relative to the imaging methods remains to be established.

GUIDELINES: HOW TO RESPOND TO PATIENTS AT INCREASED CARDIAC RISK

The possible responses to the classification of patients into high-risk subgroups are limited. In patients undergoing elective surgery, surgical cancelation on the grounds of unacceptable risk is an option, but most consultations for medical clearance are obtained in circumstances where the operation is essential. Stringent monitoring may be undertaken (including the insertion of arterial and pulmonary artery catheters, and transesophageal probes during and after surgery), and to the extent that this may alert the anesthesia team to correct minor hemodynamic disturbances before they become life-threatening, this may prevent cardiovascular events. Once an ischemic event occurs, medical therapy may be initiated, and if necessary,

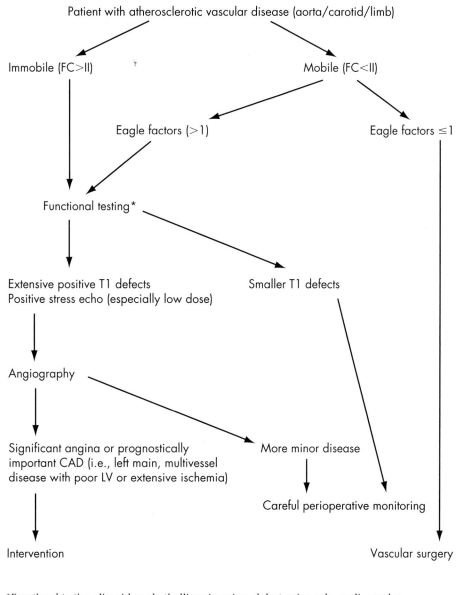

Functional testing, dipyridamole thallium imaging, dobutamine echocardiography (exercise testing is sometimes appropriate). The noninvasive test used should be dependent on the institution's expertise. Patients with asthma should not be given dipyridamole, and those with rhythm problems or hypertension should avoid dobutamine.

Fig. 13-1. Algorithm for preoperative risk stratification of patients undergoing vascular surgery.

an urgent coronary intervention may be obtained early postoperatively.

Prevention of ischemic events may also be achieved by myocardial revascularization or antianginal therapy. The efficacy of the latter is not clearly established, but preliminary (nonrandomized) studies suggest that β-blockers may be effective.[111] Certainly if patients are receiving antianginals, it is prudent to restart them as soon as possible postoperatively, as ischemic episodes occur most commonly 2 to 3 days postoperatively, reflecting pain, tachycardia, fever, and hypercoagulability.[112] The performance of myocardial revascularization before or at the time of the

planned surgery is the final option, but the risk of this in subgroups such as diabetics and the elderly may compromise its benefit in reducing the cardiac risks of major surgery.

SUMMARY

The requisite management decisions to provide for optimal survival and reduced perioperative risk in patients undergoing vascular reconstructive surgery are complex. An algorithm for perioperative risk stratification of patients undergoing vascular surgery is outlined in Fig. 13-1.

Strategies to assess risk are imperfect at best, and there is no one algorithm that is universally applicable. Assessment needs to be individualized based on the patient's clinical status. The specific modality of testing needs to be tailored to the resources available that can provide the highest degree of sensitivity and specificity at defining the extent of coronary artery disease. Often the most compelling indication to initiate cardiac evaluation is in the patient who presents with a problem that requires surgical intervention. If cardiac evaluation is reserved only for this group, a large number of patients with peripheral vascular disease will not realize the potential benefit of longer-term survival that early recognition of coronary artery disease may afford.

REFERENCES

1. Juergens JOL, Barker NW, and Hines EA: Arteriosclerosis obliterans: review of 520 cases with special reference to pathogenic and prognostic factors, Circulation 21:188, 1960.
2. DeBakey ME et al: Aneurysm of abdominal aorta. Analysis of results of graft replacement therapy one to eleven years after operation, Ann Surg 160:622, 1964.
3. DeBakey ME et al: Cerebral arterial insufficiency: one- to 11-year results following arterial reconstructive operation, Ann Surg 161:921, 1965.
4. Baker AG et al: Risk of excision of abdominal aortic aneurysm, Surgery 68:1129, 1970.
5. Tomatis LA, Fierens EE, and Verbrugge GP: Evaluation of surgical risk in peripheral vascular disease by coronary arteriography: a series of 100 cases, Surgery 71:429, 1972.
6. Thompson JE et al: Surgical management of abdominal aortic aneurysms: factors influencing mortality and morbidity—a 20-year experience, Ann Surg 181:654, 1975.
7. Malone JM, Moore WS, and Goldstone J: Life expectancy following aortofemoral arterial grafting, Surgery 81:551, 1977.
8. Young AE, Sandberg GW, and Couch NP: The reduction of mortality of abdominal aortic aneurysm resection, Am J Surg 134:585, 1977.
9. Cooperman M et al: Cardiovascular risk factors in patients with peripheral vascular disease, Surgery 84:505, 1978.
10. Ennix CL et al: Improved results of carotid endarterectomy in patients with symptomatic coronary disease: an analysis of 1546 consecutive carotid operations, Stroke 10:122, 1979.
11. Szilagyi DE et al: Autogenous vein grafting in femoropopliteal atherosclerosis: the limits of its effectiveness, Surgery 86:836, 1979.
12. Grindlinger GA et al: Volume loading and vasodilators in abdominal aortic aneurysmectomy, Am J Surg 139:480, 1980.
13. Hertzer NR: Fatal myocardial infarction following abdominal aortic aneurysm resection: three hundred and forty-three patients followed 6-11 years postoperatively, Ann Surg 192:667, 1980.
14. Whittmore AD et al: Aortic aneurysm repair. Reduced operative mortality associated with maintenance of optimal cardiac performance, Ann Surg 192:414, 1980.
15. Brown OW et al: Abdominal aortic aneurysm and coronary artery disease. A reassessment, Arch Surg 116:1484, 1986.
16. Crawford ES et al: Infrarenal abdominal aortic aneurysm. Factors influencing survival after operation performed over a 25-year period, Ann Surg 193:699, 1981.
17. Crawford ES et al: Aortoiliac occlusive disease: factors influencing survival and function following reconstructive operation over a twenty-five year period, Surgery 90:1055, 1981.
18. Cutler BS et al: Applicability and interpretation of electrocardiographic stress testing in patients with peripheral vascular disease, Am J Surg 141:501, 1981.
19. McCabe CJ et al: The value of electrocardiogram monitoring during treadmill testing for peripheral vascular disease, Surgery 89:183, 1981.
20. Jamieson WRE et al: Influence of ischaemic heart disease on early and late mortality after surgery for peripheral occlusive vascular disease, Circulation 66(suppl I):192, 1982.
21. Arous EJ, Baum PL, and Cutler BS: The ischemic exercise test in patients with peripheral vascular disease: implications for management, Arch Surg 119:780, 1984.
22. Hertzer NR et al: Coronary artery disease in peripheral vascular patients. A classification of 1000 coronary angiograms and results of surgical management, Ann Surg 199:223, 1984.
23. Hollier LH et al: Late survival after abdominal aortic aneurysm repair: influence of coronary artery disease, J Vasc Surg 1:290, 1984.
24. Rudy ST et al: Coronary artery disease in patients requiring abdominal aortic aneurysm repair: selective use of a combined operation, Ann Surg 201:758, 1985.
25. Von Knorring J and Lepantalo M: Prediction of perioperative cardiac complications by electrocardiographic monitoring during treadmill exercise testing before peripheral vascular surgery, Surgery 99:610, 1986.
26. Yeager RA et al: Application of clinically valid cardiac risk factors to aortic aneurysm surgery, Arch Surg 121:278, 1986.
27. Blombery PA et al: The role of coronary artery disease in complications of abdominal aortic aneurysm surgery, Surgery 101:150, 1987.
28. Cutler BS and Leppo JA: Dipyridamole thallium 201 scintigraphy to detect coronary artery disease before abdominal aortic surgery, J Vasc Surg 5:91, 1987.
29. Forssell C et al: Long-term results after carotid artery surgery, Eur J Vasc Surg 2:93, 1988.
30. Hanson P et al: Arm exercise testing for coronary artery disease in patients with peripheral vascular disease, Clin Cardiol 11:70, 1988.
31. Perry MO and Calaegno D: Abdominal aortic aneurysm surgery: the basic evaluation of cardiac risk, Ann Surg 208:738, 1988.
32. Sachs RN et al: Assessment by dipyridamole-thallium 201 myocardial scintigraphy of coronary risk before peripheral vascular surgery, Surgery 103:584, 1988.
33. Campbell JB, Baker J, and Morris DM: Cardiac complications of aneurysm repair, South Med J 82:458, 1989.
34. Fletcher JP et al: Risk of aortic aneurysm surgery as assessed by preoperative gated heart pool scan, Br J Surg 76:26, 1989.
35. Goodman S et al: Arm exercise testing with myocardial scintigraphy in asymptomatic patients with peripheral vascular disease, Chest 95:740, 1989.
36. Lundqvist BW et al: Cardiac risk in abdominal aortic surgery, Acta Chir Scand 155:321, 1989.
37. McPhail NV et al: A comparison of dipyridamole-thallium imaging and exercise testing in the prediction of postoperative cardiac complications in patients requiring arterial reconstruction, J Vasc Surg 10:51, 1989.
38. Raby KE et al: Correlation between preoperative ischemia and major cardiac events after peripheral vascular surgery, N Engl J Med 321:1296, 1989.

39. Ameli FM et al: Predictors of surgical outcome in patients undergoing aortobifemoral bypass reconstruction, J Cardiovasc Surg (Torino) 31:333, 1990.

40. Hendel RC et al: Dipyridamole thallium imaging predicts both perioperative and late cardiac events in vascular patients, Circulation 82(suppl III):111, 1990.

41. Levinson JR et al: Usefulness of semiquantitative analysis of dipyridamole-thallium 201 redistribution for improving risk stratification before vascular surgery, Am J Cardiol 66:406, 1990.

42. McEnroe CS et al: Comparison of ejection fraction and Goldman risk factor analysis to dipyridamole-thallium 201 studies in the evaluation of cardiac morbidity after aortic aneurysm surgery, J Vasc Surg 11:497, 1990.

43. Nesto RW et al: Silent myocardial ischemia with peripheral vascular disease: assessment by dipyridamole thallium 201 scintigraphy, Am Heart J 120:1073, 1990.

44. Younis LT et al: Perioperative and long-term prognostic value of intravenous dipyridamole thallium scintigraphy in patients with peripheral vascular disease, Am Heart J 119:1287, 1990.

45. Lette J et al: Multivariate clinical models and quantitative dipyridamole-thallium imaging to predict cardiac morbidity and death after vascular reconstruction, J Vasc Surg 14:160, 1991.

46. Bunt TJ: The role of a defined protocol for cardiac risk assessment in decreasing perioperative myocardial infarction in vascular surgery, J Vasc Surg 15:626, 1992.

47. Kalra M et al: Myocardial infarction after reconstruction of the abdominal aorta, Br J Surg 80:28, 1993.

48. McPhail NV et al: Cardiac risk stratification using dipyridamole myocardial perfusion imaging and ambulatory ECG monitoring prior to vascular surgery, Eur J Vasc Surg 7:151, 1993.

49. Gajraj H and Jamieson CW: Coronary artery disease in patients with peripheral vascular disease, Br J Surg 81:333, 1994.

50. Gersh BJ et al: Evaluation and management of patients with both peripheral vascular and coronary artery disease, JACC 18:203, 1991.

51. Hertzer NR: Basic data concerning associated coronary artery disease in peripheral vascular patients, Ann Vasc Surg 1:616, 1987.

52. Hertzer NR et al: Late results of coronary bypass in patients with peripheral vascular disease. Five year survival according to age and clinical cardiac status, Cleve Clin Q 53:133, 1986.

53. Young JR et al: Coronary artery disease in patients with aortic aneurysm: a classification of 302 coronary angiograms and results of surgical management, Ann Vasc Surg 1:36, 1986.

54. Hertzer NR and Arison R: Cumulative stroke and survival ten years after carotid endarterectomy, J Vasc Surg 2:661, 1985.

55. Jamieson WRE et al: Influence of ischemic heart disease on early and late mortality after surgery for peripheral vascular disease, Circulation 66(suppl I):I-92-7, 1982.

56. Roger VL et al: Influence of coronary artery disease on morbidity and mortality after abdominal aortic aneurysmectomy: a population based study 1971-1987, J Am Coll Cardiol 14:1245, 1989.

57. Reigel MM et al: Late survival in abdominal aortic aneurysm patients: the role of selective myocardial revascularization on the basis of clinical symptoms, J Vasc Surg 5:222, 1987.

58. Krupski WC et al: Comparison of cardiac morbidity rates between aortic and infrainguinal operations: two-year follow up, J Vasc Surg 18:609, 1993.

59. Smith GD, Shipley MJ, and Rose G: Intermittent claudication, heart disease risk factors, and mortality: the Whitehall study, Circulation 82:1925, 1990.

60. Langer RD et al: Isolated small vessel peripheral arterial disease is associated with future cardiovascular events, Circulation 81:724, 1990 (abstract).

61. Criqui MH, Coughlin SS, and Fronek A: Noninvasively diagnosed peripheral arterial disease as a predictor of mortality: results from a prospective study, Circulation 72:768, 1985.

62. Hertzer NR et al: Late results of coronary bypass in patients presenting with lower extremity ischemia: the Cleveland Clinic Study, Ann Vasc Surg 1:411, 1986.

63. Hertzer NR et al: Late results of coronary artery bypass in patients with peripheral vascular disease. II: five-year survival according to sex, hypertension and diabetes, Cleve Clin J Med 54:15, 1987.

64. Farkouh ME et al: Influence of coronary heart disease on morbidity and mortality after lower extremity revascularization surgery: a population-based study in Olmsted County Minnesota 1970-1987, JACC 24:1290, 1994.

65. Crawford ES et al: Operative risk in patients with previous coronary artery bypass, Ann Thorac Surg 26:215, 1978.

66. Mahar LJ et al: Perioperative myocardial infarction in patients with coronary artery disease with and without aorto-coronary bypass grafts, J Thorac Cardiovasc Surg 76:533, 1978.

67. Jain KM et al: Preoperative cardiac screening before peripheral vascular operations, Am Surg 51:77, 1985.

68. Foster ED et al: Risk of noncardiac operation in patients with defined coronary disease: the Coronary Artery Surgery Study (CASS) Registry experience, Ann Thorac Surg 41:42, 1986.

69. European Coronary Surgery Study Group: Prospective randomised study of coronary artery bypass surgery in stable angina pectoris: second interim report, Lancet 2:491, 1980.

70. Goldman L et al: Cardiac risk factors and complications in non-cardiac surgery, Medicine 57:357, 1978.

71. Jeffrey CC et al: A prospective evaluation of cardiac risk index, Anesthesiology 58:462, 1983.

72. Freeman WK, Gibbons RJ, and Shub C: Preoperative evaluation of the cardiac patient undergoing non-cardiac surgery, Mayo Clin Proc 64:1105, 1989.

73. Mangano DT et al: Association of peri-operative myocardial ischemia with cardiac morbidity and mortality in men undergoing non-cardiac surgery, N Engl J Med 323:1781, 1990.

74. Yeager MP: Regional anesthesia for the patient with heart disease, J Cardiovasc Anesth 3:793, 1989.

75. Diamond GA and Forrester JS: Analysis of probability as an aid in the clinical diagnosis of coronary artery disease, N Engl J Med 300:1350, 1979.

76. Pryor DB et al: Estimating the likelihood of significant coronary artery disease, Am J Med 75:771, 1983.

77. Cooperman M et al: Cardiovascular risk factors in patients with peripheral vascular disease, Surgery 84:505, 1978.

78. Rao TL, Jacobs KH, and El Etr AA: Reinfarction following anesthesia in patients with myocardial infarction, Anesthesiology 59:499, 1983.

79. O'Keefe JH, Shub C, and Rettke SR: Can patients with significant aortic stenosis undergo noncardiac surgery safely? Mayo Clin Proc 64:400, 1989.

80. Goldman L et al: Multifactorial index of cardiac risk in

noncardiac surgical procedures, N Engl J Med 297:845, 1977.

81. Goldman L: Assessment of the patient with known or suspected ischemic heart disease for non-cardiac surgery, Br J Anesth 61:38, 1988.

82. Detsky AS et al: Predicting cardiac complications in patients undergoing vascular surgery, J Gen Intern Med 1:211, 1986.

83. Gerson MC et al: Cardiac prognosis in noncardiac geriatric surgery, Ann Intern Med 103:832, 1985.

84. Ashton CM et al: The incidence of perioperative myocardial infarction in men undergoing noncardiac surgery, Ann Intern Med 118:504, 1993.

85. Eagle KA et al: Combining clinical and thallium data optimizes preoperative assessment of cardiac risk before major vascular surgery, Ann Intern Med 110:859, 1989.

86. Lette J et al: Postoperative myocardial infarction and cardiac death: predictive value of dipyridamole thallium imaging and five clinical scoring systems based on multifactorial analysis, Ann Surg 211:84, 1990.

87. Gage AA et al: Assessment of cardiac risk in surgical patients, Arch Surg 42:1488, 1977.

88. Pasternack PF et al: The value of the radionuclide angiogram in the prediction of perioperative myocardial infarction in patients undergoing lower extremity revascularization procedures, Circulation 72(suppl II):13, 1985.

89. Franco CD et al: Resting gated blood pool ejection fraction: a poor predictor of perioperative myocardial infarction in patients undergoing vascular surgery for infrainguinal bypass grafting, J Vasc Surg 10:656, 1989.

90. Kotler TS and Diamond GA: Exercise thallium-201 scintigraphy in the diagnosis and prognosis of coronary artery disease, Ann Intern Med 113:684, 1990.

91. Iskandrian AS et al: Effect of exercise level on the ability of thallium-201 tomographic imaging in detecting coronary artery disease, J Am Coll Cardiol 14:1477, 1989.

92. Boucher CA et al: Determination of cardiac risk by dipyridamole thallium imaging before peripheral vascular surgery, N Engl J Med 12:389, 1985.

93. Eagle KA et al: Dipyridamole thallium scanning in patients undergoing vascular surgery. Optimizing perioperative evaluation of cardiac risk, JAMA 257:2185, 1987.

94. Lette J et al: Usefulness of the severity and extent of reversible perfusion defects during thallium-dipyridamole imaging for cardiac risk assessment before noncardiac surgery, Am J Cardiol 64:276, 1989.

95. Marwick T and Underwood DA: Dipyridamole thallium imaging may not be a reliable screening test for coronary disease in patients undergoing vascular surgery, Clin Cardiol 13:14, 1990.

96. Mangano DT et al: Dipyridamole thallium-201 scintigraphy as a preoperative screening test: a reexamination of its predictive potential, Circulation 84:493, 1991.

97. Hendel RC et al: Prediction of late cardiac events by dipyridamole thallium imaging in patients undergoing elective vascular surgery, Am J Cardiol 70:1243, 1992.

98. Cambria RP et al: The impact of selective use of dipyridamole thallium scans and surgical factors on the current morbidity of aortic surgery, J Vasc Surg 15:43, 1992.

99. Takase B et al: Comparative prognostic value of clinical risk indexes, resting two-dimensional echocardiography, and dipyridamole stress thallium-201 myocardial imaging for perioperative cardiac events in major nonvascular surgery patients, Am Heart J 126:1099, 1993.

100. Younis LT et al: Preoperative clinical assessment and dipyridamole thallium-201 scintigraphy for prediction and prevention of cardiac events in patients having major noncardiovascular surgery and known or suspected coronary disease, Am J Cardiol 74:311, 1994.

101. Baron JF et al: Dipyridamole thallium scintigraphy and gated radionuclide angiography to assess cardiac risk before abdominal aortic surgery, N Engl J Med 330:663, 1994.

102. Marwick T et al: Use of positron emission tomography for prediction of perioperative and late events prior to vascular surgery, Am Heart J 1995 (in press).

103. Marwick T et al: Selection of the optimal non-exercise stress for the evaluation of ischemic regional myocardial dysfunction and malperfusion: comparison of dobutamine and adenosine using echocardiography and Tc-99m MIBI single photon emission computed tomography, Circulation 87:345, 1993.

104. Tischler MD et al: Prediction of major events after peripheral vascular surgery using dipyridamole echocardiography, Am J Cardiol 68:593, 1991.

105. Lane RT et al: Dobutamine stress echocardiography for assessment of cardiac risk before noncardiac surgery, Am J Cardiol 68:976, 1991.

106. Lalka SG et al: Dobutamine stress echocardiography as a predictor of cardiac events associated with aortic surgery, J Vasc Surg 15:831, 1992.

107. Davila-Roman VG et al: Dobutamine stress echocardiography predicts surgical outcome in patients with an aortic aneurysm and peripheral vascular disease, J Am Coll Cardiol 21:957, 1993.

108. Poldermans D et al: Dobutamine stress echocardiography for assessment of perioperative cardiac risk in patients undergoing major vascular surgery, Circulation 87:1506, 1993.

109. Ouyang P et al: Frequency and significance of early postoperative silent myocardial ischemia in patients having peripheral vascular surgery, Am J Cardiol 64:1113, 1989.

110. Pasternack RF et al: The value of silent myocardial ischemia monitoring in the prediction of perioperative myocardial infarction in patients undergoing peripheral vascular surgery, J Vasc Surg 10:617, 1989.

111. Pasternack RF et al: Beta blockade to decrease silent myocardial ischemia during peripheral vascular surgery, Am J Surg 158:113, 1989.

112. Mangano DT et al: Perioperative myocardial ischemia in patients undergoing noncardiac surgery. Incidence and severity during the first week after surgery, J Am Coll Cardiol 17:851, 1991.

CHAPTER FOURTEEN

ATHEROMATOUS EMBOLIZATION

John R. Bartholomew
Jeffrey W. Olin

The atheromatous embolization syndrome has received little attention in most major medical textbooks. It is a frequently misdiagnosed and unrecognized disorder that was initially believed to be little more than a curiosity to pathologists.[1,2] It is now recognized to cause significant morbidity and mortality. Atheromatous embolization may present clinically in a variety of ways, and physicians in many specialties see patients with this disorder. A failure to recognize this entity exposes patients to undue risk, since the diagnostic workup and treatment often aggravate the condition. Therefore the importance of recognizing the atheromatous embolization syndrome cannot be overemphasized.

HISTORICAL BACKGROUND

Panum[3] is credited with the first description of atheromatous embolization in 1862. He described a case involving the famous Danish sculptor Thorwaldsen in which atheromatous material was found at autopsy. The first American report, noted by Doch in 1896,[4] involved coronary occlusion and death from multiple, cholesterol-rich emboli. By 1915 there was enough awareness of this syndrome that it was included in a textbook on diseases of the arteries,[5] although atheromatous embolization was still believed to be little more than an incidental finding at autopsy.

Flory[6] drew attention to atheromatous emboli in 1945 after reviewing 267 autopsies. He suggested that emboli containing cholesterol crystals produced infarction in multiple organs such as the kidney, spleen, or pancreas. He also speculated that atheroemboli may cause gangrenous changes in the lower extremities. Experimentally he injected human atheromatous material into rabbit ears and found cholesterol crystals in the animals' arteries similar to those lesions he had earlier described in his autopsy studies. This work rekindled interest in atheromatous embolization.

Other investigators have played an important role in the recognition of this condition. Snyder and Shapiro[7] injected 16 rabbits and 9 dogs with cholesterol crystal suspensions. All animals were later sacrificed and examined for the presence of cholesterol crystals. These studies demonstrated the persistence of arterial occlusions for extended periods (up to 160 days) and noted that these occlusions caused ischemia. Gore and Collins[8] reviewed the literature and reported 16 additional cases. They suggested that spontaneous atheromatous embolization was not an unusual complication of advanced atherosclerosis. Hoye et al[9] are credited with the first histologically proven case of peripheral atheromatous embolism. This patient developed gangrene that resulted in amputation. The source of the gangrene was either the abdominal aorta or the iliofemoral arteries. Handler[10] stressed the importance of atheromatous embolization that involved the kidney as a potential factor in the pathogenesis of hypertension.

PATHOGENESIS

Atheroembolization may be spontaneous, although it occurs more often after surgery, arteriography, or anticoagulation therapy (see box below). Arteriography is invalu-

---

PRECIPITATING FACTORS IN ATHEROEMBOLIC DISEASE*

1. Arteriography
2. Surgery
3. Anticoagulants
4. Thrombolytic agents

*Atheromatous embolization may also occur spontaneously.

able in the diagnosis and evaluation of the patient with vascular disease. Unfortunately it is not without complications, including the potential to cause atheromatous embolization. This condition usually develops during or moments after the angiographic procedure. It may be heralded by an increase in blood pressure, pain, livedo reticularis pattern on the abdomen and lower extremities, or renal failure. Harrington, Sommers, and Kassirer[11] reported two cases in which progressive renal failure developed following retrograde renal arteriography. Others have reported similar findings with different techniques, including translumbar aortography and transaxillary angiography.[12-17] In a retrospective study of 71 autopsies, Ramirez et al[18] reported a 27% incidence of cholesterol embolization in patients who had arteriography performed before death, compared with a 4.3% incidence of spontaneous cholesterol emboli in an age- and disease-matched control group who did not undergo angiography. When atheroemboli occur after arteriography, the risk of death increases considerably.[15,16,19,20] Whether the rigidity of the catheter or the force of contrast injection plays a role is unclear, but some have suggested that a softer, more flexible catheter may result in a lower incidence.[13,19] Probably the most important factor that determines who will or will not develop emboli is the severity of the atherosclerotic disease in the aorta[21] (Fig. 14-1).

Other invasive procedures that may lead to the atheromatous embolization syndrome include cardiac catheterization, percutaneous transluminal coronary angioplasty (PTCA), and peripheral angioplasty.[14,15,22,23] In a review of

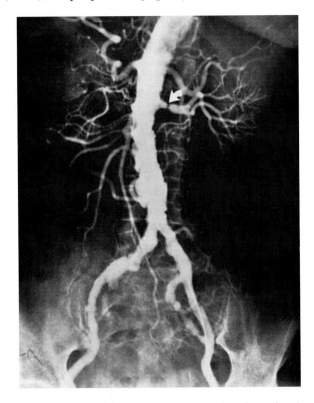

Fig. 14-1. Aortogram demonstrates severe erosive atherosclerosis of the aorta in a patient with atheromatous emboli. Note occlusion of the right renal artery and subtotal occlusion of the left renal artery (arrow).

4587 cardiac catheterizations, Drost et al[14] found seven cases of clinical cholesterol embolization (0.15%). Colt et al[15] found eight cases after heart catheterization, PTCA, and intraaortic balloon pumping involving 3733 procedures (0.2%). They also noted that there was no case reported of cholesterol embolization after cardiac catheterization when the brachial artery was used. These figures probably underestimate the true incidence in patients who undergo cardiac catheterization. Most likely only the severe cases were diagnosed, and many milder ones were not.

Atheroembolism has been associated with the use of anticoagulant and thrombolytic therapy.[24-31] "Purple or blue toes" may occur at any time during anticoagulant therapy but typically occur within 4 to 12 weeks after therapy has been initiated. For years the relationship between purple toes and warfarin was believed to be the result of a direct toxic effect on the capillaries or a drug-induced vasculitis.[31] Moldveen-Geronimus and Merriam[1] postulated that the purple toe syndrome was caused by cholesterol embolization as a result of the anticoagulant. They believed that anticoagulants prevented clot formation over ulcerated plaques, thus allowing embolization to occur. Baumann et al[32] have suggested that anticoagulants potentiate hemorrhage into plaques, leading to its disruption. Bruns, Segel, and Adler[26] noted clinical improvement in a patient when anticoagulants were discontinued. Most investigators recommend that warfarin be discontinued in patients who have an episode of cholesterol embolization.[24] However, the data suggesting that anticoagulants cause atheromatous embolization is not overwhelming. In fact, patients with "crescendo" transient ischemic attacks (TIAs) are often treated with anticoagulants. Therefore if a patient has a compelling reason to continue warfarin or heparin, as in venous thromboembolism or atrial fibrillation, we continue anticoagulation therapy while searching for the source of atheroemboli. Atheromatous emboli have also been associated with thrombolytic agents.[27-29] Other precipitating factors include surgery[33-35] due to manipulation and/or cross-clamping of the vessel and blunt trauma. Emboli may also occur spontaneously or after lifting or coughing.[36]

PATHOLOGY

Two different types of atheroemboli may lead to this syndrome. Some investigators refer to this as a noncardiac embolization of one or more large atheromatous plaques that contain red blood cells, fibrin, platelet aggregates, and cholesterol crystals. These are often called *macroemboli*. Others refer to the atheromatous embolization syndrome as a showering of multiple smaller cholesterol crystals or fibrin platelet aggregates. This is called *microembolization* or *cholesterol embolization*. Both macroemboli and microemboli originate from ulcerated or stenotic atherosclerotic plaques, or aneurysms of both the larger and smaller arteries.

CLINICAL PRESENTATION (Table 14-1)

Patients with atheromatous embolization usually have a history of atherosclerosis manifested clinically by angina, myocardial infarction, TIA, stroke, intermittent claudication, or gangrene. Atheromatous embolization may occur in any individual with advanced atherosclerosis. Almost always the patient is a heavy smoker. A race predilection has been reported, as atheroemboli are less likely to occur in black patients although this may be a failure to recognize the classic features because of skin pigmentation.[37] Clinical signs and symptoms may be nonspecific and varied, depending on the number, size, and site of origin of the atheromatous material as well as on the end organ(s) affected. Patients with macroemboli may present with a catastrophic event such as an acutely ischemic leg, whereas those with microemboli may have milder localized signs or a clinical picture that suggests a systemic illness. Signs and symptoms suggestive of a multisystemic illness include fever, weight loss, anorexia, fatigue, myalgias, headache, nausea, vomiting, or diarrhea. Occasionally the signs and symptoms may suggest necrotizing vasculitis, infective endocarditis, or malignancy.[31,37-42]

Skin Manifestations

One of the most common clinical manifestations of atheromatous embolization is changes in the skin. These changes, generally found on the lower abdomen and legs, include livedo reticularis, gangrene, cyanosis, purple or blue toes, ulcerations, nodules, and petechiae (Figs. 14-2 and 14-3). In a review of 221 histologically proven cases of cholesterol crystal embolization, cutaneous manifestations were noted in over one third of patients.[43] This high incidence was confirmed in a recent review by Falanga, Fine, and Kapoor[44] in which cutaneous manifestations were the most common physical findings.

Livedo reticularis, a red-blue mottling or discoloration of the skin that occurs in a netlike fashion, is a common manifestation of atheromatous emboli.[45,46] Generally seen on the buttocks, thighs, or legs, it represents embolization to the dermal blood vessels (Fig. 14-3). Livedo reticularis is not pathognomonic of atheroemboli, since it may occur in young healthy females or in other conditions, including vasculitis, particularly leukocytoclastic vasculitis. Livedo reticularis has also been reported to be position dependent.[47] Livedo reticularis secondary to atheroemboli is rarely seen in the upper extremity.

Blue, cyanotic, or purple toes are frequently encountered and are usually painful (Fig. 14-2). Purple or violaceous discoloration may also be seen on the sole of the foot (Figs. 14-2 and 14-3). These findings in the presence of palpable foot pulses are highly suggestive of atheromatous embolization. Ischemic or necrotic changes and frank gangrene of the lower extremities and toes are also common.

Necrosis of the penis and scrotum has been reported.[41] Nodules may occur on the calves and thighs.[45,48] They are painful, violaceous in appearance with a necrotic center, and they may mimic a necrotizing vasculitis such as

Table 14-1. Clinical Manifestations of Atheromatous Embolization

Skin	Purple or blue toes
	Gangrenous digits
	Livedo reticularis
	Nodules
Kidney	Uncontrolled hypertension
	Renal failure
Neurologic	Transient ischemic attack
	Amaurosis fugax
	Stroke
	Hollenhorst plaque
Cardiac	Myocardial infarction or ischemia
Gastrointestinal	Abdominal pain
	GI bleeding
	Ischemic bowel
	Acute pancreatitis
Constitutional symptoms	Fever
	Weight loss
	Malaise
	Anorexia

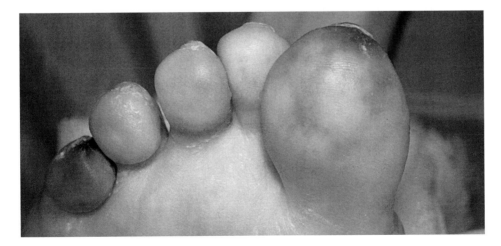

Fig. 14-2. The first, second, and third toes show patchy distribution of erythema and cyanosis, in a patient with atheromatous emboli. The fifth toe is "blue" or cyanotic.

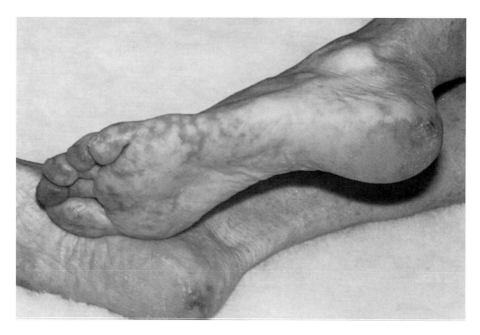

Fig. 14-3. Classic appearance of atheromatous emboli, with livedo reticularis on the lateral aspect of the foot and heel. The second toe is blue.

polyarteritis nodosa. Other manifestations include muscle tenderness and burning, throbbing, or numbness of the feet or toes. Muscle cramps, nocturnal aching, and rare cases of restless leg syndrome secondary to atheromatous emboli have been reported.[49] Splinter hemorrhages may occasionally be present secondary to atheromatous embolization.[50]

Gastrointestinal Tract

Atheroemboli may also involve the gastrointestinal tract. Frequently this site is overlooked since clinical manifestations may be varied. Gore and Collins[8] have estimated that approximately 20% of patients with widespread atheromatous emboli have gastrointestinal involvement. Even more often the pancreas may be involved.[8,51,52] Patients may complain of generalized abdominal or periumbilical pain, nausea, vomiting, melena, or hematochezia. A guaiac-positive stool may be noted. In severe cases frank bowel infarction may occur.[53] Cholesterol emboli to the gallbladder may cause acute gangrenous cholecystitis.[54]

Central Nervous System and Eye

The central nervous system and the retina may be involved with atheromatous emboli. Patients may develop visual disturbances such as amaurosis fugax or blindness caused by retinal artery occlusion. A Hollenhorst plaque may be seen on ophthalmoscopic examination as yellow, highly refractile atheromatous material that classically lodges in areas where vessels bifurcate (Fig. 14-4). TIA, stroke, headache, confusion, organic brain syndrome, dizziness, and spinal cord infarction are other manifestations of central nervous system atheroemboli. The central nervous system is discussed further in Chapter 16.

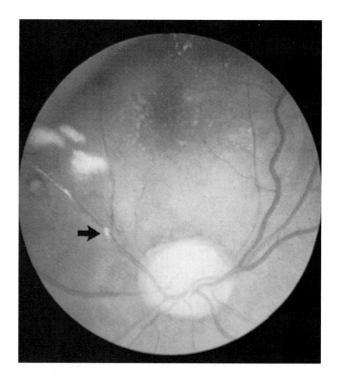

Fig. 14-4. Fundus shows a bright yellow refractile Hollenhorst plaque *(arrow)* representing atheromatous embolization to the retina.

Cardiac Manifestations

Cardiac manifestations of atheroemboli, including angina pectoris and myocardial infarction, should be suspected in any high-risk patient, especially if other clinical findings suggest atheroemboli. Spontaneous atheroemboli

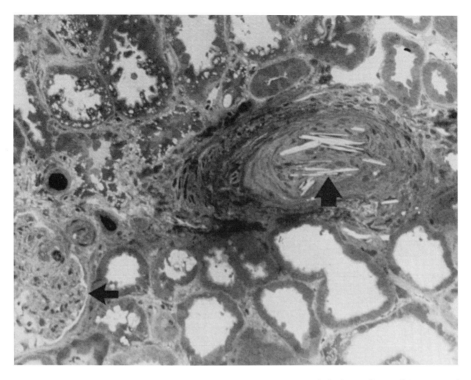

Fig. 14-5. Light microscopy shows multiple biconvex, needle-shaped cholesterol crystals in an arteriole in the kidney *(large arrow)*. A glomerulus is seen in the left lower portion *(small arrow)*. (Courtesy Gordon Gephardt, MD.)

to the coronary arteries have been reported. Intraoperative atheromatous embolization following coronary artery bypass surgery may also occur.[55-57]

Other Areas

Atheromatous emboli have also been demonstrated in the spleen, bone marrow, muscle, and prostate.

Atheroembolic Renal Disease

When atheroembolic disease involves the kidneys, occlusion of multiple small arteries is seen leading to ischemic atrophy of segments of the kidney. This small-vessel occlusive disease eventually may lead to uncontrolled hypertension, advanced renal failure, or end-stage renal disease. This disease differs from renal infarction from large *thrombo*emboli originating from the heart or from emboli from a thrombus lining an aneurysm. Renal atheroemboli originate from disease of the suprarenal aorta. The lining of the aorta may be covered with friable, shaggy cholesterol-rich atherosclerotic material (Fig. 14-1). This material may be dislodged mechanically or spontaneously and lodge in the small arteries and arterioles of the kidney.

Pathologically the interlobular and afferent arterioles (150 to 200 μm in size) are usually involved. The material demonstrated in these arterioles is a biconvex cholesterol crystal. During histologic preparation crystals dissolve and leave a space where the cholesterol crystals used to be (Fig. 14-5). Cholesterol embolization produces a foreign body reaction within the kidney. The full-blown syndrome of renal failure and accelerated hypertension may take weeks or months to develop. Initially polymorphonuclear leuko-

cytes, macrophages, and multinucleated giant cells appear several days to several weeks after the inciting event. Eventually this cellular infiltrate leads to thickening and fibrosis of the arterioles. Total occlusion of the blood vessel results from accumulation of fibrous material and connective tissue material. When large segments of small arterioles are occluded, ischemic atrophy of large portions of the kidney occurs. As glomerular filtration declines, the renin-angiotensin-aldosterone system is activated, and hypertension accelerates.[58-61]

The precipitating events associated with atheroembolic renal disease are identical to the precipitating events of atheromatous emboli, elsewhere in the body (see the box, p. 261).

Clinically this disease occurs in the elderly who have evidence of atherosclerosis elsewhere in the body. Other evidence of atheroemboli may include livedo reticularis, stroke, amaurosis fugax, a Hollenhorst plaque, gastrointestinal bleeding, pancreatitis, or myocardial infarction. Some patients may exhibit multisystem failure, which suggests a necrotizing vasculitis.

Since patients with atheroembolic renal disease have many of the same precipitating factors as patients who develop acute tubular necrosis, other features may help to differentiate atheroembolic renal disease (Table 14-2). As a general rule, the urine sediment in patients with atheroembolic renal disease is benign or shows microhematuria with or without leukocyturia. Rarely eosinophiluria may be present.[62] By contrast, the urine sediment in patients with acute tubular necrosis often demonstrates pigmented granular casts (dirty brown casts) and renal tubular cells.

Table 14-2. Differentiating Acute Tubular Necrosis from Atheroembolic Renal Disease

	Acute Tubular Necrosis	Atheroembolic Renal Disease
Precipitating factors	Hypotension Surgery Arteriography Drugs	Arteriography Surgery Anticoagulants Spontaneous
Urine sediment	Renal tubular cells Pigmented granular casts (dirty brown casts)	Benign or hematuria ± leukocyturia Rarely eosinophiluria
Other associated laboratory findings	None	Eosinophilia and/or hypocomplementemia in some patients
Hypertension	None or mild	Often present, severe, and quite difficult to control; may be an early clue to atheroembolic renal disease
Rise in serum creatinine	1-2 days after insult, peak in 4-14 days	Usually begins 7-10 days after insult and slowly rises over weeks to months (Fig. 14-6)
Renal outcome	Full recovery is the rule if underlying precipitating factor is corrected	Progression to end-stage renal disease or advanced renal failure; stabilization or recovery of renal failure may sometimes occur

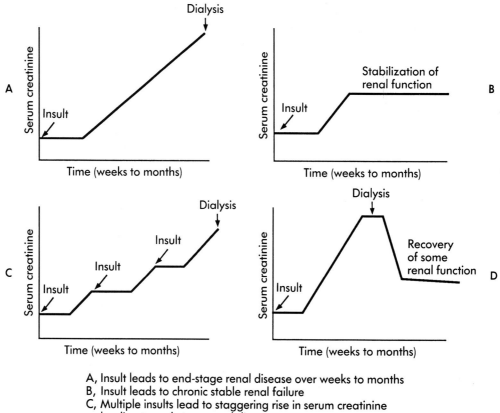

A, Insult leads to end-stage renal disease over weeks to months
B, Insult leads to chronic stable renal failure
C, Multiple insults lead to staggering rise in serum creatinine leading to end-stage renal disease
D, Insult leading to dialysis treatments and the eventual recovery of renal function to some degree

Fig. 14-6. Several patterns of renal failure in patients with atheroembolic renal disease.

Patients who develop acute tubular necrosis may have no hypertension or mild hypertension only, whereas patients with atheroembolic renal disease often experience an acceleration of their hypertension, which is often difficult to control. The hypertension is thought to be mediated through the renin-angiotensin-aldosterone system. In patients with acute tubular necrosis, the serum creatinine level usually begins to rise soon after the insult, peaks in 4 to 14 days, and often returns to normal if the precipitating event is corrected. On the other hand, in patients with atheroembolic renal disease the rise in serum creatinine level is often delayed for 7 to 10 days. It is not uncommon for a patient to have an angiographic procedure performed, and to be discharged from the hospital only to return several weeks later with a markedly elevated serum creatinine level. The serum creatinine level may rise slowly, and end-stage renal disease is not unusual.

Various patterns of renal insufficiency may occur in atheroembolic renal disease (Fig. 14-6). In the past it was thought that patients always progressed to end-stage renal disease that required dialytic support. However, in 1981 Smith, Ghose, and Henry[63] reported several cases in which renal function stabilized or even improved to the point where the patient no longer required dialysis. Since this report others have also demonstrated that renal insufficiency may not always progress to end-stage renal disease.[2,22,64,65]

No laboratory tests uniformly help in the diagnosis of atheroembolic renal disease. Kasinath et al[66] and Kasinath and Lewis[67] described eosinophilia as a clue that occurs in 80% of cases of atheroembolic renal disease. However, this effect is transient and may last for only a few days. It is thus important to check the patient's white blood cell count with a differential count early in the course if atheroembolic renal disease is suspected.

Others have suggested that hypocomplementemia may occur in patients with atheroembolic renal disease.[68,69] In one series of nine patients whose complement was measured, the C3 complement level was low in seven.[68] In rats injected with homogenized human atheromatous plaque, five of eight animals had decreased C3 complement.[68] Others have suggested that the contrast medium itself may transiently decrease serum complement, thus decreasing the sensitivity of this test for patients with atheroembolic renal disease.[70] Whether hypocomplementemia is important in the pathogenesis of renal injury or whether a foreign body reaction is a more important pathogenetic factor is unclear at the present time. Since hypocomplementemia is not a universal finding in patients with advanced atheroembolic renal disease, the foreign body hypothesis seems more likely.

The diagnosis of atheroembolic renal disease before death requires a high index of suspicion. Although a precipitating event may occur in many patients, in a review of 221 cases from the English literature[43] only 31% had at least one precipitating event. Evidence of atheroembolic disease elsewhere is helpful in making the diagnosis. Other disease entities such as atherosclerotic renal artery stenosis, renal artery thrombosis, infective endocarditis, vasculitis (such as polyarteritis nodosa), and

other forms of acute renal failure need to be considered in the differential diagnosis. A definitive diagnosis of atheroembolic renal disease requires a renal biopsy specimen in which cholesterol clefts are demonstrated. Since the atheromatous emboli are patchy in distribution, they may be missed on a needle biopsy. When a biopsy is indicated, an open renal biopsy may need to be performed.

Once an episode of atheromatous emboli to the kidney has occurred, no direct treatment is able to reverse the damage already done. The best treatment is prevention. If a patient has evidence of atheromatous emboli, that segment of aorta thought to be the source of the emboli should be replaced if feasible. The patient should be dialyzed as necessary, and blood pressure should be meticulously controlled. Anticoagulants should be avoided since they may precipitate more atheroembolic events.

Atheroembolic renal disease carries a particularly poor prognosis since it is indicative of generalized atherosclerosis. In one series[43] 179 of 221 patients (81%) died. The most common causes of death were cardiac, renal, or multisystem illness.

INCIDENCE

The exact incidence of atheroemboli is unknown. The presence of atheromatous emboli in an autopsy series or in a biopsy specimen merely indicates how often this entity is demonstrated pathologically but does not indicate how important it is clinically. Since the late 1960s, numerous clinical pathologic conferences reported in the *New England Journal of Medicine*[71-79] illustrated different aspects of atheromatous embolization, suggesting that this disease was considered a curious or uncommon entity. Recently, however, there have been more studies that have been published with larger numbers of patients,[2,43,63,80-83] showing that clinical cholesterol embolization is not as rare as previously believed.

Atheromatous embolization is reported to be a common occurrence in individuals with advanced atherosclerosis.[6] The incidence clearly differs if patients with spontaneous embolization are compared with patients in autopsy series or with patients following surgery or other invasive procedures. In Flory's series[6] the incidence of atheromatous embolization was 3.4% of 267 patients with advanced atherosclerosis at autopsy. The degree of aortic atherosclerosis predicted the likelihood of atheromatous emboli, and in those with the most severe degree of atherosclerosis, the incidence was 12.3%. In 100 consecutive autopsy cases, Maurizi, Barker, and Trueheart[84] examined the microscopic sections of muscles of the lower extremities and demonstrated atheromatous emboli in four patients (4%). In 25 patients with documented atheromatous emboli at autopsy, all patients had clinical features suggestive of atheromatous emboli (in retrospect), yet the diagnosis was not made until autopsy in 21 patients (84%).[84] When Wagner and Martin[85] reviewed 4635 cases of peripheral arterial emboli, they found only 1.4% attributed to atheroemboli. In a review of 2126 autopsies involving patients over 60 years of age, Kealy[86] found the incidence of atheroemboli to be 0.79%, although he suspected that this was probably an underestimation. Handler[10] reviewed 70 consecutive autopsies for evidence of cholesterol crystal embolization and found an incidence of 8.6%. In a review of 1352 autopsies, Sieniewicz et al[87] found atheromatous emboli in the kidneys of 3.47% of patients. The incidence clearly increased with age since the incidence was 11.76% in patients 80 to 89 years old. More recent studies[18,63,88] suggest that atheromatous embolization of the kidneys is a common histologic finding and may approach 15% to 30% in patients with severe aortic atherosclerosis or aneurysms of the abdominal aorta.[18,63,88] Clinical manifestations are clearly less common.

Over 30 years ago Thurlbeck and Castleman[33] demonstrated that 77% of patients who died after abdominal aortic aneurysm resection had atheromatous emboli in the kidney. In addition, 13 of 42 patients (31%) who were not operated on for abdominal aortic aneurysm and 6 of 38 patients (15.8%) with severe aortoiliac occlusive disease had atheromatous emboli at autopsy. More recently an autopsy study of 221 patients who had undergone myocardial revascularization or valve operations found that 21.7% of patients demonstrated atheroemboli.[57]

DIAGNOSIS OF ATHEROEMBOLI

Several studies have demonstrated that the atheromatous embolization syndrome is frequently overlooked and diagnosed only at autopsy. Maurizi, Barker, and Trueheart[84] noted that in 84% of their autopsy cases atheroemboli were not diagnosed before death, despite clinical features corresponding to pathologic findings. Falanga, Fine, and Kapoor[43] noted that only 30% of the cases they reviewed were diagnosed before death. A high index of suspicion and a thorough understanding of the possible clinical manifestations are needed in this condition because prompt diagnosis and treatment can be lifesaving.

No single laboratory test is diagnostic. Some patients merely have an elevated erythrocyte sedimentation rate, leukocytosis, or anemia, but these are common findings in any systemic illness. Elevations in levels of serum amylase, hepatic transaminases, blood urea nitrogen (BUN), and creatinine are seen if the pancreas, liver, or kidney are involved. Elevations in creatinine phosphokinase and aldolase reflect muscle involvement. The urine sediment may be abnormal. Eosinophilia and hypocomplementemia may be present.[66-69]

Biopsy remains the most effective way to make the diagnosis.[48,58,64,89,90] In one series[89] random biopsies of the gastrocnemius and quadriceps muscles were helpful in diagnosing atheroemboli, although skin or muscle biopsy from an involved area is preferred. Biopsies should be deep and should be examined in multiple sections. Other involved areas that may be biopsied include the kidney, bone marrow, amputated extremities, or gangrenous toes. The pathognomonic finding is the needle-shaped cholesterol cleft within the small vessels (Fig. 14-5).

In the appropriate clinical setting, arteriography can assist in confirming the suspected diagnosis. Generally a markedly irregular and shaggy aorta is demonstrated (Fig. 14-1). If lesions involving the lower extremity are bilateral, an attempt should be made to obtain thoracic and abdominal aortography with run-offs to each leg. Noninvasive tests such as magnetic resonance imaging, computed tomography, and ultrasound may also be helpful. These are especially valuable in confirming the presence of aneurysms or in demonstrating calcified plaques. Several recent publications have stressed the benefits of transesophageal echocardiography in detecting the source of embolization.[91,92] These articles point out that this technique not only is important for identifying potential cardiac sources of embolization but also abnormalities in the thoracic aorta that may also lead to strokes, TIA, and peripheral emboli[91,92] (Fig. 14-7).

DIFFERENTIAL DIAGNOSIS

The differential diagnosis may be quite extensive and depends on the end organs involved. Atheromatous em-

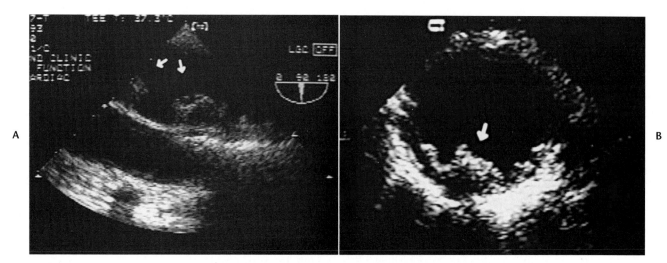

Fig. 14-7. Transesophageal echocardiography demonstrating protruding aortic etheromas (arrows) in the descending thoracic aorta in a long axis view (**A**) and short axis view (**B**).

boli may mimic a vasculitis such as polyarteritis nodosa, leukocytoclastic vasculitis, or cryoglobulinemia.[42] The clinical manifestation may also suggest an underlying malignancy, nonbacterial thrombotic endocarditis, subacute bacterial endocarditis, multiple myeloma, the antiphospholipid antibody syndrome, or atrial myxoma. A cardiac source of emboli should always be excluded.

TREATMENT

Treatment should be directed toward three goals:

1. Removal of the source of atheromatous material, usually by surgery
2. Symptomatic care of the end organ where the emboli are located
3. Risk factor modification to prevent progression of the disease

If embolization to the lower extremities has occurred, local care of ischemic ulcers is important. If significant gangrene is present, amputation may be required. However, if the amount of tissue loss is equivocal, local care with soaking in tepid soapy water and good skin care may expedite healing. Heel protectors should be used and lamb's wool placed between the toes. In some cases a chemical or surgical sympathectomy may be helpful. After the acute episode has stabilized, surgical replacement of the aorta or section of the artery that was the source of embolization should be strongly considered.

Medical Therapy

The most accepted form of therapy for atheromatous embolization is surgical removal of the source where the emboli originated. However, under certain circumstances medical therapy is indicated. Medical therapy should be considered if the source of embolization cannot be identified with certainty or if the patient is at a markedly increased surgical risk.

Anticoagulants, including heparin and sodium warfarin, should be avoided in patients who have suspected atheromatous embolization, unless there are overwhelming indications for their use. Antiplatelet agents such as aspirin and dipyridamole have been advocated as the best available medical therapy. Unfortunately there are no controlled studies demonstrating their efficacy. Morris-Jones et al[93] described reversal of pregangrenous changes in the toes in 19 of 35 patients who were treated with aspirin and dipyridamole. When antiplatelet therapy was discontinued, five patients had a recurrence of their symptoms. Walden, Adar, and Mozes[94] noted improvement in the pregangrenous changes of the toes of 10 patients treated with aspirin and/or dipyridamole. Not all patients in these studies had atheroemboli; some had fibrinoplatelet platelet emboli, and although it is probably unreasonable to expect antiplatelet therapy itself to improve ischemia, it may prevent further episodes of embolization.

Other forms of therapy have been advocated such as corticosteroids, low-molecular-weight dextran, lipid-lowering agents, intraarterial papavarine, other vasodilatory agents, pentoxifylline,[95] and the use of platelet infusions to help stabilize the source of atheroemboli.[96] However, no controlled trials have shown that any of these forms of therapy are of benefit, and we do not recommend them.

Surgical Therapy

Surgical therapy is the preferred method of removing the source of proximal atheromatous embolic material. When the source is in the aortoiliac region, replacement of that segment of aorta or iliac arteries is warranted. When the atheromatous material is infrarenal, an aortobiiliac or aortobifemoral bypass is indicated. However, if the suprarenal aorta is the source of atheromatous emboli, aortic replacement significantly increases the risk of surgical morbidity and mortality. In this situation the potential benefits of surgery must be weighed against the known risks.

Patients who are poor surgical risks for aortic replacement may be candidates for ligation of the common femoral arteries followed by an extraanatomic bypass, such as an axillobifemoral bypass.[35] The ligation prevents further embolization from reaching the legs, although embolization to the intestines and kidney may still occur. The prognosis for patients undergoing axillobifemoral bypass has often been poor. In one study[35] of 4 patients, all were dead within 6 months of this surgical procedure. However, in other studies the results have been reported to be better. In a series of 7 patients involving extraanatomic bypass with ligation of the distal external iliac arteries, only one death was reported.[97] In another series of 6 patients, all did well with a mean follow-up of almost 2½ years.[98]

No well-designed trials have compared medical and surgical therapy for treatment of atheromatous embolization. The most common types of surgery are resection and graft replacement or thromboendarterectomy. Several reports have suggested that these surgical procedures will prevent recurrences of atheromatous embolization.[99-101] In a recent series involving 62 patients with cutaneous manifestations of atheroemboli, Baumann et al[32] noted no further episodes during a mean follow-up of 20.2 months. However, not all reports show a correlation between therapeutic intervention (surgical, medical, or none) and results. Wingo et al[102] showed that surgical therapy did not predict whether the patient would suffer further atheroembolic episodes. They studied 67 extremities in 48 patients and observed these patients from 1 to 84 months (mean, 26 months). Only 28 patients (44%) manifested an uncomplicated outcome, whereas 38% had evidence of tissue loss, and 14% had recurrent digital ischemia. Amputation was required for 14 limbs (22%), and 20% of the patients died. The outcomes did not correlate at all with the type of treatment, medical or surgical. A well-controlled trial is needed to compare the various treatment modalities for this condition.

Another complicating feature is the difficulty in determining the exact source of the atheromatous emboli. Many patients have involvement of the aortoiliac segments of the arterial tree as well as more distal disease, such as in the superficial femoral artery. When there is evidence of atheromatous embolization in both lower extremities, the lesion is generally in the aorta. However, when only one extremity is involved, it is often difficult to determine whether the emboli originate at the more proximal or the more distal site. Fisher et al[103] studied this question in six patients who developed unilateral blue toe syndrome. In each case the peripheral distal lesion was corrected first by either localized thromboendarterectomy or short reverse saphenous vein grafting. Two patients had concomitant moderately severe aortoiliac atherosclerosis and four patients had mild aortoiliac disease. Only one patient had recurrent embolization during a follow-up period of 8 to 24 months. These results suggest that if there is combined peripheral and aortoiliac atherosclerosis and the embolization is confined to one extremity, the more distal lesion should be corrected first. Only if the patient continues to embolize, should the aortic lesion be corrected.[40,103]

If areas of significant digital gangrene or ischemia occur, sympathectomy may be combined with the surgical procedure to remove the source of the emboli.[35,40,99-103] A lumbar sympathectomy may relieve pain and minimize loss of lower-extremity tissue by improving blood flow and therefore tissue perfusion. Lee et al[101] demonstrated that the group who underwent concomitant sympathectomy had better healing of distal digital ischemic ulcers compared with a group of patients who did not undergo sympathectomy. Amputation may also be required for patients who have atheromatous emboli to the toes or feet. Although thromboendarterectomy or bypass surgery may prevent future embolization, these procedures do nothing to correct the ischemia from a previous embolic event. Therefore when the ischemia is extensive and the chance of healing is minimal with a sympathectomy, an amputation should be performed to relieve pain and remove gangrenous tissue.

Other Interventional Procedures

Recently several investigators[104-107] have recommended percutaneous transluminal angioplasty, laser angioplasty, or percutaneous atherectomy for patients with atheromatous embolization. However, most of these reports are anecdotal, and many patients had fibrinoplatelet emboli rather than atheroemboli. Brewer et al[104] advocated pretreatment with anticoagulants followed by percutaneous transluminal angioplasty for short-segment stenosis or occlusions distal to the aortic bifurcation. In the six patients who underwent this procedure, rest pain was relieved, and peripheral pulses were reestablished. Most of the patients did not develop further evidence of atheromatous embolization. Kumpe, Zwerdlinger, and Griffin[105] have similarly treated 10 patients with "classical blue digit syndrome" by percutaneous transluminal angioplasty. Nine patients demonstrated clinical improvement and showed no evidence of recurrent embolization during a follow-up period of 7 to 86 months (mean, 28 months). Several recent reports have suggested the removal of peripheral atheromatous plaques by means of an atherectomy device.[106,107] The short-term results in these studies are at least as good as those in patients who undergo percutaneous transluminal angioplasty or surgery. Percutaneous atherectomy makes more physiologic sense than percutaneous transluminal angioplasty for treating atheromatous embolization. In percutaneous transluminal angioplasty, the intima is cracked and remolded, and thus theoretically the chance of distal embolization should be increased. However, with percutaneous atherectomy, the plaque is actually shaved off the wall of the vessel and removed through a collection device.

It seems reasonable to try nonsurgical intervention for atheromatous embolization that arises from the vessels distal to the aortic bifurcation. If this intervention fails, surgery can then be considered. However, for most patients with atheromatous embolization the aortoiliac segments are the source of emboli, and surgery is the procedure of choice.

REFERENCES

1. Moldveen-Geronimus M and Merriam JC: Cholesterol embolization: from pathological curiosity to clinical entity, Circulation 35:946, 1967.
2. Dahlberg PJ, Frecentese DF, and Cogbill TH: Cholesterol embolism: experience with 22 histologically proven cases, Surgery 105:737, 1989.
3. Panum PL: Experimentelle Beitrage Zur Lehre Von der Embolie, Arch Pathol Anat Physiol Klin Med 25:308, 1862.
4. Doch G: Some notes on coronary arteries, MS Reporter 75:1, 1896.
5. Albutt TC: Diseases of the arteries, including angina pectoris, London, 1915, MacMillan and Company.
6. Flory CM: Arterial occlusions produced by emboli from eroded aortic atheromatous plaques, Am J Pathol 21:549, 1945.
7. Snyder HE and Shapiro JL: A correlative study of atheromatous embolism in human beings and experimental animals, Surgery 49:195, 1961.
8. Gore I and Collins DP: Spontaneous atheromatous embolization: review of the literature and a report of 16 additional cases, Am J Clin Pathol 33:416, 1960.
9. Hoye SJ et al: Atheromatous embolization: a factor in peripheral gangrene, N Engl J Med 261:128, 1959.
10. Handler FP: Clinical and pathologic significance of atheromatous embolization, with emphasis on an etiology of renal hypertension, Am J Med 20:366, 1956.
11. Harrington JT, Sommers SC, and Kassirer JP: Atheromatous emboli with progressive renal failure: renal arteriography as the probable inciting factor, Ann Intern Med 68:152, 1968.
12. Pollitt J and Lee BM: Renal failure from atheroembolism after translumbar aortography, J Am Geriatr Soc 19:989, 1971.
13. Gaines PA et al: Cholesterol embolization: a lethal complication of vascular catheterisation, Lancet 1:168, 1988.
14. Drost H et al: Cholesterol embolization as a complication of left heart catheterization: report of 7 cases, Br Heart J 52:339, 1984.
15. Colt HG et al: Cholesterol emboli after cardiac catheterization: eight cases and a review of the literature, Medicine 67:389, 1988.
16. Nawar T et al: Widespread atheromatous emboli following abdominal aortography, Can Med Assoc J 100:1005, 1969.
17. Kennedy A, Cumberland D, and Gaines P: The pathology of cholesterol embolism arising as a complication of intra-aortic catheterization, Histopathology 15:515, 1989.
18. Ramirez G et al: Cholesterol embolization: a complication of angiography, Arch Intern Med 138:1430, 1978.
19. Rosansky SJ and Deschamps EG: Multiple cholesterol emboli syndrome after angiography, Am J Med Sci 288:45, 1984.
20. Gjesdal K, Orning OM, and Smith E: Fatal atheromatous emboli to the kidneys after left heart catheterization, Lancet 2:405, 1977.

21. Fisher ER, Hellstrom R, and Myers JD: Disseminated atheromatous emboli, Am J Med 29:176, 1960.
22. Tilley W et al: Renal failure due to cholesterol emboli following PTCA, Am Heart J 110:1301, 1985.
23. Labs JD, Merillat JC, and Williams GM: Analysis of solid phase debris from laser angioplasty: potential risks of atheroembolism, J Vasc Surg 7:326, 1988.
24. Hyman BT et al: Warfarin-related purple toes syndrome and cholesterol microembolization, Am J Med 82:1233, 1987.
25. Brenowitz JB and Edwards WS: The management of atheromatous emboli to the lower extremities, Surg Gynecol Obstet 143:941, 1976.
26. Bruns FJ, Segel DP, and Adler S: Control of cholesterol embolization by discontinuation of anticoagulant therapy, Am J Med Sci 275:105, 1978.
27. Ridker PM and Michel T: Streptokinase therapy and cholesterol embolization, Am J Med 87:357, 1989.
28. Shapiro LS: Cholesterol embolization after treatment with tissue plasminogen activator, N Engl J Med 321:1270, 1989 (letter).
29. Schwartz MW and McDonald GB: Cholesterol embolization syndrome: occurrence after intravenous streptokinase therapy for myocardial infarction, JAMA 258:1934, 1987.
30. Perdue GD and Smith RB: Atheromatous microemboli, Ann Surg 169:954, 1969.
31. Feder W and Auerbach R: "Purple toes": An uncommon sequelae of oral coumarin drug therapy, Ann Intern Med 55:911, 1961.
32. Baumann DS et al: An institutional experience with arterial atheroemboli, Ann Vasc Surg 8:258, 1994.
33. Thurlbeck WM and Castleman B: Atheromatous emboli to the kidneys after aortic surgery, N Engl J Med 257:442, 1957.
34. Mashiah A et al: Massive atheromatous emboli to both kidneys: a fatal complication following aortic surgery, J Cardiovasc Surg 29:60, 1988.
35. Kaufman JL, Stark K, and Brolin RE: Disseminated atheroembolism from extensive degenerative atherosclerosis of the aorta, Surgery 102:63, 1987.
36. Elliot RS, Kanjuh VI, and Edwards JE: Atheromatous embolism, Circulation 30:611, 1964.
37. Saklayen MG: Atheroembolic renal disease: preferential occurrence in whites only, Am J Nephrol 9:87, 1989.
38. Cappiello RA et al: Cholesterol embolism: a pseudovasculitic syndrome, Semin Arthritis Rheum 18:240, 1989.
39. Fischer DA and Kistner RL: Atherothrombotic emboli in the lower extremities, Arch Dermatol 104:533, 1971.
40. Karmody AM et al: "Blue toe" syndrome: an indication for limb salvage surgery, Arch Surg 111:1263, 1976.
41. Rosansky SJ: Multiple cholesterol emboli syndrome, South Med J 75:677, 1982.
42. Olin JW: Syndromes that mimic vasculitis, Curr Opin Cardiol 6:765, 1991.
43. Fine MJ, Kapoor W, and Falanga V: Cholesterol crystal embolization: a review of 221 cases in the English literature, Angiology 38:769, 1987.
44. Falanga V, Fine MJ, and Kapoor WN: The cutaneous manifestations of cholesterol crystal embolization, Arch Dermatol 122:1194, 1986.
45. Deschamps P et al: Livedo reticularis and nodules due to cholesterol embolism in the lower extremities, Br J Dermatol 97:93, 1977.
46. Kalter DC, Rudolph A, and McGavran M: Livedo reticularis due to multiple cholesterol emboli, J Am Acad Dermatol 13:235, 1985.
47. Sheehan MG, Condemi JJ, and Rosenfeld SI: Position dependent livedo reticularis in cholesterol emboli syndrome, J Rheumatol 20:1973, 1993.
48. Richards AM et al: Cholesterol embolism: a multiple-system disease masquerading as polyarteritis nodosa, Am J Cardiol 15:696, 1965.
49. Harvey JC: Cholesterol crystal microembolization: a cause of the restless leg syndrome, South Med J 69:269, 1976.
50. Turakhiak KA: Splinter hemmorhages as a possible clinical manifestation of cholesterol crystal embolization, J Rheumatol 17:1083, 1990.
51. Probstein JG, Jostic RA, and Blumenthal HT: Atheromatous embolization: etiology in acute pancreatitis, Arch Surg 75:566, 1957.
52. Orvar K, Johlin FC: Atheromatous embolization resulting in acute pancreatitis after cardiac catheterization and angiographic studies, Arch Intern Med 154:1755, 1994.
53. Hendel RC et al: Multiple cholesterol emboli syndrome: bowel infarction after retrograde angiography, Arch Intern Med 149:2371, 1989.
54. Thomas W and Zaret P: Cholesterol emboli causing acute gangrenous cholecystitis, Mt Sinai J Med 51:716, 1984.
55. Keon WJ, Heggtveit HA, and Leduc J: Perioperative myocardial infarction caused by atheroembolism, J Thorac Cardiovasc Surg 84:849, 1982.
56. FitzGibbon GM and Keon WJ: Atheroembolic perioperative infarction during repeat coronary bypass surgery: angiographic documentation in a survivor, Ann Thorac Surg 43:218, 1987.
57. Blauth CI et al: Atheroembolism from the ascending aorta, J Thorac Cardiovasc Surg 103:1104, 1992.
58. Humphreys MH: Thromboembolic disorders of the major renal vessels. In Brenner BM and Rector FC, eds: The kidney, Philadelphia, 1981, WB Saunders.
59. Otken IB: Experimental production of atheromatous embolization, Arch Pathol 68:685, 1959.
60. Warren BA and Vales O: The ultrastructure of the stages of atheroembolic occlusion of renal arteries, Br J Exp Pathol 54:469, 1973.
61. Jones DB and Iannaccone PM: Atheromatous emboli in renal biopsies: an ultrastructural study, Am J Pathol 78:261, 1975.
62. Wilson DM, Salazer TL, and Farkouh ME: Eosinophiluria in atheroembolic renal disease, Am J Med 91:186, 1991.
63. Smith MC, Ghose MK, and Henry AR: The clinical spectrum of renal cholesterol embolization, Am J Med 71:174, 1981.
64. McGowan JA and Greenberg A: Cholesterol atheroembolic renal disease: report of 3 cases with emphasis on diagnosis by skin biopsy and extended survival, Am J Nephrol 6:135, 1986.
65. Ho Sw-C, Thatcher GN, and Matz LR: Reversible renal failure due to renal cholesterol embolism, Aust N Z J Med 12:531, 1982.
66. Kasinath BS et al: Eosinophilia in the diagnosis of atheroembolic renal disease, Am J Nephrol 7:173, 1987.
67. Kasinath BS and Lewis EJ: Eosinophilia as a clue to the diagnosis of atheroembolic renal disease, Arch Intern Med 147:1384, 1987.
68. Cosio FG, Zager RA, and Sharma HM: Atheroembolic renal disease causes hypocomplementaemia, Lancet 2:118, 1985.
69. Firth JD and North JP: Does atheroembolic renal disease cause hypocomplementemia? Lancet 2:1133, 1985.
70. Gonsette R and Delnotte P: In vitro activation of serum complement by contrast media: a clinical study, Intervent Radiol 15(suppl):26, 1980.
71. Case Records of the Massachusetts General Hospital (Case 23-1974), N Engl J Med 290:1365, 1974.

72. Case Records of the Massachusetts General Hospital (Case 49-1975), N Engl J Med 293:1308, 1975.

73. Case Records of the Massachusetts General Hospital (Case 25-1967), N Engl J Med 276:1368, 1967.

74. Case Records of the Massachusetts General Hospital (Case 50-1977), N Engl J Med 297:1337, 1977.

75. Case Records of the Massachusetts General Hospital (Case 33-1974), N Engl J Med 291:406, 1974.

76. Case Records of the Massachusetts General Hospital (Case 4-1984), N Engl J Med 310:244, 1984.

77. Case Records of the Massachusetts General Hospital (Case 21-1972), N Engl J Med 286:1146, 1972.

78. Case Records of the Massachusetts General Hospital (Case 8-1972), N Engl J Med 286:422, 1972.

79. Case Records of the Massachusetts General Hospital (Case 38-1993), N Engl J Med 329:948, 1993.

80. Rosman HS et al: Cholesterol embolization: clinical findings and implications, J Am Coll Cardiol 15:1296, 1990.

81. Vidt DG et al: Atheroembolic renal disease: association with renal artery stenosis, Cleve Clin J Med 56:407, 1989.

82. Kassirer JP: Atheroembolic renal disease, N Engl J Med 280:812, 1969.

83. Meyrier A et al: Atheromatous renal disease, Am J Med 85:139, 1988.

84. Maurizi CP, Barker AE, and Trueheart RE: Atheromatous emboli: a postmortem study with special reference to the lower extremities, Arch Pathol 86:528, 1968.

85. Wagner RB and Martin AS: Peripheral atheroembolism: confirmation of a clinical concept, with a case report and review of the literature, Surgery 73:353, 1973.

86. Kealy WF: Atheroembolism, J Clin Pathol 31:984, 1978.

87. Sieniewicz DJ et al: Atheromatous emboli to the kidneys, Radiology 92:1231, 1969.

88. Retan JW and Miller RE: Microembolic complications of atherosclerosis, Arch Intern Med 118:534, 1966.

89. Anderson WR and Richards AM: Evaluation of lower extremity muscle biopsies in the diagnosis of atheroembolism, Arch Pathol 86:535, 1968.

90. Carvajal JA et al: Atheroembolism: an etiologic factor in renal insufficiency, gastrointestinal hemorrhages, and peripheral vascular diseases, Arch Intern Med 119:593, 1967.

91. Tunick PA, Perez JL, and Kronzon I: Protruding atheromas in the thoracic aorta and systemic embolization, Ann Intern Med 115:423, 1991.

92. Karalis DG et al: Recognition and embolic potential of intraaortic atherosclerosis debris, J Am Coll Cardiol 17:73, 1991.

93. Morris-Jones W et al: Gangrene of the toes with palpable peripheral pulses: response to platelet suppressive therapy, Ann Surg 193:462, 1981.

94. Walden R, Adar R, and Mozes M: Gangrene of toes with normal peripheral pulses, Ann Surg 185:269, 1977.

95. Carr ME, Sanders K, and Todd WM: Pain relief and clinical improvement temporally related to the use of pentoxifylline in a patient with documented cholesterol emboli, Angiology 45:65, 1994.

96. Turnbull RG, Hayashi AH, and McLean DR: Multiple spontaneous intestinal perforations from atheroemboli after thrombolytic therapy: a case report, Can J Surg 37:325, 1994.

97. Kazmier FJ and Hollier LH: The shaggy aorta, Heart Dis Stroke 2:131, 1993.

98. Friedman SG and Krishnasatry KV: External iliac ligation and axillary-bifemoral bypass for blue toe syndrome, Surgery 115:27, 1994.

99. Kempczinski RF: Lower-extremity arterial emboli from ulcerating atherosclerotic plaques, JAMA 241:807, 1979.

100. Mehigan JT and Stoney RJ: Lower extremity atheromatous embolization, Am J Surg 132:163, 1976.

101. Lee BY et al: Blue digit syndrome: urgent indication for digital salvage, Am J Surg 147:418, 1984.

102. Wingo JP et al: The blue toe syndrome: hemodynamics and therapeutic correlates of outcome, J Vasc Surg 3:475, 1986.

103. Fisher DF et al: Dilemmas in dealing with blue toe syndrome: aortic versus peripheral source, Am J Surg 148:836, 1984.

104. Brewer ML et al: Blue toe syndrome: treatment with anticoagulants and delayed percutaneous transluminal angioplasty, Radiology 166:31, 1988.

105. Kumpe DA, Zwerdlinger S, and Griffin DJ: Blue digit syndrome: treatment with percutaneous transluminal angioplasty, Radiology 166:37, 1988.

106. Hofling B et al: Percutaneous removal of atheromatous plaques in peripheral arteries, Lancet 1:384, 1988.

107. Dolmatch BL et al: Blue toe syndrome: treatment with percutaneous atherectomy, Radiology 172:799, 1989.

CHAPTER FIFTEEN

ACUTE ARTERIAL OCCLUSION

Anthony J. Comerota
Russell N. Harada

An *acute arterial occlusion* is the abrupt interruption of blood flow within an artery. Manifestations of acute arterial occlusion reflect the pathophysiologic consequences of the end organ supplied by the involved artery. Acute occlusion of a coronary artery can result in myocardial infarction; occlusion of a carotid or intracranial artery can result in stroke; occlusion of a renal artery results in severe hypertension associated with renal dysfunction; and mesenteric arterial occlusion is associated with severe abdominal pain and intestinal ischemia and/or infarction. This chapter addresses only acute arterial occlusion of the extremities. Although the lower extremity is specifically addressed, upper-extremity ischemia follows precisely the same principles.

The consequences of acute arterial occlusion depend on the degree of occlusion and the patient's underlying collateral circulation. Since acute arterial occlusion is usually indicative of significant underlying pathology (either of the blood vessel or the heart), it is important for the physician to diagnose the event properly and to identify its etiology since appropriate therapy can have a profound effect on long-term outcome.

ETIOLOGY

Acute arterial occlusions can be categorized as either extrinsic or intrinsic. The former is usually traumatic and the latter embolic or thrombotic. The ischemic consequences of acute arterial occlusion of both categories can be similar, but the treatment of the underlying lesion varies considerably.

It is beyond the scope of this chapter to deal but briefly with extrinsic occlusions. Either blunt or penetrating injuries can result in extrinsic occlusions, which often occur when the interstitial pressure within an enclosed tissue space compromises the circulation of the extremity, causing a compartment syndrome. The compartmental pressures may be acutely increased because of hemorrhage within the compartment, crush injury, thermal injury, or direct muscle trauma. Elevated compartment pressures also occur following a prolonged period of muscle ischemia and are likely secondary to cell swelling and increased capillary permeability, resulting in an increase in interstitial fluid and pressure.[1,2] The anterior compartment of the leg, through which the peroneal nerve passes, is the most vulnerable muscle compartment. Tenderness over this compartment, pain with dorsiflexion and hypoesthesia of the skin between the first and second toes are helpful in making the diagnosis. Ischemic injury can occur despite the presence of distal pulses and commonly occurs with compartment pressures of 40 to 50 mm Hg.[3]

Acute venous obstruction on rare occasion can manifest as acute arterial insufficiency when massive venous occlusion causes venous pressures to rise to exceptionally high levels, thereby compromising arterial perfusion. This begins as a "physiologic occlusion" and is most commonly seen following iliofemoral deep vein thrombosis. Limb swelling that precedes the signs of acute arterial insufficiency is a clue that acute venous obstruction may be responsible.

The dissecting hematoma of an acute aortic dissection can initially be seen as an acute arterial occlusion that obstructs flow through any branch of the aorta. The diagnosis is generally made through the associated extreme hypertension and by the tearing back and abdominal pain that usually begins in the interscapular area.

The overwhelming majority of acute occlusions are either thrombotic or embolic. Acute thrombosis that occurs in a severely diseased artery because of atherosclerotic disease can be minimally symptomatic or asymptomatic; thus the actual acute occlusion may not be recognized.[4] Emboli, on the other hand, are much more likely to be acutely symptomatic since they can suddenly occlude minimally diseased or normal arteries (Table 15-1). Seventy-five percent to ninety percent of emboli originate in the heart.[4-8] The most common underlying cardiac pathology is atrial fibrillation, which occurs in up to 75% of patients with peripheral emboli.[4,9] Myocardial infarc-

Table 15-1. Acute Arterial Occlusion: Embolism vs. Thrombosis

Characteristics of Occlusion	Embolus	Thrombosis
Onset of symptoms	Rapid/immediate	Slower/insidious
Prior symptoms	Infrequent	Frequent
Duration of symptoms before presentation	Shorter	Longer
Opposite leg	Frequently normal examination	Frequently abnormal examination
Recent heart disease (artrial fibrillation, myocardial infarction)	Frequent	±
Goal of immediate therapy	Eliminate embolus	Correct underlying disease
Long-term pharmacologic prescription	Anticoagulation (if cardiac source)	Platelet inhibition (± anticoagulation)
Results of thromboembolectomy	Good	Poor
Amputation risk	Lower	Higher
Cause of subsequent mortality	Cardiac disease	Related to persistent limb ischemia

tion with mural thrombi ranks second. Less common cardiac sources include prosthetic valves, dyskinetic cardiomyopathic ventricles, and ventricular aneurysms. Rarer causes of cardiac-derived emboli include atrial myxoma, cardioversion, marantic endocarditis, diseased cardiac valves, and paradoxic emboli.[10]

Arterial emboli may also originate from proximal ulcerated arterial plaque or thrombus, the so-called arterioarterial occlusion, and frequently are associated with digital ischemia or necrosis. Patients may have associated areas of painful but punctate necrosis of the skin, with a surrounding area of cyanosis. The frequent confusion involved with the diagnosis and treatment of atheromatous emboli results from a poor understanding of its pathophysiology. In general, patients with an atherothrombotic microembolism should not be considered in the same category as those with an acute large-vessel occlusion. These patients most frequently have transient focal ischemia associated with minor tissue loss but no major foot or limb ischemia and should not be considered with those in the threatened limb categories.

Acute arterial thrombosis is the other common form of acute arterial ischemia. It generally is superimposed on a low-flow state during which the thrombotic threshold of a vessel is surpassed. Underlying atherosclerotic disease is the most commonly associated pathology. It is generally believed that limbs suffering acute ischemia after a thrombotic occlusion are associated with higher amputation rates than those with an embolic cause.[11,12] This observation is based on the results of surgical thromboembolectomy in which removal of an acute occluding embolus opens the majority of the occluded arterial tree and, in the absence of additional emboli, restores perfusion through a relatively nondiseased artery. On the other hand, removal of a thrombus from a diseased artery without definitive reconstruction leaves the pathology in place, usually resulting in reocclusion and progression of the ischemic process.[13] The clinical distinction between arterial embolism and arterial thrombosis is often difficult to make; however, a concerted effort must be made because of the short- and long-term therapeutic implications.

PATHOPHYSIOLOGIC CONSEQUENCES OF ACUTE ARTERIAL OCCLUSION

The consequences of an acute arterial occlusion hinge on several factors. Foremost is the degree of collateral circulation supplied to the tissue by the involved vessel.[14] If sufficient collateral flow is present, no clinical sequelae are discernible. This situation may occur when an acute thrombosis is superimposed on a chronic stenosis. A slowly progressing atherosclerotic stenosis allows time for the development of collaterals. An example is the patient without symptoms who is incidentally noted to have a superficial femoral artery thrombosis superimposed on chronic atherosclerotic disease. At the other extreme is the patient without peripheral vascular disease in whom an embolus suddenly moves from the heart to the femoral artery without the patient having had the opportunity to develop collaterals. This scenario almost certainly leads to acute symptoms and a threatened limb. Between these extremes is a wide range of collateralization that permits the clinical spectrum of signs and symptoms that occur with acute occlusions.

If insufficient collaterals exist, tissue susceptibility to ischemia over time assumes paramount significance. It is well established that different tissues vary in their ability to tolerate ischemia. Nerve and skeletal muscle can suffer ischemia for only 4 to 6 hours before histologically demonstrable changes occur.[15] Skin will tolerate ischemia for 10 hours or more before irreversible changes become evident microscopically. Subcutaneous tissue resists ischemia even longer since it can be nourished by interstitial fluid. These susceptibilities are presumably a measure of the oxygen demand of the various tissues.

Blebea et al[16] demonstrated the duration of ischemia required to induce irreversible injury in the gracilis muscle of a dog. They isolated the dog's gracilis muscle, leaving it attached only to its nutrient artery and vein. After arterial occlusion for 4, 6, or 8 hours, the accumulation of technetium 99m (Tc 99m) pyrophosphate in the injured muscle was measured. Only 8% more Tc 99m pyrophosphate accumulated after 4 hours of occlusion than in controls, with 215% at 6 hours, and 400% to 500% at 8 hours.

Histologic examination confirmed that irreversible cellular damage occurred after 6 hours of occlusion and reperfusion; however, the injury was reversible after 4 hours. Most of the observed injury centered around the gracilis arteries, suggesting that reperfusion may play a role in inducing injury after acute occlusion.

Abundant recent evidence suggests that a substantial component of tissue injury occurs following reperfusion of ischemic tissue. Oxygen free radicals (OFRs), the toxic metabolites of molecular oxygen generated when oxygen is supplied at the time of reperfusion, are believed to be the primary mediators of reperfusion injury. These unstable and thus highly reactive oxygen intermediates include hydrogen peroxide (H_2O_2), superoxide (O_2^-) and the hydroxyl radical ($^\bullet OH$). Because of unstable electron configurations, OFRs will react with adjacent molecules causing damage to membrane lipids, nucleic acids, proteins, and enzymes, which will lead to increased vascular permeability, edema, and muscle necrosis.[17-21] The enzyme xanthine oxidase appears to be the major source of OFR production in ischemia/reperfusion injury. This enzyme exists predominately as xanthine dehydrogenase. However, under hypoxic conditions it is rapidly converted to xanthine oxidase. Hypoxanthine is produced in large amounts in ischemic tissue from the catabolism of adenosine monophosphate (AMP). When reperfusion occurs, xanthine oxidase converts hypoxanthine to xanthine, with the production of excess O_2^- radical. Xanthine oxidase is ubiquitous throughout the body, but its highest concentrations are found in capillary endothelial cells and intestinal mucosal cells.[22,23] Although the activity of xanthine oxidase is low under resting conditions, a rapid increase in activity has been documented after the onset of ischemia in certain tissues.[23-25] Furthermore, pretreatment of isolated rat hind limbs with an inhibitor of xanthine oxidase (allopurinol) reduces lipid peroxidation, suggesting that a reduction in antioxidant production occurs with xanthine oxidase inhibition.[25]

The most compelling evidence that OFRs are involved in reperfusion injury of skeletal muscle is that scavengers of OFR have a protective effect against reperfusion injury. Walker[26] studied the effects of controlled oxygen delivery and free radical scavengers on reperfusion injury in the isolated canine gracilis muscle. The gracilis muscle was made ischemic for 5 hours, after which controlled reperfusion with reduced oxygen alone or in combination with free radical scavengers was performed. In both groups muscle necrosis was significantly reduced over the control group. However, a greater reduction in muscle necrosis was seen in the free radical scavenger treated group. In another study Ricci et al[27] studied the effect of free radical scavengers on the isolated anterior compartment of the dog hind limb after 8 hours of acute ischemia. Thirty minutes before reperfusion they administered either superoxide dismutase or mannitol (a scavenger of the –OH radical) intravenously. One hour after reperfusion Tc 99m pyrophosphate accumulation was assessed. There was significantly less muscle injury in the dogs receiving free radical scavengers than in the control animals. Muscle function studied 16

hours after reperfusion, however, demonstrated abnormal contractions even in the scavenger group. Thus free radical scavengers may decrease the muscle injury after acute arterial occlusion and reperfusion, but they did not appear to preserve normal muscle function.

The neutrophil may play an important role in ischemia/reperfusion injury. They are well equipped to produce large quantities of OFRs and a significant influx of neutrophils has been seen following reperfusion in affected tissues.[28] In vivo experiments have shown that neutrophils are sequestered in skeletal muscle following ischemia for the first 48 hours of reperfusion,[29] and ischemia followed by reperfusion in canine gracilis muscle increases O_2^- production by directly activating neutrophils.[30] Leukocyte depletion[31] and inhibition of leukocyte adherence to the endothelial cell by monoclonal antibodies directed against adhesion molecules[32] have significantly reduced microvascular permeability following reperfusion. Additionally Rubin et al[29] have shown that reperfusion with blood free of leukocytes and complement significantly reduced muscle necrosis when compared with unaltered reperfusion in a canine gracilis model.

Subfascial pressure may rise precipitously after reperfusion, resulting in a compartment syndrome that may limit capillary perfusion and eventually result in muscle necrosis. As mentioned previously, Ricci et al[27] were unable to preserve muscle function using free radical scavengers despite their decreasing the extent of necrosis. Using fasciotomy after controlled arterial occlusion, however, they decreased muscle necrosis as measured by Tc 99m pyrophosphate scanning and preserved normal muscle contraction. They concluded that early fasciotomy is the treatment of choice for reperfusion compartment syndrome. These experimental observations fit well with the clinical findings of Lim et al,[33] who treated vascular trauma of the popliteal artery by performing routine fasciotomy before vascular repair. In this traditionally morbid injury associated with a 20% to 30% limb loss, they found that early fasciotomy followed by careful vascular repair offered significantly better limb salvage than previously reported.

Beyersdorf et al[34] focused attention on the effects of reperfusion versus the direct effects of ischemia caused by acute arterial occlusion. Using the amputated hind legs of rats, they studied the effects of standard uncontrolled reperfusion through the rat femoral arteries versus controlled reperfusion. Standard reperfusion was performed using Krebs-Hanseleit buffer at 37° C at a pressure of 100 mm Hg for 60 minutes. Controlled reperfusion was performed with a substrate-enriched modified perfusate at 37° C and a pressure of 50 mm Hg for 30 minutes. Thereafter this group was further perfused with standard Krebs-Hanseleit buffer at 100 mm Hg for 30 minutes. Uncontrolled reperfusion resulted in severe injury involving massive edema and the loss of contractile function, whereas controlled reperfusion preserved near-normal leg volume and contractile function. The authors emphasize maintaining the following three conditions for performing controlled reperfusion: (1) gentle perfusion pressures (50 mm Hg), (2) normothermia, and (3) prolonged duration of controlled reperfusion. Additionally they emphasize that injury results directly from uncontrolled reperfusion, and perhaps more importantly injury can be diminished significantly by decreasing reperfusion pressure. Their argument would be more convincing if they had used the same solution to reperfuse both limbs instead of adding a substrate-enriched solution to the controlled reperfused limb.

Anoxia impairs cellular metabolism as anaerobic glycolysis assumes the burden of adenosine triphosphate (ATP) formation. The lack of energy results in the loss of biocellular functions, including the active extrusion of sodium from cells. The increased intracellular sodium leads to cellular edema. If the ischemia is reversed before irreversible injury occurs, a reactivated sodium pump will reextrude the sodium from the cell, thereby restoring normal cell volume. It has been suggested that the cellular edema may obstruct capillaries, thereby perpetuating cellular ischemia despite the restoration of blood flow.[35] This has been referred to as the *no-reflow phenomenon*. Experimentally use of intravenous hypertonic mannitol has been effective in decreasing cellular edema following ischemia by reducing the degree of tissue injury that follows transient compression of the renal artery.

The depletion of erythrocyte ATP by ischemia leads to loss of red cell deformability, which may also impair the restoration of flow in ischemic tissues with edematous cells.[36]

In addition to cellular edema, distal propagation of thrombus, particularly within arterioles and capillaries, can prevent perfusion of tissue despite restoration of blood flow through major arteries.[37] Belkin, Valeri, and Hobson[38] studied the effect of urokinase on the acute occlusion of an isolated gracilis muscle preparation. After 5 hours of acute clamp occlusion of the gracilis artery, urokinase was injected into the artery for 5 minutes and was allowed to incubate in the gracilis muscle preparation for 15 minutes before reperfusion. The contralateral canine gracilis muscle exposed to the same degree of ischemia was used as a control.

Triphenyltetrazolium chloride staining of the muscle preparation demonstrated 20.2% (±8.1%) infarction in the control muscle versus 8.6% (±6.2%) in the urokinase-infused preparations. There was a 33.6-g gain (±5.9) in weight in the control muscle versus an 18.2-g gain (±4.1) in the urokinase-treated preparation. Both findings were statistically significant. Although gracilis muscle blood flow was better in the experimental group compared with the control group, the difference was not statistically significant. Overall blood flow per se may not be a good indicator of the success of reperfusion since overall flow does not reflect the distribution of flow through the ischemic tissue.

In addition to the local consequences of acute arterial occlusion, toxic metabolites distal to the occlusion may enter the systemic circulation, particularly during reperfusion, leading to systemic consequences. Restoration of flow to a profoundly ischemic limb results in the sudden overloading of the systemic circulation with lactate, potassium, myoglobin, and sometimes bacterial toxins. The consequence is a metabolic derangement, resulting in cardiovascular depression and renal impairment.[39-41] In 1960 Haimovici[39] reported two cases of acute massive muscle ischemia associated with myoglobinuria. Since then myoglobinuria with renal failure caused by muscle necrosis after acute arterial occlusion has been well described. Myoglobin released from necrotic muscle precipitates in renal tubules and may result in renal failure. Alkalinization of urine with a bicarbonate infusion and adequate hydration accompanied by administration of a loop diuretic help keep myoglobin soluble, thereby decreasing its likelihood of precipitation in the renal tubules.

In 1970 Fisher, Fogarty, and Morrow[42] reported the biochemical effects of prolonged transient acute femoral occlusion in four patients. Each artery was occluded by an embolus for at least 12 hours. The venous efflux of the ipsilateral femoral vein was assayed for partial pressure of oxygen (P_{O_2}), creatine phosphokinase (CPK), pH, partial pressure of carbon dioxide (P_{CO_2}), and potassium. These values were compared with those of systemic venous blood. The average venous P_{O_2} in the ischemic leg was significantly lower (18, ±8 mm Hg) than the systemic venous value (40, ±3 mm Hg). Five minutes after restoration of flow the venous P_{O_2} returned to normal in all four ischemic limbs. The average venous P_{CO_2} in the ischemic legs was 40 (±5 mm Hg), and the systemic value was 32 (±3 mm Hg) before restoration of flow. Although the venous pH was lower in all four ischemic legs compared with systemic values, 5 minutes after reperfusion the pH fell further to an average value of 7.07 (±0.13). Potassium levels were normal and similar in both the ischemic leg and the systemic circulation before reperfusion. However, 5 minutes after reperfusion there was a marked increase in the venous potassium of the ischemic leg (6.2 and 6.6 mEq in two patients whose duration of occlusion exceeded 100 hours). Systemic venous CPK concentrations were elevated in all four patients before reperfusion (average, 26 U). The venous CPK in the ischemic legs was more remarkable (average, 190 U). Five minutes after restoration of flow, the CPK of the ischemic leg rose to an average of 456 U.

We have measured the degree and duration of hyperkalemia and acidosis following reperfusion of profoundly ischemic limbs. The magnitude of metabolic abnormalities was similar to that previously reported; however, the hyperkalemia and acidosis persisted well beyond the 15-minute period of monitoring. The biochemical effects of an acute arterial occlusion can be profound, and the release of by-products of cellular necrosis into the systemic circulation following reperfusion can itself be life-threatening. These metabolic abnormalities can persist for a prolonged period after revascularization.

CLINICAL MANIFESTATIONS

The classic presentation of acute arterial occlusion is described by the six "*p*'s": pain, pallor, paresthesias, pulselessness, paralysis, and polar (cold) sensation.

History

The patient frequently complains of a sudden onset of pain, coldness, and paresthesias distal to the site of occlusion. Occasionally patients remember the precise instant the pain occurred. In such cases embolic arterial occlusion at a major bifurcation has occurred. As the peripheral nerves become affected by the ischemic process, paresthesias and then numbness develop. Finally, with severe occlusion paralysis occurs.

Physical Examination

Signs of ischemia generally are observed one joint distal to the level of arterial occlusion. A superficial femoral artery occlusion, for example, will generally cause ischemia distal to the knee joint. If examined within the first 8 hours of acute occlusion, the involved extremity will often be pale (pallor) because of the acute spastic reaction of the distal arterial tree following acute occlusion. After 12 to 24 hours the extremity may become cyanotic and mottled with intermittent patches of pallor. Spasm resolves with dilation of the involved arteries. Because of profound stasis, prograde thrombosis is likely to continue, further jeopardizing the limb.

The acutely ischemic limb may appear withered and "doughy" to the touch. Palpable pulses are absent distal to the occlusion. A Doppler device is useful in verifying any pulsatile velocity signals within the distal arterial tree. The extremity is generally cold, and as one examines the more proximal limb, an area of temperature demarcation can be appreciated.

As the peripheral nerves suffer the consequences of ischemia, loss of light-touch sensation and/or position sense occurs. With more prolonged and severe ischemia the position sense becomes abolished, with loss of sensation to pinpricks and ultimately weakness and paralysis. Once paralysis occurs, the prognosis is poor, and irreversible ischemia is imminent if reperfusion is delayed. If ischemia progresses, the muscles become painful and firm and subsequently rigid. If these signs are present, the likelihood of successful revascularization with limb salvage is small, and if attempted, the patient's life may be placed in jeopardy because of the severe metabolic derangement that will follow revascularization.

The Ad Hoc Committee on Reporting Standards of the Society for Vascular Surgery and the North American Chapter of the International Society for Cardiovascular Surgery have suggested guidelines for identifying and reporting patients with acute ischemia.[43] The following categories of acute diffuse limb ischemia have been recommended (Table 15-2).

1. *Viable: extremity not immediately threatened.* The patient does not complain of ischemic rest pain, there is no neurologic deficit, and the skin capillary circulation appears adequate. On examination there are clearly audible Doppler pulsatile flow signals in the pedal arteries, with ankle pressures above 30 mm Hg.
2. *Threatened viability: implies reversible ischemia and a foot that is salvageable without major amputation if the arterial obstruction is promptly relieved.* These patients complain of ischemic rest pain and have mild or incomplete neurologic defects (sensory loss involving vibration, light touch, position, or weakness of toes or foot on dorsiflexion). Audible arterial Doppler signals are not present in pedal arteries; however, venous signals, especially with augmentation maneuvers, are demonstrable.
3. *Major, irreversible ischemic change: frequently requires major amputation of limb.* Findings include profound sensory loss and muscle paralysis, absent capillary skin blood flow, or evidence of more advanced ischemia such as muscle rigor or skin marbling. Neither arterial nor venous Doppler flow signals are audible.

Diagnostic Studies

In general, patients presenting with acute arterial ischemia undergo the routine blood studies evaluating renal and electrolyte status, blood cell count, cardiac enzymes, and blood gas determinations. An electrocardiogram and chest x-ray are also part of the routine evaluation. A rapid Doppler survey of the involved extremity and contralateral extremity is performed, and segmental pressures and pulse waveforms, if rapidly obtained, lend additional objective evidence about the severity of ischemia and may be of some predictive value as well as serving as the patient's baseline.

Table 15-2. Clinical Categories of Acute Limb Ischemia

Category	Description	Capillary Return	Muscle Weakness	Sensory Loss	Doppler Signals	
					Arterial	Venous
Viable	Not immediately threatened	Intact	None	None	Audible (AP >30 mm Hg)	Audible
Threatened	Salvageable if promptly treated	Intact	Mild, partial	Mild, incomplete	Inaudible	Audible
Irreversible	Major tissue amputation regardless of treatment	Absent (marbling)	Profound, paralysis (rigor)	Profound anesthetic	Inaudible	Inaudible

(From Ad Hoc Committee on Reporting Standards, SVS/NAISCVS: Suggested standards for reports dealing with lower extremity ischemia, J Vasc Surg 4:80, 1986.)

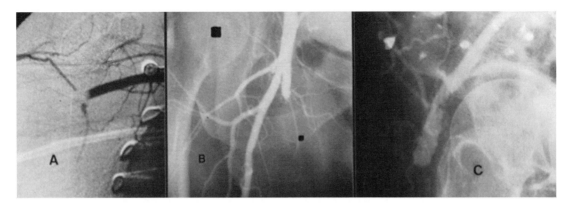

Fig. 15-1. Angiographic demonstration of three different types of acute arterial occlusion. **A,** Acute embolic occlusion of the axillary artery (note classical meniscus sign). **B,** Acute thrombotic occlusion of the superficial femoral artery. **C,** Acute iatrogenic occlusion of right common femoral artery caused by production of an atherosclerotic intimal flap during cardiac catheterization.

Angiography

The use of angiography is not always advocated. When the site of an acute occlusion is clinically apparent and is surgically accessible and the cause is obviously embolic with the limb severely ischemic, no further diagnostic studies other than those that can be done at the bedside are indicated, and a surgical embolectomy is warranted. It might be judged that no additional information of therapeutic importance will likely be obtained from an angiogram. Additionally the fear of delaying a needed embolectomy becomes real if angiography facilities or personnel are not readily available. Most patients, however, do not have a clear-cut presentation, and we generally recommend complete angiography. Examples of three different types of acute arterial occlusion are shown angiographically in Fig. 15-1.

Our preference for preoperative angiography is based on its track record of safety, its ready availability, and its usefulness in helping to establish the diagnosis and in planning therapy. In recent years angiography has become important in evaluating and preparing the patient for percutaneous intraarterial thrombolytic therapy, which has evolved as an important therapeutic adjunct in many of these patients.[44]

In addition to helping differentiate embolic occlusion from thrombotic occlusion, the angiogram can identify instances of multiple-vessel occlusions, which often indicate an underlying embolic process. Angiography localizes the occlusion, which in some cases can be atypical, especially in patients with extensive atherosclerosis, and offers important information about patent distal vessels should a bypass be required. Additionally, unusual causes of acute ischemia such as giant cell arteritis, dissecting aneurysms, and low-flow states can be appropriately identified.

Management

The most appropriate management of patients with acute arterial occlusion can be offered if the underlying cause (thrombosis vs. embolus) is delineated.[7,13,45-49]

On presentation the patient is given a bolus of heparin, followed by a heparin infusion to maintain therapeutic anticoagulation. Data suggest that higher doses of heparin (2000 to 4000 U/hr) are more effective than standard doses without increasing the risk of bleeding complications.[50]

Rapid anticoagulation is important to interrupt prograde and retrograde thrombosis, and also to minimize the risk of additional embolic episodes; therefore our suggested bolus dose is 5000 to 20,000 U, depending on the degree of ischemia, the timing of arteriography, and other patient care considerations.

The introduction of the Fogarty catheter[51] ushered in the modern era of vascular surgery and gave surgeons an important new technique for arterial thromboembolectomy. Seldom has a technical advance improved the surgical results of a procedure as has the Fogarty catheter. Good to excellent results increased by 75%, fair results decreased by 66%, and the death and amputation rates fell by 35% to 50%.[45,51-54]

Embolic Occlusion

Compared to the experience with a single-extremity embolus, surgical treatment of carotid and visceral emboli continues to be poor.[45] The results in patients with simultaneous multiple emboli continue to carry an unfavorable prognosis, resulting in a 60% to 100% mortality rate.

As stated previously, although the differentiation between embolic occlusion and thrombotic occlusion may be difficult, it remains important because of the short- and long-term therapeutic implications. Early opinions stated that it was easy to differentiate embolic versus thrombotic occlusion since years ago acute embolic occlusion mainly occurred in patients with rheumatic heart disease. These patients were generally younger with much less associated vascular disease; therefore the acute occlusion of peripheral vessels was dramatic and instantly recognized, and treatment was instituted with frequent confirmation of the diagnosis. During the last 2 decades atherosclerotic heart disease occurring in an older population has become a more common source of embolism than rheumatic heart disease. Therefore the current principal source of emboli, atherosclerotic heart disease, occurs in patients likely to have existing peripheral vascular disease. Likewise, because of the increasing age of the U.S. population, patients requiring intervention for thrombotic arterial occlusion frequently have associated heart disease, contributing further to the dilemma of accurately differentiating between embolic and thrombotic occlusion.

Numerous factors are used to differentiate between embolic and thrombotic occlusions (Table 15-1). Cambria and Abbott[11] stated that atrial fibrillation was the only sign of discriminating value to differentiate acute embolic from thrombotic occlusion. Limb salvage clearly depends on the severity of ischemia. In Cambria's series 11% of patients who had moderate ischemia lost their limb compared with 40% who had severe ischemia.

In general terms patients with an acute embolic occlusion have a higher mortality rate, reflecting the severity of their underlying cardiac condition. On the other hand, patients with an acute thrombotic occlusion have a higher limb-loss rate, indicative of the more severe underlying vascular disease and the inability to restore perfusion adequately with simple thrombectomy techniques. The mortality rate associated with acute arterial thrombosis apparently correlates with ongoing peripheral arterial ischemia and progression to gangrene.[4,7,11,12]

Jivegard, Holm, and Schersten[13] clearly demonstrated that surgical thrombectomy without definitive reconstruction for acute arterial thrombosis was associated with unacceptably high morbidity and mortality rates. These observations are supported by Field, Littoy, and Baker[46] who significantly improved limb salvage by performing a definitive reconstructive procedure at the time of initial exploration for acute limb ischemia after a thrombotic occlusion became evident. On the other hand, those patients having appropriate thromboembolectomy for acute embolic occlusion have significantly lower limb loss, and their mortality rate, as mentioned, is directly related to their underlying cardiac disease.

Thus attention to the underlying cardiac disease is critical. There is stratification of cardiac mortality, however, within the group of patients suffering embolic occlusion. Patients with emboli resulting from acute myocardial infarction have a 40% mortality rate compared with a 9% mortality rate in those suffering emboli from atrial fibrillation not associated with acute myocardial infarction.[12]

After performing the expedient patient evaluation previously mentioned, the patient is prepared for angiography. Unless there is clear-cut evidence of a large-vessel acute embolic occlusion that is surgically accessible, angiography is routinely performed before intervention. The urgency of intervention is based on the severity and extent of ischemia. Most femoral emboli can be approached through an inguinal incision, exposing the common femoral, profunda, and superficial femoral arteries. Fogarty catheter embolectomy of these vessels remains the procedure of choice in most patients. A completion arteriogram is routinely performed to evaluate the distal vessels for occlusion and residual thrombus. If the popliteal artery and its terminal branches are involved, performing a complete embolectomy is difficult if not impossible through a femoral approach.[55] In such instances exposure of the popliteal artery and embolectomy of the popliteal trifurcation is suggested. This approach has resulted in improved limb-salvage rates compared with the inadequate results obtained with a femoral exposure.

When failure of revascularization occurs after occurrence of an acute arterial embolus, it is usually due to distal small-vessel occlusion that defies removal by the Fogarty catheter. Additionally, Spencer and Eisman[56] noted extensive side-branch propagation of the clot occurring in patients having embolectomy more than 10 hours after the acute occlusion. Additionally the presence of a residual clot after thromboembolectomy is common.[57] In such instances we have found the intraoperative, intraarterial infusion of thrombolytic agents highly beneficial in regaining patency of side branches and in clearing the distal circulation following performance of mechanical thrombectomy.[58] Our current recommendation is to infuse up to 250,000 U of urokinase over 30 minutes through a distal arteriotomy either through a continuous infusion or with a repeated bolus technique over the same period. This method has proven safe in a prospective, randomized, blinded and placebo-controlled trial of intraoperative intraarterial urokinase infusion during lower-extremity revascularization.[59] One of three bolus doses of urokinase (125,000, 250,000, 500,000 U) or placebo (saline solution) was infused into the distal circulation before lower-extremity bypass for chronic limb ischemia. Blood was sampled from the femoral vein of the involved limb and the arm for plasma levels of fibrinogen, fibrin degradation products, fibrin breakdown products, and plasminogen. Although dose-related plasminogen activation resulted in significant breakdown in cross-linked fibrin systemically, there was no significant fibrinogen depletion or increased blood loss or wound hematoma formation.

In some instances the extent of distal thrombosis may be so extensive that it is not amenable to a single- or multiple-bolus technique, or the patient may have multivessel involvement and an absolute contraindication to any risk from systemic fibrinolysis. In these instances performing an isolated limb perfusion with high-dose urokinase (1,000,000 U) may be effective (Fig. 15-2). Since regional drainage of the venous effluent is part of this technique, there is no danger of systemic fibrinolysis. This technique is particularly effective in patients suffering distal arterial occlusion with propagation of thrombus, which requires higher doses and more prolonged exposure to the lytic agent than can be obtained with a single or double bolus.

Patients with multiple arterial emboli, distal emboli, and those who are poor operative risks should be considered for catheter-directed thrombolysis. We have found that intraarterial thrombolytic therapy is highly successful in patients with acute embolic arterial occlusion and restores perfusion more rapidly than in patients who suffer acute arterial thrombosis. The current technique and recent results are reviewed in the following section.

Judgment must be shown when the profoundly ischemic limb is revascularized. Gregg et al[12] reported that patients with embolic occlusion who had "recoverable" ischemia had a 90% limb-salvage rate and a mortality rate of 16% after embolectomy. On the other hand, those patients with rigidity of their involved muscles, indicating irreversible ischemia, uniformly lost their limbs and had an

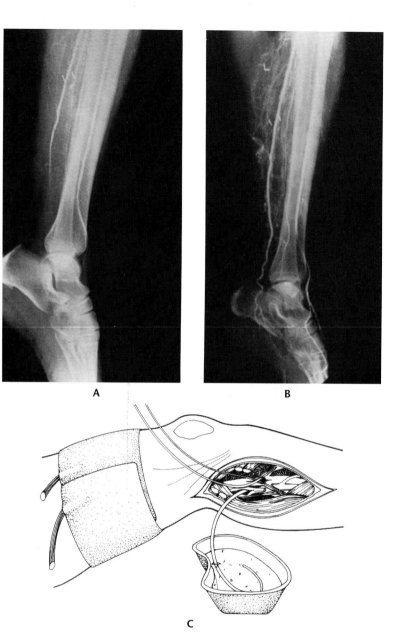

Fig. 15-2. Description of the intraoperative high-dose, isolated limb perfusion of urokinase for the treatment of multivessel distal acute arterial occlusion. This patient underwent an emergency coronary artery bypass and required the use of an intraaortic balloon for hemodynamic stabilization. Three days postoperatively the intraaortic balloon was percutaneously removed. Shortly thereafter the patient lost her previously palpable posterior tibial pulse, then lost her dorsalis pedis pulse, and finally lost her popliteal pulse. Her leg was profoundly ischemic. The patient was taken to the operating room where exposure of the distal popliteal artery and trifurcation was performed. Inflow to the popliteal artery was easily achieved. Direct thrombectomy of the anterior tibial, posterior tibial, and peroneal arteries was performed. After complete balloon catheter thrombectomy was performed, an intraoperative completion arteriogram was obtained. **A,** No contrast material reached the foot despite direct injection into the anterior and posterior tibial arteries. Thinking that this condition would necessitate a major amputation, an isolated limb perfusion of high-dose urokinase was performed. The limb was raised, venous blood was exsanguinated with the use of an Esmarch bandage, and a thigh blood pressure cuff was applied and inflated to 300 mm Hg pressure. The popliteal vein was isolated and a venotomy performed, with a red rubber catheter placed distally to allow drainage of the venous effluent. Through the small Silastic catheters in the anterior tibial and posterior tibial arteries, 1,000,000 U of urokinase dissolved in 1000 L of saline solution were infused (500,000 U each through the anterior tibial and posterior tibial arteries). **B,** After the urokinase was infused, the limb was flushed with heparinized saline solution. The venotomy was closed primarily and the arteriotomy closed with a small PTFE patch. **C,** An intraoperative completion arteriogram was again obtained, demonstrating flow into the foot through both the anterior and posterior tibial arteries. The patient had a palpable dorsalis pedis pulse, and the foot was pink and warm at the completion of the procedure.

exceptionally high mortality rate (73%). Therefore there are instances when primary amputation is justified. These instances occur in patients with profound ischemia in whom revascularization carries an exceptionally high risk to life and in those who are bedridden and unlikely to walk again.

Following restoration of perfusion to the ischemic limb after embolic occlusion, long-term anticoagulation therapy is mandatory unless the source of the embolus (e.g., proximal aneurysm) has been removed. The benefits of long-term anticoagulation therapy have been shown by Elliott et al[45] and Silvers, Royster, and Mulcare.[60] Permanent anticoagulation therapy has been associated with substantially lower mortality and recurrence rates (Fig. 15-3).

Thrombotic Occlusion

Patients presenting with acute arterial thrombosis should be initially treated with full anticoagulation

therapy as previously described. The important underlying principle of operative revascularization is that the underlying arterial segments (which are thrombosed) are diseased, and a bypass (or endarterectomy if a short segment of artery is involved) is required for definitive revascularization. Simple thrombectomy is inadequate and usually leads to recurrent thrombosis. Therefore the use of arteriography is important in all these patients to properly identify the site of occlusion, the involved vessels, and the proper outflow vessels. Revascularization with autogenous saphenous vein is our preferred surgical approach in the majority of patients with infrainguinal arterial thrombosis. In some, however, if a localized lesion can be identified and corrected, a less extensive procedure such as an endarterectomy can be performed with excellent long-term results (Fig. 15-4).

During the past decade intraarterial infusion of thrombolytic agents has offered an important alternative therapeutic approach that has obvious advantages for many

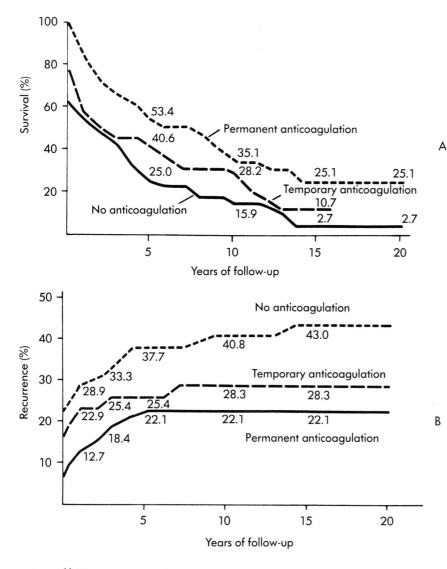

Fig. 15-3. **A,** Cumulative survival experience of 215 patients after the initial embolic episode treated with permanent anticoagulation (*n* = 97), temporary anticoagulation (*n* = 19), and no anticoagulation (*n* = 69). **B,** Cumulative rate of recurrence of embolization in 215 survivors of an initial acute embolic episode treated with permanent anticoagulation (*n* = 97), temporary anticoagulation (*n* = 19), and no anticoagulation (*n* = 69). (From Elliott JP et al: Arterial embolization: problems of source, multiplicity, recurrence and delayed treatment, Surgery 88:833, 1980.)

patients.[44] The concept is that segmental atherosclerotic disease, when severe enough, will precipitate thrombosis involving substantially longer segments of the arterial tree. Lysis of the thrombus with subsequent identification of the underlying atherosclerotic disease allows a more directed correction, whether with percutaneous balloon dilation, stenting techniques, endarterectomy, or a limited bypass. Guidewire passage is attempted through the occluded arteries at the time of the initial arteriogram in all patients judged candidates for lytic therapy. Passage of the guidewire predicts a high likelihood of successful lysis. Shortell and Ouriel[61] evaluated 80 patients with acute (< 14 days) limb ischemia treated with intraarterial thrombolysis. Successful lysis was achieved in 92% of those in whom successful guidewire passage was achieved as compared with only 10% of those in whom the guidewire did not pass.

The patient is then prepared for the direct intrathrombus infusion of urokinase, which has been shown to be important for the success of lytic therapy. Shortell and Ouriel,[61] found that intrathrombus infusion was associated with successful lysis in 85% of patients, whereas thrombolysis was unsuccessful in all 13 patients in whom

the catheter was not placed in the clot. We generally follow the technique established by McNamara and Fisher[62]; however, we have more recently been infusing higher initial doses (6000 U/min) and lacing the thrombus with urokinase before beginning the continuous infusion. With this method of patient selection lytic therapy is usually completed within 24 hours and frequently within 12 hours. If definitive correction of the underlying atherosclerotic lesion is not accomplished with percutaneous techniques at the time of the completion arteriogram, the patient is given anticoagulation therapy until definitive surgical repair is achieved.

Fig. 15-5 provides an example of treating a patient with a 5-day thrombotic occlusion of his superficial femoral artery. This patient underwent recanalization and percutaneous balloon dilation in 1982. At his most recent follow-up office visit 13 years later, he has palpable distal pulses and an ankle-brachial index of 0.90. Proper patient selection is critical for successful lytic therapy, and the guidewire test has been most helpful in this regard. If the guidewire cannot be passed through the occluded vessel, lytic therapy is not offered, and the most appropriate surgical reconstruction is planned.

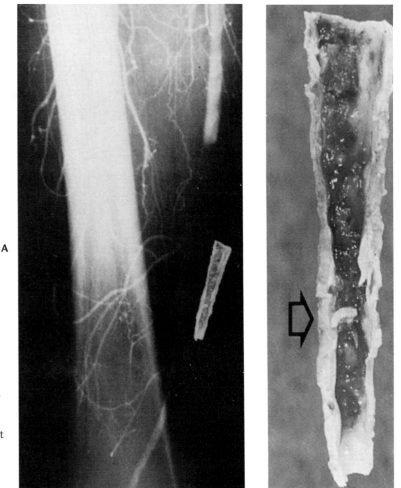

A

B

Fig. 15-4. A, Lower-extremity angiogram shows occlusion (thrombosis) of patient's superficial femoral artery. The focal plaque causing the acute thrombosis is juxtaposed to the arteriogram, showing that long-segment occlusion can be caused by short, focal lesions. **B,** Close-up of the excised atherosclerotic plaque shows small focal defect *(arrow)* responsible for the longer-segment acute arterial thrombosis.

Two recent randomized trials comparing lytic therapy to surgery for ischemia of the lower extremities have been completed. Ouriel et al[63] reported on 114 patients with ischemia of less than 7 days' duration, equally randomized to receive either intraarterial catheter-directed urokinase or operative revascularization. The ischemia was due to acute thrombosis in 80% and embolic occlusion in 20% of the patients. The limb salvage rate was 82% at 12 months in both groups of patients. However, the cumulative survival rate was significantly improved in those patients randomized to thrombolysis (84% vs. 58% at 12 months, $P = 0.01$). The increased mortality with surgery was attributed to the greater incidence of cardiopulmonary complications occurring after surgery. However, in a previously published study of the hematologic effects of intraoperative, intraarterial urokinase infusion, a significant survival benefit was observed in patients receiving urokinase compared with saline solution controls.[59] Since this was a prospective, randomized, blinded, and placebo-controlled trial and since all patients underwent surgery, the survival benefit may be related to the temporary fibrinolytic state.

The surgery versus thrombolysis for the ischemic lower extremity (STILE) trial was a prospective, randomized, multicenter trial evaluating optimal surgical treatment versus intraarterial catheter-directed thrombolysis for is-

chemia of the lower extremity due to nonembolic arterial and graft occlusion.[64] Patients with progression of ischemic symptoms during the prior 6 months were eligible for randomization. Although 30-day outcomes demonstrated significant benefit to surgical therapy compared with thrombolysis ($P < 0.001$), when stratified by duration of ischemia, patients with acute ischemia (less than 14 days) had significantly lower amputation rates ($P = 0.052$) and shorter hospital stays ($P < 0.04$) than those treated surgically. Patients presenting with chronic ischemia (14 to 180 days) had a better outcome when treated surgically, with less ongoing/recurrent ischemia ($P < 0.001$) and a trend toward lower morbidity ($P = 0.1$). At 6-month follow-up, those presenting with acute ischemia showed a significant improvement in amputation rate when treated with thrombolysis ($P < 0.01$), whereas those with ischemia of greater than 2 weeks had a significantly better amputation rate when treated surgically ($P = 0.01$). Additionally thrombolysis reduced the magnitude of the surgical procedure in 55.8% of patients. The investigators concluded that the best overall results are obtained by combining a treatment strategy of catheter-directed thrombolysis for acute limb ischemia with surgical revascularization for chronic limb ischemia.

It is revealing that in contemporary, randomized studies

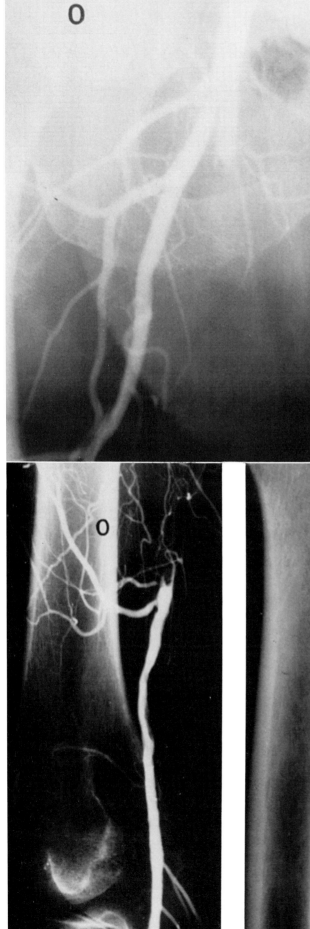

A

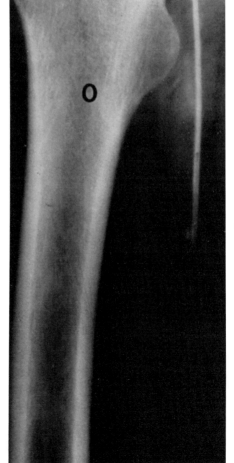

Fig. 15-5. Demonstration of the use of intraarterial delivery of thrombolytic therapy to dissolve the occluding thrombus and to identify and correct an underlying lesion. **A,** Arteriogram demonstrates acutely thrombosed superficial femoral artery in a letter carrier who complained of intolerable intermittent claudication. **B,** A patent popliteal artery; distal run-off was provided by all three intrapopliteal vessels. **C,** Infusion catheter threaded from the contralateral femoral artery and embedded 6 to 8 inches into the occluding thrombus. Following infusion of the fibrinolytic agent, the thrombus was lysed and a stenosis demonstrated at the proximal superficial femoral artery.

B

C

Continued.

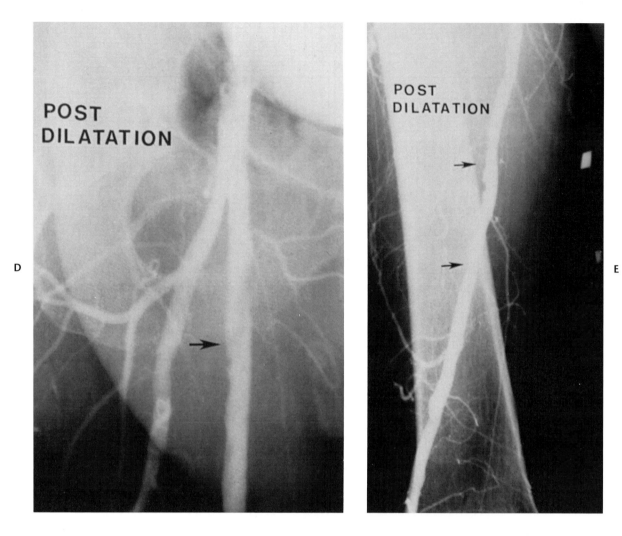

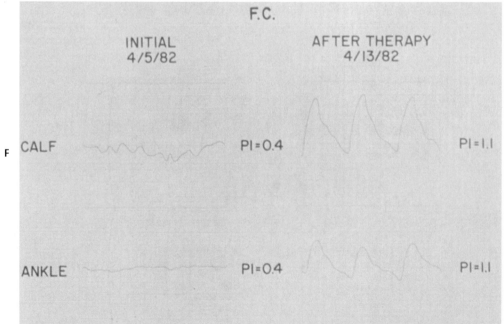

Fig. 15-5, cont'd. **D,** The stenosis *(arrow)* was dilated with good results. **E,** Two additional stenotic lesions *(arrows)* in the distal superficial femoral artery were likewise dilated with good results. **F,** Patient's initial pulse waveforms and ankle indexes on presentation and after therapy. Thirteen years after treatment the patient continues to have palpable distal pulses, nearly normal pulsewave forms, and an ankle index of 0.90.

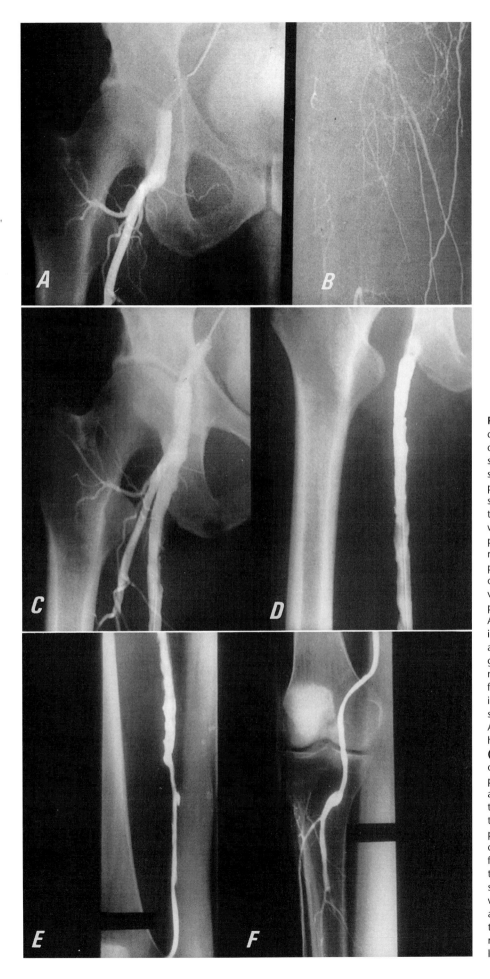

Fig. 15-6. This series of angiograms demonstrates the utility of catheter-directed thrombolysis in a patient presenting with acute occlusion of his superficial femoral artery and femoral-popliteal bypass graft **(A)** with extension of the thrombus into and through the popliteal artery **(B)**. The bypass was performed 18 months earlier as part of treatment of a popliteal aneurysm. The patient had ischemic rest pain and no audible Doppler signals on presentation. All superficial leg veins were previously used, and the patient's arm veins were diminutive. A multi-sidehole catheter and coaxial infusion guidewire were advanced into and through the occluded artery and graft. A bolus of 500,000 U of urokinase was injected into the thrombus followed by 2000 U/min of urokinase infused through the catheter and a similar dose through the guidewire. After 36 hours patency was restored to his ectatic superficial femoral artery **(C,D)** and the saphenous vein femoral-popliteal bypass graft **(E,F)**. A proximal graft stenosis was identified and underwent successful balloon dilation **(E)**. Following treatment, the patient had a palpable dorsalis pedis pulse with a normal ankle-brachial index. This allowed a Brescia-Cimino fistula (radial artery to cephalic vein at the wrist) to be constructed with subsequent maturation of a cephalic vein, which then could be used as a good autogenous conduit, bypassing his ectatic superficial femoral artery and replacing his diseased femoral-popliteal graft.

of patients with acute limb ischemia, those who are treated by initial surgical revascularization continue to be associated with high amputation rates. Acute arterial occlusion is a vascular emergency in many patients; however, others can tolerate such occlusion without limb-threatening consequences. The physician who can obtain a complete and careful history, is aware of the subtle (and obvious) physical findings as well as their evolution, can accurately identify the cause, and can put into perspective the spectrum of therapeutic options, will salvage the majority of involved limbs with the least morbidity and mortality (Fig. 15-6). These patients require the interdisciplinary efforts of a team of physicians. The cooperative efforts of the vascular surgeon, radiologist, cardiologist, and coagulation expert are important in the successful therapy of these patients. As new technology is developed, such interdisciplinary approaches will become even more important.

REFERENCES

1. Perry MO, Shires GT III, and Albert SA: Cellular changes with graded limb ischemia in reperfusion, J Vasc Surg 1:536, 1984.
2. Perry MO and Fantini G: Ischemia: profile of an enemy, J Vasc Surg 6:231, 1987.
3. Matsen FA, Winquist RA, and Krugmire RB: Diagnosis and management of compartmental syndromes, J Bone Joint Surg 62A:286, 1980.
4. Abbott WM et al: Arterial embolism: a 44 year perspective, Am J Surg 143:460, 1982.
5. Conett MC, Murray DA, and Wenneker WW: Peripheral arterial emboli, Am J Surg 148:14, 1984.
6. Cranley JJ et al: Peripheral arterial embolism: changing concepts, Surgery 55:57, 1964.
7. Dale WA: Differential management of the acutely ischemic leg, Trans South Surg 84:259, 1972.
8. Darling RC, Austen WG, and Linton RR: Arterial embolus, Surg Gynecol Obstet 124:106, 1967.
9. Balas P et al: Occlusion of the extremities, J Cardiovasc Surg 26:262, 1985.
10. Meister SG et al: Paradoxical embolism. Diagnosis during life, Am J Med 53:292, 1972.
11. Cambria RP and Abbott WM: Acute arterial thrombosis of the lower extremity, Arch Surg 119:784, 1984.
12. Gregg RO et al: Embolectomy or heparin therapy for arterial emboli? Surgery 93:377, 1983.
13. Jivegard L, Holm J, and Schersten T: The outcome in arterial thrombosis misdiagnosed as arterial embolism, Acta Chir Scand 152:251, 1986.
14. Stallone RJ et al: Analysis of morbidity and mortality from arterial embolectomy, Surgery 65:207, 1969.
15. Malan E and Tattori Q: Physio- and anatomo-pathology of acute ischemia of the extremities, J Cardiovasc Surg 4:212, 1963.
16. Blebea J et al: Technetium 99m pyrophosphate quantitation of skeletal muscle ischemia and reperfusion injury, J Vasc Surg 8:117, 1988.
17. Lindsay T et al: Measurement of hydroxy conjugated dienes after ischemia/reperfusion in canine skeletal muscle, Am J Physiol 254:H578, 1988.
18. McCord J: Oxygen-derived free radicals in postischemic tissue injury, N Engl J Med 312:159, 1985.
19. Granger DN, Hollwarth ME, and Parks DA: Ischemia-reperfusion injury: role of oxygen-derived free radicals, Acta Physiol Scand Suppl 548:47, 1988.
20. Korthuis RJ et al: The role of oxygen derived free radicals in ischemia induced increases in canine skeletal muscle vascular permeability, Circ Res 57:599, 1985.
21. Harris K et al: Metabolic response of skeletal muscle to ischemia, Am J Physiol 250(Heart Circ Physiol 19):H213, 1986.
22. Jarasch ED, Bruder G, and Heid HW: Significance of xanthine oxidase in capillary endothelial cells, Acta Physiol Scand 548:39, 1986.
23. Batelli MG, Della Corte E, and Stirpe F: Xanthine oxidase type D (dehydrogenase) in the intestine and other organs of the rat, Biochem J 126:747, 1972.
24. Roy RS and McCord JM: Ischemia-induced conversion of xanthine dehydrogenase to xanthine oxidase, Fed Proc 41:767, 1982.
25. Punch J et al: Xanthine oxidase: its role in the no-reflow phenomenon, Surgery 111:169, 1992.
26. Walker PM: Salvage of skeletal muscle with free radical scavengers, J Vasc Surg 5:68, 1987.
27. Ricci MA et al: Are free radical scavengers beneficial in the treatment of compartment syndrome after acute arterial ischemia? J Vasc Surg 9:244, 1989.
28. Granger DN: Role of xanthine oxidase and granulocyte in ischemia-reperfusion injury, Am J Physiol 255:H1269, 1988.
29. Rubin B et al: A clinically applicable method for long-term salvage of postischemic skeletal muscle, J Vasc Surg 13:58, 1991.
30. Cambria RA et al: Leukocyte activation in ischemia-reperfusion injury of skeletal muscle, J Surg Res 51:13, 1991.
31. Korthuis RJ, Grisham MB, and Granger DN: Leukocyte depletion attenuates vascular injury in postischemic skeletal muscle. Am J Physiol 254:H823, 1988.
32. Oliver MG et al: Morphologic assessment of leukocyte-endothelial cell interactions in mesenteric venules subjected to ischemia and reperfusion, Inflammation 1:331, 1991.
33. Lim LT et al: Popliteal artery trauma, Arch Surg 115:1307, 1980.
34. Beyersdorf F et al: Avoiding reperfusion injury after limb revascularization: experimental observations and recommendations for clinical application, J Vasc Surg 9:757, 1989.
35. Leaf A: Cell swelling: a factor in ischemic tissue injury, Circulation 47:455, 1973.
36. Summers WK and Jamison RL: The no reflow phenomenon in renal ischemia, Lab Invest 25:635, 1971.
37. Dunant JH and Edwards WS: Small vessel occlusion in the extremity after various periods of arterial obstruction: an experimental study, Surgery 73:240, 1973.
38. Belkin M, Valeri CR, and Hobson RW: Intra-arterial urokinase increases skeletal muscle viability after acute ischemia, J Vasc Surg 9:161, 1989.
39. Haimovici H: Arterial embolism with acute massive ischemic myopathy and myoglobinuria, Surgery 47:739, 1960.
40. Haimovici H: Myopathic-nephrotic-metabolic syndrome associated with massive arterial occlusion, J Cardiovasc Surg 14:589, 1973.
41. Haimovici H: Muscular, renal and metabolic complications of acute arterial occlusions. Myonephropathic-metabolic syndrome, Surgery 85:461, 1979.
42. Fisher RD, Fogarty TJ, and Morrow AG: Clinical and biochemical observation of the effect of transient femoral artery occlusion in man, Surgery 68:323, 1970.
43. Ad Hoc Committee on Reporting Standards, SVS/NAISCVS: Suggested standards for reports dealing with lower extremity ischemia, J Vasc Surg 4:80, 1986.
44. Comerota AJ and White JV: Overview of catheter-directed thrombolytic therapy for arterial and graft occlusion. In

Comerota AJ, ed: Thrombolytic therapy for peripheral vascular disease, Philadelphia, 1995, JB Lippincott.

45. Elliott JP et al: Arterial embolization: problems of source, multiplicity, recurrence and delayed treatment, Surgery 88:833, 1980.

46. Field T, Littoy FN, and Baker WH: Immediate and long-term outcome of acute arterial occlusion of the extremities. The effect of added vascular reconstruction, Arch Surg 117:1156, 1982.

47. Hight DW, Tilney NL, and Couch NP: Changing clinical trends in patients with peripheral arterial emboli, Surgery 79:172, 1976.

48. McPhail NV et al: The management of acute thromboembolic limb ischemia, Surgery 93:381, 1983.

49. Murray DWG: Embolism in peripheral arteries, Can Med Assoc J 35:61, 1936.

50. Blaisdell FW, Steele M, and Allen RE: Management of acute lower extremity ischemia due to embolism and thrombosis, Surgery 84:822, 1978.

51. Fogarty TJ et al: A method for extraction of arterial emboli and thrombi, Surg Gynecol Obstet 116:241, 1963.

52. Cranley JJ et al: Catheter technique for arterial embolectomy: a seven-year experience, J Cardiovasc Surg 5:44, 1969.

53. Green RM, DeWeese JA, and Rob CG: Arterial embolectomy before and after the Fogarty catheter, Surgery 77:24, 1975.

54. Thompson JE et al: Arterial embolectomy. A 20 year experience, Surgery 67:212, 1970.

55. Short D et al: The anatomic basis for the occasional failure of transfemoral balloon catheter thromboembolectomy, Ann Surg 190:555, 1979.

56. Spencer RC and Eisman B: Delayed arterial embolectomy. A new concept, Surgery 55:64, 1964.

57. Greep JM et al: A combined technique of peripheral arterial embolectomy, Arch Surg 105:869, 1972.

58. Comerota AJ, White JV, and Grosh JD: Intraoperative, intra-arterial thrombolytic therapy for salvage of limbs in patients with distal arterial thrombosis, Surg Gynecol Obstet 169:283, 1989.

59. Comerota AJ et al: A prospective, randomized, blinded and placebo-controlled trial of intraoperative intra-arterial urokinase infusion during lower extremity revascularization: regional and systemic effects, Ann Surg 218:534, 1993.

60. Silvers LW, Royster TS, and Mulcare JR: Peripheral arterial emboli and factors in their recurrence rate, Ann Surg 192:232, 1980.

61. Shortell CK and Ouriel K: Thrombolysis in acute peripheral arterial occlusion: predictors of immediate success, Ann Vasc Surg 8:59, 1994.

62. McNamara TO and Fischer JR: Thrombolysis of peripheral arterial and graft occlusions: improved results using high dose urokinase, AJR 144:769, 1985.

63. Ouriel K et al: A comparison of thrombolytic therapy with operative revascularization in the initial treatment of acute peripheral arterial ischemia, J Vasc Surg 19:1021, 1994.

64. STILE Investigators: Results of a prospective randomized trial evaluating surgery versus thrombolysis for ischemia of the lower extremity: the STILE trial, Ann Surg 220:251, 1994.

CHAPTER SIXTEEN

EXTRACRANIAL CEREBROVASCULAR DISEASE

Timothy M. Sullivan
Norman R. Hertzer

Cerebrovascular disease is a problem of enormous magnitude. Cerebrovascular accident (CVA) is the third leading cause of death in the United States, surpassed only by heart disease and malignancy.[1] Stroke accounts for 10% to 12% of all deaths in industrialized countries. Almost one in four men and one in five women aged 45 years can expect to have a stroke if they live to age 85. In a population of 1 million, 1600 people will have a stroke each year. Only 55% of these will survive 6 months, and a third of the survivors will have significant problems caring for themselves. As our population ages, the total number of people afflicted with stroke will continue to rise unless historic stroke rates decline in the future.[2]

The etiology of stroke is multifactorial. Ischemic stroke accounts for about 80% of all first-ever strokes, whereas intracerebral hemorrhage and subarachnoid hemorrhage are responsible for 10% and 5%, respectively.[3] Of those strokes that are ischemic in nature, the majority are linked to complications of atheromatous plaques. The most frequent site of such an atheroma is the carotid bifurcation.[4] Although the prevention of stroke in the general population has largely focused on the control of hypertension,[5] a substantial number of strokes are preventable by the identification and treatment of carotid disease, especially as the population ages.

This chapter concentrates on the diagnosis of carotid artery disease, including its medical and surgical treatment for both symptomatic and asymptomatic lesions. In addition, the results of several contemporary prospective randomized trials are reviewed. With this information practicing clinicians can evaluate and rationally advise their patients who present for evaluation of cerebrovascular disease.

HISTORICAL BACKGROUND

The ancient Greeks were well aware of the importance of the great vessels in the neck providing blood flow to the brain; they named the carotids after the symptoms that followed their obstruction—asphyxia or stupor.[6] In 1875,[7] Gowers was the first to link stroke with carotid disease; he reported on a patient with hemispheric stroke secondary to ipsilateral carotid occlusion. The neurologist Hunt[8] emphasized this point and in addition recognized that "cerebral intermittent claudication" was a precursor of subsequent stroke. In 1937 Moniz, Lima, and de Lacerda[9] reported that carotid artery occlusion could be diagnosed by angiography.

The first elective attempt at restoring cerebral blood flow by carotid reconstruction was reported by Strully, Hurwitt, and Blankenberg[10] in 1953, who unsuccessfully endarterectomized a totally occluded carotid artery in the neck. The first successful carotid reconstruction is credited to Eastcott, Pickering, and Robb,[11] who reported their results in 1954. They described a patient suffering from transient ischemic attacks (TIAs) secondary to an atherosclerotic lesion at the carotid bifurcation; this was treated by resection and primary anastomosis. In 1951 Carrea performed the first carotid reconstruction by resecting the diseased proximal internal carotid and restoring flow by direct anastomosis to the external carotid.[12] The results were not reported, however, until 1955. DeBakey[13] and Cooley[14] independently performed successful carotid endarterectomy before Carrea and Eastcott but did not report their results until 1975 and 1956, respectively. Other investigators, including Whisnant, Matsumoto, and Eleback,[15] Julian et al,[16] and Moore and Hall,[17] elucidated the role of cerebral embolization from carotid bifurcation plaques in the etiology of ischemic stroke, providing the basis for carotid surgery. Despite reports documenting the effectiveness of carotid endarterectomy, this procedure has been the source of heated debate and controversy for the past 2 decades. Recent reports, however, including the North American Symptomatic Carotid Endarterectomy Trial[18] (NASCET) and the Asymptomatic Carotid Atherosclerosis Study (ACAS),[19] have identified carotid endarterectomy as the treatment of choice for symptomatic and asymptomatic high-grade carotid stenosis.

ANATOMY AND PHYSIOLOGY OF THE CEREBRAL VASCULATURE

Anatomy

Despite comprising only 2% of total body weight, the brain consumes 25% of inspired oxygen and receives 15% of the total cardiac output.[20] The carotid and vertebral arteries supply blood to the anterior and posterior portions of the brain, respectively; they coalesce via the anastomotic pathways of the circle of Willis within the brain (Fig. 16-1).

Theoretically the entire brain can be adequately supplied by one of the four extracranial cerebral arteries via the circle of Willis. Autopsy studies, however, have shown that the circle of Willis is incomplete in up to 50% of humans.[21-24] A number of collateral pathways exist to provide blood to the brain in cases of major vessel stenosis or occlusion. The circle of Willis is the major collateral pathway. When incomplete, one of the communicating arteries usually is absent. Other anastomotic pathways include (1) branches around the orbit that connect the external carotid and ophthalmic arteries, (2) occipital and ascending pharyngeal branches of the external carotid that may connect to the distal vertebral artery via muscular branches, (3) retrograde flow in the external carotid (from the contralateral external carotid or ipsilateral subclavian

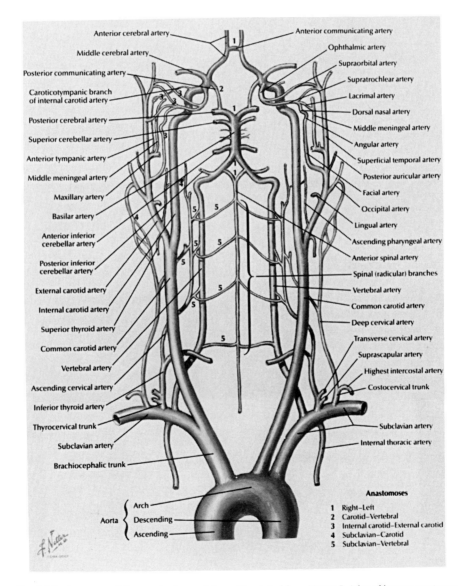

Fig. 16-1. Anatomy of the cerebral vasculature. *(Reprinted from Netter F: Atlas of human anatomy, Plate 131, Summit, NJ, 1992, CIBA-GEIGY Corporation.)*

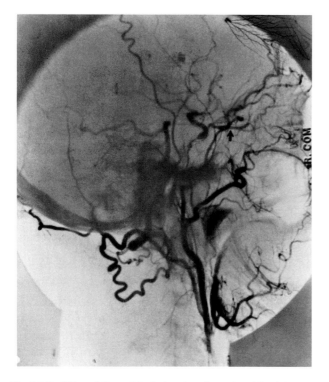

Fig. 16-2. Filling of the ophthalmic artery (arrow) and the intracranial internal carotid artery via supraorbital collaterals of the superficial temporal artery in a patient with occlusion of the extracranial internal carotid.

arteries) that may provide flow to the internal carotid in cases of common carotid occlusion, (4) leptomeningeal and dural anastomoses that may develop to supply cortical branches of the major cerebral vessels (Fig. 16-2).[25]

Physiology

Cerebral blood flow in humans is about 50 ml/100 g of brain per minute. Cerebral blood flow and cerebral energy metabolism are higher in gray matter than in white matter, whereas the ability of the brain to extract oxygen from the blood is relatively constant throughout.[26] Cerebral blood flow is influenced by minute changes in partial pressure of carbon dioxide (Pco_2) and by large drops in arterial partial pressure of oxygen (Pao_2). An acute rise in Pco_2 of 1 mm Hg causes an increase in cerebral blood flow by about 5%, secondary to cerebral vasodilatation.[27] An increase in the functional activity of the brain causes an increase in metabolic activity that is related to an increase in cerebral blood flow. The converse is also true. Cerebral blood flow remains constant when systolic blood pressure is between 60 and 160 mm Hg, secondary to autoregulation. As cerebral perfusion pressure falls, compensatory cerebral vasodilatation causes an increase in cerebral blood flow and maintains perfusion pressure. If the cerebral vasculature reaches a state of maximal dilatation and cerebral perfusion continues to fall, the brain tissue is able, at least to some extent, to increase the extraction of oxygen from the available limited blood supply. Below this level, the patient becomes symptomatic. The nature of these symptoms depends on which area or areas of the brain are ischemic.[28]

Once cerebral blood flow falls below 20 ml/100 g of

brain tissue per minute, brain tissue becomes ischemic. At this level restoration of normal flow may allow recovery of function. Levels of flow below 10 ml/100 g of brain tissue per minute will lead to irreversible cell death and cerebral infarction.[29] Flattening of the electroencephalogram (EEG) occurs when hemispheric blood flow falls below 16 to 17 ml/100 g of brain tissue per minute.[30,31] Below a value of 15 ml/100 g of brain tissue per minute, evoked somatosensory potentials are abolished. This level is thought to be critical and is referred to as the flow threshold of electrical failure in the cerebral cortex.[32-34] It is not known in humans what degree and duration of ischemia is reversible and what is irreversible, nor is it known at what point reperfusion of ischemic tissue is actually harmful. Morawetz et al[35] found that in the monkey recovery was possible following 2 to 3 hours of ischemia if local blood flow was maintained above 12 ml/100 g of brain tissue per minute. This was presumably above a level below which irreversible cellular energy failure occurred.

In addition, the process of autoregulation is lost in ischemic and infarcted brain; restoration of flow to injured tissue may lead to cerebral edema and possibly intracerebral hemorrhage without the ability of the brain to autoregulate. This concept has important ramifications in the treatment of patients with acute stroke. For example, surgical revascularization of patients with acute stroke may actually worsen the situation by converting a "bland" ischemic stroke into a hemorrhagic stroke with resultant cerebral edema.

PATHOPHYSIOLOGY OF CEREBROVASCULAR DISEASE

Atherosclerosis obliterans, although it can affect any artery, has a predilection for certain vessels, including the coronary arteries, the infrarenal abdominal aorta, the superficial femoral artery at the adductor canal, and the carotid bifurcation (Fig. 16-3). These areas seem to predominate at branch points in the arterial circulation. In the carotid circulation the common carotid and the distal internal carotid are usually spared, whereas the carotid bulb is generally involved. These observations have led to hypotheses that suggest that hemodynamic forces are in part responsible for the development of atherosclerotic plaques in certain locations.

A number of investigators, most notably Zarins et al[36] and Ku et al[37] have studied the role of hemodynamic factors in the development of atherosclerosis at the carotid bifurcation. The unique anatomic design of the carotid bulb and bifurcation causes variations in blood flow patterns, including flow separation and stasis along the outer wall of the carotid sinus opposite the flow divider between the internal and external carotid arteries. This pattern of flow has been demonstrated in glass flow models, angiographic studies,[38] and with Doppler ultrasound.[39] This area is exposed to low and oscillating shear stress and is in fact the location of atherosclerotic plaque development in the carotid bifurcation. The same area is the site of development of plaque ulceration, which may also be related to these unusual flow patterns.

Atherosclerotic lesions of the extracranial cerebral vas-

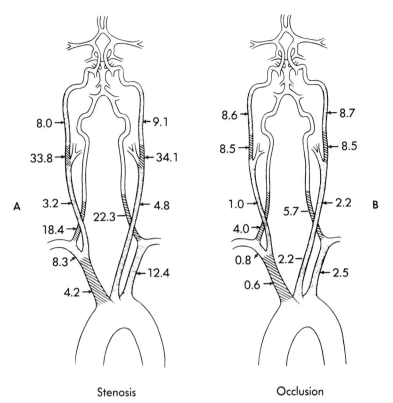

Fig. 16-3. Frequency of stenoses **(A)** and occlusions **(B)** in the surgically accessible extracranial arteries. *(Reprinted from Hass WK et al: Joint study of extracranial arterial occlusion. II. Arteriography, techniques, sites, and complications, JAMA 203:961, 1968.)*

culature may produce cerebral ischemia by a number of mechanisms. The most common of these is embolic occlusion of one or more intracranial vessels (artery to artery embolization), as first recognized by Fisher in 1951.[40,41] The emboli originate from irregularities on the inner surface of the artery, usually secondary to atherosclerotic plaque. These emboli likely consist of thrombus and platelet aggregates formed at critical points of arterial narrowing, where turbulent or stagnant blood flow has stimulated platelet aggregation, or consist of atheromatous debris from an ulcerated atherosclerotic lesion. They can originate from lesions in any of the extracranial vessels but most commonly from the carotid bifurcation. Other investigators, including Hollenhorst[42] and Russell,[43] identified patients with transient monocular blindness secondary to cholesterol crystals or thrombus that had embolized to the retinal vessels. Russell postulated that the same embolic material might be responsible for TIAs. Pathologic evidence was later obtained from the retina of a patient with monocular blindness. The debris within the retinal vessels was found to contain platelets and lipid.[44] Moore and Hall[45,46] were the first to demonstrate that surgical removal of ulcerative, nonstenotic carotid atheromata was successful in treating patients with TIA in the carotid distribution. Thus symptoms were relieved by removal of the offending embolic source, not by improving cerebral blood flow by removing an occluding lesion.

A number of changes in carotid atheromata have been related to cerebral embolization, including intraplaque hemorrhage with and without thrombosis and ulceration, simple ulceration of plaque with exposure of the underlying debris to the arterial circulation, and the formation of smooth cul-de-sacs within plaques, allowing deposition of thrombus. Interestingly these particles tend to embolize to the same terminal cerebral vessels; hence a patient with multiple TIAs will consistently have symptoms in the same neurologic distribution. This phenomenon has been attributed to the characteristics of laminar flow in the cerebral circulation and has been demonstrated in an experimental model.[47] Other less common sources of emboli include arterial irregularities from fibromuscular disease, carotid aneurysm, and arterial dissection.

Carotid plaque hemorrhage has been implicated in the development of cerebrovascular symptoms by a number of investigators.[48,49] Imparato, Riles, and Gorstein[50] were among the first to recognize the importance of carotid plaque hemorrhage in the development of symptomatic carotid disease. In pathologic examination of 69 symptomatic carotid arteries, they found stenoses due to simple fibrous thickening in only 20%. They concluded that carotid plaques start as fibrointimal thickening and evolve to symptomatic lesions by a variety of processes, most importantly intraplaque hemorrhage. Ammar et al[51] found that 82% of symptomatic carotid lesions were associated with intraplaque hemorrhage. They suggested that if a connection developed between the intraplaque hemorrhage and the arterial lumen, the patient may experience TIA or embolic stroke. Intraplaque hemorrhage may also cause thrombotic occlusion of the internal carotid artery and subsequent stroke, as documented by Ogata et al.[52]

A second, less common mechanism by which atherosclerotic carotid artery disease can produce symptoms is related to arterial thrombosis. When the lumen of any artery reaches a critical level of narrowing, the artery may ultimately thrombose. The thrombosis is thought to originate at the critical stenosis and propagate proximally and distally to the level of a major collateral; the collateral, if large enough, will provide enough flow through the remainder of the native artery to maintain patency. In the case of the internal carotid artery, the thrombus originates near its origin and propagates proximally to the origin of the external carotid and distally to the ophthalmic artery. If flow through the ophthalmic artery is adequate, the thrombus will not continue into the middle cerebral artery (MCA), and the patient may not experience any symptoms, depending on the adequacy of the intracranial collateral circulation. On the other hand, if flow via the ophthalmic collateral is insufficient, the thrombus will propagate into the MCA and the patient will suffer a cerebral ischemic event, likely a stroke. It is estimated that 25% of patients with internal carotid artery thrombosis will suffer a clinical stroke.[53,54] The largest series reported to date, which followed 38 patients from stenosis to occlusion, found that internal carotid occlusion occurred *without* symptoms in 70%. Twelve percent of patients suffered TIAs, and eighteen percent suffered a stroke.[55] The percentage of patients with computed tomographic (CT)-documented subclinical stroke was significantly higher in those evaluated for amaurosis fugax (58%) or TIA (75%) who were subsequently found to have an occluded internal carotid.[56]

Although it is now clear that emboli cause the majority of cerebral ischemic events, this view was not universally accepted in the past. A number of investigators espoused the theory that reduction in cerebral flow secondary to carotid artery stenosis was the cause of TIA and stroke.[57-59] In fact, early in the history of carotid endarterectomy, a stenosis of 50% or greater with an associated pressure gradient was considered a sufficient indication for surgery. The converse was also true, in that symptomatic lesions without a pressure gradient were not considered for endarterectomy, regardless of the characteristics of the underlying atherosclerotic lesion.[60]

The least common mechanism by which TIA and ischemic stroke can occur is by reduction in total cerebral blood flow. Patients may present with nonlateralizing cerebral ischemic attacks, including ataxia, bilateral motor or sensory disturbances, homonymous hemianopsia, or bilateral lower-extremity paralysis without loss of consciousness (so-called "drop attacks"). These symptoms are secondary to ischemia of the posterior circulation, and are thought to be flow related. Because of the rich collateral circulation to the brain via the circle of Willis, either three of the four extracranial cerebral vessels must be diseased, or the circle of Willis must be incomplete for these symptoms to occur. An even more rare situation is one in which patients may experience hemispheric TIA ipsilateral to an occluded internal carotid secondary to postural changes in systemic blood pressure. In these cases the cerebral bed distal to the carotid occlusion is marginally perfused to begin with; systemic hypotension simply exacerbates the situation.

A unique anatomic situation that may cause symptoms of vertebrobasilar insufficiency is the subclavian steal syndrome. In these cases stenosis or occlusion of either subclavian artery (or on the right, the brachiocephalic artery) proximal to the origin of the vertebral artery may produce a pressure gradient that favors retrograde flow in the ipsilateral vertebral. Blood is actually siphoned from the basilar artery and the posterior circulation via the vertebral. Neurologic symptoms may include vertigo, limb paresis, paresthesias, visual disturbance, ataxia, and syncope. Symptoms may be exacerbated by upper-extremity exercise, which in the presence of a critical proximal arterial stenosis causes a further pressure drop in the distal subclavian, thereby aggravating the siphon effect. In most cases the subclavian steal merely represents an incidental angiographic finding and is not clinically significant, given the rich collateral network in the brain.[61-65]

NEUROVASCULAR EVALUATION IN PATIENTS WITH CEREBROVASCULAR DISEASE

The key to preventing stroke or recurrent stroke is recognition of the prodromes and risk factors for stroke. The astute clinician will identify these risk factors and symptom complexes and correlate them with the specific anatomic region in the brain that is affected. Only then can appropriate investigational studies be performed and a working diagnosis entertained that will lead to appropriate treatment. As is the case in most disease states, the history and physical examination is the clinician's most important investigational tool. A number of terms require definition.[66]

Transient Ischemic Attack

A *TIA* is defined as an episode of focal cerebral dysfunction due to a vascular cause with rapid onset and complete resolution within 24 hours. The time from the onset of symptoms to their peak is usually about 10 minutes. Most TIAs last only a few minutes; events that last several hours usually leave some residua beyond 24 hours. A TIA may be single or multiple. They are usually considered to be anterior (carotid territory) or posterior (vertebrobasilar). As discussed previously, these events are generally secondary to embolization of atheroma, platelets, or fibrin from a central arterial source. *Crescendo TIA* is used to describe multiple TIAs in close proximity, usually increasing in frequency, duration, and severity with time. This pattern of TIA is thought to herald imminent cerebral infarction.[67,68]

TIA must be differentiated from other central neurologic events, such as migraine and seizure. Migraine is usually encountered in younger individuals. The neurologic deficit is of 10 to 20 minutes' duration and is usually followed by unilateral headache and nausea as the deficit resolves. Migraine is often preceded by a visual or olfactory prodrome, or "aura." Seizure disorders may mimic TIA, as they may occur without a convulsion. The peripheral signs are generally of 1 to 3 minutes' duration and are generally consistent. A jacksonian march, where symptoms spread in a sequential fashion, is readily differentiated from TIA, where the entire extremity is affected at one time.

Stroke-In-Evolution

Stroke-in-evolution refers to the progression of cerebral ischemic symptoms over time, implying progression of infarction. The evolution of infarction differs in the carotid and vertebral-basilar territories. Therefore the clinician should allow 24 hours in the carotid and 72 hours in the vertebrobasilar distributions before defining a stroke as completed.[69,70]

Completed Stroke

In *completed stroke* no further deterioration in neurologic function has occurred; the neurologic status remains stable after 24 to 72 hours. The majority of strokes are ischemic in nature; a proportionately smaller number are secondary to intracerebral hemorrhage. The differentiation between ischemic and hemorrhagic stroke must be made before decisions regarding therapy can be made. The most prominent symptom associated with intracerebral hemorrhage is headache, especially when associated with early vomiting. The onset of symptoms during activity, a history of hypertension, and the use of anticoagulants is characteristic. The presence of TIA preceding an event, the onset of symptoms during sleep, and late onset of headache is more characteristic of infarction. Although history may be helpful in differentiating ischemic from hemorrhagic stroke, the diagnosis must be confirmed by CT scan or by magnetic resonance imaging (MRI) before instituting definitive therapy.

The heart remains a significant source of emboli causing ischemic stroke, accounting for 20% of strokes in adults age 45 to 60. The percentage is even higher in young individuals with ischemic stroke.[71] Cardiac risk factors that favor embolism include valvular heart disease, prosthetic heart valve, recent myocardial infarction, cardiac dysrhythmia, cardiomyopathy, and endocarditis.

Reversible Ischemic Neurologic Deficit

That which causes TIA may cause stroke if more severe or prolonged; the converse is also true. This has led to the concept of *reversible ischemic neurologic deficit (RIND)*, which is defined as an ischemic event that lasts more than 24 hours but less than 72 hours. The definition of RIND is somewhat arbitrary; it likely represents a small cerebral infarct.

CLINICAL NEUROLOGIC SYNDROMES OF CEREBRAL INFARCTION

Internal Carotid Artery

Hemispheric cerebral ischemia is usually the result of ischemia in the distribution of the MCA. This results in contralateral hemiplegia and hemihypesthesia. Four patterns in carotid disease have been described: (1) total MCA infarction (55%) with associated anterior cerebral artery (ACA) infarction (65%), (2) infarction in the proximal MCA (21%), (3) watershed infarcts (19%), and (4) deep white matter infarcts (5%).[72] In addition to hemiplegia and hypesthesia, homonymous hemianopsia or superior quandrantanopsia may manifest in cases of involvement of the optic radiations deep in the temporal lobe. Facial weakness and suppression of the corneal reflex may also be seen. Ischemia of the dominant hemisphere causes aphasia. Ischemia of the nondominant hemisphere results in defects in body image and the inability to perform specific tasks (apraxia). The patient may deny that the affected limb is his or hers (denial or anosognosia). Two types of apraxia are most commonly seen: (1) the inability to construct three-dimensional objects (construction apraxia) and (2) the inability to dress oneself (dressing apraxia). When the entire internal carotid territory is affected, stupor and coma are likely.

Ophthalmic Artery

The ophthalmic artery is the first major branch of the internal carotid artery, and therefore the eye is often involved in neurologic symptoms that reflect disease of the internal carotid artery. Amaurosis fugax, or monocular blindness, is secondary to embolization to the retinal vessels, most commonly from the internal carotid via the ophthalmic. It is a common symptom in patients with disease of the internal carotid; as many as 50% to 70% of patients with amaurosis will have significant disease in the ipsilateral internal carotid. Amaurosis fugax occurs in approximately 30% of symptomatic cases of total internal carotid artery occlusion. Amaurosis fugax may also occur secondary to embolization from the external carotid in cases of internal carotid occlusion, as described by Barnett, Peerless, and Kaufmann.[73] Patients will often describe a dark "shade or shutter" that obscures the vision in one eye; the shade invariably begins in the upper visual field and progresses in a caudad direction. Although the visual loss is usually temporary, permanent visual loss may occur with large occlusive emboli. If collateral circulation is insufficient, high-grade internal carotid stenosis may cause relative ischemia of the retina and progressive visual loss.[74]

So-called "bright-light" amaurosis occurs when the eye is exposed to very bright light, which overcomes the ischemic retina's ability to sense light. The patient experiences temporary visual loss in the affected eye until the retina is able to recover.

Visual loss that may be confused with amaurosis can be caused by giant cell (temporal) arteritis, polycythemia, thrombocythemia, hypotension, drusen of the optic disc, and migraine.

Lacunar Transient Ischemic Attack and Stroke

Occlusion of penetrating end-arterial branches of the basilar artery and the anterior, middle, and posterior cerebral arteries may produce infarction in the internal capsule and thalamus. These infarctions are called *lacunar strokes,* or "lacunes." The name refers to the cavity or hole that remains after the infarcted tissue is removed by macrophages. They are usually small, on average 2 mm in size, and are located almost exclusively in the deep parts of the brain. They most commonly occur in hypertensive and diabetic patients and are preceded by TIA in 20% of cases. A striking finding is their leisurely mode of onset; they may develop over 36 hours, as compared with the usually rapid onset of other types of ischemic stroke. The clinical features of a lacune include pure motor hemiplegia and pure sensory stroke, as distinguished from sensorimotor stroke in MCA occlusion. Pure motor stroke is the most common presentation (60%). Classically the stroke will affect the face, arm, and leg on the same side, whereas sensation, language, and vision are not affected. Other symptom complexes include dysarthria–clumsy hand syndrome and pseudobulbar palsy (dysarthria, dysphagia, emotional lability). The diagnosis is made by CT scan or by MRI, although CT may miss small lacunes (less than 2 mm) and those in the pons (because of brainstem artifact). Treatment involves control of hypertension after stabilization of the neurologic deficit.[75]

PHYSICAL EXAMINATION

Physical examination, accompanied by a thorough history, is extremely important in making a correct diagnosis in patients who present with cerebrovascular symptoms. Neurologic symptoms may be secondary to primary neurologic diseases but more commonly are the manifestations of a systemic disease process. As atherosclerosis may affect portions of the entire vascular tree, a thorough cardiac and vascular examination is imperative in any patient who presents with cerebrovascular symptoms. Indeed, the examiner should take the opportunity to elicit symptoms in the cardiac and pulmonary systems when a patient presents for evaluation.

Physical examination should begin with evaluation of blood pressure in both arms, in both the supine and standing positions. Orthostatic hypotension may be the cause of global cerebrovascular symptoms and syncope or near-syncope and can be documented on physical examination. A difference in the systolic blood pressure of 15% from one extremity to another, accompanied by diminished pulses and pulse delay, is suggestive of subclavian artery stenosis. A further fall in pressure with ipsilateral arm exercise, associated with arm claudication and vertebrobasilar symptoms, is highly suggestive of symptomatic subclavian steal syndrome. The cardiac rate and rhythm are important to document on examination. Although cardiac dysrhythmia is rarely responsible for focal cerebrovascular symptoms in the absence of embolism, it is the usual culprit in patients with syncope or near-syncope. If a rhythm disturbance is suspected but not readily appreciated on examination, Holter monitoring may be indicated. The dysrhythmias most commonly responsible for cerebral symptoms are paroxysmal atrial fibrillation, paroxysmal ventricular tachycardia, atrioventricular block, sinoatrial block, and sinus bradycardia. Careful auscultation of the heart may reveal murmurs associated with valvular heart disease (particularly the aortic and mitral valves) or septal defects, which can cause TIA and embolic stroke. The pansystolic murmur of valvular aortic stenosis is best heard at the right second intercostal space and may radiate into the right and left carotid arteries.

The examiner should then carefully palpate the pulses in the upper and lower extremities and in the cervical region. The subclavian artery can usually be appreciated in the supraclavicular and infraclaviclar fossae. The axillary, brachial, radial, and ulnar pulses should be recorded on a 0 to 4+ scale, with 4+ being normal. With practice, the examiner can easily distinguish these five levels of pulse strength. Pulses should be compared with those in the contralateral extremity. The carotid pulse should be *gently* palpated in the lower neck, midneck, and at the angle of the jaw, along the anterior border of the sternocleidomas-

toid muscle. One may even be able to appreciate a thrill over the carotid artery, suggesting underlying pathology. A pulsatile mass at the angle of the jaw suggests primary atherosclerotic carotid aneurysm, carotid body tumor, or false aneurysm in a patient with prior carotid endarterectomy. The patency of the external carotid artery may be ascertained by palpation of the superficial temporal artery anterior to the tragus of the ear.

Finally, auscultation should be performed over the vessels of the head and neck with both the diaphragm and bell of the stethoscope. The subclavian arteries are auscultated in the supraclavicular and infraclavicular fossae. The carotid and vertebral arteries are auscultated both anterior and posterior to the sternocleidomastoid muscle with the patient holding her breath. In addition, the orbits and the skull should be auscultated, especially in those patients who complain of noises in the ears and head. The examiner should note the location, intensity, radiation, and pitch of any bruits, as well as their relationship to the cardiac cycle. Bruits located low in the neck are usually secondary to transmitted murmurs of cardiac origin, subclavian bruits, or from lesions of the aortic arch. Supraclavicular bruits are present in a significant number of normal young adults. A low-pitched, continuous bruit with diastolic accentuation is often heard in young persons. This so-called "cervical venous hum" may be obliterated by a Valsalva maneuver or by jugular venous compression, and augmented by rotating the neck away from the side of the bruit. It is generally of no pathologic significance, although it may identify a hyperdynamic circulatory state. Subclavian bruits may alert the examiner to significant stenosis in the subclavian artery, especially when accompanied by other signs and symptoms of arterial insufficiency.

Of specific significance is the midcervical or upper cervical bruit. As the external carotid artery is a high-resistance vessel, flow is abolished or reversed during diastole. A bruit in the external carotid artery is therefore a purely systolic bruit. A bruit that continues into diastole must originate from the common or internal carotid arteries, whose flow continues into diastole. A diastolic bruit generally indicates a high-grade carotid stenosis. In particular, a high-pitched, low-intensity bruit that continues into diastole is highly suggestive of a high-grade internal carotid stenosis (greater than 80%) and demands further attention. Although the presence of a cervical bruit is a helpful diagnostic sign, the absence of a bruit should not dissuade the examiner from further evaluation of the symptomatic patient. Only 40% of patients with significant internal carotid artery stenosis have an audible bruit, and of those patients with a bruit, only 20% will have a hemodynamically significant stenosis of the internal carotid artery.[76,77]

The remainder of the physical examination should concentrate on a detailed neurologic examination, including a funduscopic examination. Embolic material may be identified in the arterioles of the retina. These are most commonly cholesterol emboli or Hollenhorst plaques. Central retinal artery occlusion results in a pale retina with a "cherry-red spot" at the fovea. All retinal infarctions should be considered embolic until proven otherwise.[78]

IMAGING MODALITIES IN CEREBROVASCULAR DISEASE

Once the clinical diagnosis of cerebrovascular disease has been made, the diagnosis must be confirmed before definitive therapy can be instituted, be it medical or surgical. Studies that are noninvasive are preferable in terms of patient comfort and in view of the potential complications incurred with invasive methods. Patients who present with crescendo TIA, stroke-in-evolution, and completed stroke should have an imaging study (CT or MRI) of the brain performed, as the size, location, and etiology of stroke will have important implications on the mode and timing of therapy. Those who present with a single, classic hemispheric TIA or who are asymptomatic do not necessarily need brain imaging, although as noted earlier, a significant percentage of these patients will have "silent" infarcts.

Duplex ultrasound of the extracranial cerebral vessels is the initial study of choice in most patients who present for evaluation of carotid disease. The modern color-enhanced duplex ultrasound study can accurately characterize the degree of stenosis and the character of an atheroma at the carotid bifurcation. A number of studies have documented the accuracy of duplex ultrasound in identifying intraplaque hemorrhage, fibrous atheroma, ulceration, and calcification, when comparing duplex ultrasound findings with surgical specimens.[79,80] Goodson et al,[81] in comparing duplex ultrasound with arteriography, found that duplex ultrasound was more accurate in characterizing surface abnormalities and ulceration; the two modalities were equal in predicting degree of stenosis. Duplex ultrasound scanning is limited, however, in its inability to accurately identify lesions of the aortic arch and the distal extracranial and intracranial internal carotid. Despite these shortcomings, a number of studies have documented the safety of performing carotid endarterectomy on the basis of duplex ultrasound findings alone.[82-85]

Currently intraarterial digital subtraction angiography remains the gold standard for evaluation of cerebrovascular disease. The quality of magnetic resonance angiography (MRA) in the cerebrovascular system continues to improve. MRA is a physiologic evaluation of blood flow and only indirectly evaluates vascular anatomy. It is somewhat limited in its ability to define vascular anatomy in the presence of complex, turbulent, or minimal flow such as that seen in the carotid bulb or in aneurysms of the carotid arteries. Lesions that are frequently missed on MRA include ulcerations, tandem lesions, and lesions of the carotid and vertebral origins. Several studies have concluded that MRA consistently overestimates the degree of carotid bifurcation stenosis.[86-88]

The advantages of MRA include the following:

1. Noninvasive
2. Less operator variability than with duplex ultrasound
3. Ability to visualize the proximal common carotid artery, the distal extracranial internal carotid, and the intracranial vessels
4. Ability to evaluate the brain during the same study

5. Avoidance of iodinated contrast medium
6. Ability to present the carotid bifurcation in a format similar to conventional contrast arteriography[89-92]

With improvements in software, MRA will continue to improve and may supplant conventional angiography as the gold standard in the evaluation of patients with cerebrovascular disease (Fig. 16-4).

NATURAL HISTORY OF CAROTID ATHEROSCLEROSIS

Before a logical treatment plan for any disease can be entertained, one must first ascertain the natural history of disease without treatment. A number of studies have outlined the natural history of carotid artery disease, in the presence and absence of symptoms.

First, what is the risk of stroke in patients with prior stroke or with TIA? According to the Framingham Study,[23] the majority of strokes (63%) are secondary to ischemic brain infarction; the annualized rate of recurrent stroke in this study was 8.4% for men and 4.8% for women, a difference not explained by age. The rate of recurrent stroke was significantly lower for those patients without comorbidity such as coronary artery disease and congestive heart failure. Whisnant et al[94] retrospectively studied patients with TIA with regard to risk for subsequent stroke. Thirty-six percent of patients with TIA suffered stroke during the follow-up period. The probability of stroke-free survival at 10 years was 50%. Using the same group of patients, Cartlidge, Whisnant, and Elveback[95] focused on the relationship between type of TIA and the risk of subsequent stroke. They found little difference between carotid distribution TIA and vertebrobasilar TIA and the risk of subsequent stroke. Dennis et al[96] reported on a prospective study of 184 patients with TIA in a rural community in England. In a follow-up period of 5 years, 31% of the deaths were secondary to stroke. The mean annual risk of stroke was 5.9% over the 5-year period, but the risk of stroke during the first year following the TIA was 11.6%. Of those who were stroke-free at 1 year, the subsequent annualized stroke risk was 4.4%.

Next, what is the risk of stroke in patients with an asymptomatic carotid bruit? Chambers and Norris[97] examined stroke risk in patients with asymptomatic bruit seen at the University of Toronto. Of 500 patients followed, there were 36 TIAs and 12 strokes at mean follow-up of 23 months. Of the 12 with stroke, 4 were preceded by TIA, while the remaining 8 had stroke without a warning TIA. In another study, from The Mayo Clinic,[98] patients with asymptomatic carotid bruit were followed for subsequent TIA or stroke. Of 566 patients, 63 had a carotid territory event; half of these were ischemic stroke, the majority being ipsilateral to the carotid bruit. The cumulative probability of stroke was 7.5% at 5 years. In a matched cohort without carotid bruit, the cumulative probability of stroke was only 2.4% at 5 years. Death in both groups was most commonly secondary to cardiovascular disease. Heyman et al[99] used logistic regression to evaluate the contribution of carotid bruit in the probability of subsequent stroke in a rural

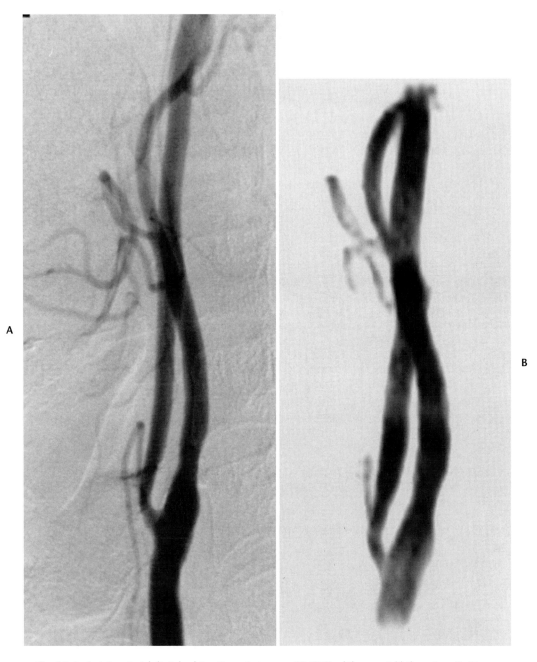

Fig. 16-4. A, Intraarterial digital subtraction arteriogram (IA-DSA) of the carotid bifurcation. **B,** Magnetic resonance angiogram (MRA) in the same patient.

population in Georgia. Among those patients with bruit, the cumulative risk of stroke was 13.9%, compared with 3.4% in those without bruit at mean follow-up of 70.5 months. Stroke risk was also increased by male gender and increasing age.

Although the preceding studies are of benefit in delineating the natural history of carotid disease and stroke, they are somewhat limited in that (1) not all strokes are ischemic or in the carotid distribution and (2) not all cervical bruits are secondary to common or internal carotid artery stenosis.

What, then, is the risk of stroke in patients with documented asymptomatic carotid artery stenosis? Roederer et al[100] pro-

spectively followed 167 asymptomatic patients with cervical bruits with carotid duplex ultrasound. During follow-up, 10 patients became symptomatic; symptoms were accompanied by progression of carotid disease in 8. The annual rate of symptom occurrence was 4% by life-table analysis. The presence of, or progression to, 80% or greater stenosis was highly correlated with the development of symptoms or with occlusion of the internal carotid. Meissner et al[101] examined the significance of abnormal ocular pneumoplethysmography (OPG) on the risk of subsequent stroke in asymptomatic patients. The annual stroke rate was 3.4%; only 4 of 29 strokes were preceded by a TIA. The "unheralded" stroke rate was 2.9%.

Of those patients studied by Chambers and Norris[97] with duplex ultrasound, the stroke incidence increased with the degree of carotid stenosis. In those patients with 75% or greater stenosis, the yearly stroke incidence was 5.3%, and the rate of unheralded strokes was 3.5%. Norris et al[102] found that in asymptomatic patients the stroke rate was negligible (1.3% annually) in those with carotid stenosis of 75% or less. With stenosis greater than 75%, however, the combined rate of TIA and stroke was 10.5%, with a combined rate of cardiac ischemia and vascular death as high as 9.9%. The vast majority (75%) of the neurologic events were ipsilateral to the stenosed artery. These data likely underestimate the true incidence of stroke ipsilateral to a high-grade internal carotid artery stenosis, as many strokes may be "asymptomatic," and TIA may actually be associated with cerebral infarction. Norris and Zhu[103] studied the relationship between silent cerebral infarction (found on CT scan) and varying degrees of carotid artery stenosis in patients with TIA or who were asymptomatic. They found CT findings of cerebral infarction in 19% of patients with asymptomatic carotid stenosis and in 47% of patients with TIA and carotid stenosis. The vast majority of infarcts (68% in asymptomatic patients, 86% in those with TIA) were ipsilateral to the carotid lesion. The higher the degree of stenosis, the higher the likelihood of cerebral infarction ipsilateral to the stenosis. They concluded that silent cerebral infarction may be an indication for prophylactic endarterectomy in asymptomatic patients. Approximately 10% of patients in the ACAS were found to have evidence of "silent" cerebral infarction on CT scan.[104]

Patients with ulcerated nonstenotic carotid atheromata are also at significant risk for ischemic stroke, as originally reported by Moore et al.[105] They grouped ulcerations into three categories: minimal ulceration (group A), large ulcers (group B), and compound ulcers (group C). In follow-up the annual stroke rate was 12.5%/yr for groups B and C. In a continuation of these data, Dixon et al[106] have reported on the natural history of 153 nonstenotic ulcerative lesions of the carotid arteries. At follow-up extending up to 10 years, 3% of patients with group A ulcers, 21% with group B ulcers, and 19% with group C ulcers had ipsilateral stroke. The annual stroke rate was 4.5% for group B ulcers and 7.5% for group C ulcers.

Symptomatic patients with high-grade internal carotid stenosis (generally considered greater than 70%) are at highest risk for subsequent ischemic stroke. In the NASCET[18] trial those patients with high-grade, symptomatic carotid stenosis randomized to best medical treatment incurred a 24% stroke rate at mean follow-up of 18 months. The stroke rate in symptomatic patients with multiple risk factors was 39% at 2 years. In the European Carotid Surgery Trial (ECST)[107] and Veterans Administration (VA)[108] trials of patients with high-grade symptomatic carotid stenosis, the rate of stroke in the nonsurgical groups was 22% and 26%, respectively. These prospective randomized trials confirm the results of previously reported clinical series that patients with symptomatic, high-grade internal carotid lesions are at high risk for subsequent ischemic stroke.

Plaque ulceration also adversely affects the risk of subsequent stroke in patients with high-grade carotid stenosis. In data gleaned from NASCET the risk of unilateral stroke at 24 months for medically treated patients with ulcerated plaques increased incrementally from 26% to 73% as the degree of stenosis increased from 75% to 95%. For patients with no ulcer, the risk of stroke remained constant at 21% for all degrees of stenosis.[109]

MEDICAL THERAPY IN CEREBROVASCULAR DISEASE

Several large trials using antiplatelet agents for the treatment of TIA and minor stroke are available for review (Table 16-1). From these data it appears that aspirin and ticlopidine have a significant impact on the clinical end points of stroke, myocardial infarction, and death from vascular causes. Although there is a theoretic benefit to adding dipyridamole (a phosphodiesterase inhibitor) or sulfinpyrazone to aspirin (a cyclooxygenase inhibitor), this potential has not been realized in clinical trials. Ticlopidine hydrochloride exerts its effect via a non-cyclooxygenase mechanism. Ticlopidine should be considered a second-line drug in the treatment of patients with TIA, reserving it for aspirin failure and in those patients unable to tolerate aspirin.[119]

Anticoagulant therapy (warfarin and heparin) is still one of the methods of treatment considered in patients with symptomatic cerebrovascular disease. There are no convincing data that anticoagulation therapy with warfarin is of benefit in the prevention of TIA or stroke in those patients with symptoms secondary to cerebrovascular disease. Warfarin is clearly beneficial, however, in preventing thromboembolic strokes in patients with atrial fibrillation.[120] Current recommendations suggest the use of therapeutic heparin anticoagulation in patients with crescendo TIA and progressing stroke in the absence of contraindications.[121,122] CT scan of the brain is mandatory to exclude hemorrhagic causes of cerebral ischemia before initiating anticoagulant therapy.

CAROTID ENDARTERECTOMY

For many years there has been considerable evidence throughout the literature suggesting that some extracranial carotid lesions simply are more dangerous than others. The addition of recent prospectively randomized trials to the countless case series preceding them hopefully will convince all parties previously involved in the long-standing controversy concerning carotid endarterectomy that their opinions with respect to treatment options are much less adversarial than they might otherwise have appeared. Surgeons, for example, are likely to recognize that antiplatelet therapy is not inappropriate as an initial approach to moderate degrees of carotid stenosis even in selected symptomatic patients. Conversely, in light of recent data from the ACAS,[19] most neurologists may be prepared to concede that surgical treatment is justified in selected asymptomatic patients having severe carotid stenosis. In retrospect, such a compromise seems to make sense. The following summary illustrates some of the data on which these new perspectives are based.

Table 16-1. Antiplatelet Agents in the Treatment of Cerebrovascular Disease

Trial (Ref.)	Indication	Agent and Dose (mg/d)	End Point	Follow-up	No. of Patients	No. of Events	P	Stroke Rate
UK-TIA ASA Trial (1991)[110]	TIA or minor stroke	ASA (1200) ASA (300) Placebo	Stroke	48 mo (mean)	815 806 814	101 100 119	NS	2.6%/yr 2.7%/yr 3.3%/yr
Reuther and Dorndorff (1978)[111]	TIA	ASA (1900) Placebo	TIA or stroke	24 mo (total)	29 29	6 13	<0.10	
SALT (1991)[112]	TIA or minor stroke	ASA (75) Placebo	TIA or stroke	32 mo (median)	676 684	101 128	0.03	
Dutch TIA Trial (1991)[113]	TIA or minor stroke	ASA (30) ASA (283)	Stroke, MI, vascular death	31 mo (mean)	1555 1576	228 240	NS	
Canadian Co-Op Study (1978)[114]	TIA	ASA (1300) ASA and sulfinpyr- azone Sulfinpyrazone (800) Placebo	TIA, stroke or death	26 mo (mean)	144 146 156 139	46/290 (all ASA) 58/302 (all sulfinpyrazone)	<0.05	7.1%/yr 4.4%/yr 8.6%/yr 6.6%/yr
Bousser et al (1983)[115]	TIA or stroke	ASA (990) ASA (990) and dipyr- idamole (225) Placebo	Stroke	36 mo (total)	198 202 204	17 18 31	<0.05 <0.05	
Persantine Aspirin Trial (1985)[116]	TIA	ASA (325) ASA (325) plus dipyridamole (75)	Stroke, retinal infarct	25 mo (median)	442 448	60 53	0.42	
Ticlopidine Aspirin Stroke Study (1989)[117]	TIA or minor stroke	Ticlopidine (500) ASA (1300)	Stroke	Range 2-6 yr	1529 1540	172 212	0.024	10%/3yr 13%/3yr
Canadian American Ticlopidine Study (1989)[118]	Thromboem- bolic stroke	Ticlopidine (500) Placebo	Stroke or stroke death	24 mo (mean)	525 528	80 98	0.063	8.5%/yr 10.7%/yr

MI, Myocardial infarction; *ASA*, acetylsalicylic acid.

Case Series

Although literally hundreds of published reports have cited the safety of carotid endarterectomy at experienced centers and its presumed favorable influence upon subsequent stroke prevention, these features have rarely been correlated with long-term outcome in contemporaneous series of comparable nonsurgical patients. Although historic controls have been employed to define the benefit of surgical intervention, they often were generic in their composition (e.g., "TIA patients" or "bruit populations") and eventually were made obsolete by the introduction of accurate noninvasive methods to document the actual severity of carotid stenosis. However, at least two case series with which the authors are particularly familiar attempted to address these issues and provided results that are remarkably similar to the available disclosures of prospectively randomized trials.

THE CLEVELAND CLINIC. Shortly before Doppler ultrasound (duplex) scanning become widely available for noninvasive carotid screening, a series of 501 patients who had greater than 50% carotid stenosis unequivocally demonstrated by diagnostic intravenous angiography was collected at the Cleveland Clinic. A total of 180 of these patients eventually underwent carotid endarterectomy, and 321 did not. During a follow-up extending to 5 years (mean, 3 years), both surgical and nonoperative management had equivalent results in the presence of moderate carotid disease (50% to 69% stenosis) irrespective of whether prior symptoms had occurred.[123,124] Nevertheless, the cumulative stroke rate after carotid endarterectomy (7%) was statistically superior ($P = 0.04$) to that associated with nonoperative management (31%) among symptomatic patients who had severe angiographic stenosis (greater than 70%). Data for patients in this investigation who had severe asymptomatic carotid stenosis are presented in Table 16-2.

THE UNIVERSITY OF WASHINGTON. Although differences in the 5-year cumulative incidence of TIA and/or stroke among asymptomatic patients in the Cleveland Clinic study did not attain statistical significance,

these trends appear to favor surgical treatment for high-grade lesions and are supported by other data in asymptomatic patients collected at the University of Washington. Using the criterion of greater than 80% stenosis confirmed by both carotid duplex scanning and angiography, Moneta et al[125] found that the 2-year results of carotid endarterectomy seemed to represent a substantial improvement over those associated with nonoperative management. Although differences in the stroke rate between the two treatment cohorts in this study did not quite attain statistical significance ($P = 0.08$), the incidence of subsequent TIA, progression to internal carotid occlusion, and all potentially unfavorable events was clearly reduced by prophylactic surgical treatment.

In another related study of long-term outcome following duplex scanning in 500 patients who had asymptomatic carotid bruits, Chambers and Norris[97] also discovered that severe stenosis (greater than 75%) is a harbinger of future neurologic complications. The 2-year incidence of stroke and/or TIA was over 20% for high-grade lesions in this series, compared with a risk slightly exceeding 5% in patients who had only moderate carotid stenosis. Despite these findings few patients with severe stenosis in this series underwent carotid endarterectomy, and the authors imply that their reluctance to consider prophylactic surgical treatment may have been related to the fact that it was associated with a perioperative stroke rate of approximately 13% at their own center. Under these circumstances their cautious approach is perfectly understandable, and it emphasizes the principle that the long-term advantages of carotid endarterectomy in asymptomatic patients are predicated on the immediate safety of the operation itself.

Randomized Trials

Although several other prospectively randomized trials of surgical versus nonoperative management of either symptomatic or asymptomatic carotid stenosis have been described, five such studies have assumed preeminence because of their size, the perceived quality of their organization, and/or the fact that at least their preliminary

Table 16-2. Cumulative Results of Surgical and Nonoperative Management of Severe Asymptomatic Carotid Stenosis (>70%) in Selected Case Series

Late Events (Cumulative)	Treatment Cohorts		
	Surgical	**Nonoperative**	
Cleveland Clinic[123,124] (5 yr)	$n = 87$	$n = 69$	
Stroke	8%	28%	($P = $ NS)
TIA or stroke	10%	44%	($P = $ NS)
Moneta et al[125] (2 yr)	$n = 56$	$n = 73$	
Stroke	4%	19%	($P = 0.08$)
TIA	5%	28%	($P = 0.008$)
ICA occlusion	0%	29%	($P = 0.003$)
All unfavorable events	9%	48%	($P = 0.0005$)

ICA, internal carotid artery.

conclusions already have been reported. Two of these are sponsored by the National Institutes of Health (NASCET and ACAS), and two others are under the direction of the VA (the VA Symptomatic Trial and Asymptomatic Trial). Recruitment for ACAS has just recently been completed, and preliminary results have been released to the lay press. Published disclosures are now available for the remaining studies by the NIH and VA, as well as for the large ECST that actually preceded them in development.[18,107,108,126]

SYMPTOMATIC TRIALS. Entry into all of the symptomatic trials was restricted to patients who had sustained either TIA or mild strokes with good functional recovery. As might have been anticipated on the basis of previous case series, the most salient results for these trials are related to outcome comparisons for high-grade carotid stenosis (greater than 70%). Only ECST randomized patients having stenosis of 29% or less—and not surprisingly, there was no superiority for surgical treatment in this cohort. Both NASCET and ECST specifically addressed patients having 30% to 69% stenosis, but each of these studies found it necessary to continue recruitment in this particular group because the results of surgical and nonoperative management have thus far been equivalent. The VA Symptomatic Trial was limited to patients having a minimum of 50% carotid stenosis, and like NASCET and ECST, no distinctions in outcome have been identified for the subset with 50% to 69% involvement.

Despite these lingering uncertainties regarding the role of carotid endarterectomy for intermediate degrees of carotid disease, enrollment of patients having stenosis of 70% or greater has been terminated by NASCET, ECST, and the VA Symptomatic Trial because of statistically significant improvement in the incidence of subsequent stroke associated with surgical intervention. A summary of these results is presented in Table 16-3.

Several features of these data should be emphasized. First, the superiority of carotid endarterectomy for symptomatic high-grade lesions was documented during relatively short follow-up intervals (12 to 18 months) in the NASCET and VA Symptomatic Trial. Second, although its perioperative stroke rate (7%) approaches the upper limit of acceptability, the ECST nevertheless confirmed benefit

of surgical management (largely relative to antiplatelet therapy) for greater than 70% stenosis within 3 years of randomization. Finally, it seems notable that the results of nonoperative management for severe, symptomatic carotid stenosis in the prospectively randomized trials are remarkably similar to those in the earlier, nonrandomized case series reported from the Cleveland Clinic and the University of Washington (Table 16-2). Caution obviously must be used in making such comparisons, but in an era in which the omission of expensive prospectively randomized trials has been implied to represent the absence of critical thought, these findings suggest that careful case series still are capable of providing important information.

ASYMPTOMATIC TRIALS. To date the VA Cooperative Study is the only major randomized trial to report its complete results for asymptomatic carotid stenosis.[9] This investigation included a total of 444 men assigned to receive either surgical treatment plus aspirin ($n = 211$) or aspirin alone ($n = 233$), 32% of whom already had undergone carotid endarterectomy on the contralateral side. The 30-day stroke (2.4%) and mortality (1.9%) rate was 4.3% in the surgical cohort, whereas the combined morbidity/ mortality rate for nonoperative management was 0.8% during the same period. After 48 months of observation, the incidence of ipsilateral stroke was 4.7% in the surgical limb of the trial, compared with 9.4% in the medical limb ($P = 0.06$). During this interval, ipsilateral TIA or amaurosis fugax occurred in 3.3% and 11%, respectively. Consequently it is necessary to combine the neurologic end points of stroke and TIA/amaurosis (8% surgical, 20% medical; $P < 0.001$) to attain solid statistical support favoring carotid endarterectomy over medical therapy in this trial.

The principal liability of the VA Cooperative Study is the fact that asymptomatic patients with as little as 50% carotid stenosis were eligible for the randomization process. Curiously its published data failed to reveal either the number of entrants with severe stenosis (greater than 70%) or the neurologic outcome in this particular subset, an oversight suggesting that severe lesions may have been relatively uncommon. Therefore although the overall implications of the VA Study are clearly favorable, it is likely

Table 16-3. Results of Surgical and Nonoperative Management of Severe Symptomatic Carotid Stenosis (>70%) in Prospective Randomized Trials

	NASCET		ECST		VA Symptomatic	
	Surgical	**Medical**	**Surgical**	**Medical**	**Surgical**	**Medical**
Patients	300	295	455	323	63	66
Follow-Up Range	30 mo		10 yr		NA	
Mean	18 mo		3 yr		12 mo	
Stroke Rates						
30-day	5%	3%	7%	NA	2%	NA
Late	7%	24%	12%	22%	8%*	26%*
	($P < 0.001$)		($P < 0.01$)		($P = 0.01$)	

*End points include stroke and crescendo TIA.

that the efficacy of "prophylactic" carotid endarterectomy will ultimately be determined by the ACAS results.

Preliminary data released from the ACAS are now available. A total of 1662 patients with asymptomatic carotid stenosis exceeding 60% were enrolled. The primary outcome was any stroke or death during the 30-day postoperative period and any ipsilateral stroke thereafter. Median follow-up was 2.7 years. The combined risk of stroke and death in the surgical group was 2.3%. The rate of primary outcome at 5 years (by Kaplan-Meyer projection) was 4.8% for the surgical group and 10.6% for the nonoperative group, a relative risk reduction of 55% in favor of surgery. Risk reduction in men was substantially greater than that for women in these preliminary results. Although results have not been stratified with respect to degree of stenosis, it is likely that the benefit incurred by surgery will be greatest for those lesions with greater than 80% stenosis.

CONCLUSIONS

In summary, the indications for carotid endarterectomy among acceptable surgical candidates at the Cleveland Clinic have remained as follows:

1. Severe carotid stenosis (≥80% by duplex ultrasound) irrespective of whether it is symptomatic or asymptomatic
2. Ulcerated or intermediate degrees of stenosis (>50% by duplex ultrasound) only if they remain (or become) symptomatic despite the use of antiplatelet therapy
3. Greater than 50% (by duplex ultrasound) if it is discovered in conjunction with contralateral internal carotid occlusion. (Although shared by many surgeons, this indication is largely intuitive and may never be proven or disproven by prospectively randomized trials.)

In the final analysis, the legitimacy of these indications and the latitude for their expansion to address atypical clinical presentations depend heavily on an acceptable incidence of perioperative complications. Carotid endarterectomy is appropriate as long as the combined morbidity and mortality is kept under 3%, 5%, and 7% for the indications of asymptomatic high-grade stenosis, TIA, and prior stroke with minimal residual deficit, respectively.[127] Accordingly the safety of carotid endarterectomy should be documented prospectively at every hospital at which it is performed.[128]

REFERENCES

1. U. S. Bureau of the Census: Statistical abstract of the United States: 1992, ed 112, Washington, DC, 1992.
2. Bonita R: Epidemiology of stroke, Lancet 339:342, 1992.
3. Bamford J et al: A prospective study of acute cerebrovascular disease in the community: the Oxfordshire Community Stroke Project, 1981-86. 2. Incidence, case fatality rates and overall outcome at one year of cerebral infarction, primary intracerebral and subarachnoid hemorrhage, J Neurol Neurosurg Psychiatry 53:16, 1990.
4. Ojemann RG: Cerebrovascular disease. In Adelman G, ed: Encyclopedia of neuroscience, Boston, 1987, Birkhauser Boston, Inc.
5. Marmot MG and Poulter NR: Primary prevention of stroke, Lancet 339:344, 1992.
6. Barker WF: A history of vascular surgery. In Moore WS, ed: Vascular surgery: a comprehensive review, ed 4, Philadelphia, 1993, WB Saunders.
7. Gowers WR: On a case of simultaneous embolism of central retinal and middle cerebral arteries, Lancet 2:794, 1875.
8. Hunt JR: The role of the carotid arteries in the causation of vascular lesions of the brain, with remarks on certain special features of the symptomatology, Am J Med Sci 147:704, 1914.
9. Moniz E, Lima A, and deLacerda R: Hemiplegies par thrombose de la carotide interne, Presse Med 45:977, 1937.
10. Strully KJ, Hurwitt ES, and Blankenberg HW: Thromboendarterectomy for thrombosis of the carotid artery in the neck, J Neurosurg 10:474, 1953.
11. Eastcott HHG, Pickering GW, and Robb CG: Reconstruction of internal carotid artery in a patient with intermittent attacks of hemiplegia, Lancet 2:994, 1954.
12. Carrea R, Mollins M, and Murphy G: Surgical treatment of spontaneous thrombosis of the internal carotid artery in the neck. Carotid-carotideal anastomosis. Report of a case, Acta Neurol Psychiatry 1:71, 1955.
13. DeBakey ME: Successful carotid endarterectomy for cerebrovascular insufficiency: nineteen year followup, JAMA 233:1083, 1975.
14. Cooley DA, Al-Naaman YD, and Carton CA: Surgical treatment of arteriosclerotic occlusion of common carotid artery, J Neurosurg 13:500, 1956.
15. Whisnant JP, Matsumoto N, and Eleback LR: Transient cerebral ischemic attacks in a community: Rochester, Minnesota, 1955 through 1969, Mayo Clin Proc 48:195, 1973.
16. Julian OC et al: Ulcerative lesions of the carotid bifurcation, Arch Surg 86:803, 1963.
17. Moore WS and Hall AD: Ulcerated atheroma of the carotid artery: a cause of transient cerebral ischemia, Am J Surg 116:237, 1969.
18. North American Symptomatic Carotid Endarterectomy Trial Collaborators: Beneficial effect of carotid endarterectomy in symptomatic patients with high-grade carotid stenosis, N Engl J Med 325:445, 1991.
19. Asymptomatic Carotid Atherosclerosis Study (ACAS): Clinical advisory: carotid endarterectomy for patients with asymptomatic internal carotid artery stenosis, Stroke 25:2523, 1994.
20. Warlow C: Disorders of the cerebral circulation. In Walton J, ed: Brain's diseases of the nervous system, ed 10, Oxford, 1993, Oxford University Press.
21. Anderson JE: Grant's atlas of anatomy, ed 7, Baltimore, 1979, Williams & Wilkins.
22. O'Mara CS: Surgical treatment of transient ischemic attack and stroke secondary to external carotid atherosclerosis. In Ernst CB and Stanley JC, eds: Current therapy in vascular surgery, ed 2, Philadelphia, 1991, BC Decker.
23. Pick TP and Howden R, eds: Gray's anatomy, ed 15, New York, 1977, Gramercy Books.
24. Sheldon JJ: Blood vessels of the scalp and brain, Summit, NJ 1981, CIBA Pharmaceutical Company.
25. Fields WS, Bruetman ME, and Weibel JW: Collateral circulation of the brain, Baltimore, 1985, Williams & Wilkins.
26. Leenders KL et al: Cerebral blood flow, blood volume and oxygen utilization, Brain 113:27, 1990.

27. Brown MM, Wade JP, and Marshall J: Fundamental importance of arterial oxygen content in the regulation of cerebral blood flow in man, Brain 108:81, 1985.

28. Powers WJ: Cerebral hemodynamics in ischemic cerebrovascular disease, Ann Neurol 29:231, 1991.

29. Wise RJS et al: Serial observations on the pathophysiology of acute stroke. The transition from ischemia to infarction as reflected in regional oxygen extraction, Brain 106:197, 1983.

30. Trojaborg W and Boysen G: Relation between EEG, regional cerebral blood flow and internal carotid artery pressure during carotid endarterectomy, Electroenceph Clin Neurophysiol 34:61, 1973.

31. Sundt TM et al: Cerebral blood flow measurements and electroencephalograms during carotid endarterectomy, J Neurosurg 41:310, 1974.

32. Branston NM et al: Relationship between the cortical evoked potential and local cortical blood flow following acute middle cerebral artery occlusion in the baboon, Exp Neurol 45:195, 1974.

33. Astrup J et al: Cortical evoked potential and extracellular K+ and H+ at critical levels of brain ischemia, Stroke 8:51, 1977.

34. Astrup J, Siesjo B, and Symon L: Thresholds in cerebral ischemia—the ischemic penumbra (editorial), Stroke 12:723, 1981.

35. Morawetz RB et al: Cerebral blood flow determined by hydrogen clearance during middle cerebral artery occlusion in unanesthetized monkeys, Stroke 9:143, 1978.

36. Zarins CK et al: Carotid bifurcation atherosclerosis. Quantitative correlation of plaque localization with flow velocity profiles and wall shear stress, Cir Res 53:502, 1983.

37. Ku DN et al: Pulsatile flow and atherosclerosis in the human carotid bifurcation. Positive correlation between plaque location and low and oscillating shear stress, Arteriosclerosis 5:293, 1985.

38. Fox JA and Hugh AE: Static zones in the internal carotid artery: Correlation with boundary layer separation and stasis in model flows, Br J Radiol 43:370, 1976.

39. Ku DN et al: Hemodynamics of the normal human carotid bifurcation: in vitro and in vivo studies, Ultrasound Med Biol 11:13, 1985.

40. Fisher M: Occlusion of the internal carotid artery, Arch Neurol Psychiatry 65:346, 1951.

41. Fisher M: Occlusion of the internal carotid artery, Arch Neurol Psychiatry 72:187, 1954.

42. Hollenhorst RW: Significance of bright plaques in the retinal arteries, JAMA 178:23, 1961.

43. Russell RWR: Observations on the retinal blood vessels in monocular blindness, Lancet 2:1422, 1961.

44. McBrien DJ, Bradley RD, and Ashton N: The nature of retinal emboli in stenosis of the internal carotid artery, Lancet 1:697, 1963.

45. Moore WS and Hall AD: Ulcerated atheroma of the carotid artery. A cause of transient cerebral ischemia, Am J Surg 116:237, 1968.

46. Moore WS and Hall AD: Importance of emboli from carotid bifurcation in pathogenesis of cerebral ischemic attacks, Arch Surg 101:708, 1970.

47. Millikan CH: The pathogenesis of transient focal cerebral ischemia, Circulation 32:438, 1965.

48. Lusby RJ et al: Carotid plaque hemorrhage. Its role in production of cerebral ischemia, Arch Surg 117:1479, 1982.

49. Persson AV, Robichaux WT, and Silverman M: The natural history of carotid plaque development, Arch Surg 118:1048, 1983.

50. Imparato AM, Riles TS, and Gorstein F: The carotid bifurcation plaque: pathologic findings associated with cerebral ischemia, Stroke 10:238, 1979.

51. Ammar AD et al: Intraplaque hemorrhage: its significance in cerebrovascular disease, Am J Surg 148:840, 1984.

52. Ogata J et al: Rupture of atheromatous plaque as a cause of thrombotic occlusion of stenotic internal carotid artery, Stroke 21:1740, 1990.

53. Bogousslavsky J, Desland P, and Regli F: Asymptomatic tight stenosis of the internal carotid artery: long-term prognosis, Neurology 36:861, 1986.

54. Nicholls SC, Bergelin R, and Strandness DE: Neurologic sequelae of unilateral carotid artery occlusion: immediate and late, J Vasc Surg 10:542, 1989.

55. Eikelboom BC, Klop RBJ, and Vrielink A: Fate of patients with high-grade carotid stenosis treated medically: outcome of progression from carotid stenosis to occlusion. In Veith FJ, ed: Current critical problems in vascular surgery, St. Louis, 1993, Quality Medical Publishing.

56. Grigg MJ et al: The significance of cerebral infarction and atrophy in patients with amaurosis fugax and transient ischemic attacks in relation to internal carotid artery stenosis: a preliminary report, J Vasc Surg 7:215, 1988.

57. DeBakey ME, Crawford ES, and Fields WS: Surgical treatment of patients with cerebral arterial insufficiency associated with extracranial occlusive lesions, Neurology 11:145, 1961.

58. Hohf RP: The clinical evaluation and surgery of internal carotid insufficiency, Surg Clin North Am 47:1, 1967.

59. DeBakey ME et al: Cerebral arterial insufficiency: one- to 11-year results following arterial reconstructive operation, Ann Surg 161:921, 1965.

60. Crawford ES et al: Hemodynamic alterations in patients with cerebral arterial insufficiency before and after operation, Surgery 48:76, 1960.

61. Contorni L: Il circolo collaterale vertebrao-vertebrale nella obliterazione dell'arterio subclavia all sua origine, Minerva Chir 15:268, 1960.

62. Parrot JD: The subclavian steal syndrome, Arch Surg 88:661, 1964.

63. Fisher CM: A new vascular syndrome—"the subclavian steal" (editorial), N Engl J Med 265:912, 1961.

64. Fields WS: Reflections of "the subclavian steal," Stroke 1:320, 1970.

65. Fields WS and Lemak NA: Joint study of extracranial arterial occlusion. VII. Subclavian steal—a review of 168 cases, JAMA 222:1139, 1972.

66. Millikan CH: A classification and outline of cerebrovascular disease, Stroke 6:564, 1975.

67. Putman SF and Adams HP: Usefulness of heparin in initial management of patients with recent transient ischemic attacks, Arch Neur 42:960, 1985.

68. Rothrock JF and Lyden PD: Unstable carotid artery syndrome: Predictive criteria, Circulation 70:136, 1984 (abstract).

69. Jones HR and Millikan CH: Temporal profile (clinical course) of acute carotid system cerebral infarction, Stroke 7:64, 1976.

70. Jones HR, Millikan CH, and Sandok BA: Temporal profile (clinical course) of acute vertebrobasilar system infarction, Stroke 11:173, 1980.

71. Easton JD and Sherman DG: Management of cerebral embolism of cardiac origin, Stroke 11:433, 1980.

72. Torvik A and Jorgensen L: Thrombotic and embolic occlusions of the carotid arteries in an autopsy series, part 2. Cerebral lesions and clinical course, J Neurol Sci 3:410, 1966.

73. Barnett HJ, Peerless SJ, and Kaufmann JC: "Stump" of in-

ternal carotid artery—a source for further cerebral embolic ischemia, Stroke 9:448, 1978.

74. Berguer R: Idiopathic ischemic syndromes of the retina and optic nerve and their carotid origin, J Vasc Surg 2:649, 1985.

75. Mohr JP: Lacunes, Stroke 13:3, 1982.

76. Ziegler DK et al: Correlation of bruits over the carotid artery with angiographically demonstrated lesions, Neurology 21:860, 1971.

77. David TE et al: A correlation of neck bruits and arteriosclerotic carotid arteries, Arch Surg 107:729, 1973.

78. Reinmuth OM and Karanjia PN: Neurological evaluation in cerebrovascular disease. In Fein JM and Flamm ES, eds: Cerebrovascular surgery, Vol I, New York, 1985, Springer-Verlag.

79. Bendick PJ et al: Carotid plaque morphology: correlation of duplex sonography with histology, Ann Vasc Surg 2:6, 1988.

80. Ricotta JJ et al: Angiographic and pathologic correlates in carotid artery disease, Surgery 99:284, 1986.

81. Goodson SF et al: Can carotid duplex scanning supplant arteriography in patients with focal carotid artery symptoms? J Vasc Surg 5:551, 1987.

82. Gelabert HA and Moore WS: Carotid endarterectomy without angiography, Surg Clin North Am 70:213, 1990.

83. Gertler JP et al: Carotid surgery without arteriography: noninvasive selection of patients, Ann Vasc Surg 5:253, 1991.

84. Moore WS et al: Can clinical evaluation and noninvasive testing substitute for arteriography in the evaluation of carotid artery disease? Ann Surg 208:91, 1988.

85. Chervu A and Moore WS: Carotid endarterectomy without arteriography, Ann Vasc Surg 8:296, 1994.

86. Litt AW et al: AJNR 12:611, 1991.

87. Masyrak AM et al: Radiology 171:801, 1989.

88. Heiserman JE et al: Radiology 182:761, 1992.

89. Mattle HP et al: Evaluation of the extracranial carotid arteries: correlation of magnetic resonance angiography, duplex ultrasonography, and conventional angiography, J Vasc Surg 13:838, 1991.

90. Edelman RR: MR angiography: present and future, AJR 161:1, 1993.

91. Polak JF et al: Carotid endarterectomy: preoperative evaluation of candidates with combined Doppler sonography and MR angiography; work in progress, Radiology 186:333, 1993.

92. Huston III J et al: Carotid artery: prospective blinded comparison of two-dimensional time-of-flight MR angiography with conventional angiography and duplex ultrasound, Radiology 186:339, 1993.

93. Wolf PA, Kannel WB, and Dawber TR: Epidemiology of stroke: the Framingham Study. In Schoenberg B, ed: Neurological epidemiology: principles and clinical applications, vol 19: advances in neurology, New York, Raven Press.

94. Whisnant JP, Cartlidge NEF, and Elveback LR: Carotid and vertebral-basilar transient ischemic attacks: effect of anticoagulants, hypertension, and cardiac disorders on survival and stroke occurence, Ann Neurol 3:107, 1978.

95. Cartlidge NEF, Whisnant JP, and Elveback LR: Carotid and vertebral-basilar transient cerebral ischemic attacks, Mayo Clin Proc 52:117, 1977.

96. Dennis M et al: Prognosis of transient ischemic attacks in the Oxfordshire community stroke project, Stroke 21:848, 1990.

97. Chambers BR and Norris JW: Outcome in patients with asymptomatic neck bruits, N Engl J Med 315:860, 1986.

98. Wiebers DO et al: Prospective comparison of a cohort with asymptomatic carotid bruit and a population-based cohort without carotid bruit, Stroke 21:984, 1990.

99. Heyman A et al: Risk of stroke in asymptomatic persons with cervical bruits. A population study in Evans County, Georgia, N Engl J Med 302:838, 1980.

100. Roederer GO et al: The natural history of carotid artery disease in asymptomatic patients with cervical bruits, Stroke 15:605, 1984.

101. Meissner I et al: The natural history of carotid artery occlusive lesions, JAMA 258:2704, 1987.

102. Norris JW et al: Vascular risks of asymptomatic carotid stenosis, Stroke 22:1485, 1991.

103. Norris JW and Zhu CZ: Silent stroke and carotid stenosis, Stroke 23:483, 1992.

104. Asymptomatic Carotid Atherosclerosis Study Group: Silent cerebral infarction in the Asymptomatic Carotid Atherosclerosis Study (ACAS), Stroke 22:147, 1991 (abstract).

105. Moore WS et al: Natural history of nonstenotic, asymptomatic ulcerative lesions of the carotid artery, Arch Surg 113:1352, 1978.

106. Dixon S et al: Natural history of nonstenotic, asymptomatic ulcerative lesions of the carotid artery. A further analysis, Arch Surg 117:1493, 1982.

107. European Carotid Surgery Trialists' Collaborative Group: MRC European carotid surgery trial: interim results for symptomatic patients with severe (70-99%) or with mild (0-29%) carotid stenosis, Lancet 337:1235, 1991.

108. Mayberg MR et al: Carotid endarterectomy and prevention of cerebral ischemia in symptomatic carotid stenosis, JAMA 226:3289, 1991.

109. Eliasziw M et al: Significance of plaque ulceration in symptomatic patients with high-grade carotid stenosis, Stroke 25:304, 1994.

110. Farrell B et al: The United Kingdom transient ischemic attack (UK-TIA) aspirin trial: final results, J Neurol Neurosurg Psychiatry 54:1044, 1991.

111. Reuther R and Dorndorf W: Aspirin in patients with cerebral ischemia and normal angiograms or non-surgical lesions. The results of a double-blind trial. In Breddin K et al, eds: Acetylsalicylic acid in cerebral ischemia and coronary heart disease, Stuttgart, 1978, FK Schattauer Verlag.

112. The SALT Collaborative Group: Swedish Aspirin Low-Dose Trial (SALT) of 75 mg aspirin as secondary prophylaxis after cerebrovascular ischemic events, Lancet 338:1345, 1991.

113. The Dutch TIA Trial Study Group: A comparison of two doses of aspirin (30 mg vs 283 mg a day) in patients after a transient ischemic attack or minor ischemic stroke, N Engl J Med 325:1261, 1991.

114. The Canadian Cooperative Study Group: A randomized trial of aspirin and sulfinpyrazone in threatened stroke, N Engl J Med 299:53, 1978.

115. Bousser MG et al: "AICLA" controlled trial of aspirin and dipyridamole in the secondary prevention of athero-thrombotic cerebral ischemia, Stroke 14:5, 1983.

116. The American-Canadian Co-Operative Study Group: Persantine aspirin trial in cerebral ischemia. Part II: endpoint results, Stroke 16:406, 1985.

117. Hass WK et al: A randomized trial comparing ticlopidine hydrochloride with aspirin for the prevention of stroke in high-risk patients, N Engl J Med 321:501, 1989.

118. Gent M et al: The Canadian American Ticlopidine Study (CATS) in thromboembolic stroke, Lancet 1:1215, 1989.

119. Ad Hoc Committee on Guidelines for the Management of Transient Ischemic Attacks of the Stroke Council of the American Heart Association: Guidelines for the management of transient ischemic attacks, Circulation 89:2950, 1994.

120. Atrial Fibrillation Investigators: Risk factors for stroke and efficacy of antithrombotic therapy in atrial fibrillation: analysis of pooled data from five randomized controlled trials, Arch Intern Med 147:1561, 1987.

121. Miller VT and Hart RG: Heparin anticoagulation in acute brain ischemia, Stroke 19:403, 1988.

122. Jonas S: Anticoagulant therapy in cerebrovascular disease: Review and meta-analysis, Stroke 19:1043, 1988.

123. Hertzer NR et al: Surgical versus nonoperative treatment of symptomatic carotid stenosis. 211 patients documented by intravenous angiography.

124. Hertzer NR et al: Surgical versus nonoperative treatment of asymptomatic carotid stenosis. 290 patients documented by intravenous angiography, Ann Surg 204:163, 1986.

125. Moneta GL et al: Operative versus nonoperative management of asymptomatic high-grade internal carotid artery stenosis: Improved results with endarterectomy, Stroke 18:1005, 1987.

126. Hobson RW et al: Efficacy of carotid endarterectomy for asymptomatic carotid stenosis, N Engl J Med 328:221, 1993.

127. Ad Hoc Committee to the Joint Council of the Society for Vascular Surgery and the North American Chapter of the International Society for Cardiovascular Surgery: Carotid endarterectomy: practice guidelines, J Vasc Surg 15:469, 1992.

128. Hertzer NR: Presidential address: outcome assessment in vascular surgery—results mean everything, J Vasc Surg 21:6, 1995.

CHAPTER SEVENTEEN

VISCERAL ISCHEMIC SYNDROMES

Richard W. Chitwood
Calvin B. Ernst

Ischemic processes within the mesenteric arterial distribution are rare when compared with ischemic syndromes that affect other regions such as the cerebrovascular, cardiovascular, and lower-extremity vascular beds. The pathologic conditions that result in mesenteric ischemia and intestinal infarction are quite varied, however, representing many of the processes of concern to physicians interested in vascular disease. Taken either independently or as a whole, these conditions result in profound morbidity and mortality. The devastating effects of systemic processes that lead to intestinal ischemia, the nonspecific signs and symptoms that often delay timely diagnosis, and the systemic effects of the ischemia itself present a formidable challenge in management and provide the basis for efforts aimed at improving outcome. If improvements in the morbidity and mortality of acute intestinal ischemic syndromes are to be made, accurate early diagnosis when remediation is feasible is paramount. Only in this setting can care that is swiftly and skillfully delivered in the intensive care unit and operating room result in success.

Acute arterial occlusion, nonobstructive mesenteric arterial insufficiency, mesenteric venous occlusion, and chronic arterial insufficiency are generally recognized as causes of mesenteric vascular insufficiency. Despite the variability of the causes of intestinal ischemia, all of the processes share a common anatomic basis. As such, a thorough understanding of mesenteric arterial anatomy is critical.

MESENTERIC VASCULAR ANATOMY AND COLLATERAL PATHWAYS

Arterial blood flow to the gastrointestinal tract, although subject to much individual variation is generally provided by three arteries: the celiac, superior mesenteric, and inferior mesenteric. Despite their separate origins from the abdominal aorta, several collateral routes serve to connect these arterial pathways. This consolidation of the mesenteric arterial supply allows adequate blood flow to the entire gastrointestinal tract even in most cases of marked vasculopathy and accounts for the rarity of the manifestations of chronic intestinal arterial insufficiency.

Celiac Artery

The celiac artery (CA) originates embryologically from the vitelline arteries, as do the other mesenteric arteries. It assumes its final position, after caudal migration during development, at the level of the lower one third of the twelfth thoracic vertebra to the upper one third of the first lumbar vertebra. It arises at a right angle from the aorta and classically terminates in three branches: the common hepatic, left gastric, and splenic arteries. This pattern, however, is present in only approximately 55% of individuals as the blood supply to the liver in particular is quite variable because of commonly occurring superior mesenteric artery (SMA) contributions.[1]

Superior Mesenteric Artery

The SMA assumes its final position opposite the body of the first lumbar vertebra and arises at a 20- to 30-degree angle in a caudal direction. The origins of the CA and SMA are 5 to 15 mm apart. In fact the two arteries can rarely arise as a single trunk from the abdominal aorta. The first branch of the SMA, the inferior pancreaticoduodenal artery, and another proximal branch, the middle colic artery, are relatively constant in location and provide important collateral circuits to the CA and inferior mesenteric artery (IMA) distributions.[2] The SMA and its branches typically supply blood to the pancreas, small bowel, and the right half of the colon.

Inferior Mesenteric Artery

The IMA arises from the most caudal vitelline elements of the developing embryo and assumes its final position opposite the body of the third lumbar vertebra 5 cm or more below the origin of the SMA. A few centimeters from its origin, the IMA gives rise to the left colic artery, then a few sigmoidal branches, and finally the superior rectal artery.[3]

Collateral Pathways

CELIAC ARTERY—SUPERIOR MESENTERIC ARTERY. The most important collateral channel between the CA and SMA is the pancreaticoduodenal arcade connecting the superior pancreaticoduodenal vessels of the CA and inferior pancreaticoduodenal vessels of the SMA (Fig. 17-1). Connections between the dorsal pancreatic branch of the splenic artery and branches of the middle colic can also be present. Last, a direct connection between the CA and SMA, the anastomotic artery of Buhler, is occasionally present as well.[4]

SUPERIOR MESENTERIC ARTERY—INFERIOR MESENTERIC ARTERY. The meandering mesenteric

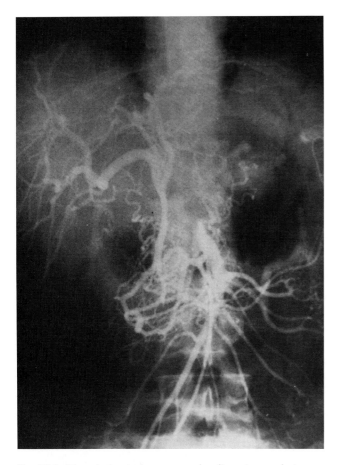

Fig. 17-1. Mesenteric arteriogram reveals celiac artery occlusion with hepatic collaterals from the SMA through the pancreaticoduodenal arcade. *(From Ernst CB: Anatomy and collateral pathways of the mesenteric circulation. In Zuidema GD, ed: Shackelford's surgery of the alimentary tract, ed 3, Philadelphia, 1991, WB Saunders.)*

artery is a direct connection between the ascending branch of the left colic artery and a branch of the SMA that originates just proximal to the middle colic artery (Fig. 17-2). It is referred to by many other names as well: arc of Riolan, mesomesenteric artery, central anastomotic artery of the colon, and arch of Treves. The marginal artery of Drummond, another collateral channel between the SMA and IMA, is more peripherally located in the colon mesentery. It connects the left branch of the middle colic artery and ascending branch of the left colic artery.

INFERIOR MESENTERIC ARTERY—HYPOGASTRIC ARTERY. An anastomotic network of vessels is formed by connections between the superior rectal artery (IMA branch) and the middle and inferior rectal arteries (hypogastric branches). Because the IMA is the most frequently occluded mesenteric artery and is often sacrificed during aortic and colonic surgical procedures, its communications with the SMA and hypogastric arteries are critical under those circumstances.[5]

ACUTE MESENTERIC ISCHEMIA

Acute mesenteric ischemia most commonly occurs as a result of embolism, acute thrombosis of preexisting atherosclerotic disease, or a low-perfusion state caused by other systemic processes. Other causes such as the inflammatory arteritides and hypercoagulable states have been reported but only in scattered cases and are thus poorly characterized. Distinct differences in demographics, pathogenesis, treatment, and prognosis exist between the various types of mesenteric ischemia. However, the diagnostic approach to the various ischemic processes is similar, and the pathophysiologic changes in the bowel wall in all forms of intestinal ischemia are identical.

Diagnosis

To detect intestinal ischemia in its early phases, a high index of suspicion is required on the part of primary care physicians and emergency department personnel. Abdominal pain is a common early manifestation of ischemia and is often described as severe. The nature of the pain can be described as crampy early in its course or constant later in its course, and rapid evacuation of the bowel sometimes occurs. Whatever the nature of the pain, few signs are noted on physical examination and can lull the clinician into a false sense that nothing serious is wrong. Indeed, pain out of proportion to the findings on physical examination should be considered a manifestation of intestinal ischemia and impending intestinal infarction until proven otherwise.

Plain abdominal radiographs are generally not helpful in reaching an early diagnosis of mesenteric ischemia because there are no specific x-ray findings associated with the process. Nonetheless, such x-ray studies should be obtained, because they can be diagnostic of other processes or document free peritoneal air, which would dictate urgent operative exploration.

Mesenteric arteriography is the diagnostic procedure of choice in the setting of suspected mesenteric ischemia when no signs of peritoneal irritation exist. Arteriography can both confirm the diagnosis and suggest a cause (em-

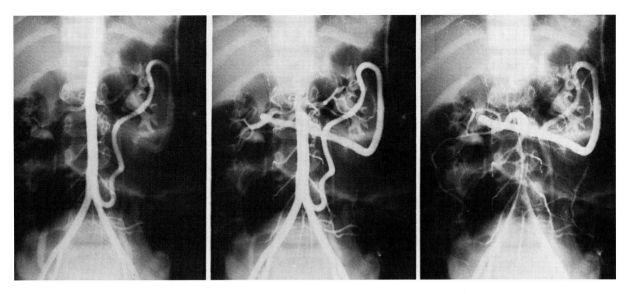

Fig. 17-2. Abdominal aortogram documents the presence of a large IMA to SMA collateral, the meandering mesenteric artery. *(From Ernst CB: Anatomy and collateral pathways of the mesenteric circulation. In Zuidema GD, ed: Shackelford's surgery of the alimentary tract, ed 3, Philadelphia, 1991, WB Saunders.)*

bolic vs. thrombotic vs. nonocclusive) in most patients. In instances of mesenteric embolism, catheter-directed therapy with thrombolytic agents may even be considered in exceptional situations as part of the procedure,[6-8] and in nonocclusive ischemia catheter-directed therapy with vasodilators is the treatment of choice.[9] Again, arteriography should not be considered in patients with peritoneal signs. Unfortunately, early diagnosis of mesenteric ischemia is not common, and the diagnosis is frequently made at operative exploration for an acute intraabdominal catastrophe rather than in the angiography suite.

Pathophysiology of Acute Intestinal Ischemia

The intestine can tolerate a 75% reduction in blood flow for 12 hours without changes detectable by light microscopy.[10] This is likely because only approximately 20% of mesenteric capillaries are open at any one time, exemplifying the tremendous blood flow reserve that the intestine receives in a resting state. In rare instances clinically, however, the oxygen and nutrient supply cannot meet the demand and ischemia ensues.[11] Regardless of the insult resulting in mesenteric ischemia, the pathophysiologic changes are the same. Predictable changes ranging from mild mucosal injury to transmural infarction occur from the mucosa outward. The rapidity with which changes develop depends on the extent that blood flow is diminished, the duration of the flow reduction, and the potential protection provided by collateral blood flow. These factors make predictions of a time course from the onset of ischemia to the development of irreversible transmural infarction difficult.

Some generalizations regarding the physiologic progression of mesenteric ischemia and pathologic progression of intestinal injury illustrate the process. The initial arterial vasomotor response to decreased blood flow is vasodilation. When no increased blood flow results, vaso-

constriction eventually ensues, often at the expense of some collateral pathways that also vasoconstrict and further decrease the potential blood flow.[12] In the intestinal wall the mucosa is the most metabolically active layer and as such is most sensitive to ischemia. This occurs despite the fact that mucosal blood flow in the bowel wall is favored during periods of ischemia.[13] The first detectable pathologic changes occur in the ultrastructure of the mucosal epithelium and are characterized by mitochondrial and endoplasmic reticulum alterations.[14] Increased capillary permeability with resultant fluid accumulation around cells and basement membranes follows. Reversible tissue loss commences with sloughing of the tips of the intestinal villi and resulting formation of a necrotic epithelial layer. Inflammatory cells and bacteria accumulate in this area of necrosis, contributing further to the progression of injury. Submucosal changes then develop characterized by edema and hemorrhage. Outward progression of cell death results until transmural necrosis occurs.[15]

To salvage ischemic bowel, reestablishment of blood flow is critical, but reperfusion of the gut after a significant period of ischemia can cause profound tissue injury as well. Parks and Granger[16] documented that the intestinal injury associated with 3 hours of ischemia followed by 1 hour of reperfusion was much greater than that associated with 4 hours of ischemia alone. Tissue injury resulting from reperfusion is caused by cytotoxic oxidation of cellular components such as membrane lipids, nucleic acids, enzymes, and receptors by reactive oxygen metabolites. Superoxide anion (O_2^-), hydrogen peroxide (H_2O_2), and hydroxyl radical ($\cdot OH$) are products of the purine degradation enzyme xanthine oxidase (XO). Following ischemia XO activity increases dramatically due to the irreversible proteolytic conversion of xanthine dehydrogenase (the normal purine degradation pathway) to XO. In addition to the direct cellular cytotoxic effects caused by formation of

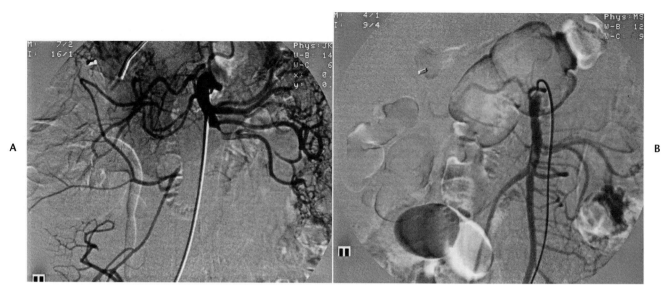

Fig. 17-3. Mesenteric arteriogram documents **(A)** typical location of a superior mesenteric artery embolus and **(B)** restored patency of SMA with minimal residual clot following thrombolysis.

the reactive oxygen free radicals, polymorphonuclear leukocyte (PMN) adherence and emigration increases because of the proinflammatory condition. PMNs cause additional cellular injury by releasing proteases and other substances that disrupt vascular integrity.[17]

Acute Embolic Mesenteric Ischemia

In 1954 Wise[18] reported that his colleague, Kean F. Westphal, had successfully performed an SMA embolectomy. The technique has remained the definitive procedure for SMA embolism consequent to that early report. Several studies of patients treated for acute mesenteric ischemia since that time have helped define this population of patients.[19-22] SMA occlusion due to embolism occurs most frequently in males in their sixth and seventh decades of life. Cases of SMA embolism slightly outnumber cases of SMA thrombosis in most reports of acute occlusive intestinal ischemia; however, nonocclusive mesenteric ischemia, SMA embolism, and SMA thrombosis occur in nearly equal proportions when pooled data from multiple reports are compiled.[23]

PATHOGENESIS. In chronic atherosclerotic disease of the SMA, collateral circulatory pathways develop with the gradual increase in severity of SMA stenosis. Acute occlusion in this setting may have little or no effect on mesenteric blood flow. Following acute mesenteric embolism, however, collateral channels are not capable of providing adequate intestinal blood supply, and profound ischemia rapidly ensues in most patients.

The acute onset of abdominal pain in a patient with cardiac disease should alert a physician to the possibility of visceral thromboembolism. Cardiac arrhythmias (particularly atrial fibrillation), cardiomyopathy, valvular disease, and acute myocardial infarction are all associated with the development of intracardiac thrombus, which can result in thromboembolic events. It has been estimated that approximately 5% of all cardiac emboli lodge in the visceral

arteries, with the vast majority lodging in the SMA.[24] The acute downward angulation of the SMA origin compared with the celiac and the size difference between the SMA and IMA probably account for this preponderance of SMA thromboemboli.[25]

Even in the absence of a cardiac source, mesenteric embolism may occur. Paradoxic venous emboli passing through a right to left cardiac shunt[26] as well as arterio-arterial atherothrombotic emboli from the proximal aorta have been reported.[27] In some patients a definable source of the mesenteric embolus can never be found.

DIAGNOSIS. The luxury of a preoperative diagnosis of SMA embolism is afforded in patients who present early enough to undergo mesenteric arteriography. Whereas atherosclerotic disease of the SMA usually results in occlusion at the ostium of the artery, emboli most frequently lodge in the vessel at the origin of the middle colic artery, approximately 3 to 8 cm from the SMA origin and beyond the origin of the inferior pancreaticoduodenal artery and a few jejunal branches (Fig. 17-3, *A*). The embolic occlusion often appears as a meniscus. Other arteriographic findings that may help confirm the diagnosis of SMA embolism include the absence of major collaterals and the presence of another embolus in the renal, celiac, or lower-extremity circulations. Peripheral location of a small SMA embolus can occur as well resulting in a limited area of threatened intestine.[25]

In patients who present late, urgent operation for an acute abdomen leads to the recognition of ischemic intestine. In these situations the cause of ischemia must be defined. Preoperative clues such as cardiac arrhythmia support SMA embolism, but the surgeon must confirm the diagnosis by evaluation of the extent of intestinal ischemia and the pulse characteristics of the SMA, since the options for treatment are quite different if thrombosis rather than embolus is present. When a SMA embolus lodges in the typical location at the middle colic artery origin, the first few centimeters of the jejunum are spared from the ischemic process. Distally the ischemia extends variably through the right half of the colon, sparing all or part of the transverse colon and the entire descending colon. Identification of the proximal SMA as it emerges from beneath the pancreas may allow pulse assessment at this site. If the embolus is lodged distal to this site, a strong pulse will be palpable. If no pulse is palpable and calcific changes of the vessel wall are identified, thrombosis should be suspected.

TREATMENT. Acute occlusive mesenteric ischemia is a surgical emergency with lethal consequences if significant delays in treatment occur. However, prompt attention should be given to several details before surgery, and the same principles of preoperative preparation apply to all forms of acute mesenteric ischemia. Hypovolemia due to intestinal sequestration of fluid, acidosis, and electrolyte abnormalities are the rule and require rapid correction and continued attention because such abnormalities are likely to persist into the operative and postoperative periods. Due to the risk of bowel necrosis and perforation, preoperative administration of parenteral broad-spectrum antibiotics is indicated. Intestinal decompression with a nasogastric tube and urine output measurement with a urinary catheter are essential. Placement of a central venous or pulmonary artery catheter will facilitate assessment of fluid resuscitation. Systemic heparinization can be instituted to prevent propagation of clot if the diagnosis is made preoperatively by arteriography.

Fortunately the classic site of SMA embolism is readily accessible. Through a midline abdominal incision, the SMA is exposed as it emerges from beneath the pancreas at the base of the transverse mesocolon (Fig. 17-4). Palpation of the artery at this site often helps to specifically locate the embolus. Care should be taken dissecting the SMA proximal and distal to the embolus to prevent fragmentation and distal embolization. Once vessel control is established, a longitudinal arteriotomy is made and gentle passage of a balloon embolectomy catheter (2 to 3 Fr) is performed to remove propagated thrombus or embolic fragments. Proximal embolectomy follows using slightly larger catheters (3 to 4 Fr) until strong pulsatile flow is obtained. After flushing the proximal and distal SMA with heparinized saline solution, the arteriotomy is closed with a fine interrupted synthetic nonabsorbable suture material such as 5-0 or 6-0 polypropylene. A vein patch should be placed if compromise of the vessel lumen is expected with primary closure.

After blood flow in the SMA is reestablished, it is advisable to wait approximately 30 minutes before assessing bowel viability to allow reperfusion to delineate any clearly unsalvageable intestine. If embolectomy has promptly followed the onset of ischemia, the intestine may rapidly return to its normal color, distal mesenteric pulsations may be easily palpable, peristalsis may be present, and viability will not be in question. Frankly necrotic intestine on the other hand may also be easily identified. It is in dusky-appearing bowel that viability must be assessed. Classic subjective evaluations of color, quality of mesenteric pulsations, and peristalsis are simple but unreliable methods of determining viability. Consequently use of a Doppler probe to detect antemesenteric pulsations[28] and/or sodium fluorescein to evaluate fluorescence patterns[29] has been suggested to increase diagnostic accuracy. Several other methods of determining bowel viability, which in general are more cumbersome or require costly special equipment, are currently under investigation.[30-33]

Unfortunately no available alternative for viability assessment can eliminate the possibility that viable bowel is being removed or nonviable bowel is being left behind. When significant bowel resection is required, preservation of intestinal length becomes critical. Second-look celiotomy 12 to 36 hours following initial exploration is indicated when intestine of questionable viability is left behind.[34] The interval between operations allows time for complete resuscitation of the patient with optimization of fluid status, cardiac function, and acid-base and electrolyte abnormalities, which may improve marginal circulation. If a decision to perform a second-look operation is made at the initial operation, this course must be followed regardless of any perceived clinical improvement in the patient's condition during the early postoperative period. In these critically ill patients, physical examination and laboratory studies cannot be relied on to assess the viability of the remaining intestine. At reoperation, intestinal viability is again assessed. Further resection is undertaken, if necessary, and reoperation planned if questionably viable intestine again remains.

Prolonged vasoconstriction can threaten the viability of intestine following revascularization for SMA embolism or thrombosis. Pharmacoangiography can be a useful adjunct under these circumstances.[9] If preoperative arteriography was performed, the angiographic catheter can be left in the SMA for postoperative infusion of vasodilators. Serial selective SMA arteriography is used in these cases to assess the effectiveness and need for continuation of the therapy.

If focal ischemic bowel segments are discovered at the time of operation, careful mesenteric pulse evaluation may document peripheral mesenteric emboli. Typically these situations are not remediable by vascular reconstruction, and bowel resection is the only option. Some peripheral mesenteric emboli undoubtedly occur without the sequelae of intestinal ischemia and threatened necrosis. Patients with asymptomatic emboli, found incidentally by arteriography performed for reasons other than abdominal symptoms, should have frequent abdominal assessments with surgical intervention only if signs or symptoms of intestinal ischemia develop.

Recent anecdotal case reports have documented the use of thrombolytic agents for lysis of SMA thromboemboli.[6-8] Although generally satisfactory results have been obtained, the potential complications and the limited number of situations in which this technique can be employed should caution against widespread application. In our single experience using SMA thrombolysis (Fig. 17-3), multiple ischemic intestinal strictures developed within 2 months following successful thrombolysis despite abdominal examinations that never suggested peritoneal inflammation (Fig. 17-4). Whether the strictures represent persistent areas of ischemia due to peripheral emboli or are manifestations of nontransmural ischemia/reperfusion injury is unclear. Whatever the cause, what is clear is that

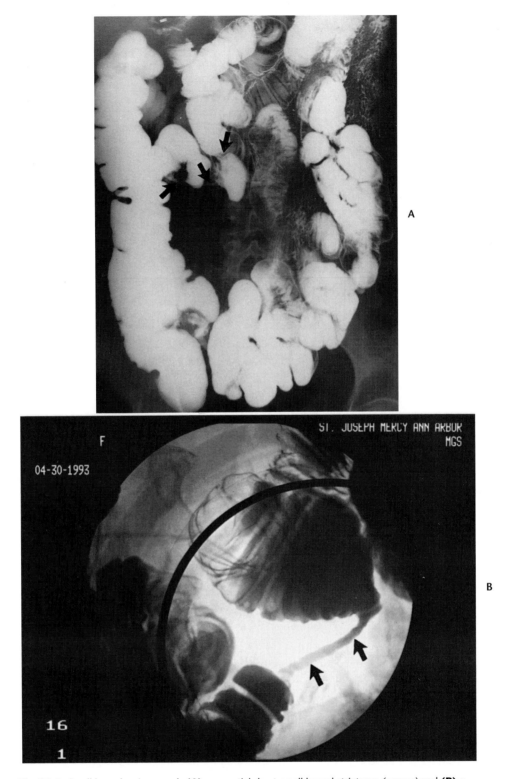

Fig. 17-4. Small bowel series reveals **(A)** sequential short small bowel strictures *(arrows)* and **(B)** a longer area of small bowel stricture *(arrows)* identified approximately 2 months following thrombolysis of an SMA embolus (Fig. 17-3). The patient required laparotomy for partial bowel obstruction.

intestine that has potentially nonreversible injury is not evaluated when thrombolysis is undertaken. Strictures or even frank intestinal necrosis with perforation may complicate the procedure. Thrombolysis may be considered in patients with SMA embolism very early in the disease when no signs of peritoneal irritation exist and there is a prohibitive surgical risk (as with recent or evolving myocardial infarction). If rapid clot lysis is not achieved, the procedure must be abandoned. Only when guidelines detailing the indications and therapeutic plan, developed by vascular surgeons and their interventional radiology colleagues, are applied and strictly adhered to can SMA thrombolysis become an acceptable alternative to surgical embolectomy.

RESULTS. SMA embolectomy in the vast majority of patients will be technically successful in restoring mesenteric pulses. Despite technical success, mortality rates remain high due to the systemic complications of intestinal ischemia and associated comorbid conditions in these patients. Mortality appears to be directly related to the length of time from onset of symptoms to treatment[35] and the extent of bowel necrosis. There are few reported survivors in whom massive small bowel resection was performed[36,37] or treatment was rendered more than 24 hours after onset of symptoms. On the other hand, reasonably good results (greater than 80% survival) can be expected in patients in whom embolectomy is performed and intestinal resection is not required.[22] The overall mortality from pooled data derived from several studies was 70% for 120 patients.[23] Recent reports of mortality rates of 50% or less are encouraging and suggest that early recognition is having an impact on survival.[22,38]

Acute Mesenteric Artery Thrombosis

Acute SMA thrombosis with development of intestinal ischemia is a devastating process that most commonly afflicts women in their sixties and seventies.[19-21] It often occurs in patients with a history of chronic abdominal pain, weight loss, or altered bowel habits suggesting chronic mesenteric ischemia.[39,40] The onset of pain may be more insidious with SMA thrombosis than SMA embolism.[41] When all causes of acute mesenteric ischemia are considered, SMA thrombosis appears to be slightly less common than SMA embolism or nonocclusive mesenteric ischemia.[23] Much of the difficulty in managing these patients is the frequent coexistence of diffuse atherosclerosis involving both the coronary and peripheral arteries. In fact, evidence of diffuse atherosclerosis may be a clue to the diagnosis of SMA thrombosis when acute mesenteric ischemia is present.

PATHOGENESIS. Acute SMA thrombosis is typically associated with proximal SMA atherosclerosis, although it has also been reported in association with fibromuscular dysplasia, hypercoagulable states, inflammatory arteritis, and aortic dissection on rare occasions.[25] A history of chronic abdominal pain in the majority of patients with acute mesenteric ischemia suggests that the SMA is frequently affected by a flow-limiting stenosis with marginal collateral flow before acute thrombosis. Flow-limiting stenosis of the SMA is well tolerated in most circumstances because of the development of collaterals from the celiac

artery and IMA. In fact occlusion of two or even all three mesenteric vessels without symptoms of intestinal ischemia is not uncommon.[42,43] Intuitively it seems unlikely that sudden occlusion of a highly stenotic SMA would result in extensive ischemia. Perhaps SMA atherosclerotic disease, like disease in the coronary and carotid arteries, is subject to destabilization and intermittent rapid progression accounting for the ischemia that develops in some patients when occlusion occurs.

DIAGNOSIS. Preoperative diagnosis using arteriography is not always possible in patients with SMA thrombosis because of delayed recognition of the manifestations of mesenteric ischemia. When arteriography can be performed, it is helpful in formulating a treatment plan. Atherosclerosis of the SMA most commonly affects the origin and proximal few centimeters of the artery. Unlike SMA embolus, proximal occlusion of the SMA without sparing of the inferior pancreaticoduodenal artery, proximal jejunal branches, or middle colic artery typifies SMA thrombosis.

Urgent surgical exploration for SMA thrombosis will typically reveal intestinal ischemia from the ligament of Treitz to the midtransverse colon. The common sparing of the proximal jejunum encountered in SMA embolism is not present. In addition, as the SMA is exposed, no proximal pulsations are palpable. Once the diagnosis is established in the operating room, SMA reconstruction is attempted if any ischemic bowel appears salvageable.

TREATMENT. If extensive intestinal necrosis is present, mortality is extreme. Massive bowel resection under these conditions rarely results in survival.[36,37] When a significant portion of small intestine appears potentially salvageable, SMA reconstruction should be performed with subsequent assessment of bowel viability and resection as indicated.

The SMA is exposed in a similar fashion as described for embolectomy. Distal balloon thrombectomy using small catheters (2 to 3 Fr) should be performed to remove distal propagated clot, which is found in approximately 20% of patients. If the infrarenal aorta is reasonably free of disease, it is dissected between the renal arteries and IMA and side clamped on the left anterolateral aspect. An aortotomy of 1 to 1.5 cm is made, and a spatulated saphenous vein graft anastomosis is constructed in an end-to-side fashion using a continuous suture technique with fine synthetic material. The anastomosis to the SMA can be performed in an end-to-side or end-to-end fashion. When constructing this aortomesenteric graft, great care must be taken to create a gentle curve (an inverted U) that will not kink and occlude when the viscera are placed into their anatomic positions.

If the aortic wall is thickened due to atherosclerotic disease, a partially occluding clamp may not be applicable, and the infrarenal aorta may require cross-clamping above and below the anticipated site of anastomosis. Atherosclerotic disease may even be so severe as to preclude placing an anastomosis in the infrarenal aorta on occasion, and antegrade bypass from the supraceliac aorta may be necessary.

As with SMA embolism, revascularization is followed by assessment of bowel viability, performance of intestinal resection as indicated, determination of the need for second-look celiotomy, and if needed, pharmacoangiographic intervention as described. Postoperative care of patients with SMA thrombosis does not differ from that for patients with SMA embolism.

RESULTS. Mortality rates for acute mesenteric thrombosis approach 90%[23] and can be correlated with the extent of bowel infarction. Even with technically successful revascularization and bowel resection, the magnitude of the surgical stress compounded by manifestations of severe concomitant systemic atherosclerotic disease results in serious, often lethal, complications.

Nonocclusive Mesenteric Ischemia

The first case of intestinal ischemia with infarction not associated with occlusive vascular disease was reported by Ende in 1958.[44] That particular patient had heart failure, which was the presumed etiology of a low-flow state. As medical science has advanced, the ability to sustain life in patients who are critically ill and those with severe cardiac disease has dramatically improved, and as such has created a population of patients susceptible to systemic low-flow states. In addition, an increasing awareness of the signs and symptoms of mesenteric ischemia has probably increased the recognition of nonocclusive mesenteric ischemia, which appears to be the most common cause of acute mesenteric ischemia in both individual reports and evaluation of pooled data.

Males and females with a mean age of 72 years are equally affected by nonocclusive mesenteric ischemia.[23] Generally, it occurs in patients with low cardiac output state or a reason for sustained mesenteric vasoconstriction.

PATHOGENESIS. Unlike acute mesenteric ischemia associated with SMA thrombosis or embolism, nonocclusive mesenteric ischemia occurs as a direct result of the effects of systemic processes on the mesenteric circulation. For ischemia to occur in the absence of a vascular occlusive lesion, either a protracted low cardiac output state, prolonged mesenteric vasoconstriction, or a combination of both must be severe enough to overwhelm compensatory mechanisms that maintain normal intestinal perfusion.

The initial splanchnic response to decreased blood flow is vasodilation, but without a resulting increase in blood flow vasoconstriction occurs. Vasoconstriction in itself is a normal compensatory mechanism; however, sustained vasoconstriction can overcompensate and injure the intestinal wall. The progression of ischemic injury is inevitable unless the vasoconstriction can be reduced and splanchnic perfusion improved. Interestingly, in some patients correction of the inciting cause does not result in resolution of pathologic mesenteric vasoconstriction, and ischemia continues due to a loss of autoregulation.[10,45]

Low cardiac output states are most frequently implicated in the development of nonocclusive mesenteric ischemia. Alone, low cardiac output can result in intestinal ischemia, but the treatment of heart failure with vasopressors and/or digitalis can aggravate the situation by direct mesenteric vasoconstriction. Mesenteric ischemia not associated with low cardiac output or pharmacologic vasoconstriction has been reported in patients with various diseases that result in mesenteric vasoconstriction including septic shock and hypovolemia (see the box, above).

CAUSES OF NONOCCLUSIVE MESENTERIC ISCHEMIA

Low Cardiac Output States
Congestive heart failure
Myocardial infarction
Cardiac arrhythmia
Cardiomyopathy
Postcardiac surgery
Aortic insufficiency

Mesenteric Vasoconstriction
Pharmacologic
Digitalis
Ergot poisoning
Cocaine abuse
Vasopressors
Nonpharmacologic
Hypovolemia
Septic shock
Postabdominal surgery
Hemoconcentration
Coarctation repair

DIAGNOSIS. As with all forms of acute mesenteric ischemia, a high index of suspicion is required for early diagnosis. Patients may present with abdominal signs and symptoms associated with systemic and/or mesenteric hypoperfusion. Unfortunately diagnosis is often delayed due to focus on the treatment of the underlying disease. Patients with nonocclusive mesenteric ischemia may also exhibit a decreased level of mentation, which complicates evaluation. An insidious rather than sudden onset of vague abdominal pain, which initially is accompanied by minimal physical findings, may suggest a diagnosis of nonocclusive mesenteric ischemia or SMA thrombosis. The identification of a low-flow state may help to differentiate occlusive and nonocclusive causes of ischemia, but the frequent concurrent cardiovascular disease that accompanies occlusive ischemia may make differentiation by history and physical examination impossible.

Arteriography is diagnostic when it can be performed.[16,46] Selective SMA study will help define the vascular pathology. A normal proximal SMA with smooth tapering of the distal artery and poor or absent opacification of distal branches suggests severe vasospasm. Although proximal SMA atherosclerosis has been identified in a number of patients, it is unusual.[47] After selective SMA arteriography has been performed and the diagnosis established, the catheter should remain in the orifice of the SMA for catheter-directed pharmacotherapy.

Intestinal ischemia ranging from patchy focal involvement of the small bowel or colon to involvement of the entire small bowel and colon can be found at exploration in nonocclusive mesenteric ischemia. If the diagnosis was not established before surgery, extensive evaluation of the SMA and its branches is indicated. A diminution of the pulse as examination proceeds from proximal to distal suggests vasoconstriction, although peripheral embolization or thrombosis due to vasculitis may be difficult to differentiate in some patients.

TREATMENT. The patient suspected of having nonocclusive mesenteric ischemia should receive rapid, aggressive treatment of the inciting process that resulted in hypoperfusion. Correction of cardiac arrhythmias, inotropic support in acute myocardial infarction, aggressive diuresis in congestive heart failure, fluid resuscitation in hypovolemia, and so on are the initial goals. Digitalis and α-agonists used for control of arrhythmias or support of blood pressure should be avoided. In all patients oxygen should be administered, nasogastric tube and urethral catheter placed, and central monitoring with a central venous pressure or pulmonary arterial catheter considered. In circumstances of mild ischemia, rapid attention to these details may be all that is required to resolve symptoms.

While underlying problems are being addressed, treatment with mesenteric vasodilators can be initiated. Selective SMA infusion of vasodilators may be started in the angiography suite. Bolus injection of tolazoline (Priscoline) 25 mg followed by continued infusion of papaverine at 30 to 60 mg/hr or the use of papaverine alone at 30 to 60 mg/hr is instituted to reduce mesenteric vasoconstriction. The effectiveness of pharmacoangiographic therapy can be evaluated as frequently as deemed necessary by repeated contrast injection through the SMA catheter in the angiography suite. Therapy is terminated when symptoms have resolved and vasoconstriction is absent on selective SMA arteriograms after vasodilator infusion is withdrawn. Continuous epidural anesthesia may also be considered to obtain mesenteric vasodilation.[48]

Advocates of this aggressive pharmacoangiographic approach suggest that arteriography should be performed for diagnostic/therapeutic purposes before abdominal exploration in all patients with suspicion of acute mesenteric ischemia. Although this may be practical when mild signs of peritoneal irritation exist, it should not be attempted in a patient who has signs of diffuse peritonitis. In these cases pharmacoangiographic therapy can be initiated after surgical exploration and resection of the nonviable intestine.

When pharmacoangiography as primary therapy for nonocclusive mesenteric ischemia does not result in rapid resolution of abdominal signs and symptoms, or signs and symptoms recur, urgent abdominal exploration is indicated.[25]

RESULTS. Mortality for nonocclusive mesenteric ischemia is 90% or greater.[19,49,50] A combination of the severity of the underlying disease process that led to nonocclusive mesenteric ischemia and the devastating systemic effects of intestinal ischemia undoubtedly led to this dismal prognosis. Dramatic improvements with mortality of less than 50% may be realized with aggressive pharmacoangiography and the improved treatment of underlying disorders.[9]

MESENTERIC VENOUS THROMBOSIS

Warren and Eberhard[51] are credited with first reporting bowel ischemia associated with thrombosis of the mesenteric veins in 1935. Early reports of mesenteric venous thrombosis (MVT) suggested a very high mortality rate. However, most patients presented late, with bowel necrosis at the time of operative diagnosis. The development of ultrasonography, computed tomography (CT), and magnetic resonance imaging (MRI) has resulted in recognition of a spectrum of MVT. MVT ranges from asymptomatic nonocclusive thrombus to portal venous occlusion with associated liver failure and extensive bowel necrosis. MVT accounts for approximately 10% of acute mesenteric ischemia cases in studies that consider all causes.[23] It can occur at any age, but most commonly from 30 to 60.[25] There appears to be a slight male preponderance.[23]

Pathogenesis

A variety of hematologic and abdominal disorders result in MVT. Hypercoagulable states including antithrombin III, protein C, and protein S deficiencies, and the myeloproliferative disorders including polycythemia vera, primary thrombocytosis have been implicated. Abdominal malignancies, prior abdominal operations, oral contraceptive use, and inflammatory abdominal conditions including acute pancreatitis and inflammatory bowel disease are suggested causes of MVT (see the box, p. 314).[52] Not surprisingly a number of instances of MVT remain labeled as idiopathic. As more coagulation abnormalities are recognized, many of those previously described as "idiopathic" may be designated as hypercoagulable disorders.

When MVT occurs, fluid begins to accumulate in the wall and lumen of the affected intestine. Hemoconcentration due to fluid sequestration is common.[53,54] If diagnosis is not made during this early phase and treatment instituted, thrombosis may extend into the vasa recti and intramural venous collaterals. When this occurs, the arterial supply is compromised due to decrease in effective perfusion pressure resulting from the increase in capillary pressure.[55] The cascade of events leading to intestinal necrosis may follow, depending on the severity of the thrombosis and compensatory capability of the splanchnic venous circulation.

Diagnosis

Vague abdominal complaints and nonspecific abdominal findings confound the early diagnosis of MVT. Fortunately the progression of MVT from symptom onset to intestinal necrosis is gradual, providing an opportunity for diagnosis before the onset of irreversible changes. The average time from the onset of symptoms to recognition of MVT exceeded 2 weeks in a recent report.[56]

Abdominal complaints range from vague epigastric pain to severe focal pain. Nausea, abdominal distention, and anorexia are frequent accompanying complaints. Physical examination does little to establish a diagnosis of MVT but is important as a guide to further diagnostic evaluation. When a patient with MVT presents with signs of an acute abdomen, urgent operation is indicated.

Routine laboratory and radiographic studies are not diagnostic in MVT. Elevation of the white blood cell count

CAUSES OF MESENTERIC VENOUS THROMBOSIS

Hematologic
Hypercoaguable states
  Antithrombin III deficiency
  Protein C deficiency
  Protein S deficiency
  Hyperfibrinogenemia
  Oral contraceptive use
  Pregnancy
Myeloproliferative disorders
  Polycythemia vera
  Primary thrombocytosis

Inflammatory
  Acute pancreatitis
  Inflammatory bowel disease
  Acute appendicitis
  Diverticulitis

Mechanical
  Volvulus
  Portal hypertension
  Abdominal malignancy

Traumatic
  Blunt abdominal injury
  Penetrating abdominal injury
  Following splenectomy
  Other previous abdominal surgery

Idiopathic

with a left shift is common but nonspecific. Other common laboratory studies including serum amylase and phosphorus concentration are frequently normal. Plain abdominal x-ray studies may show an ileus pattern, evidence of bowel wall edema, and ascites, but all are nonspecific findings.[54]

MVT is most commonly diagnosed by abdominal ultrasound, CT, or at the time of abdominal exploration for an acute abdomen.[56] Abdominal ultrasound can be performed with pulsed Doppler (duplex) or without (B-mode). The ascites and intestinal edema that accompany MVT are easily identified by either technique. Portal vein thrombosis is recognized without difficulty; however, recognition of superior mesenteric and splenic venous thrombosis may be problematic, especially with the B-mode technique alone.[57] CT has better resolution of the superior mesenteric and splenic veins than ultrasound, allowing accurate detection of thrombus in these vessels. Ascites and bowel wall edema are easily identified by CT.[58,59] Overall, CT and duplex sonography should be considered equivalent for identification of large-vessel MVT. MRI may prove to be accurate in the diagnosis of MVT, but to date there is little experience with its use.

Before CT and ultrasound technology developed, mesenteric arteriography was the gold standard for diagnosis of MVT. SMA arteriography classically reveals distal arterial spasm, stretching of peripheral vessels secondary to bowel wall edema, and prolongation of the capillary phase of the study. A venous phase may or may not be present, depending on the extent of thrombosis.[60] CT, duplex ultrasound, and SMA arteriography can be complementary in MVT when the diagnosis cannot be established with a single modality.

Massive bowel wall edema, the presence of intraabdominal fluid, and ischemic intestinal changes noted in conjunction with palpable mesenteric arterial pulsations at the time of surgical exploration suggest MVT. Peripheral arterial embolism with resulting focal areas of ischemia and absent distal pulsations can be difficult to differentiate late in the course of MVT if arteriolar thrombosis occurs due to diminished capillary blood flow. Blood clot extruding from ligated veins during intestinal resection may lead to the diagnosis of MVT when it is not otherwise suspected.

Treatment

Rapid restoration of intravascular fluid volume should be a priority in the patient diagnosed with MVT. Nasogastric tube intestinal decompression and urethral catheterization should be established early as well. Acute abdominal findings mandate administration of parenteral broad-spectrum antibiotics.

Incidental recognition of MVT by ultrasound or CT in patients with only mild to moderate abdominal symptoms presents a treatment dilemma. There are reports in which some patients with MVT who were left untreated did not develop any adverse sequelae.[56] In our opinion any patient with recognized MVT and the absence of indications for surgery should undergo extensive evaluation for a cause of MVT if none has previously been identified. In addition, systemic heparinization should be instituted with plans for warfarin anticoagulation therapy for at least 3 months. If a specific coagulation abnormality is recognized, permanent anticoagulation therapy may be indicated.

When symptoms of peritoneal irritation are present requiring surgical exploration, compromised intestine is almost always found. Wide resection of the involved bowel and mesentery is indicated. Constructing intestinal anastomoses can be difficult because of bowel wall edema. Consideration should be given to exteriorization of bowel ends or second-look celiotomy when bowel of questionable viability is left in the abdomen. Systemic heparin sodium anticoagulation therapy, unless contraindicated, should be instituted when MVT is diagnosed and continued into the postoperative period. At least 3 months of postoperative anticoagulation therapy is indicated.

Mesenteric venous thrombectomy has been described for large vein thrombosis.[61,62] Although there is some suggestion that intestinal length may be salvaged by this technique, the difficulty of performing complete thrombectomy and the inherent endothelial damage associated with manipulation have limited its use.

Results

At one extreme, untreated massive MVT results in 100% mortality. Mortality in patients with incidentally detected MVT or mildly symptomatic MVT should approach zero. The spectrum of this disease makes estimates of morbidity and mortality difficult without an acceptable classification. In general the outcome for MVT is more favorable than for the other causes of acute mesenteric ischemia. This probably relates to the broader diagnostic window afforded by slower progression of symptoms, the less frequent occurrence of concomitant disease processes, and less extensive intestinal involvement.

The other issue regarding MVT is the risk of recurrent thrombosis or extension of existing thrombosis. Since recurrence is associated with increased mortality, prevention is important. Most reports of MVT note a substantial reduction in morbidity and mortality in patients treated with perioperative heparin sodium.[63,64] Long-term warfarin anticoagulation therapy is not as well established in reducing mortality but is advocated by most investigators including the authors.

CHRONIC MESENTERIC ISCHEMIA

A syndrome of intermittent abdominal pain attributed to intestinal ischemia was first described by Klein in 1921.[65] Dunphy in 1936 recognized that both acute infarction and intermittent postprandial pain are associated with visceral artery stenoses and/or occlusions.[39] In fact, he found that about half of the patients who developed acute intestinal infarction had prior abdominal symptoms. Later the term *intestinal angina,* to describe this postprandial abdominal pain syndrome associated with chronic visceral atherosclerosis, was coined by Mikkelsen.[66]

Despite the association of visceral atherosclerotic disease with the syndrome of intestinal angina, it should be emphasized that many individuals who have significant visceral stenoses do not suffer from intestinal angina because of abundant collateral circulation. The ramifications of symptomatic chronic visceral atherosclerosis are serious, however, particularly the potential progression to acute intestinal infarction.

When intestinal angina is suggested by symptoms, and compatible visceral occlusive disease is discovered, intestinal revascularization is indicated to prevent secondary acute thrombosis and to correct symptoms that often lead to malnutrition, weight loss, and disability. Revascularization can be accomplished by a variety of techniques depending on the clinical situation. Many of the procedures are technically demanding, but in the hands of experienced vascular surgeons they can be performed with good results.

Revascularization under elective circumstances relies on recognition of symptoms, exclusion of other potential causes, systematic evaluation of concomitant disease states that can complicate major surgical procedures, and formulation of a plan that fits the clinical circumstances. Only when each of these factors is considered and a technically sound revascularization is performed can the best results be attained.

Pathogenesis

Emphasis has been placed on atherosclerosis as the cause of chronic mesenteric ischemia (CMI), but rare cases have been described following traumatic injuries and with extensive fibromuscular disease.[67] CA, SMA, and IMA atherosclerosis are generally ostial diseases, often contiguous with aortic atherosclerosis. Occlusions are typically found in the proximal few centimeters of these arteries. Due to the extraordinary compensatory ability of the mesenteric collateral circulation, significant disease of two or even all three mesenteric vessels can be tolerated without development of symptoms.

Presumably, at rest, patients with CMI have enough intestinal blood flow to maintain gut viability and prevent symptoms. It has been postulated that the increase in blood flow required in the mesenteric vascular bed after eating overwhelms the compensatory ability of the collateral circulation, and pain develops because of the release of undefined humoral substances much like classic angina from coronary disease.[66]

Diagnosis

Atherosclerosis is generally a disease of the aged, and visceral atherosclerosis is no exception. However, symptomatic splanchnic ischemia occurs in slightly younger patients than other forms of symptomatic atherosclerosis. CMI is most commonly diagnosed in patients in their fifties and sixties. Females are more commonly affected than males, perhaps as much 3:1.[23] The constellation of accompanying atherosclerotic disorders including coronary artery disease, cerebrovascular disease, and peripheral arterial occlusive disease are predictably associated with CMI.

The most common complaint in patients with CMI is postprandial abdominal pain. The classic description is crampy or colicky pain located in the epigastric area that begins 15 to 30 minutes following eating, lasts for 2 to 3 hours, and then gradually subsides. In a short time patients may begin to eat smaller and smaller meals in response to the pain, and fear of food (sitophobia) may develop. This results in weight loss, which can eventually become quite marked.

Physical examination reveals weight loss as well as findings associated with generalized atherosclerosis. Diminished peripheral pulses or even more serious signs of lower-extremity arterial occlusive disease may be noted. An epigastric abdominal bruit, although admittedly nonspecific, may suggest visceral arterial stenosis when associated with marked weight loss.

Although the classic findings of weight loss, postprandial pain, sitophobia, and stigmata of systemic atherosclerosis strongly suggest the diagnosis of CMI, this may go unrecognized due to suspicion of occult malignancy or other gastrointestinal disorders. As with all forms of mesenteric ischemia, a high index of suspicion is required to make early diagnosis.

Although plain abdominal x-ray studies, endoscopy, CT, and gastrointestinal contrast studies only serve to exclude other diagnoses, duplex ultrasound may be used in the appropriate clinical setting as a screening examination to determine the presence or absence of proximal CA and

SMA stenosis or occlusion. Visceral duplex imaging requires a skilled technologist and a well-prepared patient if adequate visualization of the mesenteric vessels is to be obtained. Vessel tortuousity, respiratory motion, and the presence of bowel gas impede visualization of either one or both vessels in 10% to 20% of patients, and this remains a significant shortcoming of the technology.[68]

Results of visceral duplex imaging are generally not highly quantitative. Velocity parameters used to determine the presence of 50% or greater stenosis[69] and 70% or greater stenosis[70] have been reported with sensitivities and specificities of near 90% when compared with biplanar arteriography. With the reasonably low incidence of false-negative studies, duplex imaging can probably be best used to exclude CMI in patients with some suspicion of the disease. Duplex imaging should not substitute for arteriography or preclude arteriography in patients in whom the diagnosis remains suspect despite negative imaging results.

Biplanar arteriography including flush aortic and selective CA, SMA, and IMA views will define the extent of visceral arterial disease. In addition, the extent and direction of collateral blood flow can be evaluated. Flow-limiting stenoses or occlusions of at least two of the three mesenteric arteries is expected if the diagnosis of CMI is to be entertained (Fig. 17-5).[42,43] Dilated collaterals may or may not be a prominent feature on arteriography, depending on the acuity of development of stenoses and individual splanchnic compensatory ability. In general, large collaterals are present and help confirm the presence of lesions that are suspected to be flow limiting.

Once the diagnosis of CMI is established using a combination of historical, physical, and radiologic data, the patient's fitness to undergo a major surgical procedure must be assessed. The anatomy of the visceral disease, nutritional status of the patient, and cardiorespiratory risk must all be considered before the best approach to revascularization can be chosen for each patient.

Treatment

To our knowledge no report of the natural history of untreated CMI exists. From data in early descriptive studies of CMI, it was recognized that perhaps 50% of patients suffering acute intestinal infarction had preceding chronic abdominal complaints.[39,40] This suggested a progression of CMI to catastrophic acute ischemia. Indeed, some patients with known CMI have developed acute ischemia before planned revascularization. In addition to the possibility of developing acute ischemia, continued weight loss, inanition, and even death can be expected in patients who are not treated for CMI. For these reasons patients diagnosed with CMI must undergo mesenteric revascularization.

Shaw and Maynard[71] reported the first successful splanchnic revascularization by visceral endarterectomy in 1958. This was followed in 1959 by the first successful autogenous vein mesenteric bypass by Derrick, Pollard, and Moore.[72] In the more than 35 years that have passed, many reports describing various techniques for mesenteric revascularization and the results have been published. Unfortunately, due to the rarity of CMI, comparisons of various techniques using prospective trials have not been

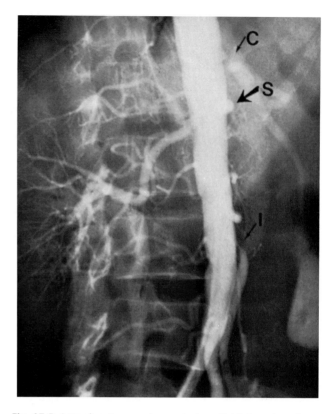

Fig. 17-5. Lateral aortogram demonstrates a tight stenosis at the celiac origin *(C),* occlusion of the superior mesenteric artery near its origin *(S),* and a tight stenosis of the inferior mesenteric artery near its origin *(I).*

performed. In addition, percutaneous angioplasty and stenting techniques await further investigation to delineate their appropriate applications. Thus the clinician is left with a perplexing variety of therapeutic options and little evidence to suggest which is superior.

Four options for visceral revascularization are available: visceral endarterectomy; antegrade supraceliac aorta to visceral bypass; retrograde infrarenal aorta to visceral bypass; and percutaneous transluminal angioplasty (PTA). Each technique has its advantages and disadvantages and should be considered part of the armamentarium of the vascular surgeon. PTA is in evolution regarding the mesenteric circulation. Whereas satisfactory long-term results of PTA have been described for iliac atherosclerotic and renal fibromuscular dysplastic lesions, limited experience with mesenteric PTA has not been as encouraging. In one representative report of 22 dilations performed in 13 patients, there was initial technical success in 20 lesions (91%), and symptom relief in 11 patients (85%). One patient died within 30 days (8%). Relief was not durable in all patients, as 5 of the 10 remaining developed recurrent symptoms. Long-term success was achieved in 6 patients (46%) with some requiring multiple dilations.[73] Other reports document similar results,[74,75] confirming the clear inferiority of PTA compared with standard surgical revascularization techniques. This is not unexpected given the experience with proximal renal artery PTA.[76] The overflow aortic atherosclerotic disease pattern in both renal and visceral arteries is not amenable to PTA. It is hoped that stenting in conjunction with PTA will improve results, but at present PTA can be recommended only in patients who are at high risk for complications of surgical revascularization.

The remaining options are surgical and represent the procedures of choice in any patient considered a reasonable operative risk. Before surgical intervention, the chronic debilitated state of many patients must be addressed. Patients who have marked weight loss and malnutrition may benefit from preoperative total parenteral nutrition (TPN). Although there is some dispute that TPN administered in this setting alters morbidity and mortality, a 7- to 10-day course before surgical intervention serves to improve overall nutritional status. In addition, nutrient delivery can be optimized in the preoperative rather than postoperative period, as TPN may be required for a significant period postoperatively while the patient overcomes the chronic enteropathic state and frequently accompanying sitophobia.

Appropriate operative monitoring depends on preoperative assessment of associated risk factors. In general, patients require at least a central venous line for ongoing evaluation of fluid status, and in many cases a pulmonary artery catheter to more directly monitor cardiac function, an arterial line for blood pressure and blood gas monitoring, a nasogastric tube for intestinal decompression, and urethral catheter for measurement of urine output. A large-bore peripheral intravenous catheter is also helpful for volume resuscitation if needed during the course of the operation.

Surgical Techniques

Transaortic visceral endarterectomy is a technically challenging procedure that requires extensive retroperitoneal vascular exposure.[77] As such, only surgeons with the necessary expertise should consider it as an option. In addition to the challenge of exposure, there may be a greater risk of paraplegia with this technique when compared with other forms of visceral revascularization because of supraceliac aortic cross-clamping. Despite these limitations, endarterectomy may be particularly suited to situations in which both visceral and renal vessels have hemodynamically significant stenoses. Alternative techniques must be considered when extensive aortic atherosclerosis is present, however, because endarterectomy may be difficult or even impossible under these circumstances.

The optimal configuration of visceral arterial bypass (antegrade vs. retrograde) remains controversial. Proponents of antegrade bypass are convinced that the quality of the aorta in the supraceliac region and the enhanced blood flow configuration of the graft are desirable.[78-80] Proponents of retrograde bypass believe that approaching the supraceliac aorta is needlessly difficult and that results of retrograde revascularization are not significantly different from those for antegrade revascularization.[40,81] There is general agreement that when marked infrarenal aortic atherosclerosis is present, antegrade bypass is the configuration of choice due to the frequent relative sparing of the aorta in the supraceliac region.

Controversy also surrounds the optimal number of visceral vessels to bypass, one or more than one. Advocates of multiple bypasses suggest that complete gastrointestinal revascularization is accomplished and there is less risk to the patient if one of the grafts fails.[42,43,82] Advocates of single-vessel revascularization suggest that if reasonable collaterals are present and the graft is well placed technically the added time of performing multiple-vessel bypass is not justified by significantly better results.[40,83]

Synthetic graft materials such as dacron or polytetrafluoroethylene are acceptable for revascularization in the absence of peritoneal contamination or bowel necrosis. These grafts are readily available and may be more resistant to kinking in certain positions than vein grafts. In addition, synthetic grafts of greater caliber than typical vein grafts are more suited to mesenteric blood flow requirements in the opinion of some investigators.[84] Because there may be some risk of peritoneal contamination, at least one groin and thigh should be prepared and draped within the operative field for vein harvest even when synthetic bypass has been planned.

Retrograde SMA bypass is the most commonly reported visceral bypass procedure. It is attractive because of the simplicity of the approach to the infrarenal aorta and infrapancreatic SMA. Application of this technique can be limited by severe atherosclerotic disease of the aorta. Technically care must be taken to configure a graft that will not kink when the abdominal contents are in place.

Retrograde celiac revascularization with bypasses to the hepatic or splenic arteries requires a complex dissection of both the infrarenal aorta and celiac branches. These grafts require tunneling beneath the pancreas as well. For surgeons who believe that celiac revascularization is critical in CMI, however, these bypasses are a reasonable alternative to antegrade celiac bypass. Retrograde celiac bypass can be performed in conjunction with SMA bypass if multiple-vessel revascularization is desired.

The supraceliac aorta used for antegrade bypass to the celiac or SMA is often relatively spared of atherosclerotic disease compared with the infrarenal segment. In addition, blood flow characteristics of an antegrade conduit may prolong graft function. On the other hand, due to the anatomic constraints posed by the costal margin of the rib cage, the esophagus, the liver, the diaphragm, and dense neural tissue in the region of the celiac axis, the supraceliac aorta, and proximal CA can be difficult to approach. Antegrade SMA bypass requires subpancreatic tunneling as well. Single-vessel bypass, end-to-end or end-to-side to the celiac or end-to-side to the SMA, or multiple-vessel bypass, both to the celiac and SMA with a bifurcated graft are options with the antegrade approach.

Results

Although mortality of SMA thrombosis is in excess of 90%, the operative mortality of elective visceral revascularization for CMI is 4% to 12%.[23] Early technical and symptomatic success of the various operations is the rule, as 95% or more of patients have pain relief and weight gain. Long-term success, defined by the absence of recurrent symptoms or acute intestinal ischemia, is 80% to 90% at 5 years.[81,84]

VISCERAL REVASCULARIZATION WITH AORTIC RECONSTRUCTION

Aortic reconstruction can lead to disruption of the collateral pathways of the mesenteric circulation and subsequent postoperative intestinal ischemia if significant visceral stenosis is present. Because of this, visceral revascularization should be considered simultaneous with aortic reconstruction even in the absence of CMI when significant visceral atherosclerosis is noted on preoperative arteriography. This can be reasonably accomplished by aortic graft to SMA bypass.[81]

When a large meandering mesenteric arterial collateral between the IMA and SMA is noted preoperatively, care must be taken to assess blood flow to the descending and sigmoid colon during reconstruction of the infrarenal aorta. Sacrifice of the IMA under these circumstances could lead to colonic ischemia and infarction. If IMA backbleeding is poor, back pressure is less than 40 mm Hg, or colonic pulsations are absent with test clamping, IMA bypass or reimplantation is indicated to prevent bowel infarction.[85,86]

CELIAC ARTERY COMPRESSION SYNDROME

The median arcuate ligament (MAL) is a fibrous thickening of the medial diaphragmatic crural borders.[87] Impingement of this structure on the CA has been reported as a variant cause of CMI. Despite clear anatomic external compression, an associated ischemic syndrome is difficult to explain because of several factors: MAL compression of the celiac axis can be noted in many asymptomatic individuals;[88,89] results of operative treatment have been inconsistent; symptoms attributed to the syndrome have been nonspecific; and the occurrence of ischemia in light of the extensive collateral intestinal circulation defies logic.[89]

Some investigators have postulated that entrapment of the celiac neural fibers rather than the CA itself by the MAL may explain the vagueness of associated symptoms and inconsistency of the results of decompression.[90] Whatever the explanation for the syndrome, the frequent lack of physical findings such as weight loss, inconsistent arteriographic findings, inconsistent treatment results, absence of a clear anatomic explanation for ischemia, and frequency of psychiatric illness and substance abuse in patients diagnosed with the disorder dispute the existence of this entity. Szilagyi et al noted:

. . . narrowing of the celiac artery is of such common occurrence as to be a normal anatomical variant, . . . [that] no objective facts have been uncovered and published to prove or even strongly suggest that isolated stenosis of the celiac artery has any pathophysiological effect on the function of the organs supplied by this vessel, . . . [and that] the association of symptoms with the presence of celiac artery narrowing, in a very large majority if not all of the cases, is a casual rather than a causal one.[89]

Despite the anecdotal reports and inconsistent defining characteristics of the syndrome in the past, there may be a population of patients in whom symptomatic celiac compression by the MAL exists. Reilly et al[91] defined a population in whom celiac compression with or without celiac revascularization had better results. Female patients with documented weight loss, postprandial abdominal pain, lack of psychiatric illness, absence of other gastrointestinal disorders, and poststenotic celiac dilation were identified as having favorable results in a retrospective study. Based on these rigid criteria, however, it is unlikely that many patients will be identified as revascularization candidates.

When operation for CA compression syndrome is undertaken, the abdomen should first be explored to rule out other causes of abdominal pain. If none is found, the supraceliac aorta is approached through the lesser space and the MAL identified. This ligament is divided and the CA is assessed for the need of revascularization. If revascularization is deemed to be necessary, a variety of techniques including operative angioplasty, celiac reimplantation, or CA bypass can be performed.[81]

REFERENCES

1. Ruzicka FF and Rossi P: Normal vascular anatomy of the abdominal viscera, Radiol Clin North Am 8:3, 1970.
2. Michels NA et al: The variant blood supply to the small and large intestines: Its import in regional resections, J Int Coll Surg 39:127, 1963.
3. Ernst CB: Colon ischemia following abdominal aortic reconstruction. In Bernhard VM and Towne JB, eds: Complications in vascular surgery, New York, 1980, Grune & Stratton.
4. Michels NA et al: Routes of collateral circulation of the gastrointestinal tract as ascertained in a dissection of 500 bodies, Int Surg 49:8, 1968.
5. Ernst CB et al: Ischemic colitis following abdominal aortic reconstruction: a prospective study, Surgery 80:417, 1976.
6. Sande E et al: Intraoperative streptokinase in the treatment of superior mesenteric artery embolisation, Eur J Surg 157:615, 1991.
7. Schoenbaum SW et al: Superior mesenteric artery embolism: treatment with intra-arterial urokinase, J Vasc Interven Rad 3:485, 1992.
8. McBride KD and Gaines PA: Thrombolysis of a partially occluding superior mesenteric artery thromboembolus by infusion of streptokinase, Cardiovasc Interven Rad 17:164, 1994.
9. Kaleya RN, Sammartano RJ, and Boley SJ: Aggressive approach to acute mesenteric ischemia, Surg Clin North Am 72:157, 1992.
10. Boley SJ, Brandt LJ, and Veith FJ: Ischemic disease of the intestine, Curr Probl Surg 15:1, 1978.
11. Bulkley GB et al: Effects of cardiac tamponade on colonic hemodynamics and oxygen uptake, Am J Physiol 244:G605, 1983.
12. Patel A, Kaleya RN, and Sammartano RJ: Pathophysiology of mesenteric ischemia, Surg Clin North Am 72:31, 1992.
13. Ahren C and Haglund U: Mucosal lesions in the small intestine of the cat during low flow, Acta Physiol Scand 88:1, 1973.
14. Brown RA et al: Ultrastructural changes in the canine ileal mucosal cell after mesentery artery occlusion, Arch Surg 101:290, 1970.
15. Chiu CJ et al: Intestinal mucosal lesions in low flow states I: a morphological, hemodynamic, and metabolic reappraisal, Arch Surg 101:478, 1970.
16. Parks DA and Granger DN: Contributions of ischemia and reperfusion to mucosal lesion formation, Am J Physiol 250:G749, 1986.

17. Zimmerman BJ and Granger DN: Reperfusion injury, Surg Clin North Am 72:65, 1992.

18. Wise RA: In discussion of: Dye WS, Olwin J, Javid H, Julian OC. Arterial embolectomy, Arch Surg 70:715, 1955.

19. Ottinger LW and Austen WG: A study of 136 patients with mesenteric infarction, Surg Gynecol Obstet 124:251, 1967.

20. Clavien PA, Muller C, and Harder F: Treatment of mesenteric infarction, Br J Surg 74:500, 1987.

21. Sachs SM, Morton JH, and Schwartz SI: Acute mesenteric ischemia, Surgery 92:646, 1982.

22. Lazaro T et al: Embolization of the mesenteric arteries: surgical treatment in twenty-three consecutive cases, Ann Vasc Surg 1:311, 1986.

23. Taylor LM and Moneta GL: Intestinal ischemia, Ann Vasc Surg 5:403, 1991.

24. Elliott JP et al: Arterial embolization: problems of source, multiplicity, recurrence, and delayed treatment, Surgery 88:833, 1980.

25. O'Mara CS and Ernst CB: Acute mesenteric ischemia. In Zuidema GD, ed: Shackelford's surgery of the alimentary tract, ed 3, Philadelphia, 1991, WB Saunders.

26. Scott WW et al: Diagnosis and pathophysiology of paradoxical embolism, Radiology 121:59, 1976.

27. Taylor LM: Treatment of acute intestinal ischemia caused by arterial occlusions. In Rutherford RB, ed: Vascular surgery, ed 4, Philadelphia, 1995, WB Saunders.

28. O'Donnell JA and Hobson RW: Operative confirmation of Doppler ultrasound in evaluation of intestinal ischemia, Surgery 87:109, 1980.

29. Bulkley GB et al: Intraoperative determination of intestinal viability following ischemic injury: a prospective controlled trial of two adjuvant methods (Doppler and fluorescein) compared to standard clinical judgement, Ann Surg 193:628, 1981.

30. Brolin RE et al: Myoelectric assessment of bowel viability, Surgery 102:32, 1987.

31. Bussemaker JB and Lindemann J: Comparison of methods to determine viability of small intestine, Ann Surg 176:97, 1972.

32. Zarins CK, Skinner DB, and James AE Jr: Prediction of the viability of revascularized intestine with radioactive microspheres, Surg Gynecol Obstet 138:576, 1974.

33. Pearce WH et al: The use of infrared photoplethysmography in identifying early intestinal ischemia, Arch Surg 122:308, 1987.

34. Shaw RS and Rutledge RH: Superior mesenteric artery embolectomy in the treatment of massive infarction, N Engl J Med 252:595, 1957.

35. Rius X et al: Mesenteric infarction, World J Surg 3:489, 1979.

36. Pierce GE and Brockenbrough ED: The spectrum of mesenteric infarction, Am J Surg 119:233, 1970.

37. Slater H and Elliott DW: Primary mesenteric infarction, Am J Surg 123:309, 1972.

38. Inderbitzi R et al: Acute mesenteric ischaemia, Eur J Surg 158:123, 1992.

39. Dunphy JE: Abdominal pain of vascular origin, Am J Med Sci 192:109, 1936.

40. Taylor LM and Porter JM: Treatment of chronic intestinal ischemia, Semin Vasc Surg 3:186, 1990.

41. Krausz MM and Manny J: Acute superior mesenteric arterial occlusion: a plea for early diagnosis, Surgery 83:482, 1978.

42. Crawford ES et al: Celiac axis, superior mesenteric artery, and inferior mesenteric artery occlusion: surgical considerations, Surgery 82:856, 1977.

43. Zelenock GB et al: Splanchnic arteriosclerotic disease and intestinal angina, Arch Surg 115:497, 1980.

44. Ende WP: Infarction of the bowel in cardiac failure, N Engl J Med 258:879, 1958.

45. Martin WB, Laufman H, and Tuell SW: Rationale of therapy in acute vascular occlusion based upon micrometric observations, Ann Surg 129:476, 1949.

46. Habboushe F et al: Nonocclusive mesenteric vascular insufficiency, Ann Surg 180:819, 1974.

47. Russ JE et al: Surgical treatment of nonocclusive mesenteric infarction, Am J Surg 134:638, 1977.

48. Britt LC and Cheek RC: Nonocclusive mesenteric vascular disease: clinical and experimental observations, Ann Surg 169:704, 1969.

49. Herr FW, Silen W, and French SW: Intestinal gangrene without apparent vascular occlusion, Am J Surg 110:231, 1965.

50. Bergan JJ et al: Revascularization in the treatment of mesenteric infarction, Ann Surg 182:430, 1975.

51. Warren S and Eberhard TP: Mesenteric venous thrombosis, Surg Gynecol Obstet 61:102, 1935.

52. Kispert JF and Kazmers A: Acute intestinal ischemia caused by mesenteric venous thrombosis, Semin Vasc Surg 3:158, 1990.

53. Schwalke MA, Rodil JV, and Vezeridis MP: Mesenteric venous thrombosis, Contemp Surg 35:95, 1989.

54. Grendell JH and Ockner RK: Mesenteric venous thrombosis, Gastroenterology 82:358, 1982.

55. Johnson CL and Baggenstoss AM: Mesenteric vascular occlusion: study of 99 cases of occlusion of veins, Mayo Clin Proc 24:628, 1949.

56. Grieshop RJ et al: Acute mesenteric venous thrombosis: revisited in a time of diagnostic clarity, Am Surg 57:573, 1991.

57. Miller VE and Berland U: Pulsed Doppler duplex sonography and CT of portal vein thrombosis, Am J Radiol 145:73, 1985.

58. Rosen A et al: Mesenteric vein thrombosis: CT identification, Am J Radiol 143:83, 1984.

59. Vogelzang RL et al: Thrombosis of the splanchnic veins: CT diagnosis, Am J Radiol 150:93, 1988.

60. Subranamyan BR et al: Portal venous thrombosis: correlative analysis of sonography, CT, and angiography, Am J Gastroenterol 79:773, 1984.

61. Inahara T: Acute superior mesenteric venous thrombosis treatment by thrombectomy, Ann Surg 174:956, 1971.

62. Bergentz SE et al: Thrombosis in the superior mesenteric and portal veins: report of a case treated with thrombectomy, Surgery 76:286, 1974.

63. Jona J et al: Recurrent primary mesenteric venous thrombosis, JAMA 227:1033, 1974.

64. Naitove A and Weismann RE: Primary mesenteric venous thrombosis, Ann Surg 161:516, 1965.

65. Klein E: Embolism and thrombosis of the superior mesenteric artery, Surg Gynecol Obstet 33:385, 1921.

66. Mikkelsen WP: Intestinal angina: its surgical significance, Am J Surg 94:262, 1957.

67. Ernst CB: Chronic mesenteric ischemia. In Zuidema AD, ed: Shackelford's surgery of the alimentary tract, ed 3, Philadelphia, 1991, WB Saunders.

68. Moneta GL et al: Duplex ultrasound criteria for diagnosis of splanchnic artery stenosis or occlusion, J Vasc Surg 14:511, 1991.

69. Bowersox JC et al: Duplex ultrasonography in the diagnosis of celiac and superior mesenteric artery occlusive disease, J Vasc Surg 14:780, 1991.

70. Lee RW et al: Mesenteric artery duplex scanning: a blinded prospective study, J Vasc Surg 17:79, 1993.

71. Shaw RS and Maynard EP: Acute and chronic thombosis of

the mesenteric arteries associated with malabsorption: a report of two cases successfully treated by thromboendarterectomy, N Engl J Med 258:874, 1958.

72. Derrick JR, Pollard HS, and Moore RM: The pattern of arteriosclerotic narrowing of the celiac and superior mesenteric arteries, Ann Surg 149:684, 1959.

73. Sniderman KW: Transluminal angioplasty in the management of chronic mesenteric ischemia. In Strandness DE and vanBreda A, eds: Vascular diseases: surgical and interventional therapy, New York, 1994, Churchill Livingstone.

74. Levy PJ, Haskell L, and Gordon RL: Percutaneous transluminal angioplasty of splanchnic arteries: an alternative method to elective revascularization in chronic visceral ischemia, Eur J Radiol 7:239, 1987.

75. McShane MD et al: Mesenteric angioplasty for chronic intestinal ischaemia, Eur J Vasc Surg 6:333, 1992.

76. Martin LG, Rees CR, and O'Bryant T: Percutaneous angioplasty of the renal arteries. In Strandness DE and vanBreda A, eds: Vascular diseases: surgical and interventional therapy, New York, 1994, Churchill Livingstone.

77. Cunningham CG et al: Chronic visceral ischemia, three decades of progress, Ann Surg 214:276, 1991.

78. McAfee MK et al: Influence of complete revascularization on chronic mesenteric ischemia, Am J Surg 164:220, 1992.

79. Rapp JH et al: Durability of endarterectomy and antegrade grafts in the treatment of chronic visceral ischemia, J Vasc Surg 3:799, 1986.

80. Beebe HG, MacFarlane S, and Raker EJ: Supraceliac aortomesenteric bypass for intestinal ischemia, J Vasc Surg 5:749, 1987.

81. Ernst CB and Shepard AD: Chronic mesenteric ischemia. In Zuidema GD, ed: Shackelford's surgery of the alimentary tract, ed 4, Philadelphia, 1995, WB Saunders.

82. Hallett JW Jr et al: Recent trends in the diagnosis and management of chronic intestinal ischemia, Ann Vasc Surg 4:126, 1990.

83. Cormier JM et al: Atherosclerotic occlusive disease of the superior mesenteric artery: late results of reconstructive surgery, Ann Vasc Surg 5:510, 1991.

84. Taylor LM and Porter JM: Treatment of chronic visceral ischemia. In Rutherford RB, ed: Vascular surgery, ed 4, Philadelphia, 1995, WB Saunders.

85. Ernst CB: Prevention of intestinal ischemia following abdominal aortic reconstruction, Surgery 93:102, 1983.

86. Ernst CB et al: Inferior mesenteric artery stump pressure: a reliable index for safe IMA ligation during abdominal aortic aneurysmectomy, Ann Surg 187:641, 1978.

87. Linder HH and Kemprud E: A clinicoanatomical study of the arcuate ligament of the diaphragm, Arch Surg 103:600, 1971.

88. Levin DC and Baltaxe HA: High incidence of celiac artery narrowing in asymptomatic individuals, Am J Roentgenol 116:426, 1972.

89. Szilagyi DE et al: The celiac artery compression syndrome: Does it exist? Surgery 72:849, 1972.

90. Carey J, Stemmer EA, and Connolly JE: Median arcuate ligament syndrome, Arch Surg 99:441, 1969.

91. Reilly LM et al: Late results following operative repair for celiac compression syndrome, J Vasc Surg 2:79, 1985.

CHAPTER EIGHTEEN

RENOVASCULAR DISEASE

Jeffrey W. Olin
Andrew C. Novick

HISTORICAL PERSPECTIVE

Richard Bright first demonstrated an association between hypertension and the kidney. This association was taken several steps forward in 1934 when Goldblatt et al[1] elucidated the pathogenesis of renovascular hypertension based on experimental renal artery constriction in animals. Shortly thereafter Page and Helmer[2] and Braun-Menendez et al[3] published reports describing a renal pressor system, which led to an early understanding of the renin-angiotensin system. Since these early times much has been learned about the pathogenesis, diagnosis, and treatment of renovascular disease, and several excellent accounts of the history are described in more detail elsewhere.[4-6] Exactly how common renovascular disease and renovascular hypertension are is a matter of dispute. The prevalence of renovascular *hypertension* varies between 0.2% and 32%.[7,8] The higher percentages occur among tertiary referral centers and highly selected populations. Renovascular hypertension is much less common in blacks than in whites.[9] It has been suggested that less than 0.5% of an entire hypertensive population has renovascular hypertension.[10]

These data on prevalence of renovascular hypertension are difficult to interpret for several reasons. The only true way to diagnose renovascular hypertension is to correct the renal artery stenosis (surgery or percutaneous transluminal angioplasty [PTA]) and demonstrate cure of the hypertension. The prevalence of renovascular *disease* is much higher than renovascular *hypertension*. To determine the prevalence of atherosclerotic renal artery stenosis (ARAS), we studied 395 consecutive patients who had atherosclerosis in other peripheral arteries.[11] There was greater than 50% renal artery stenosis in 38% of patients with abdominal aortic aneurysms, 33% in patients with aortoocclusive disease, and 39% in patients with lower-extremity occlusive disease. These patients did not have the usual clinical clues to suggest renal artery stenosis. High-grade bilateral disease was present in approximately

13% of patients. Others have demonstrated a similarly high prevalence of atherosclerotic renal artery disease in patients who have concomitant peripheral vascular disease.[12-14] Similar associations have been documented in patients with coronary disease.[15]

The average age of patients with generalized atherosclerosis is approximately 65 to 70 years. The prevalence of hypertension among this age group is approximately 65%. Thus there is a high prevalence of renovascular disease and a high prevalence of hypertension in the elderly population. However, renovascular hypertension per se is much less common. Some patients have renal artery stenosis and essential hypertension. Also, not all patients who have anatomic evidence of renal artery stenosis have hypertension. Dustan et al[16] demonstrated that only 50% of the people with significant renal artery stenosis in fact had hypertension.

With the advent of newer and more potent antihypertensive agents, control of blood pressure is not as much of a problem as it was in the past. However, with the higher prevalence of unilateral and bilateral significant renovascular disease, patients now undergo intervention more often for preservation of renal function than they do for control of blood pressure.[17,18]

CLASSIFICATION OF RENOVASCULAR DISORDERS

Atherosclerosis

Approximately 65% to 70% of all renovascular lesions are caused by atherosclerosis. This disease may be limited to the renal artery but more commonly is a manifestation of generalized atherosclerosis involving the abdominal aorta and coronary, cerebral, and lower-extremity vessels. Atherosclerotic stenosis usually occurs in the proximal 2 cm of the renal artery, and distal arterial or branch involvement is distinctly uncommon (Fig. 18-1).

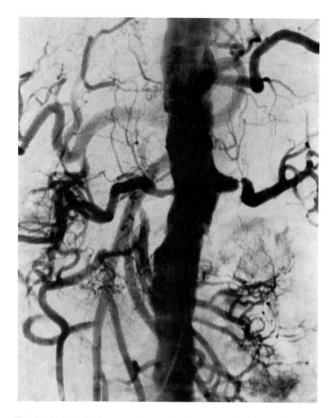

Fig. 18-1. This aortogram demonstrates a severely atherosclerotic aorta. The right renal artery demonstrates an osteal lesion that reduces the lumen by 50% to 60%. The left renal artery shows an atherosclerotic lesion several centimeters distal to the takeoff in which the lumen is reduced by >95%. This is a typical nonostial lesion.

Because of the proximal location of these lesions, oblique aortic views are often needed to adequately visualize the area of stenosis. The lesion involves the intima of the artery and in two thirds of the cases appears as an eccentric plaque. In the remainder the vessel is circumferentially involved with narrowing of the lumen and destruction of the intima. Dissecting hematomas may complicate this disease, sometimes resulting in thrombosis of the entire vessel.

There have been relatively few published reports on the natural history of atherosclerotic lesions in patients managed nonoperatively. The available data suggest that progressive arterial stenosis, occasionally resulting in total occlusion, is a relatively common sequela of this disease. In 1968 Wollenweber, Sheps, and Davis[19] reviewed 30 patients with atherosclerotic renovascular disease who had been followed up with serial renal arteriograms from 3 to 88 months apart; progressive renal artery stenosis was observed unilaterally in 13 patients (43%) and bilaterally in 6 patients (20%). Also in 1968 Meaney, Dustan, and McCormack[20] reported progression of ARAS in 14 of 39 patients (36%) followed with serial arteriography during intervals ranging from 6 months to 7 years. Schreiber, Novick, and Pohl[21] reviewed the outcome of atherosclerotic renovascular disease in 85 patients treated medically and followed with sequential renal arteriography during

intervals of 3 to 172 months. The mean angiographic follow-up interval was 52 months, and the mean clinical follow-up period in these patients was 87 months. Progressive renal artery obstruction from atherosclerosis was observed in 37 patients (44%), including 14 patients (16%) who developed complete arterial occlusion. Clinical follow-up checks revealed that serial decreases in both overall renal function ($P < 0.02$) and the size of the involved kidney ($P < 0.001$) occurred more commonly in patients who developed progressive renovascular disease than in those who did not. However, serial blood pressure control was no different in these two groups, and therefore it was not a useful marker for progressive disease. This study indicates not only that atherosclerotic renal artery disease progresses in a large number of patients, but also that such progression is commonly associated with clinically detectable loss of functioning renal parenchyma.

Tollefson and Ernst[22] studied 194 sequential aortograms in 48 patients to better define the natural history of renal artery stenosis associated with concomitant aortic disease. The disease progressed in 42 arteries (53%) and 7 arteries developed occlusion. Zierler et al[23] prospectively studied 80 patients with serial duplex ultrasound. None of the renal arteries initially classified as normal progressed over the follow-up period. However, the cumulative incidence of progression from less than 60% to 60% or greater renal artery stenosis was 23% (±9%) at 1 year and 42% (±14%) at 2 years. Four renal arteries progressed to occlusion, and all had 60% or greater stenosis at the initial visit. The cumulative incidence of progression to occlusion was 5% (±3%) at 1 year and 11% (±6%) at 2 years. Progression of renal artery stenosis occurs at a rate of approximately 20%/yr, and progression leading to occlusion is associated with a marked decrease (mean, 1.8 cm) in kidney length.[23,24]

Fibrous Dysplasia

Fibrous dysplasias comprise approximately 40% of all renovascular disorders. These lesions are considered to be congenital dysplasias with maldevelopment of the fibrous, muscular, and elastic tissues of the renal artery. They are subcategorized according to the layer of the arterial wall involved.[25] This classification is important since each type of fibrous dysplasia has distinct histologic and angiographic features, and each type occurs in a different clinical setting.

Primary intimal fibroplasia occurs in children and young adults and accounts for approximately 10% of the total number of fibrous lesions. This lesion is characterized by a circumferential accumulation of collagen inside the internal elastica lamina. Disruption and duplication of the elastica interna occur more often in younger patients, with dissecting hematomas as a complication in some patients. Intimal fibroplasia with complicating medial dissection is characterized pathologically by large dissecting channels in the outer half of the media. These lesions are thought to develop because of defects in the internal elastica with resultant medial dissection and aneurysmal dilation.

Arteriography in primary intimal fibroplasia reveals a smooth, fairly focal stenosis, usually involving the midportion of the vessel or its branches (Fig. 18-2). Dissecting

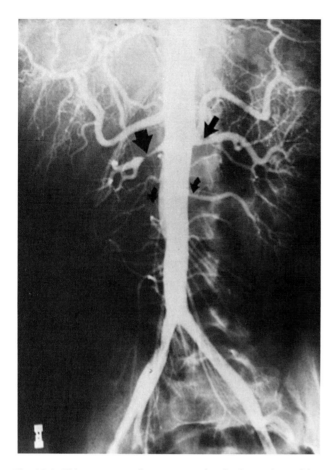

Fig. 18-2. This aortogram demonstrates the classic arteriographic appearance of intimal fibroplasia. The left renal artery stenosis demonstrates a focal area of narrowing simulating a band around the renal artery *(arrow)*. The right renal artery demonstrates a long smooth area of narrowing *(large arrow)*. The lower pole renal arteries bilaterally also demonstrate smooth long areas of narrowing *(small arrows)*.

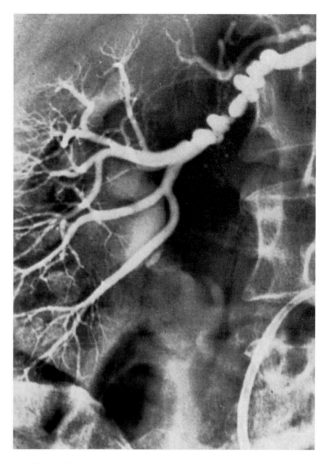

Fig. 18-3. This renal arteriogram demonstrates typical medial fibroplasia of the renal artery. The "string of beads" appearance of the renal artery involves the distal portion of the main renal artery, and the "beads" are larger than the normal diameter of the artery.

hematomas may distort the area of the stenosis. With nonoperative management, progressive renal artery obstruction and ischemic atrophy of the involved kidney invariably occur. Severe intimal fibroplasia may subsequently develop de novo in the contralateral renal artery. Although primary intimal fibroplasia most commonly affects the renal arteries, this may also occur as a generalized disorder with concomitant involvement of the carotid, upper and lower extremities, and mesenteric vessels.

Medial fibroplasia is the most common of the fibrous lesions, making up 75% to 80% of the total number. It tends to occur in 25- to 50-year-old women and often involves both renal arteries. It may involve other vessels in the body, most notably the carotid, mesenteric, and iliac arteries. Microscopically the internal elastic membrane is focally variably thinned and lost. Within the alternating thickened areas much of the muscle is replaced by collagen, hence the term *medial fibroplasia*. In other areas thinning of the media occurs to the point of complete loss, and microaneurysms can be seen as saccules lined by only the external elastica. In extreme cases giant aneurysms may be found in association with medial fibroplasia.

Arteriographically medial fibroplasia demonstrates a typical "string of beads" appearance involving the distal two thirds of the main renal artery and branches (Fig. 18-3). The areas of stenosis are often overshadowed by contrast medium in the microaneurysms, making the degree of actual stenosis difficult to assess. The aneurysms themselves are greater in diameter than the normal renal artery proximal to the disease, and extreme collateral circulation is absent. These are important features in differentiating the lesion from perimedial fibroplasia.

Schreiber, Novick, and Pohl[21] studied the natural history of renal artery disease caused by medial fibroplasia in 66 patients who had follow-up serial angiograms. Progressive renal artery stenosis occurred in 22 patients (33%), and contrary to an earlier report, this occurrence was no different in patients 40 years of age or older. Significantly there were no cases of progression to total arterial occlusions in this group. Also, clinical follow-up studies revealed that serial decreases in either overall renal function or the size of the involved kidney seldom occurred in patients with progressive medial fibroplasia, suggesting that the risk of losing renal function is relatively small in patients with this disease who are managed medically.

Perimedial fibroplasia occurs predominantly in 15- to 30-year-olds and therefore has been referred to as "girlie

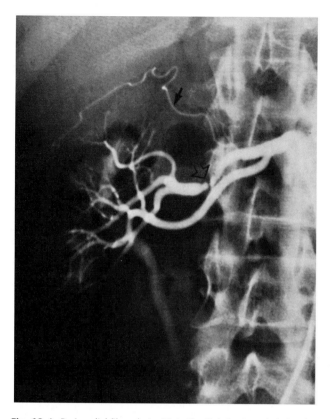

Fig. 18-4. Perimedial fibroplasia. Note the tightly stenotic lesion in the distal right renal artery. One may appreciate the appearance of arterial beading but the "bead" is smaller than the normal vessel (open arrow). A collateral vessel is noted (closed arrow).

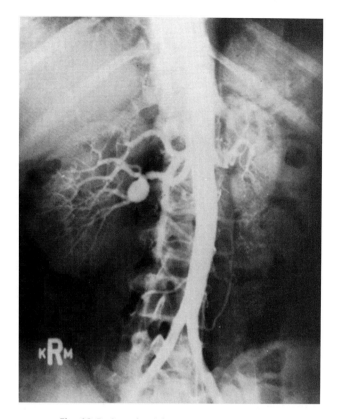

Fig. 18-5. Saccular right renal artery aneurysm.

disease." Of all fibrous lesions 10% to 15% are perimedial fibroplasias. These tightly stenotic lesions only occur in the renal artery and consist pathologically of a collar of dense collagen enveloping the renal artery for variable lengths and thicknesses. The collagen is deposited in the outer border of the media and usually replaces a considerable portion of the media; in some areas it may completely replace the media. Islands of smooth muscle are occasionally seen trapped within the collagenous ring. Special stains show that the lesion is confined within the external elastic lamina and contained in all cases by intact adventitial connective tissue. The arterial lumen may be further compromised by a process of secondary intimal fibroplasia. It has been suggested that this secondary thickening of the intima is related to slowing of blood flow through a narrowed arterial segment, with resultant platelet and fibrin deposition and subsequent fibrous organization.

The arteriogram of perimedial fibroplasia may give the appearance of arterial beading, but careful observation shows that the caliber of the normal segment of the vessel is not exceeded by the "bead." This fact, along with the frequent occurrence of external collateral circulation, differentiates this lesion angiographically from that of medial fibroplasia (Fig. 18-4). Perimedial fibroplasia produces severe stenosis, and although complicating thrombosis or dissection is relatively uncommon, progressive obstruction with ischemic renal atrophy occurs in almost all patients managed nonoperatively.

Fibromuscular hyperplasia is an extremely rare disease, comprising only 1% to 2% of fibrous lesions and tends to occur in children and young adults. This is the only renal arterial disease in which true hyperplasia of the smooth muscle cells is present. The renal artery shows a concentric thickening of its wall with a mixture of proliferating smooth muscle and fibrous tissue in variable quantity. Arteriographically, fibromuscular hyperplasia appears as a smooth stenosis of the renal artery or its branches and from a radiographic standpoint may be indistinguishable from intimal fibroplasia. Follow-up serial angiographic studies have shown that most patients with this disease have developed progressive vascular obstruction.

Renal Artery Aneurysms

Renal artery aneurysms may require surgical treatment when they are the cause of significant hypertension or to obviate the risk of rupture. The latter is of greatest concern with aneurysms that are larger than 2 cm in diameter and noncalcified, particularly when they occur in premenopausal women because of the predisposition for aneurysmal rupture during pregnancy.[26] According to the classification of Poutasse,[27] there are four basic types of renal artery aneurysms: saccular, fusiform, dissecting, and intrarenal. Saccular aneurysms, which account for about 75% of renal artery aneurysms, are the most common. They generally occur at the bifurcation of the renal artery, perhaps due to an inherent weakness in the wall of the artery at this point (Fig. 18-5). Because of this location, branch arterial involvement is common. These aneurysms may become involved with secondary atherosclerotic degeneration and/or intramural calcification. Saccular aneurysms may be causally related to hypertension by several mechanisms including compression or displacement of renal artery branches with resulting ischemia, aneurysmal erosion into a renal vein with formation of an arterial venous fistula, mural thrombus formation within the aneurysm with peripheral renal embolization, and the association of some aneurysms with stenosing fibrous renal artery disease. It is also well appreciated that saccular aneurysms can cause hypertension in the absence of these sequelae, most likely because of relative renal ischemia caused by the turbulent flow of blood as it passes through the aneurysmally dilated arterial segment. Saccular aneurysms may be quite variable in their location and extent. The incidence of bilateral and multiple renal aneurysms is approximately 25%. Fusiform renal artery aneurysms are almost always associated with stenosing fibrous renal artery disease. The latter is the cause for the severe hypertension generally seen in these patients. Fusiform aneurysms actually represent a severe poststenotic dilation of the renal artery. Dissecting renal artery aneurysms are most often a complication of primary intimal fibroplasia or atherosclerosis. These are often manifested clinically by the sudden onset of pain that stimulates renal colic. In some patients the dissection in the wall of the vessel may reenter the lumen more distally. In other patients total arterial occlusion with renal infarction may ensue. Intrarenal arterial aneurysms are of mixed origin and may be congenital, post-traumatic, iatrogenic, neoplastic, or associated with polyarteritis nodosa. Intrarenal aneurysms that occur following blunt trauma or closed renal biopsy will occasionally resolve spontaneously with expectant management. Intrarenal aneurysms do have the propensity for rupture, and surgical treatment may be indicated if their diameter is greater than 2 cm.

Renal Arteriovenous Fistulas

Renal arteriovenous fistulas are relatively uncommon lesions that are generally discovered during the course of angiographic evaluation for suspected renal or renovascular disease.[26] The most common clinical symptoms are hematuria, high-output cardiac failure, and diastolic hypertension. Congenital or cirsoid fistulas comprise approximately 25% of these lesions and are the result of a developmental anomaly of the involved renal vessels. The angiographic appearance is one of multiple small interconnecting arterial and venous channels with impaired distal renal parenchymal vascularity and early filling of the renal vein. Idiopathic fistulas make up only 3% to 5% of these lesions and have no apparent cause. They are considered to develop as a result of venous erosion by a preexisting arterial aneurysm. Acquired fistulas are the most common type, accounting for 70% to 75% of all renal arteriovenous fistulas. By far the most common cause is iatrogenic trauma resulting from needle biopsy of the kidney. The majority of the latter will close spontaneously. Fistulas may also be acquired through blunt or penetrating trauma, tumor, inflammation, or prior renal surgery.

Renal Artery Thrombosis or Embolism

Acute occlusion of the renal artery or its branches may result from thrombosis or embolism. Embolic occlusions may occur as a complication of rheumatic heart disease, infective endocarditis, cardiac operations, saccular aneurysm of the renal artery, or renal artery catheterization. Thrombosis of the renal artery is somewhat less common and is associated with a variety of diseases such as intimal fibroplasia, segmental arteritis, polycythemia vera, tumors, trauma, or umbilical arterial catheterization. Blunt trauma to the renal artery may result in disruption of the intima with subsequent dissection and thrombotic occlusion.

Miscellaneous

Middle aortic syndrome, Takayasu's arteritis, and neurofibromatosis are all associated with renal artery stenosis. External compression or obstruction of the renal arteries by neural tissue, musculocutaneous fibers, or diaphragmatic crura rarely occur.

PATHOGENESIS OF RENOVASCULAR HYPERTENSION

In 1934 Goldblatt et al[1] first demonstrated that constriction of the main artery in dogs produced elevation in blood pressure, which was sustained. The mechanism of the hypertension was not known at the time of these experiments. Since then a number of humoral factors have been shown to play an important role in the generation and maintenance of hypertension. Animal models for renovascular hypertension include the two kidney–one clip (2K-1C) model, which is a model for unilateral renal artery stenosis and the one kidney–one clip (1K-1C) model of renovascular hypertension, which is the model for renal artery stenosis to a solitary functioning kidney or bilateral renal artery stenosis. Although the acute phases of both of these models are similar, different events occur in the chronic phase.

In the 2K-1C model (unilateral renal artery stenosis) decreased renal blood flow stimulates the production of renin (Fig. 18-6, A). Renin cleaves the proenzyme angiotensinogen to form angiotensin I and in the presence of angiotensin-converting enzyme (ACE) is converted to angiotensin II. Angiotensin II has several important functions: (1) It elevates blood pressure directly by causing systemic vasoconstriction. (2) It stimulates aldosterone secretion, causing sodium reabsorption and potassium and hydrogen ion secretion in the cortical collecting duct. (3) It changes the intrarenal hemodynamics, such as diminishing glomerular filtration, by decreasing glomerular capillary surface area and redistributing intrarenal blood flow. The salt and water retention caused by excess aldosterone production is rapidly excreted by the contralateral (normal) kidney by pressure natriuresis. This produces a cycle of renin-dependent hypertension.[28-32] Administration of an ACE inhibitor blocks the vicious cycle and early in the course of renovascular hypertension returns the blood pressure to normal. There is decreased blood flow to the kidney with the clipped (stenotic) artery, increased renin secretion from the ischemic kidney, and suppressed renin secretion from the contralateral kidney in the 2K-1C model.

In the 1K-1C model of renovascular hypertension, there is a similar decrease in blood flow to the affected kidney(s),

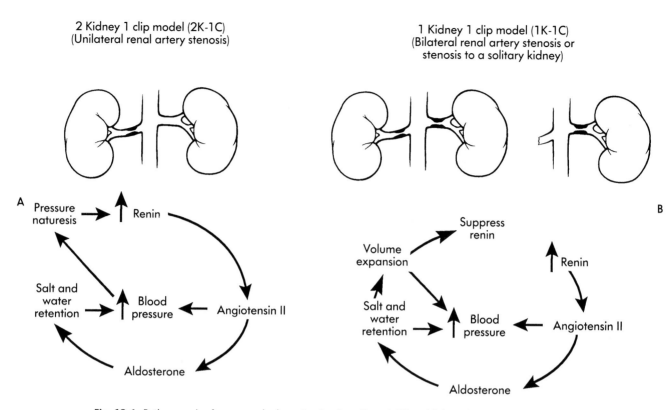

2 Kidney 1 clip model (2K-1C)
(Unilateral renal artery stenosis)

1 Kidney 1 clip model (1K-1C)
(Bilateral renal artery stenosis or
stenosis to a solitary kidney)

Fig. 18-6. Pathogenesis of renovascular hypertension in unilateral (**A**) and bilateral (**B**) renal artery stenosis.

acutely causing the secretion of renin and synthesis of angiotensin II and aldosterone (Fig. 18-6, *B*). Angiotensin II directly elevates blood pressure and aldosterone causes salt and water retention. Now there is not a normal kidney that can *sense* the elevated blood pressure; therefore no pressure natriuresis occurs. The increased aldosterone causes sodium and water retention and volume expansion. The expanded plasma volume suppresses plasma renin activity, thus converting the animal from renin-mediated hypertension to volume-mediated hypertension.[30,31,33] At this stage, administration of an ACE inhibitor or angiotensin II antagonist does not decrease blood pressure or change renal blood flow.[33] Dietary restriction of sodium or administration of diuretics will convert the animal to a renin-mediated form of hypertension, and the animal will then become sensitive to an ACE inhibitor or an angiotensin II antagonist. As discussed later in this chapter, functional renal insufficiency may occur in humans when ACE inhibitors are administered to patients with bilateral renal artery stenosis or renal artery stenosis to a solitary kidney.

The time course for the chronic phase to occur may be weeks in the 1K-1C rat model, whereas it may take up to 4 months in the 2K-1C rat model.[34] In the 2K-1C model, loss of renin sensitivity in the chronic state may also occur and is caused by an inability of the contralateral (normal) kidney to excrete an increased sodium load when the blood pressure is increased (pressure natriuresis). This attenuation is thought to be produced by changes in intrarenal hemodynamics and structural changes in the microvasculature of the kidney.[35] A whole host of other mechanisms and other systems have been shown to be important to

varying degrees in the generation and maintenance of hypertension in animals and patients with renal artery stenosis.[36] These include prostaglandins, thromboxane, renal medullary vasodepressor system (nonprostanoic vasodilator lipids), the sympathetic nervous system, renal nerves, vasopressin, atrial natriuretic factor and the kallikrein-bradykinin system.[36,37]

Several newer concepts regarding the renin-angiotensin system have emerged over the last several years. These include local production of angiotensins in various vascular beds, the discovery of biologically active peptides other than angiotensin II, and the identification of multiple angiotensin receptor subtypes.[38] These concepts have allowed a clearer understanding of the mechanisms involved in hypertension and renal insufficiency in patients with renovascular disease. It is hoped that a better understanding of the pathophysiology will lead to improved treatment strategies in patients with renovascular disease.

CLINICAL MANIFESTATIONS OF RENOVASCULAR DISEASE

A number of clinical features may be present in patients with renovascular disease (see the box, p. 327). None of these features alone can be used with certainty to make the diagnosis. However, the presence of one or more of these features will increase the likelihood of finding renal artery stenosis. In a series of 76 patients with one or more of the following clinical clues, renal arteriography demonstrated significant renal artery stenosis to be present in 70% of patients.[11]

CLINICAL CLUES TO SUGGEST RENOVASCULAR DISEASE

1. Onset of hypertension before the age of 30 or after the age of 55
2. Hypertension that was well controlled and has become difficult to control
3. Malignant or accelerated hypertension
4. Resistant hypertension
5. Epigastric bruit (systolic/diastolic)
6. Atrophic kidney or discrepancy in size between the two kidneys
7. Azotemia while receiving angiotensin-converting enzyme (ACE) inhibitors
8. Azotemia in the elderly patient with atherosclerosis elsewhere
9. Patients with generalized atherosclerosis

Onset of Hypertension Before the Age of 30 or After the Age of 55 Years

The onset of primary (essential) hypertension is usually between the ages of 30 and 55. When hypertension begins below the age of 30, secondary causes should be sought, and fibromuscular dysplasia would be one of the more common secondary causes in this age group. When hypertension appears for the first time in a patient over the age of 55, a likely diagnosis is atherosclerotic renovascular disease.

Hypertension that was Well Controlled and has Become More Difficult to Control

When the blood pressure has been reasonably well controlled on a particular blood pressure regimen and the blood pressure suddenly becomes more difficult to control, one should suspect a secondary cause. Often the secondary cause, such as renovascular disease, is superimposed on previously diagnosed essential hypertension.

Malignant or Accelerated Hypertension

Patients with grade III or grade IV hypertensive retinopathy have an extremely high prevalence of renovascular disease.[39] Davis et al[8] demonstrated that renovascular hypertension was present in 32% of 76 white patients and 11% of 29 black patients studied with arteriography.

Resistant Hypertension

Renovascular disease and renovascular hypertension occur in patients with mild, moderate, or severe hypertension. As discussed earlier, patients with renal artery stenosis may also have normal blood pressure.[16] The likelihood of having renal artery stenosis is increased in patients with truly resistant hypertension. In one study 72% of patients with atherosclerotic renovascular disease and 65% of patients with fibromuscular dysplasia had increased blood pressure despite a good medical regimen.[40] This report was published before many of the newer antihypertensive agents were available, leading some investigators to believe

that normalization of blood pressure may occur as frequently in patients with renovascular disease as it does in patients with essential hypertension.[41]

Resistant hypertension is defined as failure to normalize blood pressure (less than 140/90 mm Hg) following a good medical regimen consisting of at least three drugs with different mechanisms of action such as a diuretic, sympathetic inhibiting agent, and a vasodilator. Under this circumstance the presence of renovascular hypertension should be strongly considered.

Epigastric Bruit

In the cooperative study of renovascular hypertension, abdominal bruits were detected in only 9% of patients with essential hypertension compared with 46% of patients with renovascular hypertension.[39] Patients with fibromuscular dysplasia were more likely to have bruits than patients with atherosclerotic renovascular disease (57% vs. 41%).

The presence of a short systolic bruit in the epigastrium is frequently not significant. However, a holosystolic epigastric bruit, or more importantly a systolic/diastolic epigastric bruit, increases the likelihood of renovascular disease. The presence of a diastolic component to the bruit indicates that the degree of narrowing of the artery under investigation is severe since there is continued flow during diastole.[42] A systolic/diastolic bruit more often occurs in patients with fibromuscular disease (53%) than in patients who have atherosclerotic disease (12.5%).[43] Hunt et al[40] found a systolic/diastolic bruit in one third of patients with atherosclerotic renovascular disease and in 75% of patients with fibromuscular disease. The presence of a bruit is helpful, but the absence does not exclude the diagnosis of either atherosclerotic renovascular disease or fibromuscular dysplasia.

Atrophic Kidney or Discrepancy in Size Between the Two Kidneys

In the past an atrophic kidney was believed to be caused by chronic pyelonephritis. Although this may be true in the pediatric population, several studies have demonstrated that a small kidney in adults is most often associated with renovascular disease.[11,44,45] Gifford, McCormack, and Poutasse[44] demonstrated total occlusion or severe stenosis of the renal artery supplying the atrophic kidney in 53 of 75 patients (71%). More importantly, 22 patients (42%) had significant stenosis of the contralateral (normal-sized kidney) renal artery. Similarly, in a group of 40 patients with a totally occluded renal artery, there was associated contralateral renal artery stenosis in 31 patients (78%).[45] If an atrophic kidney or a discrepancy in size between the kidneys is discovered in an adult, a thorough investigation for the presence of renovascular disease should be undertaken.

Azotemia While Receiving Angiotensin-Converting Enzyme Inhibitors

Numerous reports suggest that patients who develop azotemia while receiving ACE inhibitors have either bilateral renal artery stenosis, renal artery stenosis to a solitary kidney, or decompensated congestive heart failure in the

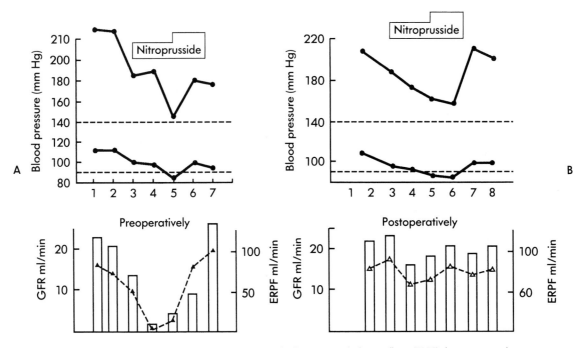

Fig. 18-7. A, Glomerular filtration rate *(GFR)* and effective renal plasma flow *(ERPF)* decreases markedly as blood pressure is lowered with sodium nitroprusside in a patient with bilateral renal artery stenosis. **B,** This is reversible following unilateral renal revascularization. (From Textor SC et al: Regulation of renal hemodynamics and glomerular filtration rate in patients with renovascular hypertension during converting enzyme inhibition with captopril, Am J Med 76[5B]:29, 1984.)

sodium-depleted state.[46-49] There are two mechanisms by which renal functional impairment may occur with the use of antihypertensive agents. The first may occur with any antihypertensive agent and occurs when a critical perfusion pressure is reached below which the kidney is no longer able to be perfused (Fig. 18-7). This has been shown by the infusion of sodium nitroprusside in patients with high-grade bilateral renal artery stenosis. When the critical perfusion pressure was reached, urine output, renal blood flow, and glomerular filtration rate declined and later returned to normal when the blood pressure increased above this critical perfusion pressure.[46] The exact pressure necessary to perfuse a kidney with renal artery stenosis varies with the degree of stenosis and is different among different patients.

The second mechanism is confined to patients receiving ACE inhibitors and may occur despite no significant change in blood pressure (Fig. 18-8). Patients with high-grade bilateral renal artery stenosis or renal artery stenosis to a solitary kidney may be highly dependent on angiotensin II for glomerular filtration. This is particularly common in patients who receive a combination of ACE inhibitor and diuretic[50] or in patients who are placed on a sodium-restricted diet.[51] Under these circumstances the constrictive effect of angiotensin II on the efferent arteriole allows for the maintenance of normal transglomerular capillary hydraulic pressure, thus allowing glomerular filtration to remain normal in the presence of markedly diminished blood flow (Fig. 18-9). In this instance glomerular filtration is highly dependent on angiotensin II, and when an ACE inhibitor is administered, the efferent arte-

riolar tone is no longer maintained and glomerular filtration is therefore decreased. A similar situation is seen in patients with decompensated congestive heart failure who are sodium depleted.[49]

Several animal studies have suggested that ACE inhibitor–induced acute renal failure may not be functional or reversible. Grone and Helmchen[52] have demonstrated that after 14 days of treatment with enalapril in rats with 2K-1C renovascular hypertension, proximal tubular atrophy occurred. This was not demonstrated in rats treated with dihydralazine. Jackson et al[53] demonstrated more marked irreversible fibrotic atrophy in the clipped kidney in animals receiving enalapril compared with those receiving minoxidil or no antihypertensive treatment. These data have led some investigators[54] to suggest that these tubular interstitial changes represent a form of "disuse atrophy" due to hypofiltration.

Azotemia in Elderly Patients with Atherosclerosis Elsewhere

It has been suggested that an elderly patient who has azotemia with no readily explainable cause should have a careful search for the presence of renovascular disease.[10,48]

EPIDEMIOLOGY

Generally fibromuscular disease occurs in a younger patient population (usually women), whereas atherosclerotic renal artery disease occurs in an older patient population. Keith[9] suggested that renovascular disease is much more common in whites than in blacks. However, Svetkey et al[55] demonstrated that in a clinically selective popula-

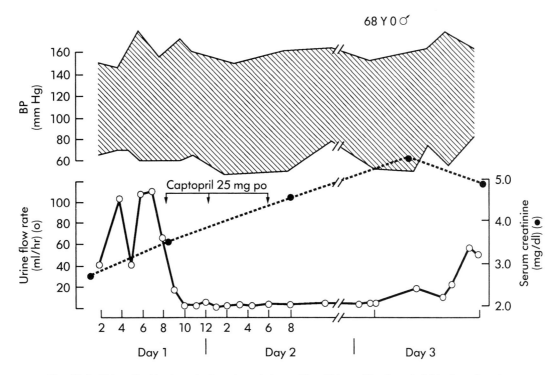

Fig. 18-8. This patient had renal artery stenosis to a solitary kidney. After the administration of captopril, the urine output decreased, and serum creatinine level increased despite no change in the systemic blood pressure. (From Textor SC et al: Regulation of renal hemodynamics and glomerular filtration rate in patients with renovascular hypertension during converting enzyme inhibition with captopril, Am J Med 76[5B]:29, 1984.)

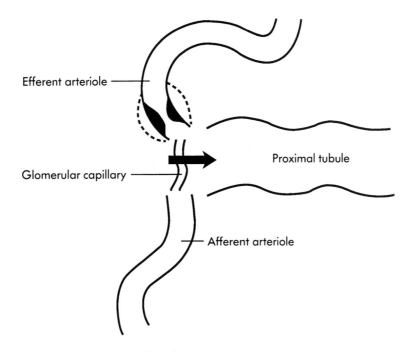

Fig. 18-9. Patients with high-grade bilateral renal artery stenosis or renal artery stenosis to a solitary kidney may be highly dependent on the efferent arteriolar constriction caused by angiotensin II in preserving transglomerular capillary hydraulic pressure *(arrow)* and glomerular filtration rate. When an ACE inhibitor is given, the efferent arteriole dilates *(dotted line),* and blood is shunted past the glomerulus.

tion, the prevalence of renovascular hypertension is similar in blacks and whites. They prospectively evaluated 167 hypertensive subjects with one or more clinical features known to be associated with renovascular hypertension. Renal artery stenosis or occlusion was found in 26 of 97 white patients (27%) and 13 of 67 black patients (19%) (P = 0.27). Blacks had much lower postcaptopril plasma renin activity (PRA) than whites. Novick et al[56] noted significant epidemiologic and clinical differences between black patients (n = 40, 4.9%) and white patients (n = 779, 95.1%) with renovascular disease. Blacks were more likely to have severe or refractory hypertension. In addition blacks had a higher prevalence of coronary artery disease, cerebrovascular disease, and peripheral vascular disease than the white patients in this series.

There is a particularly strong correlation between cigarette smoking and renovascular disease.[57,58] This is not surprising since cigarette smoking is quite prevalent in all forms of atherosclerosis. There are no good studies that evaluate the role of hypercholesterolemia in patients with ARAs, but there is one report suggesting that aggressive control of hyperlipidemia may allow for regression of an atherosclerotic renal artery lesion.[59] In all likelihood hypercholesterolemia is as strong a risk factor for atherosclerotic renal artery stenosis as it is for all other forms of atherosclerosis.

DIAGNOSTIC STUDIES FOR RENOVASCULAR DISEASE

There are numerous screening tests for renovascular disease.[60-63] These have differing sensitivities and specificities and are discussed in detail in the following section. These include newer noninvasive techniques that either directly visualize the renal arteries (i.e., duplex scanning) or use pharmacologic agents to exaggerate the stimulation of the renin-angiotensin-aldosterone system or decrease in renal blood flow and glomerular filtration rate in the kidney with renal artery stenosis. Arteriography, however, remains the gold standard.

It is important to keep in mind that the mere presence of renal artery stenosis does not mean that the renal artery lesion is functionally significant. It may not be causing the high blood pressure, and it may not be causing a decrement in renal function. It is hoped that some of these newer diagnostic tests will not only define the anatomy but also will sort out which lesions are functionally important and which are not.

Intravenous Urography

Maxwell et al[64] described the rapid-sequence intravenous pyelogram as a useful screening procedure in the early 1960s. Since that time many studies have demonstrated an unacceptably high false-positive and false-negative rate. In the cooperative study of renovascular hypertension[65] 11.4% of patients with essential hypertension had an abnormal intravenous urogram, and 17% of patients with documented significant renal artery stenosis by arteriography had a normal intravenous urogram. A false-positive rate of up to 41% has been reported.[66,67]

Nuclear Imaging Modalities

Radionuclide imaging techniques are a noninvasive and relatively safe way of evaluating renal blood flow and excretory function. However, they have similar degrees of sensitivity as the intravenous urogram and are much less specific in that many patients with essential hypertension or glomerular or tubulointerstitial diseases have abnormal radionuclide studies.[17,66] When an ACE inhibitor such as captopril is added to the standard nuclear medicine studies, the sensitivity and specificity increase considerably especially for unilateral renal artery stenosis.[68-70] This technique involves using glomerular radionuclide tracers such as technetium-99m diethylenetriamine pentaacetic acid (DTPA) and performing dynamic renal scintigraphy before and 1 hour after the administration of captopril, 25 mg. The captopril produces an acute and reversible decrement in renal function on the ipsilateral side to the renal artery stenosis, whereas renal function (glomerular filtration) will remain normal on the contralateral (nonstenotic) side. The Working Party on Captopril Renography[71] concluded that both scintigraphic images and computer-generated time-activity curves provided useful information about renal size, perfusion, and excretory capacity. Abnormalities that were important to the Working Party included the following:

1. A delayed time to maximal activity (T_{max} of 11 minutes or more after captopril administration)
2. Significant asymmetry of peak activity of each kidney
3. Marked cortical retention of radionuclide after captopril
4. Marked reduction in the calculated glomerular filtration rate of the ipsilateral kidney after the administration of an ACE inhibitor

Examples of these abnormalities are demonstrated in Fig. 18-10.

The sensitivity of captopril renography identifying patients with renovascular disease is approximately 90% (range, 83% to 94%) and the specificity is approximately 93% (range, 85% to 100%). Unfortunately the sensitivity of this screening test diminishes markedly in the presence of bilateral renal artery stenosis[73] or in patients who have significant degrees of azotemia (serum creatinine level exceeding 2.5 mg/dl). It is that very population of patients in whom a good noninvasive screening test is needed most. The ACE inhibitor needs to be discontinued several days before the captopril-stimulated renal flow scan. However, other antihypertensive agents are often allowed.[74]

Numerous investigators[75-77] have demonstrated that a positive captopril renogram is predictive of a cure or improvement of hypertension in 80% to 90% of cases after surgical or nonsurgical intervention. A positive captopril renogram did not correlate with improved blood pressure control in a series by Mann and Pickering.[60] There are no data available on a positive captopril renogram and improvement in renal function following interventional therapy for ARAS.

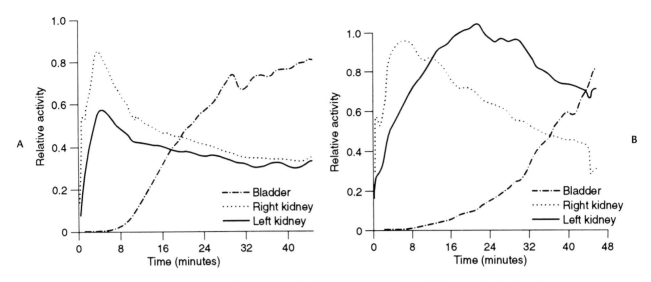

Fig. 18-10. Unilateral left renal artery stenosis. **A,** Tc-99m DTPA time-activity curves during baseline. **B,** Tc-99m DTPA time-activity curves following captopril stimulation. (From Nally JV: Provocative captopril testing in the diagnosis of renovascular hypertension, Urol Clin North Am 21:232, 1994.)

Duplex Scanning of the Renal Arteries

Standard ultrasonic imaging provides an accurate assessment of renal size and contour. However, patients with renal artery stenosis may not demonstrate an atrophic kidney or a discrepancy in renal size. Duplex scanning of the renal arteries is an excellent noninvasive test for the detection of renal artery stenosis. It combines direct visualization of the renal artery (B-mode imaging) with a measurement of the velocity of blood flow (Doppler) providing a useful anatomic and functional assessment of the degree of renal artery stenosis. Duplex scanning of the renal arteries is discussed in detail in Chapter 3. As opposed to other noninvasive diagnostic tests, duplex ultrasound scanning is not affected by various antihypertensive agents that the patient may be taking, whether or not the renal artery disease is unilateral or bilateral, or the degree of azotemia present.[78] The B-mode image is used to identify the renal artery and a Doppler sample is taken from the origin, midsection, and distal renal artery. If the ratio of the renal peak systolic velocity to the aortic peak systolic velocity (renal aortic ratio [RAR]) is 3.5 or greater, this signifies 60% to 99% stenosis of the renal arteries. Using these criteria, several studies have demonstrated a sensitivity from 83% to 98% and specificity of 95% to 100%.[78-81] We prospectively studied 102 patients who underwent duplex ultrasound examination of the renal arteries who had concomitant renal arteriography (Table 18-1). The sensitivity was 98%, specificity 98%, positive predictive value 99%, and negative predictive value 97%.[79] Accessory renal arteries can be difficult to image and the sensitivity of detecting them was approximately 67% in one series.[80] Duplex ultrasound is also useful in following patients after PTA, stent placement, or surgical revascularization to screen for restenosis.[82,83]

Duplex ultrasound is particularly attractive because it is safe and noninvasive. The limitations are that its quality is highly dependent on the expertise of the physician or technician performing the study and at times the study can be time-consuming. Excessive weight and bowel gas may limit the quality of the study. As ultrasonic equipment continues to improve, this technique will play a more prominent role in screening for renovascular disease.

Table 18-1. Comparison of Duplex Ultrasound with Arteriography

	% Stenosis by Arteriogram				
Ultrasound	0-59	60-79	80-99	100	TOTAL
0-59	62	0	1	1	64
60-99	1	31	67	0	99
100	0	1	1	22	24
TOTAL	63	32	69	23	187

Arteriography

Several angiographic techniques have been used to visualize the renal arteries. These include intravenous digital subtraction, intraarterial digital subtraction, or standard cut film arteriography.

The intravenous digital subtraction arteriogram has been used by many as an initial screening test for renovascular disease.[84] This technique is noninvasive in that the contrast medium is injected directly into a peripheral vein or into a catheter advanced into a more central vein such as the superior vena cava. The distal renal arteries are usually not well visualized with intravenous digital subtraction arteriography and thus are poor in patients who have fibromuscular disease. Even the proximal renal arteries are not visualized with the same resolution as one encounters with intraarterial digital subtraction arteriography or standard cut film arteriography. The amount of contrast medium needed is much more than that for an intraarterial digital subtraction arteriogram and often approaches that necessary for standard cut film arteriography. Havey et al[84] reviewed the literature of 406 hypertensive patients who had intravenous digital subtraction arteriograms and standard arteriograms. They found a sensitivity and specificity of the intravenous digital subtraction arteriogram to be 87.6% and 89.5%, respectively. In this same report 7.4% of 965 intravenous digital subtraction arteriograms were considered uninterpretable because of technical problems. With the advent of better noninvasive tests such as duplex ultrasound of the renal arteries and captopril renography, there really is no need for intravenous digital subtraction arteriograms any longer. In addition, with better catheterization techniques, softer and more flexible catheters, improved digitalized equipment, intraarterial digital subtraction arteriography is now relatively safe and provides superior images.

Intraarterial digital subtraction arteriography is performed by inserting a catheter into the femoral artery by the Seldinger technique and injecting contrast medium. A digital computer allows subtraction of the bone and soft tissues. This technique provides excellent resolution of the aorta, main renal arteries, and its branches. There are several advantages of this technique. An aortogram with visualization of the main renal arteries can be accomplished with much smaller amounts of contrast medium than standard cut film arteriography. The resolution is much better than with intravenous digital subtraction arteriography and is at least as good as cut film arteriography for the aorta and main renal arteries. With the advent of sophisticated digitalized equipment, standard cut film arteriography no longer is performed in many institutions.[85]

When patients undergo arteriography, a lateral view of the aorta should be obtained to assess the origin of the celiac and superior mesenteric arteries if surgical revascularization is contemplated and a hepatorenal or splenorenal bypass is considered. It is important to know the status of inflow (proximal celiac artery) before either of these operations is performed.

Magnetic Resonance Angiography and Spiral Computed Tomographic Scanning

Magnetic resonance angiography (MRA) has emerged as an excellent noninvasive method of visualizing the aorta and its major branches including the renal arteries. The two main techniques that are used are time-of-flight sequences and phase-contrast sequences.[86]

One may visualize the renal arteries two dimensionally, in which one slice is excited at a time, or three dimensionally, in which a whole volume is excited at the same time. In a series of 55 renal arteries in 25 patients, Kim et al[87] demonstrated that MRA had a sensitivity of 100% for detecting renal artery stenosis of 50% or greater and a specificity of 92%. Debatin et al[88] likewise showed that when using two-dimensional (2D) time-of-flight angiography and three-dimensional (3D) phase-contrast angiography the combined sensitivity and specificity were 87% and 97%, respectively. Other series[89,90] have shown similar excellent results. Major drawbacks of MRA at the current time include limited availability in some medical

centers, expense, and time to perform the examination. Larger prospective series will be required to determine the exact role of MRA in screening for renal artery stenosis.

Several reports have recently been published on spiral computed tomographic angiography (spiral CT scanning) for imaging for the abdominal aorta and its branches.[91,92] Spiral CT scanning allows 360-degree gantry rotation with continuous scanning of a defined volume of interest once the patient is transported through the gantry during a 30-second scan.[91] The material obtained in the scan can be reconstructed to form a 3D surface-shaded display or 2D maximum-intensity projection. The quality of these images is excellent, and the images clearly visualize the aorta and its major branches. There are three major drawbacks of spiral CT scanning: (1) expense; (2) the large volume of intravenous contrast material administered as a bolus (which may be undesirable as a screening test in patients with azotemia); and (3) the necessity for patients to breath-hold for 30 seconds (which may be difficult in elderly, debilitated patients). Nonetheless, CT spiral scanning appears to be an exciting noninvasive modality to visualize the aorta and its major branches.

DETERMINING THE FUNCTIONAL SIGNIFICANCE OF A STENOTIC RENAL ARTERY

Once renal artery stenosis is demonstrated on arteriography, it becomes important to determine whether it is functionally significant. In other words, is the lesion causing the patient's hypertension or leading to a decrement in renal function?

Plasma Renin Activity

Maxwell, Rudnick, and Waks[93] reviewed 540 patients reported in the literature to assess the value of PRA in the diagnosis of renovascular hypertension. There was a sensitivity of 57% and a specificity of 66%. The false-negative (43%) and false-positive (34%) rates were extremely high. The PRA did not predict which patients benefited from renal revascularization. Elevated PRA may be present in 15% of patients with essential hypertension.

In an attempt to increase the usefulness of measuring PRA, Muller et al[94] administered captopril, 50 mg orally, and obtained PRA 60 minutes later. In patients with normal renal function, the test correctly identified all 56 patients with proven renovascular disease. False-positive results occurred in only 2 of 112 patients (1.8%) with essential hypertension. The role of baseline PRA and captopril-stimulated PRA (the captopril test) in screening for and determining the significance of renal artery stenosis is summarized in several excellent reviews.[60,63,95]

Renal Vein Renin Ratios

Measurement of renin produced from the renal vein of the kidney with renal artery stenosis compared with the renal vein of the "normal" kidney has been used as a method for predicting which patients may benefit from intervention such as surgery, PTA, or stent placement. A number of factors can interfere with renin measurements, which will limit the usefulness of this particular test. If patients are not receiving any medications that suppress renin production, and if furosemide or ACE inhibitors are administered before blood is taken from the renal vein, the test may be accurate in predicting those in whom a cure of renovascular hypertension may occur.[70,96]

A renal vein renin ratio of 1.5:1 or greater with suppression of renin production by the contralateral (nonstenotic) kidney is considered a positive renal vein renin response. Hughes et al[97] demonstrated that when a renal vein renin ratio greater than 1.4:1 was combined with a duration of hypertension of less than 5 years, 19 out of 20 patients (95%) had a cure of their renovascular hypertension. Several reports have now been published that show that renal vein renin lateralization does not predict which patient will have an improvement in blood pressure after surgical revascularization or nonsurgical intervention.[98-101] The renal vein renin ratio may be helpful in selecting a patient in whom one can expect a cure in hypertension, but it does not predict which patient will show an improvement after interventional therapy. Therefore this test is somewhat limited in its overall usefulness.

TREATMENT OF RENOVASCULAR DISEASE

The three modalities available for the treatment of renovascular disease include medical therapy, surgical therapy, and nonsurgical intervention (PTA and endovascular stent placement).

The best treatment for renovascular disease is not known because there have been no controlled prospective randomized trials comparing medical therapy with either surgical therapy or nonsurgical intervention. Currently a study is under way at our institution in which patients with high-grade bilateral ARAS are randomly assigned either medical therapy or surgical therapy. It is hoped that this study will provide an answer to this very important question.

The usual reasons for intervention in renal artery disease include failure to adequately control blood pressure, despite a good antihypertensive regimen, or renal artery lesions, which have the potential to jeopardize or already have jeopardized renal function. Failure to control blood pressure may appear as truly drug-resistant hypertension (elevated blood pressure despite maximal doses of a good triple-drug regimen), intolerable side effects to antihypertensive medications, noncompliance, or the opinion that it may not be desirable to keep a young person on antihypertensive medications for the next 30 or 40 years.

An emerging indication for intervention is in patients with recurrent episodes of "flash" pulmonary edema, which may or may not be associated with blood pressure surges. Many of these patients have a normal left ventricle on echocardiography but have severe bilateral renal artery stenosis or renal artery stenosis to a solitary functioning kidney.[102,103] The exact pathogenesis of the pulmonary edema is not clearly delineated. Surgical revascularization[104] and renal artery stent placement[105] can ameliorate many episodes of pulmonary edema.

The therapeutic options available are discussed in the following sections for two of the most common underlying types of renovascular disease—atherosclerosis and fibromuscular disease.

Medical Therapy

The same principles apply to treating patients medically with renovascular disease as they do to treating patients with essential (primary) hypertension. With a few minor modifications, the principles of drug therapy are the same as those discussed in Chapter 17. One should begin with one antihypertensive agent. If the blood pressure is not controlled, a second agent of a different pharmacologic class should be added, and a third agent with a different mechanism of action added if necessary.

If the patient has a known unilateral renal artery stenosis, an ACE inhibitor either alone or with a diuretic is the preferred initial therapy. If, however, the patient has high-grade bilateral renal artery stenosis or significant renal artery stenosis to a solitary functioning kidney, an ACE inhibitor should either not be used or should be used with great caution because of the possibility of causing renal insufficiency. Case et al[106] demonstrated the long-term efficacy of captopril in renovascular hypertension in approximately 90% of patients. Havelka et al[107] have demonstrated that captopril plus a diuretic and β-blocker was more effective at 1 month and 30 months in patients with atherosclerotic renovascular disease than was standard triple therapy of a diuretic, a sympathetic inhibiting agent, and a direct vasodilator.

In addition to simply treating the blood pressure, all cardiovascular risk factors need to be modified. Almost all patients with atherosclerotic renal artery disease die from complications of atherosclerosis such as myocardial infarction and stroke. The same approach should be taken with these patients as with patients who have atherosclerosis elsewhere. The incidence of coronary artery disease is very high in this patient population; therefore, the presence of coronary artery disease should be carefully searched for. Patients should be encouraged to stop smoking; diabetes and lipid disturbances should be aggressively treated.

SURGICAL RENAL REVASCULARIZATION. Advances in both surgical renovascular reconstruction and medical antihypertensive therapy have limited the role of total or partial nephrectomy in the management of patients with renal artery disease. These operations are only occasionally indicated in patients with severe arteriolar nephrosclerosis, severe renal atrophy, noncorrectable renovascular lesions, and renal infarction.

A variety of surgical revascularization techniques are available for treating patients with significant renal artery disease. Aortorenal bypass with a free graft of autogenous hypogastric artery or saphenous vein remains a popular method in patients with a nondiseased abdominal aorta.[108,109] Polytetrafluoroethylene aortorenal bypass grafts have been successfully employed by some surgeons, usually when an autogenous graft is not available.[110-112] Renal endarterectomy also continues to be used to treat atherosclerotic renal artery disease. Patients with complex branch renal artery lesions are managed with extracorporeal microvascular reconstruction and autotransplantation.[113-115]

In older patients severe atherosclerosis of the abdominal aorta may render an aortorenal bypass or endarterectomy technically difficult and potentially hazardous to perform. In such cases several investigators prefer alternate surgical approaches that allow renal revascularization to be safely and effectively accomplished while avoiding surgery on a badly diseased aorta. The most effective alternate bypass techniques have been a splenorenal bypass for left renal revascularization,[116,117] and a hepatorenal bypass for right renal revascularization.[118] The absence of occlusive disease involving the origin of the celiac artery is an important prerequisite for these operations. A recent study indicated the presence of significant celiac artery stenosis in 50% of patients with ARAS.[119] This information underscores the importance of obtaining preoperative lateral aortography to evaluate the celiac artery origin in patients who are being considered for hepatorenal or splenorenal bypass.

Use of the supraceliac or lower thoracic aorta for renal revascularization is a new surgical alternative in patients with significant atherosclerosis of the abdominal aorta and its major visceral branches.[120,121] The supraceliac aorta is often relatively disease-free in such patients and can be used to achieve renovascular reconstruction with an interposition saphenous vein graft. Simultaneous aortic replacement and renal revascularization have been associated with an increased risk of operative mortality,[122,123] and this approach is best reserved for patients with an indication for aortic replacement such as an aortic aneurysm or symptomatic aortoiliac occlusive disease.

Recent reports from several centers indicate that the techniques previously described for surgical renovascular reconstruction can be safely performed with a high technical success rate.[17,124-129] Patients with fibrous dysplasia are usually otherwise healthy, and operative morbidity and mortality following revascularization in this group have been minimal.[17,124] Operative mortality rates of 2.1%,[17] 3.1%,[124] 3.4%,[125] and 6.1%[126] have been reported following surgical revascularization in patients with atherosclerotic renal artery disease. An increased risk of operative mortality has been observed with bilateral simultaneous renal revascularization,[130] or when renal revascularization

is performed in conjunction with another major vascular operation such as aortic replacement.[129] Most studies have indicated a high technical success rate for surgical vascular reconstruction with postoperative thrombosis or stenosis rates of less than 10%.[17,126,128]

In evaluating the results of surgical revascularization for renovascular hypertension, most studies have considered patients as cured if the blood pressure is 140/90 mm Hg or less postoperatively. Patients have been considered improved if they have either shown a reduction in diastolic pressure 10 to 15 mm Hg or more or become normotensive on medication. Failures have been those who have not qualified for either of the aforementioned categories. The results of surgical treatment for renovascular hypertension vary according to the underlying pathologic diagnosis. In patients with fibrous dysplasia, 50% to 60% are cured, 30% to 40% are improved, and the failure rate is less than 10%.[17,124] In patients undergoing revascularization for atherosclerotic renovascular hypertension (Table 18-2), the failure rate is approximately the same; however, fewer patients are cured and more patients are improved postoperatively. The explanation for this is that renovascular hypertension is often superimposed on existing essential hypertension in older patients. A recent study by Van Bockel et al[128] highlighted the excellent long-term results following reconstructive surgery for atherosclerotic renovascular hypertension; with a mean follow-up of 8.9 years, postoperative hypertension was cured or improved in 83 of 105 patients (79%).

In recent years more centers have been performing surgical revascularization to preserve renal function in patients with high-grade atherosclerotic arterial occlusive disease affecting both kidneys or a solitary kidney. These are generally older patients with diffuse atherosclerosis, ostial renal artery lesions, and varying degrees of renal functional impairment. Studies from several centers (Table 18-3) have indicated improvement or stabilization of renal function postoperatively in 75% to 89% of patients. Con-

Table 18-2. Results of Surgical Revascularization for Atherosclerotic Renovascular Hypertension

Series	No. of Patients	No. Cured (%)	No. Improved (%)	No. Failed (%)
Van Bockel et al (1987)[128]	105	19 (18)	64 (61)	22 (21)
Novick et al (1987)[17]	180	55 (31)	110 (61)	15 (8)
Libertino et al (1988)[127]	86	38 (44)	44 (51)	4 (5)
Hansen et al (1992)[124]	152	22 (15)	116 (75)	14 (10)

Table 18-3. Results of Surgical Revascularization for Atherosclerotic Ischemic Nephropathy

Series	No. Patients	No. Improved (%)	No. Stable (%)	No. Deteriorated (%)
Novick et al (1987)[17]	161	93 (58)	50 (31)	18 (11)
Hallet et al (1987)[130]	91	20 (22)	48 (53)	23 (25)
Hansen et al (1992)[124]	70	34 (49)	25 (36)	11 (15)
Bredenberg et al (1992)[125]	40	22 (55)	10 (25)	8 (20)
Libertino et al (1992)[126]	91	45 (49)	31 (35)	15 (16)

sidering the significant risks of progressive occlusive disease and renal failure that have been associated with medical management of such patients, these results demonstrate a favorable influence of revascularization on the natural history of untreated atherosclerotic renal artery disease.

PATIENT SELECTION FOR INTERVENTION TO PRESERVE RENAL FUNCTION

Anatomic Severity and Extent of Renal Artery Disease

Following angiographic diagnosis of ARAS, and with knowledge of the natural history of this disease, one can identify those patients in whom such disease poses a significant threat to overall renal function. This designation applies to patients with high-grade arterial stenosis (greater than 75%) affecting their entire renal mass—namely, where such stenosis is present bilaterally or involves a solitary kidney. In these patients the risk of complete renal arterial occlusion is significant, and if this occurs, the clinical outcome is a critical decrease in functioning renal mass with resulting renal failure. Intervention to restore normal renal arterial blood flow is indicated in such patients for the purpose of preserving renal function. In a study from the Cleveland Clinic, surgical revascularization for preservation of renal function was performed in 161 patients with ARAS bilaterally or in a solitary kidney.[17] Postoperatively renal function was improved in 93 patients (58%), stable in 50 patients (31%), and deteriorated in only 18 patients (11%).

The benefit of undertaking revascularization for preservation of renal function in patients with unilateral ARAS and an unobstructed contralateral renal artery is not established. If the contralateral kidney is anatomically and functionally normal, revascularization for this purpose is clearly not warranted. If the opposite kidney is functioning but involved with some type of parenchymal disorder, revascularization of the ischemic kidney may benefit some patients, but specific indications for this approach are not well defined. Dean et al[131] reviewed the renal functional outcome following surgical revascularization in 53 patients with ischemic nephropathy. The postoperative estimated glomerular filtration rate (EGFR) was improved significantly in 41 patients treated for bilateral ARAS but was unaltered in 12 patients with unilateral ARAS.

Complete occlusion of the renal artery most often eventuates in irreversible ischemic damage of the involved kidney. However, in some patients with gradual arterial occlusion, the viability of the kidney can be maintained through the development of collateral arterial supply.[132-134] Helpful clinical clues suggesting renal salvageability in such cases include the following: (1) angiographic demonstration of late filling of the distal renal arterial tree by collateral vessels on the side of total arterial occlusion, (2) a renal biopsy showing well-preserved glomeruli, (3) kidney size greater than 9 cm, and (4) function of the involved kidney on isotope renography or intravenous pyelography. When such criteria are present, restoration of normal renal arterial flow can lead to recovery of renal function.

Level of Renal Function

In general, revascularization to preserve renal function in patients with ARAS is most likely to be beneficial in those who have not yet sustained severe, permanent impairment of overall renal function. In a study from the Cleveland Clinic, we evaluated the effect of baseline renal function on the outcome of surgical revascularization in elderly patients with ARAS.[135] The majority of these patients had preoperative serum creatinine levels of less than 3.0 mg/dl; postoperative renal function was stable or improved in 89% of patients in this category.

Revascularization to preserve renal function is generally not worthwhile in patients with severe azotemia (serum creatinine level greater than 4.0 mg/dl), because advanced underlying renal parenchymal disease is inevitably present and obviates improvement in renal function with restored perfusion. This observation has been recorded by several groups including our own.[136,137] Severe nephrosclerosis is the most common form of renal parenchymal disease in such patients; however, renal cholesterol embolization may be an additional complicating feature.[138] In patients with atherosclerotic ischemic renal disease and a serum creatinine level greater than 4.0 mg/dl, our policy is to perform a renal biopsy to evaluate the severity of renal parenchymal involvement from one or both of these disorders.

Some patients present with severe impairment of overall renal function that has developed acutely following initiation of medical antihypertensive therapy.[51,139] Such rapidly progressive renal insufficiency may be a manifestation of perfusion-dependent renal function due to underlying ARAS. If this problem is detected promptly, renal function will often improve following discontinuation of the offending antihypertensive medications. Intervention to relieve renal arterial obstruction can prevent permanent renal damage in patients with this type of severe acute renal insufficiency.

In addition to the absolute level of renal function, the rate of decline in overall renal function is an important determinant of the outcome following intervention in atherosclerotic ischemic renal disease. In a study by Dean et al[131] patients with a rapid rate of deterioration in EGFR during the 6 months preceding surgical revascularization achieved the greatest benefit in terms of postoperative improvement of EGFR. Unfortunately their data precluded definition of a critical rate of decline in EGFR that would predict retrieval of renal function by revascularization. Nevertheless, rapid deterioration of overall renal function in association with ARAS suggests a strong possibility of retrieval of function by intervention to restore normal renal arterial flow.

Patients with end-stage renal disease (ESRD) from ischemic nephropathy have been encountered in whom renal function has been salvageable with revascularization.[140,141] The basis for this has been the presence of chronic bilateral total renal arterial occlusion where, fortuitously, the viability of one or both kidneys has been maintained through collateral vascular supply. In such cases revascularization can yield dramatic recovery of renal function. Unfortunately this clinical presentation is rare and a less favorable outcome of bilateral arterial occlusion on renal viability is far more common.

Finally, it is important to emphasize that patients with ESRD and ARAS without complete occlusion are not appropriate candidates for revascularization to restore function. In such cases main renal arterial blood flow is preserved, albeit at a reduced level, and yet the supplied renal parenchyma is without function. The basis for this is the presence of severe unalterable parenchymal damage that precludes recovery of renal function with improved perfusion.

Renal Histopathology

Evaluation of renal histopathology can help to determine the presence of salvageable renal function in selected patients with atherosclerotic renal ischemic disease. In patients with ARAS and severe existing impairment of overall renal function (serum creatinine level greater than 4.0 mg/dl), renal biopsy findings can help to predict whether revascularization is likely to forestall further progressive renal insufficiency. In patients with atherosclerotic renal artery occlusion, renal biopsy findings can indicate whether the involved kidney is viable and functionally salvageable on the basis of collateral vascular supply. The two predominant morphologic lesions in such patients are arteriolar nephrosclerosis and atheroembolic renal disease, with the former being more often encountered. Both of these diagnoses can be established upon a frozen-section histopathologic examination, and therefore the renal biopsy can be done at the same time as surgical revascularization, if the biopsy findings are favorable. In patients with arteriolar nephrosclerosis, the most important favorable criterion is histologic evidence that a majority of examined glomeruli are intact and viable.[133,134] The presence of tubular atrophy, interstitial fibrosis, and arteriolar sclerosis are of lesser importance and do not necessarily preclude recovery of renal function; these findings may merely reflect the histologic changes of chronic reversible renal ischemia. However, the finding of widespread glomerular hyalinization indicates irreversible ischemic renal injury that obviates any benefit from relief of renal arterial obstruction. The finding of extensive atheroembolic disease would also preclude renal revascularization. With respect to the technique for renal biopsy in such patients, a more representative specimen of renal tissue is obtained with an open surgical wedge biopsy than with a closed needle biopsy.

Percutaneous Transluminal Angioplasty

PTA for renal artery stenosis was first reported by Grüntzig et al[142] in 1978 when they successfully dilated a 61-year-old patient with hypertension. PTA is quite effective in treating patients with fibromuscular disease. However, its use in treating ARAS has been disappointing.[143,144] Hayes et al[143] reported on 55 patients with ARAS who underwent PTA. A successful clinical outcome was achieved in only 12 patients (26.1%) with atherosclerotic disease. The nonostial lesions fared better than ostial lesions (50% improvement vs. 15.4%).

Cicuto et al[145] have demonstrated that patients with ostial lesions fare much worse than those who have lesions distal to the takeoff of the renal artery. Sos et al[144] reported that when angioplasty was technically successful, 84% of patients with atheromatous disease demonstrated a cure or improvement in blood pressure control. Unfortunately these data are misleading in that only 57% of patients with unilateral atheromatous disease had technically successful angioplasty, and only 10% of patients with bilateral disease had a technically successful angioplasty. Therefore when all patients are considered, of the 51 patients with ARAS, only 33.3% had either a cure or improvement in blood pressure control. Those with bilateral disease fared worse than those with unilateral disease, and those with ostial lesions did worse than those with nonostial lesions.

In one recent report[146] there were technical success rates of 76.2%, 74.1%, and 67.7% for unilateral renal artery disease ($n = 42$), bilateral disease ($n = 27$), and disease in a solitary kidney ($n = 31$). Of those patients who had technical successes, 43 of 73 patients (59%) demonstrated significant improvement in blood pressure control. These patients were observed for a mean period of 29 months. As in most other series, ostial lesions fared worse than those that were nonostial. Another recent report has suggested that if patients demonstrate sustained reduction in blood pressure on ACE inhibitors and have a renal vein renin ratio greater than 1.5:1, the chance of successful blood pressure lowering with PTA is much greater than if neither of these features is present.[147]

Rimmer and Gennari[18] (Table 18-4) summarized the results of preservation of renal function after PTA. Improvement or stabilization occurred in a large number of patients. There are reports of restoration of renal function after dilation of an occluded renal artery.[153,154] However, the high rate of recurrence of disease may necessitate repeat dilatation of the renal artery. Duplex ultrasound scanning of the renal arteries has been of enormous benefit in following patients after PTA or endovascular stent placement to look for restenosis. By performing duplex ultrasound every 3 to 6 months, restenosis can be identified and corrected before occlusion of the renal artery occurs.[82,83]

Weibull et al[155] performed a prospective randomized study comparing percutaneous renal angioplasty versus surgical reconstruction in a small number of patients. Twenty-nine patients were randomized to each group. PTA of the renal arteries was successful in 83% of patients and surgical revascularization in 97% of patients. The primary patency rate after 24 months was 75% in the PTA group and 96% in the operative group. The secondary patency rate was 90% and 97%, respectively. Four patients in the PTA group required future operation. Hypertension was cured or improved in 90% of the PTA group and 86% of the surgical group. Renal function was stable in 83% of the PTA group and 72% of the surgery group. Seventeen percent of patients treated with PTA eventually required surgical revascularization.

Complications can occur with PTA. In the Sos et al[144] series of 51 patients (70 arteries) undergoing angioplasty, 3 patients required surgery for puncture site trauma, 4 patients had nonocclusive renal artery dissection, of which 3 underwent a successful renal revascularization. Two patients had transient acute renal failure and one patient had transient myocardial ischemia. Acute rupture of the renal artery at the time of renal artery angioplasty[156] and

Table 18-4. Results of Percutaneous Transluminal Angioplasty for Atherosclerotic Ischemic Nephropathy

Series (Ref.)	No. of Patients	No. Improved (%)	No. Stable (%)	No. Worse* (%)	No. of Deaths (%)
Luft, Grim, and Weinberger (1983)[148]	12	3 (25)	5 (42)	4 (33)	0
Pickering et al (1986)[149]	55	26 (47)	19 (35)	10 (18)	NA
Bell, Reid, and Buist (1987)[150]	20	7 (35)	10 (50)	3 (15)	0
O'Donovan et al (1992)[151]	17	9 (53)	2 (12)	6 (35)	5 (29)
TOTAL	104	45 (43)	36 (35)	23 (22)	5 (10)
Canzanello et al (1989)[146]	69	36 (52)†		33 (48)	2 (3)
Martin, Casarela, and Gaylord (1988)[152]	79	34 (43)	45 (57)‡		1 (1)
TOTAL and Canzanello et al	173	117 (68)†		56 (32)	7 (6)
TOTAL and Martin, Casarela, and Gaylord[152]	183	79 (43)	104 (57)‡		6 (5)

(From Rimmer M and Gennari J: Atherosclerotic renovascular disease in progressive renal failure, Ann Intern Med 118:712, 1993.)
*Includes all deaths.
†Sum of improved and stable.
‡Sum of stable and worse.

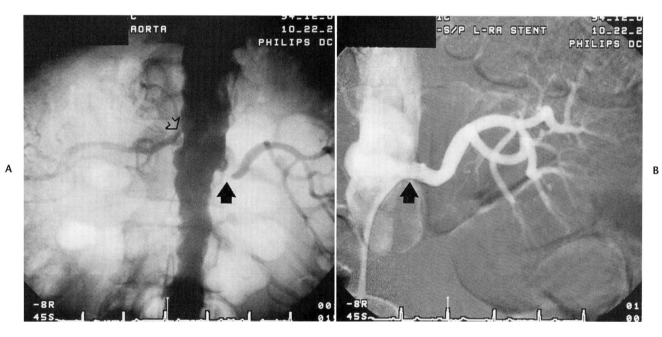

Fig. 18-11. A, Aortogram shows subtotal occlusion of the left renal artery *(arrow)* and stenosis of an upper-pole right renal artery *(arrowhead)*. The lower-pole artery to the right kidney is occluded. **B,** The left renal artery is now widely patent after stent placement *(arrow)*.

delayed rupture of the renal artery up to 9 days after PTA[157] have been reported.

We use PTA for atherosclerotic renovascular disease in focal nonostial renal artery lesions and only dilate patients with diffuse disease or ostial lesions if no other options are available. However, the focal lesions are clearly less common than ostial lesions or more diffuse atherosclerosis. Therefore the usefulness of PTA in atherosclerotic renovascular disease is limited.

Due to the inability of angioplasty to have any mean-ingful, long-term benefit for osteal renal artery stenosis, several groups of investigators have used endovascular stenting for osteal renal artery stenosis[158-162] (Fig. 18-11). In an initial series reported by Rees et al[158] using the Palmaz stent for osteal ARAS, technical success was achieved in 27 of 28 patients. Sixty-four percent of patients had blood pressure cured or improved, and 10 of 14 patients had stabilization of renal function. However, restenosis occurred in 7 of the 18 patients studied (39%). In patients with greater than 15% residual stenosis, all 4 patients restenosed, whereas in patients with less than 15% residual stenosis, only 3 of 14 patients (21%) restenosed. We reported 77 patients (98 renal arteries) who underwent endovascular stenting for ARAS.[162] Technical success was 98%. Angiographic patency was available in 33 patients (43%), and the duration of follow-up was a mean of 8 months. Cumulative patency at 6 months was 93% and at 10 months was 81%. The primary assisted patency was 100%. This was achieved by using surveillance duplex scanning to identify restenosis.

It is unclear what the long-term restenosis rate will be for renal artery stenting for osteal disease. However, some investigators believe that the results will be improved by overexpanding the renal artery stent, using intraarterial ultrasound to make sure that the stent is properly deployed. Renal artery stenting is an excellent procedure for the patient with advanced atherosclerosis who is at high risk for surgical revascularization.

Nine patients in our series developed pseudoaneurysm at the catheter entry site, and this was repaired by ultrasound-guided compression in seven patients. Three patients developed acute tubular necrosis and three atheromatous embolization.

Hennequin et al[160] placed wall stents in 21 patients who had unsuccessful result or restenosis after transluminal angioplasty. Using follow-up angiography, the cumulative primary patency rate was 95%, 85%, and 77% at 7, 9, and 15 months, respectively. Hypertension was cured in three patients and improved in eighteen.

PTA is the preferred modality in many patients with fibromuscular disease. The results are superior to, and the complication rate less than, the results in patients with atherosclerosis.[144] In the Sos et al series of 31 patients, 27 (87.1%) had a technically successful dilation. Of those who were successfully dilated, 16 of the patients (59.3%) had a cure in their blood pressure, 9 patients (33.3%) had improvement, and 2 patients (7.4%) failed to improve. When there was a successful response in lowering blood pressure, it was usually sustained. Although recurrence of stenosis is common in atherosclerotic disease, it is particularly uncommon in patients with fibromuscular disease. In a series of 31 patients in whom 34 arteries were dilated, there was no mortality, one nonocclusive renal artery dissection, and one occlusive renal artery dissection. Similar good results have been reported in other series in which patients underwent PTA for fibromuscular disease.[163,164]

The main limitation of percutaneous transluminal renal angioplasty for patients with fibromuscular disease is that it is usually effective only for patients who have disease in the main renal arteries. Medial fibroplasia and perimedial fibroplasia often involve the branches of the renal artery, and these may be technically difficult or impossible lesions to dilate. Therefore patients with branch disease often must undergo extracorporeal reconstruction and autotransplantation.

In summary, PTA is the procedure of choice for patients who have main renal artery disease secondary to fibromuscular dysplasia. However, if branch disease is involved, surgical revascularization may be necessary.

REFERENCES

1. Goldblatt H et al: Studies in experimental hypertension. I. The production of persistent elevation of systolic blood pressure by means of renal ischemia, J Exp Med 59:347, 1934.
2. Page IH and Helmer M: A crystalline pressor substance (angiotonin) resulting from the reaction between renin and renin activator, J Exp Med 71:29, 1940.
3. Braun-Menendez E et al: The substance causing renal hypertension, J Physiol 98:283, 1940.
4. Dustan HP: History of clinical renovascular hypertension. In Stanley JC et al, eds: Renovascular hypertension, Philadelphia, 1984, WB Saunders Co.
5. Hoobler SW: History of experimental renovascular hypertension. In Stanley JC et al, eds: Renovascular hypertension, Philadelphia, 1984, WB Saunders Co.
6. Page IH: Hypertension research: a memoir 1920, New York, 1988, Pergamon Press.
7. Gifford RW Jr: Evaluation of the hypertension patient with emphasis on detecting curable causes, Milbank Memorial Fund Q 47:170, 1969.
8. Davis BA et al: Prevalence of renovascular hypertension in patients with grade III or IV hypertensive retinopathy, N Engl J Med 301:1273, 1979.
9. Keith TA: Renovascular hypertension in black patients, Hypertension 4:438, 1982.
10. Working Group on Renovascular Hypertension: Detection, evaluation and treatment of renovascular hypertension, Arch Intern Med 147:820, 1987.
11. Olin JW et al: Prevalence of atherosclerotic renal artery stenosis in patients with atherosclerosis elsewhere, Am J Med 88:46N, 1990.
12. Missouris CG et al: Renal artery stenosis: a common and important problem in patients with peripheral vascular disease, Am J Med 96:10, 1994.
13. Valentine RJ et al: Detection of unsuspected renal artery stenosis in patients with abdominal aortic aneurysms: redefined indications for preoperative aortography, Ann Vasc Surg 7:220, 1993.
14. Choudhri AH et al: Unsuspected renal artery stenosis in peripheral vascular disease, Br Med J 301:1197, 1990.
15. Harding MB et al: Renal artery stenosis: prevalence and associated risk factors in patients undergoing routine cardiac catheterization, J Am Soc Nephrol 2:1608, 1992.
16. Dustan HP et al: Normal arterial pressure in patients with renal arterial stenosis, JAMA 187:1028, 1964.
17. Novick AC et al: Trends in surgical revascularization for renal artery disease: ten years experience, JAMA 257:498, 1987.
18. Rimmer JM and Gennari J: Atherosclerotic renovascular disease in progressive renal failure, Ann Intern Med 118:712, 1993.
19. Wollenweber J, Sheps SG, and Davis GD: Clinical course of atherosclerotic renovascular disease, Am J Cardiol 21:60, 1968.
20. Meaney TF, Dustan HP, and McCormack LJ: Natural history of renal arterial disease, Radiology 91:881, 1968.
21. Schreiber MJ, Novick AC, and Pohl MA: The natural history of atherosclerotic and fibrous renal artery disease, Urol Clin North Am 116:1408, 1981.
22. Tollefson DFJ and Ernst CB. Natural history of atherosclerotic renal artery stenosis associated with aortic disease, J Vasc Surg 14:327, 1991.
23. Zierler RE et al: Natural history of atherosclerotic renal artery stenosis: a prospective study with duplex ultrasonography, J Vasc Surg 19:250, 1994.

24. Guzman RP et al: Renal atrophy and arterial stenosis. A prospective study with duplex ultrasound, Hypertension 23:346, 1994.

25. Harrison HG and McCormack LJ: Pathologic classification of renal artery disease in renovascular hypertension, Mayo Clin Proc 46:161, 1971.

26. Novick AC: Renal artery aneurysm and arteriovenous malformation. In Novick AC and Straffon RA, eds: Vascular problems in urologic surgery, Philadelphia, 1982, WB Saunders Co.

27. Poutasse EF: Renal artery aneurysms, J Urol 113:443, 1975.

28. Gross F: The renin-angiotensin system in hypertension, Ann Intern Med 75:777, 1971.

29. Mohring J et al: Salt and water balance and renin activity in renal hypertension of rats, Am J Physiol 228:1847, 1975.

30. Dzau VJ, Gibbons GH, and Leven DC: Renovascular hypertension: an update on pathophysiology, diagnosis and treatment, Am J Nephrol 3:172, 1983.

31. Vaughan ED: Renovascular hypertension, Kidney Int 27:811, 1985.

32. Brunner HR et al: Hypertension of renal origin: evidence for two different mechanisms, Science 174:1344, 1971.

33. Vaughan ED Jr et al: Renovascular hypertension: renin measurements to indicate hypersecretion and contralateral suppression, estimate renal plasma flow and score for surgical curability, Am J Med 55:402, 1973.

34. Dzau VJ et al: Sequential renal hemodynamics in experimental, benign and malignant hypertension, Hypertension 3(suppl I):63, 1981.

35. Rostrand SG et al: Attenuated pressure natriuresis in hypertensive rats, Kidney Int 21:330, 1982.

36. Martinez-Maldonado M: Pathophysiology of renal vascular hypertension, Hypertension 17:707, 1991.

37. Gavras H et al: Angiotensin-sodium interaction and blood pressure maintenance of renal hypertensive and normotensive rats, Science 180:1369, 1973.

38. Goldfarb DA: The renin-angiotensin system. New concepts in regulation of blood pressure and renal function, Urol Clin North Am 21:187, 1994.

39. Simon N et al: Clinical characteristics of renovascular hypertension: cooperative study of renovascular hypertension, JAMA 220:1209, 1972.

40. Hunt JC et al: Renal and renovascular hypertension, Arch Intern Med 133:988, 1974.

41. Gifford RW Jr: Epidemiology and clinical manifestations of renovascular hypertension. In Stanley JC, Ernst CB, and Fry WJ, eds: Renovascular hypertension, Philadelphia, 1984, WB Saunders Co.

42. Olin JW: Evaluation of the peripheral circulation. In Izzo JL and Black HR, eds: Hypertension Primer, Dallas, 1993, American Heart Association.

43. Eipper DF et al: Abdominal bruits in renovascular hypertension, Am J Cardiol 37:48, 1976.

44. Gifford RW Jr, McCormack LJ, and Poutasse EF: The atrophic kidney: its role in hypertension, Mayo Clin Proc 40: 834, 1965.

45. Lawrie GM, Morris GC, and Debakey ME: Long-term results of treatment of the totally occluded renal artery in 40 patients with renovascular hypertension, Surgery 88:753, 1980.

46. Textor SC et al: Regulation of renal hemodynamics and glomerular filtration rate in patients with renovascular hypertension during converting enzyme inhibition with captopril, Am J Med 76(5B):29, 1984.

47. Silas JH et al: Captopril induced reversible renal failure: a marker for renal artery stenosis affecting a solitary kidney, Br Med J 286:1702, 1983.

48. Jacobson HR: Ischemic renal disease: an overlooked clinical entity? Kidney Int 34:729, 1988.

49. Packer M et al: Functional renal insufficiency during long-term therapy with captopril and enalapril and severe congestive heart failure, Ann Intern Med 106:346, 1987.

50. Watson ML et al: Captopril/diuretic combinations in severe renovascular disease: a cautionary note, Lancet 2:404, 1983.

51. Hricik D et al: Captopril-induced functional renal insufficiency in patients with bilateral renal-artery stenosis or renal-artery stenosis to a solitary kidney, N Engl J Med 308:373, 1983.

52. Grone H and Helmchen U: Impairment and recovery of the clipped kidney in two kidney, one clip hypertensive rats during and after antihypertensive therapy, Lab Invest 54:645, 1986.

53. Jackson B et al: Pharmacologic nephrectomy with chronic angiotensin converting enzyme inhibitor treatment in renovascular hypertension in the rat, J Lab Clin Med 115:21, 1990.

54. Hricik DE and Dunn MJ: Angiotensin-converting enzyme inhibitor-induced renal failure: causes, consequences and diagnostic uses, J Am Soc Nephrol 1:845, 1990.

55. Svetkey LP et al: Similar prevalence of renovascular hypertension in selected blacks and whites, Hypertension 17: 678, 1991.

56. Novick AC et al: Epidemiologic and clinical comparison of renal artery stenosis in black patients and white patients, J Vasc Surg 20:1, 1994.

57. Nicholson JP et al: Cigarette smoking and renovascular hypertension, Lancet 2:765, 1983.

58. Black HR and Cooper KA: Cigarette smoking and atherosclerotic renal artery stenosis, J Clin Hyper 4:322, 1986.

59. Basta LL et al: Regression of atherosclerotic stenosing lesions of the renal arteries and spontaneous cure of systemic hypertension through controlled hyperlipidemia, Am J Med 61:420, 1976.

60. Mann SJ and Pickering TG: Detection of renovascular hypertension. State of the art, Ann Intern Med 117:845, 1992.

61. Davidson RA and Wilcox CS: Newer diagnostic tests for the diagnosis of renovascular disease, JAMA 268:3353, 1992.

62. Nally JV, Olin JW, and Lammert GK: Advances in noninvasive screening for renovascular disease, Cleve Clin J Med 61:328, 1994.

63. Canzanello VJ and Textor SC: Noninvasive diagnosis of renal vascular disease, Mayo Clin Proc 69:1172, 1994.

64. Maxwell MH et al: Use of the rapid sequence intravenous pyelogram: the diagnosis of renovascular hypertension, N Engl J Med 270:213, 1964.

65. Bookstein JJ et al: Radiologic aspects of renovascular hypertension. II. The role of urography and unilateral renovascular disease: cooperative study of renovascular hypertension, JAMA 220:1225, 1972.

66. Kaufman JJ: Renovascular hypertension: the UCLA experience, J Urol 121:139, 1979.

67. Thornbury JR, Stanley JC, and Fryback DG: Hypertensive urogram: a nondiscriminatory test for renovascular hypertension, AJR 138:43, 1982.

68. Fommei E et al: Renal scintigraphic captopril test in the diagnosis of renovascular hypertension, Hypertension 10:212, 1987.

69. Nally JV et al: Captopril renography for the detection of renovascular hypertension, Cleve Clin J Med 55:311, 1988.

70. Wilcox CS et al: Diagnostic uses of angiotensin-converting enzyme inhibitors in renovascular hypertension, Am J Hypertens 1:344S, 1988.

71. Nally JV et al: Diagnostic criteria of renovascular hypertension with captopril renography. A consensus statement, Am J Hypertens 4(suppl):749S, 1991.

72. Nally JV: Provocative captopril testing in the diagnosis of renovascular hypertension, Urol Clin North Am 21:227, 1994.

73. Nally JV: Renal scintigraphy in the evaluation of renovascular hypertension: a note of optimism yet caution, J Nucl Med 28:1501, 1987.

74. Sheps SG et al: Radionuclide scintigraphy in the evaluation of patients with hypertension, J Am Coll Cardiol 21:838, 1993.

75. Elliott WJ: Comparison of two noninvasive screening tests for renovascular hypertension, Arch Intern Med 153:755, 1993.

76. Setaro JF et al: Simplified captopril renography in diagnosis and treatment of renal artery stenosis, Hypertension 18:289, 1991.

77. Geyskes GG et al: Renography with captopril: changes in a patient with hypertension and unilateral renal artery stenosis, Arch Intern Med 146:1705, 1986.

78. Olin JW: The role of duplex ultrasonography and screening for significant renal artery disease, Urol Clin North Am 21:215, 1994.

79. Olin JW et al: Utility of duplex scanning of the renal arteries for diagnosing significant renal artery stenosis, Ann Intern Med 122:833, 1995.

80. Hansen KJ et al: Renal duplex sonography: evaluation of clinical utility, J Vasc Surg 12:227, 1990.

81. Taylor DC et al: Duplex ultrasound scanning in the diagnosis of renal artery stenosis: a prospective evaluation, J Vasc Surg 7:363, 1988.

82. Taylor DC, Moneta GO, and Strandness DE Jr: Follow up of renal artery stenosis by duplex ultrasound, J Vasc Surg 9:410, 1989.

83. Hudspeth DA et al: Renal duplex sonography after treatment of renovascular disease, J Vasc Sug 18:381, 1993.

84. Havey RJ et al: Screening for renovascular hypertension: is renal digital-subtraction angiography the preferred noninvasive test? JAMA 254:388, 1985.

85. Kim D et al: Renal artery imaging: A prospective comparison of intra-arterial digital subtraction angiography with conventional angiography, Angiology 5:345, 1991.

86. Gedroyc WMW: Magnetic resonance angiography of renal arteries, Urol Clin North Am 21:201, 1994.

87. Kim D et al: Abdominal aorta and renal artery stenosis: evaluation with MR angiography, Radiology 174:727, 1990.

88. Debatin JF et al: Imaging of the renal arteries: value of MR angiography, AJR 157:981, 1991.

89. Loubeyre P et al: Screening patients for renal artery stenosis: value of three dimensional time-of-flight MR angiography, AJR 162:847, 1994.

90. Hertz SM et al: Evaluation of renal artery stenosis by magnetic resonance angiography, Am J Surg 168:140, 1994.

91. Rubin GD et al: Three-dimensional spiral computed tomographic angiography: an alternative imaging modality for the abdominal aorta and its branches, J Vasc Surg 18:656, 1993.

92. Galanski M et al: Renal arterial stenosis: spiral CT angiography, Radiology 189:185, 1993.

93. Maxwell MH, Rudnick M, and Waks AU: New approaches to the diagnosis of renovascular hypertension, Adv Nephrol 14:285, 1985.

94. Muller FB et al: The captopril test in identifying renovascular disease in hypertensive patients, Am J Med 80:633, 1986.

95. Wilcox CS: Use of angiotensin converting enzyme inhibitors for diagnosing renovascular hypertension, Kidney Int 44:1379, 1993.

96. Re R et al: Inhibition of angiotensin-converting enzyme for diagnosis of renal artery stenosis, N Engl J Med 298:582, 1978.

97. Hughes JS et al: Duration of blood pressure elevation in accurately predicting surgical cure of renovascular hypertension, Am Heart J 101:408, 1981.

98. Maxwell MH et al: Predictive value of renin determinations in renal artery stenosis, JAMA 238:2617, 1977.

99. Marks LS et al: Renovascular hypertension: does the renal vein renin ratio predict operative results? J Urol 115:365, 1976.

100. Novick AC et al: Diminished operative morbidity and mortality in renal revascularization, JAMA 246:749, 1981.

101. Olin JW et al: Renovascular disease in the elderly: an analysis of 50 patients, J Am Coll Cardiol 5:1232, 1985.

102. Pickering TG et al: Recurrent pulmonary oedema in hypertension due to bilateral renal artery stenosis: treatment by angioplasty or surgical revascularization, Lancet 2:5512, 1988.

103. Diamond JR: Flash pulmonary edema and diagnostic suspicion of occult renal artery stenosis, Am J Kidney Dis 21:328, 1993.

104. Messina LM et al: Renal revascularization for recurrent pulmonary edema in patients with poorly controlled hypertension and renal insufficiency: a distinct subgroup of patients with atherosclerotic renal artery occlusive disease, J Vasc Surg 15:73, 1992.

105. Olin JW, Graor RA, and Bacharach JM: Renal artery stenting for control of congestive heart failure, J Am Coll Cardiol 23(suppl):96A, 1994 (abstract).

106. Case DB et al: Long-term efficacy of captopril in renovascular and essential hypertension, Am J Cardiol 49:1440, 1982.

107. Havelka et al: Long-term experience with captopril in severe hypertension, Br J Pharmacol 14(suppl 2):71S, 1982.

108. Ernst CB et al: Autogenous saphenous vein aortorenal autografts: a ten-year experience, Arch Surg 105:855, 1972.

109. Stoney RJ and Olofsson PA: Aortorenal arterial autografts: the last two decades, Ann Vasc Surg 2:169, 1988.

110. Khauli RB, Novick AC, and Coseriu CV: Renal revascularization and polytetrafluoroethylene grafts, Cleve Clin Q 51:365, 1984.

111. Cormier JM et al: Renal artery revascularization with polytetrafluoroethylene bypass graft, Ann Vasc Surg 4:471, 1990.

112. Lagenau P, Michel JB, and Charrat JM: Use of polytetrafluoroethylene grafts for renal bypass, J Vasc Surg 5:738, 1987.

113. Novick AC, Jackson CL, and Straffon RA: The role of renal autotransplantation in complex urologic reconstruction, J Urol 143:45, 1990.

114. Dubernard JM et al: Renal autotransplantation versus bypass techniques for renovascular hypertension, Surgery 97:529, 1985.

115. Van Bockel JH et al: Extracorporeal renal artery reconstruction for renovascular hypertension, J Vasc Surg 13:101, 1991.

116. Brewster DC and Darling RC: Splenorenal arterial anastomosis for renovascular hypertension, Ann Surg 189:353, 1979.

117. Khauli R, Novick AC, and Ziegelbaum W: Splenorenal bypass in the treatment of renal artery stenosis: experience with 69 cases, J Vasc Surg 2:547, 1985.

118. Chibaro EA, Libertino JA, and Novick AC: Use of hepatic circulation for renal revascularization, Ann Surg 199:406, 1984.

119. Valentine RJ et al: Asymptomatic celiac and superior mesenteric artery stenoses are more prevalent among patients with unsuspected renal artery stenosis, J Vasc Surg 14:195, 1991.

120. Fry RE and Fry WJ: Supraceliac aortorenal bypass with saphenous vein for renovascular hypertension, Surg Gynecol Obstet 168:181, 1989.

121. Novick AC et al: Use of the thoracic aorta for renal arterial reconstruction, J Vasc Surg 19:605, 1994.

122. Shahian DM et al: Simultaneous aortic and renal artery reconstruction, Arch Surg 115:1491, 1980.

123. Tarazi RY et al: Simultaneous aortic reconstruction and renal revascularization: risk factors and late results in 89 patients, J Vasc Surg 5:709, 1987.

124. Hansen KJ et al: Contemporary surgical management of renovascular disease, J Vasc Surg 16:319, 1992.

125. Bredenberg CE et al: Changing patterns in surgery for chronic renal artery occlusive diseases, J Vasc Surg 15:1018, 1992.

126. Libertino JA et al: Renal revascularization to preserve and restore renal function, J Urol 147:1485, 1992.

127. Libertino JA et al: Changing concepts in surgical management of renovascular hypertension, Arch Int Med 148:357, 1988.

128. Van Bockel JH et al: Surgical treatment of renovascular hypertension caused by arteriosclerosis: influence of preoperative factors on blood pressure control early and late after reconstructive surgery, Surgery 101:698, 1987.

129. Lawrie GM et al: Renovascular reconstruction: factors affecting long-term prognosis in 919 patients followed up in 31 years, Am J Cardiol 63:1085, 1989.

130. Hallett JW Jr et al: Renovascular operations in patients with chronic renal insufficiency: do the benefits justify the risks? J Vasc Surg 5:622, 1987.

131. Dean RH et al: Evolution of renal insufficiency in ischemic nephropathy, Ann Surg 213:446, 1991.

132. Morris GC, Heider CF, and Moyer JH: The protective effect of subfiltration arterial pressure on the kidney, Surg Forum 6:623, 1956.

133. Zinman L and Libertino JA: Revascularization of the chronic totally occluded renal artery with restoration of renal function, J Urol 118:517, 1977.

134. Scheeft P et al: Renal revascularization in patients with total occlusion of the renal artery, J Urol 124:184, 1980.

135. Bedoya L et al: The effect of baseline renal function on the outcome following renal revascularization, Cleve Clin J Med 56:415, 1989.

136. Mercier C et al: Occlusive disease of the renal arteries and chronic renal failure: the limits of reconstructive surgery, Ann Vasc Surg 4:166, 1990.

137. Chaikof EL et al: Ischemic nephropathy and concomitant aortic disease: a ten-year experience, J Vasc Surg 19:135, 1994.

138. Vidt DG et al: Atheroembolic renal diseases: an association with renal artery stenosis, Cleve Clin J Med 56:407, 1988.

139. Textor SC et al: Renal function limiting antihypertensive therapy as an indication for renal revascularization, Arch Intern Med 143:2208, 1983.

140. Wasser WG et al: Restoration of renal function after bilateral renal artery occlusion, Arch Intern Med 141:1647, 1981.

141. Kaylor W et al: Reversal of end-stage renal failure with surgical revascularization in patients with atherosclerotic renal artery occlusion, J Urol 141:486, 1989.

142. Grüntzig A et al: Treatment of renovascular hypertension with percutaneous transluminal dilatation of renal/artery stenosis, Lancet 1:801, 1978.

143. Hayes JM et al: Experience with percutaneous transluminal angioplasty for renal artery stenosis at the Cleveland Clinic, J Urol 139:488, 1988.

144. Sos TA et al: Percutaneous transluminal renal angioplasty in renovascular hypertension due to atheroma or fibromuscular dysplasia, N Engl J Med 309:274, 1983.

145. Cicuto KP et al: Renal artery stenosis: anatomic classification for percutaneous transluminal angioplasty, AJR 137:599, 1981.

146. Canzanello VJ et al: Percutaneous transluminal renal angioplasty in management of atherosclerotic renovascular hypertension: result in 100 patients, Hypertension 13:163, 1989.

147. Staessen J et al: Blood pressure during long-term converting enzyme inhibition predicts the curability of renovascular hypertension by angioplasty, Am J Hypertens 1:208, 1988.

148. Luft FC, Grim, and Weinberger MH: Intervention in patients with renovascular hypertension and renal insufficiency, J Urol 130:654, 1983.

149. Pickering TG et al: Renal angioplasty in patients with azotemia and renovascular hypertension, J Hypertens 4(suppl 6):S667, 1986.

150. Bell BM, Reid J, and Buist TA: Percutaneous transluminal angioplasty improves blood pressure and renal function in renovascular hypertension, Q J Med 63:393, 1987.

151. O'Donovan RM et al: Preservation of renal function by percutaneous renal angioplasty in high-risk elderly patients: short-term outcome, Nephron 60:187, 1992.

152. Martin LG, Casarela WJ, and Gaylord GM: Azotemia caused by renal artery stenosis: treatment by percutaneous transluminal angioplasty, AJR 150:839, 1988.

153. Gutierrez OH, Izzo JL, and Burgener FA: Transluminal recanalization of an occluded renal artery: reversal of anuria in a patient with a solitary kidney, AJR 137:1254, 1981.

154. Mann JFE et al: Dilatation to avoid dialysis: angioplasty of an occluded renal artery with a coronary guiding catheter, Lancet 1:579, 1985.

155. Weibull H et al: Percutaneous transluminal angioplasty vs surgical reconstruction of atherosclerotic renal artery stenosis: a prospective, randomized trial, J Vasc Surg 18:841, 1993.

156. Dixon GD, Anderson S, and Crouch TT: Renal arterial rupture secondary to percutaneous transluminal angioplasty treated without surgical intervention, Cardiovasc Intervent Radiol 9:83, 1986.

157. Olin JW and Wholey M: Rupture of the renal artery 9 days after percutaneous transluminal angioplasty, JAMA 257:518, 1987.

158. Rees CR et al: Palmaz stent in atherosclerotic stenosis involving the ostia of the renal arteries: preliminary report of a multicenter study, Radiology 181:507, 1991.

159. Wilms GE et al: Renal artery stent placement with use of the wall stent endoprosthesis, Radiology 179:457, 1991.

160. Hennequin LM et al: Renal artery stent placement: Long-term results with the Wallstent endoprosthesis, Radiology 191:713, 1994.

161. Joffre F et al: Midterm results of renal artery stenting, Cardiovasc Intervent Radiol 15:313, 1992.
162. Bacharach JM et al: Patency and clinical experience with endovascular stents for the treatment of osteal renal artery stenosis, J Vasc Surg 1994 (abstract).
163. Tegtmeyer CJ et al: Percutaneous transluminal angio-plasty: treatment of choice for renovascular hypertension due to fibromuscular dysplasia, Radiology 143:631, 1982.
164. Archibald GR, Beckmann CF, and Libertino JA: Focal renal artery stenosis caused by fibromuscular dysplasia: treatment by percutaneous transluminal angioplasty, AJR 151:593, 1988.

CHAPTER NINETEEN

ARTERIAL ANEURYSMS

Patrick J. O'Hara

GENERAL CONSIDERATIONS

Definition

An *aneurysm* is defined as a circumscribed dilation of an artery, or a blood-containing swelling connecting directly with the lumen of an artery. Aneurysms may be classified according to their shape, such as saccular or fusiform, or their etiology. They are also subclassified according to their location. Although there is no universal agreement regarding the precise size of arterial enlargement required to qualify for the designation of aneurysm, a widely accepted view holds that a dilation of an artery to twice the maximum transverse diameter of the adjacent, uninvolved artery should be defined as an aneurysm. Similar dilation that is less than twice normal should be described as arterial ectasia. Histologically a true aneurysm involves the entire arterial wall and contains all three microscopic arterial layers. In contrast, *pseudoaneurysms,* which may be anastomotic or traumatic, are localized, contained disruptions of the native artery, and their walls are formed only by fibrous tissue.

Classification

From a practical perspective the classification of an arterial aneurysm according to its assumed etiology and observed location offers the most usefulness in planning effective management. Traditionally aneurysms have been classified according to their presumed pathogenesis as either atherosclerotic, mycotic, traumatic, dissecting, congenital, or inflammatory (see the box, on this page). The pathogenesis of most aneurysms is a matter of conjecture, however, and some of the traditional classifications may be misleading. For example, although atherosclerotic arterial occlusive disease and arterial aneurysms may coexist in some patients, a causal relationship has yet to be established. Zarins et al[1] have reasoned that aneurysmal dilation may be an adaptive mechanism used to compensate for diminished arterial flow secondary to occlusive disease but this view is still speculative. Consequently those aneu-rysms traditionally considered atherosclerotic in origin are currently more precisely described by the term *degenerative aneurysms.* Similarly the term *mycotic,* commonly used to describe an infected aneurysm, is more precisely applied to aneurysms caused by fungal sepsis. The term inflammatory aneurysm is usually used clinically to describe a particular variation of abdominal aortic aneurysm, often involving the iliac arteries, in which the aneurysm is surrounded by a dense fibrous reaction that is often adherent to adjacent structures.[2,3] Confusion may arise because the inflammatory arteritides may be associated with the formation of aneurysms presumably caused by weakening of the arterial wall by inflammation not associated with microorganisms. Traumatic aneurysms are pseudoaneurysms that are due to direct arterial damage. They may be iatrogenic, such as those caused by catheter injuries, or noniatrogenic, such as those associated with thoracic aortic deceleration injuries. Congenital aneurysms are rare and may be associated with developmental abnormalities involving the arterial wall leading to weakness and subsequent dilatation.[4] Finally, dissecting aneurysms, although uncommon, are recognized with increasing frequency and are probably associated with a biochemical or mechanical defect involving the arterial media.

CLASSIFICATION OF ARTERIAL ANEURYSMS

Atherosclerotic (degenerative)

Mycotic (infected)

Inflammatory

Arteritis

Traumatic

Congenital

Dissecting

Natural History and Clinical Manifestations

The natural history of arterial aneurysms varies with the etiology and location of the aneurysm and is probably related to some extent to the size of the artery involved and the time the lesion has been present. Progressive expansion with eventual rupture is most commonly associated with aneurysms involving larger arteries, such as the aorta, but may occur in any location. When large arteries are involved, untreated rupture is associated with pain, exsanguination, and death. Embolization of thrombotic or atheromatous debris originating in the aneurysm or thrombosis of the aneurysm with associated distal ischemia may also originate from aortic aneurysms but is more commonly observed in aneurysms involving smaller arteries such as the popliteal or carotid arteries. Larger aneurysms, especially in confined spaces such as the neck, mediastinum or axilla may cause symptoms from space occupation and pressure on adjacent structures. Finally, the presence of a pulsatile mass may alert the patient or the clinician to the presence of an aneurysm. The diagnosis should generate a careful search for the presence of other aneurysms that may coexist in approximately 5% to 50% of patients presenting with an aortic or peripheral aneurysm.[5-7]

Therapeutic Objectives

For all aneurysms the therapeutic objectives are twofold: to eliminate the inherent risks of the aneurysm itself, which are rupture, thrombosis, or the production of emboli, and to maintain adequate arterial perfusion.

Relative Frequency by Location

The distribution of 1449 true aneurysms surgically treated at the Cleveland Clinic in the Department of Vascular Surgery from January 1, 1989 through June 1, 1995 are illustrated in Fig. 19-1 (Departmental Vascular Registry, unpublished data). The most commonly encountered aneurysms involved the infrarenal aortoiliac arteries, accounting for approximately two thirds of the total true aneurysms treated during the interval. Suprarenal and thoracoabdominal aortic aneurysms comprised 10% (151 of 1449) of true aneurysms, whereas femoral (8%), popliteal (4%), visceral (3%), and carotid (1%) aneurysms were less commonly encountered. Eighty-seven true aneurysms (6%) encompassed a miscellaneous group consisting of brachiocephalic aneurysms and other rare lesions. Although the precise distribution may vary among centers, the relative frequency of occurrence of aneurysmal disease in each arterial segment depicted in Fig. 19-1 is probably reasonably representative of the relative prevalence and recognition of each lesion.

ANEURYSMS INVOLVING THE INFRARENAL AORTOILIAC ARTERIES

The majority of aortic aneurysms involve the infrarenal aorta. Among 1136 aneurysms involving the aorta that were operated on at the Cleveland Clinic Foundation between January 1, 1989 and June 1, 1995, 985 (87%) involved the infrarenal aortoiliac arteries, whereas 151 (13%) involved the suprarenal or thoracoabdominal aorta (Fig. 19-2).

Incidence and Prevalence

Incidence is defined as the rate at which an event occurs and is expressed as the number of new cases observed during a defined interval of time. *Prevalence*, in contradistinction, is defined as the total number of cases observed in a population at a specific time. The incidence of an event or observation may vary with the time period sampled,

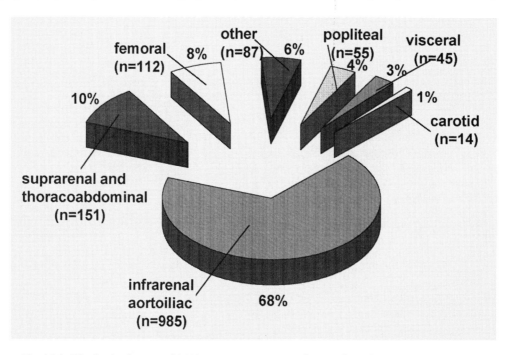

Fig. 19-1. Distribution by type of 1449 true aneurysms treated surgically in the Department of Vascular Surgery at the Cleveland Clinic from 1/1/89 through 6/1/95.

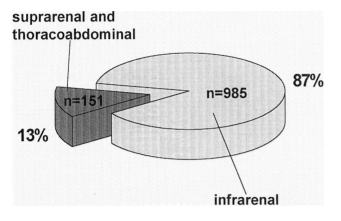

suprarenal and thoracoabdominal

n=151

13%

n=985

87%

infrarenal

Fig. 19-2. Distribution by extent of 1136 true aneurysms involving the aorta treated surgically in the Department of Vascular Surgery at the Cleveland Clinic from 1/1/89 through 6/1/95.

whereas its prevalence depends on the characteristics of the population sampled.

A survey of the Rochester, Minnesota, population over the three decades from 1951 through 1980 demonstrated an incidence of 21 abdominal aortic aneurysms per 100,000 person-years. Furthermore, an absolute increase in the number of aneurysms in each decade of the study was noted. The male-to-female ratio in this study was 2:1 compared with the 5:1 ratio observed among referral patients.[8] Large autopsy surveys reported the discovery of an abdominal aortic aneurysm in approximately 2% of postmortem examinations.[9]

The prevalence of abdominal aortic aneurysms reported in several recent studies varies from 1% to 16%, depending on the age and sex distribution of the particular population surveyed as well as the density of preselected comorbidities such as hypertension or atherosclerotic occlusive disease.[10] An apparent increase in the prevalence of abdominal aortic aneurysms among some families and among the siblings of patients with aneurysms has been reported, an observation supporting the influence of genetic factors in aneurysm pathogenesis.[10-13] Among the siblings of patients presenting with abdominal aortic aneurysms, 25% to 29% of their male and 6% to 7% of their female siblings also had aneurysms.[10,14,15]

Although screening of unselected populations for the presence of abdominal aortic aneurysms is probably not cost-effective, the survey of selected populations of patients in which the prevalence of aneurysms is likely to be high may have merit. Considering patients presenting with aortic aneurysms, screening of first-degree relatives over the age of 55 years has been advocated.[10,15]

Natural History

The natural history of an abdominal aortic aneurysm is one of progressive enlargement to eventual rupture. Although the rate of enlargement varies among individuals, abdominal aortic aneurysms have been reported to enlarge at a mean rate of 0.39 cm/yr.[16,17] The reported cumulative 5-year survival rate for patients with unresected atherosclerotic infrarenal aneurysms larger than 6 cm is 6%.[18]

Numerous studies have demonstrated the single greatest risk factor associated with aneurysm rupture is its size factor associated with aneurysm rupture is its size on presentation.[19-21] In a study by Crane[22] aneurysms less than 6 cm in diameter had a 4% rupture rate, whereas those greater than 6 cm in diameter had an 82% rupture rate. Other work by Szilagyi et al[18] has confirmed these results. More recent data suggest that the risk of rupture with time increases when the aneurysm diameter at presentation exceeds 5 cm as measured by ultrasonography or computed tomography (CT) scans.[21,23] Small aneurysms can also rupture and should not be regarded as innocuous. Szilagyi et al[18], in 1966, demonstrated that 19.5% of unrepaired aneurysms less than 6 cm in diameter ruptured with a mortality rate of 55%. Among aneurysms discovered at autopsy, 18% of those found ruptured at postmortem examination were less than 5 cm in diameter.[19] In another report by Cronenwett et al,[24] 18% of unrepaired aneurysms that were less than 6 cm in diameter at the time of discovery eventually ruptured. This event was associated with a 66% mortality rate. The actuarial rupture rate in this series was 6%/yr.

Clinical Manifestations

An asymptomatic abdominal aortic or iliac aneurysm may present as a pulsatile abdominal mass that is found either by the patient or is discovered as an incidental finding on physical examination. Increasingly, asymptomatic aortic aneurysms are diagnosed as unsuspected lesions detected by abdominal ultrasound examinations or CT scans performed for the investigation of unrelated problems.

In contrast, symptomatic aortic or iliac aneurysms typically present with severe lumbar, flank, or abdominal pain probably caused by stretching of the peritoneum as the aneurysm expands. The aneurysm may be tender to palpation at this time. Although some patients with acutely symptomatic aneurysms may stabilize for a short time because their ruptures are contained by the retroperitoneal structures, others may rapidly advance to free rupture. This progression is accompanied by the development of signs of peritoneal irritation by intraperitoneal blood and is usually rapidly followed by collapse and profound hypovolemic shock. Because of the frequent association of severe coronary disease among patients with aortic aneurysms, the hypoperfusion associated with aneurysm rupture can occasionally precipitate myocardial ischemia, which may complicate the presentation and delay diagnosis. Rarely aortic aneurysms can rupture into the vena cava and lead to fulminant high-output congestive heart failure or evidence of venous hypertension in the lower extremities. Subsequent venous hemorrhage into the urinary bladder has produced gross hematuria.

Less commonly, aortic aneurysms may be the source of atheromatous emboli, which may lead to digital gangrene and limb loss.[25] In a series of 1034 aortic aneurysms operated on at the Cleveland Clinic Foundation from January 1, 1989 through February 28, 1995, only 9 (1%) were resected because of the presenting symptom of atheromatous embolization (Departmental Vascular Registry, unpublished data).

AORTIC IMAGING TECHNIQUES

Lateral lumbar spine x-ray films

Ultrasonography

CT scan

MRI scan

Angiography

    Conventional

    Digital subtraction

Diagnosis

With an adequate level of awareness, the diagnosis of abdominal aortic aneurysm should be made on the basis of a good history and physical examination alone in the majority of patients. Recent studies have suggested, however, that a substantial number of asymptomatic abdominal aortic aneurysms may be missed on the basis of physical examination alone.[26]

Because of the importance of early diagnosis and accurate size assessment in the successful management of abdominal aortic and iliac aneurysms, a variety of imaging techniques have been developed to facilitate their detection of and to permit an accurate determination of their sizes. These imaging methods are summarized in the box on this page. Historically, lateral lumbar spine x-ray films have long been recognized to provide an inexpensive means to measure the diameter of the abdominal aorta. However, with this method, the image is magnified by approximately 25% and calcification in the aortic wall, present in only about 60% of the population at risk for aneurysm development, is required for visualization. Abdominal ultrasonography is inexpensive, well tolerated, and usually accurate. It has become the preferred method for diagnosis, size determination, and sequential follow-up examinations of most aneurysms involving the infrarenal aortoiliac arterial segments. Accuracy is degraded, however, by obesity. Furthermore, visualization of the thoracic and visceral aorta is obscured by the gas in the thoracic cavity, and bowel gas may limit visualization of the iliac vessels in the pelvis. CT scans offer excellent visualization of the entire aortoiliac system and are currently the preoperative imaging technique of choice when aneurysm resection is indicated or when ultrasound images are inadequate. Angiography is useful in selected patients to define the arterial anatomy before resection. However, because mural thrombus lines the aneurysm sack, aortography is not a reliable means to diagnose an aneurysm or to accurately determine its size. Aortography is not absolutely necessary unless findings on the CT scan suggest proximal extension of the aneurysm to involve the visceral vessels or is required to delineate associated occlusive disease.[27] Occasionally the CT scan may suggest suprarenal extension of the aneurysm in the presence of a tortuous proximal neck. In this situation a lateral aortogram will usually define the proximal extent of the aneurysm. Magnetic resonance imaging (MRI) scans are emerging as the modality of choice, especially for determining the anatomic details of aortic dissections. Future imaging techniques include variations of the CT scan such as spiral CT, ultrafast CT with an electron beam imaging, or bolus dynamic slip-ring cine CT scans as well as magnetic resonance angiography (MRA) incorporating three-dimensional imaging software. The development of faster acquisition times for MRI scanning should provide better images of aortic aneurysms that may be rotated in space to provide more accurate assessment of the pathoanatomy of the aneurysms. The development of software to allow computer-assisted reconstruction of digitized images acquired by CT and MRI scans holds the promise of producing dynamic and multidimensional reproductions of aneurysms that may facilitate unprecedented views of these lesions and permit more effective approaches to treatment.[27]

Important anatomic factors that commonly influence the management of an aortic aneurysm include its proximal and distal extent, the presence of associated arterial occlusive disease, especially involving the visceral or lower-extremity arteries, and the presence of associated aneurysms. Although less frequently encountered, situations such as the presence of a contained rupture, aortic dissection, infection, or atheroemboli also significantly influence surgical strategy. Unusual but important considerations include atypical anatomy associated with inflammatory aneurysms, venous anomalies, aortocaval fistulas, and previous arterial or colon surgery. The presence of horseshoe kidney is often associated with anomalies of both the arterial anatomy and urinary collecting systems as well. If a horseshoe kidney is discovered preoperatively, the coexisting aneurysm is most expeditiously repaired using a left thoracoabdominal retroperitoneal approach.[28,29]

Comorbidities and Preoperative Evaluation

The predictable risk factors associated with the repair of abdominal aortic aneurysms include advanced stage, the presence of coronary artery disease, chronic obstructive pulmonary disease, impaired renal function, hypertension, diabetes mellitus, and smoking.[30] The coexistence of severe, correctable coronary artery disease in patients presenting with aortic aneurysms has been documented by coronary angiography in 29% of 530 patients, as part of a preliminary assessment before abdominal aortic aneurysm repair at the Cleveland Clinic Foundation. These findings led to myocardial revascularization by coronary bypass in 22% and coronary angioplasty in 4% of these patients.[31-34] Preliminary treatment of severe correctable coronary artery disease has been shown to reduce early mortality following aneurysm repair to that of patients without associated coronary artery disease, and has been also shown to decrease cardiac mortality and prolong 5-year survival at late follow-up, especially among nondiabetic men.[34-36] Consequently at the Cleveland Clinic Foundation we currently recommend a cardiac stress test, such as thallium stress or dobutamine stress echo, for patients with no clinical evidence of coronary artery disease who are under serious consideration for abdominal aortic aneurysm repair. If the stress test is abnormal, then coronary angiography and appropriate intervention are recommended

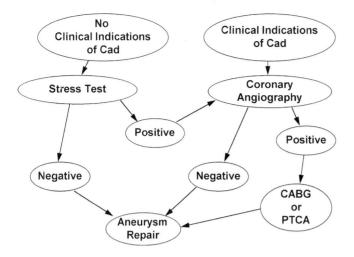

Fig. 19-3. Algorithm for the management of associated coronary artery disease before aortic aneurysm resection at the Cleveland Clinic. (*Cad,* Coronary artery disease; *CABG,* coronary artery bypass grafting; *PTCA,* percutaneous transluminal coronary angioplasty.)

before aneurysm repair. Patients who present with traditional indications of coronary artery disease—such as a convincing history of myocardial infarction, angina pectoris, or electrocardiographic changes suggesting myocardial ischemia—are evaluated by coronary angiography. This approach is diagramed in the algorithm illustrated in Fig. 19-3.

Indications for Repair

Currently surgical repair is indicated for all ruptured or symptomatic abdominal aortic aneurysms provided that the patient does not have an underlying preexisting medical condition that would preclude meaningful survival. Asymptomatic aneurysms should be repaired when the risk of the operation is less than the risk of aneurysm rupture. Although the decision to operate must be individualized according to the age and general condition of the patient and the rate of expansion of the aneurysm, the usual threshold for aneurysm repair is 5 cm.[37]

Surgical Management

Currently, direct surgical repair of the aneurysm by means of replacement with a synthetic graft is the treatment of choice for aneurysms involving the aortoiliac arteries. Advances in anesthetic management, most notably the adjunctive use of continuous epidural anesthesia in conjunction with general endotracheal anesthesia, have improved the pulmonary management of these patients and allowed for a less protracted period of ventilator dependence in most patients.[38] Improvements in the preoperative evaluation and, when necessary, the correction of coexisting coronary artery disease as well as improvements in perioperative cardiac monitoring, fluid management, and physiologic support have allowed even the very elderly to undergo safe aneurysm repair in most instances.[39]

Attempts to avoid an intraabdominal procedure by inducing thrombosis of the aneurysm by means of iliac ligation and adjunctive extraanatomic bypass have now been abandoned for the most part because of the persisting risk of aneurysm rupture, which usually occurs near the proximal neck.[40-43] Innovative attempts to develop a system that will allow the repair of aortoiliac aneurysms without the need for laparotomy are currently under way. These systems employ synthetic grafts that are delivered intraluminally under radiographic guidance and anchored by means of intraluminal, catheter-delivered, balloon expandable stents.[44-49] These systems currently have significant limitations including the risk of atheroembolization, the size of the delivery system required, the durability of the lightweight graft materials employed, problems with correct sizing, the delivery of bifurcated grafts, and persisting problems with the anchoring systems employed. Until the development of systems that can deliver bifurcated grafts, only approximately one in seven aortoiliac aneurysms have anatomy suitable for consideration of stent graft placement.[48,50] Clinical trials with an anchoring system have recently been halted because of materials failure involving the anchoring strut hooks used to attach the stent graft to the aortic wall. A potentially difficult problem is likely to be dislodgement of the stent attachments over time because of continued enlargement of the previously normal adjacent artery, which is commonly observed.

Currently surgical repair of aortoiliac aneurysms is most often accomplished by means of a midline or transverse abdominal incision with exposure of the aortoiliac system in the retroperitoneum after retracting the viscera laterally. Other maneuvers, such as medial visceral rotation, have been proposed to allow better exposure of the proximal infrarenal and visceral aorta.[51] Some surgeons prefer to use a retroperitoneal approach through the left flank or via a low left thoracoabdominal incision with equally good results.[52-54] Each approach has advantages and disadvantages depending on the particular anatomic features encountered, and each should be part of the armamentarium of the experienced vascular surgeon.

The usual aortoiliac aneurysm is currently repaired by replacement with a synthetic graft. After heparinization and the application of inflow and outflow arterial clamps, the aneurysm is incised, mural thrombus is removed, and lumbar arterial back bleeding is controlled. The synthetic graft, usually dacron or polytetrafluoroethylene (PTFE), is inserted by suturing it from within the aneurysm using the method described by Creech.[55] An end-to-end proximal anastomosis is required and is usually preferred distally. The autonomic plexus crossing the left iliac artery is preserved whenever possible, especially in sexually active male patients, and an attempt is made to preserve hypogastric perfusion to diminish problems with impotence in males and colon ischemia in both sexes.[56,57] On occasion, implantation of the inferior mesenteric artery is required if the colon circulation is compromised.[56] The aneurysm sac is closed over the graft, the heparin is neutralized with protamine sulfate, and the abdominal incision is closed after hemostasis has been attained. The patient is transferred to the intensive care unit for close monitoring and support only after the surgeon is assured that distal perfusion is adequate.

Adjuncts to Aortic Aneurysm Repair

The routine use of intraoperative autotransfusion has been demonstrated to result in a reduction in the perioperative homologous blood requirement at the time of aortic aneurysm repair and is now accepted by most vascular surgeons.[58] In the elective situation the preoperative donation of autologous blood is feasible in most patients and results in further reduction of the banked blood requirement associated with aneurysm repair, especially when combined with intraoperative autotransfusion.[59] Preoperative autologous blood donation has the further advantages of providing fresh coagulation factors and lessening the drain on homologous blood supplies.

Results

It is generally agreed that common factors influencing early postoperative mortality following abdominal aortic aneurysm repair are the necessity for emergency operation, advanced age of the patient, and the presence of associated comorbidities especially coronary artery, pulmonary, and renal disease.

The early postoperative mortality rates following abdominal aortic aneurysm repair are dramatically lower for elective operations than for emergency operations.[60] Representative early mortality rates for the emergency repair of symptomatic or ruptured abdominal aortic aneurysms range from 19% to 50%.[7,60] This wide variation probably reflects the condition of the patient at the time the emergency operation is undertaken. Patients who are moribund with profound hypotension and active intraperitoneal hemorrhage at the time of operation are less likely to survive than those who have had their retroperitoneal hemorrhages temporarily tamponaded and arrive in the operating room in a relatively stable hemodynamic condition. In contrast, representative early mortality rates for elective infrarenal aortic aneurysm repair has been reported to range from 3.5% to 11%.[7,60] More recently the elective postoperative mortality rate for infrarenal abdominal aortic aneurysm repair has continued to improve.[60] At our own center a steady decline in early postoperative mortality has been observed, from 9.6% from 1968 through 1973, to 1.8% in the most recent era. The current mortality for 887 infrarenal abdominal aortic aneurysms operated on at the Cleveland Clinic Foundation from January 1, 1989 through February 28, 1995 is 1.8% for asymptomatic aneurysms and 15% for symptomatic aneurysms, a figure that includes symptomatic intact aneurysms as well as those that are freely ruptured (Fig. 19-4, Departmental Vascular Registry, unpublished data).

The cumulative 6-year survival of patients who survive repair of ruptured abdominal aortic aneurysms (22%) is less than that of patients who undergo elective repair of their aneurysms (60%). Furthermore, cardiac complications account for most of the late deaths. These and other data suggest that an aggressive approach to the detection and treatment of severe associated coronary artery disease is warranted to enhance late survival, especially among nondiabetic men.[34-36]

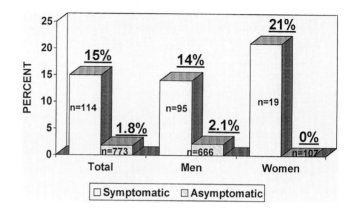

Fig. 19-4. Hospital mortality rates according to presentation and gender for 887 infrarenal abdominal aortic aneurysms repaired at the Cleveland Clinic from 1/1/89 through 2/28/95.

Early and Late Results of Aortic Aneurysm Repair in Octogenarians

The early and late results of 106 infrarenal and 8 juxtarenal abdominal aortic aneurysm repairs performed in 114 consecutive octogenarians (mean age, 83 years) during 10 years (1984 through 1993) at the Cleveland Clinic were reported recently.[61]

The 30-day mortality rate for the entire series was 14%, but it declined from 23% (11 of 48) during the first 5 years to 8% (5 of 66) during the second 5 years of the study ($P = 0.028$). Fatal complications occurred in 9 of the 94 patients (9.6%) with asymptomatic abdominal aortic aneurysms, and in 7 (35%) of the 20 patients who had symptomatic abdominal aortic aneurysms ($P = 0.008$). Considering only patients with asymptomatic abdominal aortic aneurysms, the early mortality rate in the second 5 years (4%) improved significantly ($P = 0.038$) compared with that for the first 5 years (17%) of the study period.

The cumulative 5-year survival rate of 48% for 97 available operative survivors was not quite so good as that (59%) for the normal male U.S. population at the age of 80 years ($P < 0.0001$). Nevertheless, the 5-year survival rate was 80% for 27 operative survivors who received previous myocardial revascularization compared with 38% for 70 others who did not ($P = 0.0077$).

Multiple Cox regression analysis suggested that the presence of abdominal aortic aneurysm symptoms and the preoperative serum creatinine level significantly influenced the initial 30-day survival rate but did not influence the long-term survival of operative survivors. Conversely a history of previous myocardial revascularization did not affect the initial postoperative survival rate, but it did favorably influence late survival. A high perioperative homologous transfusion requirement had a deleterious effect on both early and late survival rates.

We concluded that repair of abdominal aortic aneurysms in properly selected octogenarians is safe and durable. When otherwise indicated, it should not be withheld on the basis of advanced age alone. Prior treatment of severe coronary artery disease is associated with enhanced late survival, but patient selection probably is an important consideration in this respect.[61]

ANEURYSMS INVOLVING THE SUPRARENAL AND THORACOABDOMINAL AORTA

Pathogenesis

Proximal extension of an aortic aneurysm to involve the visceral segment of the abdominal aorta and the thoracic aorta is relatively uncommon, comprising only 10% of all true aneurysms treated surgically in the Department of Vascular Surgery from January 1989 through June 1995 (Fig. 19-1). By convention this consideration excludes aneurysms involving the aortic arch as well as those confined exclusively to the thoracic aorta.

Thoracoabdominal aortic aneurysms, which involve the thoracic as well as the abdominal aorta, are classified according to their extent according to a system proposed by Crawford et al.[62] Group I aneurysms involve all of the descending thoracic and upper abdominal aorta; group II aneurysms involve all of the descending thoracic aorta and all of the abdominal aorta; group III aneurysms involve the distal descending thoracic aorta and the abdominal aorta; group IV aneurysms involve most or all of the abdominal aorta distal to the diagphram including the segment from which the visceral vessels arise (see the box, this page).

The etiology of the extensive aneurysms is most commonly degenerative disease in approximately 80% to 88% of patients and aortic dissection in most (12% to 17%) of the remainder.[62-64] The natural history of patients with untreated thoracoabdominal aortic aneurysms is usually one of eventual rupture with exsanguination and death. The actuarial survival of 94 patients with thoracoabdominal aortic aneurysms who did not undergo surgical repair has been reported to be only 24% at 2 years, and half of the deaths were due to aneurysm rupture.[65]

Indications for Intervention

Because the morbidity associated with thoracoabdominal aortic aneurysm repair is substantially greater than that associated with the treatment of infrarenal aneurysms, the indications for thoracoabdominal repair should be more conservative. Furthermore, the accepted diameter at which an asymptomatic thoracoabdominal aortic aneurysm is likely to rupture is not as well established as that for infrarenal aneurysms. The thoracic aorta is normally larger than the infrarenal abdominal aorta, commonly measuring nearly 3 cm in transverse diameter. Aneurysms that are enlarging, symptomatic, or have evidence to suggest contained rupture on CT or MRI scans should be repaired because the risk of rupture is presumably imminent. Asymptomatic aneurysms should be seriously considered for repair when their diameters exceed twice the normal aortic diameter (6 cm).[66]

Surgical Management

Surgical replacement of the aneurysmal thoracoabdominal aorta is best accomplished through a left thoracoabdominal approach as described by Crawford et al.[62] For group I and II aneurysms an incision through the left fifth intercostal space and extended to a midline or left paramedian abdominal incision usually is required for adequate exposure. For group III and IV aneurysms an

CLASSIFICATION OF THORACOABDOMINAL AORTIC ANEURYSMS

Group I
Involves all of the descending thoracic aorta and the proximal abdominal aorta

Group II
Involves all of the descending thoracic aorta and all of the abdominal aorta

Group III
Involves the distal descending thoracic aorta and the abdominal aorta

Group IV
Involves all of the abdominal aorta distal to the diaphragm

approach through the eighth or ninth interspace, which is similarly extended to a midline or left paramedian abdominal incision. Exposure is facilitated by the use of a split endotracheal tube, which allows selective collapse of the left lung during the thoracic portion of the procedure. The diaphragm is incised radially through the crus to preserve as much phrenic innervation as possible, and the viscera are rotated to the patient's right to expose the left lateral and posterior aspects of the aorta. The aorta is clamped proximally, opened along its posterior aspect, and mural thrombus is removed. Back bleeding from the visceral vessels as well as the iliac arteries is usually controlled from within the aneurysm by means of balloon occlusion catheters. An albumin-coated knitted dacron graft of suitable size is sewn into place from within the aneurysm using a continuous nonabsorbable suture. Following completion of the proximal anastomosis, large intercostal vessels are identified and attached to the graft as a button using the inclusion technique. Perfusion is reestablished to the intercostal vessels and the visceral vessels are attached in a similar manner. Often the celiac, superior mesenteric and right renal arteries can be incorporated in one button. Subsequently the left renal artery can be reconstructed by means of a short dacron graft from the aortic graft or reimplanted into the aortic graft as the situation dictates. Perfusion is reestablished to the visceral vessels, and the rest of the reconstruction is carried out as is done for a standard infrarenal aortic aneurysm.

Complications and Special Considerations

One of the most dreaded complications of thoracoabdominal aortic aneurysm repair is paraplegia, which is reported to occur in 4% to 40% of patients who survive long enough to be neurologically evaluated.[62-64] This complication ultimately results from spinal cord ischemia secondary to hypoperfusion at the cellular level. Multiple factors probably play a role in the development of spinal cord ischemia. Its incidence is roughly proportional to proximal extent of the aortic cross-clamp level and the clamp time required for graft placement.

Cerebrospinal fluid (CSF) pressure rises with aortic cross-clamp application. Since spinal cord perfusion pressure is influenced by the gradient between the arterial pressure and the CSF pressure, some investigators have proposed CSF drainage during aortic cross-clamping to augment spinal cord perfusion. Although the effectiveness of this maneuver is controversial, some surgeons use CSF drainage to maintain the CSF pressure below 10 cm H_2O during the perioperative period.[67] Epidural cooling of the spinal cord has also been proposed as a method of spinal cord preservation during thoracoabdominal aortic aneurysm repair.[68] To date, this method has been used in only a small number of patients, and its clinical effectiveness has not yet been adequately demonstrated. The use of pharmacologic agents such as naloxone and intrathecal papaverine has also been proposed.[69,70]

Coagulopathy that results in massive hemorrhage has also been observed during the perioperative period following thoracoabdominal aortic aneurysm repair. This complication is also probably related to several factors including hypothermia, acidosis, dilution of coagulation factors associated with high-volume transfusion requirements and the release of fibrinolytic metabolic products associated with visceral ischemia. Aggressive and preemptive replacement of coagulation factors and platelets, minimizing clamp time, and careful attention to core body temperature have been helpful but have not eliminated the problem.

In an effort to minimize these complications, more surgeons are using a combined approach involving CSF drainage, atriofemoral bypass, and sequential aortic clamping with retrograde perfusion during the repair of extensive thoracoabdominal aortic aneurysms.[71] The theoretic advantages of this approach are diminished spinal cord and visceral ischemic times, better temperature control, improved autotransfusion capabilities, and better left ventricular decompression. Whether these potential advantages will overshadow the disadvantages associated with systemic heparinization, the management of cannulation sites, and the potential for atheromatous embolization during retrograde perfusion remain to be demonstrated.

Results

Contemporary hospital mortality data for 147 aortic aneurysm repairs involving the suprarenal and thoracoabdominal aorta performed at the Cleveland Clinic from January 1989 through February 1995 are illustrated in Fig. 19-5 (Departmental Vascular Registry, unpublished data). As expected, the early postoperative mortality rate for elective procedures (11%) is superior to that of emergency operations (38%). The published results of thoracoabdominal aortic aneurysm repair reported in three large selected series are summarized in Table 19-1.[62-64] Early overall postoperative mortality rates ranged from 9% to 35%. Actuarial 5-year survival of operative survivors was 60%, which was superior to that of patients with thoracoabdominal aortic aneurysms who did not undergo surgical repair. Neurologic deficits, defined as paraplegia or paraparesis, calculated for operative survivors ranged from 11% to 21% for the entire patient populations and were severalfold higher for the extensive aneurysms treated in groups I and II.

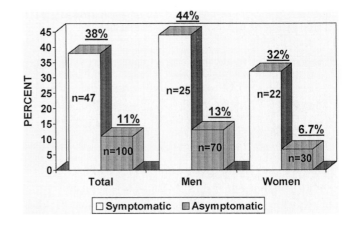

Fig. 19-5. Hospital mortality rates according to presentation and gender for 147 suprarenal and thoracoabdominal aortic aneurysms repaired at the Cleveland Clinic from 1/1/89 through 2/28/95.

Table 19-1. Representative Mortality and Morbidity Following Thoracoabdominal Aortic Aneurysm Repair

	Series		
	Crawford et al[62]	Cox et al[64]	Cambria et al[63]
Date published	1986	1992	1989
No. of patients	605	129	55
Early mortality			
Overall	9	35	35
Elective	9	15	24
Nonelective	19	63	80
Late survival (actuarial)	60	NA	NA
Neurologic deficit (% survivors)			
Overall	12	21	11
Groups I + II	38	39	NA
Groups III + IV	5	12	NA

NA, Not available.

ANEURYSMS INVOLVING THE FEMORAL AND POPLITEAL ARTERIES

Incidence

True aneurysms involving the femoral and popliteal arteries are relatively rare, comprising 8% and 4% of the true aneurysms treated surgically in the Department of Vascular Surgery at the Cleveland Clinic from January 1989 through June 1995. Nevertheless, when considered together, femoral and popliteal aneurysms encompassed 53% (167 of 313) of all surgically treated true aneurysms not involving the aortoiliac arteries (Fig. 19-1; Departmental Vascular Registry, unpublished data).

In contrast, pseudoaneurysms commonly involve the femoral artery but are relatively unusual in the popliteal location. Pseudoaneurysms of the femoral arteries, which

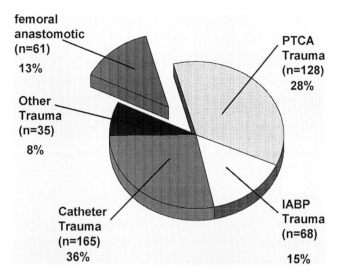

Fig. 19-6. Distribution by type of 457 femoral pseudoaneurysms treated surgically in the Department of Vascular Surgery at the Cleveland Clinic from 1/1/89 through 6/1/95.

are often related to either iatrogenic or noniatrogenic trauma, are now being encountered with increasing frequency, probably because of an increase in the number of catheter-mediated intervention procedures performed via the femoral arteries. Furthermore, anastomotic pseudoaneurysm formation may complicate vascular reconstruction involving the femoral artery. During the same period, 457 femoral pseudoaneurysms were treated at our center (unpublished data, Departmental Vascular Registry); 87% were due to trauma, whereas only 61 (13%) were anastomotic femoral pseudoaneurysms (Fig. 19-6).

Natural History and Clinical Manifestations

The natural history of both femoral and popliteal true aneurysms is not known with certainty since reports to date are retrospective and therefore subject to selection bias. In a series of 100 patients presenting with 172 femoral aneurysms, 40 patients were asymptomatic on presentation. One hundred and five aneurysms in this series were initially treated conservatively with a mean follow-up interval of 28 months. The overall thrombosis rate was about 3%, and the overall rupture rate was 2%.[6,72,73] In a series of 100 popliteal aneurysms in 69 patients followed for a mean of 50 months, 23% of the involved extremities that were not surgically treated eventually required amputation, most often above the knee.[72,74,75]

Most true aneurysms involving the femoral or popliteal arteries are either asymptomatic on presentation or cause ischemic symptoms by local thrombosis or distal embolization. Rupture of true aneurysms involving these arteries is rare, occurring in up to 5% of limbs.[6,72,73,76-79] Although pseudoaneurysms can also thrombose or be a source of emboli, they are more likely than true aneurysms to present with symptoms of expansion or rupture. Both varieties can cause symptoms by compression of adjacent structures.

Diagnosis

The diagnosis of femoral and popliteal aneurysms can usually be made on the basis of history and physical examination. Symptomatic lesions may present with associated limb ischemia from aneurysm thrombosis or with evidence of peripheral embolization. An asymptomatic pulsatile mass presenting in the groin or popliteal fossa can be confirmed to be an aneurysm by ultrasound examination. CT and MRI scans can also visualize femoral and popliteal aneurysms but are more expensive and only infrequently are required for diagnosis. Ultrasonography can also differentiate between other common mass lesions in the popliteal or femoral areas, such as Baker's cyst, femoral hernia, or lymphocele formation, which may transmit underlying arterial pulsations. Arteriography is usually necessary to define the arterial anatomy and to plan repair.

Treatment

Because of their benign natural history, asymptomatic femoral aneurysms are probably best treated conservatively unless they significantly enlarge.[73] Symptomatic femoral aneurysms, in contrast, are best treated by direct surgical repair using interposition grafts. Autogenous saphenous vein is the material of choice, but synthetic grafts may be required if vein is either unavailable or its diameter is inadequate.

Since the available information suggests that untreated, asymptomatic, popliteal aneurysms are associated with substantial late morbidity, they are best treated agressively.[6,72-79] Small popliteal aneurysms are best treated by ligation and bypass with autogenous saphenous vein. Synthetic grafts may be required if autogenous vein is unavailable or inadequate, but their long-term patency rates are inferior. Large popliteal aneurysms may require evacuation of mural thrombus and interposition grafting to eliminate the mass effect of the aneurysm.

Thrombosed aneurysms may require adjunctive thrombectomy or, if time permits, preoperative thrombolytic therapy to restore an obliterated outflow bed.

Results

The early and late results of the surgical treatment of atherosclerotic femoral aneurysms is largely anecdotal because of the relative rarity of these lesions. A cumulative 5-year patency rate of 83% for autogenous saphenous vein and dacron interposition grafts has been reported.[80]

In contrast, the operative mortality associated with popliteal aneurysm repair ranges from 0% to 2%.[74,76-78,81] The 5-year cumulative patency rates for popliteal aneurysm repair range from 77% to 100% for saphenous vein grafts to 29% to 74% for synthetic grafts.[74,76-78,81] Late patency is also better among patients treated for asymptomatic aneurysms, presumably because the run-off has not yet been compromised by distal embolization.[72]

ANEURYSMS INVOLVING THE BRACHIOCEPHALIC ARTERIES

General Considerations

The material in the following section has been published previously[82] and is summarized and shortened. The essential, original articles are listed in the references.

Incidence

Aneurysmal degeneration of the innominate, extracranial carotid, subclavian, and axillary arteries is rare.[83,84] Reliable data regarding the natural history of these lesions are unavailable because no large series of untreated cases has been published. Definitive guidelines for the optimal treatment of these rare aneurysms await the accumulation of data regarding sufficiently large numbers of patients with brachiocephalic aneurysms to allow statistical analysis. Because these lesions are rare, the development of large patient registries probably will be required to provide such data.

Etiology

The etiologies usually proposed for brachiocephalic aneurysms are atherosclerosis, trauma, or infection.[83,84] In the preantibiotic era, mycotic aneurysms secondary to syphilitic arteritis were the most common type observed. Luetic aneurysms are now extremely rare, and mycotic aneurysms are more likely to be related to infected arterial puncture sites associated with parenteral drug abuse.[85] Other less common etiologies include various forms of medial degeneration,[86] fibromuscular disease, arteritis, and congenital aneurysms.[86]

Pathophysiology

The pathophysiology of these lesions has certain common features. In general, rupture is rare, although it has been reported in each location, usually associated with catastrophic consequences.[6,83,84,87] Depending on the location, size, and rate of expansion of the aneurysm, symptoms of nerve, tracheal, esophageal, or venous compression from its mass effect may prevail. The most threatening aspect of these aneurysms is the propensity for embolism and thrombosis leading to end-organ ischemia or infarction.[83,84]

Therapeutic Objectives

The therapeutic objectives for all brachiocephalic aneurysms involve common priorities. Foremost is the preservation of life and neurologic function, followed closely by preservation or restoration of end-organ function. Optimally the embolic source is eliminated or excluded, and perfusion is maintained by resection and arterial reconstruction or ligation and bypass. Recent progress in the development of endovascular catheter techniques for the placement of intraluminal prosthetic grafts may considerably simplify the treatment of brachiocephalic aneurysms.[45,49,88] The placement of a transluminal prosthetic graft stent device for treatment of a subclavian artery aneurysm has been reported.[46] The applicability of this approach to the treatment of many aneurysms may currently be limited, but further refinements of this technique seem likely to permit its more widespread application.

CAROTID ANEURYSMS

Incidence

The true prevalence of extracranial carotid aneurysms is unknown because most early reports are anecdotal, and more recent series from single institutions contain relatively few patients. There is general agreement that the incidence, especially of nontraumatic carotid aneurysms, is probably low.

Etiology

The most common causes of extracranial carotid aneurysms are atherosclerosis and trauma.[13,89-93] Other less common causes include infection, cystic medial necrosis, dissection, fibromuscular dysplasia, and congenital anomalies.[94]

Clinical Manifestations

Symptomatic extracranial carotid aneurysms most commonly present with stroke, focal transient ischemic attacks, amaurosis fugax, or evidence of retinal infarction—all of which are manifestations of the propensity for embolization from these lesions. The reported incidence of associated focal neurologic symptoms is 15% to 67%.* A pulsatile neck mass is commonly observed, whereas rupture is particularly uncommon. Other less commonly reported symptoms include dysphagia, respiratory stridor, Horner's syndrome, and symptoms of cranial nerve compression, presumably from the mass effect of large aneurysms.[84] Associated abdominal aortic and peripheral arterial aneurysms are reported in about one patient in four.[89,93,97,98,101]

Diagnosis

The presence of a pulsatile mass in the neck on physical examination should raise the suspicion of aneurysmal disease, although the most frequent explanation for this finding is a prominent, tortuous carotid artery, commonly observed in elderly, hypertensive women.[84] The differential diagnosis also includes carotid body tumors, lymphadenopathy, cystic hygromas, salivary gland tumors, metastatic tumors, cervical lymphoma, lipomas, peritonsillar abscess, and brachial cleft cysts.[84] Careful examination usually is sufficient to distinguish these entities from aneurysm, and duplex scanning or intraarterial digital subtraction angiography usually provides the definitive diagnosis. Until arterial pathology has been ruled out, biopsy of a neck mass is unwise because of the risk of hemorrhage, which may be substantial and difficult to control.

Indications for Intervention

Because of the rarity of these lesions, definitive data about the natural history of untreated extracranial carotid aneurysms are unavailable. In a recent report atherosclerotic extracranial carotid artery aneurysms treated nonoperatively and followed over a mean interval of 6.3 years were associated with a 50% ipsilateral stroke rate in three of six patients.[93] Two of these strokes were preceded by focal transient ischemic attacks, although one patient had an asymptomatic carotid aneurysm on initial presentation. Because of the significant potential for neurologic morbidity, extracranial carotid aneurysms should be treated when the diagnosis is made.

*References 13, 89, 90, 92, 93, 95-101.

Treatment Options

The procedure of choice for the treatment of extracranial carotid aneurysms is direct reconstruction.[89,93,99] Reconstructive methods include resection of the aneurysm and primary anastomosis with reimplantation of the external carotid artery if the carotid bifurcation is involved. A saphenous vein interposition graft may be used in a variety of configurations when required. Although synthetic grafts may be employed for this purpose, we believe that autogenous reconstruction is usually preferable.

Aneurysmorrhaphy or resection with patch angioplasty may be applicable to the reconstruction of some saccular aneurysms.[89,98,101] Transposition of the distal internal carotid artery to the transected external carotid artery is another alternative.[93,101] Rarely, ligation of the internal carotid artery or balloon catheter occlusion may be required for the management of nonreconstructible aneurysms extending to the base of the skull or beyond. Although this approach may have an occasional role, it has been associated with substantial mortality and morbidity.[89,99,101] Extracranial to intracranial bypass may have a role in the management of these unusual patients.

Results

Data regarding the early and late results of the treatment of extracranial carotid aneurysms are sparse. The collected early results of 66 procedures performed from 1972 to 1985 for the correction of atherosclerotic extracranial carotid aneurysms reported that ligation appears to be associated with a 40% incidence each of mortality and morbidity, although only 5 patients were treated in this manner.[99] Considering the 61 patients who underwent direct carotid reconstruction, 13 (8%) sustained transient neurologic deficits and 8 (5%) had permanent strokes. The single death in this subset yielded a mortality rate of 1.6%. One patient in the collected series was reported to exhibit late postoperative ipsilateral hemispheric transient ischemic attacks.[93,99]

AXILLOSUBCLAVIAN ANEURYSMS

Incidence

Aneurysms of the subclavian and axillary arteries are unusual, and for this reason accurate data regarding the prevalence of these lesions in the general population are unavailable.

Etiology

Axillosubclavian aneurysms are most commonly caused by trauma or atherosclerosis, although other less common etiologies such as infection (especially syphilis in the past), arteritis, medial degeneration, fibromuscular disease, and congenital anomalies account for occasional aneurysms.[83,87,102] Among axillosubclavian aneurysms, about half are thought to result from atherosclerosis, and chronic trauma or extrinsic compression are also frequent etiologies.[6,83,103,104] Chronic injury of the arterial wall by a cervical rib or fibrous band at the thoracic outlet or from improper crutch use may lead to poststenotic dilatation or frank aneurysm formation.[83,105-108] Aneurysms involving an aberrant right subclavian artery are now recognized with increasing frequency.[109-112]

Clinical Manifestations

Axillosubclavian aneurysms may be asymptomatic but are usually associated with symptoms of peripheral embolism or pressure from the presence of a pulsatile mass against surrounding neurovascular structures.[83,87,102,113] Rupture is relatively uncommon.[83,87,102] Rarely, dysphagia or respiratory distress can occur from esophageal or tracheal compression secondary to atherosclerotic aneurysmal degeneration of an aberrant right subclavian artery originating from the distal aortic arch.[114-118]

Thirty-three percent (7 of 21) of the patients with true axillosubclavian aneurysms had other associated aneurysms.[87]

Diagnosis

A careful history and physical examination coupled with a high index of suspicion should yield the diagnosis in most instances. Among patients presenting with symptoms of upper-extremity ischemia or embolism, small-vessel involvement may be demonstrated by noninvasive arterial studies. Cervical spine x-ray films should be obtained to identify a cervical rib. Ultrasound examination may identify dilatation and intimal injury in the extrathoracic subclavian and axillary arteries. Arteriography is required to confirm the diagnosis and define the extent of the aneurysm as well as the state of the outflow bed. As technology improves, MRI and MRA will probably play an increasingly important role in the definition of these lesions in the future.

Treatment Options

Because of their associated risks, it is generally agreed that surgical repair of axillosubclavian aneurysms is indicated if the patient's general medical condition is acceptable.[83,87,102]

The surgical procedure required depends on the etiology, size, and location of the aneurysm. Although resection of the aneurysm with end-to-end anastomosis is preferred, arterial interposition grafting or bypass is usually required.[83,87,102,119,120] We believe that autogenous saphenous vein is the graft material of choice, but vein availability or size discrepancy may dictate the need for synthetic graft placement. Concomitant thoracic outlet decompression and adjunctive peripheral embolectomy may also be needed. If an associated vasospastic disorder is present or if symptomatic irretrievable small-vessel emboli are present, a sympathectomy may be considered.[87] Perioperative thrombolytic therapy in this setting is probably associated with an increased risk of hemorrhage, but it may be a consideration in the treatment of the patient with small-vessel embolism and limb-threatening ischemia unresponsive to conventional therapy. Arterial ligation may be required for infected aneurysms or in other situations where reconstruction is not feasible but is accompanied by a 25% incidence of upper-extremity claudication.[87]

Patients who have required repair of axillary aneurysms for chronic crutch trauma should be retrained to use the

Canadian-style, elbow-supporting crutches to avoid further trauma to the arterial reconstruction.[105]

Results

Late follow-up (mean, 9.2 years) of 31 patients in one series included 3 patients who were not operated on and 28 who underwent operative repair. Of the 27 operative survivors, 1 required a forearm amputation 6 days after aneurysm repair because of distal arterial thrombosis. Eighteen other operative survivors who underwent aneurysm repair and arm revascularization had no recurrence of aneurysm or signs of ischemia at late follow-up. The 4 remaining patients who underwent thoracic outlet decompression alone had no late evidence of embolism or aneurysm rupture.[87] Cumulative 5- and 10-year survival rates for patients who underwent axillosubclavian aneurysm repair have been reported to be 87% and 62%, respectively.[121]

INNOMINATE ANEURYSMS

Incidence and Etiology

The actual incidence of innominate artery aneurysms is unknown since there are only a few cases reported.

Clinical Manifestations

Patients with innominate artery aneurysms are either asymptomatic, have chest discomfort, or have hoarseness caused by recurrent laryngeal nerve dysfunction. Dysphagia, mediastinal mass, and a right hemispheric stroke has been reported.[122,123] Emboli from innominate aneurysms theoretically may cause right upper-extremity ischemic symptoms.

Diagnosis

The diagnosis is usually made during the investigation of a mediastinal mass revealed on chest x-ray. MRI or contrast-enhanced CT scanning may differentiate aneurysm from tumor mass. Arch aortography confirms the diagnosis and is required to plan surgical reconstruction.

Treatment

Surgical repair is indicated, especially if the aneurysm is symptomatic, large or enlarging, and the patient is an acceptable surgical risk.

Optimal therapy involves excision of the aneurysm and restoration of upper-extremity and cerebral perfusion. Resection of a small aneurysm with end-to-end anastomosis has been reported, but direct replacement of the aneurysmal innominate artery with an interposition graft or a bifurcated graft to the right common carotid and subclavian arteries is usually necessary.[122,123] Synthetic grafts are usually required since the caliber of autogenous saphenous vein is probably inadequate. Ligation is rarely performed and intuitively seems less preferable than direct reconstruction.

Results

Data regarding early and late results of treatment of these rare lesions are largely anecdotal. In a recent report there were no operative deaths among six innominate

artery reconstructions for aneurysm, although one patient with preoperative neurologic symptoms sustained a postoperative brainstem infarct. The cumulative 5-year survival rate for patients who underwent innominate aneurysm reconstructions in this series was 63%.[121]

ANEURYSMS INVOLVING THE VISCERAL ARTERIES

Definition

Visceral aneurysms refer to those involving the celiac, superior, and inferior mesenteric arteries and their branches as well as the renal arteries. For the purposes of this review, however, renal artery aneurysms are considered separately in Chapter 18.

Incidence and Natural History

True aneurysms involving the nonrenal visceral arteries are relatively rare, involving only 1% (19 of 1449) of the true aneurysms treated surgically in the Department of Vascular Surgery at the Cleveland Clinic from January 1989 through June 1995. Among these patients, nonrenal visceral aneurysms comprised only 6% (19 of 313) of the aneurysms that did not involve the aortoiliac arteries but 42% (19 of 45) of those involving all visceral arteries.

Splenic artery aneurysms are reported to be the most common of the visceral aneurysms, followed by those involving the hepatic artery.[124-127] Little is known with certainty about the natural history of untreated visceral artery aneurysms. Splenic artery aneurysms are thought to be associated with female gender, portal hypertension, and multiple pregnancies.[126,128-130] Rupture is thought to occur infrequently, but most of the splenic artery aneurysms reported to occur in pregnant women had already ruptured by the time of their diagnosis.[125-130] Similarly, among those hepatic aneurysms reported, 20% to 44% had ruptured before their discovery.[127,128,131]

Diagnosis and Indications for Treatment

Surgical intervention is indicated for patients with symptomatic visceral artery aneurysms. Such patients usually present with abdominal pain because of rapid expansion or rupture of the aneurysm. Peritoneal signs and hemodynamic instability may quickly develop because of associated intraperitoneal hemorrhage. Often the diagnosis is made intraoperatively at the time of urgent laparotomy.

Asymptomatic visceral artery aneurysms are sometimes detected as incidental findings on angiograms, abdominal ultrasound examinations, and CT or MRI scans performed to evaluate other abdominal problems. Because the natural history of untreated visceral artery aneurysms is unclear and rupture is associated with substantial risk for mortality and morbidity, it seems justified to recommend intervention if the aneurysm is large and the patient is an acceptable surgical candidate.

Treatment

Splenic artery aneurysms are usually treated by ligation without arterial reconstruction since the spleen usually has adequate collateral circulation to maintain its viability. In contrast, hepatic artery aneurysms often require arterial reconstruction to maintain adequate perfusion to the liver parenchyma, since collateral circulation may be inadequate, especially if the gastroduodenal artery collateral is interrupted.[127,128,131] Other less common visceral aneurysms are managed with ligation and arterial reconstruction or ligation alone as the clinical situation dictates. In general, however, arterial continuity should be maintained if this is feasible. Excision of a saccular aneurysm with vein patch angioplasty, aneurysmorrhaphy, or autogenous interposition grafting may be used to maintain arterial continuity, depending on the intraoperative findings. Preoperative arteriography is required to assess collateral circulation and to plan reconstruction. In general, autogenous graft material is preferred because of the risk of graft sepsis in the setting of visceral ischemia.

The development of interventional catheter techniques that induce aneurysm thrombosis or, alternatively, allow the deployment of stent grafts may simplify the management of some visceral artery aneurysms.[132,133]

REFERENCES

1. Zarins CK et al: Differential enlargement of artery segments in response to enlarging atherosclerotic plaques, J Vasc Surg 7:386, 1988.
2. Crawford JL et al: Inflammatory aneurysms of the aorta, J Vasc Surg 2:113, 1985.
3. Pennell RC et al: Inflammatory abdominal aortic aneurysm: a thirty-year review, J Vasc Surg 2:859, 1985.
4. O'Hara PJ et al: Medial agenesis associated with multiple extracranial peripheral and visceral arterial aneurysms, J Vasc Surg 2:298, 1985.
5. Johnston KW and Scobie TK: Multicenter prospective study of nonruptured abdominal aortic aneurysms. I. Population and operative management, J Vasc Surg 7:69, 1988.
6. McCann RL: Basic data related to peripheral artery aneurysms, Ann Vasc Surg 4:411, 1990.
7. Taylor LM and Porter JM: Basic data related to clinical decision making in abdominal aortic aneurysms, Ann Vasc Surg 1:502, 1986.
8. Bickerstaff LK et al: Abdominal aortic aneurysms, the changing natural history, J Vasc Surg 1:6, 1984.
9. Carlson J and Sternby NH: Aortic aneurysm, Acta Chir Scand 127:466, 1964.
10. Webster MW et al: Ultrasound screening of first-degree relatives of patients with an abdominal aortic aneurysm, J Vasc Surg 13:9, 1991.
11. Tilson DM and Seashore MR: Fifty families with abdominal aortic aneurysms in two or more first-order relatives, Am J Surg 147:551, 1984.
12. Verloes A et al: Aneurysms of the abdominal aorta: familial and genetic aspects in three hundred thirteen pedigrees, J Vasc Surg 21:646, 1995.
13. Welling RE et al: Extracranial carotid artery aneurysms, Surgery 93:319, 1983.
14. Bengtsson H, Bergqvist D, and Sternby NH: Increasing prevalence of abdominal aortic aneurysms: a necropsy study, Eur J Surg 158:19, 1992.
15. Webster MW et al: Abdominal aortic aneurysm: result of a family study, J Vasc Surg 13:366, 1991.
16. Bernstein EF et al: Growth rates of small abdominal aortic aneurysms, Surgery 80:765, 1976.
17. Wolf YG and Bernstein EF: A current perspective on the natural history of abdominal aortic aneurysms, Cardiovasc Surg 2:16, 1994.
18. Szilagyi DE et al: Contribution of abdominal aortic aneurysmectomy to prolongation of life, Ann Surg 164:678, 1966.
19. Darling RC et al: Autopsy study of unoperated abdominal aortic aneurysms, Circulation 56(suppl II):161, 1977.
20. Johansson G et al: Survival in patients with abdominal aortic aneurysms: comparison between operative and nonoperative management, Eur J Vasc Surg 5:497, 1990.
21. Nevitt MP, Ballard DJ, and Hallett JW: Prognosis of abdominal aortic aneurysm: a population based study, N Engl J Med 321:1009, 1989.
22. Crane C: Arteriosclerotic aneurysm of the abdominal aorta, N Engl J Med 253:954, 1955.
23. Hallett JW Jr: Abdominal aortic aneurysm: natural history and treatment, Heart Dis Stroke 1:303, 1992.
24. Cronenwett JL et al: Actuarial analysis of variables associated with rupture of small abdominal aortic aneurysms, Surgery 98:472, 1985.
25. Lord JW et al: Unsuspected abdominal aortic aneurysms as the cause of peripheral arterial occlusive disease, Ann Surg 177:767, 1973.
26. Chervu A et al: Role of physical examination in detection of abdominal aortic aneurysm, Surgery 117:454, 1995.
27. O'Hara PJ: Preoperative arteriography versus other imaging techniques before elective abdominal aortic aneurysm repair. In Veith FJ, ed: Current critical problems in vascular surgery, vol 6, St Louis, 1994, Quality Medical Publishing.
28. Crawford ES et al: The impact of renal fusion and ectopia on aortic surgery, J Vasc Surg 8:375, 1988.
29. O'Hara PJ et al: Surgical management of abdominal aortic aneurysm and coexistent horseshoe kidney; review of a 31 year experience, J Vasc Surg 17:940, 1993.
30. Hertzer NR: Fatal myocardial infarction following abdominal aortic aneurysm resection, Ann Surg 192:667, 1980.
31. Hertzer NR et al: Routine coronary angiography prior to elective aortic reconstruction, Arch Surg 114:1336, 1979.
32. Hertzer NR et al: Coronary artery disease in peripheral vascular patients. A classification of 1000 coronary angiograms and results of surgical management, Ann Surg 199:223, 1984.
33. Young JR et al: Coronary artery disease in patients with aortic aneurysm: a classification of 302 coronary angiograms and results of surgical management, Ann Vasc Surg 1:36, 1986.
34. Hertzer NR et al: Late results of coronary bypass in patients with infrarenal aortic aneurysms. The Cleveland Clinic Study, Ann Surg 205:360, 1987.
35. Hertzer NR et al: Late results of coronary bypass in patients with peripheral vascular disease. I. Five-year survival according to age and clinical cardiac status, Cleve Clin Q 204:154, 1986.
36. Hertzer NR et al: Late results of coronary bypass in patients with peripheral vascular disease. II. Five-year survival according to sex, hypertension, and diabetes, Cleve Clin J Med 54:15, 1987.
37. Hollier LH, Taylor LM, and Ochsner J: Recommended indications for operative treatment of abdominal aortic aneurysms. Report of a subcommittee of the Joint Council of the Society for Vascular Surgery and the North American Chapter of the International Society for Cardiovascular Surgery, J Vasc Surg 15:1046, 1992.
38. Gottlieb A: Aortic reconstructive surgery: anesthetic considerations, Curr Opin Anesthesiol 6:35, 1993.
39. Hallett JW Jr et al: Subspecialty clinics: surgery. Selection and preparation of high risk patients for repair of abdominal aortic aneurysm, Mayo Clin Proc 69:763, 1994.

40. Inahara T et al: The contrary position to the nonresective treatment for abdominal aortic aneurysm, J Vasc Surg 2:42, 1985.

41. Karmody AM et al: The current position of non-resective treatment for abdominal aortic aneurysm, Surgery 94:591, 1980.

42. Pevec WC, Holcroft JW, and Blaisdell FW: Ligation and extraanatomic arterial reconstruction for the treatment of aneurysms of the abdominal aorta, J Vasc Surg 20:629, 1994.

43. Schwartz RA, Nichols WK, and Silver D: Is thrombosis of the infrarenal abdominal aortic aneurysm an acceptable alternative? J Vasc Surg 3:348, 1986.

44. Lazarus HM: Endovascular grafting for the treatment of abdominal aortic aneurysms, Surg Clin North Am 72:959, 1992.

45. Marin ML et al: Transluminally placed endovascular stented graft repair for arterial trauma, J Vasc Surg 20:446, 1994.

46. May J et al: Transluminal placement of a prosthetic graft-stent device for treatment of subclavian artery aneurysm, J Vasc Surg 18:1056, 1993.

47. Moore WS and Vescera CL: Repair of abdominal aortic aneurysm by transfemoral endovascular graft placement, Ann Surg 220:331, 1994.

48. Parodi JC: Endovascular repair of abdominal aortic aneurysms and other arterial lesions, J Vasc Surg 21:549, 1995.

49. Sayers RD, Thompson MM, and Bell PRF: Endovascular stenting of abdominal aortic aneurysms, Eur J Vasc Surg 7:225, 1993.

50. Cauter TA et al: Infrarenal aortic aneurysm structure: implications for transfemoral repair, J Vasc Surg 20:44, 1994.

51. Reilly LM et al: Optimal exposure of the proximal abdominal aorta: a critical appraisal of transabdominal medial visceral rotation, J Vasc Surg 19:375, 1994.

52. Cambria RP et al: Transperitoneal versus retroperitoneal approach for aortic reconstruction: a randomized prospective study, J Vasc Surg 11:314, 1990.

53. Leather RP et al: Comparative analysis of retroperitoneal and transperitoneal aortic replacement for aneurysm, Surg Gynecol Obstet 168:387, 1989.

54. Sicard GA et al: Comparison between the transabdominal and retroperitoneal approach for reconstruction of the infrarenal abdominal aorta, J Vasc Surg 5:19, 1987.

55. Creech O Jr: Endo-aneurysmorrhaphy and treatment of aortic aneurysm, Ann Surg 164:935, 1966.

56. Brewster DC et al: Intestinal ischemia complicating abdominal aortic surgery, Surgery 109:447, 1991.

57. O'Hara PJ: Aortoiliac revascularization in disorders of male sexual function. In Montague DK, ed: Disorders of male sexual function, Chicago, 1987, Year Book Medical Publishers.

58. O'Hara PJ et al: Intraoperative autotransfusion during abdominal aortic reconstruction, Am J Surg 145:215, 1983.

59. O'Hara PJ et al: Reduction in the homologous blood requirement for abdominal aortic aneurysm repair by the use of preadmission autologous blood donation, Surgery 115:69, 1994.

60. Katz DJ, Stanley JC, and Zelenock GB: Operative mortality rates for intact and ruptured abdominal aortic aneurysm in Michigan: an eleven-year statewide experience, J Vasc Surg 19:804, 1994.

61. O'Hara PJ et al: Ten-year experience with abdominal aortic aneurysm repair in octogenarians: early results and late follow-up, J Vasc Surg 21:830, 1995.

62. Crawford ES et al: Thoracoabdominal aortic aneurysms: preoperative and intraoperative factors determining immediate and long-term results of operations in 605 patients, J Vasc Surg 3:389, 1986.

63. Cambria RP et al: Recent experience with thoracoabdominal aneurysm repair, Arch Surg 124:620, 1989.

64. Cox GS et al: Thoracoabdominal aneurysm repair: a representative experience, J Vasc Surg 15:780, 1992.

65. Crawford ES and DeNatale RW: Thoracoabdominal aortic aneurysm: observations regarding the natural course of the disease, J Vasc Surg 3:578, 1986.

66. Williams GM: Management of thoracoabdominal aortic aneurysm. In Ernst CB and Stanley JC, eds: Current therapy in vascular surgery, ed 3, Philadelphia, 1995, Mosby–Year Book.

67. Murray MJ et al: Effects of cerebrospinal fluid drainage in patients undergoing thoracic and thoracoabdominal aortic surgery, J Cardiothorac Vasc Anesth 7:266, 1993.

68. Davison JK et al: Epidural cooling for regional spinal cord hypothermia during thoracoabdominal aneurysm repair, J Vasc Surg 20:304, 1994.

69. Acer CW et al: Combined use of cerebral spinal fluid drainage and naloxone reduces the risk of paraplegia in thoracoabdominal aneurysm repair, J Vasc Surg 19:236, 1994.

70. Svensson LG et al: Appraisal of cerebrospinal fluid alterations during aortic surgery with intrathecal papaverine administration and cerebrospinal fluid drainage, J Vasc Surg 11:423, 1990.

71. Safi HJ et al: Neurologic deficit in patients at high risk with thoracoabdominal aortic aneurysms: the role of cerebrospinal fluid drainage and distal aortic perfusion, J Vasc Surg 20:434, 1994.

72. Breslin DJ and Jewell ER: Peripheral aneurysm, Cardiol Clin 9:489, 1991.

73. Graham LM et al: Clinical significance of arteriosclerotic femoral artery aneurysms, Arch Surg 115:502, 1980.

74. Anton GE et al: Surgical management of popliteal aneurysms. Trends in presentation, treatment, and results from 1952-1984, J Vasc Surg 3:125, 1986.

75. Gifford RW Jr, Hines EA Jr, and Janes JM: An analysis and follow-up study of one hundred popliteal aneurysms, Surgery 33:284, 1953.

76. Dawson I et al: Popliteal artery aneurysms: long term follow-up of aneurysmal disease and results of surgical treatment, J Vasc Surg 13:398, 1991.

77. Inahara T and Toledo AC: Complications and treatment of popliteal aneurysms, Surgery 84:775, 1978.

78. Reilly MK, Abbott WM, and Darling RC: Aggressive surgical management of popliteal artery aneurysms, Am J Surg 145:498, 1983.

79. Whitehouse WM et al: Limb-threatening potential of arteriosclerotic popliteal artery aneurysms, Surgery 93:694, 1983.

80. Cutler BS and Darling RC: Surgical management of arteriosclerotic femoral artery aneurysms, Arch Surg 74:764, 1973.

81. Szilagyi DE, Schwartz RL, and Reddy DJ: Popliteal artery aneurysms, Arch Surg 116:724, 1981.

82. O'Hara PJ: Extracranial carotid, innominate, subclavian and axillary artery aneurysms. In Greenfield L, ed: Textbook of surgery: scientific principles and practice, Philadelphia, 1992, JB Lippincott.

83. Hobson RW, Israel MR, and Lynch TG: Axillosubclavian arterial aneurysms. In Bergan JJ and Yao JST, eds: Aneurysms: diagnosis and treatment, New York, 1982, Grune & Stratton.

84. Trippel OH et al: Extracranial carotid aneurysms. In Bergan JJ and Yao JST, eds: Aneurysms: diagnosis and treatment, New York, 1982, Grune & Stratton.

85. Miller CM et al: Infected false aneurysms of the subclavian artery: a complication in drug addicts, J Vasc Surg 1:684, 1984.

86. Fee HJ et al: Bilateral subclavian artery aneurysm associated with idiopathic cystic medial necrosis, J Thorac Cardiovasc Surg 26:387, 1978.

87. Pairolero PC et al: Subclavian-axillary artery aneurysms, Surgery 90:757, 1981.

88. Parodi JC, Palmaz JC, and Barone HD: Transfemoral intraluminal graft implantation for abdominal aortic aneurysms, Ann Vasc Surg 5:491, 1991.

89. Busuttil RW et al: Selective management of extracranial carotid arterial aneurysms, Am J Surg 140:85, 1980.

90. Krupski WC et al: Aneurysms of the carotid arteries, Aust N Z J Surg 53:521, 1983.

91. Morki B et al: Subject review. Extracranial internal carotid artery aneurysms, Mayo Clin Proc 57:310, 1982.

92. Sahlman A et al: Extracranial carotid artery aneurysms, Vasa 20:369, 1991.

93. Zwolak RM et al: Atherosclerotic extracranial carotid artery aneurysms, J Vasc Surg 1:415, 1984.

94. Hammon JW, Silver D, and Young WG Jr: Congenital aneurysm of the extracranial carotid arteries, Ann Surg 176:777, 1971.

95. Bour P et al: Aneurysm of the extracranial internal carotid artery due to fibromuscular dysplasia: results of surgical management, Ann Vasc Surg 6:205, 1992.

96. Dehn TCB and Taylor GW: Extracranial carotid artery aneurysms, Ann R Coll Surg 66:247, 1984.

97. Kaupp HA et al: Aneurysms of the extracranial carotid artery, Surgery 72:946, 1972.

98. McCollum CH et al: Aneurysms of the extracranial carotid artery: twenty-one years' experience, Am J Surg 137:196, 1979.

99. Painter TA et al: Extracranial carotid aneurysms: report of six cases and review of the literature, J Vasc Surg 2:312, 1985.

100. Pratschke E et al: Extracranial aneurysms of the carotid artery, Thorac Cardiovasc Surg 28:354, 1980.

101. Rhodes EL et al: Aneurysms of extracranial carotid arteries, Arch Surg 111:339, 1976.

102. Hobson RW et al: Atherosclerotic aneurysms of the subclavian artery, Surgery 85:368, 1979.

103. Israel M et al: Subclavian and axillary aneurysms: etiology, manifestations and management, J Med Soc N J 78:173, 1981.

104. McCollum CH et al: Aneurysm of the subclavian artery, J Cardiovasc Surg 20:159, 1979.

105. Abbott WM and Darling RC: Axillary artery aneurysms secondary to crutch trauma, Am J Surg 125:515, 1973.

106. Cormier JM et al: Arterial complications of the thoracic outlet syndrome: fifty-five operative cases, J Vasc Surg 9:778, 1989.

107. Mathes SJ and Salam AA: Subclavian artery aneurysm: sequela of thoracic outlet syndrome, Surgery 76:506, 1974.

108. Sanders RJ and Haug C: Review of arterial thoracic outlet syndrome with a report of five new instances, Surg Gynecol Obstet 173:415, 1991.

109. Esposito RA, Khalil I, and Spencer FC: Surgical treatment for aneurysm of aberrant subclavian artery based on a case report and review of the literature, J Thorac Cardiovasc Surg 95:888, 1988.

110. Harrison LH, Batson RC, and Hunter DR: Aberrant right subclavian artery aneurysm: an analysis of surgical options, Ann Thoracic Surg 57:1012, 1994.

111. Kieffer E, Bahnini A, and Koskas F: Aberrant subclavian artery: surgical treatment in thirty-three adult patients, J Vasc Surg 19:100, 1994.

112. Kiernan PD et al: Aneurysm of an aberrant right subclavian artery: case report and review of the literature, Mayo Clin Proc 68:468, 1993.

113. Salo JA et al: Diagnosis and treatment of subclavian artery aneurysms, Eur J Vasc Surg 4:271, 1990.

114. Austin EH and Wolfe WG: Aneurysm of aberrant subclavian artery with a review of the literature, J Vasc Surg 2:571, 1985.

115. Langman J: Arterial system. In Medical embryology: human development—normal and abnormal, Baltimore, 1963, Williams & Wilkins.

116. Poker N, Finby N, and Steinberg I: The subclavian arteries: roentgen study in health and disease, AJR 80:193, 1958.

117. Schmidt FE, Hewitt RL, and Flores AA: Aneurysm of anomalous right subclavian artery, South Med J 73:255, 1980.

118. Stone WM et al: Aberrant right subclavian artery: varied presentations and management options, J Vasc Surg 11:812, 1990.

119. Coselli JS and Crawford ES: Surgical management of aneurysms of the intrathoracic segment of the subclavian artery, Chest 91:704, 1987.

120. Neumayer LA et al: Atherosclerotic aneurysms of the axillary artery, J Cardiovasc Surg 33:172, 1992.

121. Bower TC et al: Brachiocephalic aneurysm: the case for early recognition and repair, Ann Vasc Surg 5:125, 1991.

122. Brewster DC et al: Innominate artery lesions: problems encountered and lessons learned, J Vasc Surg 2:99, 1985.

123. Schumacher PD and Wright CB: Management of arteriosclerotic aneurysm of the innominate artery, Surgery 85:489, 1979.

124. Jorgensen BA: Visceral artery aneurysms. A review, Dan Med Bull 32:237, 1985.

125. Stanley JC: Abdominal visceral aneurysms. In Haimovici H, ed: Vascular emergencies, New York, 1981, Appleton-Century-Crofts.

126. Stanley JC and Fry WJ: Pathogenesis and clinical significance of splenic artery aneurysms, Surgery 76:898, 1974.

127. Stanley JC, Thompson NW, and Fry WJ: Splanchnic artery aneurysms, Arch Surg 101:689, 1970.

128. Busuttil RW and Brin BJ: The diagnosis and management of visceral artery aneurysms, Surgery 88:619, 1980.

129. Trastek VF et al: Splenic artery aneurysms, Surgery 91:694, 1982.

130. de Vries JE, Schattenkerk ME, and Malt RA: Complications of splenic artery aneurysm other than intraperitoneal rupture, Surgery 91:200, 1982.

131. Weingarten MS and Nosher JL: Combined hepatic and gastric artery aneurysms: a case report and review of the literature, Ann Vasc Surg 1:598, 1987.

132. Baker JS et al: Splanchnic artery aneurysms and pseudoaneurysms: transcatheter embolization, Radiology 163:135, 1987.

133. Okazaki M et al: Percutaneous embolization of ruptured splanchnic artery pseudoaneurysms, Acta Radiol 32:349, 1991.

134. Johnston KW and the Canadian Society for Vascular Surgery Aneurysm Study Group: Nonruptured abdominal aortic aneurysm: six-year follow-up results from the multicenter prospective Canadian aneurysm study, J Vasc Surg 20:163, 1994.

135. Johnston KW and the Canadian Society for Vascular Surgery Aneurysm Study Group: Ruptured abdominal aortic aneurysm: six-year follow-up results of a multicenter prospective study, J Vasc Surg 19:888, 1994.

CHAPTER TWENTY

DISSECTION OF THE AORTA AND OTHER PERIPHERAL ARTERIES

Michael R. Jaff
Jeffrey W. Olin

Dissection of the aorta is one of the most catastrophic vascular events facing the clinician today. Despite heightened awareness of this disorder, the presenting symptoms and signs are myriad and often nonspecific, making the diagnosis difficult. There are few, if any, other conditions that require as prompt a diagnosis and treatment as aortic dissection, since the mortality rate of untreated aortic dissection within the first 48 hours may be as high as 1%/hr. The mortality rate is 80% at 14 days and 90% at 3 months.[1]

HISTORICAL PERSPECTIVE

Although autopsy confirmation of aortic dissection was made in 1761, Laennec in 1819 used the term "aneurysme dissequant," which translates to "dissecting aneurysm."[2] It has increasingly been recognized that the pathophysiology involves a hematoma that dissects rather than actual aneurysm formation. Therefore the term *aortic dissection* should be used instead of dissecting aneurysm. In the mid-1900s, investigators began to recognize the increased occurrence of aortic dissection.[1,3,4] Newer diagnostic modalities were developed, more potent antihypertensive agents became available to medically treat patients with aortic dissection, and innovative and more effective surgical techniques were employed in an attempt to lower the extremely high morbidity and mortality that occurred in untreated aortic dissection.

PATHOGENESIS AND ETIOLOGIC FACTORS

The inciting event in aortic dissection is a transverse tear in the aortic intima.[5] Blood within the true aortic lumen is then forcefully propelled through this intimal tear into the outer or middle layer of aortic media, forming a second, or false, lumen.[2] The dissection may propagate proximally

(retrograde) and/or distally (antegrade) and may narrow or occlude the origin of any branch arising from the aorta. Antegrade dissection is most common.

It is not uncommon for the dissection to "spiral," so that some aortic branches are supplied by the true lumen, whereas others are supplied by the false lumen. The false lumen may compress portions of the true lumen or vice versa.

The intimal tear most commonly involves approximately 50% of the aortic circumference. This gives rise to the appearance of an "intimal flap," a criterion often used for diagnosis during objective testing. Rarely circumferential dissection occurs and an intimal flap is not found.[6] The intimal tear originates in the ascending aorta in 65% of cases, transverse arch in 10%, the upper descending aorta (just distal to the origin of the left subclavian artery) in 20%, and more distally in the aorta in 5% of cases.[5] The false lumen may terminate at any point along the aorta, iliac or femoral arteries. Multiple intimal flaps and reentry sites may be found. The false lumen can thrombose, rupture, organize and form a pseudoaneurysm, compress the true lumen, or dissect in retrograde fashion. In the latter scenario the coronary ostia may occlude, the aortic valve may disrupt, or extension into the heart and pericardial space may occur, leading to pericardial effusion and tamponade.

The most feared complication of aortic dissection is aortic rupture. Retrograde dissection and rupture into the pericardial space, with resulting cardiac tamponade can occur. Antegrade dissection and rupture can lead to hemorrhage into the left pleural space, mediastinum, or abdomen. In patients with indications for surgical treatment, acute rupture before surgery occurs in approximatley 3% of cases. In 25 patients who underwent surgical repair for proximal dissections, no early rupture occurred, and only two ruptures developed in late follow-up. In 59 patients surgically treated for distal dissections, there was one early rupture and four late ruptures.[7] DeBakey et al[8] reported on the 20-year follow-up of 527 patients with aortic dissection. They noted that 29.3% of the late deaths were caused by the development and rupture of an aneurysm.

Aortic dissection occurs more often in males than in females, with a 2 to 3:1 male preponderance.[9] The disorder is more common in the sixth and seventh decades of life.

Systemic hypertension is the major predisposing risk factor for the development of aortic dissection. Patients with distal aortic dissection are more likely to have hypertension than those with proximal dissection. Spittell et al[9] reported that 86% of 88 patients with distal dissection had hypertension, whereas only 71% to 73% with proximal dissection had a documented history of hypertension.

Marfan's syndrome, a heritable disorder of connective tissue, has a high incidence of aortic dilatation, dissection, and rupture. In a large retrospective series of patients with Marfan's syndrome, 48% died as a result of aortic dissection or rupture.[10] Traditionally patients with Marfan's syndrome with aortic dilatation have been observed until hemodynamic changes became evident. However, as these changes were often unpredictable and life-threatening, the current approach is surgical intervention, even for distal dissection once the diagnosis is made.[11] Early surgical intervention of thoracic aortic aneurysms in Marfan's syndrome prolonged life expectancy 30 years in contrast to patients with Marfan's syndrome who did not receive such therapy.[12] Cosselli, Le Maire, and Büket[13] suggest that patients with Marfan's syndrome and asymptomatic thoracic or thoracoabdominal aneurysms should have elective surgical repair when the aortic diameter is greater than 5.5 cm.

Bicuspid aortic valve is a risk factor for aortic dissection, possibly as a result of abnormal shear forces on the proximal aorta.[14] Aortic dissection may occur in pregnancy, often in the third trimester. Underlying causes, such as hypertension or cystic medial necrosis, may be contributing factors in pregnancy.[15-17] Aortic dissection has been iatrogenically induced after angiographic procedures[18,19] and surgical vascular procedures.[20] Giant cell arteritis, Erdheim's cystic medial necrosis, aortic coarctation, and aortic trauma are other less likely causes of aortic dissection.[9] Rarely both ascending[21] and descending[22] aortic dissection have occurred in young weight lifters.

Isolated aortic dissections arising from the abdominal aorta are quite uncommon, with an incidence of 2.5% of all aortic dissections.[23] Hypertension occurs in 70% of cases of abdominal aortic dissections. Acute and chronic complications are comparable to those dissections arising in the thoracic aorta.

Another similar pathologic condition, the penetrating atherosclerotic aortic ulcer, may mimic or even cause aortic dissection. The penetrating aortic ulcer is "an ulcerating atheromatous lesion that disrupts the internal elastic lamina and burrows deeply into the media."[24] In 684 aortograms performed to diagnose aortic dissection, the incidence of a penetrating aortic ulcer was 2.3%.[25] The differences between an aortic ulcer and a dissection are subtle but important. Patients with penetrating ulcers are often elderly hypertensives with sudden back or chest pain. No intimal flap is seen, as a hematoma develops in the wall of the aorta. Large atheromas are present at the site of the ulcer, a finding uncommonly seen in the area of an intimal flap of a dissection.[25] Correct diagnosis of this condition is critical so that appropriate therapy and recommendations can be made. Surgery should be offered to any patient with hemodynamic instability, pseudoaneurysm formation, or rupture.[26] In the absence of the previously mentioned complications, the prognosis of penetrating aortic ulcers without surgical intervention may be quite good. In a small series of five patients followed medically, all five were alive at 30 months after the diagnosis.[27]

CLINICAL PRESENTATION

Although multiple classification schemes have been suggested for aortic dissection, the DeBakey et al[8,28] and Daily et al[29] methods have been most widely accepted (Table 20-1). These classifications are based on the location of the inciting intimal tear and dissection.

The most common symptom at presentation of aortic dissection is chest pain.[2] The sudden onset of ripping, tearing, shearing chest or upper back pain is a classic description. Although not diagnostic, the pain associated with aortic dissection often migrates as the dissection propagates from proximal (chest pain) to distal (back pain) sites. Back pain is more common in distal dissections (Table 20-2). Painless aortic dissection is uncommon, occurring in only 15% of patients in one large clinical series.[9]

Transient cerebral ischemia or completed stroke results from involvement of the carotid or vertebral arteries by the dissection and can be found in 2% to 8% of cases (Table 20-2). Syncope may be a manifestation of stroke or decreased cardiac output from acute aortic insufficiency or

Table 20-1. Classification of Aortic Dissection

DeBakey et al[8,28]		Daily et al[29]	
Type I	Ascending, transverse, descending aorta	Type A	All dissections involving the ascending aorta
Type II	Ascending aorta	Type B	All other dissections
Type III			
A	Descending aorta to the diaphragm		
B	Descending aorta to and below the diaphragm		

pericardial tamponade. Interruption of circulation to the spinal cord can lead to paraparesis or paraplegia.[33] Overall 15% to 20% of patients will have some neurologic abnormality. Acute lower-extremity ischemia from dissection involving the iliac or femoral arteries has been reported in approximately 20% of cases.[34,35] Unusual symptoms at presentation may include hoarseness of voice, hematochezia, and dysphagia.[9]

Physical examination can often be helpful in supporting the suspicion of aortic dissection. Although hypertension is the most commonly found physical finding, shock and cardiovascular collapse may be present in 3% to 18% of patients (Table 20-2). Hypertension may be a result of preexisting hypertension, previously undiagnosed renal artery stenosis,[36] involvement of the renal arteries by the dissection itself,[37] or a result of a response to pain. A diminished or absent pulse is a helpful finding, if present, and can be detected in the carotid,[38] subclavian, axillary, radial, ulnar, and femoral arteries.[9]

The new onset of a diastolic murmur of aortic valve insufficiency can be an important clue to the diagnosis of aortic dissection. Aortic insufficiency is a common finding, especially in proximal dissection, and has been reported in 11% to 55% of cases (Table 20-2). Cardiac dysrhythmias and myocardial infarction may occur because of extension of the dissection into the coronary arteries or the region of the atrioventricular node.[2] Physical findings suggestive of a pericardial effusion such as soft, muffled cardiac tones, distended neck veins, and a paradoxic pulse may be seen in a minority of patients.[39]

DIAGNOSIS

Since aortic dissection can mimic other diseases, the clinician needs a high index of suspicion for this disorder.

Because of the increasing mortality rates of untreated aortic dissection with time, a prompt and accurate diagnosis must be made. Some simple diagnostic tests are used to exclude other causes of the symptoms.

An electrocardiogram must be performed to exclude acute myocardial infarction, as thrombolytic therapy mistakenly administered in acute aortic dissection carries a high mortality rate.[40-42]

Laboratory studies such as hematocrit, serum creatinine, and blood urea nitrogen levels are nonspecific. However, abnormalities of these parameters in the face of aortic dissection may suggest the extent of the dissection. Elevated serum creatinine kinase (CK) levels are seen in many patients with aortic dissection. However, the isoenzyme pattern of CK elevation is predominantly CK-MM, indicating a nonspecific marker of skeletal muscle damage.[43] This is in contrast to the CK elevation in acute myocardial infarction, in which at least 15% of the isoenzyme elevation is CK-MB.

Chest radiography is nonspecific but may also exclude other causes of chest pain including pneumothorax. The most common radiographic findings on chest roentgenography include widening of the superior mediastinum (Fig. 20-1), pleural effusion, or displacement of the aortic intimal calcification by 10 mm or more.[44,45] Although chest radiography in some series may have a sensitivity of 81% and specificity of 89% in aortic dissection diagnosis, it cannot be used as the sole diagnostic test.[46]

Computed tomography (CT) has been considered a reliable, rapid, and safe diagnostic method. The primary diagnostic criterion for the diagnosis of aortic dissection with CT is the demonstration of two contrast-filled lumens separated by an intimal flap. One recent series reported a sensitivity and specificity of greater than 95%.[47] However, several pitfalls can occur including inadequate contrast

Table 20-2. Clinical Symptoms/Signs on Presentation with Aortic Dissection

	Proximal (Type I, II, A)				Distal (Type IIIB)			
	Investigator (Ref.)				Investigator (Ref.)			
Symptom/Sign (%)	Crawford et al[30] (n = 229)	Glower et al[31] (n = 52)	Fradet et al[32] (n = 156)	Spittell et al[9] (n = 102)	Crawford et al[30] (n = 317)	Glower et al[31] (n = 69)	Fradet et al[32] (n = 103)	Spittell et al[9] (n = 66)
Chest pain	66*	NA	51	59	79*	NA	43	29
Back pain	NA	NA	18	12	NA	NA	42	52
Abdominal pain	NA	NA	7	8	NA	NA	14	15
Cerebrovascular accident	7	5	6†	2	3	8	NA	0
Renal insufficiency	10	8	NA	NA	12	0	NA	NA
Shock	NA	18	18	3	NA	8	3	1
Aortic insufficiency	55	31	11†	16	NA	25	NA	0
Rupture	4	35	30†	NA	8	0	NA	NA

NA, Not available.
*No differentiation into type/location of pain.
†No differentiation between location of dissection.

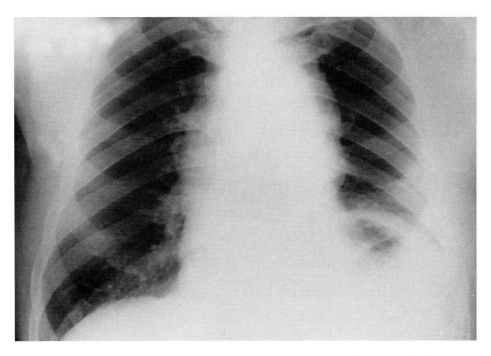

Fig. 20-1. Chest radiograph demonstrates a widened mediastinum and a left pleural effusion.

Table 20-3. Comparison of Diagnostic Methods in Aortic Dissection

Series (Ref.)	No. of Patients	Sensitivity/Specificity (%)			
		CT	**MRA/MRI**	**TTETEE**	**Aortography**
Erbel et al (1989)[52]	82	83/100	NA	99/98	88/94
Nienaber et al (1993)[48]	110	93.8/87.1	98.3/97.8	97.7/76.9	NA
Nienaber et al (1992)[59]	53	NA	100/100	100/68.2	NA
Chirillo et al (1994)[58]	70	NA	NA	97.5/96.7	87.5/96.7

NA, Not available; *CT,* computerized tomography; *TTE,* transthoracic echocardiography; *TEE,* transesophageal echocardiography; *MRA,* magnetic resonance angiography; *MRI,* magnetic resonance imaging.

opacification of the lumens, nonvisualization of the intimal flap, "streak artifact" (artifacts extending across the aortic lumen, simulating an intimal flap), adjacent veins or arteries mistaken for the intimal flap, prominent sinus of Valsalva, atelectatic lung, pleural thickening, and complete thrombosis of the false lumen.[47]

A more recent comparison of multiple methods used to diagnose aortic dissection found a sensitivity of 93.8% but a specificity of only 87% when CT scanning was performed[48] (Table 20-3). Aside from errors that may occur in making the diagnosis of aortic dissection with CT scanning, the technique is unable to detect aortic insufficiency, delineate involvement of the coronary arteries, and intravenous contrast material must be used.

Color-enhanced duplex ultrasonography, combining real-time two-dimensional imaging with pulsed Doppler waveform analysis may be useful in selected cases where involvement of the abdominal aorta is suspected[49] (Fig. 20-2, *A* and *B*).

Aortography was previously considered to be the best method of accurately diagnosing aortic dissection before newer modalities became available. Aortography can accurately locate the site of the intimal tear, the presence of two lumens, the degree of aortic insufficiency, and can clearly delineate the branches of the aorta[50] (Figs. 20-3 and 20-4).

Although earlier reports noted diagnostic accuracy of aortography of 95% to 99%,[51] comparative studies revealed an 88% sensitivity and 94% specificity in aortic dissection[52] (Table 20-3). Inability to diagnose dissection when there is thrombosis of the false lumen, inability to identify the intimal tear when there is a circumferential dissection, the need to use intraarterial contrast material, the invasive nature of the examination, and the potential delay in performing the test while the angiography suite is being prepared are all real limitations of aortography.[53]

Transthoracic echocardiography has several limitations, most often related to inadequate image acquisition

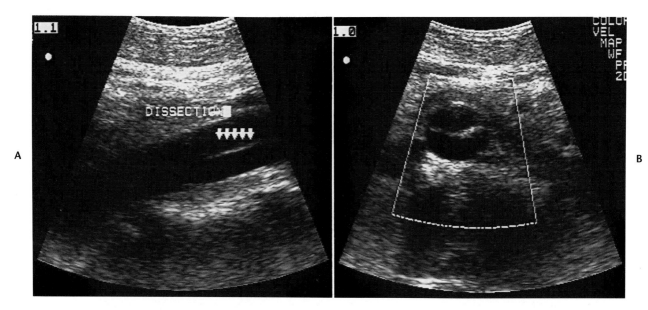

Fig. 20-2. B-Mode ultrasound study in the longitudinal (long) axis **(A)** and the transverse (short) axis **(B)** demonstrates a dissection of the abdominal aorta *(arrows)*.

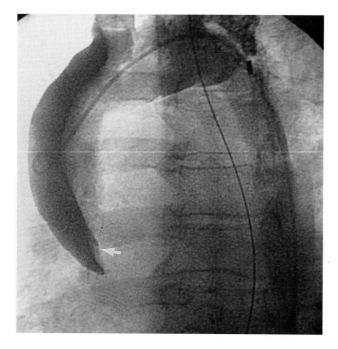

Fig. 20-3. Aortogram demonstrates an ascending aortic dissection. The intimal flap is clearly seen *(arrow)*.

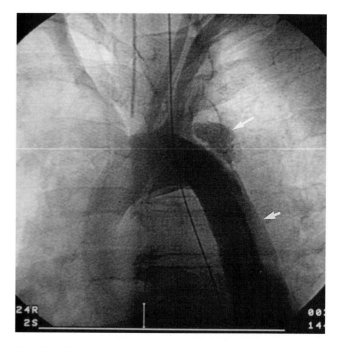

Fig. 20-4. Aortogram of the transverse and descending aorta shows the false lumen *(arrows)*.

caused by poor acoustic windows and inability to visualize the ascending and transverse aorta well.[54] Sensitivity and specificity of 79% and 91%, respectively, has been reported.[55]

Biplane and multiplane transesophageal echocardiography (TEE) has emerged as an excellent noninvasive diagnostic test in aortic dissection (Fig. 20-5). The TEE probe allows for three-dimensional imaging of the aorta and an assessment of flow dynamics.[56] The examination can be safely and rapidly performed, even in the most

critically ill patients.[57] The test itself consumes significantly less time than contrast aortography and CT imaging and has a higher sensitivity and negative predictive value than that of aortography.[58] The high sensitivity and specificity[48,54,59,60] has made TEE the diagnostic test of choice in many centers (Table 20-3). TEE is also quite useful in the diagnosis of circumferential aortic dissection[61] and penetrating aortic ulcers.[62] One of the difficulties with TEE is defining the true lumen from the false lumen. Recently fibroelastic cords (aortic cobwebs) have been described in

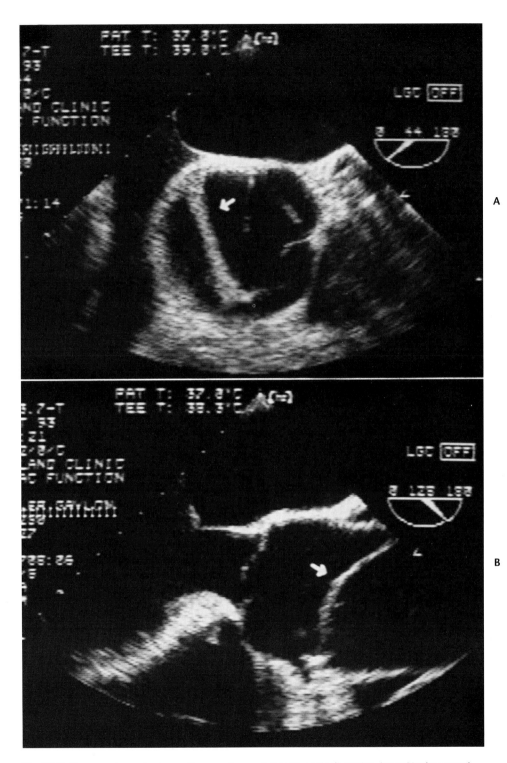

Fig. 20-5. Transesophageal echocardiogram demonstrates an aortic dissection *(arrow)* in the ascending aorta. The transverse view **(A)** and longitudinal view **(B)** clearly show the intimal flap *(arrow)* just superior to the noncoronary cusp and right coronary cusp. The aortic valve architecture is normal.

the false lumen and may improve the differentiation of the true and false lumens.[63] Aortic cobwebs are fibroelastic strands that project from the false lumen wall.

Magnetic resonance imaging (MRI) and magnetic resonance angiography (MRA) are newer diagnostic modalities that are very sensitive (100%) and specific (100%)[59] in the

diagnosis of aortic dissection (Table 20-3). MRI and MRA are effective because of the characteristics of blood and surrounding tissue. Using standard spin-echo technology, rapidly flowing blood produces a signal void, allowing for clear and direct visualization of the aortic lumen and wall, whereas sluggish blood flow (i.e., false lumen flow) pro-

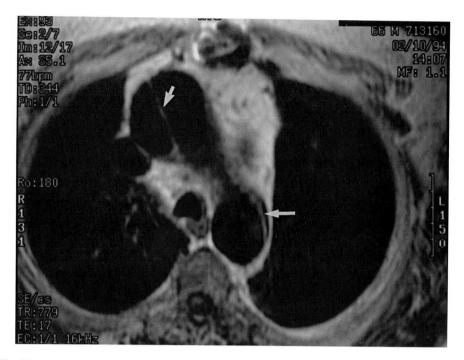

Fig. 20-6. Magnetic resonance image *(transverse view)* shows an intimal flap in the ascending aorta *(short arrow)* and descending aorta *(long arrow).*

duces a signal and image.[53] No iodinated contrast material is required, a particularly appealing aspect of MRI (Fig. 20-6). Real-time cine MRA is a significant advance in that the direction of blood flow can be determined and entry and exit sites can be more easily visualized.

MRI can also measure blood flow velocity in both the true and false lumens.[64-66] Several pitfalls have been identified in MRI. When the false lumen is thrombosed, the dissection may appear to be an aneurysm.[53] Other limitations include structures that can be mistaken for aortic dissection such as the left brachiocephalic vein, arch arteries, superior pericardial recess, azygos vein, and aortic plaque.[67] Other obvious shortcomings of MRI include inaccessibility to patients for 30 to 60 minutes; inability to use MRI in patients with pacemakers and implantable cardioverter defibrillators; and the inability to provide continuous intravenous hydration, medication, and close hemodynamic monitoring during the examination.[53]

Although invasive, recent use of intravascular ultrasonography with high-frequency ultrasound transducers has proved quite promising. This technology can accurately assess the location and extent of the dissection and interrogate branch vessels for involvement by the dissection. It is useful for differentiating aortic dissection from a penetrating atherosclerotic ulcer.[68-71] Intravascular ultrasonography as a diagnostic test may become more important in the future.

Each diagnostic method offers advantages and disadvantages. Table 20-3 compares the sensitivity and specificity of each test. There are several approaches to the diagnosis of aortic dissection, and variables include the hemodynamic status of the patient, availability and skill of the technicians and physicians in performing and interpreting the tests, and the speed with which the test can be performed. A diagnostic algorithm that we use is shown in Fig. 20-7.

DIFFERENTIAL DIAGNOSIS

It is not surprising that many other medical conditions often mimic aortic dissection. The symptoms of aortic dissection are often nonspecific and can suggest other disease processes. In one recent series 28% of patients with aortic dissection were not accurately diagnosed antemortem.[9]

Conditions that may appear initially as aortic dissection include acute myocardial infarction, thoracic aortic aneurysm without dissection, musculoskeletal chest wall or thoracic spine pain, mediastinal tumors, pericarditis, unstable angina pectoris, acute cholecystitis or cholelithiasis, pleuritis, pulmonary embolus, acute aortic valvular insufficiency, pneumothorax, ureteral colic, acute appendicitis, acute mesenteric ischemia unrelated to aortic dissection, pyelonephritis, stroke, transient ischemic attacks, and acute extremity ischemia.

Given the extensive differential diagnosis, it is apparent that objective diagnostic testing must be performed when aortic dissection is considered. As a clinical clue, however, the presence of known systemic hypertension and migratory chest and back pain of less than 24 hours' duration have occurred with greater prevalence in patients with documented aortic dissection.[72]

TREATMENT

Since the mortality rate during the acute phase of aortic dissection is high and increases with time, medical therapy must commence as soon as possible, often before a definite

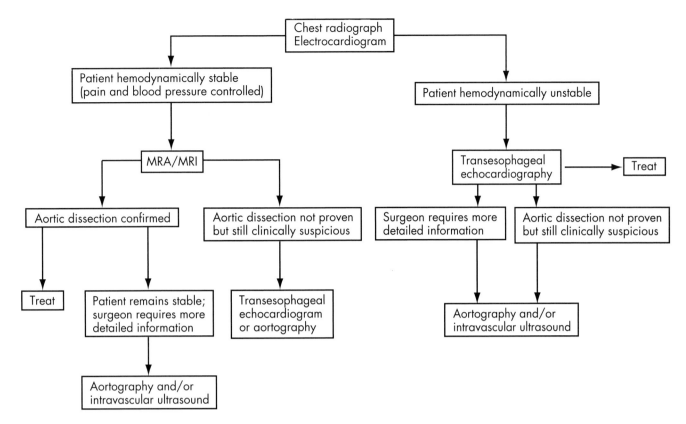

Fig. 20-7. Diagnostic algorithm for aortic dissection.

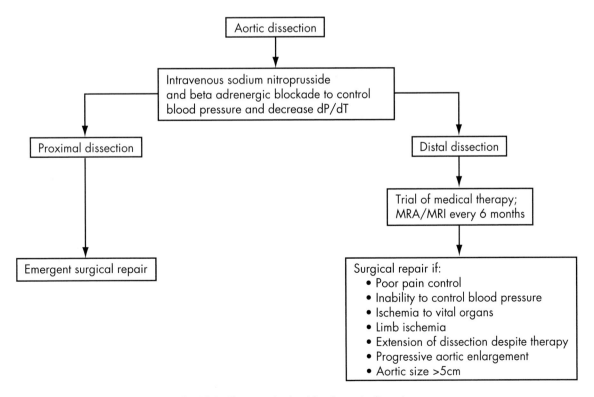

Fig. 20-8. Therapeutic algorithm in aortic dissection.

diagnosis is made. The goals of acute medical therapy include reducing the blood pressure, reducing the velocity of contraction of the left ventricle (thereby reducing shear forces on the aorta), and treating the pain. Initially, supplemental oxygen, an indwelling arterial cannula insertion for close monitoring of blood pressure, a pulmonary artery catheter placement, indwelling bladder catheterization for hourly urine volumes, and intravenous morphine sulfate are all provided for the patient. An algorithm illustrating the management of patients with aortic dissection is shown in Fig. 20-8.

A reduction in the velocity of ventricular contraction (dP/dT), or shear forces, is critical, and has been shown to lessen the rate of expansion of the dissection.[73] The shear forces exerted on the aorta have been implicated as the major cause of progression of the dissection.[74] Both high blood pressure and tachycardia contribute to an increase in dP/dT, promoting extension of the intimal defect and propagation of the dissection. These two variables must be rapidly modified in order to decrease dP/dT. A reduction in heart rate must occur before or simultaneous to reductions in blood pressure. β-Adrenergic antagonists are considered the first line of medical therapy. Intravenous (IV) propranolol (1 to 5 mg) is most commonly used. However, in patients with chronic lung disorders or asthma, a cardioselective β-blocking agent (i.e., metoprolol 5 mg) should be administered. Labetalol, an α- and β-adrenergic antagonist, has also been reported to be effective in doses of 10 to 20 mg as a bolus or as a continuous IV drip. The heart rate may not decrease as much as desired with labetalol in some patients. The target heart rate is approximately 60 beats/min. An ultra-short-acting β₁ selective antagonist, esmolol, is quite effective in lowering heart rate in patients with aortic dissection. A 500-μg/kg/min bolus IV dose is given, and a 50-μg/kg/min continuous infusion follows. This agent can be titrated to control heart rate.

Concomitant IV administration of sodium nitroprusside is used to rapidly and reliably lower blood pressure. Doses of 0.5 to 10 μg/kg/min IV are often used. The goal is to lower the systolic blood pressure to the lowest limits possible without compromising arterial perfusion to vital organs, usually 90 to 110 mm Hg. Sodium nitroprusside is susceptible to degradation after exposure to light, and therefore should be protected by aluminum foil. After 48 hours of use, patients may experience nausea, along with central nervous system irritability, which may represent early thiocyanate toxicity. However, it is unusual in patients with normal renal function. This can be reversed with hydroxocobalamin, if needed. Because sodium nitroprusside does not lower heart rate, a β-blocking agent must be used along with this agent.

In patients with preexisting cardiac conduction system abnormalities, reactive airway disease, or congestive heart failure who cannot tolerate β-blockade, reserpine, clonidine, or calcium channel blockers may be helpful. Trimethaphan camsylate is an alternative agent to nitroprusside, used as a continuous IV infusion at a rate of 1 to 4 mg/min. Tachyphylaxis is a significant problem with this agent, limiting the duration of infusion to 48 to 72 hours. Patients must be in a reverse Trendelenburg position because this antihypertensive agent acts by causing significant postural hypotension. Urinary retention, bowel and bladder atony, and pupillary dilatation are significant side effects of trimethophan camsylate.

Once the patient has been medically treated and the diagnosis is secure, surgical intervention may be warranted. Medical management has been considered a reasonable therapeutic alternative in patients with DeBakey type III dissection.[75] A direct comparison of surgical versus medical therapy for type III aortic dissections reveals comparable survival rates at 1, 5, and 10 years.[76] However, survival rates for medically treated proximal aortic dissections (DeBakey type I, II) is poor, with 2-week, 5- and 10-year survival rates of 43%, 34%, and 28%.[77]

The surgical procedure most recommended to repair an ascending aortic dissection is replacement of the aortic segment involved by the intimal tear and aneurysmal dilatation with a tubular interposition graft.[5] The mortality rate of emergent aortic dissection surgery has dramatically decreased over the past 30 years and now ranges from 5%[5] to 32%.[78] The factors that have contributed to this improved survival include greater surgical experience, advances in anesthetic and surgical technique, and improved postoperative care.[7]

If the aortic valve is involved or incompetent at the time of repair of the ascending aorta, combined aortic valve–ascending aorta replacement is completed, despite an 8-year survival after emergent repair of only 44 (±17)%.[79] Of aortic dissections that extend beyond the ascending aorta and involve the arch, the perioperative mortality increases. However, operative techniques to reimplant the great vessels and the coronary arteries has improved.

The cornerstone of long-term treatment in patients with distal dissection is β-adrenergic blockade. Any β-blocker can be used, although those with "intrinsic sympathomimetic activity" (i.e., pindolol, acebutolol) may not decrease dP/dT effectively. Direct arteriolar vasodilators such as hydralazine and minoxidil should not be used if at all possible, as these agents may increase dP/dT, especially if the patient is not adequately treated with β-blockers. Angiotensin-converting enzyme inhibitors (e.g., captopril, enalapril, lisinopril), calcium channel antagonists (e.g., nifedipine, diltiazem, verapamil), and diuretics (hydrochlorothiazide, furosemide, bumetanide) are all effective agents along with β-blockers for the treatment of chronic hypertension associated with aortic dissection.

Long-term follow-up should be performed with MRA/MRI evaluations every 6 months. A clinical event or significant radiographic change in the location of the dissection or size of the aorta may warrant surgical repair (Fig. 20-8).

Several events mandate surgical intervention for distal (DeBakey type III) aortic dissections. These include evidence of leak or rupture, organ or limb ischemia due to arterial compromise from the dissection, persistent pain, extension of the dissection despite adequate therapy, or poorly controlled hypertension.[2] Some researchers believe that an aortic size greater than 5 cm warrants surgical repair.[5]

More recently, endovascular therapy has been used to repair predominantly distal thoracic aortic dissection with the use of endoluminal stent graft devices, along with percutaneous transluminal angioplasty and endovascular septal fenestration.[80] A recent series was reported using transluminally placed endovascular stent graft devices in 13 patients with thoracic aortic aneurysms, 9 of which had dissection or penetrating atherosclerotic ulceration. All procedures were successful, and after 11.6 months of follow-up, all patients remained alive without major complication.[81] The future of this therapy is promising.

DISSECTION OF PERIPHERAL ARTERIES

Although generally considered unusual, spontaneous dissection of peripheral arteries has been recognized with increasing frequency over the past decade.[82] Increasing awareness of this disorder, along with frequent use of duplex ultrasonography and contrast arteriography has aided in the diagnosis.

Any peripheral artery can develop a dissection. Dissection of the cervical arteries (carotid, vertebrobasilar) and renal arteries occur most commonly, followed by mesenteric, pulmonary and upper- and lower-extremity vessels.

Atherosclerosis is an uncommon finding in peripheral arterial dissections, and often no obvious arterial abnormality is demonstrated on radiographic studies. Although spontaneous dissections can occur, trauma (often minor) and other arteriopathies (e.g., fibromuscular disease, Marfan's syndrome, and Ehlers-Danlos syndrome) are frequent underlying factors.

Dissection of renal arteries is discussed in Chapter 18.

Cervical Artery Dissection

Patients who present with carotid and vertebrobasilar artery dissections are young in comparison to the population most often associated with cerebral ischemia.[83] The mean age is generally in the fourth and fifth decades. Patients may suffer ipsilateral headache followed by either transient ischemic attacks or completed strokes.[84] Oculosympathetic paresis, or incomplete Horner's syndrome, can also be observed.[85] In a series of internal carotid artery dissection in 163 patients, 72% presented with headache, 63% demonstrated evidence of cerebral ischemia, and oculosympathetic palsy was present in 37% of patients.[86] Vertebral artery dissection often occurs in the distal one third of this vessel and causes neck or occipital skull pain followed by signs of brainstem ischemia.[87] Symptoms suggestive of subarachnoid hemorrhage may be present.[88] Patients may present with nonspecific symptoms of neck pain and dizziness.

Cervical artery dissections are often spontaneous. Minor trauma including nose-blowing,[89] coughing,[90] vigorous flexion and extension of the neck,[91] and chiropractic manipulation[92,93] has been reported. Fibromuscular dysplasia,[86] major trauma, both iatrogenic and noniatrogenic,[94] and very unusual causes such as polyarteritis nodosa,[95] α_1-antitrypsin deficiency,[96] and moyamoya disease,[97] have all been described.

Duplex ultrasonography[98] may be very helpful in establishing the diagnosis of cervical artery dissection, but arteriography remains the standard examination. Classic

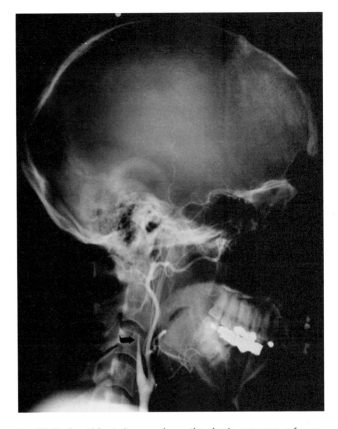

Fig. 20-9. Carotid arteriogram shows the classic appearance for carotid dissection. The internal carotid artery tapers to a point where it then occludes (arrow).

arteriographic findings include elongated, irregular, tapering stenoses[82] (Fig. 20-9), and/or pseudoaneurysm formation.[83] Resolution or improvement of a stenosis often occurs on serial arteriographic studies.[87] Intracranial saccular aneurysms appear to occur with greater frequency in patients with cervical artery dissection.[99] MRA has recently demonstrated utility in diagnosing cervical artery dissection.[100-102]

Although the initial presentation of patients with cervical artery dissection can be quite disturbing, the prognosis is often good. Although a uniform approach to treatment has not been established, observation, either with or without concomitant anticoagulation therapy, is often recommended as first-line therapy.[82] Antiplatelet therapy has also been used.[83] Surgical therapy is reserved for recurrent dissection or deterioration of neurologic status due to extension of the dissection. The majority of the dissections have improved or resolved on follow-up arteriography.[82] Recurrent dissections occur in only a minority of patients, noted in only 8% of patients during 1472 patient-years of follow-up.[86] Endovascular occlusion of the dissecting site in vertebral artery dissection has been safely and effectively used in some patients.[103]

Mesenteric Artery Dissection

Dissection of the superior mesenteric artery (SMA), hepatic arteries, and other mesenteric arteries are rare in the absence of coexistent aortic dissection. Until recently dissection of an SMA was uniformly fatal. Prompt diagnosis and aggressive surgical treatment are the cornerstones of successful management. Patients present with symptoms of acute mesenteric ischemia. Arteriography, with attention to a lateral view of the aorta, remains the diagnostic test of choice. Emergent surgical exploration is often necessary in the face of abdominal pain and hemodynamic instability. Surgical techniques include transposition of the SMA to the infrarenal aorta, endoaneurysmorrhaphy, intimectomy with patch closure,[104] and various bypass procedures.[104,105] There has been some preliminary work with stenting of the SMA.

Scattered case reports of hepatic artery dissection have been described. Fibromuscular dysplasia[106] and cystic medial necrosis[107] are underlying pathologic arteriopathies seen. The dissection occurs between the media and the external elastic lamina, which is different from the pathology of aortic dissection.[108] Signs and symptoms are often nonspecific,[109] and the diagnosis must be suspected promptly, as hemorrhage, shock, and death may ensue rapidly.

Upper- and Lower-Extremity Artery Dissection

Subclavian and iliac artery dissections are extremely rare. Excluding type 4 Ehlers-Danlos syndrome, iliac artery dissections present after trauma or are rarely caused by an unusual coexistent illness such as α_1-antitrypsin deficiency[110] or in association with exercise.[111] Subclavian artery dissections almost always occur as a result of trauma, and a pulsatile supraclavicular mass may be palpable. Shoulder and ipsilateral extremity pain may occur. Surgical repair is the treatment of choice.

REFERENCES

1. Hirst AE et al: Dissecting aneurysms of the aorta: a review of 505 cases, Medicine 37:217, 1958.
2. DeSanctis RW et al: Aortic dissection, N Engl J Med 317:1060, 1987.
3. Cooke JP and Safford RE: Progress in the diagnosis and management of aortic dissection, Mayo Clin Proc 61:147, 1986.
4. DeBakey ME, Cooley DA, and Creech O: Surgical considerations of dissecting aneurysm of the aorta, Ann Surg 142:586, 1955.
5. Crawford ES: The diagnosis and management of aortic dissection, JAMA 264:2537, 1990.
6. Lijoi A et al: Circumferential dissection of the ascending aorta with intimal intussusception, Tex H Inst J 21:166, 1994.
7. Svensson LG et al: Dissection of the aorta and dissecting aortic aneurysm: improving early and long-term surgical results, Circulation 82(suppl IV):IV-24, 1990.
8. DeBakey ME et al: Dissection and dissecting aneurysms of the aorta: twenty-year follow-up of five hundred twenty-seven patients treated surgically, Surgery 92:1118, 1982.
9. Spittell PC et al: Clinical features and differential diagnosis of aortic dissection: experience with 236 cases (1980 through 1990), Mayo Clin Proc 68:642, 1993.
10. Marsalese DL et al: Marfan's syndrome: natural history and long-term follow-up of cardiovascular involvement, J Am Coll Cardiol 14:422, 1989.
11. Kunz R and Valentine R: Marfan's syndrome presenting as a type 3 aortic dissection, Chest 88:463, 1985.
12. Finkbohner R et al: Marfan syndrome: long-term survival and complications after aortic aneurysm repair, Circulation 91:728, 1995.
13. Coselli JS, Le Maire SA, and Büket S: Marfan syndrome: the variability and outcome of operative management, J Vasc Surg 21:342, 1995.
14. Larson EW and Edwards WD: Risk factors for aortic dissection: a necropsy study of 161 cases, Am J Cardiol 53:849, 1984.
15. Chow SL: Acute aortic dissection in a patient with Marfan's syndrome complicated by gestational hypertension, Med J Aust 159:760, 1993.
16. Pumphrey CW, Fay T, and Weir I: Aortic dissection during pregnancy, Br Heart J 55:106, 1986.
17. Wahlers T et al: Repair of acute type A aortic dissection after cesarian section in the thirty-ninth week of pregnancy, J Thorac Cardiovasc Surg 107:314, 1994.
18. Moles VP et al: Aortic dissection as complication of percutaneous transluminal coronary angioplasty, Cathet Cardiovasc Diag 26:8, 1992.
19. Sakamoto I et al: Aortic dissection caused by angiographic procedures, Radiology 191:467, 1994.
20. Strichartz SD, Gelabert HA, and Moore WS: Retrograde aortic dissection with bilateral renal artery occlusion after repair of infrarenal aortic aneurysm, J Vasc Surg 12:56, 1990.
21. DeVirgilio et al: Ascending aortic dissection in weight lifters with cystic medial degeneration, Ann Thorac Surg 49:638, 1990.
22. Schor JS, Horowitz MD, and Livingstone AS: Recreational weight lifting and aortic dissection: case report, J Vasc Surg 17:774, 1993.
23. Becquemin JP et al: Acute and chronic dissections of the abdominal aorta: clinical features and treatment, J Vasc Surg 11:397, 1990.
24. Cooke JP, Kazmier FJ, and Orszulak TA: The penetrating aortic ulcer: pathologic manifestations, diagnosis, and management, Mayo Clin Proc 63:718, 1988.
25. Stanson AW et al: Penetrating atherosclerotic ulcers of the thoracic aorta: natural history and clinicopathologic correlations, Ann Vasc Surg 1:15, 1986.
26. Movsowitz HD et al: Penetrating atherosclerotic aortic ulcers, Am Heart J 128:1210, 1994.
27. Hussain S et al: Penetrating atherosclerotic ulcers of the thoracic aorta, J Vasc Surg 9:710, 1989.
28. DeBakey ME et al: Surgical management of dissecting aneurysms of the aorta, J Thorac Cardiovasc Surg 49:130, 1965.
29. Daily PO et al: Management of acute aortic dissections, Ann Thorac Surg 10:237, 1970.
30. Crawford ES et al: Aortic dissection and dissecting aortic aneurysms, Ann Surg 208:254, 1988.
31. Glower DD et al: Management and long-term outcome of aortic dissection, Ann Surg 214:31, 1991.
32. Fradet G et al: Aortic dissection: current expectations and treatment. Experience with 258 patients over 20 years, Can J Surg 33:465, 1990.
33. Strouse PJ et al: Aortic dissection presenting as spinal cord ischemia with a false-negative aortogram, Cardiovasc Intervent Radiol 13:77, 1990.
34. Cambria RP et al: Vascular complications associated with spontaneous aortic dissection, J Vasc Surg 7:199, 1988.
35. Raby N, Giles J, and Walters H: Aortic dissection presenting as acute leg ischaemia, Clin Radiol 42:116, 1990.
36. Rackson ME, Lossef SV, and Sos TA: Renal artery stenosis in patients with aortic dissection, increased prevalence, Radiology 177:555, 1990.

37. Gates JD, Clair DG, and Hechtman OH: Thoracic aortic dissection with renal artery involvement following blunt thoracic trauma: case report, J Trauma 36:430, 1994.

38. Bensard J, Dany F, and Hammel J: The carotid pulse in dissecting aneurysms of the aorta, Angiology 36:846, 1985.

39. Isselbacher EM, Cigarroa JE, and Eagle KA: Cardiac tamponade complicating proximal aortic dissection: is pericardiocentesis helpful? Circulation 90:2375, 1994.

40. Butler J, Davies AH, and Westaby S: Streptokinase in acute aortic dissection, Br Med J 300:517, 1990.

41. Kahn JK: Inadvertent thrombolytic therapy for cardiovascular diseases masquerading as acute coronary thrombosis, Clin Cardiol 16:67, 1993.

42. Marian AJ et al: Inadvertent administration of rtPA to a patient with type 1 aortic dissection and subsequent cardiac tamponade, Am J Emerg Med 11:613, 1993.

43. Davidson E et al: Elevated serum creatinine kinase levels: an early diagnostic sign of acute dissection of the aorta, Arch Intern Med 148:2184, 1988.

44. Earnest F, Muhm JR, and Sheedy PF: Roentgenographic findings in thoracic aortic dissection, Mayo Clin Proc 54:43, 1979.

45. Petasnick JP: Radiologic evaluation of aortic dissection, Radiology 180:297, 1991.

46. Jaganrath AS et al: Aortic dissection: a statistical analysis of the usefulness of plain chest radiographic findings, AJR 147:1123, 1986.

47. Thorsen MK, Lawson TL, and Foley WD: CT of aortic dissections, Crit Rev Diagn Imaging 26:291, 1986.

48. Nienaber CA et al: The diagnosis of thoracic aortic dissection by non-invasive imaging procedures, N Engl J Med 328:1, 1993.

49. Thomas EA and Dubbins PA: Duplex ultrasound of the abdominal aorta: a neglected tool in aortic dissection, Clin Radiol 42:330, 1990.

50. Soto B et al: Angiographic diagnosis of dissecting aneurysm of the aorta, Surgery 116:146, 1972.

51. Mast HL, Gordon DH, and Kantor AM: Pitfalls in diagnosis of aortic dissection by angiography: algorithmic approach utilizing CT and MRI, Comput Med Imaging Graph 15:431, 1991.

52. Erbel R et al: Echocardiography in diagnosis of aortic dissection, Lancet 1:457, 1989.

53. Cigarroa JE et al: Diagnostic imaging in the evaluation of suspected aortic dissection, N Engl J Med 328:35, 1993.

54. Ballal RS et al: Usefulness of transesophageal echocardiography in assessment of aortic dissection, Circulation 84:1903, 1991.

55. Khandheria BK et al: Aortic dissection: review of value and limitations of two-dimensional echocardiography in a six-year experience, J Am Soc Echocardiogr 2:17, 1989.

56. Omoto R et al: Evaluation of biplane color Doppler transesophageal echocardiography in 200 consecutive patients, Circulation 85:1237, 1992.

57. Pearson AC, Castello R, and Lebovitz AJ: Safety and utility of transesophageal echocardiography in the critically ill patient, Am Heart J 119:1083, 1990.

58. Chirillo F et al: Comparative diagnostic value of transesophageal echocardiography and retrograde aortography in the evaluation of thoracic aortic dissection, Am J Cardiol 74:590, 1994.

59. Nienaber CA et al: Diagnosis of thoracic aortic dissection: magnetic resonance imaging versus transesophageal echocardiography, Circulation 85:434, 1992.

60. Wiet SP et al: Utility of transesophageal echocardiography in the diagnosis of disease of the thoracic aorta, J Vasc Surg 20:613, 1994.

61. Farah MG and Suneja R: Diagnosis of circumferential dissection of the ascending aorta by transesophageal echocardiography, Chest 103:291, 1993.

62. Mohr-Kahaly S et al: Aortic intramural hemorrhage visualized by transesophageal echocardiography: findings and prognostic implications, J Am Coll Cardiol 23:658, 1994.

63. Buonavolonta J, O'Connor W, and Weiss R: Transesophageal echocardiography identification of the false lumen in thoracic aortic dissection by aortic cobwebs, Chest 106 (suppl):49S, 1994.

64. Bogren HG et al: Magnetic resonance velocity mapping in aortic dissection, Br J Radiol 61:456, 1988.

65. Chang JM et al: MR measurement of blood flow in the true and false channel in chronic aortic dissection, J Comput Assist Tomogr 15:418, 1991.

66. Mitchell L et al: Case report: aortic dissection: morphology and differential flow velocity patterns demonstrated by magnetic resonance imaging, Clin Radiol 39:458, 1988.

67. Solomon SL et al: Thoracic aortic dissection: pitfalls and artifacts in MR imaging, Radiology 177:223, 1990.

68. Pande A et al: Intravascular ultrasound for diagnosis of aortic dissection, Am J Cardiol 67:662, 1991.

69. Weintraub AR et al: Evaluation of acute aortic dissection by intravascular ultrasonography, N Engl J Med 323:1566, 1990.

70. Weintraub AR et al: Intravascular ultrasound imaging in acute aortic dissection, J Am Coll Cardiol 24:495, 1994.

71. Yamada E et al: Usefulness of a prototype intravascular ultrasound imaging in evaluation of aortic dissection and comparison with angiographic study, transesophageal echocardiography, computed tomography, and magnetic resonance imaging, Am J Cardiol 75:161, 1995.

72. Eagle KA et al: Spectrum of conditions initially suggesting acute aortic dissection but with negative aortograms, Am J Cardiol 57:322, 1994.

73. Wheat MW et al: Treatment of dissecting aneurysms of the aorta without surgery, J Thorac Cardiovasc Surg 50:364, 1965.

74. Prokop EK, Palmer RF, and Wheat MW: Hydrodynamic forces in dissecting aneurysms: in-vitro studies in a tygon model and in dog aortas, Circ Res 27:121, 1970.

75. Wheat MW et al: Acute dissecting aneurysms of the aorta: treatment of results in 64 patients, J Thorac Cardiovasc Surg 57:344, 1969.

76. Glower DD et al: Comparison of medical and surgical therapy for uncomplicated descending aortic dissections, Circulation 82(suppl IV):IV-39, 1990.

77. Masuda Y et al: Prognosis of patients with medically treated aortic dissections, Circulation 84(suppl III):III-7, 1991.

78. Ikonomidis JS et al: Thoracic aortic surgery, Circulation 84(suppl III):III-1, 1991.

79. Taniguchi K et al: Long-term survival and complications after composite graft replacement for ascending aortic aneurysm associated with aortic regurgitation, Circulation 84(suppl III):III-31, 1991.

80. Walker PJ et al: The use of endovascular techniques for the treatment of complications of aortic dissection, J Vasc Surg 18:1042, 1993.

81. Dake MD et al: Transluminal placement of endovascular stent-grafts for the treatment of descending thoracic aortic aneurysms, N Engl J Med 331:1729, 1994.

82. Mokri B et al: Spontaneous dissection of the cervical internal carotid artery: presentation with lower cranial nerve palsies, Arch Otolaryngol Head Neck Surg 118:431, 1992.

83. Biller J et al: Cervicocephalic arterial dissections: a ten-year experience, Arch Neurol 43:1234, 1986.

84. Ehrenfeld WK and Wylie EJ: Spontaneous dissection of the internal carotid artery, Arch Surg 111:1294, 1976.

85. Vanneste JAL and Davies G: Spontaneous dissection of the cervical internal carotid artery, Clin Neurol Neurosurg 86:307, 1984.

86. Schievink WI, Mokri B, and O'Fallon WM: Recurrent spontaneous cervical-artery dissection, N Engl J Med 330:383, 1994.

87. Hart RG: Vertebral artery dissection, Neurology 38:987, 1988.

88. Shimoji T et al: Dissecting aneurysm of the vertebral artery: report of seven cases and angiographic findings, J Neurosurg 61:1038, 1984.

89. Roome NS and Aberfeld DC: Spontaneous dissecting aneurysm of the internal carotid artery, Arch Neurol 34:251, 1977.

90. Kiely MJ: Neuroradiology case of the day, AJR 160:1336, 1993.

91. Jackson MA et al: "Headbanging" and carotid dissection, Br Med J 287:1262, 1983.

92. Cashley MAP: Cervicocephalic artery dissections and chiropractic manipulations, Lancet 341:1213, 1993.

93. Mas JL et al: Dissecting aneurysm of the vertebral artery and cervical manipulation: a case report with autopsy, Neurology 39:512, 1989.

94. Zelenock GB et al: Extracranial internal carotid artery dissections: noniatrogenic traumatic lesions, Arch Surg 117:425, 1982.

95. Lomeo RM, Silver RM, and Brothers M: Spontaneous dissection of the internal carotid artery in a patient with polyarteritis nodosa, Arthritis Rheum 32:1625, 1989.

96. Schievink WI et al: Alpha-1-antitrypsin deficiency in intracranial aneurysms and cervical artery dissection, Lancet 343:452, 1994.

97. Yamashita M et al: Cerebral dissecting aneurysms in patients with moyamoya disease, J Neurosurg 58:120, 1983.

98. Sturzenegger M: Ultrasound findings in spontaneous carotid artery dissection: the value of duplex sonography, Arch Neurol 48:1057, 1991.

99. Schievink WI, Mokri B, and Peipgras DG: Angiographic frequency of saccular intracranial aneurysms in patients with spontaneous cervical artery dissection, J Neurosurg 76:62, 1992.

100. Levy C et al: Carotid and vertebral dissections: three-dimensional time-of-flight MR angiography and MR imaging versus conventional angiography, Radiology 190:97, 1994.

101. Long TD, Carter MP, and Reynolds T: Spontaneous internal carotid artery dissection shown by magnetic resonance imaging, South Med J 84:1140, 1991.

102. Quint DJ and Spickler EM: Magnetic resonance demonstration of vertebral artery dissection: report of two cases, J Neurosurg 72:964, 1990.

103. Halbach VV et al: Endovascular treatment of vertebral artery dissections and pseudoaneurysms, J Neurosurg 79:183, 1993.

104. Cormier F et al: Dissecting aneurysms of the main trunk of the superior mesenteric artery, J Vasc Surg 15:424, 1992.

105. Vignati PV et al: Acute mesenteric ischemia caused by isolated superior mesenteric artery dissection, J Vasc Surg 16:109, 1992.

106. Patchefsky AS and Paplanus SH: Fibromuscular hyperplasia and dissecting aneurysm of the hepatic artery, Arch Pathol 83:141, 1967.

107. Hill DE, Lobell M, and Edwards JE: Primary dissecting aneurysm of the hepatic artery, Arch Intern Med 133:471, 1974.

108. Callicott JH and Hoke HF: Dissecting aneurysm of the common hepatic artery, Arch Pathol 85:681, 1968.

109. James AW: Primary dissecting aneurysm of the hepatic artery simulating acute myocardial infarction, Can Med Assoc J 114:110, 1976.

110. Cattan S et al: Iliac artery dissection in alpha-1-antitrypsin deficiency, Lancet 343:1371, 1994.

111. Declemy S et al: Spontaneous dissecting aneurysm of the common iliac artery, Ann Vasc Surg 5:549, 1991.

THROMBOANGIITIS OBLITERANS (BUERGER'S DISEASE)

John W. Joyce

After decades of controversy thromboangiitis obliterans (Buerger's disease) has emerged as a well-defined, distinctive clinicopathologic entity that causes claudication and a significant incidence of digit and limb loss in youthful tobacco users. It is a vasculopathy involving distal arteries and veins of both upper and lower extremities with a distinctive thrombus at sites of vessel wall inflammation in its acute phase and is often classified as a vasculitis, in the generic sense of the term. It is a disease of the second through fourth decades seen predominantly in men, although the incidence of women is increasing. Tobacco use is universally associated with the active phase of the disease, but the exact etiologic mechanisms are not defined.

The evolution of our current knowledge of thromboangiitis obliterans (TAO) has been slow. Felix von Winiwarter,[1] an Austrian surgeon working with Billroth, described the cellular thrombus and adjacent wall pathology of a single patient in 1879. The eponym "von Winiwarter-Buerger's Disease" is commonly used in Europe. It was in 1908 that Leo Buerger[2] of New York published his first observations on a small group of patients, defining the disease and naming it "thromboangiitis obliterans." His description of the clinical features is superb and remains valid to this day. In this and several subsequent reports, culminating in a monograph, he detailed the histopathology of acute and healing arterial lesions, superficial phlebitis, the focal and segmental distribution of lesions, and the clinical course that became the foundation for recognition and further study of the disease.[3] He did not appreciate the relationship of tobacco to TAO. However, the wording of Buerger's differentiation of TAO from atherosclerotic gangrene caused confusion, resulting in the overdiagnosis of TAO for many years.[4,5]

Wessler et al[6] challenged these original observations in 1960. They noted a dramatic drop in the diagnosis of Buerger's disease at their hospital, at a time when tobacco use had clearly increased. After careful retrospective reviews of both clinical and pathology material, they correctly concluded that premature atherosclerosis was greatly underappreciated and found that histopathologic criteria were not specific as being applied. They asked if idiopathic thrombosis and systemic embolization might not explain most of the cases studied and, indeed, questioned if TAO as a distinct entity existed.[6]

The original report and the following essay by Wessler et al[6,7] resulted in better recognition of premature atherosclerosis and other mechanisms of distal ischemia. His writings gave impetus to several studies that defined Buerger's disease more precisely. McPherson, Juergens, and Gifford[8] noted that the survival of patients with TAO approximated that of an age/sex-matched population without the disease, in contrast to a third group with premature atherosclerosis whose survival was significantly shorter because of atherosclerotic cardiac and cerebral events. McKusick et al[9,10] reconfirmed both the clinical profile and the histopathology of TAO. They carefully pointed out that interpretation of tissue specimens was dependent on the site of the biopsy and the stage of the disease at that time and site. Then, of prime importance, angiography was established as the third modality for diagnosing TAO. The work of McKusick et al,[10] particularly of Szilagyi, DeRusso, and Elliot,[11] and several subsequent European authors correlated clinical and histologic features with radiographic images and established clear, diagnostic criteria for angiographic correlation with the diagnosis.

It remains an observation of referral practice that the diagnosis of TAO continues to be either ignored or invoked too readily. Vascular disease in general is not fully taught clinically in most medical schools, and the incidence of TAO is small, perhaps two to four cases each year in active vascular practices.[12,13] These observations help explain underdiagnosis. In turn, the diagnosis is often invoked almost automatically for young male smokers with claudication or ischemia, when other conditions causing digital microcirculatory or distal arterial disease should be considered. These are delineated in the discussion of differential diagnosis. Diagnostic criteria have been proposed by Shionoya,[14] Mills, Taylor, and Porter,[15] and Papa and Adar.[16] All list clinical features of age, tobacco use, and distal disease; the characteristic histology of the acute lesion; various angiographic details; and the exclusion of other diseases, as well as patients with significant manifestations of atherosclerosis or its risk factors, other than smoking. The author is in agreement with Mills and Porter[17] that upper-extremity involvement, superficial phlebitis, and foot claudication are minor criteria that strongly support but are not essential for the diagnosis. These events are not seen in every patient, or may occur after the original presentation. The diagnosis of TAO is established by knowledge of the natural history of the disease, exclusion of other entities, supported by angiography, and confirmed by the acute histopathologic lesion when feasible. The reader is referred to several excellent contemporary reviews.[16-19]

PATHOGENESIS

Early studies supported that TAO occurred exclusively in males, most of Jewish heritage, and Buerger suspected it was of infectious origin. Each of these concepts has been altered by subsequent observations. Buerger did not appreciate the relationship of TAO to tobacco, and the role of smoking was subsequently noted by others and has remained a constant observation since.[20,21]

Buerger's report indicated that TAO was primarily a disease of Jews, but clearly this reflected the population he attended. Of 112 patients treated at the Cleveland Clinic 90% were white and less than 8% ethnic Jews.[18] The disease has a broad ethnic base and occurs worldwide, with a greater incidence apparent in the Orient, Southeast Asia, India, and Israel.[16,22-25] Blacks have a low rate of reported occurrence, but a contemporary study is desirable.[26]

Women constitute only 1% to 2% of the patients in early reports. This has increased to 11% to 23% from 1971 to 1990.[13,15,18] This may indicate that women now have better access to health care, or that the accuracy of diagnosis has improved in the face of the long-standing belief that TAO is a male disease. It should also represent, however, the increased use of tobacco by women in America in recent decades. TAO is equally as severe in women as in men.[13]

The prevalence of TAO diagnosed has dropped most significantly in recent decades. At The Mayo Clinic the diagnosis per 100,000 patients per year was 114.3 in 1947, 61.1 in 1956, 18.8 in 1966, 9.9 in 1976, and 12.6 in 1986.[27] Although this may represent a change in referral patterns, perhaps an appreciation of premature atherosclerosis and other causes of distal ischemia since the challenge of Wessler, and the common use of angiography account for this manifold drop in the incidence of TAO. In Japan, where care is more centralized and less subject to referral bias, a similar dramatic reduction has taken place, and the current incidence is 5 cases per 100,000 patients each year.[28]

The definitive etiology of TAO is unknown, but it is universally observed that the disease and its exacerbations occur in active smokers and that cessation of smoking brings remission. Most reports document use of 20 to 40 cigarettes daily. The author has noted exacerbation of TAO in patients acknowledging only 4 to 8 cigarettes in a few days each week for 3 years. McKusick et al[10] have made a similar observation. The disease has been reported in pipe smokers and in a patient using only chewing tobacco.[29,30] In the face of continued smoking, progression is usual but not inevitable.[4,31]

The effect of passive exposure to smoke is an intriguing and frequent question. Matsushito, Shionoya, and Matsumoto[32] noted that quantitation of urinary cotinine could separate active smokers, nonsmokers, and those exposed to passive inhalation, and that the values accurately reflected both the number of cigarettes used and disease activity. Levels were diagnostically low in those experiencing passive exposure to smoke and in nonsmokers, of whom only 1 of 18 had worsening of the disease. This suggests that passive exposure to smoke has minimal effect, yet it should probably be avoided by the patient with TAO.

The fact that only a minuscule percentage of smokers develop TAO in contrast to the almost inevitable multiple manifestations of atherosclerosis obliterans in heavy smokers, and in the face of the observation that the disease can occasionally occur unrelated to a large volume or long duration of smoking, again true of atherosclerosis, strongly suggests that an additional factor specific to these patients is present. Both genetic predisposition and immunologic mechanisms have been implicated to explain the pathogenesis of TAO.

Histocompatibility leukocyte antigen (HLA) typing has been conducted in several countries. A modest increase or decrease in various A, B, and DR antigens has been identified. Patterns vary with ethnic populations, asymptomatic controls overlap with those having TAO, and not all patients with the disease show the antigenic marker. Further study may define a genetic substrate for TAO, but the presence of an antigen in a lesser but significant number of controls suggests that yet another factor must be present to trigger the disease.[15,16,33]

The small subset of smokers who develop TAO, the specific distribution of focal segmental lesions, and the intense cellular response of the thrombus and the adjacent vessel point to a biocellular mechanism. Autoimmune disease remains the most plausible cause, but data thus far have been modest although supportive. A specific antigen or immune complex similar to ANA or rheumatoid factor has not been identified. Antineutrophilic cytoplasmic antibodies (ANCAs) have not been found.[34] Adar et al[35] have identified an increased sensitivity of leukocytes in TAO patients to collagens I and III and modest increase in anticollagen antibody in their sera. In another study lymphocytes were challenged with tobacco glycoprotein antibody; nonsmokers did not respond whereas smokers did, but there was no distinction between smokers with and without TAO.[36] Gulati et al[37] have demonstrated an increase in precipitated immunoglobulins and increased complement consumption in patients with TAO when compared with smoking and nonsmoking controls, but there was considerable overlap between groups. Of importance, they noted deposition of immune complexes on normal arteries treated with immunoglobulins from patients with TAO. It is somewhat surprising that there are so few immunologic studies of this important disease.

No evidence for a hypercoagulable state was found in a small group of patients, using contemporary hematologic tests.[15] Increases of D-dimer and fibrin-split products can be expected with an acute thrombotic flare but are not specific. At this time the specific cause of TAO cannot be found, but tobacco use is clearly a contributing factor.

PATHOLOGY

The gross pathologic features of TAO in amputated limbs are focal, segmental, and sometimes long thrombotic occlusions of arteries and the adjacent vein, involvement of digital arteries, presence of normal vessels proximally, and absence of atherosclerosis.

Much of the controversy surrounding TAO has centered on the microscopic findings. Buerger[3] identified acute, subacute, and chronic phases of the process and considered the acute lesion essential for the diagnosis. Considering the protracted course of the disease before amputation is required, it is logical that chronic lesions will predominate, and that subacute and acute lesions must be sought, correlating the specimen site with recent disease activity or angiographic detail. Given these difficulties, and because arterial biopsy would further jeopardize flow, observations of the acute lesion are limited. Nonetheless, Buerger's findings have been confirmed definitively and in the clinical setting he described.[3,5,10]

The acute lesion is considered diagnostic.[3,5,10,13] The artery or vein is modestly swollen, and there is a moderate infiltrate of the adventitia and media. The lumen is occluded by a highly cellular, unique thrombus, with characteristic microabscesses. Lymphocytes exceed neutrophils, and occasional giant cells, and some eosinophils may be seen (Fig. 21-1). In the subacute phase cellularity of the vessel wall and thrombus is less, microabscesses have disappeared, and recanalization has begun (Fig. 21-2). Late

lesions consist of organized and recanalized thrombus in fibrotic, small vessels. These lesions are compatible with several forms of vascular injury. The architecture of the vessel wall, including the internal elastic membrane, re-

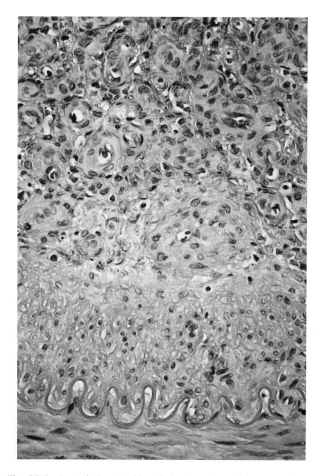

Fig. 21-1. Acute lesion. Highly cellular thrombus with giant cells, no recanalization. Note the intact internal elastic membrane.

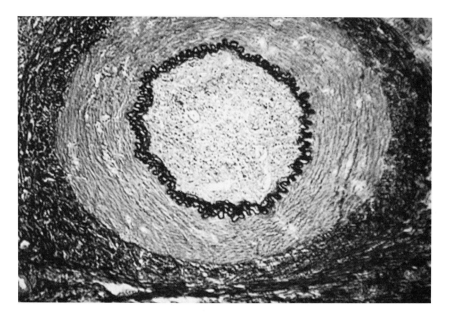

Fig. 21-2. Artery, dorsum of foot. Organizing, highly cellular thrombus with early recanalization; subacute stage; mild infiltrated media. Note the intact elastic membrane. (Elastin stain; ×40.)

mains essentially intact in all stages, and no necrosis is seen.

Buerger[2] reported skip areas of normal vessel between involved segments as Shionoya et al[38] emphasized in their angiographic observations. Buerger[39] also noted bland thrombi, without cellular involvement, and he considered the acute phase in superficial veins as "typical and diagnostic." Bearing on these references Lie[5] provided three provocative photomicrographs taken from different segments of an acutely inflamed superficial vein. One showed acute phlebitis without thrombus, another phlebitis with bland thrombus, and the third phlebitis with the typical acute thrombus of Buerger. That bland thrombus can occur in an inflamed vessel is not surprising, but the finding of vasculitis without thrombus supports the hypothesis that TAO begins with a reaction of the vessel wall or endothelium. Specimens from an acutely inflamed superficial vein are an excellent source of diagnostic biopsy. TAO has also been diagnosed in acutely inflamed temporal and epididymal arteries.[10,40,41] Acute occlusion of an ectatic or frankly aneurysmal popliteal artery, with additional distal manifestations, is an occasional manifestation of TAO. When a youthful smoker has such an event, both the thrombus and a portion of the arterial wall warrant histologic study.[19,29,30] It is also important to examine multiple specimens of mesenteric vessels when bowel ischemia occurs in TAO of the limbs.[42]

CLINICAL ASPECTS

The diagnosis of Buerger's disease should be considered in all tobacco users, both male and female, presenting with digital ischemia of the feet or hands, distal claudication, migratory superficial thrombophlebitis, or Raynaud's phenomenon. The diagnosis of a typical case can be made on clinical assessment alone and other diseases excluded by selected laboratory testing. Angiography and biopsy, when feasible, are used for confirmation or for clarification of difficult problems. Several features help distinguish it from premature atherosclerosis. The disease is always bilateral, often involving three or all four limbs. It begins distally and progresses cephalad. The tempo is brisk, the interval from onset to tissue loss often only 2 to 5 years. In TAO, foot claudication, involvement of the upper extremity, superficial phlebitis, and Raynaud's phenomenon are common; each of these events is rare in atherosclerotic disease of the limbs.

Major reports cite the onset of TAO as between the ages of 19 and 45 years of age, with a median age of 30 to 35 years.[3,8,14-16] Many studies arbitrarily exclude the diagnosis by age 45 or 50. In a summary of reported series, Vink[43] identified less than 2% of patients with onset beyond 50 years. However, Olin et al[18] identified a surprising incidence of 29% of 112 patients exceeding 50 years of age when diagnosed. The study defined accepted clinical criteria for diagnosis, and arteriography or tissue diagnosis was available in 79% of the total group. It is not clear if these older patients started smoking later or how intensively blood studies were pursued early in the study. These observations, made by competent clinicians, await further confirmation but impose a need for vigilance in the differential diagnosis of occlusive disease beyond age 45.

Although the patient may present with complaints of one limb, examination will always show additional involvement. In an analysis of 255 patients, Shionoya[19] observed involvement of all four limbs in 40%, of three limbs in 43%, and of only two limbs in the remaining 17%. The disease begins in the digital and pedal vessels and later involves the distal tibioperoneal system. Initial presentations include complaints of cold sensitivity, dysesthesias, coolness and rubor or cyanosis of the foot in 33%; rest pain in 10% to 80%; digital ulceration or gangrene in 18% to 60%; and pedal claudication in 15% to 25%.[19] Claudication of the foot is almost pathognomonic of Buerger's disease.[44] Ulceration and gangrene may appear spontaneously but most often is induced by trauma such as nail trimming or pressure from footwear, and secondary infection can cause further loss of the ischemic tissues (Fig. 21-3). Claudication levels increase as the disease extends cephalad in contiguous or skipping fashion, involving the femoropopliteal system in about 40% over 1 to 2 years, and later the external iliac artery in 8%.[19,38,45] Aortic involvement is rare and is probably due to proximal propagation of bland thrombus.[46]

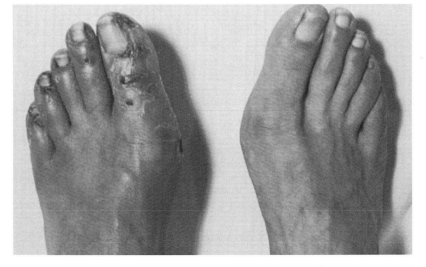

Fig. 21-3. Man, 36. Recurrent crops of nodular phlebitis of the calves, 4 years earlier. Claudication of pedal arches, 2 years. Hand claudication while water skiing, 6 months. Rest pain has occurred in the left foot since new boots induced skin lesions. Absent wrist and pedal pulses. Note the multiple ulcers at sites of pressure, left foot.

Reports of upper-extremity involvement show great variability, the incidence ranging from 15% to 100% (the latter figure noted when this was a criterion of diagnosis). When the wrist pulses are routinely examined and an inquiry of Raynaud's phenomenon is made, upper-extremity TAO at the time of diagnosis is noted in 45% to 60% of patients[10,16,17,19] and over the course of the disease in 90%.[19] Olin et al[18] reported a representative experience: upper extremity digital ischemia occurred in 54% and Raynaud's phenomenon in 44% of 112 patients when initially seen.

The value of a careful clinical assessment is brought out by the observations of Hirai and Shinoya:[47] of 34 patients with TAO of the legs, only 6 complained of upper-extremity involvement, but 22 were found to have pulse deficits or Raynaud's phenomenon when examined. All patients underwent brachial angiography, and the incidence of arterial involvement increased to 91%. Digital artery lesions were the most common, with subsequent involvement of the radial and ulnar arteries at the wrist. Lesions later extended up the forearm, frequently sparing the interosseous, but disease above the elbow was rare. Angiographic findings were identical to those of the leg. The absence of clinical manifestations in patients with angiographic evidence of the disease early in their course is explainable by the dual, parallel circulation of the hand and each digit.

The majority of patients with Buerger's disease present with symptoms of lower-extremity disease, or simultaneous involvement of the arms and legs. Goodman et al[12] noted that 5% of 80 patients had their initial symptoms in the hands. Mills, Taylor, and Porter,[15] with a special interest and expertise in upper-extremity problems, noted that 34% of their patients presented with upper-extremity manifestations.

Raynaud's phenomenon of the fingers, with or without digital ischemia, is noted during the course of TAO in 30% to 45% of patients.[14,17,19] Shionoya[14] notes an incidence of 3% at the time of presentation and 43% over the course of the disease.

Superficial thrombophlebitis, usually migratory and recurrent, is seen in the zones of arterial involvement of both arms and legs of patients with TAO. The lesions are usually linear or branched, but may be round nodules 1 to 2 cm in diameter and are frequently forgotten by the patient when presenting later and preoccupied with ischemic pain. Superficial thrombophlebitis occurs in 30% to 45% of patients[11,12,18,19,48] and has been observed as the presenting complaint in 3% to 27%.[12,19,48]

Buerger's disease is a significant cause of limb loss in these youthful patients, but death from the disease is rare. Finger amputations are reported in 3% to 15%; toe and forefoot amputations in 19% to 23%; and leg amputations, mostly below the knee, in 3% to 30% of patients. Arm removal is rarely required.[8,15,18,49] These amputation rates reflect the duration of follow-up, the effectiveness of local care of ischemic digits, and whether the patients have stopped tobacco use. Interruption of the disease is uniformly reported with abstinence from tobacco, but it is most interesting that Ohta and Shionoya[49] noted disease stability in almost half of the patients who continued

smoking. This raises the question of whether TAO is a self-limiting disease, as is seen in some forms of vasculitis.

TAO is not a lethal disease, and McPherson noted a survivorship equal to a matched control group of non-smokers.[8] Shionoya[19] reported only 5 deaths in 255 patients followed for several years. Death from coronary events and mesenteric insufficiency were noted by both and in other random case reports—raising the question whether these and cerebral events are coincidental or rare manifestations of TAO. When this small literature is reviewed, the evidence for peripheral TAO is not always classic, cerebral involvement is documented chiefly by angiography, histology is not always convincing, and other mechanisms can be postulated in some.[42,50,51] However, Lie[5] provided a photomicrograph typical of an acute Buerger lesion in a patient with mesenteric ischemia and peripheral disease, and collected series suggested that abdominal pain in the Buerger patient should alert the clinician to the possibility of mesenteric ischemia.[52,53]

Laboratory Tests

An appropriate workup should exclude the risk factors of hyperlipidemia and diabetes mellitus. Collagen-vascular disease can be evaluated both clinically and by testing for ANA, complement, erythrocyte sedimentation rate, and using the VDRL (Veneral Disease Research Laboratory) test. Several clotting disorders and the dysproteinemias can cause distal ischemia. Serum protein electrophoresis, erythrocyte and platelet counts, antiphospholipid antibody, and sometimes proteins C and S and antithrombin III are appropriate.

The vascular laboratory can document and quantitate occlusive disease with standard techniques of digital artery pressures and waveforms, and segmental Doppler pressures and waveforms of the limbs. Of importance, ankle and wrist pressures may be normal early in the course when the disease is confined to the toes, foot, or fingers. Laser flow velocities, where available, are useful in assessing occlusive disease of the fingers and their potential response to sympathetic block. Ohta[54] has introduced thallium-202 scanning to determine the healing potential of distal ischemia.

Angiographic Correlations

Arteriography has played an essential role in the contemporary understanding and definition of TAO.[10,11] It is considered diagnostic by some, supportive by others, and some suggest it is not essential when the clinical features are classical. An argument can be made for its routine use: first, there remains a need for further study of the disease; on clinical grounds the diagnosis is uncommon enough that full study may preclude other diagnostic searches in these often migratory patients; and angiography can identify patients amenable to bypass surgery extending to the distal calf and foot and the occasional patient with a popliteal aneurysm. Last, it is important to rule out a proximal site of atherosclerosis.

The essential findings are multiple, bilateral focal segments of stenosis or occlusion with normal intervening and proximal vessels. Stenoses may be a few millimeters or several centimeters long, and occlusions may be abrupt or tapering. Collaterals are usually generous and can be "tree-root," spiderlike, or corkscrew. The latter term variously is used to describe what are clearly nearby serpentine collaterals but also named, involved vessels that are apparently recanalizing. It is debated if the corkscrew appearance of some vessels represents vasa vasorum. Involved digital arteries are attenuated, may be tortuous, and have abrupt cutoffs[10,11,25,55,56] (Figs. 21-4, 21-5, and 21-6).

The patterns of occlusive disease seen by angiography parallel both the distribution and severity of the clinical picture. Digital, pedal, and low-calf vessel involvement is almost universal.[25,56] Bilateral infrapopliteal occlusive disease was seen in all of 210 limbs studied by Shionoya: 90% of anterior tibial, 80% of posterior tibial, and 50% of peroneal arteries were diseased. The peroneal often serves as an important collateral. He observed that toe ulceration occurred in 57% of patients with three obstructed infrapopliteal vessels but that ulcers occurred in only 7% when at least one vessel reached the foot. An additional "skip area" of the disease at the femoropopliteal segment was noted at the time of diagnosis in 41% of patients, and an additional 40% of patients later showed progression at that level.[25] Ectasia of the popliteal segment is an occasional finding.[19,29,30] Involvement of the common and profunda femoris arteries is seen in about 10% of patients and the external iliac in 6%[19,45] (Fig. 21-7).

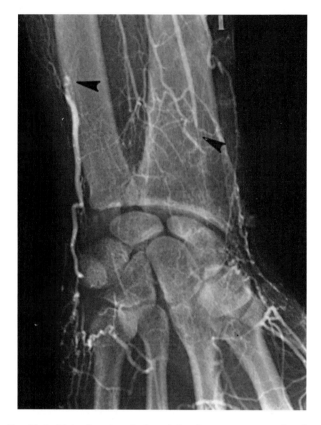

Fig. 21-5. Note abrupt occlusion of the ulnar artery, tapered occlusion of the radial artery. "Tree-root" collaterals emanate from the interosseous artery. Note the multiple areas of stenoses in the distal vessels of the hand.

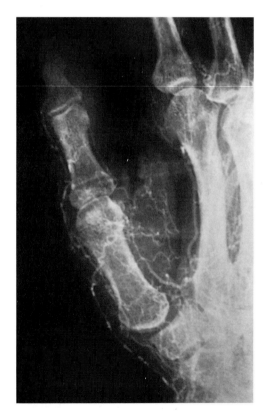

Fig. 21-4. Woman, 41. Bilateral arch claudication, 6 years. Presented with cyanosis and rest pain at left second, third, and fourth fingers. Note the multiple smooth stenosis, numerous occluded vessels.

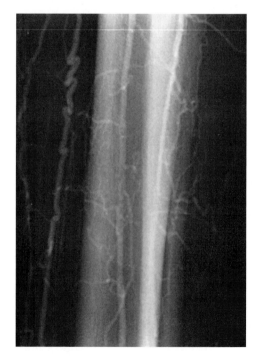

Fig. 21-6. Classic "corkscrew" changes of the posterior tibial artery with segmental occlusion of the peroneal and anterior tibial arteries. This type of corkscrewing is believed to represent the primary disease process in the lumen of the vessel with areas of inflammation.

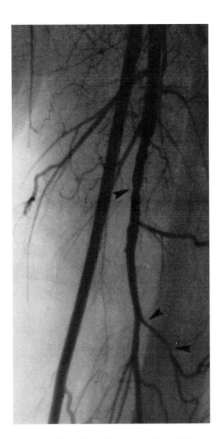

Fig. 21-7. Man, 29. Veins of both calves stripped 6 years earlier for recurrent phlebitis. Bilateral foot, calf claudication, 4 years. Left thigh claudication, 1 year. Acrocyanotic left foot with rest pain. Pedal pulses absent bilaterally. Note the focal stenosis in the left profunda femoris artery *(upper arrow)* and focal smooth zones of narrowing in branches *(lower arrows)*; these latter lesions may represent spasm or disease.

Differential Diagnosis

Premature atherosclerosis is the most common cause of leg claudication and ischemia in young men and women. Pairolero et al[57] studied 50 consecutive patients under age 35 whose symptoms warranted arteriography: 24 had premature atherosclerosis, 14 had TAO, and 12 had a diversity of other problems. It was striking that all but one of those with premature atherosclerosis were heavy smokers. Diabetes was also present in 10 patients, and increased lipids, or hypertension, was present in 8 patients.

Patients with premature atherosclerosis are identified by their more proximal symptoms, associated risk factors, and characteristic angiographic findings. Patients with embolic occlusive disease almost always have an acute onset and an obvious source for the embolus. Rare sources of either progressive claudication and/or distal emboli are the popliteal entrapment syndrome, thoracic outlet entrapment, and cystic disease of the popliteal or common femoral artery, all of which occur in the age range of TAO. The unusual heritable disorders of connective tissue, Ehlers-Danlos syndrome and pseudoxanthoma elasticum, can manifest themselves in the young. The former can occlude arteries both by rupture with thrombosis or aneu-

rysm with embolization, and pseudoxanthoma elasticum can cause chronic occlusion of the forearm, thigh, and calf arteries. Pseudoxanthoma elasticum is diagnosed by its specific cutaneous manifestations and Ehlers-Danlos syndrome by its cutaneous, ocular, and musculoskeletal defects.

Digital occlusive disease is often a major manifestation of collagen-vascular and hematologic disorders. Scleroderma, polyarteritis nodosa, and systemic lupus erythematosus are each accompanied by other manifestations and yield to clinical diagnosis, supported by laboratory testing or biopsy. However, lupus may be initiated by a specific clotting problem, a circulating inhibitor, that causes thrombus in veins, and large digital arteries. Anticardiolipin antibodies or plasma clot time support the diagnosis. It should be noted that serologic and immunologic tests are normal in TAO.[15] Thrombocytosis, polycythemia, intravascular coagulopathy, and dysproteinemia can also be associated with major and microcirculatory occlusion. These are uncommon in the young, and each can be tested for. In essence, the clinical picture of TAO, knowledge of the natural history of the other lesions listed (with selective testing when indicated), and angiography will establish the diagnosis of TAO in most instances.

THERAPY

Only total abstinence from tobacco use will halt the progress and prevent recrudescence of TAO. This cornerstone of therapy must be conveyed clearly and unequivocally to the patient and supporting family or friends. Firmness should be matched with concern and patience in seeking the patient's motivation. Many patients with TAO have well-developed denial patterns and skip from one source of care to another seeking pain medications. Continuity of care in a single, supportive setting is highly desirable and use of a smoking clinic, sometimes on an inpatient basis, can reinforce and increase compliance and aid withdrawal.

Adequate pain control is an essential first step, using whatever drugs and dosages required to achieve this goal. Patients with dysesthesias and minor lesions can be treated as outpatients, but those with rest pain, ulceration, or infection warrant hospitalization. Continuous intravenous narcotics by pump or epidural anesthesia are often required. Wound debris and eschar is removed by gentle, periodic debridement. Topical medications are avoided because of skin reactions they may induce. Infection is treated by drainage and removal of nail beds when subungual abscess is present. Antibiotic therapy is based on culture and sensitivity data.

The success of both medical and surgical therapy relate to the degree of ischemia and pattern of occlusive disease in a given patient. The use of vasodilating agents, currently calcium channel blockers and α-adrenergic blockers, has its greatest impact on vasomotor changes, and the efficacy on ischemic pain and wound healing is not documented by controlled studies. Because thrombus formation is a major component of TAO, it is logical to consider heparinization in those who present with an acute exacerbation or show fresh cutoffs on angiograms. But one can only hope to prevent further clot propagation, just as long-term antiplatelet agents might do for chronic cases. Information on both agents is anecdotal and not convincing. However, given clinical or angiographic evidence of a recent clot, the concept of lysis is attractive and some limited success has been reported on focal lesions.[58] Prostaglandins provide the dual benefits of vasodilation and antiplatelet activity, and in a controlled study showed benefit in patients with chronic rest pain, some gain being maintained for 6 months.[59] The drug requires intravenous administration daily over several weeks, and the requirements for retreatment have not been established. An ideal drug would stop the disease process, even in the face of continued tobacco use. Steroids given in years past showed no benefit, but should TAO be proven a vasculitis, trials with higher dosages combined with newer cytotoxic or immunosuppressive agents would be justified.

Shionoya et al[60] found bypass surgery precluded by extensive distal disease in most patients but reported on 44 patients who had distal segments suitable for grafting. Patency rates for suprainguinal (aortofemoral or iliofemoral) grafts were 90% at 1 year, 70% at 2 years, and 70% at 10 years. The patency rates of femoropopliteal or tibioperoneal grafts were 56%, 48%, and 32%, respectively.[14] Sasajima et al[61] found 15 patients with pedal ischemia suitable for pedal bypass. Their three earlier failures were attributed to technical problems and three later failures from disease progression in patients who continued smoking. Nine grafts remained patent at 4 to 9 years of follow-up. Although these results do not approach those achieved in atherosclerosis, surgery would seem justified in these small subsets of patients if wound healing occurred, rest pain cleared, or amputation was avoided. When ischemic rest pain, ulceration, or gangrene cannot be improved by the measures discussed within 3 to 4 weeks, early amputation should be considered as a positive tool of rehabilitation.

Sympathectomy has a long tradition of use for TAO, yet proof of its efficacy is lacking; results are disappointing and hard to evaluate. It may relieve vasomotor symptoms of coolness and mild pain in early TAO, but a controlled study with attention to the extent of the disease and the status of tobacco use is needed to clearly define its value.

Progress in the therapy of Buerger's disease is dependent on unveiling its etiology and evaluation of past and future therapy with proper controls that relate to the stage of the disease and status of tobacco use.

REFERENCES

1. von Winiwarter F: Ueber eine eigenthumliche Dorm von Endarteritis und Endophlebitis mit Gangran des Fusses, Arch Klin Chirur 13:202, 1879.
2. Buerger L: Thrombo-angiitis obliterans: a study of the vascular lesions leading to presenile spontaneous gangrene, Am J Med Sci 136:567, 1908.
3. Buerger L: The circulatory disturbances of the extremities; including gangrene, vasomotor, and trophic disorders, Philadelphia, 1924, Saunders.
4. Eastcott HHG: Buerger's disease. In Bergan JJ and Yao JST, eds: Evaluation and treatment of upper and lower extremity circulatory disorders, New York, 1984, Grune & Stratton.
5. Lie JT: II. Thromboangiitis obliterans (Buerger's disease) revisited, Pathol Annu 23:257, 1988.
6. Wessler S et al: A critical evaluation of thromboangiitis obliterans: the case against Buerger's disease, N Engl J Med 262:1149, 1960.
7. Wessler S: Buerger's disease revisited, Surg Clin North Am 49:703, 1969.
8. McPherson JR, Juergens JL, and Gifford RW: Thromboangiitis obliterans and arteriosclerosis obliterans: clinical and prognostic differences, Ann Intern Med 59:288, 1963.
9. McKusick VA and Harris WS: The Buerger syndrome in the Orient, Bull Johns Hopkins Hosp 109:241, 1961.
10. McKusick VA et al: Buerger's disease: a distinct clinical and pathologic entity, JAMA 181:5, 1962.
11. Szilagyi ED, De Russo FJ, and Elliot JP Jr: Thromboangiitis obliterans: clinico-angiographic correlations, Arch Surg 88:824, 1964.
12. Goodman RM et al: Buerger's disease in Israel, Am J Med 39:601, 1965.
13. Lie JT: Thromboangiitis obliterans (Buerger's disease) in women, Medicine (Baltimore) 66:65, 1987.
14. Shionoya S: What is Buerger's disease? World J Surg 7:544, 1983.
15. Mills JL, Taylor LM Jr, and Porter JM: Buerger's disease in the modern era, Am J Surg 154:123, 1987.
16. Papa MZ and Adar R: A critical look at thromboangiitis obliterans (Buerger's disease). In Goldstone J, ed: Perspectives in vascular surgery, St. Louis, 1992, Quality Medical Publishing.
17. Mills JL and Porter JM: Buerger's disease: a review and update, Semin Vasc Surg 6:14, 1993.
18. Olin JW et al: The changing clinical spectrum of thromboangiitis obliterans (Buerger's disease), Circulation 82(suppl IV):3, 1990.
19. Shionoya S: Buerger's disease (thromboangiitis obliterans). In Rutherford RB, ed: Vascular surgery, ed 4, Philadelphia, 1994, Saunders.
20. Lilienthal H: Thrombo-angiitis obliterans: multiple ligation of varicose veins of leg, Ann Surg 59:796, 1914.
21. Meyer W: Etiology of thromboangiitis obliterans (Buerger), JAMA 71:1268, 1918.
22. Hill GL and Smith AH: Buerger's disease in Indonesia: clinical course and prognostic factors, J Chronic Dis 27:205, 1974.
23. Kjeldsen K and Mozes M: Buerger's disease in Israel, Acta Chir Scand 135:495, 1969.
24. Rao AS, Rao GN, and Vasantha VC: Thromboangiitis obliterans: a clinicopathologic study, J Indian Med Assoc 66:98, 1976.
25. Shionoya S, Hiari M, and Kawai S: Pattern of arterial occlusion in Buerger's disease, Angiology 33:375, 1982.
26. Davis HA and King LD: A comparative study of thromboangiitis in white and negro patients, Surg Gynecol Obstet 85:597, 1947.
27. Lie JT: The rise and fall and resurgence of thromboangiitis obliterans (Buerger's disease), Acta Pathol Jpn 39:153, 1989.
28. Kimoto S: The history and present status of aortic surgery in Japan particularly for aortitis syndrome, J Cardiovasc Surg 20:101, 1979.
29. Case Records of the Massachusetts General Hospital (Case 16-1989), N Engl J Med 320:1068, 1989.
30. Lie JT: Thromboangiitis obliterans (Buerger's disease) and smokeless tobacco, Arthritis Rheum 31:812, 1988.
31. Schatz IJ, Fine G, and Eyler WR: Thromboangiitis obliterans, Br Heart J 28:84, 1966.
32. Matsushita M, Shionoya S, and Matsumoto T: Urinary coti-

nine measurements in patients with Buerger's disease—effect of active and passive smoking on the disease process, J Vasc Surg 14:53, 1991.

33. Numano F et al: HLA in Buerger's disease, Clin Immunogenet 3:195, 1986.
34. Schellong SM et al: No ANCA in thromboangiitis obliterans (Buerger's disease). In Gross WL, ed: ANCA-associated vasculitides: immunologic and clinical aspects, New York, 1993, Plenum Press.
35. Adar R et al: Cellular sensitivity to collagen in thromboangiitis obliterans, N Engl J Med 308:1113, 1983.
36. Papa M et al: Autoimmune mechanisms in thromboangiitis obliterans (Buerger's disease): the role of tobacco antigen and the major histocompatability complex, Surgery 111:527, 1992.
37. Gulati SM et al: Significance of circulatory immune complexes in thromboangiitis obliterans (Buerger's disease), Angiology 35:276, 1984.
38. Shionoya S et al: Pattern of arterial occlusion in Buerger's disease, Angiology 33:375, 1982.
39. Buerger L: Recent studies in the pathology of thromboangiitis obliterans, J Med Res 31:181, 1914.
40. Ferguson GT and Starkebaum G: Thromboangiitis obliterans associated with idiopathic hypereosinophilia, Arch Intern Med 145:1726, 1985.
41. Lie JT and Michet CJ Jr: Thromboangiitis obliterans with eosinophilia (Buerger's disease) of the temporal arteries, Hum Pathol 19:598, 1928.
42. Wolf EA, Sumner DS, and Strandness DE Jr: Disease of the mesenteric circulation in patients with thromboangiitis obliterans, Vasc Surg 6:218, 1973.
43. Vink M: Symposium on Buerger's disease, J Cardiovasc Surg 14:1, 1973.
44. Hirai M and Shionoya S: Intermittent claudication in the foot and Buerger's disease, Br J Surg 65:210, 1978.
45. Shionoya S et al: Involvement of the iliac artery in Buerger's disease: a pathogenesis and arterial reconstruction, J Cardiovasc Surg 19:69, 1978.

46. Ishikawa A: Annual report on Buerger's disease, Tokyo, 1970, Japanese Ministry of Health and Welfare.
47. Hirai M and Shinoya S: Arterial obstruction of the upper limb in Buerger's disease: its incidence and primary lesion, Br J Surg 66:124, 1979.
48. Schatz IJ, Fine G, and Eyler WR: Thromboangiitis obliterans, Br Heart J 28:84, 1966.
49. Ohta T and Shionoya S: Fate of the ischemic limb in Buerger's disease, Br J Surg 75:259, 1988.
50. Biller J et al: A case for cerebral thromboangiitis obliterans, Stroke 12:686, 1981.
51. Drake ME: Winiwarter-Buerger disease (thromboangiitis obliterans) with cerebral involvement, JAMA 246:1170, 1982.
52. Ito M et al: Intestinal ischemia resulting from Buerger's disease: report of a case, Jpn J Surg 23:988, 1993.
53. Kempczinski RF et al: Intestinal ischemia secondary to thromboangiitis obliterans, Ann Vasc Surg 7:354, 1993.
54. Ohta T: Noninvasive technique using thallium-201 for predicting ischemic ulcer healing of the foot, Br J Surg 72:892, 1985.
55. Hagen B and Lohse S: Clinical and radiologic aspects of Buerger's disease, Cardiovasc Intervent Radiol 7:283, 1984.
56. Suzuki S et al: Buerger's disease (thromboangiitis obliterans): an analysis of the arteriograms of 119 cases, Clin Radiol 33:235, 1982.
57. Pairolero PC et al: Lower limb ischemia in young adults: prognostic implications, J Vasc Surg 1:459, 1984.
58. Hussein EA and El Dorri A: Intra-arterial streptokinase as adjuvant therapy for complicated Buerger's disease, Int Surg 78:54, 1993.
59. Fiessinger JN and Schafre M: Trial of illprost versus aspirin for critical limb ischemia of thromboangiitis obliterans, Lancet 335:555, 1990.
60. Shionoya S et al: Vascular reconstruction in Buerger's disease, Br J Surg 63:841, 1976.
61. Sasajima T et al: Plantar or dorsalis pedis artery bypass in Buerger's disease, Ann Vasc Surg 8:248, 1994.

CHAPTER TWENTY-TWO

SYSTEMIC VASCULITIS

Leonard H. Calabrese

Gary S. Hoffman

John D. Clough

While the vast majority of patients with ischemic vascular disease have conditions that are noninflammatory in nature, no textbook of peripheral vascular disease would be complete without a thorough consideration of inflammatory vascular disease as well. The term *vasculitis* is generally used interchangably with the term *necrotizing vasculitis,* which refers to a heterogeneous group of disorders all sharing in varying degrees the pathologic features of vascular inflammation and vascular necrosis. Generally speaking, while inflammation may accompany a wide variety of vascular syndromes, the term necrotizing vasculitis is not used to refer to the incidental inflammatory reactions that may occur in other vascular diseases or to vascular inflammation resulting from simple mechanical or chemical trauma. The vasculitides encompass those syndromes that are either suspected or proven to be immune mediated and frequently with distinctive clinical pictures.

The clinical approach to vascular inflammatory disease has been evolving since the first detailed description of polyarteritis nodosa over 100 years ago. This approach has been influenced by our improved understanding of these disorders, particularly in the following areas:

1. Immune mechanisms responsible for these diseases
2. Pathologic spectrum of the disorders
3. Identification of certain etiologic agents
4. Promising therapies for what used to be considered frequently fatal disorders

This chapter will review our current understanding of the pathogenesis, classification, and clinical spectrum of these disorders and will also provide a practical diagnostic and therapeutic approach.

PATHOGENESIS

Over the past decade there has been considerable progress in the understanding of vascular inflammation.

Before the mid 1980s most pathogenetic theories centered on the role of immune complexes (ICs). Unfortunately, the early enthusiasm for IC-mediated theories of vascular inflammation has been limited by the appreciation of the low specificity IC detection. As a result, broader mechanisms of vascular inflammation have been searched for and elucidated. Although specific etiologies are rare, there is clinical and experimental support for at least four separate mechanisms involved in vasculitic diseases. These mechanisms include (1) IC, (2) antibody-mediated, (3) cell-mediated or endothelial focus, and (4) immunproliferative processes.

IMMUNE COMPLEXES

Supporting evidence for circulating immune complexes (CICs) in a limited number of vasculitic conditions include (1) animal models of IC disease, (2) identification of IC in tissues, (3) identification of IC in the sera of patients with necrotizing vasculitis, and (4) identification of discrete antigens responsible for certain IC disorders.[1] In humans both identification of IC in sera and tissues are supportive of their importance in certain diseases. In particular, the diseases within the hypersensitivity vasculitis group (see the box, p. 381) have the strongest support for an IC-mediated pathogenesis. Infectious diseases that may mediate vascular inflammatory disease include hepatitis B and C. In certain patients with hepatitis B infection arthritis, vasculitis, and glomerulonephritis (GN) can be seen. In this disease hepatitis viral antigens, specific antibodies, and resultant ICs have been identified in both the circulation and in inflamed tissues. The majority of cases of mixed cryoglobulinemia, which previously were considered idiopathic or essential have now been linked to hepatitis C.[2] True hypersensitivity vasculitis, which generally follows exposure to an antigenic trigger such as a drug, also appears to be IC mediated. In this condition small-vessel vasculitis follows the exposure to a discrete

CLASSIFICATION OF NECROTIZING VASCULITIS

Polyarteritis Nodosa Group of Systemic Necrotizing Vasculitis
Classic polyarteritis nodosa
Allergic granulomatosis (Churg-Strauss syndrome)
Microscopic polyarteritis

Hypersensitivity Vasculitis Group
True hypersensitivity vasculitis
Henoch-Schönlein purpura
Mixed cryoglobulinemia with vasculitis
Vasculitis with connective tissue disease
Urticarial vasculitis (hypocomplementemic vasculitis)
Vasculitis associated with other primary disorders

Wegener's Ganulomatosis Group
Classical Wegener's granulomatosis
Limited Wegener's granulomatosis

Giant Cell Arteritis
Temporal arteritis
Takayasu's arteritis

Angiocentric Immunoproliferative Disorders
Benign lymphocytic angiitis
Lymphomatoid granulomatosis
Angiocentric lymphoma

Miscellaneous Vasculitides

antigen by 7 to 10 days and is often accompanied by evidence of complement activation and immunoglobulin and/or complement deposition in involved tissues. Strong evidence for humoral immunity also is shared by Henoch-Schönlein purpura, urticarial vasculitis, and a fraction of patients with polyarteritis nodosa (PAN).

ANTIBODY-ASSOCIATED DISEASE

Perhaps the greatest breakthrough in the past several decades has been the discovery of antineutrophil cytoplasmic antibodies (ANCAs). In the early part of the 1980s ANCAs were identified by immunofluorescent technique in a small number of patients with crescentic GN and vasculitis. This was followed by the observations of many others that ANCAs were frequently present in patients with Wegener's granulomatosis (WG) and often appeared to correlate with disease activity. Since then numerous investigators have confirmed and extended these findings as well as documented their presence in patients with several other conditions including crescentic GN of the pauci immune variety, microscopic polyarteritis, and subsets of patients with PAN and Churg-Strauss syndrome.[3]

It is uncertain at the present time whether ANCAs are

directly pathogenic, but there is growing evidence suggesting this to be the case. The antigens responsible for the ANCA reaction include proteinase-3 (C-ANCA) and myeloperoxidase (P-ANCA) as well as others. Under certain circumstances involving neutrophil and monocyte activation, these antigens may become expressed on the surface of these cells. ANCAs are then capable of binding to neutrophils, causing release of their toxic products. Myeloperoxidase and proteinase-3 (PR3) may also bind to endothelial cells and serve as "innocent bystanders" for ANCA-mediated injury. If such a mechanism is true, strategies to reduce ANCA levels by selective techniques may afford an additional treatment option for these diseases.

Additional antibodies that may be involved in the pathogenesis of certain vasculitic syndromes include anti-endothelial antibodies and a number of other autoantibodies without organ specificity.

CELL-MEDIATED/ENDOTHELIAL FOCAL DISEASE

Several vasculitic syndromes including giant cell arteritis (GCA) and Takayasu's disease demonstrate little evidence for either CIC or specific antibodies, and their pathology is more suggestive of cell-mediated processes. The ability of endothelial cells to become "activated" and serve as antigen-presenting cells and sources of cytokine production suggests their ability to interact with immunocompetent cells even in the absence of injury. Endothelial cells also express multiple adhesion molecules, which have the ability to interact with complementary ligands on immunocytes, including both polymorphonuclear leukocytes as well as lymphocytes, leading to leukocyte binding and emigration. Endothelial cells may also become the targets for cell-mediated immune damage including cytotoxic T cells and natural killer (NK) cells since both have been demonstrated capable of such activity in vitro. Endothelial cells are also important in initiating and controlling coagulation pathways.[4]

IMMUNOPROLIFERATIVE DISORDERS

Several vascular inflammatory disorders demonstrate strong evidence of being lymphoproliferative disorders, in particular the syndromes of benign lymphocytic angiitis and lymphomatoid granulomatosis/polymorphic reticulosis. These conditions are angiocentric and predominantly T cell in nature with little propensity for vessel necrosis. Frequently they are the forerunners of frank T cell lymphomas within the vascular wall (i.e., angiocentric lymphoma). Recent studies using gene rearrangement have demonstrated the clonal nature of many of these cases even in the presence of morphologically benign disease.[5]

Finally, it should be appreciated that most vasculitic syndromes represent admixtures of these proposed mechanisms. For example, endothelium initially injured by antibody or IC may then become activated, secrete cytokines, and/or display adhesion molecules and become the focus for cell-mediated pathologic damage. Other conditions such as Kawasaki disease demonstrate strong evidence of endothelial activation and cytokine release, but also are associated with ANCAs. A clearer understanding of the pathologic mechanisms involved in discrete syndromes will facilitate more specific therapies including biologic response modifiers.

CLASSIFICATION

Since the earliest descriptions of necrotizing vasculitis in the nineteenth century, numerous attempts have been made to classify these disorders and thus provide clinicians a useful basis for approaching them. The desire to separate these disorders on some rational basis has been limited by the simple fact that the vascular system has a limited range of responses to noxious stimuli and that the resultant end-organ damage caused by vasculitis is not unique but simply that of vascular ischemia, regardless of the underlying vascular pathology. As a result, attempts to separate these disorders by various criteria or variables has been problematic.

Early classification schemes were based on a variety of factors such as the pathologic picture including the presence or absence of fibrinoid necrosis, giant cells, granulomas, eosinophils or other morphologic features. Unfortunately, many diseases such as Henoch-Schönlein purpura, systemic lupus erythematosus, hepatitis B associated vasculitis, and vasculitis associated with malignancies frequently yielded the identical histopathologic picture. Other more specific morphologic findings such as those found in allergic granulomatous angiitis and Wegener's granulomatosis may at times be distinct but do not assist in the separation of the remainder of the vasculitic syndromes.

Classification schemes have also been proposed based on characteristic distribution of target organ damage, but these, too, have not been uniformly successful. For example, most cases of polyarteritis nodosa appear to spare the lungs, but the now recognized overlap syndrome or polyangiitis may demonstrate lung involvement as well as the other clinical and pathologic features identical to classic polyarteritis nodosa.[6] Classification schemes based purely on laboratory findings such as the presence or absence of immune complexes or based on identification of etiologic agents have been less rewarding.

In 1978 Fauci, Haynes, and Katz at the National Institutes of Health proposed a classification scheme[7] based on an admixture of clinical, pathologic, immunologic and therapeutic variables that yield a scheme that is not only approachable in its clarity but clinically useful. This classification, with several modifications, is displayed in the box, p. 381. Diseases are grouped into headings that frequently serve as points of differential diagnosis and thus assist diagnostic and therapeutic decision-making by clinicians. For example, the hypersensitivity group all share the features of near-universal involvement of the skin and the fact that these diseases tend to involve the smallest branches of the vascular system though etiologically they are diverse. When confronted with such a patient with a small-vessel cutaneous vasculitis, this group of disorders forms a logical starting place in the differential diagnostic process. The remainder of this chapter will discuss the clinical and pathologic features of the main forms of necrotizing vasculitis as well as provide a diagnostic and therapeutic approach to their management.

POLYARTERITIS NODOSA

Polyarteritis nodosa (PAN) was first described by the term periarteritis nodosa by Kussmaul and Maier over 100 years ago. The prefix "peri" referred to the fact that the disease could be identified grossly by the presence of visible nodules found along the course of muscular arteries. Over the ensuing years many similar cases were described by the same gross appearance. These cases all shared the clinical features of a general sparing of the tissues of the lungs and the microscopic features of tendencies of involving the bifurcations of the muscular arteries as well as sparing the smallest branches of the intrinsic vascular system. Unfortunately, because of a lack of appreciation of the broader spectrum of necrotizing vasculitis, the term polyarteritis, or periarteritis, was also applied to other vasculitic syndromes, both primary and secondary, not recognized to be nosologically distinct. Rheumatic fever, syphilis, Wegener's granulomatosis, hypersensitivity vasculitis, and others were all included under the same heading, thus leaving considerable confusion and controversy in subsequent attempts to classify these disorders. In the 1970s the recognition that the hepatitis B virus was etiologically responsible for some cases of PAN gave new insight into the pathogenesis of the disorder and new controversy about whether it represented a single entity or was multifactorial in its origin.

Clinical Features

Though the incidence of PAN is not precisely known, it is generally considered to be clinically rare. There is a sex predilection for males over females of approximately 2-3:1. The disease has been recognized in virtually all age groups but appears to peak in the fourth and fifth decades.[8,9]

The most common signs of PAN relate to its devastating multisystem inflammatory nature. Constitutional symptoms including malaise and weakness accompanied by varying degrees of fever and weight loss are common. Other clinical findings depend on the distribution of target organ involvement, which may be highly variable. Musculoskeletal symptoms including inflammatory polyarthritis mimicking rheumatoid disease is not uncommon. Muscle involvement characterized by either muscle pain and/or proximal weakness mimicking polymyositis can also be observed. Symptoms relating to the presence of a sensory and/or motor neuropathy are also quite common. Abdominal pain, which may be mild to severe, may represent gastrointestinal involvement.[8,9]

KIDNEYS. The kidneys are involved in the vast majority of patients estimated to be between 75% and 85%. The renal manifestations of PAN are varied and may consist of glomerulonephritis, renal vasculitis or aneurysms of the renal vascular system. The clinical sequelae of this pathologic involvement can be asymptomatic or life-threatening. The glomerular disease of PAN is that of focal segmental necrotizing glomerulonephritis.[9] Immunoglobulin or complement deposition is variably present.

Necrotizing vasculitis of the renal vessels is found in over half of autopsied cases but is rarely encountered in percutaneous renal biopsies. This finding is frequently misinterpreted by clinicians as a strong negative indicator of disease presence. Microaneurysms identified by arteriography when present in medium or small caliber vessels are considered almost pathognomonic of polyarteritis nodosa, but they may be observed in other types of vasculitis and rarely in nonvasculitic conditions such as atrial myxoma.[10]

The clinical sequelae of renal involvement include hypertension, which is seen in the majority of patients and, at times, can be clinically severe. The mechanism of this hypertension appears to be renin mediated from diffuse intrarenal vascular disease and may persist after the disease is adequately treated. Renal failure is seen in a varying number of patients and may be responsible for death in up to 50% of patients with PAN.[9]

NEUROLOGIC SYSTEM. The central nervous system is involved in as many as 25% of patients with PAN when it is assessed by clinical findings or autopsy results. This may be manifested by strokes, altered mental status, cognitive impairment, seizures, or hemorrhage.[9]

Peripheral neurologic lesions are seen in nearly half the patients with PAN. Several patterns of clinical involvement of the peripheral nerves have been reported including mononeuritis multiplex (the most characteristic), symmetric sensory involvement (glove and stocking neuropathy) and a lesion known as dense mononeuritis multiplex resulting from the infarction of multiple peripheral nerves in one extremity leading to profound weakness of the affected limb.[11] Isolated mononeuropathies may be observed as well. The new appearance of mononeuritis multiplex in the absence of diabetes or trauma should be considered presumptive evidence of necrotizing vasculitis until proven otherwise.

MUSCULOSKELETAL SYSTEM. PAN may appear as a symmetric polyarthritis mimicking rheumatoid arthritis. The differential diagnosis is further complicated by the fact that many patients with PAN may have elevated sedimentation rates and rheumatoid factors. There is generally a discordance between the amount of systemic disease and the amount of arthritis in PAN as opposed to rheumatoid. In PAN there is often prominent constitutional symptoms from the outset in the presence of arthritis that is nonerosive. In rheumatoid arthritis, on the other hand, the arthritis is usually the earliest manifestation of the disease and significant constitutional symptoms usually arise further along in the clinical course.

Muscle involvement may be manifested by simple myalgias or a proximal myopathy mimicking polymyositis. Muscle enzymes may be slightly elevated and electromyographic examination may be consistent with a patchy inflammatory myopathy. Rarely does PAN cause dramatic proximal muscle weakness, but because of clinical similarities, it is important to differentiate these conditions because of differences in therapy and prognosis.

GASTROINTESTINAL SYSTEM. Gastrointestinal involvement is present in nearly half the patients with PAN. The clinical manifestations relate to underlying ischemia, which may involve the mucosa, submucosa, or the entire thickness of the bowel. Other organs within the gastrointestinal system may be involved including the liver and pancreas. Occasionally, in patients with PAN with gastrointestinal involvement there will be the typical symptoms of "intestinal angina." This symptom complex consists of postprandial abdominal pain and cramping. The most severe complication of gastrointestinal involvement by PAN is visceral perforation. This is a catastrophic complication because it generally occurs when the underlying disease is uncontrolled and in need of immunosuppressive therapy, and the resultant complication is a septic process in need of strengthened host defenses.

Virtually every part of the gastrointestinal tract can be involved by PAN and the diagnosis has occasionally been made by biopsy of gastric polyps, cholecystectomy, and appendectomy. Of important clinical note is the syndrome of isolated gallbladder or appendiceal involvement by PAN. In this clinical situation the histopathology of the resected gallbladder or appendix is typical of PAN with fibrinoid necrosis of medium-sized muscular arteries, but there is no evidence of systemic disease, and long-term follow-up care of several of these patients has revealed a benign prognosis.

CARDIAC INVOLVEMENT. Cardiac involvement occurs in up to 80% of patients with PAN and is second only to renal disease as a cause of death.[9] Cardiac involvement is generally difficult to detect and the most common expression of its presence is congestive heart failure. All anatomic areas of the heart including the endocardium, myocardium, and pericardium may be involved by the vasculitic process. Conduction abnormalities have been observed and are clinically rare.

MISCELLANEOUS FINDINGS. Skin involvement in PAN is relatively infrequent when compared to other categories of systemic vasculitis (e.g., hypersensitivity vasculitis). The most common cutaneous manifestations are nonspecific vascular rashes, such as palpable purpura, nonblanching maculopapular lesions or urticaria. This may cause some confusion with diseases within the hypersensitivity vasculitis group, but the presence of extensive involvement of larger caliber vessels should help clarify the situation. The most characteristic cutaneous finding is the subcutaneous inflammatory nodule, which may occur in as many as 10% to 15% of patients. The syndrome of subcutaneous PAN is characterized by skin lesions that are highly inflammatory and painful and pathologically display necrotizing vasculitis of muscular vessels within the subcutaneous tissue but are unassociated with systemic disease.[12]

Ocular involvement can be seen in 10% to 15% of cases. This may be manifested by hemorrhages, conjunctivitis, iritis, or also by involvement of the corroid leading to retinal detachment.

Testicular involvement has been mentioned as a common clinical finding and a source of diagnostic material. Orchitis occurs in approximately 10% to 15% of male patients and, when present, may be useful as a source for pathologic documentation.

Involvement of the lungs is distinctly uncommon in classic PAN and usually suggests another form of angiitis such as Wegener's granulomatosis. The involvement of the lungs in the overlap syndrome or polyangiitis representing an admixture of the clinical findings of several different vasculitic syndromes should be kept in mind.[6] While the pulmonary circulation is generally spared, the bronchial circulation may be affected in classic PAN and secondary pulmonary disease such as infection complicating immunosuppressive therapy may be seen.

Laboratory

There is no specific laboratory test for PAN and the most sensitive laboratory findings in this disease are elevation of the erythrocyte sedimentation rate, white blood cell count, and the presence of anemia.[9] The absence of all of these findings in an individual suspected of having PAN would be strong evidence of its absence. The presence of elevated circulating immune complexes and hypocomplementemia are helpful when present but are absent in the majority of patients. Rheumatoid factor may be found in a sizable number of patients with PAN. The remainder of the laboratory studies reflect the presence or absence of various target organ damage including kidneys, central nervous system, gastrointestinal, etc. ANCA, either of the C or P variety, may be present in less than 50%.

Pathophysiology

In the 1970s it was reported that hepatitis B surface antigen could be found in the majority of patients with PAN. This finding prompted an aggressive search for other etiologic agents that could explain this disease. Unfortunately, current estimates suggest that only about 15% of patients with PAN have evidence of hepatitis B infection with the remaining patients representing an admixture of idiopathic disease and those associated with a variety of other findings. Other underlying diseases and problems that have been associated with the presence of a PAN-like syndrome include hairy cell leukemia, endocarditis, connective tissue disease, and drug abuse.[9] The presence of ANCAs in a minority of patients is of uncertain significance.

Diagnosis

The diagnosis of PAN can be highly problematic but must first start with a high suspicion of its presence. Fever of unknown origin, unexplained multisystem disease, mononeuritis multiplex, unexplained inflammatory disease of muscle or joints may all be the initial manifestations of PAN. There are no laboratory tests that can diagnose the presence of this condition, though, as stated previously, a normal hemoglobin, white count, and sedimentation rate strongly suggest its absence. The presence of numerous symptoms or signs consistent with PAN in conjunction with elevated circulating immune complexes and hypocomplementemia would strongly support its presence.

The diagnosis of the condition must be based on either tissue evidence of necrotizing vasculitis or angiographic evidence of multiple microaneurysms. The pathologic lesion is characterized by a predilection for medium-sized muscular arteries with a tendency to involve the bifurcations (Fig. 22-1). There is significant debate as to which is the first test to choose when trying to diagnose this condition, but several generalizations can be made. First in the absence of any obvious target organ involvement, such as renal, gastrointestinal, or neurologic, panabdominal arteriography is the diagnostic mode of choice. Approximately 70% to 80% of patients with PAN will have

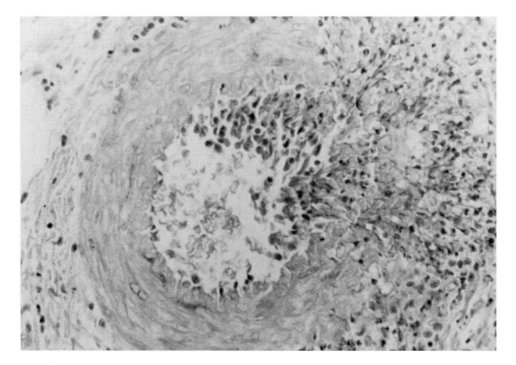

Fig. 22-1. Vessel biopsy from a patient with PAN demonstrates vascular wall necrosis and acute inflammation.

abnormal abdominal arteriograms with three fourths of these patients demonstrating classic multiple microaneurysms (Fig. 22-2).[10] In the presence of documented peripheral neurologic disease by either clinical examination or EMG, a sural nerve biopsy has extremely high yield.[13] Blind biopsies of the muscle, kidney, and testicle in the absence of clinical signs or symptoms of their involvement is rarely productive. Skin biopsy alone is inadequate evidence of the presence of PAN. Percutaneous renal biopsies may be employed with the recognition that they will rarely demonstrate extraglomerular vasculitis, but rather a segmental necrotizing glomerulonephritis.

Treatment

Untreated, the 5-year survival rate for PAN is 10% to 15%. With the use of corticosteroids the 5-year survival rate was noted to improve to nearly 50%. In recent years, the use of combination therapy with cyclophosphamide and high-dose steroids has been reported to increase the 5-year survival rate to 80% or more.[14] Treatment of this condition is generally instituted with doses of cyclophosphamide in a range of 1 to 2 mg/kg/day and prednisone 1 mg/kg/day. Milder cases (i.e., without renal, pulmonary, or central nervous system [CNS] involvement) may be at times treated with corticosteroids alone. Treatment is prolonged, and it may require several years to allow for total control of the disease.

The treatment of PAN associated with hepatitis B is a special and complicated situation. Recent investigations have suggested that a program combining corticosteroids, plasma exchange, and an antiviral agent (α-interferon or vidarabine) may be efficacious.[15]

ALLERGIC GRANULOMATOUS ANGIITIS AND ALLERGIC GRANULOMATOSIS (CHURG-STRAUSS SYNDROME)

In 1951 Churg and Strauss described 13 cases of systemic necrotizing vasculitis that had a variety of distinguishing features from classic PAN.[16] These patients had a predominance of involvement of the pulmonary circulation, a frequent history of adult onset asthma, and striking peripheral eosinophilia. It also bore a variety of similarities to classic PAN, including the predominance of medium-sized vessel involvement and, with the exception of the lungs, a similar array of target organ involvement.

The syndrome is clinically rare and in the largest series of patients reported from the Mayo Clinic there was a predominance of males over females by a 2:1 ratio. The mean age is approximately 47 years but has been reported in both children and the elderly.[17]

The lungs are nearly always involved with x-ray changes being noted in over 90% of patients. Skin involvement is also present in approximately two thirds of patients manifested by palpable purpura or inflammatory nodules. Peripheral neurologic involvement as seen in classic PAN is also frequently observed with mononeuritis multiplex being the most common complication. Involvement of the gastrointestinal, cardiac, and renal systems are also not infrequent.[17]

There is a striking history of asthma in the vast majority of patients with the symptoms often antedating the vasculitis by approximately 2 years. We have noticed that in several patients with the disorder, the asthma may actually become less severe or go into a clinical remission at the time of the onset of the vasculitis.

The laboratory hallmark of this disorder is a striking degree of peripheral eosinophilia, generally in excess of 1500 cells/mm^3. Elevation of IgE has also been described. The pathology of the disorder is a necrotizing vasculitis involving medium- and small-sized muscular arteries. In distinction to PAN, eosinophils and granulomata are seen in and around the vascular infiltrates.

The prognosis of this disorder is not as well documented as that of classic PAN, though some observers have considered it similar. The initial treatment of the disorder is generally with high-dose corticosteroids. For those failing to respond to corticosteroids alone or those with unacceptable toxicities from these agents, the use of additional immunosuppressive drugs such as cyclophosphamide has been reported to be successful.[14]

MICROSCOPIC POLYARTERITIS—POLYANGIITIS OVERLAP SYNDROMES

In addition to classic PAN and allergic granulomatosis, the polyangiitis, or overlap syndrome, has been included under the heading of systemic necrotizing vasculitis. The legitimization of this disorder as a distinct nosologic entity

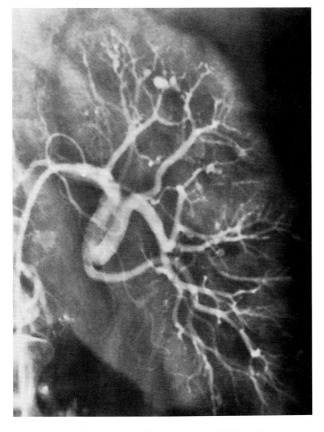

Fig. 22-2. Renal arteriogram demonstrates multiple microaneurysms.

within the necrotizing vasculitides is supported by the recognition that there are patients with both classic PAN and Churg-Strauss syndrome bearing features of each condition but not precisely fitting the clinical descriptions of either.[6,7]

In addition to bearing features of each of these conditions, patients with polyangiitis may demonstrate clinical features of other vasculitic syndromes such as hypersensitivity vasculitis or giant cell arteritis.[6,7]

Examples of patients with polyangiitis may be individuals with classic PAN without lung involvement but with a high degree of peripheral eosinophilia. Alternatively, patients with a classic picture of Churg-Strauss syndrome with multiple microaneurysms on abdominal angiography may also fit this description. In a series of 10 patients with this disorder reported from the National Institutes of Health, cutaneous disease was the most common feature frequently and mistakenly diagnosed as a disorder from the hypersensitivity vasculitis group.[6] While many of these patients displayed features of either PAN or Churg-Strauss syndrome, others had features of disorders such as temporal arteritis, Takayasu's arteritis, Henoch-Schönlein purpura or Wegener's granulomatosis.

The prognosis of this disorder is unclear at the present time. Patients fitting this description should be approached diagnostically and therapeutically in a similar fashion to PAN or Churg-Strauss syndrome. Overall, in the National Institutes of Health experience, the mean duration of remission was 45.9 months with a mean follow-up period of 58.4 months. All patients were treated with a combination of cyclophosphamide and corticosteroids.[6]

The term *microscopic polyarteritis* or *microscopic polyangiitis* is often used to describe a form of necrotizing vasculitis with few or no immune deposits, affecting primarily the small vessels (i.e., capillaries, venules, or arterioles). Necrotizing GN is common as well as pulmonary small-vessel involvement. The majority of patients with microscopic polyarteritis with GN are ANCA positive. The syndrome is differentiated from classic PAN by the presence of small-vessel predominance and pulmonary involvement and from other forms of small-vessel disease such as Henoch-Schönlein purpura by its lack of immune deposits.

THE HYPERSENSITIVITY VASCULITIS GROUP

The concept of vasculitis secondary to allergic or hypersensitivity mechanisms was first proposed by Zeek, Smith, and Weeter in 1948.[18] Support for this rationale included a series of experimental and clinical observations distinguishing this disorder from other recognized vasculitic conditions. These distinguishing features included the frequent precipitation by a drug or serum, prominent involvement of the skin and pathologically the tendency to involve the small vessels and display leukocytoclasis (nuclear fragmentation).

Despite the distinguishing features of hypersensitivity vasculitis, it has subsequently been recognized that many patients with these clinical and pathologic findings have no history of exposure to drugs or toxins. Additionally, a wide variety of disorders with mechanisms other than

hypersensitivity have also been noted to have the same clinical and pathologic picture. These conditions include certain cases of vasculitis secondary to connective tissue disease (e.g., rheumatoid arthritis, Sjögren's syndrome, and systemic lupus erythematosus), Henoch-Schönlein purpura, certain malignancies, the presence of mixed cryoglobulins in the serum and even occasional patients with systemic necrotizing vasculitis. At present the term hypersensitivity vasculitis group (HVG) refers to a heterogeneous group of disorders all displaying the clinical and pathologic features previously referred to. The presence of these findings (i.e., vasculitic rash, which upon biopsy displays a small vessel vasculitis with leukocytoclasia) should serve as a clinical starting point for a differential diagnosis of those disorders referred to in the classification scheme under this heading (see the box, p. 381).

Pathogenesis

The causes of the disorders within the hypersensitivity vasculitis group are diverse, but there is strong evidence that they all share a similar mechanism of vascular inflammatory disease; namely, that mediated by immune complexes. Evidence supporting an immune complex pathogenesis includes the experimental model of serum sickness elucidated by Dixon over 20 years ago. In this model rabbits immunized with a nontoxic protein antigen develop specific antibodies to the antigen resulting in soluble circulating immune complexes. At the point in time where the concentration of these soluble circulating immune complexes is maximal, evidence of complement activation and the coincidental production of a variety of target organ manifestations including carditis, glomerulonephritis, arthritis, and vasculitis is observed. In humans with small vessel vasculitis caused by hypersensitivity to proteins or drugs, there has been identification of soluble circulating immune complexes both in the peripheral blood and in the tissues. While these findings are not universal, this is understandable since detection of circulating immune complexes is greatly influenced by detection techniques as well as the timing and nature of the biopsy sample.[19]

Specific Diseases

Diseases that frequently share the cardinal features of the hypersensitivity vasculitis group (cutaneous involvement, small vessel vasculitis, and leukocytoclasis) are listed below:

1. True hypersensitivity vasculitis. This term should be limited to those conditions strongly linked to exposure to an exogenous antigen (e.g., drug, serum, toxin, infection).
2. Henoch-Schönlein purpura.
3. Cryoglobulinemia of essential origin.
4. Vasculitis associated with certain connective tissue disease (e.g., rheumatoid arthritis, systemic lupus erythematosus, Sjögren's syndrome).
5. Vasculitis associated with malignancies.
6. Urticarial vasculitis (hypocomplementemic vasculitis).
7. Vasculitis associated with systemic diseases. These diseases include, but are not limited to, inflamma-

ANTIGENIC EXPOSURES CAUSING HYPERSENSITIVITY VASCULITIS

I. Drugs
Penicillin

Sulfa

Iodides

Griseofulvin

Quinidine

Tetracycline

Dilantin

Phenylbutazone

Allopurinol

ASA phenacetin

Phenothiazine

II. Infections
Streptococcus

Staphylococcus

Subacute bacterial endocarditis

Meningococcus

Leprosy

Malaria

Tuberculosis

HIV

Hepatitis B

Cytomegalovirus

Epstein-Barr virus

Others

III. Chemicals
Insecticides

Herbicides

IV. Immunizations
Influenza

Allergy

V. Miscellaneous
Foreign protein

Insect bites

Others

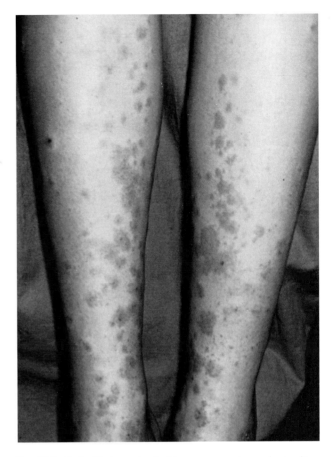

Fig. 22-3. Typical lesions of palpable purpura and maculopapular rash in a patient with hypersensitivity vasculitis.

listed in the accompanying box. The typical case of hypersensitivity vasculitis occurs 7 to 10 days following the initial exposure to incriminate antigen. The disease is frequently heralded by the development of the characteristic rash. The most common rash is palpable purpura (Fig. 22-3), though a variety of other cutaneous findings such as ulcers, nodules, bullae or urticaria may be seen. All the lesions tend to be at one anatomic stage and, when biopsied, display typical histopathologic features. These include the presence of polymorphonuclear leukocytes and associated leukocytoclasis, but at times the infiltrates may be predominantly mononuclear in nature (Fig. 22-4). Immunofluorescent studies often demonstrate the deposition of complement and immunoglobulins in vessel walls. The laboratory examination may reveal evidence of soluble immune complexes detected by a variety of techniques as well as evidence of complement activation.[20] These laboratory findings, however, are neither universal nor necessary for the diagnosis.

The clinical course of patients with hypersensitivity vasculitis is variable, but is usually self-limited. Varying degrees of constitutional symptoms including fever, malaise, and weight loss may be observed. Occasionally, more significant target organ involvement may be present including the muscle, joint, renal, pulmonary, and central nervous systems. At times the disorder may become chronic or recurrent. The treatment of true hypersensitiv-

tory bowel disease, primary biliary cirrhosis, Behçet's syndrome, Goodpasture's syndrome, and retroperitoneal fibrosis.

TRUE HYPERSENSITIVITY VASCULITIS. True hypersensitivity vasculitis, which is caused by exposure to an exogenous antigen, is the most common syndrome within the hypersensitivity vasculitis group. Incriminate antigens that have been associated with this syndrome are

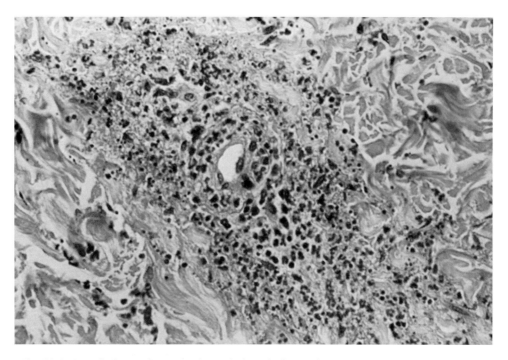

Fig. 22-4. Acute leukocytoclastic vasculitis with dense leukocytoclasia. (From Calabrese LH and Clough JD: Hypersensitivity vasculitis group [HVG]: a case-oriented review of a continuing clinical spectrum, Cleve Clin Q 49:17, 1982.)

ity vasculitis should focus primarily on removal of the inciting antigen. If the antigen is a drug, it should be discontinued, and if there is an incriminate infection, it should be treated. Mild cases may require no treatment at all while more advanced cases may require the use of a variety of modalities including antihistamines, colchicine, corticosteroids, and for severe cases, cytotoxic drugs.[20] In fulminant hypersensitivity vasculitis caused by an exogenous antigen, plasmapheresis has been occasionally reported to be of dramatic benefit, though there are no controlled studies of this or any other modality in this disorder.[21]

HENOCH-SCHÖNLEIN PURPURA. Henoch-Schönlein purpura is a syndrome characterized by the presence of palpable purpura and varying degrees of gastrointestinal ischemia and glomerulonephritis. Other symptoms such as arthritis, fever, and constitutional symptoms are not uncommon. Typically, the lesions of Henoch-Schönlein purpura may be identical to true hypersensitivity vasculitis and the conditions may be confused since Henoch-Schönlein purpura is frequently reported following an upper respiratory infection, and children are often given an antibiotic incriminated in hypersensitivity vasculitis for their condition.[19] Useful points of differentiation include the facts that Henoch-Schönlein purpura occurs most often in the spring, displays a high frequency of gastrointestinal involvement including colicky abdominal pain and gastrointestinal bleeding, and occurs in individuals under 18 years of age, though adults may occasionally be affected.[22] Immunopathologically, Henoch-Schönlein purpura is distinguished by the presence of IgA containing circulating immune complexes and the deposition of IgA containing immune complexes within the vasculitic tis-

sues.[23] An IgA associated glomerulonephritis is identified in about half the patients, and while generally mild and self-limiting, may infrequently be severe and persistent. The treatment of Henoch-Schönlein purpura depends upon the severity of the syndrome with mild disease requiring essentially no therapy while life-threatening visceral disease may require high-dose corticosteroids and possibly the addition of cytotoxic drugs.

CRYOGLOBULINEMIC VASCULITIS. *Cryoglobulinemia* refers to the presence of serum immunoglobulins and other proteins that precipitate at temperatures at below 37° C. Cryoglobulins are classified based on their composition. Type I cryoglobulins are monoclonal and are usually found in the presence of hematologic malignancies. Type III cryoglobulins are polyclonal and generally represent immune complexes and are found in the presence of a variety of disorders including connective tissue disease, chronic infections, and inflammatory disorders. Type II cryoglobulins contain both mixed and monoclonal components and are rarely seen in connective tissue disease or with malignancy. Until recently most type II cryoglobulins were classified as idiopathic and referred to as "essential." An association of type II cryoglobulins with hepatitis C has now been established.[2]

The clinical findings in patients with cryoglobulinemia are variable.[19,20] In patients with extremely high levels of cryoglobulins, generally type I or II, profound cold-induced symptoms resulting in vasoocclusion with stroke or necrosis of the skin or even an entire extremity may occur. In patients with type III cryoglobulins, the findings are generally of a small-vessel vasculitis reflective of the underlying disorder. The clinical findings in most patients with type II cryoglobulins are distinctive. The skin, joints, peripheral nerves, liver, and kidney are most frequently involved. Renal involvement occurs in 30% to 50% of patients and may be associated with hypertension, azotemia, or nephrosis. The natural history of type II cryoglobulinemia is variable, and rare spontaneous remissions have been reported. Renal disease has been considered a poor prognostic marker with 5-year survival of approximately 60%. Death is frequently related to cardiovascular, cerebrovascular, infectious, and vasculitic complications. A high incidence of transformation to non-Hodgkin's lymphoma has been reported, suggesting that type II cryoglobulinemia is a premalignant condition. It is difficult to interpret some of these older reports since cases were not identified as to whether they were associated with hepatitis C.

The therapy of most patients with cryoglobulinemic vasculitis (generally type I or III) is first directed at the underlying disorder, such as connective tissue disease or malignancy. In those with type II cryoglobulinemia, previously labeled as "essential" (now largely associated with hepatitis C), the mainstays of therapy for the past several decades have been apheresis and immunosuppression.[24] The goals of therapy have been to control the formation, deposition, and inflammatory effects of the cryoglobulins. All reported therapies with these drugs and modalities have been empiric, and there have been no controlled trials. Treatment of nonacute disease, in the absence of visceral target organ involvement, should generally be conservative. For more serious disease, treatment generally involves the use of steroids either as oral or intravenous pulse therapy. Cytotoxic drugs including the use of alkylators have also been used with varying reported success.[19,20,24] Enthusiasm for the long-term use of such drugs should be tempered by the potential for malignant transformation of the disease.

The discovery that most cases of type II cryoglobulinemia previously considered essential are associated with hepatitis C infection has introduced a rationale for more specific therapy with antiviral drugs, in particular α-interferon.[24] Unfortunately, although some therapeutic success has been reported, relapse is common after the therapy has been discontinued.

VASCULITIS ASSOCIATED WITH CONNECTIVE TISSUE DISEASE. Small vessel vasculitis may be observed in association with a variety of connective tissue diseases.[19] Though this presentation is not the only manifestation of vasculitis in this disorder, it is probably the most frequent. Patients with rheumatoid arthritis, systemic lupus erythematosus and Sjögren's syndrome may occasionally display cutaneous vasculitic involvement, including palpable purpura. These disorders, however, may also be associated with larger vessel disease reminiscent of systemic necrotizing vasculitis. The identification of these disorders as a cause for hypersensitivity vasculitis is generally readily apparent on clinical and serologic grounds. The treatment for hypersensitivity vasculitis in patients with connective tissue disease is based on control of the underlying connective tissue disease.

HYPERSENSITIVITY VASCULITIS ASSOCIATED WITH MALIGNANCY. Occasionally vasculitis may be a manifestation of an underlying malignancy. Those conditions most frequently associated with vasculitis include lymphoproliferative or myeloproliferative disorders.[19,25] In the majority of cases the vasculitis antedates the malignancy by many months, but occasionally the vasculitis may appear after the malignancy. The most common manifestations include palpable purpura, petechial lesions, maculopapular rashes, and ulcers. Though systematic investigations for the deposition of immunoglobulin and complement have been largely unrevealing, we have identified the presence of a paraprotein within the vascular lesions in a patient with chronic lymphocytic leukemia. The symptoms of vasculitis associated with malignancy are generally poorly responsive to therapy but may remit with the underlying therapy of the condition.

URTICARIAL VASCULITIS. While the most classic cutaneous manifestation of small vessel vasculitis is palpable purpura, a variety of other cutaneous findings may occasionally be encountered. A syndrome predominantly associated with urticaria, which upon biopsy reveals leukocytoclastic vasculitis, has been named urticarial vasculitis or hypocomplementemic vasculitis.[26,27] While hypocomplementemia is a prominent part of this disorder, it should be noted that complement levels may be normal in some cases of urticarial vasculitis and that hypocomplementemia may readily be observed in cutaneous vasculitis without urticaria. Patients with this syndrome clinically have attacks of urticaria that frequently last for greater than 24 hours at a time. Constitutional symptoms including arthralgias and low-grade fever are prominent features. Angioneurotic edema of the face and bowel may occasionally be encountered. Renal disease is not generally observed though occasionally cases of glomerulonephritis are reported. A unique syndrome of urticarial vasculitis, membranoproliferative glomerulonephritis and pseudotumor cerebri has been reported in six patients and is not completely understood.[28] Many patients with urticarial vasculitis have many features of systemic lupus erythematosus but do not satisfy the American College of Rheumatology criteria for the diagnosis.[29]

Laboratory studies in patients with this disease frequently reveal evidence of hypocomplementemia with marked depressions of C1 through C3. It should be noted that urticaria may also be observed in a variety of other immune complex conditions including serum sickness, Henoch-Schönlein purpura, connective tissue disease, and hepatitis B. Therefore the presence of urticaria and immune complexes is not specific for this disease but depends on a careful exclusion of a variety of other conditions and appropriate documentation by biopsy. The treatment of this disorder is generally accomplished by a combination of medications including antihistamines, colchicine and corticosteroids.

HYPERSENSITIVITY VASCULITIS ASSOCIATED WITH SYSTEMIC DISEASES. As previously mentioned the presence of a cutaneous vasculitic condition associated with leukocytoclasis should aid the clinician in formulating a differential diagnosis that centers around the classification scheme (see the box, p. 381). While the vast majority of these cases may be caused by conditions such as hypersensitivity to drugs, infections, toxins, Henoch-Schönlein purpura, or connective tissue disease, it must be

MISCELLANEOUS CONDITIONS ASSOCIATED WITH CUTANEOUS VASCULITIS MIMICKING HYPERSENSITIVITY VASCULITIS

Celiac disease

Inflammatory bowel disease

Primary biliary cirrhosis

Behçet's syndrome

Goodpasture's syndrome

Retroperitoneal fibrosis

Transplant vasculitis

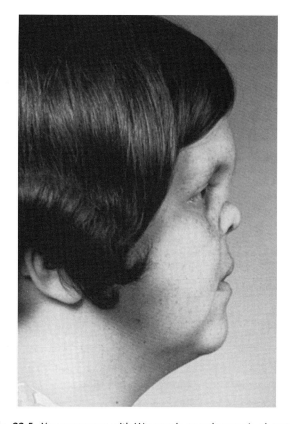

Fig. 22-5. Young woman with Wegener's granulomatosis, shows the typical "saddle-nose" deformity, seen in patients with extensive destruction of nasal cartilage and loss of the nasal septum. (From Orlowski JP, Clough JD, and Dyment PG: Wegener's granulomatosis in the pediatric age group, Pediatrics 61:83, 1978.)

noted that there are a variety of systemic diseases that have been reported in association with small vessel vasculitis similar to that reported in these conditions.[19,30,31] The box on this page contains a partial list of those disorders that must be searched for when confronted with a patient with a small vessel vasculitic condition with prominent skin involvement.

WEGENER'S GRANULOMATOSIS

Wegener's granulomatosis (WG) is a granulomatous inflammatory disease of unknown cause. It affects small- and medium-sized blood vessels throughout the body with major manifestations in the upper and lower respiratory tract and the kidneys. It was definitively described in 1939[32] and was more recently subdivided into "classical" and "limited" forms, the difference being absence of renal manifestations in the latter form.[33] Until recognition that alkylating agents, especially cyclophosphamide, could be used to control the disease in most patients, WG was always fatal. Although the cause remains unknown, recent developments in both diagnosis and therapy of WG offer the clinician powerful tools for early recognition and management of this disease.

Clinical Aspects

Although WG can begin at any age, onset most commonly occurs in the fifth decade. Males and females are affected with approximately equal frequency.[34,35] No racial or geographic predilections have been reported, although the majority of reported patients are white. Despite a few reports of familial occurrence of the disease, little evidence of a genetic pattern has emerged; furthermore, there appear to be no HLA linkages or associations.[36] The leading candidates for etiology are autoimmunity and infection. Although there is circumstantial evidence that disrupted immune mechanisms play a role in pathogenesis, the cause of this disruption has not been defined.

In classical WG all three target areas (upper airways, lungs, and kidneys) are typically involved at onset or soon thereafter, with upper airway involvement being the most common[34]; however, cases have been reported in which delays of up to several years occurred between the onset of disease and involvement of all three areas. On the other

hand, WG may present in other organ systems, making diagnosis more difficult. There have been reports of patients presenting with breast mass, prostatic nodule, gastrointestinal hemorrhage or diarrhea, palpable purpura, cranial nerve palsies, scleritis, unilateral parotid enlargement, or erosive arthritis. Since an infectious process is often suspected initially, the correct diagnosis is often delayed, especially when the presentation is unusual.

Upper airway involvement, which occurs in 90% of patients[34] and may be the sole initial site of disease in 12%,[35] is often destructive; the nasal mucosa is obscured by purulent crusts, and perforation of the nasal septum may soon follow, with collapse of the nose resulting in the typical "saddle-nose" deformity (Fig. 22-5). Nasal drainage is often bloody or tarry in appearance. Chronic sinusitis is frequent and often painful. Even when the sinuses are asymptomatic, x-ray studies often reveal opacification of the sinuses. The middle ear may be involved, presenting as otitis media. Damage to the inner ear may result in sensorineural hearing loss and/or vertigo; this results from vasculitic involvement of the vessels of the endolymphatic sac.[37] Oral involvement is uncommon, most frequently manifested by hypertrophic gingivitis ("strawberry gums") with loosening of the teeth. Subglottic stenosis is a particularly troublesome complication that may require surgical correction.[38]

Upper airway involvement must be differentiated from malignancy or idiopathic midline destructive disease (IMDD). Biopsy is the usual method for this, although less invasive procedures, such as magnetic resonance imaging (MRI), may be helpful.

Pulmonary involvement, present eventually in 85%[34] and the only site of disease in 10% initially,[35] usually produces symptoms suggestive of pneumonia including fever, cough, and often chest pain. The cough may be productive, but sputum cultures grow normal flora. Chest x-ray studies typically show nodules or infiltrates, which are often bilateral, with a tendency to cavitate. Occasionally WG presents as diffuse alveolar hemorrhage with massive hemoptysis[39]; in the presence of renal involvement, this clinical picture resembles Goodpasture's syndrome, and antibodies against glomerular basement membrane have been rarely reported in this setting. A less dramatic presentation is that of a pleural mass. Confirmation of the diagnosis of WG requires biopsy, and the lung is the site most likely to yield definitive histopathology in WG. Tissue may be obtained either by thoracotomy or bronchoscopy, although the former method is more likely to be successful.

Renal disease is the third component of the classical triad, eventually found in 77% of patients[34]; if it is absent, the condition is referred to as limited WG.[33] A recent report has documented late onset (1 to 4 years after diagnosis) of renal disease in 14% of patients initially presenting with limited WG.[40] Symptoms and signs of renal involvement are those of rapidly progressive GN. They include malaise, edema, proteinuria, active urinary sediment, and rising serum creatinine levels. Even in the face of severe renal disease, biopsy of the kidney may not produce diagnostically specific findings, and the kidney is not the ideal biopsy site if WG is suspected.

Arthritis and other rheumatic complaints are common (67% of patients), but they are usually mild.[34] Patients often complain of arthralgias when the disease is active. Erosive arthritis has been rarely described. Joint pain, especially in the hips, may also result from avascular necrosis of bone in patients treated with corticosteroids (CSs); it is important to distinguish this from arthritis because of therapeutic implications.

Skin lesions are present in 46% of patients at some time during their course, and occasionally (15%) these are among the initial manifestations.[34] Several types of lesions have been described, ranging from palpable purpura typical of leukocytoclastic angiitis to pyoderma-like skin ulcerations resembling Weber-Christian panniculitis. Skin biopsy is unlikely to yield a definitive diagnosis.

Ocular manifestations are common, occurring eventually in 52% of the patients.[34] Most ominous is the appearance of an orbital mass with the potential to displace and destroy the eyeball; this usually presents as painful unilateral or asymmetrically bilateral proptosis with impaired vision on the involved side. Computed tomography of the orbits is helpful in detecting and monitoring this condition. Most frequently seen are episcleritis and scleritis. Uveitis can also occur. Lacrimal gland involvement has been described as well.

The nervous system may be affected either centrally (8%) or peripherally (mononeuritis multiplex, 15%).[34] Both cerebral infarction and diffuse cerebritis have been described. Multiple cranial nerve palsies have also been observed.

Gastrointestinal manifestations are less common in WG than in other forms of necrotizing arteritis, but they may be severe and life-threatening when they occur. Abdominal pain is the most frequent symptom of intestinal vasculitis, followed by diarrhea and hemorrhage. Abnormal liver function tests[41] and findings suggestive of pancreatitis[42] have also been described. Colonic lesions may be identified and biopsied endoscopically.

Cardiovascular involvement may occur in the form of myocardial infarction, cardiomyopathy, conduction system abnormalities, aortitis, or valvulitis. Although significant cardiac symptoms are uncommon, like gastrointestinal WG, they may be quite severe.[34]

Finally, WG may present as a mass in almost any location. There have been several reports of breast masses, identified either at examination or mammography, found to be WG by biopsy. WG also occasionally presents as a prostatic lesion, sometimes causing gross hematuria. Splenic involvement has also been described.

Pathology

The histopathologic hallmarks of WG are granuloma formation and necrotizing vasculitis of small- and medium-sized arteries. This picture is seen in its most complete and diagnostically useful form in the lung (Fig. 22-6), which is the preferred biopsy site for this reason.[43] Recent studies of involved lung tissue suggest that although vasculitis is an important component of WG, the disease has a significant extravascular component, and vasculitic lesions are not always found. Both vascular and extravascular collagen and reticulum are affected. The granulomas, which often contain giant cells, differ from the compact granulomata typically seen in infectious processes (such as tuberculosis) and sarcoidosis in that the cells are lined up in palisades. The lesions pass through stages of micronecrosis with neutrophilic microabscesses, then macronecrosis, which is more widespread, and finally fibrosis.[44] Not all patients show these findings to the same degree, and the findings can be classified into four histologic types that have prognostic significance: (1) the fulminant type (most severe, poorest prognosis); (2) the granulomatous type (little evidence of vasculitis in some cases); (3) the fibrous scar type (most protracted course); and (4) the mixed type.[45] Criteria for the histopathologic differentiation of WG from other forms of vasculitis have recently been proposed.[46]

Renal biopsies often show evidence of crescentic GN. Granuloma formation may not be evident, and specimens often have little diagnostic specificity for WG. The characteristic lesion is focal in distribution, often involving less than half the glomeruli; it is a segmental necrotizing GN (SNGN). Most studies show little or no evidence of IC deposition using immunohistochemical methods and/or electron microscopy, although fibrin deposition is usually present. Findings have been interpreted as suggesting that glomerulothrombosis, rather than IC deposition, is the primary event.[47]

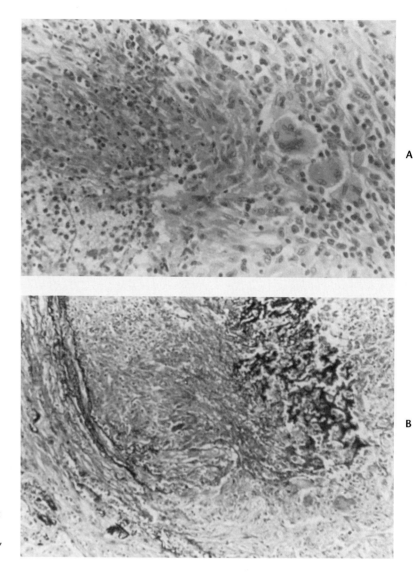

A

B

Fig. 22-6. Lung biopsy from a patient with Wegener's granulomatosis showing **(A)** a lymphocytic/histiocytic infiltrate with multinucleated giant cells adjacent to a necrotic area at the lower left (hematoxylin-eosin stain; ×340) and **(B)** destruction of elastin in an arterial wall (Van Gieson stain; ×140). (Courtesy GN Gephardt, MD, Cleveland Clinic Foundation.)

Diagnosis

WG is suspected in patients presenting with fever, malaise, and multisystem disease with prominent lung and upper airway symptoms. Physical examination will often disclose crusts on the nasal mucosa and sometimes perforation of the nasal septum.

Routine laboratory studies suggest acute and chronic inflammation. Anemia, leukocytosis, thrombocytosis, polyclonal hypergammaglobulinemia, and elevated acute-phase reactants are usually found; C-reactive protein has been reported to be a more sensitive indicator of active inflammation in WG than the erythrocyte sedimentation rate (ESR). In the majority of cases CICs are not detected by the Raji cell assay, cryoglobulin assay, or the C1q-binding assay. Complement levels are usually normal.

The American College of Rheumatologists adopted diagnostic criteria for WG in 1990.[48] These criteria include (1) nasal inflammation, manifested by purulent or bloody nasal discharge, or oral inflammation with oral ulcers, which may be painful or painless; (2) abnormal chest radiograph showing nodules, fixed infiltrates, or cavitation; (3) urinary sediment with microhematuria or red cell

casts; and (4) biopsy evidence of granulomatous inflammation within the wall of an artery or in the perivascular or extravascular area surrounding an artery or arteriole. If no biopsy data are available, hemoptysis may serve as a surrogate for this criterion. The presence of any two of these criteria carries a sensitivity of 88.2% and specificity of 92.0% for WG.

Antibodies against components of neutrophilic cytoplasm (ANCAs) are usually found in patients with WG.[49] These antibodies, which were originally detected by indirect immunofluorescence using ethanol-fixed human neutrophils as substrate (Fig. 22-7), have a high degree of specificity (greater than 90%) for WG, although they are occasionally found in a wide variety of other inflammatory conditions. Sensitivities vary in different studies from 58% to 96%, primarily depending on whether the patients have active or inactive disease. It was recognized relatively early that specificity for WG was greatest when the immunofluorescence was diffusely distributed throughout the cytoplasm and slightly granular (C-ANCA) rather than perinuclear in distribution (P-ANCA). The latter appearance is usually produced by antibody against myeloperoxidase,[50]

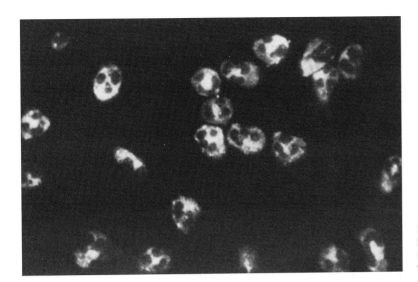

Fig. 22-7. Detection of antineutrophil cytoplasm antibody (ANCA) by indirect immunofluorescence. This antibody is a marker for diagnosis and disease activity in Wegener's granulomatosis.

whereas the former is generally associated with specificity for the cellular enzyme PR3.[51] Antibodies specific for PR3 can also be measured by ELISA. Of great interest also is the finding that C-ANCA titers correlate with disease activity better than other parameters that have commonly been used for this in WG.

The diagnosis of WG is confirmed by ruling out infection and by obtaining appropriate histologic confirmation through biopsy of involved areas. As previously noted, if there is clinical evidence of lung involvement, the lung is the most appropriate biopsy site. However, biopsies may be obtained from upper airways or other locations if the lung is not considered practical. The kidney is usually not a suitable site. An unequivocally positive ANCA test may greatly supplement or at times substitute for histopathology if the clinical likelihood for disease is high.

Three major categories of disease constitute the bulk of the differential diagnosis of WG: (1) infection, (2) malignancy, and (3) connective tissue disease, including other forms of vasculitis. Chronic infections have many features in common with WG, and there is, in fact, some evidence that WG itself is an infection with an as yet unidentified agent. Mycobacterial and fungal infections must be differentiated by appropriate cultures and immunologic methods. Malignant diseases, such as lymphomatoid granulomatosis, Hodgkin's disease, and IMDD are typically distinguished by biopsy. Other forms of vasculitis and connective tissue disease, such as PAN, allergic granulomatous vasculitis, GCA with pulmonary nodules, Goodpasture's syndrome, and bronchocentric granulomatosis can be differentiated by a combination of histologic, serologic, and clinical criteria. Antibodies against PR3 (C-ANCA) have become a useful differentiating factor.

Immunology and Pathogenesis

The recognition of c-ANCA in WG and its later characterization as antibody against PR3 sparked interest in the possibility that immune mechanisms might be involved in the pathogenesis of WG. Numerous studies have shown evidence of activation of the immune system through demonstration of elevated plasma levels of soluble interleukin-2 receptor as well as the inflammatory cytokines (tumor necrosis factors α and β, interleukin-6, and interleukin-8) and the appearance of lymphocyte surface activation markers, such as CD25, HLA-DR, CD29, and the adhesion molecules ICAM-1 and LFA-3. Furthermore, it has been shown that the inflammatory cytokines (tumor necrosis factor α, interleukin-1 α/β, and gamma interferon) provoke increased expression of PR3 on the surface of both vascular endothelial cells and neutrophils (priming), which is thus accessible to circulating ANCAs, leading to increased neutrophil adhesion to endothelium.[52] ANCA reacts with neutrophil PR3 and has been shown to produce an oxidative burst with neutrophil degranulation.[53] It is thus tempting to speculate that the release of lysosomal enzymes and the production of toxic reactive oxygen intermediates as a result of this activity may play a role in the vasculitic endothelial damage that occurs in WG. None of this explains why anti-PR3 activity appears in the first place or how the immune system becomes activated, and more work will need to be done in this exciting area to unravel the whole sequence of events.

Treatment

Three important developments in the treatment of WG have occurred during the past 15 years. The first was the recognition that cyclophosphamide has a potent suppressive effect on WG.[54] The second was recognition that trimethoprim-sulfamethoxazole appears to be able to induce remission in at least some patients with WG.[55] The third was the discovery that methotrexate (MTX) may also be effective in certain patients.[56]

Based on the widely held concept that WG is an autoimmune disease as well as the recognition that corticosteroids alone are ineffective in the long-term management of WG, several immunosuppressive agents have been tried, and anecdotal reports of response to a variety of drugs including azathioprine, chlorambucil, MTX, and cyclophosphamide have been published. Fauci et al[54] assembled a convincing, though uncontrolled, body of data on the favorable response to cyclophosphamide from the NIH series, which led to the widespread acceptance of this modality. The preferred regimen is daily oral cyclophosphamide 100 to 150 mg/day for 1 year, with or without low-dose prednisone, followed by taper and discontinuance. We have found that rapid control of the disease may be achieved by preceding the initiation of cyclophosphamide therapy with a course of intravenous nitrogen mustard (0.3 mg/kg)[57]; unlike cyclophosphamide, this drug is not affected by impaired renal function, a considerable advantage in classical WG. Although the early results suggested that remissions induced in this way might be permanent, it has since become clear that many patients relapse after periods of a few months to a few years. There are, moreover, significant short- and long-term adverse effects associated with the use of cyclophosphamide including marrow suppression, increased susceptibility to infection, hemorrhagic cystitis, sterility, alopecia, and malignancy.

The initial report of efficacy of trimethoprim-sulfamethoxazole in WG was greeted with some skepticism, but subsequent confirmatory studies from a number of different centers have supported the original findings of DeRemee, McDonald, and Weiland.[55] Most, but not all, reported cases of successful use of this drug combination have been in patients who had already had one or more courses of cytotoxic drug treatment; the success rate in such patients is impressive, and it warrants consideration of this approach in patients with WG. The usual course of treatment is trimethoprim 160 mg/day and sulfamethoxazole 800 mg/day.

Hoffman et al[56] reported favorable results in an open-label pilot study of MTX and prednisone given to 29 WG patients who had either failed another form of therapy, had relapses during a period of no treatment, or had made an initial response to cyclophosphamide. Of these 29 patients, 22 (76%) responded to treatment. Although the major advantage of MTX over cyclophosphamide is greater long-term safety, nine of these patients experienced significant side effects attributed to the drug combination, including abnormal liver function tests, *Pneumocystis carinii* pneumonia (fatal in 2 of 3 cases), MTX pneumonitis, oral ulcers, or rash. MTX was administered orally in doses not exceeding 15 mg/week. Initial prednisone doses were 1 mg/kg/day followed by tapering dosages as the patients improved.

High-dose corticosteroid therapy is the treatment of choice for serious ocular problems,[58] although the process may recur when the steroid dose is lowered. A granulomatous mass behind the eyeball can cause excruciating pain, which can be temporarily relieved with the use of corticosteroids. Surgical decompression may be necessary, but this is technically difficult and may result in further loss of vision.

Other treatments include intensive plasmapheresis for patients with severe active GN, intravenous administration of immunoglobulins, and the use of other cytotoxic agents and cyclosporin, although none of these has widespread application at present. Progressive multifocal encephalopathy has been reported as a side effect of cyclosporin in WG.[59] No controlled trials of any form of treatment for WG are available.

GIANT CELL ARTERITIS

The term giant cell arteritis (GCA) is commonly used to refer to granulomatous arteritis of unknown cause, predominantly affecting large arteries with prominent destruction of the internal elastic lamina. Giant cells are often but not invariably present in positive biopsies. Moreover, giant cells are also frequently found in other forms of granulomatous vaculitis, such as Wegener's granulomatosis. Thus the term GCA is a something of a misnomer.

Two syndromes have been recognized under the general heading of GCA, temporal arteritis[60] and Takayasu's arteritis.[61] The major differences between these syndromes are the age at which they occur (temporal arteritis generally occurs in individuals over 50), the distribution and severity of vascular involvement (more widespread and severe for Takayasu's arteritis), and the racial distribution (predominantly white for temporal arteritis and oriental for Takayasu's arteritis). During the past few years increasing numbers of cases have been recognized in which these distinctions are blurred,[62] and it is not at all clear that these are two separate entities.

It may be more sensible to view GCA as a spectrum of disease severity with temporal arteritis (with or without polymyalgia rheumatica) at the mild end and Takayasu's arteritis at the more severe end. Other presentations of GCA, not easily classified under either syndrome, would occupy positions along the spectrum determined by the systems or organs affected and the patient's responsiveness to treatment.

Temporal Arteritis

The most common syndrome of GCA is temporal arteritis. Its major importance stems from its threat to vision. It is frequently seen in association with the clinical syndrome of polymyalgia rheumatica (PMR), but the basis for this association is unknown.

CLINICAL ASPECTS. Temporal arteritis affects the elderly and increases in frequency with age. It is seldom seen before the age of 50. It has a predilection for whites of northern European descent; the largest demographic studies have been done in Scandinavia and Minnesota, where large numbers of Americans of Scandinavian descent reside.[62] The disease is uncommon in blacks, but it has been reported.

Classic symptoms are persistent headache, often in the temporal areas, which may be locally tender over the superficial temporal arteries; transient visual disturbances (amaurosis fugax), usually manifested by dimming or "graying" of vision but sometimes by blurring or diplopia; and jaw claudication. This picture is even more characteristic when it occurs in a patient with PMR, a clinical syndrome characterized by acute onset of proximal muscular stiffness and pain on active motion.[63] The relationship between these two conditions has never been satisfactorily explained, but it is close enough that asymptomatic temporal arteritis is often sought and sometimes found in patients with PMR. Temporal arteritis may also be identified without typical symptoms in up to one sixth of elderly patients with fever of unknown origin.

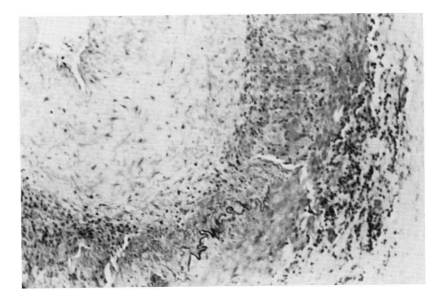

Fig. 22-8. Biopsy of the superficial artery from a patient with temporal arteritis shows disruption of the internal elastic lamina, granulomatous infiltrate, and giant cells. (Silver stain; ×140.)

On physical examination tenderness and swelling are often found in the temporal arteries, which may be pulseless, but these findings are not invariable, and the physical examination is frequently normal. If the patient has PMR, active motion of limb and pelvic girdle muscles is usually more painful than passive motion; muscle strength is not affected but may be difficult to test because of pain.

Complications are more common in males than females. These include permanent partial or complete visual loss (the most frequent complication), necrosis of the tongue, paresthesias of the face, multiple cranial nerve palsies, hearing loss, diabetes insipidus, stroke, and other ischemic phenomena in the head and neck region. Blindness can result from occlusion of the central retinal artery.

Involvement outside the area of the head and neck may occur in patients with or without temporal arteritis. Unless the temporal arteries are involved, this is more properly referred to as GCA or, in the proper clinical setting, as Takayasu's arteritis (see next section).

In temporal arteritis, the characteristic lesion is granulomatous inflammation of the arterial wall with destruction of the internal elastic lamina and giant cell formation (Fig. 22-8). Immunoglobulin deposits in the region of the internal elastic lamina have been detected in some patients by direct immunofluorescence. The cellular infiltrate contains many lymphocytes, which have been characterized as CD4-positive T cells, an elevated percentage of which bear class II histocompatibility antigens and interleukin-2 receptors, indicating activation. Activated macrophages are also present. Smooth muscle cells have been shown not to express class II antigens; this suggests that these cells are not functioning as antigen-presenting cells.[64]

Although there is some controversy over the distribution of the granulomatous lesion, most authorities agree that it is a skip lesion and that small biopsy specimens may not show evidence of disease in affected individuals. Another area of controversy is the ability to diagnose "healed" temporal arteritis from biopsy material; most authorities now believe that the findings on which such conclusions are based are too nonspecific to warrant this.

DIAGNOSIS. Biopsy of the temporal artery is the "gold standard" for the diagnosis of temporal arteritis. However, in clinical situations where the degree of certainty about the diagnosis before biopsy is high, it is reasonable to make the diagnosis tentatively and begin treatment without the biopsy result. Prednisone therapy changes the biopsy findings relatively slowly, and there is evidence of active arteritis in specimens obtained up to 7 weeks after initiation of treatment.[65] The improvement of symptoms after initiation of treatment, however, is rapid in most cases, and the observation of rapid disappearance of headache and PMR (generally within 24 hours) provides additional support for the diagnosis. Patients failing to respond rapidly to prednisone and ultimately having negative biopsies have turned out most frequently to have either malignancy or diabetes mellitus.

The only helpful laboratory test is the erythrocyte sedimentation rate (ESR), which is usually markedly elevated. Although cases of otherwise typical temporal arteritis with normal ESR have been described, this test has such a high sensitivity for temporal arteritis that other diagnostic possibilities should be strongly considered when it is normal. The role of the ESR in monitoring patients for response to treatment and relapse is controversial. Although ESR is widely used for this, some authorities recommend monitoring clinical symptoms only, since it may rise again without clinical relapse.[65] Other acute phase reactants (fibrinogen, C-reactive protein, haptoglobin) have been found not to be as useful or dependable as ESR. The von Willebrand factor is often elevated in temporal arteritis, and levels have been reported higher in GCA than in "pure" PMR and certain other rheumatic conditions, but this has no recognized diagnostic utility at present.[66]

HLA-DR4, a class II histocompatibility antigen associated with several "autoimmune" diseases (most notably rheumatoid arthritis), has been found with increased frequency in patients with temporal arteritis (40%, compared to 20% of controls). This increased frequency is almost entirely segregated to the group with PMR, 59% of whom have HLA-DR4, compared to the group without PMR, 19% of whom are positive for this antigen.[67]

The differential diagnosis of temporal arteritis depends on the clinical presentation. Classically the presentation is so typical that other explanations are unlikely. Occasionally systemic lupus erythematosus presents a PMR-like picture that may be associated with headache and retinal vasculitis leading to visual symptoms. The presence of other features of lupus as well as the typical serologic findings can usually make this distinction. Malignancy and diabetes mellitus have already been referred to. Patients who have fever of unknown origin, infections, and other connective tissue diseases also become part of the differential diagnosis.

TREATMENT. Prednisone remains the treatment of choice. Classically the recommendation was low-dose prednisone (15 mg/day) for PMR without evidence of temporal arteritis but much higher doses (60 to 100 mg/day) for patients with temporal arteritis. High-dose prednisone would be continued for 6 weeks, then tapered to the lowest dose that would maintain freedom from symptoms (with or without maintenance of normal ESR). Low-dose prednisone would be continued for as long as necessary to prevent relapse upon discontinuing the drug.

Prednisone, however, has many side effects, not the least of which is osteoporosis in the elderly, predominantly female population. There has been considerable interest in minimizing exposure to prednisone to the least necessary amount, and some investigators have shown results equal to those obtained with high-dose prednisone using more moderate doses (20 to 40 mg/day) with considerable reduction of side effects.[68] However, temporal arteritis has developed in some patients with "clinically pure" PMR while on treatment with low-dose prednisone with good control of symptoms and normal ESR. Furthermore, development of ischemic optic neuropathy has been reported despite high-dose prednisone treatment. An alternative approach is to take advantage of the steroid-sparing potential of certain chemotherapeutic agents such as azathioprine[69] in clinical situations that warrant it (e.g., preexisting osteoporosis or severe diabetes mellitus).

The relapse rate on discontinuing prednisone is high; in several studies it approached 50% whether high- or low-dose prednisone was used. Approximately 40% of patients required prednisone for more than 4 years. Reported mean durations of therapy ranged from 2 to 6 years, but many patients required treatment for more than 10 years. Fortunately, once the disease is controlled, the required dose is generally low enough not to pose much of a problem for most patients (less than 10 mg/day).

TAKAYASU'S ARTERITIS

Background

Takayasu's arteritis (TA) is an idiopathic systemic inflammatory disease that characteristically includes the aorta and its primary branches (Figs. 22-9 and 22-10).

Women of reproductive age are most often affected. Inflammation may produce either arterial stenoses, occlusion, dilation and/or aneurysms. Previous beliefs that TA evolves from an early systemic inflammatory phase to a late inactive stage with fixed "burned-out" lesions have been challenged. Increasing numbers of studies suggest that this is a simplistic model.[70-74] Most reports have failed to either define and document what was considered evidence of systemic inflammation. Many studies have not included criteria for active disease. Nonetheless, unsubstantiated statements abound regarding the excellent reliability of the ESR.[75-78] These observations have suggested that a normal ESR almost always precludes progressive inflammatory vascular changes, a concept that has been recently refuted.[70,71,80]

In spite of the fact that TA is a multifocal disease that may include numerous clinically silent as well as obvious lesions, many studies have either not required patients to have angiography, or have included patients with limited aortic arch studies. Consequently the effect of TA on major components of the vascular tree remained undefined. Most studies have also not documented disease status with sequential angiography. Histopathologic proof of vasculitis is the gold standard in other vasculitides; however, the size of the vessels affected in TA makes diagnostic biopsies impractical. Outcome analyses have been difficult because of variable therapies and variable access to medical and surgical care in different countries. Consequently TA disease mortality has been estimated from 2%[80,81] to 35%[82] over 5 years.

This critique should not be considered an indictment of prior studies. The dilemmas and controversies that affect TA are common to many rare diseases. By necessity, rare illnesses are often retrospectively characterized, without benefit of diagnostic criteria, reliable parameters of active disease, or uniformly applied treatment interventions.

Differential Diagnosis

TA can resemble a variety of conditions associated with congenital and acquired diseases (Table 22-1). Infectious processes and congenital abnormalities of collagen production most often produce aneurysms and not stenoses. In TA, stenoses are generally at least fourfold more common than aneurysms.[70,83] Progression of certain infectious angiopathies may be subtle (e.g., tuberculosis, mycoses, and syphilis).[84,85] Indolent infection-related vascular lesions are most often single aneurysms. Suspicion of infection should lead to a search for a primary source, PPD skin testing with control antigens, and serologic studies for syphilis. Inappropriate treatment of such patients with corticosteroids could contribute to vascular rupture and death. Acquired idiopathic inflammatory syndromes may produce aneurysms and/or stenosis that can be confused with TA. However, these disorders (e.g., Cogan's and Behçet's syndromes, GCA of the elderly, and Kawasaki disease) are associated with other features that allow distinction from TA. Sarcoidosis has been noted to be complicated by vasculitis that may affect a range of vessels from those of microscopic size[86-88] to the pulmonary arteries[89] and aorta.[70,90] When larger vessels are affected, the angiographic appearance of lesions may be indistin-

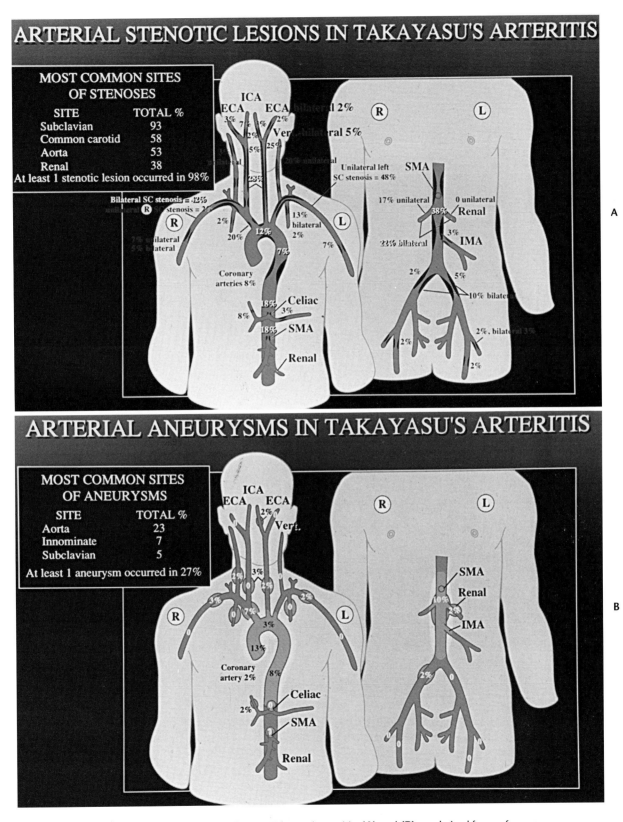

Fig. 22-9. Angiographic abnormalities in Takayasu's arteritis; **(A)** and **(B)** are derived from reference 70 (Kerr et al [1994]). These composite diagrams summarize the frequency and distribution of vascular lesions among 60 patients in the National Institutes of Health 20-year prospective study. (*ICA*, Internal carotid artery; *ECA*, external carotid artery; *SMA*, superior mesenteric artery; *IMA*, inferior mesenteric artery.)

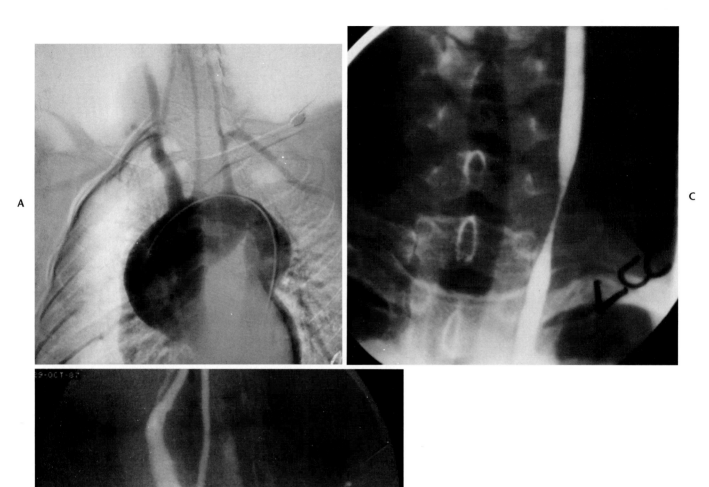

Fig. 22-10. The angiographic images demonstrate **(A)** aortic root dilatation and diffuse narrowing of the left common carotid artery, **(B)** aneurysmal dilatation of the innominate artery, and common carotid arteries, and threadlike narrowing of the left vertebral artery. In image **(C)** left common carotid stenosis was associated with a subsequent fatal stroke.

guishable from TA. This observation raises questions about whether TA is a syndrome that may have numerous different precipitants.

The fibrous dysplasias are thought to be congenital proliferative abnormalities that most often affect the medial or perimedial layers of large- and medium-sized vessels in children and young adults.[91,92] Females are affected more often than males. The most frequently affected sites are the renal arteries, although other vessels such as the carotid, mesenteric, and iliac arteries can also be involved.[93] Stenotic lesions are most common, and aneurysms are seen in a minority of cases. The arteriographic appearance of these lesions may be identical to TA. The pathogenesis of the fibrous dysplasias is thought to be noninflammatory proliferation. In some cases the only clear difference between fibrous dysplasias and TA has been the lack of fever and systemic symptoms and a normal ESR.

However, in the absence of histologic proof of a bland proliferative lesion and knowing that TA may be active in as many as 50% of patients who lack clinical and serologic evidence of inflammation,[70] the distinction between these diseases may be difficult.[71]

Patients with noninflammatory lesions due to Ehlers-Danlos syndrome, Marfan syndrome, or fibrous dysplasia would not be expected to experience improvement if misdiagnosed and treated with corticosteroids. In fact, if fibrous dysplasia was a cause of renal artery stenosis and hypertension, corticosteroid therapy may exacerbate hypertension.

TREATMENT. Hypertension complicates the course of TA in 32% to 93% of patients* and may be present regardless of disease activity.[94] Most TA-related deaths are

*References 70, 73, 74, 77, 78, 80, 93.

Table 22-1. Takayasu's Arteritis

Differential Diagnosis	Comment
Tuberculous, mycotic, or syphilitic arteritis	Aneurysms, stenoses rare
Ehlers-Danlos syndrome	Aneurysms
Marfan syndrome	Aortic root dilatation
Spondyloarthropathies	Aortic root dilatation (uncommon)
Vasculitides: Cogan's syndrome, Behçet's syndrome, GCA of elderly, and Kawasaki disease	Unique disease features
Sarcoid vasculopathy	Aneurysms and stenoses, vessels of any size
Fibromuscular dysplasia	Stenoses >> aneurysms, noninflammatory

(Reprinted with permission from Hoffman GS: Treatment of resistant Takayasu's arteritis, Rheum Dis Clin North Am 21:73, 1995.)

INDICATIONS FOR ANGIOPLASTY OR REVASCULARIZATION IN TAKAYASU'S ARTERITIS

1. Hypertension in the setting of renal artery stenosis
2. Extremity ischemia limiting routine activities of daily living
3. Clinical features of cerebral ischemia and/or critical stenosis of at least three cerebral vessels.*
4. Moderate aortic regurgitation
5. Coronary artery stenosis leading to ischemia

(Reprinted with permission from Hoffman GS: Treatment of resistant Takayasu's arteritis, Rheum Dis Clin North Am 21:1995.
*Whether bypass is indicated in the setting of asymptomatic critical stenosis in three primary cerebral vessels (e.g., both carotid arteries and one vertebral artery) is controversial.

due to congestive heart failure, ischemic or hemorrhagic strokes, or renal failure.[†] Because subclavian artery stenosis is common and may be bilateral,[70,94,95] in some patients upper-extremity blood pressures may be unreliable. Normal or low pressures in the arms may provide a false sense of security in a patient with deteriorating cardiac or renal function or a stroke. Although renal artery stenosis is the most common cause of high-renin hypertension in TA, the same sequence of events can complicate suprarenal aortic stenosis. Knowing the distribution and severity of vascular anatomic lesions is essential to good management. Arteriographic studies should be performed with pressure transducers, so that aortic pressures can be compared with extremity pressures. This is particularly important in the setting of hypertension and one or more stenoses in the subclavian, iliac, or femoral arteries or the aorta. Such pressure recordings will allow the physician to know which extremity accurately reflects the pressures in the aortic arch and should be used to monitor antihypertensive therapy. In worst case examples, none of the extremities are reliable and antihypertensive therapy becomes a very dangerous endeavor.

Immunosuppressive therapy may restore or improve vascular patency in some patients whose inflammatory lesions are of recent onset and have not become fibrotic. However, for most individuals with TA, such reversibility is uncommon. Critical stenoses, such as those leading to renovascular hypertension, coronary artery ischemia, or extremity claudication curtailing normal activities of daily living, are best treated by surgical revascularization or angioplasty (see box on this page). It is preferable for these interventions to be undertaken during periods of disease remission.

In brief, aggressive assessment and treatment of hypertension is a pivotal element in the therapy of TA. Deterioration in cardiac, cerebral, and renal function may be due

to fixed "burned-out," or active inflammatory lesions of vessels that affect renal perfusion. Damaged, uninflamed vessels may later undergo progressive narrowing due to secondary atheromatous disease. In the setting of "failing therapy" or clinical deterioration, it is essential to determine whether end-organ damage is at least in part due to hypertension, whether blood pressure measurements are being determined in an extremity that accurately reflects aortic arch pressures, and whether anatomic abnormalities could be improved by vascular surgery or angioplasty as adjuncts to, or in place of, medical therapies.

IMMUNOSUPPRESSIVE THERAPY. Corticosteroids have been the mainstay of therapy for active TA. Cumulative observational data have demonstrated dramatic improvement in many patients with unequivocal active progressive disease. Because TA is uncommon, corticosteroid dose and duration comparison studies have not been performed. In an attempt to standardize treatment, the Systemic Vascular Disorders Research Committee of the Ministry of Health and Welfare of Japan was formed to seek consensus regarding corticosteroid therapy for TA.[96] The committee suggested that active TA be defined by fever, pain of vascular origin, and an elevated ESR or CRP. If active disease was present, the committee recommended therapy with daily prednisolone, about 30 mg, followed by tapering after active TA remitted. Cytotoxic agents were recommended if active disease persisted or corticosteroid withdrawal was difficult. Surgical treatment of hypertension was advised whenever possible. The committee then retrospectively analyzed the outcome of 150 patients treated in this fashion. It was concluded that quality of life improved in 51% of patients, 37% experienced no change, and 12% became worse. Among 28 patients treated with either adjunctive azathioprine, cyclophosphamide, or mercaptopurine, the following responses were noted: excellent, 0%; good, 29%; fair, 33%; and ineffective, 29%.

A recent report[70] of TA from the National Institutes of Health (NIH) spans 20 years and is unique in several

[†]References 57, 73, 74, 82, 93-95.

TAKAYASU'S ARTERITIS: NIH CRITERIA FOR ACTIVE DISEASE

1. New onset or worsening of at least two features: Vascular ischemia or inflammation: either extremity claudication, decreased or absent extremity pulse or blood pressure, bruit, or vascular pain (e.g., carotidynia)
2. Angiographic abnormalities
3. Systemic symptoms not attributable to other events (e.g., fever, polyarthralgias, polymyalgias)
4. Elevated ESR

(Reprinted with permission from Hoffman GS: Treatment of resistant Takayasu's arteritis, Rheum Dis Clin North Am 21:73, 1995.)

---

respects: (1) Patients were prospectively studied. (2) Angiographic proof of diagnosis was required in all patients. All patients had sequential angiographic follow-up, regardless of disease activity status. Angiograms included the entire aorta and its primary branches. (3) Treatment was standardized to NIH-approved protocols. (4) Criteria for active disease were delineated as noted in the box on this page. (The authors note that the criteria to measure TA disease activity were intuitively derived, based on prior experience.)

Treatment protocols for active disease included daily prednisone in doses of 1 mg/kg, up to 60 mg for 1 to 3 months, followed by a slow taper if disease remained quiescent. Barring recrudescence of illness, corticosteroid tapering and discontinuance was attempted over 6 to 12 months. If corticosteroid tapering was not successful or the patient relapsed shortly after corticosteroid discontinuance, the individual became eligible for daily cyclophosphamide 2 mg/kg or weekly MTX 0.15 to 0.3 mg/kg.

Sixty patients entered the NIH studies and were followed over a median period of 5.3 years. Twenty percent of patients did not meet criteria for active disease and did not require immunosuppressive therapy of any kind. Of the 48 patients who appeared to have active TA, 60% achieved remission with corticosteroid therapy alone. Patients who did not achieve a remission that allowed for subsequent successful corticosteroid tapering, and those who relapsed, received additional cytotoxic therapy. Only 40% of these more treatment-resistant patients achieved sustained remissions with addition of cytotoxic therapy. Twenty-three percent of the 48 treated patients never achieved "drug-free" remissions, and in 45% whose disease remitted, relapse occurred at least once. Twenty-six percent of the complete cohort (60 patients) became either partially (26%) or completely (47%) vocationally disabled. It is clear from both this experience, as well as that from Japan,[96] that outcome is less optimistic than some authors have previously suggested.

An earlier NIH study[97] had suggested that cyclophos-phamide may improve outcome in selected patients who had failed corticosteroid therapy. However, extended experience with cyclophosphamide in both TA[70] and other systemic vasculitides[34] has led to concerns about the long-term risks of cystitis, bladder cancer, other malignancies, and infertility. This has encouraged enrollment in alternative therapy protocols, particularly those using weekly MTX.[56,98] In a recent study of corticosteroid-resistant or relapsing patients with severe TA, weekly MTX (mean dose, 17.1 mg; range, 10 to 25 mg) produced remissions in 81% of patients. Fifty percent sustained corticosteroid-free remissions over a mean period of 14.4 months. Half of those patients remained in remission after MTX was later tapered and stopped. In spite of these encouraging results, 19% of patients failed to sustain remission regardless of therapy.

These recent experiences from Japan and the NIH indicate that a minority of patients (approximately 20%) appear to have self-limiting or monophasic disease that may not require treatment. About half of all TA patients with active disease may respond to corticosteroid and will be able to eventually discontinue treatment without relapse. Half of corticosteroid-treated patients will not be able to sustain remission without continuing potentially toxic doses of corticosteroid. Such patients may benefit from addition of a cytotoxic agent. Most patients treated with cytotoxic agents will improve, but they may again relapse with subsequent tapering of medications. Because TA may eventually remit spontaneously and because such therapies carry significant risks, periodic tapering is necessary to minimize toxicity, expense, and reassess disease activity.

Do Clinical Parameters Accurately Reflect Disease Activity?

The clinical and laboratory markers that are listed in the box on this page have been conventionally accepted as reliable measures of active TA. However, in recent years, observations from vascular specimens obtained at the time of bypass surgery and sequential angiographic studies,[70] have led investigators to question the usefulness of these parameters in TA. Lagneau, Michel, and Vuong,[79] Kerr et al,[70] and Kieffer et al[99] have all recognized patients who were thought to be in remission at the time of bypass surgery, but in whom vascular specimens revealed histopathologic evidence of acute and/or chronic inflammation. These disappointing observations were noted in as many as 44% of patients[70,79] and correlate with clinical angiographic data. The recent NIH series required that all patients undergo sequential angiography.[70] As expected, the great majority of patients (88%) who had clinically persistent, active disease had new lesions demonstrated in sequential studies. However, 61% of patients who were clinically judged to have prolonged remission also had new lesions by angiography. The following conclusions can be derived from these observations: (1) When symptoms and signs of vascular inflammation are present, they usually predict vascular injury. (2) However, vascular inflammation may be present in about 50% of patients who lack symptoms of active inflammation or have a normal ESR. (3) Currently employed surrogate markers of vascular inflammation may be inadequate guides to the clinical decision-making process in TA.

The recognition of clinically "silent" active disease adds another dimension to the treatment of TA and raises the following questions: Should all surgical candidates receive a limited course of corticosteroid during the perioperative period? Should subsequent therapy in the "clinically inactive" patient be determined by histopathologic findings? Should patients with radiographic progression, absence of constitutional symptoms, and normal ESR/CRP receive corticosteroids? What dose of corticosteroid should be employed and how long should treatment continue? And, most important of all, would such an approach change outcome?

We have learned a great deal about TA in recent years. Much of this knowledge has emphasized our limitations in monitoring disease activity, understanding pathophysiology, and providing effective treatment. For those patients in whom disease is clearly active, treatment with immunosuppressive agents is often palliative. Medical and surgical treatment of hypertension, if present, is essential. Vascular bypass procedures or angioplasty may substantially reduce morbidity from ischemia or infarction. Aortic arch and valve surgery for aortic regurgitation may be lifesaving. Vascular procedures are best performed during periods of remission,[79,100] although clinical and laboratory definitions of remission are imperfect.

Improved care and outcomes for TA can be expected with discovery of better surrogate markers of vascular inflammation and development of high-resolution vascular imaging techniques that permit sequential studies with minimal radiation exposure.

BEHÇET'S DISEASE

Behçet's disease is a chronic inflammatory disease manifesting in its classic form recurrent aphthous stomatitis along with two or more of the following: genital ulcerations; ocular inflammation, most commonly uveitis; skin manifestations including erythema nodosum or pustules; meningoencephalitis and synovitis. The diagnosis is often delayed because of the intermittent nature of the various forms of target organ involvement that are frequently separated by months to years. Although the etiology of Behçet's disease is unknown, an important part of the underlying pathology is vascular inflammation.[101]

Pathologic lesions occur in both the arterial and venous systems and are often the source of major morbidity and mortality. Arterial vascular lesions include small-vessel involvement in the skin that may range from lymphocytic perivasculitis to frank necrotizing lesions. Large artery aneurysms and occlusions are also well described. In a recently reported series of 250 patients with Behçet's disease, 15 had arterial lesions the majority of which were aneurysmal with or without thrombosis. Concomitant venous disease was present in nine of the patients.[102] In general, larger arterial trunks are involved more than distal and may resemble Takayasu's disease. Common locations include pulmonary, subclavian, and femoral arteries. The underlying pathology includes vasculitis of the vasa vasorum causing medial fragmentation and rupture. The clinical manifestations reflect ischemia and infarction in involved tissues and may produce claudication in the extremities and pulmonary hemorrhage and infarction caused by bronchial arterial fistula.

Venous disease may also be the source of significant morbidity, and its frequency in Behçet's disease exceeds that seen in systemic lupus erythematosus. Thrombosis of superficial or deep veins in the extremities as well as occlusions of the superior and inferior vena cavas can be seen. Well-defined syndromes include Budd-Chiari syndrome or thrombosis of the intracranial venous sinuses presenting with increasing headache and visual blurring with or without papilledema. Collectively arterial and venous disease in Behçet's disease is a major source of morbidity and mortality.

Treatment of Behçet's disease in general includes the use of corticosteroids to reduce inflammation as well as the use of immunosuppressives such as chlorambucil and cyclosporine for more serious and possibly life-threatening complications such as severe eye inflammation or central nervous system involvement or for major arterial disease.[101] Venous complications can often be prevented by anticoagulation therapy in appropriate patients, but this should probably be avoided in patients with active arteritis particularly of the pulmonary arteries. Antiplatelet therapy is widely used, but there are no controlled trials supporting its efficacy.

CLINICAL APPROACH

Diagnosis

The vasculitides as a group of disorders remain a formidable challenge to clinicians from both the diagnostic and therapeutic perspectives. Diagnostically, the signs and symptoms of vasculitis are generally nonspecific since they represent those of vascular ischemia regardless of the cause. Certain vasculitic syndromes represent greater diagnostic challenges than others because of the nature and distribution of their target organ involvement. For example, when the skin is involved, such as in the hypersensitivity vasculitides, it is generally apparent that vasculitis is the underlying process, but a greater challenge is to determine the precise cause and thus the prognosis and treatment. In the absence of topical signs of vasculitis such as a characteristic rash or signs of peripheral ischemia, systemic vasculitis may mimic a wide variety of nonvasculitic diseases.

The box on p. 42 enumerates a series of warning signs or symptoms of systemic vasculitis. These findings should alert clinicians to the possibility of systemic vasculitis when a careful workup for other causes is unrevealing. Clearly, certain of these signs or symptoms have greater degrees of sensitivity or specificity depending upon the clinical situation. The following is a brief description of the significance of these warning signs or symptoms:

1. Fever of unknown origin. Virtually all the vasculitic syndromes are capable of producing fever. The differential diagnosis of fever of unknown origin centers around infections, malignancies, and connec-

WARNING SIGNS AND SYMPTOMS OF VASCULITIS

1. Fever of unknown origin
2. Unexplained multisystem disease
3. Mononeuritis multiplex
4. Unexplained inflammatory arthritis
5. Unexplained inflammatory myositis
6. Unexplained glomerulonephritis
7. Unexplained cardiac, gastrointestinal, or CNS ischemia

CONDITIONS MIMICKING SYSTEMIC VASCULITIS

Cholesterol embolism

Atrial myxoma

Sarcoidosis

Fibromuscular dysplasia

Angioendotheliomatosis

Ergotism

Neuroectodermal dysplasia

tive tissue diseases. Among the connective tissue diseases, systemic vasculitis remains among the most prominent possibilities.

2. Unexplained multisystem disease. Because of the potential widespread distribution of vascular inflammatory disease, multisystem organ dysfunction is not uncommon in systemic vasculitis. While there are many other diagnostic considerations including disseminated infection, disseminated cancer, and other infiltrating and inflammatory diseases (e.g., amyloidosis or sarcoidosis), systemic vasculitis should be kept in mind.

3. Mononeuritis multiplex. The clinical involvement of isolated peripheral nerves in differing anatomic sites is probably the most specific warning sign of underlying systemic vasculitis. Mononeuritis multiplex may be seen in a variety of vasculitic syndromes. While other patterns of peripheral neurologic involvement may be seen including symmetric polyneuropathy, pure sensory neuropathy, or the diffuse involvement of peripheral nerves in a single limb, mononeuritis multiplex is the most common problem. In the absence of diabetes or trauma, mononeuritis multiplex should be considered vasculitic until proven otherwise.

4. Unexplained inflammatory arthritis. Associated with a number of the vasculitic syndromes including polyarteritis nodosa, Wegener's granulomatosis, certain of the hypersensitivity vasculitides, and others, articular disease may be prominent. In general the arthritic picture associated with systemic vasculitis is one of a symmetric polyarthritis that is nonerosive and may be clinically severe. Because of the frequent presence of rheumatoid factor, it is not uncommon for inflammatory arthritis to be misdiagnosed as rheumatoid arthritis. The presence of severe constitutional signs and symptoms in the presence of unexplained inflammatory arthritis should always raise the diagnostic possibility of systemic vasculitis.

5. Unexplained inflammatory myositis. Muscle is a frequent target organ of systemic vasculitis and may produce an angiocentric myositis. The myositis of systemic vasculitis may be associated with elevated

muscle enzymes and varying degrees of muscle pain or weakness. Electromyographic studies of these patients will usually reveal evidence of a patchy inflammatory myopathy, which may be confused with idiopathic polymyositis. In our experience the primary muscle weakness associated with vasculitic muscle involvement is generally not as severe as that seen in polymyositis, and the symptoms of muscular pain and tenderness are somewhat more prominent.

6. Unexplained glomerulonephritis. Glomerulonephritis can be caused by a variety of systemic and immunologic diseases. There is no specific finding in the urinary sediment or in the associated laboratory tests that has a high degree of predictive value for the presence of systemic vasculitis. Frequently, patients with renal involvement and systemic vasculitis develop severe hypertension or a syndrome of rapidly progressive glomerulonephritis.

7. Unexplained cardiac, gastrointestinal, or CNS ischemia. This is probably the least specific of all the warning signs or symptoms of vasculitis but still must be considered in appropriate clinical context. Obviously, a stroke in an octagenerian would not raise a high degree of suspicion regarding the possibility of CNS angiitis, but a TIA in a 15-year-old girl certainly would. Similarly, ischemic events involving the cardiovascular or gastrointestinal systems should be considered potentially vasculitic if no other causes are apparent after careful investigation.

Conditions Mimicking Vasculitis

It should be kept in mind that there are a variety of conditions that can closely mimic the presence of systemic vasculitis. These conditions can lead to vascular occlusion, and thus ischemic symptomatology, but are generally noninflammatory. A partial listing of these mimicking syndromes is listed in the box on this page.

Among these syndromes cholesterol embolization perhaps represents the greatest challenge at differentiation from systemic vasculitis. Cholesterol microembolization may produce a variety of signs or symptoms resembling a multisystem disorder by virtue of its involvement of the nervous system, skin, heart, muscle, kidney, and gastrointestinal systems. Laboratory abnormalities may include leukocytosis, eosinophilia, hypocomplementemia, and elevated erythrocyte sedimentation rates. A recent study by Cappiello[103] has revealed the occasional presence of antinuclear antibodies and rheumatoid factors. To diagnose cholesterol embolization, a high degree of suspicion must exist based upon the clinical findings. The definitive diagnosis depends on histologic demonstration of needle-shaped cholesterol clefts on biopsy of an affected target organ. The amputated tissue may be a prime source for this characteristic finding. The condition should be suspected when a patient develops signs or symptoms of multifocal vascular ischemia and occlusion following an arteriographic procedure or while on warfarin therapy.

DIAGNOSTIC APPROACH

The diagnosis of the systemic vasculitides represents a formidable challenge in both recognition that a syndrome exists, and also in its precise nosologic classification. The precise approach is highly dependent on which syndrome is primarily suspected. Certain vasculitic syndromes such as hypersensitivity vasculitis are not difficult to recognize because of their prominent cutaneous involvement, but further identification of the precise cause and therefore prognosis, and appropriate treatment may be quite challenging. Giant cell arteritis is generally diagnosed by a temporal artery biopsy and Takayasu's arteritis is generally diagnosed by angiography for obvious reasons.

The overlap of the systemic necrotizing vasculitides, polyarteritis nodosa, Churg-Strauss syndrome, and polyangiitis is most challenging to diagnose. Numerous algorithms have been proposed based on a series of laboratory tests, organ biopsies, and the use of visceral angiography. There are no laboratory tests that have an extremely high predictive value in diagnosing these conditions, but certain combinations of tests may be extremely helpful. For example, the presence of elevated circulating immune complexes and a depressed level of serum complement in the presence of mononeuritis multiplex would certainly strongly suggest an underlying vasculitic condition, whereas the same laboratory findings in a person with merely a fever of unknown origin may not be nearly as predictive. Generally speaking, biopsies in patients suspected of having systemic necrotizing vasculitis are best directed at obvious clinically involved organs. Blind biopsies of asymptomatic tissues such as muscle, nerve, kidney, or testicle are generally unrewarding.[104] Recent studies have suggested that a clinically or electrically documented involved sural nerve may yield an extremely high sensitivity for picking up systemic necrotizing vasculitis.[105]

Visceral abdominal angiography has been reported to be abnormal in up to 70% to 80% of patients with PAN though not all patients have equally characteristic findings. The presence of multiple saccular aneurysms in the distribution of the renal arteries or celiac axis is highly predictive of PAN while the presence of isolated vessel cutoff or mild luminal irregularities is far less specific.[10]

The diagnosis of Wegener's granulomatosis is basically a clinical pathologic one based on the characteristic distribution of target organ involvement. The diagnosis is secured when the characteristic histopathology is identi-fied in the appropriate clinical setting. The development of the ANCA test has provided a powerful adjunct in the diagnosis of Wegener's granulomatosis and related conditions. Even in the absence of confirmatory histology, an unequivocally positive ANCA (confirmed by specific antigenic reactivity to myeloperoxidase or PR3) in a patient with a high pretest probability of vasculitis may be sufficient to secure the diagnosis. Of course in such instances it is extremely important to rule out the possibility of mimicking or concomitant infection before commencing therapy.

Pitfalls in the Diagnosis of Systemic Necrotizing Vasculitis

Since there is no single test or combination of tests that is totally sensitive for the presence of systemic vasculitis, the clinician must be both patient and persistent to secure the diagnosis. Since most vasculitic lesions may be patchy by their nature, false negative biopsies are not uncommon. Certain tissues such as muscle, nerve, temporal artery, kidney, and testicle are well known for this problem. Certain organs such as the kidney may reveal nonvascular pathology that must be appropriately interpreted. For example, a closed-needle biopsy of a kidney in a patient with PAN or Wegener's granulomatosis is more likely than not to *fail* to reveal frank vasculitis of the renal vasculature. Similarly, the same technique is likely to yield evidence of a focal segmental necrotizing glomerulitis in the presence of an active urinary sediment or azotemia. Thus recognizing the characteristic finding of glomerulonephritis as opposed to vasculitis of the renal vasculature may secure the diagnosis. Another situation that is frequently encountered is a false negative nasal biopsy in patients with Wegener's granulomatosis. Because of the highly destructive nature of the lesions, the pathology may reveal only inflammation and necrosis. This should not be cast off as evidence of a nonvasculitic cause but should stimulate the clinician to further pursue securing the diagnosis of Wegener's granulomatosis if clinical suspicion is high. Collectively, the diagnosis of vasculitis remains clinically and pathologically based on a combination of history and physical findings, laboratory data, organ biopsy, and the selected use of vascular imaging studies.

REFERENCES

1. Gauthier J and Mannik M: Immune complexes in the pathogenesis of vasculitis. In Carivile Le Roy E, ed: Systemic vasculitis, New York, 1992, Marcel Dekker.
2. Abel G, Zhang Q, and Agnello V: Hepatitis C virus in type II mixed cryoglobulinemia, Arthritis Rheum 10:1341, 1993.
3. Jeannette JC: Antineutrophil cytoplasmic antibody associated disease: a pathologist's perspective, Am J Kidney Dis 2:164, 1991.
4. Oppenheimer-Marks N and Lipsky P: Transendothelial migration of T cells in chronic inflammation, The Immunol 2:58, 1994.
5. Lipford EH et al: Angiocentric immunoproliferative lesions: a clinicopathologic spectrum of post-thymic T cell proliferations, Blood 72:1674, 1988.
6. Leavitt RY and Fauci AS: Polyangiitis overlap syndrome, Am J Med 81:79, 1986.

7. Fauci AS, Haynes B, and Katz P: The spectrum of vasculitis: clinical pathologic, immunologic and therapeutic considerations, Ann Intern Med 89:660, 1978.

8. Guillevin L et al: Clinical findings and prognosis of polyarteritis nodosa and Churg-Strauss angiitis: a study of 165 patients, Br J Rheumatol 27:258, 1988.

9. Cupps TR and Fauci AS: The vasculitides. Chapter 4: Systemic necrotizing vasculitis of the polyarteritis nodosa group, Philadelphia, 1981, WB Saunders Co.

10. Travers RL et al: Polyarteritis nodosa: a clinical angiographic analysis of 17 cases, Semin Arthritis Rheum 8:184, 1979.

11. Moore PM and Fauci AS: Neurologic manifestations of systemic necrotizing vasculitis: a retrospective and prospective analysis of the clinical pathologic features and responses to therapy in 25 patients, Am J Med 71:517, 1981.

12. Diaz-Perez JL and Winkelman RK: Cutaneous periarteritis nodosa: a study of 33 patients. In Wolf K and Winkelman RK, eds: Vasculitis, Philadelphia, 1980, WB Saunders Co.

13. Wees SJ, Sunwoo IN, and Oh SJ: Sural nerve biopsy in systemic necrotizing vasculitis, Am J Med 71:525, 1981.

14. Cupps TR and Fauci AS: Management and treatment. In Cupps R and Fauci AS, eds: The vasculitides, Philadelphia, 1981, WB Saunders Co.

15. Guillevin L et al: Treatment of polyarteritis nodosa related to HBV with interferon alpha and plasma exchanges: results in 6 patients, Ann Rheum Dis 53:334, 1994.

16. Churg J and Strauss L: Allergic granulomatosis, allergic angiitis and periarteritis nodosa, Am J Pathol 27:277, 1951.

17. Chumbley LC, Harrison EG, and DeRemee RD: Allergic granulomatosis and angiitis (Churg-Strauss syndrome): report and analysis of 30 cases, Mayo Clin Proc 52:477, 1977.

18. Zeek PM, Smith CC, and Weeter JC: Studies on periarteritis nodosa. III. The differentiation between the vascular lesions of periarteritis nodosa and of hypersensitivity, Am J Pathol 24:889, 1948.

19. Calabrese LH and Clough JD: Hypersensitivity vasculitis group (HVG): a case-oriented review of a continuing clinical spectrum, Cleve Clin Q 49:17, 1982.

20. Cupps TR and Fauci AS: Hypersensitivity vasculitis. In Cupps TR and Fauci AS, eds: The vasculitides, Philadelphia, 1981, WB Saunders Co.

21. Wysenbeck AJ et al: Limited plasmapheresis in fulminant leukocytoclastic vasculitis, J Rheumatol 9:315, 1982.

22. Cream JJ, Gumpel JM, and Peachy AOG: Schönlein Henoch purpura in the adult: a study of 77 adults, Q J Med 39:461, 1970.

23. Levy M et al: Anaphylactoid purpura nephritis in children: natural history and immunopathology, Adv Nephrol 6:183, 1976.

24. Calabrese LH, Hoffman GS, and Guillivan L: Therapy of treatment resistant systemic necrotizing vasculitis: Churg-Strauss, Wegener's granulomatosis and hypersensitivity vasculitis group disorders, Rheum Clin North Am 21:41, 1995.

25. Greer JM et al: Vasculitis associated with malignancy, Medicine 67:220, 1988.

26. Zeiss CR et al: A hypocomplementemic vasculitic urticarial syndrome: report of four new cases and definition of the disease, Am J Med 68:867, 1980.

27. McDuffie FC et al: Hypocomplementemia with cutaneous vasculitis and arthritis: possible immune complex syndrome, Mayo Clin Proc 48:340, 1973.

28. Lieberman J, Gephardt G, and Calabrese LH: Chronic urticarial disease associated with pseudotumor cerebri membranoproliferative glomerulonephritis and hypocomplementemia: case report and review of the literature, Cleve Clin J Med 57:197, 1990.

29. Agnello V: Complement deficiency states, Medicine (Baltimore) 57:1, 1978.

30. Ekenstam EA and Callen JP: Cutaneous leukocytoclastic vasculitis: clinical and laboratory features of 82 patients seen in private practice, Arch Dermatol 120:484, 1984.

31. Gilliam JN and Smiley JD: Cutaneous necrotizing vasculitis and related disorders, Ann Allergy 37:328, 1976.

32. Wegener F: Über eine eigenartige rhinogene Granulomatose mit besonderer Beteiligung des arteriensystems und der Nieren, Beitr Pathol Anat Allgemein Pathol 102:36, 1939.

33. Carrington CB and Liebow AA: Limited forms of angiitis and granulomatosis of the Wegener's type, Am J Med 41:497, 1966.

34. Hoffman GS et al: Wegener granulomatosis: an analysis of 158 patients, Ann Intern Med 116:488, 1992.

35. Anderson G et al: Wegener's granuloma. A series of 265 British cases seen between 1975 and 1985. A report by a sub-committee of the British Thoracic Society Research Committee, Q J Med 83:427, 1992.

36. Papiha SS et al: Association of Wegener's granulomatosis with HLA antigens and other genetic markers, Ann Rheum Dis 51:246, 1992.

37. Leone CA, Feghali JG, and Linthicum FH Jr: Endolymphatic sac: possible role in autoimmune sensorineural hearing loss, Ann Otol Rhinol Laryngol 93:208, 1984.

38. Lebovics RS et al: The management of subglottic stenosis in patients with Wegener's granulomatosis, Laryngoscope 102:1341, 1992.

39. Haworth SJ et al: Pulmonary hemorrhage complicating Wegener's granulomatosis and microscopic polyarteritis, Br Med J 290:1775, 1985.

40. Luqmani RA et al: Classical versus non-renal Wegener's granulomatosis, Q J Med 87:161, 1994.

41. Camiller M et al: Gastrointestinal manifestations of systemic vasculitis, Q J Med 52:141, 1983.

42. Kemp JA, Arora S, and Fawaz K: Recurrent acute pancreatitis as a manifestation of Wegener's granulomatosis, Dig Dis Sci 35:912, 1990.

43. Churg J and Churg A: Idiopathic and secondary vasculitis: a review, Mod Pathol 2:144, 1989.

44. Mark EJ et al: The pulmonary biopsy in the early diagnosis of Wegener's (pathergic) granulomatosis: a study based on 35 open lung biopsies, Hum Pathol 19:1065, 1988.

45. Yoshikawa Y and Watanabe T: Pulmonary lesions in Wegener's granulomatosis: a clinicopathologic study of 22 autopsy cases, Hum Pathol 18:401, 1984.

46. Lie JT: American College of Rheumatology Subcommittee on Classification of Vasculitis. Illustrated histopathologic classification criteria for selected vasculitis syndromes, Arthritis Rheum 33:1074, 1990.

47. Weiss MA and Crissman JD: Renal biopsy findings in Wegener's granulomatosis: segmental necrotizing glomerulonephritis with glomerular thrombosis, Hum Pathol 15:943, 1984.

48. Leavitt RY et al: The American College of Rheumatology 1990 criteria for the classification of Wegener's granulomatosis, Arthritis Rheum 33:1101, 1990.

49. Van der Woude FJ et al: Antibodies against neutrophils and monocytes: tool for diagnosis and marker of disease activity in Wegener's granulomatosis, Lancet 1:425, 1985.

50. Falk RJ and Jeannette JC: Anti-neutrophil cytoplasmic antibodies with specificity for myeloperoxidase in patients

with systemic vasculitis and idiopathic necrotizing and crescentic glomerulonephritis, N Engl J Med 318:1651, 1988.

51. Niles JL et al: Wegener's granulomatosis autoantigen is a novel neutrophil serine protease, Blood 74:1888, 1989.

52. Mayet WJ and Meyer zum Buschenfelde KH: Antibodies to proteinase 3 increase adhesion of neutrophils to human endothelial cells, Clin Exp Immunol 94:440, 1993.

53. Brouwer E et al: Neutrophil activation in vitro and in vivo in Wegener's granulomatosis, Kidney Int 45:1120, 1994.

54. Fauci AS et al: Wegener's granulomatosis: prospective clinical and therapeutic experience with 85 patients for 21 years, Ann Intern Med 98:76, 1983.

55. DeRemee RA, McDonald TJ, and Weiland LH: Wegener's granulomatosis: observations on treatment with antimicrobial agents, Mayo Clin Proc 60:27, 1985.

56. Hoffman GS et al: The treatment of Wegener's granulomatosis with glucocorticoids and methotrexate, Arthritis Rheum 35:1322, 1992.

57. Orlowski JP, Clough JD, and Dyment PG: Wegener's granulomatosis in the pediatric age group, Pediatrics 61:83, 1978.

58. Alloway JA and Cupps TR: High dose methylprednisolone for retroorbital Wegener's granulomatosis, J Rheumatol 20:752, 1993.

59. Ettinger J et al: Progressive multifokale Leukoenzephalopathie bei Wegener'scher Granulomatose unter Therapie mit Cyclosporin A, Klin Wochenschr 67:260, 1989.

60. Hamilton CR Jr, Shelley WM, and Tumulty PA: Giant cell arteritis: including temporal arteritis and polymyalgia rheumatica, Medicine (Baltimore) 50:1, 1971.

61. Ishikawa K: Natural history and classification of occlusive thromboarthropathy (Takayasu's disease), Circulation 57:27, 1978.

62. Klein RG: Large artery involvement in giant cell (temporal) arteritis, Ann Intern Med 83:808, 1975.

63. Harmin B: Polymyalgia arteritica, Acta Med Scand Suppl 533:1, 1972.

64. Andersson R et al: HLA-DR expression in the vascular lesion and circulating T lymphocytes of patients with giant cell arteritis, Clin Exp Immunol 73:82, 1988.

65. McDonnell PJ et al: Temporal arteritis: a clinico-pathologic study, Ophthalmology 83:518, 1986.

66. Healey LA and Wilske KR: Polymyalgia rheumatica and giant cell arteritis, West J Med 141:64, 1984.

67. Cid MC et al: Polymyalgia rheumatica: a syndrome associated with HLA-DR4 antigen, Arthritis Rheum 31:678, 1988.

68. Delecoeuillerie G et al: Polymyalgia rheumatica and temporal arteritis: a retrospective analysis of prognostic features and different corticosteroid regimens (11 year survey of 210 patients), Ann Rheum Dis 47:733, 1988.

69. DeSilva M and Hazleman BL: Azathioprine in giant cell arteritis/polymyalgia rheumatica: a double-blind study, Ann Rheum Dis 45:136, 1986.

70. Kerr GS et al: Takayasu's arteritis, Ann Intern Med 120:919, 1994.

71. Hoffman GS: Treatment of resistant Takayasu's arteritis, Rheum Dis Clin North Am 21:73, 1995.

72. Giordano JM, Hoffman GS, and Leavitt RY: Takayasu's disease. In Rutherford surgical textbook, 1994.

73. Hong CY et al: Takayasu arteritis in Korean children: clinical report of seventy cases, Heart Vessels 7(suppl):91, 1992.

74. Sharma BK et al: Takayasu arteritis in India, Heart Vessels 7(suppl):37, 1992.

75. Fraga A et al: Takayasu's arteritis: frequency of systemic manifestations (study of 22 patients) and favorable response to maintenance steroid therapy with adrenocorticosteroids (12 patients), Arthritis Rheum 15:617, 1972.

76. Hall SH and Buchbinder R: Takayasu's arteritis, Rheum Dis Clin North Am 16:411, 1990.

77. Nakao K et al: Takayasu's arteritis. Clinical report of eighty-four cases and immunologic studies of seven cases, Circulation 35:1141, 1967.

78. Hall S et al: Takayasu's arteritis. A study of 32 North American patients, Medicine 64:89, 1985.

79. Lagneau P, Michel J-B, and Vuong PN: Surgical treatment of Takayasu's disease, Ann Surg 205:157, 1987.

80. Koide K: Takayasu arteritis in Japan, Heart Vessels 7(suppl):48, 1992.

81. Sekiguchi M and Suzuki J: An overview on Takayasu's arteritis, Heart Vessels 7(suppl):6, 1992.

82. Morales E, Pineda C, and Martinez-Lavin M: Takayasu's arteritis in children, J Rheumatol 18:1081, 1991.

83. Cho YD and Lee KT: Angiographic characteristics of Takayasu arteritis, Heart Vessels 7(suppl):97, 1992.

84. Goldbaum TS et al: Tuberculous aortitis presenting with an aortoduodenal fistula: a case report, Angiology 37:519, 1986.

85. Leavitt AD and Kauffman CA: Cryptococcal aortitis, Am J Med 85:108, 1988.

86. Banford WA, Farr PM, and Porter DI: Annular vasculitis of the head and neck in a patient with sarcoidosis, Br J Dermatol 106:713, 1982.

87. Bottcher E: Disseminated sarcoidosis with a marked granulomatous arteritis, Arch Pathol 68:419, 1959.

88. Johnston C and Kennedy C: Cutaneous leukocytoclastic vasculitis associated with acute sarcoidosis, Postgrad Med J 60:549, 1984.

89. Michaels L, Brown NJ, and Cory-Wright M: Arterial changes in pulmonary sarcoidosis, Arch Pathol 69:741, 1960.

90. Maeda S et al: Generalized sarcoidosis with sarcoid aortitis, Acta Pathol Jpn 33:183, 1983.

91. Gray GH, Young JR, and Olin JW: Miscellaneous arterial diseases. In Young JR et al, eds: Peripheral vascular diseases, St Louis, 1991, Mosby–Year Book.

92. Olin JW and Novick AC: Renovascular disease. In Young JR et al, eds: Peripheral vascular diseases, St Louis, 1991, Mosby–Year Book.

93. Deyu Z, Dijun F, and Lisheng L: Takayasu arteritis in China: a report of 530 cases, Heart Vessels 7(suppl):32, 1992.

94. Chugh KS and Sakhuja V: Takayasu's arteritis as a cause of renovascular hypertension in Asian countries, Am J Nephrol 12:1, 1992.

95. Ueda H et al: Clinical and pathological studies of aortitis syndrome. Committee report, Jpn Heart J 9:76, 1968.

96. Ito I: Medical treatment of Takayasu arteritis, Heart Vessels 7(suppl):133, 1992.

97. Shelhamer JH et al: Takayasu's arteritis and its therapy, Ann Intern Med 103:121, 1985.

98. Hoffman GS et al: Treatment of glucocorticoid-resistant or relapsing Takayasu's arteritis with methotrexate, Arthritis Rheum 37:578, 1994.

99. Kieffer E et al: Reconstructive surgery of the renal arteries in Takayasu's disease, Ann Vasc Surg 4:156, 1990.

100. Giordano JM et al: Experience with surgical treatment of Takayasu's disease, Surgery 109:252, 1991.

101. O'Duffy JD: Vasculitis in Behçet's disease, Rheum Dis North Am 16:423, 1990.

102. Du LTH et al: Arterial manifestations in Behçet's disease: fifteen cases in a series of 250 patients. In Duffy JD and Kokmen, eds: Behçet's disease, New York, 1991, Marcel Dekker.

103. Cappiello RA: Cholesterol embolism: a pseudovasculitic syndrome, Semin Arthritis Rheum 18:240, 1989.

104. Dahlberg PJ, Lockhart JM, and Overholt EL: Diagnostic studies for systemic necrotizing vasculitis, Arch Intern Med 149:161, 1989.

105. Wees SH, Sunwoo IN, and OH SJ: Sural nerve in systemic necrotizing vasculitis, Am J Med 71:525, 1981.

CHAPTER TWENTY-THREE

VASOSPASTIC DISEASES

Jay D. Coffman

Vasospastic diseases of the extremities include Raynaud's phenomenon, acrocyanosis, and livedo reticularis. Vasospasm implies reversible localized or diffuse vasoconstriction of arteries or smaller blood vessels. If the vasospasm is short-lived, the ischemia is reversible, and permanent damage does not result. Therefore patients may have vasospastic attacks for many years with no trophic changes of the digits. However, prolonged vasospasm with ischemia may lead to tissue damage with loss of subcutaneous tissue, ulcers, or gangrene. Raynaud's phenomenon, acrocyanosis, and livedo reticularis each occur in an idiopathic or primary form—that is, the underlying cause cannot be found. Usually the idiopathic varieties are benign and little permanent ischemic damage results. However, each of the entities may occur secondary to underlying conditions, and then the tissue damage can be extreme. Evidently any disease, persistent vasoconstrictor stimulus, or constant trauma that causes damage to blood vessels or tissue may lead to one of the vasospastic syndromes, perhaps by the common mechanism of ischemia.

PRIMARY RAYNAUD'S DISEASE

Maurice Raynaud[1] described Raynaud's phenomenon in 1888. The clinical picture is characteristic with the occurrence of episodic attacks of well-demarcated discoloration of the digits brought on by cold. Between attacks, the digits appear normal, or they may be cool and moist.

Sex and Age

Women are predominantly affected in a ratio of four females to one male.[2,3] The onset of the disease usually occurs in the second to fourth decade in both sexes.[2-4]

Prevalence

Studies of the prevalence of Raynaud's phenomenon in a general population have yielded estimates of 3.7% to 30% of randomly questioned people.[5-8] The most recent study affirms a higher prevalence in cooler climates compared with warmer climates.[8] The prevalence in Charles-ton, South Carolina, was 5% compared with 16.8% in Tarentaise, Savoie, France. One study reported that 89% of the cases had primary Raynaud's phenomenon and 11% had secondary Raynaud's phenomenon.[5]

Pathology

There are few studies on the pathology of primary Raynaud's phenomenon. Lewis[9] found no abnormalities in the digital arteries in two patients with mild disease. In patients with more severe disease intimal hyperplasia, narrowing or total occlusion of the digital arteries, or thrombi were present. Other studies[10,11] describe inflammatory destruction of the capillary bed or fibrinoid degeneration of the capillaries and various abnormalities at the cellular level and in the basement membranes, but whether these were primary or secondary changes caused by the ischemic episodes is unknown. There are conflicting reports of abnormalities in the digital arteries by arteriography in patients with primary Raynaud's disease with some studies finding normal vasculature[12] and others reporting digital artery stenoses and occlusions.[13,14] It is probable that the digital arteries are normal in early primary Raynaud's disease.

Pathophysiology

In normal subjects digital blood flow is primarily controlled by the sympathetic nervous system. It is decreased by activation of the sympathetic nerves and increased by withdrawal of sympathetic activity. Reflex sympathetic digital vasoconstriction results from body cooling or application of cold to other parts of the body, which is absent in sympathectomized or nerve-blocked digits. In vitro experiments using pharmacologic agonists and antagonists on hand arteries and veins have shown that α_1-adrenoceptors and α_2-adrenoceptors are present.[15,16] In human subjects intraarterial phenylephrine, an α_1-adrenoceptor agonist, and clonidine, an α_2-adrenoceptor agonist, produce dose-related decreases in total finger blood flow and increases in vascular resistance.[17] These responses are blocked by the appropriate antagonists. The

α_2-adrenoceptors have been shown to be most important during reflex sympathetic vasoconstriction induced by body cooling.

In addition to the capillary circulation, human digits contain a large number of arteriovenous anastomoses, which directly connect the arterial with the venous circulation, bypassing the capillary bed. These shunts allow a very large blood flow to pass through the digits in a warm environment and to close during cold exposure, allowing the body to regulate its core temperature. They are mainly under the control of the sympathetic nervous system via the α_2-adrenoceptors.[17] During body cooling the arteriovenous shunts constrict, but capillary or nutritional blood flow is maintained in normal subjects.[18]

Serotonin may also be important in reflex sympathetic vasoconstriction induced by body cooling in normal subjects. In vitro pharmacologic studies have shown that 5-hydroxytryptamine$_2$ (5-HT$_2$) receptors are present in human hand arteries and veins.[16] In normal subjects intraarterial 5-HT produces a dose-dependent decrease in total finger blood flow and an increase in vascular resistance, which is blocked by a specific 5-HT$_2$ antagonist, ketanserin.[19] Ketanserin also causes a large increase in total finger blood flow during reflex sympathetic vasoconstriction, which is not related to α_1-adrenoceptor or α_2-adrenoceptor antagonism.

As is true of most vascular beds, digital blood flow is integrated and regulated by the central nervous system via the sympathetic nervous system. The arteriovenous anastomoses are controlled by the hypothalamus to regulate body temperature; emotional responses also occur through the hypothalamus. The latter receives messages from the cerebral cortex and passes them on to the pressor and depressor vasomotor centers in the medulla oblongata. Baroreceptors, chemoreceptors, and somatic afferent nerves also influence the vasomotor centers. Messages from the medulla travel in the intermediolateral cell columns to the sympathetic ganglia and then to the sympathetic nerves.

In a 28.3° C or 20° C room total finger blood flow is decreased in patients with primary Raynaud's disease compared with normal subjects.[20] The hand blood flow is also abnormally low in a 20° C room with the hand in 32° C water, but hand blood flow rises to normal levels with body warming with the hand in 42° C water.[21,22] Capillary blood flow in the finger is significantly less in both warm and cool environments in patients with primary and secondary Raynaud's phenomenon compared with that in normal subjects.[20] A decrease in capillary blood flow with body cooling in these patients contrasts with the lack of change in normal subjects. This decrease is very important since capillary flow provides the nutritional support for the tissues.

The cause of the decreased finger blood flow or vasospastic attacks of the digits in primary Raynaud's phenomenon is unknown. The two classic theories are a local fault—that is, an abnormality at the level of the digital artery and an overactivity of the sympathetic nervous system. Lewis[23] proposed the local fault theory after finding that local cooling produced ischemic attacks in a single finger and that attacks could be produced in sym-

pathetically blocked fingers. He also showed that an ulnar nerve block, which blocks the sympathetic nerves, did not relieve vasospasm in the fifth finger. Jamieson, Ludbrook, and Wilson[24] found an enhancement by local cooling of the hand of reflex sympathetic vasoconstriction produced by ice application to the neck in patients with primary Raynaud's disease or scleroderma compared with normal subjects. They postulated that cold sensitized the α-adrenoceptor–mediated vasoconstriction of vascular smooth muscle. In support of this hypothesis increased levels of α_2-adrenoceptors of platelets have been reported in patients with primary Raynaud's disease compared with normal subjects or patients with secondary Raynaud's phenomenon.[25] Furthermore, patients with primary Raynaud's disease have a greater vasoconstrictor response to an α_2-adrenoceptor agonist than normal subjects[26]; cooling may also potentiate this vasoconstrictor response.[27] However, patients also show an increased vasoconstrictor response to serotonin.[26] The local fault theory is logical but remains to be proved.

Lewis[23] also presented evidence that the vasospasm occurred in the digital arteries and not the arterioles. Cooling the proximal finger with the distal finger kept warm induced vasospastic attacks, and resolution of attacks occurred by proximal and not distal warming of the finger. Digital artery vasospasm is substantiated by a fall in digital systolic pressure to zero after fingers are cooled to temperatures below 15° C during occlusion of blood flow in most patients with primary Raynaud's disease, whereas normal subjects show a gradual reduction in systolic pressure.[28]

Raynaud[1] considered that an overactivity of the sympathetic nervous system was the cause of vasospastic attacks in Raynaud's phenomenon. In support of this theory is the fact that patients attain normal hand blood flow during body and hand warming[21,22] and have an exaggerated vasoconstrictor response of digital blood flow to changes in body posture, which is a sympathetic nervous system response.[29] In some patients emotional stress induces attacks that could be explained by this theory but not by the local fault theory. Evidence against overactivity of the sympathetic nervous system is the recording by microelectrodes of normal sympathetic nerve activity with and without sympathetic stimulation,[30] a normal vasoconstriction of the ipsilateral hand to cooling of the opposite hand,[31] and normal blood and urine catecholamine levels in patients with primary Raynaud's disease.[32,33]

Associated factors are also important in either helping to induce or maintain digital vasospastic attacks but are probably not the definitive abnormality. Patients with primary Raynaud's disease have a lower brachial and finger systolic blood pressure and fingertip perfusion pressure than normal subjects.[34] This would result in a decreased arterial transmural distending force, and less external pressure would be required to stop blood flow. However, not all subjects with low finger blood pressure have vasospastic attacks.

Increased blood or plasma viscosity has been investigated as a causative factor in primary Raynaud's disease, but studies have been conflicting.[35-38] Viscosity is probably not of pathogenetic significance in the primary disease but may be important in secondary Raynaud's phenomenon because of cryoglobulinemia, polycythemia, and cold agglutinins by decreasing digital blood flow or occluding small blood vessels. Serotonin has been implicated in vasospasm in some vascular beds in humans and animals and may be involved in the pathogenesis of Raynaud's phenomenon.[39] It may be important in persistence of vasospastic attacks but is probably not the instigating factor.[40]

Endothelin-1 levels have been reported increased in patients with Raynaud's phenomenon and to rise with a cold stimulus.[41,42] Levels were higher in diffuse as compared with limited scleroderma and were inversely correlated with the carbon monoxide–diffusing capacity.[41] However, other investigators have not found elevated levels of endothelin-1 in patients with Raynaud's phenomenon.[43] The pathophysiologic importance of endothelin is unknown.

A significant correlation of Raynaud's phenomenon and migraine headaches in patients with variant angina pectoris, which is considered to be caused by coronary artery vasospasm, has been reported.[44] Another study reported an increased prevalence of migraine headaches in patients with Raynaud's phenomenon; nonspecific or musculoskeletal chest pains were common especially in patients with migraine.[45] Vasospasm has also been reported in the pulmonary,[46] renal,[47] and macular capillary circulation.[48] Another example of possible vasospasm in more than one vascular bed is the rare condition of primary pulmonary hypertension and Raynaud's phenomenon with no underlying disease. A blood-borne or neurologic factor or a generalized functional abnormality of vascular smooth muscle has been postulated to explain generalized vasospasm.[49]

In secondary causes of Raynaud's phenomenon, decreased blood flow or blood pressure in the digits is usually present, which accounts for the vasospastic attacks. Low blood pressure occurs distal to digital or larger vessel obstructions or stenoses in connective tissue diseases, vinyl chloride disease, and obstructive arterial diseases. A decreased blood flow would occur from hyperviscosity in cryoglobulinemia and other blood abnormalities or from persistent vasoconstriction with drug therapy or sympathetic nerve irritation in the thoracic outlet syndrome. With a low digital blood flow or blood pressure, a normal sympathetic stimulus or external pressure on the digits could induce abrupt closure of blood vessels.

Clinical Picture

Most patients have vasospastic attacks only in the fingers.[4] Less than half the patients also have attacks in the toes. Only a few patients have only the toes involved. The nose, ears, face, chest, and lips have been affected in some patients. When the disease first appears, only one or two fingers may be affected. Later, more fingers become involved and sometimes the toes; the thumbs are often spared.

Classically the digits turn white or sometimes yellow and numb because of the cessation of blood flow (Fig. 23-1). The hands are not involved. As slow blood flow returns, the digits turn blue because of the desaturation of the blood. When the digital arteries fully reopen, the digits become red from reactive hyperemia. During this last phase, a throbbing pain may occur. Pallor is often the only color change; the three-phase color change has been reported to occur in 4% to 65% of patients.[2,4] Exposure to cold is the precipitating factor of vasospastic attacks in all patients, but emotions may also cause attacks in some patients. In a large study reported in 1957, 13% of patients had ulcerations, chronic paronychia, necrosis, scarring, or fissuring of the fingers; sclerodactyly occurred in 12%.[4]

The patient's physical examination is normal except for cool digits and sometimes excess sweating of the hands. Radial, ulnar, dorsalis pedis, and posterior tibial pulses are present.

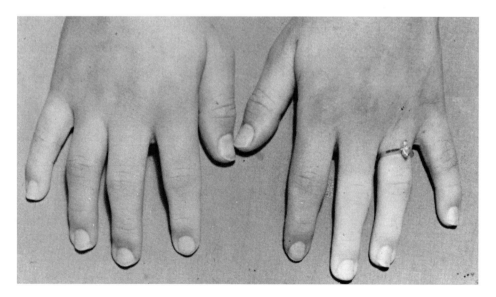

Fig. 23-1. Pallor phase of Raynaud's phenomenon in a young woman with Raynaud's disease.

Diagnosis

The diagnosis of Raynaud's phenomenon can usually be made from the patient's description of the attacks. In primary Raynaud's disease vasospastic attacks are usually difficult to induce in the physician's office. Well-demarcated, episodic white or blue discoloration of one or more digits or digital segments on exposure to cold is characteristic. The fingers may first turn white and numb, then blue, and finally bright red with throbbing pain as the circulation returns. This classic triad of colors is not always present; only one of the ischemic phases may occur or only two of the color changes.

After the physician is satisfied that a patient has Raynaud's phenomenon, then it must be determined if there is a secondary cause or if the syndrome is primary (idiopathic). In 1932 Allen and Brown[50] proposed the following criteria to distinguish primary from secondary Raynaud's phenomenon:

1. Vasospastic attacks precipitated by exposure to cold or emotional stimuli
2. Bilateral involvement of the extremities
3. Absence of gangrene or if present, limited to the skin of the fingertips
4. No evidence of an underlying disease that could be responsible for vasospastic attacks
5. A history of symptoms for at least 2 years

These criteria may help in the diagnosis of primary Raynaud's disease, but connective tissue diseases, such as scleroderma, can develop several years after the onset of Raynaud's phenomenon. Involvement of the hands may occur in secondary cases of Raynaud's phenomenon but not in the primary disease. The criteria can be strengthened by measurement of antinuclear antibodies, erythrocyte sedimentation rate, and examination of nail fold capillaries. Secondary causes of Raynaud's phenomenon should be more actively sought in men, in women who develop vasospastic attacks after age 40, and in patients with sclerodactyly, ulcers, or gangrene.

Measurement of finger systolic blood pressure during ischemia combined with local cooling is a useful diagnostic test for Raynaud's phenomenon.[28] The digit is cooled by circulating water through a cuff around the proximal finger at 20° C, 15° C, 10° C, and 5° C for 5-minute intervals. To aid the finger to approximate the external temperature, blood flow is stopped by inflating another digital cuff to suprasystolic pressure during cooling. Patients with Raynaud's phenomenon have a greater reduction in finger systolic pressure or digital arterial closure at higher pressures than normal subjects following ischemic cooling. If the body is also cooled during the test, about 80% of patients show a positive response.[51] This test does not help differentiate primary from secondary Raynaud's phenomenon.

The capillaries of the skin of the nail fold can be visualized using a microscope or even an ophthalmoscope. They are spaced regularly with hairpin loops aligned along the axis of the digit. Patients with primary Raynaud's disease usually have a normal nail fold capillary pattern. In scleroderma, mixed connective tissue disease, and dermatomyositis there are a decreased number of capillaries that are enlarged and deformed, and avascular areas are present.[52] In systemic lupus erythematosus abnormal capillary loops are present and the subpapillary venous plexus is more prominent than in normal subjects. Other diseases may also have abnormal capillaries. The value of this test is that an abnormal capillary pattern indicates a secondary cause of Raynaud's phenomenon; a normal pattern is not diagnostic but favors the primary disease.

The erythrocyte sedimentation rate is normal in patients with primary Raynaud's disease and often elevated in the connective tissue diseases. However, it can be normal in the latter diseases. Therefore the value of measuring the erythrocyte sedimentation rate is to determine if it is elevated and then secondary causes of Raynaud's phenomenon should be sought.

The presence of antinuclear antibodies in patients with Raynaud's phenomenon usually indicates that a systemic disease is present or will manifest itself later. Elderly patients may have a titer as high as 1:64 without systemic disease, but younger patients rarely exceed 1:16. A speckled pattern is often present in scleroderma. Anticentromere antibodies are present in the majority of patients with CREST (*c*alcinosis, *R*aynaud's phenomenon, *e*sophageal involvement, *s*clerodermatous skin thickening, and *t*elangiectasia) syndrome.[53] A homogeneous pattern of antinuclear antibodies with antibodies to desoxyribonucleic acid is often present in systemic lupus erythematosus. Antinuclear antibodies and rheumatoid factor may be present in other connective tissue diseases and can also be induced by some drugs. The detection of antinuclear antibodies by immunofluorescence and immunoblotting has a positive predictive value of 65% and 71% and a negative predictive value of 93% and 83%, respectively, for the development of a connective tissue disease.[54] Immunoblotting is especially useful in predicting systemic sclerosis, the CREST syndrome, and mixed connective tissue disease.

Since the majority of patients with Raynaud's phenomenon have the benign, primary disease, a young woman with no other symptoms and a normal physical examination should have a minimum laboratory workup.[55] If a complete blood cell count, erythrocyte sedimentation rate, urinalysis, and chest x-ray film show any abnormalities, a more extensive workup searching for a secondary cause should be instituted.

Prognosis

In a long-term study[4] of 307 patients with Raynaud's phenomenon, primary by the criteria of Allen and Brown,[50] 38% had stable disease, 36% improved, 16% became worse, and the syndrome disappeared in 10%. Sclerodactyly disappeared in 19 of 27 patients and was unchanged in 7 patients; it developed in 3.3%. Only 0.4%, or 2 patients, had digital amputations, but 13% had ulceration, chronic paronychia, necrosis of the skin, scarring, or fissuring. Tobacco smoking did not affect the prognosis. Symptoms were alleviated in just over half of the 44 patients who moved to a warmer climate. In another study[3] that included surgically treated patients, 40% remained the same, 48% had slight to severe progression, and 12% had regression or disappearance of vasospastic attacks. Medical or surgical treatment did not affect the prognosis.

The presence of sclerodactyly with Raynaud's phenomenon does not predict an adverse prognosis.[56] Of 71 patients with sclerodactyly and primary Raynaud's disease by the Allen and Brown criteria,[50] 28% improved, 22.5% deteriorated, and 40.8% were unchanged over an average 10-year follow-up study. Six patients died of unrelated causes. Scleroderma developed in only 4% (3 patients).

Evidently connective tissue disease does not frequently develop over the ensuing years in patients diagnosed as having primary Raynaud's disease. Of 87 patients followed for an average of 5.1 years after the onset of symptoms, 5% developed scleroderma of the CREST variety, although 17% of these patients had antinuclear antibodies.[57]

SECONDARY CAUSES OF RAYNAUD'S PHENOMENON

Raynaud's phenomenon may be caused by drugs; connective tissue diseases; constant trauma to the fingers; compression of nerves or blood vessels; obstruction of blood vessels; increased blood viscosity, or sludging of blood; vasculitis; or endocrine disorders. The most common causes are drugs and the connective tissue diseases.

Drugs

β-Adrenoceptor antagonists are the most common drugs inducing Raynaud's phenomenon. Both nonselective and cardioselective agents have been implicated,[58] although β_2-adrenoceptors predominate in the peripheral circulation. Unlike primary Raynaud's disease, males and females are equally afflicted, and all ages may be affected.[59,60] There is no apparent relationship to dose. The incidence has been reported as 4.1% to 40% of patients taking these agents.[59-61] Almost every β-adrenoceptor blocking drug has been reported to cause vasospastic attacks. Substitution with β-blocking drugs with α-adrenoceptor antagonist[62] or intrinsic sympathetic activity does not always alleviate the syndrome. However, administration of β-adrenoceptor blocking agents to patients who already have Raynaud's phenomenon does not appear to aggravate the vasospastic attacks.[62,63] How these agents induce Raynaud's phenomenon is unknown, but the phenomenon may be caused by unopposed α-adrenoceptor vasoconstrictor activity, a decrease in cardiac output or blood volume with reflex vasoconstriction, or central cardiovascular depressant effects with increased reflex sympathetic vasoconstriction.

Ergot produces intense vasospasm of the digits and large blood vessels by stimulation of α-adrenoceptors. Ergot intoxication can occur from ingestion of rye contaminated with the fungus, *Claviceps purpurea,* but the most common cause is the use of ergotamine preparations for migraine headaches. Pathologic studies in humans have shown proliferation of the endothelium, thrombosis, hyaline degeneration, and fibrosis of the vascular wall in severe cases. Vasospasm occurs from excess doses of the drugs, usually greater than 10 mg/week.[64] Females are affected more frequently than males; the incidence of toxicity is 0.01% of patients using the drug. Digital, carotid, axillary,

renal, coronary, ophthalmic, and splanchnic vessels may be involved.[65] Patients develop painful, cold, discolored extremities or intermittent claudication. Occasionally an intense burning pain in the extremities called St. Anthony's fire occurs.[64] Only the large-vessel pulses may be palpable. Gangrene may occur. The diagnosis is usually easily made by a careful history and physical examination. Arteriograms show uniform smooth tapering of large- and medium-size arteries, and the vessels often disappear at the forearm or calf level.[66] In patients who do not have limb-threatening vasospasm, conservative therapy with heparin and bed rest is the best course since the blood vessels usually relax within 3 days. Many drugs have been recommended for the more severe cases; intraarterial or intravenous nitroprusside with or without oral nifedipine is as successful as any regimen.[67,68]

Methysergide is a congener of lysergic acid diethylamide, which has both serotonin antagonist and agonist activity. About 3% of patients who take this drug for migraine headaches develop ischemia of the upper and lower extremities.[69] This complication may occur with as small a dose as 1 mg. The clinical manifestation and treatment are similar to ergot toxicity.

Vinblastine and bleomycin therapy for a variety of tumors may induce Raynaud's phenomenon in 2.6% to 37% of patients.[70,71] It is not known whether one or both agents is the cause. Vinblastine can cause neuropathy and bleomycin can cause cutaneous toxicity. Symptoms usually appear after 10 months of therapy. Arteriograms show diffuse digital arterial narrowing or multiple digital or palmar arterial occlusions. Symptoms may improve when chemotherapy is terminated, but many patients continue to have vasospastic attacks.[71]

Other drugs that have rarely been reported to induce Raynaud's phenomenon are bromocriptine, clonidine, imipramine, amphetamine, cyclosporine, and withdrawal from chronic nitroglycerin exposure. Oral contraceptives have also been incriminated, but the data are inconclusive.[72]

Connective Tissue Diseases

SCLERODERMA. Approximately 90% of patients with scleroderma (systemic sclerosis) have Raynaud's phenomenon or persistent digital vasospasm.[73] It is the initial complaint in almost 50% of patients. In the CREST syndrome Raynaud's phenomenon accompanies subcutaneous calcifications, esophageal motility abnormalities, skin thickening or tightness, and telangiectasias (Fig. 23-2). More advanced cases of scleroderma may also have sclerodactyly, arthralgias or arthritis, and pulmonary or renal involvement. Digital ulcerations from ischemia of the fingertips is common in scleroderma (Fig. 23-3) but may also be caused by subcutaneous diffuse or localized calcifications. The claw finger deformity of the hands, caused by thickened skin and contracture of the phalangeal joints, is not diagnostic of scleroderma since only 3 of 71 patients with sclerodactyly observed for an average of 10 years developed the systemic disease.[56]

Laboratory studies in scleroderma can be normal. The erythrocyte sedimentation rate is increased in about two thirds of patients. Antinuclear antibodies are usually

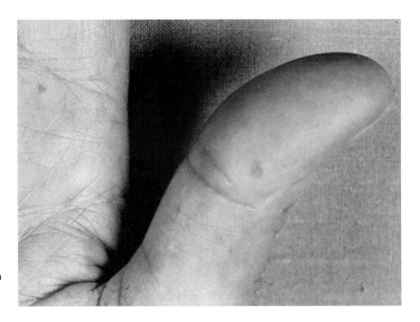

Fig. 23-2. Telangiectasias of the thumb and palm of a patient with Raynaud's phenomenon associated with the CREST syndrome.

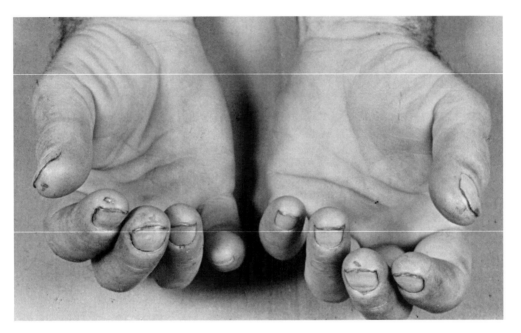

Fig. 23-3. Small-healed fingertip ulcers in a patient with scleroderma and Raynaud's phenomenon.

present in the advanced disease and are directed against a soluble nuclear antigen called SCL-70, nucleolar ribonucleic acid, or the centromere of chromosomes. The CREST syndrome usually has the anticentromere antibody,[74] whereas the other antibodies occur in the systemic disease. Barium swallow examination or esophageal manometry may reveal the motor abnormality, which is limited to the lower smooth muscle part of the esophagus. Chest x-ray films may show linear streaks of fibrosis in the basal areas of the lungs. Nailbed microscopic examination may reveal sparse, dilated, and convoluted capillaries and avascular areas. The cause of scleroderma is unknown. Pathologic studies show cutaneous edema and chronic inflammatory cells with homogeneous, acellular deposits

of collagen in indistinct bundles. Capillaries may be sparse and arterioles may show hyaline. The cause of Raynaud's phenomenon is unknown, but the walls of small arteries and arterioles may be thickened, and also the blood vessels may be entrapped in nondistensible fibrous tissue.

SYSTEMIC LUPUS ERYTHEMATOSUS. Raynaud's phenomenon has been reported in 10% to 44% of patients with systemic lupus erythematosus.[75,76] Systemic lupus erythematosus occurs mostly in women in their third to fourth decade, and the disease is more common in blacks than whites. The vasospastic attacks may precede other disease manifestations but usually develop later in the course of the disease. This multisystem disease should be suspected in young women with Raynaud's phenomenon who have a photosensitive rash on the face in a butterfly pattern, arthralgias or arthritis, seizures, psychosis, alopecia, pericarditis, or nephritis. Anemia, leukopenia, and thrombocytopenia are common. A circulating anticoagulant may cause a prolongation of the partial thromboplastin time. The erythrocyte sedimentation rate is usually elevated. Complement levels are often low. A large number of antibodies to nuclear and cytoplasmic constituents may be present and are usually homogeneous. Antibodies to double-stranded deoxyribonucleic acid (DNA) and Sm antigen are characteristic. The cause of systemic lupus erythematosus is unknown, but it is considered to be an autoimmune disease. Immune complexes are deposited in various organs and tissues, producing an inflammatory response. The pathologic picture is that of a vasculitis affecting arterioles and venules; fibrinoid necrosis of blood vessels is commonly present. In most cases it is believed the patient is reacting against his or her own tissues. Many popular drugs including procainamide, isoniazid, and hydralazine can induce a similar disease.

RHEUMATOID ARTHRITIS. Raynaud's phenomenon may occur in rheumatoid arthritis. Focal ischemic lesions and microinfarctions also occur in the periungual areas and digital pulp. Pathologically there may be an obliterative intimal proliferation of the digital arteries,[77] and arteriograms often show occlusions of one or more digital arteries.[78]

SJÖGREN'S SYNDROME. Patients who develop Raynaud's phenomenon and who have dry eyes and mouth with enlargement of the salivary or lacrimal glands should be investigated for primary or secondary Sjögren's syndrome. The secondary syndrome occurs most frequently in rheumatoid arthritis and systemic lupus erythematosus. The majority of patients with primary Sjögren's syndrome have antibodies to Sjögren's syndrome A antigen (SS-A), and about 50% have antibodies to Sjögren's syndrome B (SS-B).[79] These antibodies are not frequent in rheumatoid arthritis but do occur in systemic lupus erythematosus. However, patients with primary Sjögren's syndrome rarely have antibodies to double-stranded DNA and lack sufficient clinical features for the diagnosis of systemic lupus erythematosus. Antibodies to salivary gland ducts occur in rheumatoid arthritis but not in primary Sjögren's syndrome.

POLYMYOSITIS AND DERMATOMYOSITIS. Polymyositis occurs more often in women in their fifth and sixth decades than it does in men, whereas dermatomyositis is more common in children. Patients develop symmetric weakness of proximal muscles but may also have arthritis or arthralgias, an erythematous skin rash, dysphagia, dysarthria, and pulmonary fibrosis. Raynaud's phenomenon occurs in about one third of patients. A heliotrope or purplish discoloration of the upper eyelids is a characteristic finding. Elevated levels of creatine phosphokinase and aldolase are usually present. In polymyositis muscle fiber degeneration, necrosis, and fibrosis with a mononuclear cell infiltrate is seen by muscle biopsy, but sclerotic changes in small vessels and arterioles may be seen in dermatomyositis.[80]

MIXED CONNECTIVE TISSUE DISEASE. Patients with mixed connective tissue disease have many features of other connective tissue diseases such as joint, muscle, pulmonary, and renal involvement.[81] Swelling of the dorsum of the hands and fingers with a sausage-shaped appearance of the digits is characteristic. Raynaud's phenomenon may precede other manifestations of the disease by many years; it may occur in up to 85% of patients. Antinuclear antibodies of a speckled pattern are often found, and a high titer of antibodies to extractable ribonuclease antigens is diagnostic. Rheumatoid factor and an increased erythrocyte sedimentation rate are also common. Raynaud's phenomenon may improve with steroid therapy.

Traumatic Vasospastic Disease

Raynaud's phenomenon may occur in people engaged in occupations in which their fingers are constantly exposed to trauma or vibratory tools. Traumatic vasospastic disease has also been called vibration-induced white fingers or Raynaud's phenomenon of occupational origin. Pneumatic hammers, chain saws, riveting machines, pounding and lasting machines, and brush saws are the most common offenders, but telephone operators, typists, pianists, meat cutters, and sewing machine operators have also been affected. Of workers who use vibratory tools 30% to 84% develop vasospastic symptoms,[82-84] usually after 6000 to 7000 hours of exposure.[85] The vasospastic attacks are manifested by blanching and numbness of the fingers, but pain and cyanosis are uncommon.[86] Both hands may be involved, but the feet are asymptomatic. Attacks are produced not only by exposure to the tools but also to cold. Gangrene or loss of fingers is rare.

Some investigators[87,88] consider that there is a syndrome of muscle and joint pain or weakness, hearing loss, headache, forgetfulness, fatigability, tinnitus, impotence, dizziness, and palmar hyperhidrosis with Raynaud's phenomenon. Pathologic studies of biopsies of fingers have shown a normal picture[86] or medial muscular hypertrophy and subintimal fibrosis of the digital vessels.[87] Angiography only showed tapered forearm arteries. The pathophysiology of traumatic vasospastic disease is unknown. Some improvement in symptoms may occur after cessation of tool exposure, but sensitivity to cold often remains.[89] Prognosis for recovery is better in brush saw than chain saw workers. Prevention of traumatic vasospastic disease includes training in the easiest way to use the tools, use of multiple layers of warm gloves inside an outer waterproof glove, and frequent changes of gloves if the hands become wet.[87] Using antivibratory saws and limiting the duration of tool use to 2 hours a day has decreased the incidence of the disease.[85] In an open study[90] diltiazem 30 mg three times a day decreased a variety of subjective symptoms and improved the rewarming time of hands immersed in 10° C water in patients with traumatic vasospastic disease.

Hypothenar Hammer Syndrome

About 2 cm distal to the wrist, the ulnar artery is protected only by skin, subcutaneous tissue, and the palmar brevis muscle. Trauma to the vessel by hammering with the palm of the hand, practicing karate, and using bowling balls or walkers may cause ulnar artery occlusion.[91-93] Patients with the hypothenar hammer syndrome can develop Raynaud's phenomenon involving one hand. Pallor or cyanosis with numbness occurs on exposure to cold, but a reactive hyperemia phase does not develop. The inciting trauma may not seem important to the patient, but calluses over the hypothenar eminences suggest the diagnosis. There may also be a tender mass in the area. Radial and ulnar pulses are normal at the wrist. An Allen test, which is done by compression of the radial artery while the patient exercises the hand above heart level, produces a pale hand that regains color on release of the radial artery. Normally the ulnar artery would supply the hand, and the hand would retain normal color with radial artery occlusion. Doppler flow examination of the superficial palmar arch during compression of the radial artery will document that flow sounds disappear. About 1.7% of patients with Raynaud's phenomenon will have this entity[92]; men are mainly afflicted in their third to fifth decade. Pathologically the ulnar artery is occluded and often aneurysmal. Angiography is diagnostic, showing thrombosis, irregularity, or aneurysm of the ulnar artery in the region of the hamate bone.[92,94] Multiple digital artery occlusions may also be present, which are probably the result of emboli. The treatment is initially conservative since symptoms often abate in a few months.[92] Resection of the diseased segment of artery,[93] sympathectomies or sympatholytic agents, and even fibrinolytic agents[95] have been used with some success.

Carpal Tunnel Syndrome

Patients with carpal tunnel syndrome complain of numbness, burning, or tingling in the first three fingers. Pain may radiate to the arm or shoulder. Symptoms are usually bilateral. Raynaud's phenomenon is commonly present and may precede other symptoms by 6 to 12 months.[96] Examination may reveal weakness and atrophy of muscles of the thenar eminence. Sensory changes only occur distal to the wrist, and usually only the first three fingers are involved. There are many causes of carpal tunnel syndrome but no underlying cause can be found in many patients. Carpal tunnel syndrome is a common occupational disease and may be induced by any job requiring constant wrist action; it is a frequent occurrence in keyboard operators. The carpal tunnel consists of the carpal bones covered by the transverse ligament running across the ventral surface of the wrist. Any increase in pressure in the tunnel by swelling, inflammation, or deposition or infiltration of tissue may compress the median nerve. The diagnosis is made by nerve conduction studies, which reveal prolonged sensory latencies of the median nerve and decrease sensory potentials in 85% to 95% of patients. Delayed motor latencies occur in few cases.[97] Reproduction of symptoms by tapping the median nerve at the wrist (Tinel's sign) or maximal wrist flexion (Phalen's sign) may be present but are not reliable tests.[98] Surgical decompression of the carpal tunnel by section of the transverse ligament is the preferred treatment with an 80% to 90% cure rate.[99] Injection of steroids into the tunnel,[100] splinting of the wrist, and vitamin B_6 have been advocated.[101] Diuretics may be of value in pregnancy.[102] The vasospastic attacks may or may not be helped by successful treatment of the entrapped nerve.

Thoracic Outlet Syndromes

As many as 38.6% of patients with the hyperabduction syndrome[103] and 5.3% of patients with different types of thoracic outlet syndromes[104] manifest Raynaud's phenomenon. The vasospastic attacks may involve one or both hands. The attacks may be caused by compression of the sympathetic nerves in the thoracic outlet, but some patients have digital arterial emboli from thrombi in the subclavian artery.[105] There may be an aneurysmal dilation with thrombi distal to the point of subclavian artery compression. The thoracic outlet syndromes may be caused by compression of the neurovascular bundle by cervical ribs or the scalenus anticus muscle, between the first thoracic rib and clavicle (costoclavicular syndrome) or by the pectoralis minor tendon (hyperabduction syndrome). Cervical ribs occur in 0.5% to 1% of the population, but only 10% cause symptoms.[106] For a more detailed description of thoracic outlet syndromes see Chapter 31.

Cryoproteinemia, Cold Agglutinins, and Polycythemia

Patients with cold agglutinins, polycythemia, or cryoproteinemia may develop Raynaud's phenomenon, probably because of the intravascular clumping of red blood cells or precipitated proteins decreasing or obstructing blood flow in small blood vessels. Of 100 patients with polycythemia vera, 3 had attacks of pallor of single digits, which were relieved by decreasing the blood volume,[107] but this is a rare cause of vasospastic attacks. Patients with Waldenström's macroglobulinemia have been reported to have Raynaud's phenomenon, but they may also have cryoglobulins.[108]

Patients with cryoglobulinemia develop purpura of the lower legs, joint pains, leg ulcers, renal failure, and occasionally Raynaud's phenomenon.[109] Ten percent of patients with essential cryoglobulinemia may have vasospastic attacks. The disease is twice as common in females as males, and symptoms usually occur in the patient's third or fourth decade. Secondary cryoglobulinemia may develop in a variety of disorders including infections, autoimmune or connective tissue diseases, lymphoproliferative disease, and liver disease. Occasionally cryofibrinogens may also cause Raynaud's phenomenon.[110] The symptoms and signs of cryoglobulinemia are evidently caused by the precipitation of the proteins at low temperatures. The precipitates then act as immune complexes inciting an inflammatory reaction. However, the cryoglobulins may also increase blood and plasma viscosity, leading to a decrease in hand blood flow.[111] Cryoglobulinemia has been successfully treated with alkylating agents plus prednisone[112] or plasmapheresis[113] but not with prednisone alone.

Raynaud's phenomenon may occur in patients with cold agglutinins. Cold agglutinins may develop in viral infections or lymphomas. In elderly patients cold agglutinins may be found with no underlying disease and may cause cyanosis, hemolytic anemia, and hemoglobulinuria.[110] Males are affected twice as commonly as females, and patients are usually 30 to 90 years of age.[114] Cold agglutinins are antibodies of the γ-IgM type and are usually present in titers greater than 1:128 when symptoms and signs occur. Although Raynaud's phenomenon may occur, pallor or cyanosis may involve the whole hand. Necrosis and gangrene of the fingers may develop. The pathophysiology is caused by intravascular clumping of red blood cells with a blockage of blood flow in small vessels.[115] Treatment is nonspecific and depends on avoidance of cold. Chlorambucil will reduce the quantity of cold agglutinins, but it must be given for prolonged periods, and toxicity is a problem.

Vinyl Chloride Disease

Vinyl chloride exposure may cause a multisystem disease resembling scleroderma with thickening of the skin of the hands and forearms, nodule formation, thinning of bones, thrombocytopenia, hepatic and pulmonary dysfunction, and angiosarcoma of the liver.[116] Raynaud's phenomenon is common. The disease occurs mainly in workers who clean autoclaves. Circulating immune complexes occur in over 60% of symptomatic workers with a polyclonal increase in immunoglobulins, usually IgG.[117] Antinuclear antibodies may be present in low titers. Their fingernail beds show dilated capillary loops, disarray of capillary polarity, and avascular areas.[118] Angiography shows stenoses or occlusions of digital arteries.[119] Skin biopsies reveal thickened dermis, nonfibrillary homogenization of collagen, and swollen, thickened collagen. Treatment is removal from exposure to polyvinyl chloride.

Obstructive Arterial Diseases

Raynaud's phenomenon may occur in limbs affected by arteriosclerosis obliterans, thromboangiitis obliterans, or arterial emboli. In arteriosclerosis obliterans usually only one or two toes of the affected extremity show attacks of pallor or cyanosis.[120] A reactive hyperemia phase does not occur. The diagnosis is made by the occurrence of vasospastic attacks only in the lower extremity of one limb, absence of pulses in the extremity, and usually a history of intermittent claudication. Raynaud's phenomenon may occur in as many as 57% of patients with thromboangiitis obliterans.[121] The cause of this disease is unknown, but it occurs most often in young male smokers, and episodes of superficial thrombophlebitis are frequent. Pathologically there is inflammation of the walls of arteries and veins with secondary thromboses. The thrombi contain foci of leukocytes surrounded by giant cells. The lower extremities are affected most often, but the upper extremities may be involved in greater than 70% of patients. Digital ulcers and gangrene are common and the pain is often excruciating. Arteriography shows segmental involvement of medium to small arteries with intervening normal areas, absence of atheroma, and a tree-root pattern of collateral vessels springing from the thrombosed end of the arteries. Blood vessel biopsy during the acute stages is required for a definite diagnosis. Raynaud's phenomenon may occur in the fingers or toes in a limb or digit that has had a previous arterial embolus.

Reflex Sympathetic Dystrophy

Extreme, constant pain that persists after the healing phase of major or minor trauma, fractures, or surgery is termed reflex sympathetic dystrophy. Initially the affected part is dry, swollen, and warm but then becomes persistently cold, swollen, and pale or cyanotic. Raynaud's phenomenon may occur in the latter stage. For a more detailed description of reflex sympathetic dystrophy see Chapter 32.

Vasculitis

Any of the many diseases causing vasculitis may also cause Raynaud's phenomenon. They may manifest immune complexes, which can induce inflammatory reactions in small vessels. The connective tissue diseases, periarteritis nodosa and hepatitis B antigenemia, are examples.[122-124]

Arteriovenous Fistula

Greater than 50% of patients with arteriovenous fistulas may manifest Raynaud's phenomenon.[125] Diminished blood flow and blood pressure distal to the fistula may result in peripheral coldness and trophic changes. Other factors than decreased blood flow may be involved, since an abnormal response of digital artery blood pressure to cooling occurs in the opposite hand.[126] Arteriovenous shunts are seen most frequently in patients who need hemodialysis. Renal transplantation has been reported to improve the cold sensitivity.

Renal Disease

Patients with severe renal disease may have cool, cyanotic hands, and gangrene may develop. These patients often have calcification of their medium-sized and digital arteries. Occlusions of radial and ulnar arteries have been shown by arteriography. The pathogenesis of the ischemia is unknown since medial calcification of blood vessels occurs in many patients with renal or other diseases without vasospastic manifestations. Parathormone, hypercalcemia, steroid or immunosuppressive therapy, and mechanical obstruction resulting from calcium deposition have been postulated as etiologically important.[127] Some patients have responded to parathyroidectomy.

Hypothyroidism

Raynaud's phenomenon is seen in some patients with hypothyroidism, and improvement has occurred with thyroid therapy.[128] The incidence may be as high as 24%.[129] The extremity blood flow is decreased in patients with myxedema. Their decreased heat production may induce peripheral vasoconstriction in an attempt to conserve body heat. It is also possible that thickening of the blood vessel walls by edema could lead to closure of blood vessels with normal sympathetic stimuli.

Neoplasms

Raynaud's phenomenon or digital ischemia and gangrene may occur in neoplastic diseases without the presence of cryoglobulinemia, cold agglutinins, carpal tunnel syndrome, or compression of the cervical sympathetic chain. The reports include cancers of the stomach, kidney, colon, ovary, cervix, and lung and leukemias. In one patient with a high level of γ-globulins, skin biopsy showed leukocytoclastic angiitis.[130] Fibrinoid necrosis, intimal proliferation, and inflammatory cell infiltration of the digital vessels, suggesting a vasculitis, were also described in another patient. Raynaud's phenomenon of 2 years' duration in a 59-year-old woman was resolved with resection of a small bowel adenocarcinoma and did not recur in the next 5 years.[131] In a review of 180 cases of malignancy associated with Raynaud's phenomenon over 6 years, 63 cases preceded tumor discovery by an average of 9.3 years.[131] Breast and lung cancer were the most common malignancies. Raynaud's phenomenon did not resolve in any patient after tumor resection. No information is given regarding abnormal proteins or metastases in these patients, so it is difficult to analyze the cause of the vasospastic attacks.

Heavy Metals

Raynaud's phenomenon has been attributed to toxicity from lead, arsenic, thallium, and mercury. Substantial evidence has not been presented that these heavy metals induce typical episodic vasospastic attacks.

Primary Pulmonary Hypertension

Several patients with primary pulmonary hypertension have been reported to have Raynaud's phenomenon but no other evidence of a systemic disease.[132,133] Marked intimal thickening or concentric proliferation has been described in pulmonary arterioles,[132] but skin or muscle biopsies have shown no vascular changes. An incidence of Raynaud's phenomenon of 10% to 30% has been reported in two series of patients with primary pulmonary hypertension.[134,135] Whether a separate disease entity of pulmonary hypertension and Raynaud's phenomenon exists is unknown, but it has been postulated that vasospasm may occur in both circulations because of a neurohumoral mechanism and that recurrent episodes of vasospasm could lead to pathologic changes in small blood vessels.[49]

Primary Biliary Cirrhosis

Patients with primary biliary cirrhosis who also have Raynaud's phenomenon, calcinosis cutis, telangiectasias, and thickened, tight skin resembling scleroderma have been described.[136,137] Skin biopsies have suggested scleroderma. Antinuclear antibodies are present in some, but not all, patients but can occur in primary biliary cirrhosis without scleroderma. Hepatitis B antigen is not present. A common immunologic mechanism has been suggested for both the liver and skin disease.

TREATMENT OF RAYNAUD'S PHENOMENON

Conservative Therapy

Many patients who experience few vasospastic attacks never seek a physician's advice. Of those who do, reassurance that the disease is benign and does not lead to loss of digits or limbs often suffices. It is always helpful to give patients a few suggestions on living with their problem. Mittens are better than gloves because the fingers can share their heat. Pressure plus cold is likely to induce attacks—for instance, holding cold steering wheels and iced drinks. Body plus hand chilling is also likely to cause attacks; shopping in the frozen food section of a supermarket is a good example. It should be explained to patients that they must keep the whole body warm, since chilling most parts of the body can lead to digital vasoconstriction. Although a connection with tobacco smoking has not been made for primary Raynaud's disease, smoking should be avoided, since nicotine causes cutaneous vasoconstriction via the sympathetic nervous system. There are various foot- or hand-warming devices, battery operated or chemical, that may be helpful to some patients.

Drug Therapy

If, despite conservative therapy, vasospastic attacks interfere with the patient's daily activities or employment or if trophic digital lesions occur, drug treatment should be considered. However, drug therapy is nonspecific and often produces intolerable side effects. The most common agents used are calcium entry blockers or sympatholytic drugs.

Nifedipine is a calcium entry blocker with a potent peripheral vasodilator action and has been shown to decrease the frequency, duration, and severity of vasospastic attacks in about two thirds of patients with Raynaud's phenomenon in several placebo-controlled studies.[138,139] Doses of 10 to 20 mg three times a day are used. Side effects include headache, dizziness, flushing, palpitations, edema, dyspepsia, and pruritus. The slow-release preparations of nifedipine are better tolerated by patients and, in our experience, are as therapeutically beneficial in doses from 30 to 90 mg. Diltiazem in doses of 30 to 120 mg three times a day has also been reported to have favorable effects,[140,141] although one study[142] failed to find a beneficial response. Side effects are fewer than with nifedipine and include headache, flushing, dizziness, nausea, and edema. Verapamil has not been shown to be of value.[143] Newer calcium entry blockers have not been adequately studied but may be beneficial. Felodipine was as effective as nifedipine in one study[144,145] and israpidine was beneficial in one small trial.[146] Side effects are similar with these agents to nifedipine.

Reserpine and guanethidine are agents that interfere with sympathetic vasoconstriction and have been shown to increase digital capillary blood flow in Raynaud's phenomenon.[147-149] Adequate placebo-controlled studies have not been performed, but these agents have been used with benefit in patients with Raynaud's phenomenon.[149] Both drugs must be carefully titrated to the relief of symptoms or the production of side effects to be sure an adequate dose is being used. For reserpine 0.125 to 0.5 mg daily is recommended. Intraarterial reserpine has also been used but probably is no more beneficial than oral administration.[150] The preparation is also no longer available in the United States. Side effects of reserpine are bradycardia, postural hypotension, dyspepsia, edema, lethargy, and depression. It should never be given to a depressed patient or a patient with a history of depression. Recommended doses of guanethidine are 10 to 50 mg daily, and side effects are diarrhea, postural hypotension, and impotence. It can be used in patients with depression.

Prazosin is an α_1-adrenoceptor antagonist that has been shown to decrease the frequency, duration, or severity of vasospastic attacks in patients with Raynaud's phenomenon in placebo-controlled studies.[151,152] The favorable effects are moderate and occur in about two thirds of patients. However, improvement may dissipate with time.[151] Recommended doses are 2 to 8 mg daily. Side effects of nausea, headache, palpitations, dizziness, fatigue, edema, dyspnea, rash, and diarrhea often prevent its use. Phenoxybenzamine is a potent α-adrenoceptor blocking agent, which has been recommended for the treatment of Raynaud's phenomenon.[153,154] Placebo-controlled studies have not been performed. Usual dosage has been 10 to 30 mg four times a day. Side effects often preclude its use and include postural hypotension, nasal congestion, palpitations, impotence, and gastrointestinal symptoms. Methyldopa, which decreases peripheral sympathetic vasoconstriction by stimulation of central inhibitory α-adrenoceptors, has been used in patients with Raynaud's phenomenon. In an uncontrolled study[155] 75% of patients improved with 1 to 2 g daily, whereas no benefit was apparent at an average dose of 704.3 mg daily in a study[156] comparing it with other drugs. Side effects are edema, drowsiness, headache, postural hypotension, diarrhea, nasal congestion, and rarely fever and hemolytic anemia.

Tolazoline is an α-adrenoceptor antagonist with a histamine-like effect, which increases skin blood flow. It has been recommended for the treatment of Raynaud's phenomenon in doses of 25 to 100 mg daily. Placebo-controlled studies have not been performed. The oral preparation of tolazoline is no longer available in the United States.

Nitroglycerin is a direct-acting vasodilator, which has been used as an ointment in the treatment of Raynaud's disease for many years. Nitroglycerin ointment, compared with lanolin placebo, improved patients in one study of patients with secondary Raynaud's phenomenon, who were on maximally tolerated doses of sympatholytic agents.[157] Reports of the use of transdermal nitropaste plasters in Raynaud's phenomenon have indicated variable results.[158,159] Headache often precludes the use of nitroglycerin preparations, and postural hypotension and paresthesias may also occur.

Prostaglandins, which induce vasodilation and inhibit platelet aggregation are being used in severe Raynaud's phenomenon, but must be given intravenously. A multicenter study of prostaglandin E_1 (PGE_1) found no benefit over placebo[160] in patients with primary or secondary Raynaud's. Studies of prostacyclin (PGI) and its analog are more promising with long-term beneficial effects after the infusions are stopped.[161,162] Hypotension, headache, facial flushing, abdominal colic, nausea, vomiting, and diarrhea may occur during the infusions.

Ketanserin is a selective 5-HT_2 antagonist and has some $α_1$-adrenoceptor blocking activity. It inhibits the vasoconstriction and platelet aggregation caused by serotonin. In several placebo-controlled studies, ketanserin in a daily dose of 80 to 120 mg orally has been reported to improve or have no benefit in patients with Raynaud's phenomenon.[163-165] In the largest multicenter study performed in patients with Raynaud's phenomenon, ketanserin significantly decreased the frequency of, but not the duration or severity of, vasospastic attacks.[166] Patients and their physicians rated the drug better than placebo.

Side effects of ketanserin are dizziness, sedation, edema, dry mouth, and anxiety. It also may prolong the QT interval.

Captopril inhibits the enzyme converting angiotensin I to angiotensin II and kinase II, allowing bradykinin to accumulate. It has been reported to improve patients with primary or secondary Raynaud's phenomenon in uncontrolled studies.[167-169] It is effective treatment for the hypertension occurring in some patients with scleroderma but needs to be studied with suitable controls in the treatment of Raynaud's phenomenon.

Other vasodilator drugs, including niacin derivatives, papaverine, cyclandelate, griseofulvin, and isoxsuprine, have not been shown to be of benefit in Raynaud's phenomenon.

Thyroid preparations have been recommended for the treatment of Raynaud's phenomenon. In a study of 18 patients with secondary Raynaud's phenomenon, 60 to 80 μg of triiodothyronine sodium daily decreased the frequency, duration, and severity of vasospastic attacks compared with placebo.[170] However, there was a high incidence of palpitations, and significant increases in pulse rate and pulse pressure.

Plasmapheresis

Plasma exchange has been reported as beneficial in patients with severe Raynaud's phenomenon.[171] In one study[172] it was superior to placebo tablets or intermittent intravenous heparin therapy. Plasma exchange has not been studied adequately by other groups.

Conditioning and Biofeedback

Pavlovian conditioning has been used to treat patients with Raynaud's phenomenon.[173] Patients immerse their hands in 43° C water while their bodies are exposed to 0° C temperature for about 30 minutes a day. Patients with Raynaud's phenomenon, compared with normal subjects, showed a significant increase in finger temperature during cold exposure. Patients also reported subjective benefit, which sometimes lasted 9 to 12 months.

Many forms of biofeedback have been used to treat patients with Raynaud's phenomenon,[174-176] and patients generally show improvement. The type of behavioral therapy does not seem to make a difference, although finger temperature feedback has been most successful in some studies. Pavlovian conditioning or biofeedback may benefit some patients and have no side effects. They are therefore worth a trial if the patient is willing to spend the time involved.

Sympathectomy

Sympathectomy of the upper extremities may benefit 50% to 60% of patients with Raynaud's phenomenon.[177-180] However, vasospastic attacks often recur within 6 months to 2 years.[181,182] More success has been reported with digital sympathectomy in small numbers of patients with severe disease.[183,184] Improvement in pain and healing of ulcers has occurred. Lumbar sympathectomy for Raynaud's phenomenon in the toes is successful in over 80% of patients and the results persist longer.[177,185] In the upper extremities, sympathetic vasoconstrictor activity often returns after sympathectomy. This has been attributed to incomplete denervation, reinnervation, or denervation hypersensitivity. The evidence is strong that sympathetic activity returns, but the mechanism is unknown.

SUMMARY

Most patients with Raynaud's phenomenon, especially the primary disease, will respond to conservative measures and reassurance. Conditioning or biofeedback may be helpful for some patients but is time-consuming. When drug therapy is necessary, nifedipine yields the most beneficial effects if the side effects can be tolerated. Guanethidine, reserpine, prazosin, diltiazem, and dibenzyline may give some relief. Ketanserin and prostacyclin are promising therapeutic agents. The benefits of plasmapheresis need more documentation. Sympathectomy is not indicated in Raynaud's phenomenon.

ACROCYANOSIS

Patients whose hands and feet became blue on exposure to cold were described by Crocq[186] in 1896. Patients with acrocyanosis have persistent cyanosis and coldness of the digits (Fig. 23-4), hands, and feet, and sometimes the distal arms, face, and ears are involved. The blueness intensifies with cold and is relieved by warming.[187,188] Trophic changes such as ulceration, severe pain, or contractures do not occur. In some patients edema and excess sweating of the hands and feet may occur.[187] Idiopathic acrocyanosis is a benign condition that is mainly a cosmetic problem to patients. Secondary acrocyanosis may occur in association with connective tissue diseases or any disease complicated by central cyanosis.

The cause of idiopathic acrocyanosis is unknown. Only one study[187] reported pathologic findings of skin biopsies. Findings were nonspecific with thickening of the medial layers of the arterioles. Nail fold capillary studies have shown dilated capillary loops, a decreased number of capillaries, and an inhomogeneous capillary flow.[189,190] The pathophysiology evidently involves arteriolar spasm, but the reason is not known. Elevation of the cyanotic hand above heart level produces pallor, ruling against venous obstruction.[191] With body heating the temperature of the fingers becomes normal and reactive hyperemia of the fingers is normal, ruling against structural arterial disease. Also, ulnar nerve blockade relieves cyanosis in the fifth finger. Since the color of the digit did not change until the temperature of the digit rose 7° C, the digital arteries probably opened before the arterioles. Patients have normal hand blood flows during local warming to 42° C but low blood flow at 32° C.[188,192] In one child the cyanotic limbs became warm and red during sleep. This was considered evidence for an abnormal vascular response originating in the central nervous system and against a local hypersensitivity of digital blood vessels to cold.[193]

The incidence of acrocyanosis is unknown, and there is no sex predominance. The age range in one study was 20 to 45 years.[187] Physical examination and laboratory studies are normal.

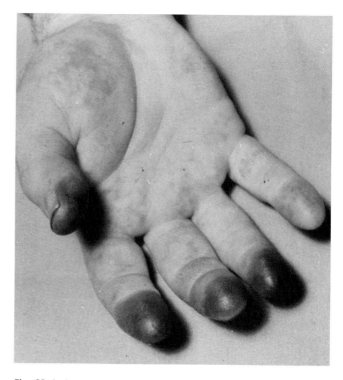

Fig. 23-4. Acrocyanosis in a young man who has had this condition since birth.

The differential diagnosis of acrocyanosis is Raynaud's phenomenon, connective tissue diseases, and central cyanosis. In Raynaud's phenomenon the vasospastic attacks are episodic, the color changes are only in the fingers and are well-demarcated, and females are predominantly affected. History, physical examination, and laboratory tests will rule out the connective tissue diseases. If central cyanosis is suspected, it can be confirmed by an arterial oxygen saturation measurement.

Treatment is usually unnecessary since this is a benign disease. For the few patients who request therapy, small doses of reserpine or guanethidine may relieve some of the manifestations.

LIVEDO RETICULARIS

There are at least three types of livedo reticularis. The benign form is a mottled discoloration of the extremities and sometimes the trunk of the body in a reticular or lacelike pattern. It is intensified by cold exposure and relieved by warming. Besides livedo reticularis this form has also been called cutis marmorata, livedo racemosa, livedo annularis, sympathetic or idiopathic livedo reticularis, and asphyxia reticularis. Livedo reticularis with ulceration (livedo vasculitis, livedoid vasculitis, atrophie blanche en plaque) is either a vasculitis or vascular thrombosis causing the same skin pattern but is usually irreversible with warming. Secondary livedo reticularis occurs in connective tissue diseases (Fig. 23-5) and with the use of amantadine hydrochloride.

Pathologic findings in the benign form are nonspecific, although increased numbers of dilated capillaries may be

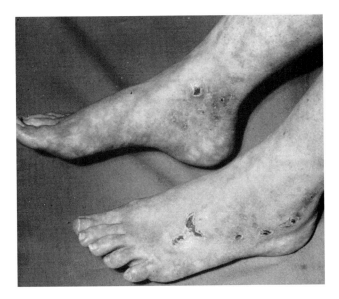

Fig. 23-5. Reticular mottling of the skin and ulcerations of the feet in a patient with livedo reticularis secondary to systemic lupus erythematosus.

present.[194,195] In livedo reticularis with ulceration, a segmental hyalinizing vasculitis affects the middle dermal vessels.[194-196] Infarcts of the skin are caused by obstructed arterioles. Some investigators believe that thrombosis of arterioles resulting from blood or tissue abnormalities causes the disease rather than vasculitis, since a defect in the fibrinolytic system and abnormalities of platelet aggregation may be present.[197-200]

The reticular pattern on the skin is considered to be secondary to vasospasm or obstruction of small perpendicular arterioles in the dermis.[201] The red to blue periphery of each reticulum is caused by deoxygenated blood in the surrounding horizontally arranged venous plexuses.[202] Increased sympathetic nervous system activity is considered to cause the benign form because it is reversible by warming and use of sympathetic blocking agents. Arteriolar obstruction caused by vasculitis or thrombosis may cause livedo reticularis with ulceration. Amantadine releases norepinephrine from nerves and enhances the action of norepinephrine and dopamine on peripheral vessels, which could cause arteriolar vasoconstriction.[203]

Benign livedo reticularis is common in women during their second to fifth decades. Livedo reticularis with ulceration is rare and also more common in women but in their third to fifth decades.[204]

Except for the rose, red, violet, or blue color of the lacelike reticular pattern and coldness of the extremities and sometimes the trunk, physical examination in benign livedo reticularis is normal. In livedo reticularis with ulceration, besides the reticular pattern, purpuric macular lesions and cutaneous nodules develop and progress to ulcers. These ulcers usually occur in the winter but some patients develop them in the summer.[196] Edema occurs in about half the patients often before ulcers appear. The ulcers are very painful and take months to heal. Most ulcers occur on the calves, ankles, and feet. Healed ulcers leave a smooth ivory-white plaque of atrophic skin surrounded by

hyperpigmented borders with telangiectatic blood vessels, which led to the name "atrophie blanche."

Secondary livedo reticularis occurs with diseases that cause decreased blood flow to the skin—for instance, connective tissue diseases, polyarteritis nodosa, hyperviscosity states, cryoglobulinemia, thrombocythemia, atheromatous emboli, obstructive arterial diseases, endocrine disorders, infections, and neurogenic diseases. Sneddon's syndrome is characterized by livedo reticularis with cerebrovascular lesions causing transient ischemic attacks or strokes.[205] Also groups of patients have been described with lupus erythematosus, arterial or venous thromboses, spontaneous abortions, livedo reticularis, and anticardiolipin antibodies.[206] Anticardiolipin antibodies may be the cause of these syndromes and precede other clinical and laboratory manifestations of lupus erythematosus by several years.[207]

Amantadine hydrochloride causes a benign form of livedo reticularis and is not a reason for stopping the medication.[208,209] It usually affects the legs of both sexes, and pedal edema may occur. It disappears 2 to 6 weeks after the drug is stopped.

There are no consistently abnormal laboratory tests in benign livedo reticularis or livedo reticularis with ulceration. The prognosis of the benign disease is excellent since it is only a cosmetic problem. Recurrent, painful ulcerations may occur for years in patients with livedo reticularis with ulceration.[210] Amputations have been rarely done for deep, nonhealing ulcers or severe pain.[194,210]

No treatment is necessary in benign livedo reticularis. Treatment for livedo reticularis from underlying diseases is that of the associated disease. Many therapies have been recommended for patients with livedo reticularis with ulceration attesting to the fact that treatment is usually unsuccessful. Antiplatelet therapy with aspirin, dipyridamole, or ticlopidine has benefited some patients[198,199] as has nicotinic acid.[200] Some patients do not respond to any therapy, and remissions often occur without treatment so that it is difficult to evaluate the uncontrolled studies. Controlled trials have not been performed because of the rarity of the disease.

REFERENCES

1. Raynaud M: On local asphyxia and symmetrical gangrene of the extremities, London, 1888, The Syndenham Society (translated by T. Barlow).
2. Hines EA Jr and Christensen NA: Raynaud's disease affecting men, JAMA 129:1, 1945.
3. Blain A, Coller FA, and Carver GB: Raynaud's disease: a study of criteria for prognosis, Surgery 29:387, 1951.
4. Gifford RW Jr and Hines EA Jr: Raynaud's disease among women and girls, Circulation 16:1012, 1957.
5. Riera G et al: Prevalence of Raynaud's phenomenon in a healthy Spanish population, J Rheumatol 20:66, 1993.
6. Olsen N and Nielsen SL: Prevalence of primary Raynaud phenomena in young females, Scand J Clin Lab Invest 37:761, 1978.
7. Heslop J, Coggon D, and Acheson ED: The prevalence of intermittent digital ischaemia (Raynaud's phenomenon) in a general practice, J R Coll Gen Pract 33:85, 1983.
8. Maricq HR et al: Geographic variation in the prevalence of Raynaud's phenomenon: Charleston, SC, USA, vs Tarentaise, Savoie, France, J Rheumatol 20:70, 1993.

9. Lewis T: The pathological changes in the arteries supplying the fingers in warm-handed people and in cases of so-called Raynaud's disease, Clin Sci 3:288, 1938.

10. Burch GE, Harb JM, and Sun CS: Fine structure of digital vascular lesions in Raynaud's phenomenon and disease, Angiology 30:361, 1979.

11. Vajda K et al: Ultrastructural investigations of finger pulp biopsies: a study of 31 patients with Raynaud's syndrome, Ultrastruct Pathol 3:175, 1982.

12. Jeune R and Thivolet J: Ètude arteriographique de la main au cours de 52 phenomenes de Raynaud d'etiologie diverse, Nouv Presse Med 7:2619, 1978.

13. Porter JM et al: The clinical significance of Raynaud's phenomenon, Surgery 80:756, 1976.

14. Laws JW, Lillie JG, and Scott JT: Arteriographic appearances in rheumatoid arthritis and other disorders, Br J Radiol 36:477, 1963.

15. Stevens MJ and Moulds RFW: Heterogeneity of post-junctional α-adrenoceptors in human vascular smooth muscle, Arch Int Pharmacodyn Ther 254:43, 1981.

16. Arneklo-Nobin B and Owman C: Adrenergic and serotonergic mechanisms in human hand arteries and veins studied by fluorescence histochemistry and in vitro pharmacology, Blood Vessels 22:1, 1985.

17. Coffman JD and Cohen RA: Role of alpha-adrenoceptor subtypes mediating sympathetic vasoconstriction in human digits, Eur J Clin Invest 18:309, 1988.

18. Coffman JD: Total and nutritional blood flow in the finger, Clin Sci 42:243, 1972.

19. Coffman JD and Cohen RA: Serotonergic vasoconstriction in human fingers during reflex sympathetic response to cooling, Am J Physiol 254:H889, 1988.

20. Coffman JD and Cohen AS: Total and capillary blood flow in Raynaud's phenomenon, N Engl J Med 285:259, 1971.

21. Peacock JH: A comparative study of the digital cutaneous temperatures and hand blood flows in the normal hand, primary Raynaud's disease, and primary acrocyanosis, Clin Sci 18:25, 1959.

22. Peacock JH: Vasodilatation in the human hand: observations on primary Raynaud's disease and acrocyanosis of the upper extremities, Clin Sci 17:575, 1957.

23. Lewis T: Experiments relating to the peripheral mechanism involved in spasmodic arrest of the circulation in the fingers, a variety of Raynaud's disease, Heart 15:7, 1929.

24. Jamieson GG, Ludbrook J, and Wilson A: Cold hypersensitivity in Raynaud's phenomenon, Circulation 44:254, 1971.

25. Edward JM et al: α_2-Adrenergic receptor levels in obstructive and spastic Raynaud's syndrome, J Vasc Surg 5:38, 1987.

26. Coffman JD and Cohen RA: α_2-Adrenergic and 5-HT$_2$ receptor hypersensitivity in Raynaud's phenomenon, J Vasc Med Biol 2:100, 1990.

27. Freedman RR et al: Cold-induced potentiation of α_2-adrenergic vasoconstriction in primary Raynaud's disease, Arthritis Rheum 36:685, 1993.

28. Nielsen SL: Raynaud phenomenon and finger systolic pressure during cooling, Scand J Clin Lab Invest 38:765, 1978.

29. Olsen N, Petring OU, and Rossing N: Exaggerated postural vasoconstrictor reflex in Raynaud's phenomenon, Br Med J 294:1186, 1987.

30. Fagius J and Blumberg H: Sympathetic outflow to the hand in patients with Raynaud's phenomenon, Cardiovasc Res 19:249, 1985.

31. Downey JA and Frewin DB: The effect of cold on blood flow in the hands of patients with Raynaud's phenomenon, Clin Sci 44:279, 1973.

32. Kontos HA and Wasserman AJ: Effect of reserpine in Raynaud's phenomenon, Circulation 39:259, 1969.

33. Nielsen SL et al: Raynaud's phenomenon: peripheral catecholamine concentration and effect of sympathectomy, Acta Chir Scand 502:57, 1980.

34. Cohen RA and Coffman JD: Reduced fingertip arterial pressures in Raynaud's disease, J Vasc Med Biol 1:21, 1989.

35. Pringle R, Walder DM, and Weaver JPA: Blood viscosity and Raynaud's disease, Lancet 1:1086, 1965.

36. Goyle KB and Dormandy JA: Abnormal blood viscosity in Raynaud's phenomenon, Lancet 1:1317, 1976.

37. McGrath MA, Peck R, and Penny R: Raynaud's disease: reduced hand blood flows with normal blood viscosity, Aust N Z J Med 8:126, 1978.

38. Ayres ML, Jarrett PEM, and Browse NL: Blood viscosity, Raynaud's phenomenon and the effect of fibrinolytic enhancement, Br J Surg 68:51, 1981.

39. Halpern A et al: Raynaud's disease, Raynaud's phenomenon, and serotonin, Angiology 11:151, 1960.

40. Seibold JR and Terregino CA: Selective antagonism of S$_2$-serotonergic receptors relieves but does not prevent cold-induced vasoconstriction in primary Raynaud's phenomenon, J Rheumatol 13:337, 1986.

41. Kanno K et al: Endothelin and Raynaud's phenomenon, Am J Med 90:130, 1991.

42. Biondi ML et al: Increased plasma endothelin levels in patients with Raynaud's phenomenon, N Engl J Med 324:1139, 1991.

43. Smith P et al: Endothelin-1 in patients with Raynaud's phenomenon, Lancet 337:236, 1991.

44. Miller D et al: Is variant angina the coronary manifestation of a generalized vasospastic disorder? N Engl J Med 304:763, 1981.

45. O'Keefe ST, Tsapatsaris NP, and Beetham WP Jr: Increased prevalence of migraine and chest pain in patients with primary Raynaud's disease, Ann Intern Med 116:985, 1992.

46. Vergnon J-M et al: Raynaud's phenomenon of the lung, Chest 101:1312, 1992.

47. Cannon PJ et al: The relationship of hypertension and renal failure in scleroderma (progressive systemic sclerosis) to structural and functional abnormalities of the renal cortical circulation, Medicine 53:1, 1974.

48. Salmerson BD et al: Macular capillary hemodynamic changes associated with Raynaud's phenomenon, Ophthalmology 99:914, 1992.

49. Coffman JD and Cohen RA: Vasospasm: ubiquitous? N Engl J Med 304:780, 1981.

50. Allen EV and Brown GE: Raynaud's disease: a critical review of minimal requisites for diagnosis, Am J Med Sci 183:187, 1932.

51. Carter SA, Dean E, and Kroeger EA: Apparent finger systolic pressures during cooling in patients with Raynaud's syndrome, Circulation 77:988, 1988.

52. Maricq HR et al: Diagnostic potential of in vivo capillary microscopy in scleroderma and related disorders, Arthritis Rheum 23:183, 1980.

53. Kallenberg CGM et al: Antinuclear antibodies in patients with Raynaud's phenomenon: clinical significance of anti-centromere antibodies, Ann Rheum Dis 41:382, 1982.

54. Wollersheim H et al: The diagnostic value of several immunological tests for anti-nuclear disease in patients presenting with Raynaud's phenomenon, Eur J Clin Invest 19:535, 1989.

55. Coffman JD: Evaluation of the patient with Raynaud's phenomenon, Postgrad Med 78:175, 1985.

56. Farmer RG, Gifford RW Jr, and Hines EA Jr: Raynaud's disease with sclerodactylia, Circulation 23:13, 1961.

57. Gerbracht DD et al: Evolution of primary Raynaud's phenomenon (Raynaud's disease) to connective tissue disease, Arthritis Rheum 28:87, 1985.

58. Wollersheim H et al: Influence of cold challenge on finger skin temperature during long-term use of beta-adrenoceptor blocking drugs in hypertensive patients, Int Angiol 6:307, 1987.

59. Marshall AJ, Roberts CJC, and Barritt DW: Raynaud's phenomenon as side effect of beta-blockers in hypertension, Br Med J 1:1498, 1976.

60. Feleke E et al: Complaints of cold extremities among patients on antihypertensive treatment, Acta Med Scand 213:381, 1983.

61. VandenBurg MJ et al: Is the feeling of cold extremities experienced by hypertensive patients due to their disease or their treatment? Eur J Clin Pharmacol 27:47, 1984.

62. Steiner JA et al: Vascular symptoms in patients with primary Raynaud's phenomenon are not exacerbated by propranolol or labetalol, Br J Clin Pharmacol 7:401, 1979.

63. Coffman JD and Rasmussen HM: Effects of β-adrenoceptor blocking drugs in patients with Raynaud's phenomenon, Circulation 72:466, 1985.

64. Cameron EA and French EB: St. Anthony's fire rekindled: gangrene due to therapeutic dose of ergotamine, Br Med J 2:28, 1960.

65. Greene FL, Ariyan S, and Stansel HC Jr: Mesenteric and peripheral vascular ischemia secondary to ergotism, Surgery 81:176, 1977.

66. Bagby RJ and Cooper RD: Angiography in ergotism, Am J Roent 116:179, 1972.

67. Carliner NH et al: Sodium nitroprusside treatment of ergotamine-induced peripheral ischemia, JAMA 227:308, 1974.

68. Dagher FJ et al: Severe unilateral ischemia of the lower extremity caused by ergotamine: treatment with nifedipine, Surgery 97:369, 1985.

69. Graham JR: Methysergide for prevention of headache, N Engl J Med 270:67, 1964.

70. Vogelzang NJ et al: Raynaud's phenomenon: a common toxicity after combination chemotherapy for testicular cancer, Ann Intern Med 95:288, 1981.

71. Teutsch C, Lipton A, and Harvey HA: Raynaud's phenomenon as a side effect of chemotherapy with vinblastine and bleomycin for testicular carcinoma, Cancer Treat Rep 61:925, 1977.

72. Birnstingl M: The Raynaud syndrome, Postgrad Med J 47:297, 1971.

73. Tuffanelli DL and Winkelmann RK: Systemic scleroderma: a clinical study of 727 cases, Arch Dermatol 84:359, 1961.

74. Fritzler MJ and Kinsella TD: The CREST syndrome: a distinct serologic entity with anticentromere antibodies, Am J Med 69:520, 1980.

75. Tuffanelli DL and Dubois EL: Cutaneous manifestations of systemic lupus erythematosus, Arch Dermatol 90:377, 1964.

76. Hochberg MC et al: Systemic lupus erythematosus: a review of clinico-laboratory features and immunogenetic markers in 150 patients with emphasis on demographic subsets, Medicine 64:285, 1985.

77. Scott JT et al: Digital arteries in rheumatoid disease, Ann Rheum Dis 20:224, 1961.

78. Laws JW, Lillie JG, and Scott JT: Arteriographic appearance in rheumatoid arthritis and other disorders, Br J Radiol 36:477, 1963.

79. Fox RI et al: Primary Sjögren syndrome: clinical and immunopathologic features, Semin Arthritis Rheum 14:77, 1984.

80. Boyland RC and Sokoloff L: Vascular lesions in dermatomyositis, Arthritis Rheum 3:379, 1960.

81. Sharp GC: Mixed connective tissue disease, Bull Rheum Dis 25:828, 1975.

82. Futatsuka M et al: Comparative study of vibration disease among operators of vibratory tools by factor analysis, Br J Ind Med 42:260, 1985.

83. Theriault G et al: Raynaud's phenomenon in forestry workers in Quebec, Can Med Assoc J 126:1404, 1982.

84. Hellstrom B and Andersen KL: Vibration injuries in Norwegian forest workers, Br J Ind Med 29:255, 1972.

85. Futatsuka M and Ueno T: Vibration exposure and vibration-induced white finger due to chain saw operation, J Occup Med 27:257, 1985.

86. Gurdjian ES and Walker LW: Traumatic vasospastic disease of the hand (white fingers), JAMA 129:668, 1945.

87. Ashe WF, Cook WT, and Old JW: Raynaud's phenomenon of occupational origin, Arch Environ Health 5:333, 1962.

88. Miyashita K et al: Epidemiological study of vibration syndrome in response to total handtool operating time, Br J Ind Med 40:92, 1983.

89. Ekenvall L and Carlson A: Vibration white finger: a follow up study, Br J Ind Med 44:476, 1987.

90. Matoba T, Ogata M, and Kuwahara H: Diltiazem and Raynaud's syndrome, Ann Intern Med 97:445, 1982.

91. Little JM and Ferguson DA: The incidence of the hypothenar hammer syndrome, Arch Surg 105:684, 1972.

92. Vayssairat M et al: Hypothenar hammer syndrome: seventeen cases with long-term follow-up, J Vasc Surg 5:538, 1987.

93. Millender LH, Nalebuff EA, and Kasdon E: Aneurysms and thromboses of the ulnar artery in the hand, Arch Surg 105:686, 1972.

94. Conn J Jr, Bergan JJ, and Bell JL: Hypothenar hammer syndrome: post-traumatic digital ischemia, Surgery 68:1122, 1970.

95. Pineda CJ et al: Hypothenar hammer syndrome. Form of reversible Raynaud's phenomenon, Am J Med 79:561, 1985.

96. Serra G, Migliore A, and Tugnoli V: Raynaud's phenomenon and entrapment neuropathies, Ann Neurol 18:519, 1985.

97. Stevens JC: The electrodiagnosis of carpal tunnel syndrome, Muscle Nerve 10:99, 1987.

98. Heller L et al: Evaluation of Tinel's and Phalen's signs in diagnosis of the carpal tunnel syndrome, Eur Neurol 25:40, 1986.

99. Taylor N: Carpal tunnel syndrome, Am J Phys Med 50:192, 1971.

100. Gelberman RH, Aronson D, and Weisman MH: Carpal-tunnel syndrome, J Bone Joint Surg 62A:1181, 1980.

101. Ellis JM et al: Survey and new data on treatment with pyridoxine of patients having a clinical syndrome including the carpal tunnel and other defects, Res Commun Chem Pathol Pharmacol 17:165, 1977.

102. Layton KB: Acroparaesthesia in pregnancy and the carpal tunnel syndrome, J Obstet Gynaec 65:823, 1958.

103. Beyer JA and Wright IS: The hyperabduction syndrome: with special reference to its relationship to Raynaud's syndrome, Circulation 4:161, 1951.

104. McGough EC, Pearce MB, and Byrne JP: Management of thoracic outlet syndrome, J Thorac Cardiovasc Surg 77:169, 1979.

105. Banis JC Jr, Rich N, and Whelan TJ Jr: Ischemia of the upper extremity due to noncardiac emboli, Am J Surg 134:131, 1977.

106. Adson AW and Coffey JR: Cervical rib: a method of anterior approach for relief of symptoms by division of the scalenus anticus, Ann Surg 85:839, 1927.

107. Brown GE and Griffin HZ: Peripheral arterial disease in polycythemia vera, Arch Intern Med 46:705, 1930.

108. Imhof JW, Boars H, and Verloop MC: Clinical haematologic aspects of macroglobulinaemia Waldenström, Acta Med Scand 163:349, 1959.

109. Invernizzi F et al: Secondary and essential cryoglobulinemias, Acta Haematol 70:73, 1983.

110. Ritzmann SE and Levin WC: Cryopathies: a review, Arch Intern Med 107:186, 1961.

111. McGrath MA and Penny R: Blood hyperviscosity in cryoglobulinemia: temperature sensitivity and correlation with reduced skin blood flow, Aust J Exp Biol Med Sci 56:127, 1978.

112. Ristow SC et al: Reversal of systemic manifestations of cryoglobulinemia, Arch Intern Med 136:467, 1976.

113. McLeod BC and Sassetti RJ: Plasmapheresis with return of cryoglobulin-depleted autologous plasma (cryoglobulinpheresis) in cryoglobulinemia, Blood 55:866, 1980.

114. Olesen H: The cold agglutinin syndrome, Dan Med Bull 14:138, 1967.

115. Marshall RJ, Shepherd JT, and Thompson ID: Vascular responses in patients with high serum titres of cold agglutinins, Clin Sci 12:255, 1953.

116. Markowitz SS et al: Occupational acroosteolysis, Arch Dermatol 106:219, 1972.

117. Ward AM et al: Immunological mechanisms in the pathogenesis of vinyl chloride disease, Br Med J 1:936, 1976.

118. Maricq HR et al: Capillary abnormalities in polyvinyl chloride production workers, JAMA 236:1368, 1976.

119. Falappa P et al: Angiographic study of digital arteries in workers exposed to vinyl chloride, Br J Ind Med 39:169, 1982.

120. Hines EA Jr and Barker NW: Arteriosclerosis obliterans: a clinical and pathologic study, Am J Med Sci 200:717, 1940.

121. Goodman RM et al: Buerger's disease in Israel, Am J Med 39:601, 1965.

122. Gocke DJ et al: Association between polyarteritis and Australian antigen, Lancet 2:1149, 1970.

123. Kim WK and Koff RS: Coexistence of Raynaud's phenomenon and chronic active hepatitis and hepatitis B antigen, Digestion 11:152, 1974.

124. Cosgriff TM and Arnold WJ: Digital vasospasm and infarction associated with hepatitis B antigenemia, JAMA 235:1362, 1976.

125. Lappchen J et al: Raynaud-Phanomen bei dialysepatienten, Dtsch Med Wochenschr 102:521, 1977.

126. Nielsen SL and Lokkegaard H: Cold sensitivity and finger systolic blood pressure in hemodialysis patients, Scand J Urol Nephrol 15:319, 1981.

127. Gipstein RM et al: Calciphylaxis in man, Arch Intern Med 136:1273, 1976.

128. Shagan BP and Friedman SA: Raynaud's phenomenon in hypothyroidism, Angiology 27:19, 1976.

129. Nielsen SL, Parving H-H, and Hansen JEM: Myxoedema and Raynaud's phenomenon, Acta Endocrinol 101:32, 1982.

130. Andrasch RH et al: Digital ischemia and gangrene preceding renal neoplasm, Arch Intern Med 136:486, 1976.

131. Wytock DH, Bartholomew LG, and Sheps SG: Digital ischemia associated with small bowel malignancy, Gastroenterology 84:1025, 1983.

132. Celoria GC, Friedell GH, and Sommers SC: Raynaud's disease and primary pulmonary hypertension, Circulation 22:1055, 1960.

133. Winters WL, Joseph RR, and Learner N: "Primary" pulmonary hypertension and Raynaud's phenomenon, Arch Intern Med 114:821, 1964.

134. Walcott G, Burchell HB, and Brown AL: Primary pulmonary hypertension, Am J Med 49:70, 1970.

135. Fuster V et al: Primary pulmonary hypertension: natural history and the importance of thrombosis, Circulation 70:580, 1984.

136. Murray-Lyon IM et al: Scleroderma and primary biliary cirrhosis, Br Med J 3:258, 1970.

137. Sherlock S and Scheuer PJ: The presentation and diagnosis of 100 patients with primary biliary cirrhosis, N Engl J Med 289:674, 1973.

138. Smith CD and McKendry RVR: Controlled trial of nifedipine in the treatment of Raynaud's phenomenon, Lancet 2:1299, 1982.

139. Rodeheffer RJ et al: Controlled double-blind trial of nifedipine in the treatment of Raynaud's phenomenon, N Engl J Med 308:880, 1983.

140. Rhedda A et al: A double blind placebo controlled crossover randomized trial of diltiazem in Raynaud's phenomenon, J Rheumatol 12:724, 1985.

141. Kahan A, Amor B, and Menkes CJ: A randomized double blind trial of diltiazem in the treatment of Raynaud's phenomenon, Ann Rheum Dis 44:30, 1985.

142. Da Costa JT et al: Inefficacy of diltiazem in the treatment of Raynaud's phenomenon with associated connective tissue disease: a double blind placebo controlled study, J Rheumatol 14:858, 1987.

143. Kinney EL et al: The treatment of severe Raynaud's phenomenon with verapamil, J Clin Pharmacol 22:74, 1982.

144. Kallenberg CCM et al: Once daily felodipine in patients with primary Raynaud's phenomenon, Eur J Clin Pharmacol 40:313, 1991.

145. Schmidt JF, Valentin N, and Nielsen SL: The clinical effects of felodipine and nifedipine in Raynaud's phenomenon, Eur J Clin Pharmacol 37:191, 1989.

146. Leppert J et al: The effect of israpidine, a new calcium-channel antagonist in patients with primary Raynaud's phenomenon: a single-blind dose-response study, Cardiovasc Drugs Ther 3:397, 1989.

147. Coffman JD and Cohen AS: Total and capillary fingertip blood flow in Raynaud's phenomenon, N Engl J Med 285:259, 1971.

148. LeRoy EC, Downey JA, and Cannon PJ: Skin capillary blood flow in scleroderma, J Clin Invest 50:930, 1971.

149. Kontos HA and Wasserman AJ: Effect of reserpine in Raynaud's phenomenon, Circulation 34:259, 1969.

150. McFadyen IJ, Housley E, and MacPherson AIS: Intra-arterial reserpine administration in Raynaud's syndrome, Arch Intern Med 132:526, 1973.

151. Nielsen SL, Vithing K, and Rasmussen K: Prazosin treatment of primary Raynaud's phenomenon, Eur J Clin Pharmacol 24:421, 1983.

152. Wollersheim H et al: Double-blind, placebo-controlled study of prazosin in Raynaud's phenomenon, Clin Pharmacol Ther 40:219, 1986.

153. Moser M et al: Clinical experience with sympathetic blocking agents in peripheral vascular disease, Ann Intern Med 38:1245, 1953.

154. Hillestad LK: Dibenzyline in vascular disease of the hands, Angiology 13:169, 1962.

155. Varadi DP and Lawrence AM: Suppression of Raynaud's phenomenon by methyldopa, Ann Intern Med 124:13, 1969.

156. Strozzi G et al: Management of Raynaud's phenomenon with drugs affecting the sympathetic nervous system, Curr Therap Res 32:225, 1982.

157. Franks AG Jr: Topical glyceryl trinitrate as adjunctive treatment in Raynaud's disease, Lancet 1:76, 1982.

158. Nahir AM, Schapira D, and Scharf Y: Double-blind randomized trial of Nitroderm TTS in the treatment of Raynaud's phenomenon, Isr J Med Sci 22:139, 1986.

159. Sovijarvi ARA, Siitonen L, and Anderson P: Transdermal nitroglycerin in the treatment of Raynaud's phenomenon: analysis of digital blood pressure changes after cold provocation, Curr Therap Res 35:832, 1984.

160. Mohrland JS et al: A multicenter placebo-controlled, double-blind study of prostaglandin E₁ in Raynaud's syndrome, Ann Rheum Dis 44:754, 1985.

161. Wigley FM et al: Intravenous iloprost infusion in patients with Raynaud's phenomenon secondary to systemic sclerosis, Ann Int Med 120:199, 1994.

162. Rademaker M et al: Comparison of intravenous infusions of iloprost and oral nifedipine in treatment of Raynaud's phenomenon in patients with systemic sclerosis: a double blind randomized study, Br J Med 298:561, 1989.

163. Roald OK and Seem E: Treatment of Raynaud's phenomenon with ketanserin in patients with connective tissue disorders, Br Med J 289:577, 1984.

164. van de Wal HJCM et al: Quantitative study of the effects of ketanserin in patients with primary Raynaud's phenomenon, Microcirc Endothelium Lymphatics 2:657, 1985.

165. Brouwer RML et al: Does serotonin receptor blockade have a therapeutic effect in Raynaud's phenomenon? Vasa (suppl 18):64, 1987.

166. Coffman JD et al: International study of ketanserin in Raynaud's phenomenon, Am J Med 87:264, 1989.

167. Lopez-Ovejero JA et al: Reversal of vascular and renal crisis of scleroderma by oral angiotensin-converting enzyme blockade, N Engl J Med 300:1417, 1979.

168. Tosi S et al: Treatment of Raynaud's phenomenon with captopril, Drugs Exp Clin Res 13:37, 1987.

169. Trubestein G et al: Behandling des Raynaud-Syndroms mit Captopril, Dtsch Med Wochenschr 109:857, 1984.

170. Dessein PH et al: Triiodothyronine treatment for Raynaud's phenomenon: a controlled trial, J Rheumatol 17:1025, 1990.

171. Talpos G et al: Plasmapheresis in Raynaud's disease, Lancet 1:416, 1978.

172. O'Reilly MJG et al: Controlled trial of plasma exchange in treatment of Raynaud's syndrome, Br Med J 1:1113, 1979.

173. Jobe JB et al: Induced vasodilation as treatment for Raynaud's disease, Ann Intern Med 97:706, 1982.

174. Surwit RS, Pilon RN, and Fenton CH: Behavioral treatment of Raynaud's disease, J Behav Med 1:323, 1978.

175. Keefe FJ, Surwit RS, and Pilon RN: Biofeedback, autogenic training and progressive relaxation in the treatment of Raynaud's disease, J Appl Behav Anal 13:3, 1980.

176. Freedman RR, Ianni P, and Wenig P: Behavioral treatment of Raynaud's disease, J Consult Clin Psych 51:539, 1983.

177. Gifford RW Jr, Hines EA Jr, and Craig WM: Sympathectomy for Raynaud's phenomenon, Circulation 17:5, 1958.

178. Tsur N et al: Upper thoracic sympathectomy, Isr J Med Sci 9:53, 1973.

179. Baddeley RM: The place of upper dorsal sympathectomy in the treatment of primary Raynaud's disease, Br J Surg 52:426, 1965.

180. Laroche GP et al: Chronic arterial insufficiency of the upper extremity, Mayo Clin Proc 51:180, 1976.

181. Felder DA et al: Evaluation of sympathetic neurectomy in Raynaud's disease, Surgery 26:1014, 1949.

182. Johnston ENM, Summerly R, and Birnstingl M: Prognosis in Raynaud's phenomenon after sympathectomy, Br Med J 1:962, 1965.

183. Eb-Gammal TA and Blair WF: Digital periarterial sympathectomy for ischemic digital pain and ulcers, J Hand Surg (Br) 16:382, 1991.

184. Drake DB, Kesler RW, and Morgan RF: Digital sympathectomy for refractory Raynaud's phenomenon in an adolescent, J Rheumatol 19:1286, 1992.

185. Janoff KA, Phinney ES, and Porter JM: Lumbar sympathectomy for lower extremity vasospasm, Am J Surg 150:147, 1985.

186. Crocq C: De l'acrocyanose, Semaine Med 16:297, 1896.

187. Stern ES: The aetiology and pathology of acrocyanosis, Br J Derm Syph 49:100, 1937.

188. Peacock JH: Vasodilatation in the human hand: observations on primary Raynaud's disease and acrocyanosis of the upper extremities, Clin Sci 17:575, 1957.

189. Jacobs MJHM et al: Nomenclature of Raynaud's phenomenon: a capillary microscopic and hemorrheologic study, Surgery 101:136, 1987.

190. Bollinger A, Mahler F, and Meier B: Velocity patterns in nailfold capillaries of normal subjects and patients with Raynaud's disease and acrocyanosis, Bibl Anat 16:142, 1977.

191. Lewis T and Landis EM: Observations upon the vascular mechanism in acrocyanosis, Heart 15:229, 1930.

192. Peacock JH: A comparative study of the digital cutaneous temperatures, and hand blood flows in the normal hand, primary Raynaud's disease and primary acrocyanosis, Clin Sci 18:25, 1959.

193. Day R and Klingman WO: The effect of sleep on the skin temperature reactions in a case of acrocyanosis, J Clin Invest 18:271, 1939.

194. Barker NW, Hines EA Jr, and Craig W: Livedo reticularis: a peripheral arteriolar disease, Am Heart J 21:592, 1941.

195. Pearce LA, Waterbury LD, and Green HD: Amantadine hydrochloride: alteration in peripheral circulation, Neurology 24:46, 1974.

196. Feldaker M, Hines EA Jr, and Kierland RR: Livedo reticularis with ulcerations, Circulation 13:196, 1956.

197. Cunliffe WJ and Menon IS: The association between cutaneous vasculitis and decreased blood fibrinolytic activity, Br J Dermatol 84:99, 1971.

198. Drucker CR and Duncan WC: Antiplatelet therapy in atrophie blanche and livedo vasculitis, J Am Acad Dermatol 7:359, 1982.

199. Yamamoto M et al: Antithrombic treatment in livedo vasculitis, J Am Acad Dermatol 18:57, 1988.

200. Milstone LM et al: Classification and therapy of atrophie blanche, Arch Dermatol 119:963, 1983.

201. Williams C and Goodman H: Livedo reticularis, JAMA 85:955, 1925.

202. Copeland PWM: Livedo reticularis, Br J Dermatol 93:519, 1975.

203. Heimans RLH, Rand MJ, and Fennessy MR: Some actions of amantadine on peripheral tissues, J Pharm Pharmacol 24:869, 1972.

204. Winkelmann RK et al: Clinical studies of livedoid vasculitis (segmental hyalinizing vasculitis), Mayo Clin Proc 49:746, 1974.

205. Sneddon IB: Cerebrovascular lesions and livedo reticularis, Br J Dermatol 77:180, 1965.

206. Hughes GRV: Autoantibodies in lupus and its variants: experience in 1000 patients, Br Med J 289:339, 1984.

207. Weinstein C et al: Livedo reticularis associated with increased titers of anticardiolipin antibodies in systemic lupus erythematosus, Arch Dermatol 123:596, 1987.

208. Shealy CN, Weeth JB, and Mercier D: Livedo reticularis in patients with Parkinsonism receiving amantadine, JAMA 212:1522, 1970.

209. Silver D and Sahs AL: Livedo reticularis in Parkinson's disease patients treated with amantadine hydrochloride, Neurology 22:645, 1972.

210. Cabbabe EB and Clift SD: Leg ulcerations in livedoid vasculitis, Plast Reconstr Surg 75:888, 1985.

CHAPTER TWENTY-FOUR

MISCELLANEOUS ARTERIAL DISEASES

Bruce H. Gray

Jess R. Young

Jeffrey W. Olin

Arteriosclerosis obliterans (ASO) causes arterial insufficiency through the accumulation of atheromatous plaque in the vessel lumen. Multiple other mechanisms can cause arterial insufficiency. In this chapter we discuss arterial entrapment, cystic degeneration of the arterial wall, fibromuscular arterial wall proliferation, and arterial calcification diseases. Disease conditions such as vasculitis, aneurysmal disease, systemic embolization, and thromboangiitis obliterans are discussed elsewhere.

POPLITEAL ARTERY ENTRAPMENT SYNDROME

Intermittent claudication is usually a warning symptom of arterial insufficiency, and when induced by compression of a peripheral vessel between musculoskeletal structures is referred to as an *entrapment syndrome*. This is more frequently seen in younger individuals, although it can occur in all age groups. Entrapment can occur at a number of sites including the axillary, brachial, celiac, common femoral, superficial femoral, and popliteal arteries. The most frequent and well-known site of entrapment is at the popliteal artery.

Historical Background
Popliteal artery entrapment was first described in 1879 by T.P. Anderson Stuart[1] in an amputated gangrenous limb. He described the abnormal path of the popliteal artery as it deviated medially around the medial head of the gastrocnemius muscle rather than coursing between the heads of the muscle. The involved muscle rose much higher on the femoral condyle than usual, allowing space for the artery to pass (Figs. 24-1 and 24-2).

In 1925 Chambardel-Dubreuil[3] described a situation in which the popliteal artery and vein were separated by an accessory slip of the gastrocnemius muscle (Fig. 24-4). It was not until 1959 that complications arising from this disease entity were successfully treated by Hamming[4] in a 12-year-old boy. Subsequent case reports then began to appear in the literature with greater frequency. Many of these had anatomic variants from the original type described by Stuart. In 1961 Hall[2] reported a case in which the site of attachment of the medial head of the gastrocnemius muscle was more lateral than usual, separating the artery medially (Fig. 24-3).

In 1964 Hall[5] described another variant, coined "intervascular gastrocnemius insertion," in which the artery courses through the body of the muscle. Later that same year the concept of bilateral occurrence of these congenital anomalies was recognized by Carter and Eban.[6] In 1965 Love and Whelan[7] labeled this disease popliteal artery entrapment syndrome (PAES). They noted that entrapment could be caused by an abnormal popliteal muscle/popliteal artery relationship (Fig. 24-5). By 1967 the first case of entrapment of both the popliteal artery and vein was described by Rich and Hughes.[8] Since then at least 18 anatomic variants have been described.[9] Furthermore, cases with an isolated popliteal vein or popliteal nerve entrapment have also been reported.[10,11]

Pathogenesis
Popliteal artery entrapment has generally been regarded as a congenital aberration. Most frequently the medial head of the gastrocnemius muscle has been the compressing structure (approximately 74%), although the involvement of a concomitant compressive popliteal muscle or band may be underestimated.[12,13] The actual ontogenic explanation for all the variants is incomplete.[13] Iatrogenic entrapment after placement of bypass grafts has also been described.[14] This technical error usually has been the result of placing the graft medial to the medial head of the gas-

Normal

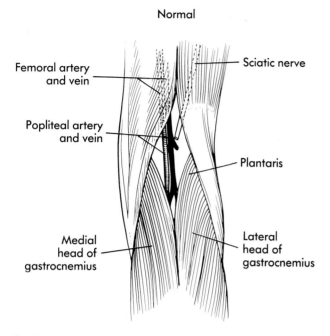

Femoral artery
and vein

Popliteal artery
and vein

Sciatic nerve

Plantaris

Medial
head of
gastrocnemius

Lateral
head of
gastrocnemius

Fig. 24-1. Normal anatomic relationship *(posterior view)* of the right popliteal space. (From Insua JA, Young JR, and Humphries AW: Popliteal artery entrapment syndrome, Arch Surg 101:771, 1970. Copyright 1970, American Medical Association.)

Type II

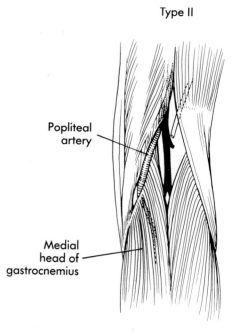

Popliteal
artery

Medial
head of
gastrocnemius

Fig. 24-3. Type II anomaly. The medial head of the gastrocnemius muscle arises more laterally on the femoral condyle, with a separation between the artery and vein. The artery may be minimally displaced on arteriogram. (From Insua JA, Young JR, and Humphries AW: Popliteal artery entrapment syndrome, Arch Surg 101:771, 1970. Copyright 1970, American Medical Association.)

Type I

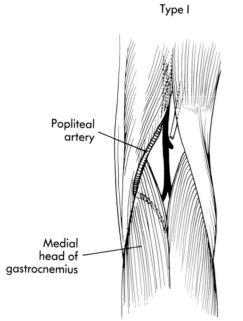

Popliteal
artery

Medial
head of
gastrocnemius

Fig. 24-2. Type I anomaly. The popliteal artery deviates medially around the medial head of the gastrocnemius muscle that arises close to its normal location. (From Insua JA, Young JR, and Humphries AW: Popliteal artery entrapment syndrome, Arch Surg 101:771, 1970. Copyright 1970, American Medical Association.)

Type III

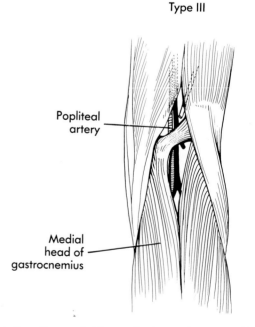

Popliteal
artery

Medial
head of
gastrocnemius

Fig. 24-4. Type III anomaly. The popliteal artery is entrapped by a lateral slip of the medial gastrocnemius muscle. The artery takes a normal course. (From Insua JA, Young JR, and Humphries AW: Popliteal artery entrapment syndrome, Arch Surg 101:771, 1970. Copyright 1970, American Medical Association.)

Type IV

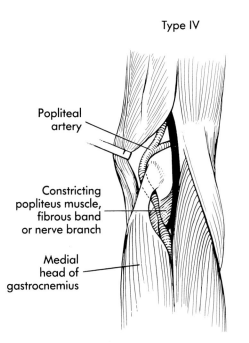

Fig. 24-5. Type IV anomaly. The popliteus muscle or a deep fibrous band compresses the popliteal artery. This anomaly can be accompanied by medial deviation of the artery around a normally arising medial head of the gastrocnemius muscle, but the site of entrapment is distal to this deviation. (Modified from Rich NM et al: Popliteal vascular entrapment. Its increasing interest, Arch Surg 114:1377, 1979. Copyright 1979, American Medical Association.)

trocnemius muscle. Perhaps most of these resulted from a failure to recognize the underlying native artery entrapment. Histologic examination of resected arterial segments has demonstrated the presence of abundant longitudinal muscle fibers in the tunica media.[15] The internal elastic lamina is disrupted with fibrous thickening of intima. It has been postulated that repetitive trauma to the arterial wall results in the development of these muscle bundles.[15,16] These muscular changes are generally seen on the arterial wall adjacent to the contracting muscle.[16] This can be a histologic feature distinguishing this condition from occlusive atherosclerotic disease.

Classification

Different classification schemes for PAES have appeared as regularly as new anatomic variants are recognized. The schemes have been based on anatomic or angiographic characteristics, because the same principles in treatment apply almost universally. Many of these classifications were proposed early in the era of clinical recognition of the disease, without the exposure to all the variants that have since been recognized.[9,17-19] There are many diverse anomalies in muscle, arterial, venous, and neural structures, making individual classification of each variant cumbersome. Therefore the specific classification schemes to date have limited usefulness in the management or prognosis of the entrapment phenomenon. A pictorial description of four of the most common types is seen in Figs. 24-2 to 24-5.

Clinical Presentation

The clinical presentation is usually that of a healthy, "athletic-type" male complaining of typical claudication symptoms in the absence of premature atherosclerosis. It is not unusual for the onset of the claudication symptoms to be sudden. Patients may also describe nocturnal cramps, numbness, paresthesias, focal ischemia in the distal digits, worsening of symptoms with knee flexion, or the sudden development of a cold leg. The degree of stenosis and the presence of collateral flow will dictate the extent of circulatory compromise and the consequent symptoms. Acute thrombosis and/or distal embolization can also occur if entrapment leads to poststenotic dilation, intraluminal thrombus, or aneurysm formation.

The incidence in the general population is unknown, but reported incidences range from 0.165% in a study of 20,000 Greek army patients[19] to 3.5% in postmortem examinations of 86 patients.[20] Males are involved predominantly by a 15:1 ratio.[9] The patient age at the time of diagnosis has ranged from 12 to 64 years, with 60% being less than 30 years of age.[9] Bilateral popliteal artery involvement has been found to be about 22% in the older literature,[9] but a more recent study reported bilateral anomalies in 67% (8 of 12 patients).[12] These higher figures could reflect a more consistent study of the contralateral side. The anatomic variant seen in bilateral disease may frequently vary from one side to another.[9]

Diagnostic Testing

Palpation of the arteries in the involved limb is the cornerstone of the initial evaluation. The timing and the quality of the pulse may suggest the level of disease, the extent of involvement, and the presence of aneurysmal dilation. The disappearance of the pulse with passive dorsiflexion of the foot or active plantar flexion against resistance may suggest the diagnosis.[21] In patients with pulses that are difficult to palpate, Doppler ultrasound increases the diagnostic yield.

Plethysmographic tests such as pulse-volume recordings have increased our diagnostic capabilities. A baseline waveform and blood pressure is established with the patient in the supine position. The foot is then put through flexion maneuvers, and changes in the flow tracing can be evaluated. Finally, the addition of stress testing with treadmill walking can elucidate not only symptoms, but also document the physiologic and functional alterations in blood flow.[22] The addition of treadmill testing should lower the false-negative rate associated with isolated supine testing. The mechanism for the change in flow characteristics with the foot put through flexion maneuvers can be explained either by direct compression of the entrapped artery or through an increase in run-off resistance secondary to contracting muscle beds.[22]

Duplex ultrasound of the popliteal artery has also been studied in asymptomatic, athletic subjects.[23] Normal popliteal fossa anatomy in these subjects was confirmed with magnetic resonance imaging (MRI). The popliteal artery became occluded in 53% of these normal limbs when put through the flexion maneuvers. Consequently, functional popliteal artery compression can occur, raising

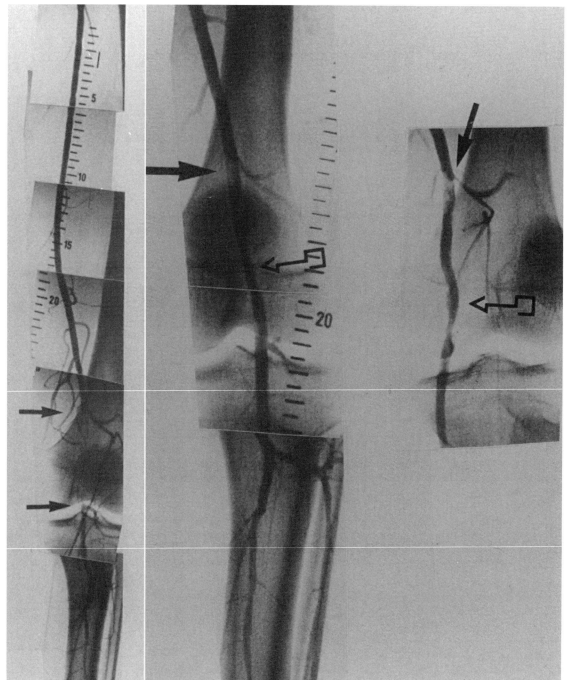

Fig. 24-6. A, Arteriogram of the left popliteal artery occlusion *(arrows)* in a 16-year-old soccer player with popliteal artery entrapment syndrome. **B,** Arteriogram after intraarterial infusion of thrombolytic therapy, showing restoration of antegrade flow.

caution with the diagnosis of PAES until anatomic confirmation of entrapment is made.

Confirmatory evidence for PAES can be provided by computed tomography (CT) or MRI scanning.[23,24] CT or MRI scanning can clearly delineate soft tissue, vascular, and bony structures, unlike ultrasound, which differentiates soft tissue structures less clearly. The relationship between the popliteal artery and vein, the architecture of the local osseus prominences, and the presence of interly-

ing muscle can be documented. Furthermore, both popliteal spaces can be evaluated at the same time. This allows for direct comparison and screening for bilateral anatomic variances. Clinically this is also useful in differentiating cystic advential disease (CAD) of the popliteal artery from PAES. With a better understanding of the anatomy, the surgeon can then decide on the best operative approach.

Arteriography remains the gold standard for evaluation

and can be done in both the neutral and flexed positions. A characteristic finding is medial deviation of the artery in the popliteal region, although the course of the artery may be normal. Poststenotic dilation and aneurysmal dilation of the midpopliteal or distal popliteal artery are also highly suggestive of popliteal entrapment but have been found in only 27% of the cases.[25] Usually atherosclerotic changes of the arterial tree are minimal in these patients, but the presence of angiographically documented atheroma should not exclude this diagnosis.

Other entities that cause midpopliteal occlusion include CAD, thrombosed popliteal aneurysm, and ASO. When faced with a thrombosed popliteal artery, the combination of ultrasound or CT scanning and arteriography is usually sufficient to make the correct diagnosis.

Treatment

Once the diagnosis of PAES is made, surgical intervention is warranted regardless of symptoms. The prevention of thrombotic and embolic complications, coupled with highly successful surgical techniques, favor this approach. The surgical approach is made either through a medial or posterior incision. The medial approach is generally used in standard bypass surgery. However, the posterior approach offers a distinct advantage in the ability to visualize many of these anatomic variants.

Once entrapment is recognized, any surgical procedure should be tailored to the specific clinical situation. Transection of the offending structure is mandatory. The artery needs to be freely mobilized. The muscle or fibrous band need not necessarily be translocated for functional integrity. Optimal results have been obtained when treated early with only musculotendinous division (94% patency at mean of 46 months) as compared with those requiring arterial grafting (58% patency at mean of 43 months).[13] The condition of the underlying vessel dictates the need for thrombectomy, lytic therapy, resection, patch angioplasty, or bypass procedure. Aneurysmal disease needs to be treated with excision or (bypass) ligation. If the artery is already thrombosed or if emboli have occurred, the surgical procedure can be preceded by attempting intraarterial thrombolytic therapy. The use of thrombolytic therapy can simplify the surgical approach and thus potentially lead to better long-term results (Fig. 24-6).[26] Operative complications can be minimized by correctly recognizing the anatomy and underlying pathology. Care must also be taken to avoid transection of the median cutaneous sural nerve in the posterior approach. Postoperative complications of infection, graft thrombosis, bleeding, and deep venous thrombosis have all been reported.[25]

CYSTIC ADVENTITIAL DISEASE

An unusual cause for arterial insufficiency stems from the accumulation of gelatinous fluid in an arterial wall cyst. The fluid builds under pressure in the cyst, encroaching upon the vessel lumen and causing stenosis or occlusion. This process has been referred to by many names including CAD, cystic adventitial degeneration, cystic mucoid degeneration, cystic myxomatous adventitial degeneration, degenerescence colloide de l'adventice, mucinous cystic

dissecting intramural degeneration, and subadventitial pseudocyst. CAD most commonly affects the popliteal artery, although it can be associated with other upper- or lower-extremity vessels. The nomenclature proposed by Ishikawa[27] separates the popliteal artery (CAD-PA) involvement from that of other vessels (CAD-non-PA).

Historical Background

CAD was first reported in 1946 by Atkins and Key[28] after finding a myxomatous tumor involving the left external iliac artery in a 40-year-old man. In 1954 Ejrup and Hiertonn[29] described a gelatinous-filled mass arising from the popliteal artery causing subtotal stenosis and calf claudication. Hiertonn, Lindberg, and Rob[30] had collected four cases of popliteal artery involvement in 1957 and noted that the process occurred particularly in young men. By 1970 approximately 40 cases had been reported in the world literature, with most involving the popliteal artery and causing either stenosis or occlusion of the affected vessel.[31]

A group at Northwestern University developed a correspondence registry of all of the reported cases in the world literature and published these data in 1979.[32] They reported a total of 115 cases involving the popliteal artery, of which 105 were acceptable for inclusion. Of these 105 cases, 83 were men and 18 were women, and in 4 the patient's gender was not reported. The mean age was 42 years (range, 11 to 70 years).

In 1987 Ishikawa[27] added 91 additional cases of CAD-PA and presented 39 CAD-non-PA cases. The other sites of involvement included vessels adjacent to joints such as the radial, ulnar, brachial, iliac, and femoral arteries. Of the cases recorded by Ishikawa,[27] 15% were documented to have an anatomic connection between the cyst and the adjacent joint capsule. Sakamoto et al[33] reported a case of bilateral popliteal artery involvement, and Ohta et al[34] presented a case of ipsilateral iliofemoral artery and vein disease. The sites of venous CAD include the femoral, external iliac, popliteal, and saphenous veins.

Pathophysiology

The cyst arises in the outer tunica media or subadventital layer with cyst expansion (or degeneration) into the adventitia of the vessel wall. The rate of growth is unknown, but once the intracystic pressure exceeds that in the lumen of the vessel, stenosis (70%) or occlusion (30%) results.[27] As a rule CAD appears as an isolated lesion devoid of a systemic process. However, CAD-PA has been reported in a 32-year-old patient with the nail-patella syndrome.[35]

The exact pathophysiologic mechanism for the development of CAD is unknown. Several authors have supported the role of repeated microtrauma to the popliteal artery leading to degenerative changes and cyst formation.[27,30,32] Two cases of CAD affecting the radial arteries 2 months after radial artery blood gas sampling were described.[36] The rarity of this disease and the fact that it is usually an isolated lesion detracts from the hypothesis of trauma as a sole factor. Another hypothesis tries to account for the disease involvement seen around adjacent joints. Robb[37] proposed that synovial membrane from a tendon sheath or joint capsule became attached to the artery either developmentally or traumatically. Ruppel et al[38] recognized the chemical and structural similarity between vascular cysts and ganglia and proposed that these are true ganglia of the vessel wall. Another theory suggests that pseudocyst formation occurred after hemorrhagic rupture of vasa vasorum. No one theory has received total support to explain the observed findings; possibly an interplay of more than one of the preceding mechanisms is responsible.

Analysis of pathologic specimens reveals a cyst arising from the subadventitial layer or the outer tunica media layer of the vessel. The cyst can be uniloculated or multiloculated and is lined by flattened cells, usually filled with clear fluid, although it can be hemorrhagic (currant jelly appearance) or even yellow. Mucoprotein and mucopolysaccharides, hyaluronic acid, and hydroxyproline have been reported as the major cystic components. Endo et al,[39] through extensive chemical evaluation, concluded that the main component was proteohyaluronic acid. The mechanism for the fluid accumulation in the cyst is unknown.

Clinical Presentation

Initially most case reports originated from Europe and Japan, but as recognition has increased, a global distribution has been seen. Men predominate by an approximate 5:1 ratio. The age ranges from 10 to 77 years, with a mean of 44.9 years. There is equal involvement of the right and left popliteal arteries.[26] The cysts can vary in length. Sizes up to 13 cm have been reported; the cysts can be adherent to adjacent structures (i.e., vein, nerve).[40]

Claudication in a younger individual in the absence of atherosclerotic risk factors should heighten the clinical suspicion of CAD. Typically the symptoms develop over several months and can wax and wane. The degree of artery narrowing, as well as the degree of collateralization, dictates the severity of claudication. In the presence of stenosis, distal pulses are frequently present but may disappear upon flexion of the knee joint (Ishikawa's sign).[27] A systolic bruit in the popliteal area has been suggested as a pertinent physical finding. Occlusion of the involved artery usually appears with absent distal pulses, but distal ischemia at rest or neurologic deficit secondary to ischemia is a rare finding.

Diagnostic Testing

Frequently CAD can be diagnosed preoperatively. Pulse-volume recordings may show the characteristic drop in blood pressure and change in waveform configuration at the affected level. These changes may not be evident at rest but can be brought out by exercise. The claudication distance depends on the degree of stenosis and the extent of collateralization.

Duplex ultrasonographic techniques can be helpful in recognizing the presence of a perivascular cystic structure. Ultrasound can demonstrate hypoechoic spaces that may be septated, and Doppler can show turbulence and an elevated shift frequency in the area of stenosis.[41] CT or MRI can provide direct evidence of adjacent masses, muscle insertions, and the course of the artery.[24,40,42] On CT the cystic contents show no enhancement and the relative attenuation value is between those of water and muscle, thus clearly delineating the soft tissue structures.

Arteriography will demonstrate the degree of stenosis and is best done by including anteroposterior and lateral projections. The arteriographic appearance is most frequently that of a scimitar, hourglass, or flute embouchure configuration but can also appear as an M-shaped or a triangular filling defect[24] (Figs. 24-7 and 24-8). Poststenotic dilation or aneurysm formation is not generally seen, and collateral channels may be well developed. Medial displacement of the artery is not seen in CAD-PA, and atherosclerotic changes of ASO are characteristically absent. Arteriographic changes seen with the calf in active or passive flexion should not dissuade against the diagnosis of CAD while also considering PAES.[23]

Treatment

An important factor in considering the best treatment option is the timing of the diagnosis. Treatment options differ on the basis of whether the artery is stenotic or occluded.[27] In the past most cases were diagnosed at the time of surgery, after the artery had occluded. Now, however, with increased awareness of the disease and with excellent noninvasive diagnostic studies available, early diagnosis allows wider therapeutic options. In the stenotic lesion ultrasound or CT-guided needle aspiration of the cyst has been attempted.[43] The multiloculated lesion coupled with the high viscosity of the gelatinous fluid may make evacuation with percutaneous techniques incomplete. Also leaving the cystic structure in place may lead to higher recurrence rates. These techniques can lower the intracystic pressure and improve the flow characteristics of the involved vessel. Percutaneous balloon angioplasty has not proven to be a viable alternative.[44]

Once arterial occlusion has occurred, intraarterial thrombolytic therapy can be considered to restore arterial patency. This can then be followed by the appropriate resection or nonresectional technique to alleviate the underlying pathology. Faced with persistent stenoses, recurrent stenosis, or persistent occlusive disease, a more definitive surgical technique should be performed.

Flanigan et al[32] provide comparative data between resectional and nonresectional therapy. Nonresectional therapy included simple evacuation, evacuation with vein patch, evacuation with synthetic patch, or simple aspiration. In this group an overall success rate of 85% (initial success, 89%) was reported. This was compared with resectional techniques using vein graft, synthetic graft, end-to-end anastomosis, or homograft placement, which revealed an overall success rate of 91% (initial success, 93%).[32] The patency of autogenous reversed saphenous vein graft after 27 to 30 years has been demonstrated in three patients who were originally operated on for complaints of intermittent claudication secondary to CAD-PA.[45] Long-term follow-up data on larger patient groups have not been available.

EXTRARENAL FIBROMUSCULAR DYSPLASIA

Fibromuscular dysplasia (FMD) is an uncommon, noninflammatory disease of the arteries. Exceedingly rare,

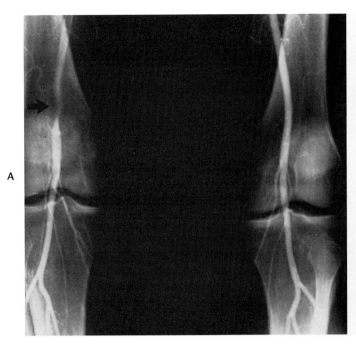
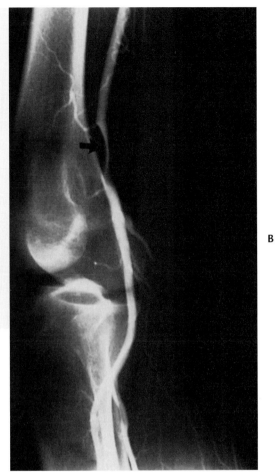

Fig. 24-7. A, Bilateral lower-extremity arteriogram demonstrates smooth area of stenosis in the right proximal popliteal artery *(arrow).* **B,** Lateral arteriogram of the right leg shows the scimitar pattern *(arrow)* characteristic of cystic adventitial disease. (From Buonocore E: Unusual cause of claudication in a 48-year-old man, Cleve Clin Q 50:46, 1982.)

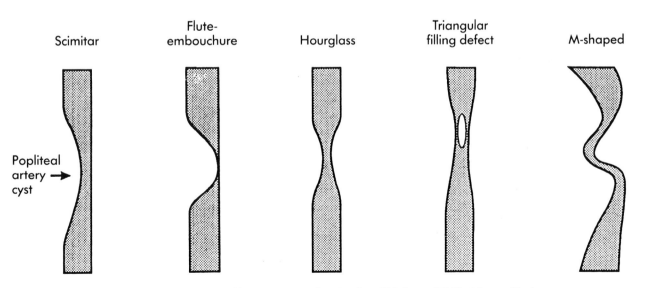

Scimitar Flute-embouchure Hourglass Triangular filling defect M-shaped

Popliteal artery cyst →

Fig. 24-8. Different arteriographic appearances of cystic adventitial disease (CAD) of the popliteal arteries. (Modified from Ishikawa K: Cystic adventitial disease of the popliteal artery and of other stem vessels in the extremities, Jpn J Surg 17:227, 1987.)

Table 24-1. Characteristics of Extrarenal Fibromuscular Dysplasia

Artery Involved	Predominant FMD Subtype	Site of Involvement	Associated Lesions	Arteriograms
Internal carotid	Intimal and medial fibroplasia	Segment adjacent to C1-2	Intracranial aneurysms Renal FMD	String of beads Tubular stenoses Dissection
Vertebral	Medial fibroplasia	Segment adjacent to C5	Carotid FMD	String of beads
Mesenteric and celiac	Intimal fibroplasia	Midvessel segment beyond orifice	Renal FMD Visceral aneurysms	Focal stenoses Long tubular stenoses
Upper extremity (subclavian, axillary)	Intimal fibroplasia	Middle or distal segments of vessel	Renal FMD	Long tubular stenoses
Lower extremity (external iliac, femoral, tibial)	Medial fibroplasia	Proximal segment of external iliac	Carotid FMD Renal FMD	String of beads

venous FMD has been histologically documented in the renal, portal, mesenteric, and peripheral veins. FMD most commonly involves the renal arteries (60% to 75%) (see Chapter 18) but has been described in almost every arterial bed, including the cervicocranial (25% to 30%), visceral (9%), and extremity arteries (5%).[46-49] Histologic confirmation of FMD has been lacking in some of the reported cases.

The histologic classification system of renal artery FMD proposed by Harrison and McCormack[50] is also used for extrarenal FMD. The authors separated FMD into subtypes according to the layers of vessel wall involved. The classification includes intimal fibroplasia, medial hyperplasia, medial fibroplasia, perimedial fibroplasia, and periarterial fibroplasia. Whether spontaneous dissection is a complication of FMD or whether it is a separate category of FMD remains controversial.[46,50]

Table 24-1 summarizes several features of extrarenal FMD. The angiographic appearance can be very suggestive of FMD, but the diagnosis is based on histologic confirmation. The appearance of concomitant atherosclerosis may make the diagnosis more difficult, particularly in the older age groups; however, classic intimal or medial changes on arteriography are highly suggestive of FMD.[51] The lesions of FMD typically arise in the middle or distal arterial segments, sparing the orificial or bifurcation sites typical of atherosclerotic disease.[46] In 24% of patients with FMD there is involvement in more than one vascular territory.[46] The workup therefore should exclude other sites of involvement, including renal FMD.

The pathogenesis of FMD remains unknown, although multiple theories exist. The genetic theory was used to explain the familial involvement seen particularly in whites. Rushton[52] observed the inheritance pattern of FMD to be consistent with an autosomal dominant trait with variable penetrance. In those patients without a family history of FMD, a new mutation was thought to have occurred.[46] The humoral theory relates the predilection of FMD in females to increased estrogen levels.[53] Mechanical factors such as local trauma, stretching, or vessel torsion have also been proposed to account for the anatomic location or topography of the disease.[54] Furthermore, some other injurious mechanisms may disrupt the

vasa vasorum of the vessel wall leading to mural ischemia.[55] Other theories take into account the possibility of exogenous toxins such as smoking, ergotamine use, or rubella syndromes as causes.[46] A combination of these mechanisms may interact in the susceptible host. The differential diagnosis of FMD should include vascular spasm, arterial hypoplasia, arteritis, or simply diminished flow leading to a decrease in the caliber of the visualized vessel. In the presence of arterial dilations, other considerations include aneurysmal disease, pseudoaneurysm, and atherosclerosis with poststenotic dilation.

Disease conditions that have been associated with FMD include coarctation of the aorta, neurofibromatosis,[56] pheochromocytoma,[57] Ehlers-Danlos syndrome type IV,[58] Alport's syndrome,[59] and cystic medial necrosis.[60]

Cervicocranial Fibromuscular Dysplasia

In 1965 Connett and Lansche[61] histologically confirmed that FMD can affect the cervicocranial arteries. It can affect any or all of the arteries supplying the central nervous system (CNS) circulation[61-66] (Fig. 24-9). The internal carotid artery is involved in approximately 90% of cases, with bilateral lesions (60% to 85%) being more common.[63-65] Vertebral artery disease is seen in a minority of cases.[62] Associated FMD of the renal arteries is present in roughly one third of the cases.[46] There is also a high association of intracranial aneurysms with FMD, with estimates ranging from 21% to 50%.[62,63] (Fig. 24-9). In one series of patients with subarachnoid hemorrhage (SAH), 31 out of 102 patients (30%) had FMD.[67]

Females are predominant among individuals with cervicocranial FMD. The disease has been reported in all age groups (4 to 86 years, mean 58).[65,66]

Cervicocranial FMD can be symptomatic or asymptomatic; however, the natural history is unknown. Asymptomatic carotid FMD is either found serendipitously or when searched for because of the presence of renal artery FMD. The symptoms associated with FMD depend on the location of the disease and the extent of ischemia induced. Specific CNS signs/symptoms include strokes, transient ischemic attacks (TIAs), SAH, Horner's syndrome, and cranial nerve paresis. Nonspecific signs/symptoms of symptomatic FMD include headache, vertigo, neck pain,

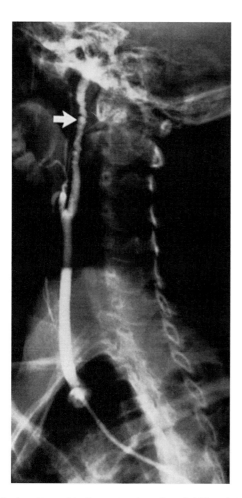

Fig. 24-9. Arteriographic demonstration of medial fibroplasia involving the right internal carotid artery in a 76-year-old woman. Note the "string-of-beads" appearance and the topographic location next to C1-2 *(arrow)*.

nausea, vomiting, disorientation, drowsiness, seizure, or loss of consciousness.[53] The incidence of major complications, stroke, TIAs, and SAH in cervicocranial FMD is estimated between 29% and 44%.[64,66] On the other hand, many patients develop nonspecific symptoms (i.e., headache, tinnitus, dizziness), and FMD is diagnosed during the workup of these symptoms.

All classic arteriographic and pathologic changes of FMD have been described in the cervicocranial arteries.[62] Subtypes of cervicocranial FMD reflect the same incidence as that in the renal circulation.[68] Topographically the lesion in the internal carotid artery is usually adjacent to the C1-2 vertebral bodies and not at the proximal origin[64] (Fig. 24-10). A "string-of-beads" appearance next to C1-2 is quite suggestive of FMD. When the "beading" is larger than the proximal caliber of the vessel, it is indicative of medial fibroplasia. The "beads" are smaller than the proximal caliber of the vessel in perimedial fibroplasia. Not uncommonly, though, the changes of concomitant ASO may be present (Fig. 24-10). The diagnosis of carotid FMD may be suspected with carotid duplex ultrasonography, but the examination is limited by the distal site of involvement in the internal carotid artery and can be missed by this technique. MRI and magnetic resonance angiography

(MRA) of cervical FMD may be useful.[69,70] The treatment of cervicocranial FMD is quite variable, ranging from observation to surgical intervention. The natural history of the disease is uncertain, particularly in asymptomatic FMD. In general, asymptomatic, nonaneurysmal FMD of the extracranial arteries should be treated with antiplatelet agents. However, the presence of concomitant intracranial aneurysms may warrant surgical intervention.

Treatment options for symptomatic (TIAs, stroke) cervicocranial FMD include medical therapy (acetylsalicylic acid, coumarin), intraoperative graduated intraluminal dilation (GID), or surgical resection or bypass.[71-78] Percutaneous balloon angioplasty has been tried in cervicocranial FMD but is not recommended based on unacceptable complication rates.[76] The expertise in the specific medical community should help dictate the procedure of choice.

Nonrenal Visceral Fibromuscular Dysplasia

FMD of the visceral arteries other than the renal arteries is uncommon. The visceral arteries most frequently affected include (in descending order of prevalence) the celiac, superior mesenteric, hepatic, splenic, and coronary arteries. Estimates range from less than 0.1%, in unselected autopsy series, to 13% in patients with splenic artery aneurysms.[77,78]

Isolated visceral arterial involvement has been reported, but multiple visceral vessels are more commonly affected. Visceral artery involvement can also be associated with generalized hypoplasia of the aorta or coarctation of the aorta.[79] The coarctation may be thoracic, suprarenal, or infrarenal with concomitant involvement of the renal, mesenteric, or carotid circulation. Infrarenal coarctation is more commonly associated with FMD than is coarctation of the suprarenal or thoracic aorta. Frequently the histologic specimens are consistent with those seen in neurofibromatosis; therefore a diagnostic workup should be performed to exclude this disease.[46,56]

Angiographically, nonrenal visceral FMD may reveal long areas of smooth narrowing rather than the classic "string-of-beads" appearance seen in FMD at other sites. This corresponds to the natural history in that arterial occlusion is a more common complication of nonrenal visceral FMD than aneurysm rupture or embolization. The histologic subtypes (intimal, medial, perimedial dysplasias) have all been described in the visceral circulation.[46-48] Intimal hyperplasia has been the predominant histologic form of FMD in the coronary circulation, but medial FMD with dissections has also been reported.[80] This exceedingly rare condition can affect all age groups, but only a handful of case reports exist.[81]

Because of the extensive collateralization normally available, mesenteric ischemia usually results only after two of the three main splanchnic vessels are occluded. Abdominal angina is usually accompanied by weight loss, fear of food secondary to postprandial pain, and sometimes a change in stool formation. Aneurysm rupture and/or arteriovenous fistula formation can be manifested as hypotension, shock, or high-output heart failure. Overall though, this is an asymptomatic disease and is most often found by chance in association with renal or carotid

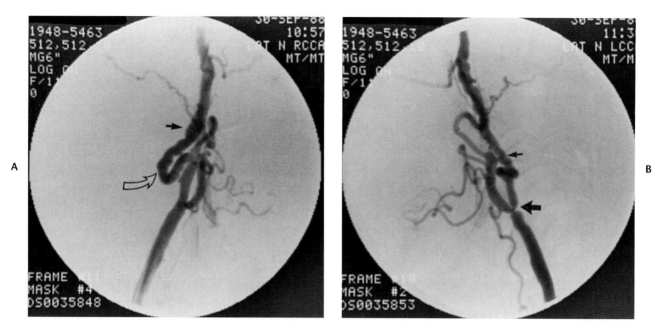

Fig. 24-10. Arteriogram of right **(A)** and left **(B)** carotid arteries in an 80-year-old woman. There appears to be arteriographic evidence of both medial fibroplasia *(small arrows)* and atherosclerosis *(large arrow)*. Note the kinking of the right ICA *(open arrow)*. She also had an asymptomatic 3-mm anterior communicating artery aneurysm (not seen). Left carotid endarterectomy was done with histologic confirmation of both medial fibroplasia and atherosclerosis.

artery FMD. To date the primary treatment of symptomatic disease has been surgical intervention.[53] Percutaneous balloon angioplasty has been reported to be successful when technically feasible. It is the most viable alternative to surgery for patients with stenotic disease, but its applicability is limited by the presence of occlusive or aneurysmal disease.[82]

Extremities

FMD has been described in all of the peripheral arteries of the extremities (iliac, superficial femoral, popliteal, tibial, subclavian, axillary, radial, and ulnar) (Figs. 24-11 and 24-12). These lesions are typically asymptomatic but can produce signs and symptoms such as a difference in blood pressure, paresthesias, claudication, or frank ischemia.[46,53,83]

To date, most studies of FMD in the extremities demonstrate a female predominance. However, Estahani et al[84] described 17 cases in Iranian men with upper- and/or lower-extremity occlusive disease (ages 22 to 45 years), but there was histologic confirmation in only 6 of these patients. Arteritis, thromboangiitis obliterans, aneurysmal disease, ASO, or vasospasm can masquerade as FMD. Histologic proof may be needed for a definite diagnosis. Most cases have been diagnosed angiographically. The symptomatic population has generally been older than 50 years of age, but complications of aneurysmal disease have been reported in the very young.[85] The older patients may have had predominantly asymptomatic FMD, but when the atherosclerotic process is superimposed on FMD, symptoms may arise. Intimal fibroplasia seems to be the most frequent histologic subtype seen in peripheral FMD,

although medial and perimedial fibroplasia have been described.[86]

The appropriate interventional therapy may be different, depending on the site, extent, and distal manifestations of the disease. Therapy should be reserved for symptomatic disease. The successful therapies reported to date include balloon dilation, GID, surgical bypass and/or resection, and sympathetic blockade or transection.[87-90] If applicable, intervention with percutaneous balloon angioplasty should probably be the procedure of choice initially, with the surgical approach reserved for refractory or technically difficult disease. Minimal follow-up data are available to compare the efficacy of each approach.

ARTERIAL CALCIFICATION DISEASES

A heterogeneous group of diseases that share a common feature, calcification, are grouped together in this section. The four disease entities include ASO; Mönckeberg's sclerosis, or medial calcinosis; idiopathic infantile arterial calcification (IIAC); and arterial calcification associated with chronic renal failure. ASO is discussed in detail in other chapters. Venous calcification is an uncommon finding when unassociated with thrombosis. The portal venous system can calcify in the setting of longstanding portal hypertension from chronic liver disease.[91]

The cellular mechanism of calcification is poorly understood and is probably dependent on the underlying disease process in which calcification is seen. The usual theory is that the calcium buildup occurs as a passive process, either through passive precipitation or adsorption. Passive precipitation results from the intracellular uptake of excessive

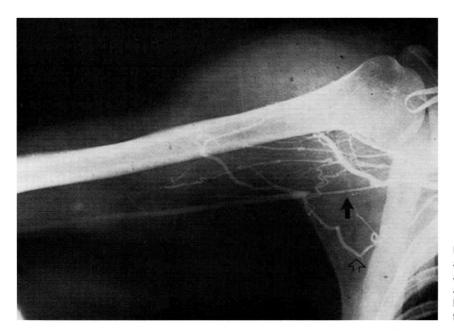

Fig. 24-11. Arteriogram of the right axillary artery with marked collaterals *(open arrow)* around an area of stenosis *(solid arrow)*. This area of smooth narrowing *(solid arrow)* was histologically confirmed to be intimal fibroplasia.

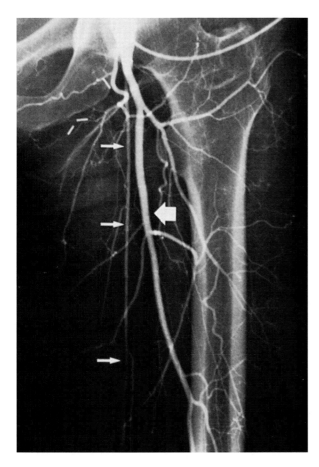

Fig. 24-12. Arteriogram of the left leg in a 58-year-old woman. Note the caliber of the superficial femoral (long smooth narrowing) *(small arrows)* compared with the normal-appearing profunda femoris *(large arrow)*. She also had internal carotid artery FMD that was confirmed to be intimal fibroplasia.

calcium at the mitochondrial level, which leads to saturation and precipitation. This imbalance in calcium regulation intracellularly may account for metastatic calcification seen in end-stage renal failure patients with elevated calcium phosphate products. "Calciphylaxis" is the term used to describe experimentally induced metastatic calcification and is also used clinically to describe patients with systemic calcinosis.[92,93] A second theory describes an extracellular matrix vesicle as a common factor in calcification.[94] These membrane-invested particles initiate calcification in a variety of sites, such as bone growth plates, cardiac prosthetic valves, and arterial vascular walls. This secondary process of dystrophic calcification usually results after ischemic or traumatic injury to the involved tissue.[95] The process or stimuli promoting vesicle formation is unknown. Newer theories of atherosclerotic calcification address the role of G1a proteins in the organization and regulation of calcium deposition. These proteins are normally associated with bone metabolism but may be part of pathologic vascular calcification.[96]

Mönckeberg's Sclerosis

In 1903 Mönckeberg described a condition of extensive calcification involving the tunica media of the large- and medium-sized arteries of the upper and lower extremities and viscera. The dense medial calcinosis produces a rigid conduit without encroachment on the vessel lumen, theoretically maintaining normal end-organ perfusion. Mönckeberg's sclerosis is distinctly different from the intimal and medial calcification seen with ASO, where plaque progression can lead to luminal narrowing and end-organ ischemia. The calcification secondary to ASO is often diffuse in distribution and frequently affects orificial and bifurcation arterial sites. Mönckeberg's sclerosis tends to spare these areas and can often be appreciated on plain radiographs of the extremities (Fig. 24-13). Histologic examination of affected arteries shows fibrotic and calcified

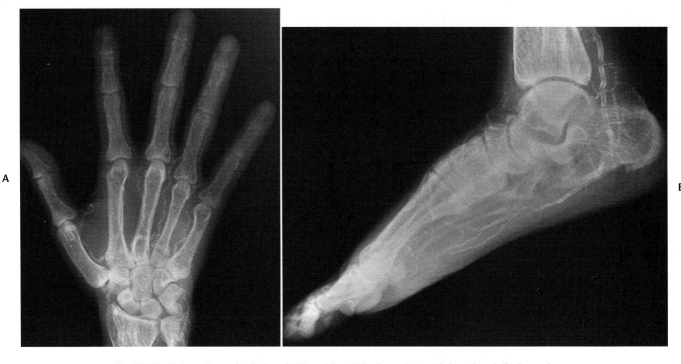

Fig. 24-13. Plain radiograph of a hand **(A)** and foot **(B)** of a patient with heavily calcified vessels secondary to end-stage renal disease and diabetes mellitus.

replacement of the tunica media. The internal and external elastic lamina may be involved in the fibrotic process, whereas the intima is normal in pure Mönckeberg's sclerosis.[97] The intimal changes of ASO can be superimposed on the medial disruption of Mönckeberg's sclerosis. This is usually present in patients over 50 years of age who may have had asymptomatic medial calcification for years.

The actual mechanism leading to medial calcification is unknown, but calcium, phosphate, and parathyroid hormone (PTH) levels are usually normal.[97] Diabetics tend to have a higher incidence of medial arterial calcification.[98] This association is believed to be related to the duration of the metabolic derangement rather than the tightness of metabolic control. Some researchers suggest that diabetics with peripheral neuropathy have an even higher incidence of calcification than those without neuropathy.[99] Others have found that those patients with autonomic neuropathy as part of their polyneuropathy have an extremely high incidence of calcification.[100] Data from the Epidemiology of Diabetes Complications Study suggest that duration of diabetes, presence of hypertension, and triglyceride to apolipoprotein A-1 ratio are the most consistent risk factors for the development of calcification.[101] Corticosteroids and immunosuppressant therapies have also been implicated in stimulating calcification. A link between Mönckeberg's sclerosis and metabolic bone disease such as osteoporosis has been suspected.

The diagnosis of Mönckeberg's sclerosis is usually made by the classic radiographic appearance on plain roentgenograms. These changes are described as ringlike calcifications against a finely granular background (Fig. 24-13).

This disease is asymptomatic unless associated with superimposed ASO.

Idiopathic Infantile Arterial Calcification

IIAC is a rare disease of unknown cause. IIAC, also known as generalized arterial calcification of infancy, is associated with widespread calcification and usually leads to early death from coronary artery occlusion.[102-108] The calcification in the tunica media is quite evident on plain roentgenograms and can affect all of the vessels including those of the heart, brain, mesentery, and extremities. Marked intimal proliferation sets this disease apart from the other calcification disorders, especially with the aggressive, progressive nature of the process. The calcification can be evident on fetal ultrasound examination and has led to more frequent prenatal diagnosis.[102] Respiratory insufficiency results from congestive heart failure and secondary hypertension results from renovascular disease. The hypertension can be refractory to aggressive medical therapy.[103] An autosomal recessive transmission pattern is believed to account for the genetic familial occurrence of the disease.[104] Biochemical tests usually are normal in the disease with appropriate levels of calcium, phosphate, and PTH.[105] Treatment has consisted of strict blood pressure control with calcium channel blockers or angiotensin-converting enzyme inhibitors.[104] Diphosphonates combined with a low-calcium diet have been shown to cause regression of the vessel calcification in some patients.[102,105,107] Despite prenatal diagnosis and initiation of therapy with improvement of vascular calcification, death from coronary artery intimal proliferation may be unpreventable.[102] One survivor has reportedly lived to age 22 despite four myocardial infarctions.[108]

Arterial Calcification Associated with Chronic Renal Failure

Arterial disease is common in patients with renal insufficiency, especially if they are also diabetic. Herman et al[109] reported that 10% of the diabetic population in Rochester, Minnesota, had peripheral vascular disease, whereas only 2.6% of the nondiabetic patients had similar symptoms. The prevalence of arterial calcification is substantially greater in the dialysis population. At least one third of dialysis patients have arterial calcification, and this number escalates to 90% of diabetic predialysis patients.[110,111]

ASO and Mönckeberg's sclerosis are the two common arterial histopathologic features seen in renal insufficiency patients. Claudication, rest pain, and gangrene associated with extensive ASO can be seen in this population. Peripheral neuropathy can be a complicating factor in the masking of clinical signs of arterial insufficiency. Generally the distribution of the disease includes a greater incidence of lower-extremity arterial involvement, especially of the profunda femoris artery and the tibial vessels. However, ASO can be diffuse and quite widespread. All these patients should be considered as having coronary artery disease, the clinical significance of which should be determined. ASO usually does not occur in the distal portion of the arms or hands. An exception to this is patients with chronic renal failure, especially those with diabetes who undergo chronic dialysis treatment or who have undergone renal transplantation. The exact pathogenesis of this involvement of the arms and hands is unknown, but it cannot be solely explained on the basis of calcium-phosphorus imbalance or hyperparathyroidism. Accelerated atherosclerosis seems to be a more likely explanation. There is progressive systemic intimal proliferation. The smaller-caliber vessels are most affected by the intimal proliferation, thus an acral distribution to the ischemia ensues.[112] There is usually calcification of the media. These patients can present in a dramatic fashion, have progressive gangrene of the fingers, and eventually lose the entire hand (Fig. 24-14). Outside of amputation there is no known treatment for this complication and amputations may be multiple as the disease progresses. Sepsis is a frequent terminal complication.[113]

Another form of calcification in end-stage renal disease patients is called systemic calcinosis, metastatic calcification, or calciphylaxis. This infrequent soft tissue and arterial calcium deposition is a result of high calcium-phosphorus product (greater than 60 to 70).[93,114] Recently Levin, Mehta, and Goldstein[115] have devised a mathematical formula ($2 \times [CaPO_4{-}5] \times$ alkaline phosphatase $\times$ PTH ratio) to help to predict which patients may develop ischemic tissue necrosis, a potentially lethal complication of hyperparathyroidism, in patients with end-stage renal disease. Long-term validation of this equation will be required to determine its true sensitivity and specificity. Significant precipitation of calcium can also occur in the connective tissue of the skin, lungs, kidneys, stomach, heart, and arteries.[116] Most patients have elevated PTH levels. Factors that exacerbate this calcification process

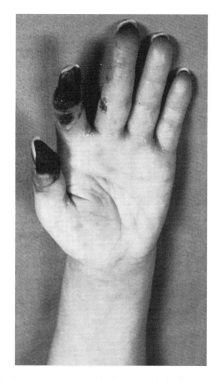

Fig. 24-14. Gangrene of several digits in a diabetic patient with end-stage renal disease.

include vitamin D, calcium carbonate, corticosteroids, immunosuppressants, and blood product therapies.[93,117] Mehta et al[118] suggested that calciphylaxis may also be a result of abnormal protein C activity in patients with renal failure.

The treatment of calciphylaxis is to lower the calcium-phosphate product and remove any aggravating factors. Parathyroidectomy has been performed with successful reversal of the calcification process in some patients.[112] However, many patients do not improve after parathyroidectomy and treatment can be problematic. One recent case report[119] described a 58-year-old woman on continuous ambulatory peritoneal dialysis who developed calciphylaxis in both lower extremities. She did not improve with the usual measures including parathyroidectomy. She received 38 sessions of hyperbaric oxygen therapy and the skin ulcers completely healed. Although there is no large series to support the use of hyperbaric oxygen, it could be considered in the patient in which no other therapeutic modalities have been beneficial. The vigilant approach to the control of infections and septic complications should be employed in all patients since this is a frequent complicating feature of calciphylaxis.

REFERENCES

1. Stuart TPA: Note on a variation in the course of the popliteal artery, J Anat Physiol 13:162, 1879.
2. Hall KV: Anomalous insertion of the medial gastrocnemic head with circulatory complications, Acta Path Microbiol Scand 148(suppl):53, 1961.
3. Chambardel-Dubreuil L: Variations des arteres du pelvis et du membre inferieur, Paris, 1925, Masson and Cie.

4. Hamming JJ: Intermittent claudication at an early age, due to an anomalous course of the popliteal artery, Angiology 10:369, 1959.

5. Hall KV: Intervascular gastrocnemic insertion, Acta Chir Scand 128:193, 1964.

6. Carter AE and Eban R: A case of bilateral developmental abnormality of the popliteal arteries and gastrocnemius muscles, Br J Surg 51:518, 1964.

7. Love JW and Whelan TJ: Popliteal artery entrapment syndrome, Am J Surg 109:620, 1965.

8. Rich NM and Hughes CW: Popliteal artery and vein entrapment, Am J Surg 113:696, 1967.

9. Cavallaro A et al: Popliteal artery entrapment: analysis of the literature and report of personal experience, Vasc Surg 20:404, 1986.

10. Connell J: Popliteal vein entrapment, Br J Surg 65:351, 1978.

11. Podore PC: Popliteal entrapment syndrome: a report of tibial nerve entrapment, J Vasc Surg 2:335, 1985.

12. Collins PS, McDonald PT, and Lim RC: Popliteal artery entrapment: an evolving syndrome, J Vasc Surg 10:484, 1989.

13. diMarzo L et al: Surgical treatment of popliteal artery entrapment syndrome: a ten-year experience, Eur J Vasc Surg 5:59, 1991.

14. Carpenter JP et al: Infrageniculate bypass graft entrapment, J Vasc Surg 18:81, 1993.

15. Inada K et al: Popliteal artery entrapment syndrome: a case report, Br J Surg 65:613, 1978.

16. Iwai T et al: Diagnostic and pathological considerations in the popliteal artery entrapment syndrome, J Cardiovasc Surg 24:243, 1983.

17. Insua JA, Young JR, and Humphries AW: Popliteal artery entrapment syndrome, Arch Surg 101:771, 1970.

18. Delaney TA and Gonzalez LL: Occlusion of the popliteal artery due to muscular entrapment, Surgery 69:97, 1971.

19. Bouhoutsos J and Daskalakis E: Muscular abnormalities affecting the popliteal vessels, Br J Surg 68:501, 1981.

20. Gibson MHL et al: Popliteal artery entrapment syndrome, Ann Surg 185:341, 1974.

21. Hamming JJ and Vink M: Obstruction of the popliteal artery at an early age, J Cardiovasc Surg 6:516, 1965.

22. McDonald PT et al: Popliteal artery entrapment syndrome: clinical non-invasive and angiographic diagnosis, Am J Surg 139:318, 1980.

23. Erdoes LS et al: Popliteal vascular compression in a normal population, J Vasc Surg 20:978, 1994.

24. Rizzo RJ et al: Computed tomography for evaluation of arterial disease in the popliteal fossa, J Vasc Surg 11:112, 1990.

25. Whelan TJ: Popliteal artery entrapment. In Rutherford RB, ed: Vascular surgery, 1989, WB Saunders.

26. The STILE Investigators: Results of a prospective randomized trial evaluating surgery versus thrombolysis for ischemia of the lower extremity, Ann Surg 220:251, 1994.

27. Ishikawa K: Cystic adventitial disease of the popliteal artery and of other stem vessels in the extremities, Jpn J Surg 17:221, 1987.

28. Atkins HJB and Key JA: A case of myxomatous tumour arising in the adventitia of the left external iliac artery, Br J Surg 34:426, 1946.

29. Ejrup B and Hiertonn T: Intermittent claudication: three cases treated by free vein graft, Acta Chir Scand 108:217, 1954.

30. Hiertonn T, Lindberg K, and Rob C: Cystic degeneration of the popliteal artery, Br J Surg 44:348, 1957.

31. Haid SP, Conn J Jr, and Bergan JJ: Cystic adventitial disease of the popliteal artery, Arch Surg 101:765, 1970.

32. Flanigan DP et al: Summary of cases of adventitial cystic disease of the popliteal artery, Ann Surg 189:165, 1979.

33. Sakamoto H et al: Bilateral cystic adventitial disease of the popliteal artery, J Jpn Coll Angiol 16:607, 1976.

34. Ohta T et al: Cystic adventitial degeneration of the ilio-femoral artery and vein, Vasc Surg 18:119, 1984.

35. Mark TM et al: Cystic adventitial degeneration of the popliteal artery, Arch Pathol Lab Med 107:186, 1983.

36. Durham JR et al: Adventitial cystic disease of the radial artery, J Cardiovasc Surg 30:517, 1989.

37. Robb D: Obstruction of popliteal artery by synovial cyst: report of a case, Br J Surg 48:221, 1960.

38. Ruppel V et al: Pathological anatomical observations in cystic adventitial degeneration of blood vessels, Beitr Path Bd 144:101, 1971.

39. Endo M et al: Isolation and identification of proteohyaluronic acid from a cyst of cystic mucoid degeneration, Clin Chim Acta 47:417, 1973.

40. Crolla RM et al: A case of cystic adventitial disease of the popliteal artery demonstrated by magnetic resonance imaging, J Vasc Surg 18:1052, 1993.

41. Bunker SR, Lauten GJ, and Hutton JE: Cystic adventitial disease of the popliteal artery, AJR 136:1209, 1981.

42. Jasinski RW et al: Adventitial cystic disease of the popliteal artery, Radiology 163:153, 1987.

43. Wilbur AC and Spigos DG: Adventitial cyst of the popliteal artery: CT-guided percutaneous aspiration, J Comput Assist Tomogr 10:161, 1986.

44. Fox RL et al: Adventitial cystic disease of the popliteal artery: failure of percutaneous transluminal angioplasty as a therapeutic modality, J Vasc Surg 2:464, 1985.

45. Hiertonn T and Hemmingsson A: The autogenous vein graft as popliteal artery substitute, Acta Chir Scand 150:377, 1984.

46. Luscher TF et al: Arterial fibromuscular dysplasia, Mayo Clin Proc 62:931, 1987.

47. Iwai T et al: Fibromuscular dysplasia in the extremities, J Cardiovasc Surg 26:496, 1985.

48. Palubinskas AJ and Ripley HR: Fibromuscular hyperplasia in extrarenal arteries, Radiology 82:451, 1964.

49. Setoyama M et al: Cutaneous arterial fibromuscular dysplasia: a case report and electron-microscopic study, J Dermatol 21:205, 1994.

50. Harrison EJ Jr and McCormack LJ: Pathologic classification of renal arterial disease in renovascular hypertension, Mayo Clin Proc 46:161, 1971.

51. McCormack LJ et al: A pathologic-arteriographic correlation of renal arterial disease, Am Heart J 72:188, 1966.

52. Rushton AR: The genetics of fibromuscular dysplasia, Arch Intern Med 140:233, 1980.

53. Luscher TF et al: Fibromuscular hyperplasia: extension of the disease and therapeutic outcome, Nephron 44(suppl 1):109, 1986.

54. Rothfield NJH: Fibromuscular arterial disease: experimental studies, Australas Radiol 14:294, 1970.

55. Sottiurai VS, Fry WF, and Stanley JC: Ultrastructure of medial smooth muscle and myelofibroblasts in human arterial dysplasia, Arch Surg 113:1280, 1978.

56. Craddock GR, Challa VR, and Dean RH: Neurofibromatosis and renal artery stenosis: a case of familial incidence, J Vasc Surg 8:489, 1988.

57. Qunibi WJ et al: Pheochromocytoma and fibromuscular hyperplasia, South Med J 72:1481, 1979.

58. Schievink WI and Limburg M: Angiographic abnormalities

mimicking fibromuscular dysplasia in a patient with Ehlers-Danlos syndrome, type IV, Neurosurgery 25:482, 1989.

59. Hodgins LB and Limbacher JP II: Fibromuscular dysplasia in Alport's syndrome, J Tenn Med Assoc 75:733, 1982.

60. Schievink WI et al: Coexistence of fibromuscular dysplasia and cystic medial necrosis in a patient with Marfan's syndrome and bilateral carotid artery dissections, Stroke 25:2492, 1994.

61. Connett MC and Lansche JM: Fibromuscular hyperplasia of the internal carotid artery: report of a case, Ann Surg 162:59, 1965.

62. Mettinger KL and Ericson K: Fibromuscular dysplasia and the brain: observations on angiographic, clinical and genetic characteristics, Stroke 13:46, 1982.

63. Mettinger KL: Fibromuscular dysplasia and the brain. II. Current concept of the disease, Stroke 13:53, 1982.

64. Houser OW et al: Cephalic arterial fibromuscular dysplasia, Radiology 101:605, 1971.

65. Osborn AG and Anderson RE: Angiographic spectrum of cervical and intra-cranial fibromuscular dysplasia, Stroke 8:617, 1977.

66. Corrin LS, Sandok BA, and Houser OW: Cerebral ischemic events in patients with carotid artery fibromuscular dysplasia, Arch Neurol 38:616, 1981.

67. George B et al: Vascular abnormalities in the neck associated with intracranial aneurysms, Neurosurgery 24:499, 1989.

68. Sato S and Hata J: Fibromuscular dysplasia: its occurrence with a dissecting aneurysm of the internal carotid artery, Arch Pathol Lab Med 106:332, 1982.

69. Heiserman JE et al: MR angiography of cervical fibromuscular dysplasia, Am J Neuroradiol 13:1454, 1992.

70. Furie DM et al: Fibromuscular dysplasia of the head and neck: imaging findings, Am J Radiol 162:1205, 1994.

71. Dublin AB, Baltaxe HA, and Cobb CA III: Percutaneous transluminal carotid angioplasty in fibromuscular dysplasia: case report, J Neurosurg 59:162, 1983.

72. Effeney DJ et al: Why operate on carotid fibromuscular dysplasia? Arch Surg 115:1261, 1980.

73. Ehrenfeld WK, Stoney RJ, and Wylie EJ: Fibromuscular hyperplasia of the internal carotid artery, Arch Surg 95:284, 1967.

74. Maiuri F et al: Fibromuscular dysplasia of the carotid arteries: clinical and radiographic considerations, Clin Neurol Neurosurg 90:57, 1988.

75. McNeill DH Jr, Dreisbach J, and Marsden RJ: Spontaneous dissection of the internal carotid artery: its conservative management with heparin sodium, Arch Neurol 37:54, 1980.

76. Hasso AN and Bird CR: Percutaneous transluminal angioplasty of carotid and vertebral arteries. In Jang GC, ed: Angioplasty, New York, 1986, McGraw-Hill.

77. Deterling RA: Aneurysm of the visceral arteries, J Cardiovasc Surg 12:309, 1971.

78. Kreel L: The recognition and incidence of splenic artery aneurysms: a historical review, Australas Radiol 16:126, 1972.

79. Connolly JE: Fibromuscular hyperplasia of the abdominal aorta, J Cardiovasc Surg 19:563, 1978.

80. Lie JT and Berg KK: Isolated fibromuscular dysplasia of the coronary arteries with spontaneous dissection and myocardial infarction, Hum Pathol 18:654, 1987.

81. James TN and Marshall TK: Multifocal stenoses due to fibromuscular dysplasia of the sinus node artery, Circulation 53:736, 1976.

82. Odurny A, Sniderman KW, and Colapinto RF: Intestinal angina: percutaneous transluminal angioplasty of the celiac and superior mesenteric arteries, Radiology 167:59, 1988.

83. Walter JF et al: External iliac artery fibrodysplasia, AJR 131:125, 1978.

84. Estahani F et al: Arterial fibrodysplasia: a regional cause of peripheral occlusive vascular disease, Angiology 40:108, 1989.

85. Stinnett DM, Graham JM, and Edwards WD: Fibromuscular dysplasia and thrombosed aneurysm of the popliteal artery in a child, J Vasc Surg 5:769, 1987.

86. van den Dungen JJAM, Boontje AH, and Oosterhuis JW: Femoropopliteal arterial fibrodysplasia, Br J Surg 77:396, 1990.

87. Wing RJ et al: Treatment of fibromuscular hyperplasia of the external iliac artery by percutaneous transluminal angioplasty, Australas Radiol 37:223, 1993.

88. Yoshida T et al: Fibromuscular disease of the brachial artery with digital emboli treated effectively by transluminal angioplasty, Cardiovasc Intervent Radiol 17:99, 1994.

89. Houston C et al: Fibromuscular dysplasia of the external iliac arteries: surgical treatment by graduated internal dilatation technique, Surgery 85:713, 1979.

90. Mashiah A, Pasik S, and David A: Phenol sympathectomy for symptomatic fibromuscular angiodysplasia of the lower limb, J Cardiovasc Surg 30:244, 1989.

91. Ayuso C et al: Calcifications in the portal venous system: comparison of plain films, sonography, and CT, Am J Radiol 159:321, 1992.

92. Selye H: Calciphylaxis, Chicago, 1962, University of Chicago Press.

93. Conn J Jr et al: Calciphylaxis: etiology of progressive vascular calcification and gangrene? Ann Surg 177:206, 1973.

94. Kim KM and Huang SN: Ultrastructural study of dystrophic calcification of human aortic valve, Lab Invest 26:481, 1972.

95. Tanimura A et al: Matrix vesicles in atherosclerotic calcification, Proc Soc Exp Biol Med 172:173, 1983.

96. Doherty TM and Detrano RC: Coronary arterial calcification as an active process: a new perspective on an old problem, Calcif Tissue Int 54:224, 1994.

97. Lachman AS et al: Medial calcinosis of Mönckeberg, Am J Med 63:615, 1977.

98. Goebel FD and Fuessl HS: Mönckeberg's sclerosis after sympathetic denervation in diabetic and non-diabetic subjects, Diabetologia 24:347, 1983.

99. Young MJ et al: Medial arterial calcification in the feet of diabetic patients and matched non-diabetic control subjects, Diabetologia 36:615, 1993.

100. Gentile S et al: Medial arterial calcification and diabetic neuropathy, Acta Diabet Latina 27:243, 1990.

101. Maser RE et al: Cardiovascular disease and arterial calcification in insulin-dependent diabetes mellitus: interrelations and risk factor profiles, Arterioscler Thromb 11:958, 1991.

102. Bellah RD et al: Idiopathic arterial calcification of infancy: prenatal and postnatal effects of therapy in an infant, J Pediatr 121:930, 1992.

103. Milner LS et al: Hypertension as the major problem of idiopathic arterial calcification of infancy, J Pediatr 105:934, 1984.

104. Juul S et al: New insights into idiopathic infantile arterial calcinosis, Am J Dis Child 144:229, 1990.

105. Moran JJ: Idiopathic arterial calcification of infancy: a clinicopathologic study, Pathol Annu 10:393, 1975.

106. Sholler GF et al: Generalized arterial calcification of infancy: three case reports, including spontaneous regression with long-term survival, J Pediatr 105:257, 1984.
107. Van Dyck M et al: Idiopathic infantile arterial calcification with cardiac, renal and central nervous system involvement, Eur J Pediatr 148:374, 1989.
108. Marrott PK et al: Idiopathic infantile arterial calcification with survival into adult life, Pediatr Cardiol 5:119, 1984.
109. Herman WH et al: Closing the gap: the problem of diabetes mellitus in the United States, Diabetes Care 8:391, 1985.
110. Meema HE et al: Arterial calcifications in severe chronic renal disease and their relationship to dialysis treatment, renal transplant and parathyroidectomy, Radiology 121:315, 1976.
111. Meema HE and Oreopoulos DG: Arterial calcifications in patients undergoing chronic peritoneal dialysis: incidence, progression and regression, PD Bull 6:241, 1985.
112. Wilkinson SP et al: Symmetric gangrene of the extremities in late renal failure: a case report and review of the literature, Q J Med 67:319, 1988.
113. Janigan DT et al: Acute skin and fat necrosis during sepsis in a patient with chronic renal failure and subcutaneous arterial calcification, Am J Kidney Dis 20:643, 1992.
114. Mallick NP and Berlyne GM: Arterial calcification after vitamin D therapy in hyperphosphatemic renal failure, Lancet 2:1316, 1968.
115. Levin A, Mehta RL, Goldstein MB: Mathematical formulation to help identify the patient at risk of ischemic tissue necrosis—a potentially lethal complication of chronic renal failure. Am J Nephrol 13:448, 1993.
116. Ross CN et al: Proximal cutaneous necrosis associated with small vessel calcification in renal failure. Q J Med 79:443, 1991.
117. Duh Q, Lim RC, Clark OH: Calciphylaxis in secondary hyperparathyroidism. Diagnosis and parathyroidectomy, Arch Surg 126:1213, 1991.
118. Mehta RL et al: Skin necrosis associated with acquired protein C deficiency in patients with renal failure and calciphylaxis, Am J Med 88:252, 1990.
119. Vassa N, Twardowski Z, Campbell J: Hyperbaric oxygen therapy in calciphylaxis-induced skin necrosis in a peritoneal dialysis patient, Am J Kidney Dis 23:878, 1994.

CHAPTER TWENTY-FIVE

VASCULOGENIC IMPOTENCE

Ralph G. DePalma

HISTORICAL BACKGROUND

Interest in vasculogenic impotence began with Leriche's[1] 1923 observation that aortoiliac atherosclerosis led to erectile failure due to inadequate cavernosal perfusion. Because aortic operations themselves often caused postoperative impotence,[2,3] in the 1970s techniques were developed to minimize this complication.[4] The use of vascular surgical procedures to revascularize the cavernous bodies became a subject of increasing interest in the late 1970s.

In 1982 stimulation of erection by intracorporal injection of the vasoactive agents papaverine[5] and phentolamine[6] changed this emphasis. Not only did the use of intracavernous injection (ICI) lead to effective methods for better delineation of erectile physiology, ICI also evolved as an important diagnostic and therapeutic tool. Although the original vasoactive substances remain valuable for certain applications, due to the risks of priapism and legal issues in the United States, prostaglandin E_1 is currently preferred for ICI.

Modern research emphasis shifted from methods to increase arterial inflow or to diminish venous outflow toward detailed study of the cavernosal smooth muscle itself. Notable advances included elaboration of the roles of nitric oxide and oxygen tension[7] on erectile function. Current diagnosis and therapy rely on noninvasive studies of blood flow as well as the effects of ICI with vasoactive drugs in planning initial treatment. However, there remains a subset of men comprising about 6% to 7% of those who present with the complaint of impotence who exhibit well-defined arterial or venous abnormalities. Depending on etiology, about 70% of this subset will respond to appropriate vascular interventions.[8]

PATHOGENESIS

Impotence is a symptom, not a disease. The box on this page classifies various causes of vasculogenic impotence. Although vasculogenic abnormalities are common, erec-

FACTORS IN VASCULOGENIC IMPOTENCE

Cavernosal

Arteriolar	Functional or anatomic
	Helicine vessel abnormalities
	Blood pressure medication
Fibrosis	Postpriapic; drug injection
Peyronie's disease	Deformity invading cavernous smooth muscle
	Venous leakage through tunica albuginea
Refractory smooth muscle	Hormonal: prolactinemia, low testosterone level
	Blood pressure medication
	Metabolic: diabetes, uremia

Venous Leakage

Acquired	Abnormal tunica albuginea; traumatic lesions
Congenital	Isolated leakage from corpora into the spongiosum

Arterial

Aortoiliac atherosclerosis

Steal due to external iliac disease

Occlusive disease of pudendal arteries

Occlusive disease of penile arteries	Atherosclerotic Idiopathic proliferative

Atheroembolization

tile failure is also caused by endocrine, metabolic, neurologic, and psychogenic factors. Any of these can coexist with vasculogenic impotence or even in a sense be etiologic, since erectile failure is a vascular dysfunction. Some form of arterial inflow abnormality is associated with the complaint of impotence in 45% of men screened noninvasively.[8,9] Endocrine causes of impotence, except for diabetes, are less common. In my experience, about 3% to 4% of men demonstrate consistently lowered testosterone levels, an experience similar to that of Keogh et al.[10] Keogh et al also noted that when thyroid hypofunction was detected, restoration to a euthyroid state failed to reverse impotence. The most common accompanying factors in men complaining of impotence are diabetes and the use of antihypertensive drugs. Overall, 28% of men tested neurologically for the complaint of impotence[11] exhibit one or more abnormalities in pudendal- or tibial-evoked potentials or in bulbocavernosal reflex times.

In understanding the pathogenesis of penile erectile dysfunction, the clinician must consider two interrelated hemodynamic processes in normal erection: (1) an adequate arterial flow increase and (2) closure or marked reduction of venous outflow. Both processes depend on relaxation of the cavernosal smooth muscle, which in turn depends on intact neural mechanisms as well as the physiology of the smooth muscle–endothelial complex comprising the cavernous tissues. To function normally, an adequate supply of oxygenated arterial flow is needed. Relaxation of the subalbugineal smooth muscle conditions closure of cavernosal outflow needed for a normal erection. The hemodynamics of the erectile process have been recently reviewed.[9] During normal erection, intracavernous pressure increases from pressure approximating venous pressure in the flaccid state to 80 to 90 mm Hg in the erect state. Higher and even suprasystolic pressures are generated by perineal muscle contraction.

PATHOLOGY

Abnormalities can exist in each of the three areas outlined in the box on p. 441. In pure arteriogenic impotence caused by macrovascular disease, the pathology of the aortoiliac system is almost always atherosclerotic, though fibromuscular hyperplasia causing a steal phenomenon has been seen.[12] Atherosclerotic involvement can be either occlusive or aneurysmal and can involve the internal iliac system itself. Another type of occlusive disease may involve the internal pudendal artery, usually in Alcock's canal, as this artery exits the pelvis. These lesions have not been characterized pathologically. Diffuse penile artery disease in young men is not atherosclerotic but rather a fibrotic obliteration of the vascular lumen. Perineal trauma or pelvic fractures cause mechanical interruption of blood supply, whereas radiation causes diffuse vascular injury in some cases.

Structural abnormalities of the cavernosal smooth muscle have proved to be difficult to define.[13] Changes in structure and function in aging human corporal smooth muscle are as yet poorly documented, though some studies suggest that these occur. In aging rats decreased nitric

oxide synthetase has been demonstrated histochemically.[14] Recent studies support the idea that endothelially derived relaxant factor (nitric oxide) is a key mediator of nonadrenergic noncholinergic neurotransmission in normal erection. Histochemically, NADH diaphorase–positive nerve fibers have been demonstrated in human penile tissue[15] along with other neurotransmitters including vasoactive polypeptide (VIP) as well as fibers positive for acetylcholinesterase. It is important to recognize that in flaccidity, the corporal smooth muscle is intensely contracted due to normally present overriding adrenergic tone.[16] Erection is accomplished by release of overriding adrenergic tone. Other receptors in penile smooth muscle include those corresponding to VIP, dopamine, prostaglandin, and other mediators. Thus abnormalities in either neurotransmitter or cell receptors can lead to failure of corporal muscle relaxation. For example, testosterone has recently been shown in experimental animals to stimulate nitric oxide synthetase activity in corporal tissue.[17]

Cigarette smoking is strongly associated with vasculogenic impotence, presumably because of its effect on accelerating atherosclerosis. This addiction caused nonresponsiveness to ICI in young men after intravenous injection of 100 mg of papaverine in volunteers previously responsive to this potent dose of vasoactive agent.[18] This dramatic effect is probably due to stimulation of adrenergic tone caused by cigarette smoke. Structural changes, notably fibrosis of the cavernous tissues, can be caused by untreated priapism, drug injection, hyperosmolar contrast media, Peyronie's disease, and trauma. Placement of conventional prostheses also causes loss of cavernous tissue.

The pathology of cavernosal leakage is difficult to document in most instances. Congenital venous leaks occur as a communication between the corpus cavernosum and the spongiosum, usually in the area of the glans penis. These can be seen by cavernosography in a young man who from the time of puberty has never had satisfactory erections. Both a large vein and tunical defect are present. Acquired cavernosal leakage is more difficult to define pathologically. As noted, cavernosal leakage can be due to failure of smooth muscle to relax from any cause. Cavernosal "leakage" is constant in the flaccid state. Causes of acquired venous leakage include Peyronie's disease, fracture of the penis, and possibly degenerative changes in albugineal structure, though convincing data to support this process are lacking. Important underlying pathology for venous leakage can relate to undiagnosed arterial disease and failure of smooth muscle relaxation. For example, among men screened for venous leakage based on a previously described noninvasive sequence[19,20] and employing dynamic cavernosometry and cavernosography (DICC), we found that 23% showed unsuspected arterial insufficiency when selective pudendal arteriography was done.[21] This led to the recommendation that both pudendal arteriography and DICC are needed before considering venous interruption or microvascular reconstruction. The etiology of cavernous leakage can be remote from the structure of the cavernous bodies themselves and relate to physiologic effects on smooth muscle.

CLINICAL PRESENTATIONS

Gradual erectile failure in the absence of traumatic life events and symptomatic lower-extremity vascular disease suggest large-vessel arteriogenic impotence. In these men both the intensity and duration of risk factors predisposing to atherosclerosis (i.e., smoking, hypertension, diabetes, and hyperlipidemia) contribute to arteriogenic impotence. Aortoiliac aneurysms or ulcerative disease can cause embolic pudendal or penile artery occlusion. A recent observation is that small aortoiliac aneurysms, particularly at the bifurcation of the distal common iliac,[8,22] can be associated with an abrupt onset of impotence due to embolic occlusion as documented by penile Doppler studies and plethysmography.

In a recent analysis of vascular interventions for impotence,[8] men with arteriogenic impotence due to aortoiliac disease averaged 61 years of age. During the same period, impotent men with small-vessel disease or venous leakage averaged 42 to 47 years of age. In this latter category of men, risk factors for atherosclerosis were less frequent. In some cases of distal arterial disease, particularly in men in their third or fourth decades, risk factors were virtually absent. Many diabetics and hypertensives taking medication present with impotence in the absence of abnormalities of penile arterial perfusion. In the diabetics neuropathy is an important factor and should be documented when possible by testing of the appropriate somatic pathways. The immediate onset of impotence following rectal, urologic, or vascular surgery is a critical historical point that requires neurovascular testing. Finally, drug or excessive alcohol use often correlates with onset of impotence.

DIAGNOSIS

History and physical examination contribute to an understanding of possible causes of impotence; in some cases, however, physical examination is often unrevealing. Preexamination vascular testing results are therefore of value at the first visit. The historical points in presentation previously described are often more important than physical findings. Clearly, absent lower-limb pulses suggest macrovascular disease, and femoral bruits are associated with pelvic arterial disease. Neuropathy can be, in some cases, detected on physical examination by sensory testing of the extremities, perineum, or glans penis. However, measurement of evoked potentials and bulbocavernosus reflex time is more sensitive. At this time the prostate is examined; palpation of the corpora cavernosa and estimation of testicular size complete the specific examination. Absence or atrophy of testicular mass suggests hypogonadism, which must be confirmed by low testosterone levels. During the initial visit laboratory studies include levels of testosterone, prolactin, prostatic specific antigen, and blood glucose. Many diabetics will be found; often men reporting diet-controlled diabetes exhibit casual blood glucose levels in excess of 300 mg/dl. Among 1145 men screened, the author found 2 prolactinomas; Keogh et al[10] reported 20 prolactinomas among 6428 men screened. Therefore although primary endocrine disorders apart from diabetes are rare, screening for these abnormalities is of value.

DIFFERENTIAL DIAGNOSIS

A variety of noninvasive or invasive alternatives are available to investigate men with erectile dysfunction. At this time no universally accepted approach exists. A limited and patient goal-directed approach that depends on initial responsiveness to therapy has been suggested.[23] Should initial medical therapy (e.g., oral medications) fail, further investigation can be done. This approach would use, for example, vacuum constrictor devices (VCDs) or ICI with no attempt to outline etiology. When these modalities fail, further invasive tests are indicated. The clinician must keep in mind that impotence may signal a lethal disorder such as abdominal aneurysm, diabetes, renal failure, or more rarely prolactinoma.

The author's approach uses previsit neurovascular testing[24,25] and ICI usually at the first visit. Depending on initial findings of noninvasive testing and patient desires, ICI with 10 to 30 μg of prostaglandin E_1[26] is used to observe the erectile response. ICI in this setting provides a measure of vascular responsiveness, may uncover Peyronie's disease, and provides an estimate of ICI as future therapy. Previsit neurovascular testing helps determine initial dosage of prostaglandin; patients with normal penile pressure and neurologic dysfunction can be exquisitely sensitive, whereas those with low pressure often need initially higher doses. Patients who ultimately fail to erect with ICI become candidates for further invasive testing to determine whether they might be candidates for vascular interventions. The details of noninvasive and invasive testing are described in the next sections.

NONINVASIVE TESTING

Penile/Brachial Indices

The penile/brachial index (PBI) is a ratio between the systolic pressure detected by a Doppler probe placed distal to a penile cuff and systemic or brachial arm pressure. In an average-sized penis a cuff of at least 2.5 cm is used. The cuff is inflated, then deflated. Reappearance of Doppler signals in the dorsal artery branches just proximal to the corona of the glans signals reflow. Normally this pressure is systemic. PBI above 0.75 suggests that no major obstacle exists between the aorta and the distal measurement point (Fig. 25-1). Generally PBI less than 0.6 relates to major vascular obstructions in the aortoiliac bed. PBI between 0.6 and 0.75 is abnormal and can occur with lesions involving the internal pudendal and the penile arteries.

Penile Plethysmographic Pulse-Volume Recording

Penile plethysmographic pulse-volume recording (PVR) is performed using a pneumoplethysmographic cuff with a contained transducer[19,27] on the penis in the flaccid state. The variables recorded are crest time, waveform, and the presence or absence of a dicrotic notch. Penile PVR

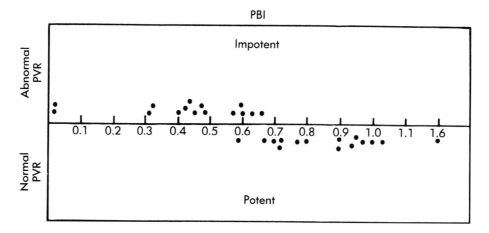

Fig. 25-1. Relationship between PBI and PVR in clinically potent and impotent men. Note the zone of overlap at PBI of 0.6 to 0.7. (Recordings obtained with Buffington Plethysmographic Cuff, Buffington Clinical Systems, Inc., P.O. Box 24241, Cleveland, OH 44124.)

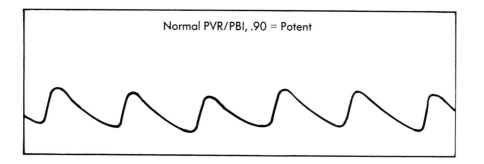

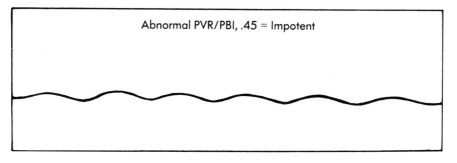

Fig. 25-2. Examples of pulse wave recordings in potent and impotent patients with arterial insufficiency.

measures total pulsation of all penile arteries as the cuff compresses the penile tissue. The cuff is applied and inflated to mean arterial pressure, which is calculated as diastolic pressure plus one third of systemic pulse pressure. Waveforms are recorded on a polygraph with a chart speed of 25 mm/sec and a sensitivity setting of 1. In normal patients the upstroke of the waveform is completed by 0.2 second (5 mm); normal waveform amplitudes vary from 5 to 6 to 30 mm in height (Fig. 25-2). These tests help detect arteriogenic impotence. However, vasculogenic impotence caused by venous leak or Peyronie's disease is not detected. The sensitivity of these tests predicted an abnormal arteriogram in 85% of the cases; specificity (i.e., percent of true negatives) was 70%.[25]

Neurologic Testing

Neural disorders frequently contribute to erectile failure. Among 290 patients evaluated in our laboratory using pudendal-evoked potentials and measuring bulbocavernosus reflex, 84 men (28%) exhibited at least one abnormality. Such subtle neurologic changes are not detected by ordinary physical examination. The use of pudendal-evoked potentials in the evaluation of impotence has shown that reproducible responses can be obtained.[11,28,29] Normal reference latencies for pudendal, lumbar, and cortical somatosensory-evoked potentials have been measured. Because many impotent patients are diabetic, pudendal responses are compared with spinal and cortical-evoked responses from posterior tibial nerve stimulation.

Bulbocavernosus reflex time after dorsal penile nerve stimulation is also measured. Mean normal bulbocavernosus reflex time in our laboratory is 28.3 to 37.5 ms. Grossly abnormal findings suggesting neurologic deficits contraindicate vascular operations for impotence.

Duplex Scanning

Color flow duplex scanning can be used to examine penile arteries at intervals after ICI or ICI combined[30,31] with visual sexual stimulation (VSS). Values for normal middle-aged men after ICI using prostaglandin E_1 and VSS have been suggested to be a 70% increase in deep cavernosal artery diameter and systolic peak blood flow velocities above 30 cm/sec. Duplex scanning might also suggest venous leakage in the presence of high diastolic cavernosal artery flow. Here the data are less secure, and ultimately the duplex scan is used to select for arteriography or DICC. If an aneurysm is suspected, an appropriate probe can be used at this time to examine the abdomen. In contrast to PBI and plethysmography, duplex scanning is time intensive and requires a physician present for ICI. Patients must be observed in the clinic to assure subsidence of the induced erection. A recent report showed the diagnostic difficulties of the use of duplex scanning to evaluate the corporal venoocclusive mechanism. False-positive results were noted in 22% of patients when compared with nocturnal penile tumescence (NPT).[32]

NPT is a useful study particularly when psychogenic impotence is likely and in cases with medicolegal problems. NPT is done optimally in a formal sleep laboratory setting using three nights of monitoring[33] and measurement of erectile rigidity during maximum tumescence. Normal penile rigidity is taken at 400 to 500 g of buckling pressure. Although NPT testing is time-consuming and expensive, a normal sleep erection virtually rules out organic erectile dysfunction.

INVASIVE TESTING

DICC provides a measure of venous efflux and localizes sites of cavernosal leakage. Flow to maintain erection (FME) is a valid measure provided complete muscular relaxation has been obtained to produce a linear pressure flow relationship as recently described.[34] ICI in this setting requires much larger doses of vasoactive agents and sometimes reinjection.

Although impotence is often caused by inadequate arterial supply, closure of the venous outflow system is also needed to achieve and maintain an erection. Arterial and venous function are thus closely interrelated. Erection begins with cavernosal smooth muscle relaxation. This in turn decreases peripheral vascular resistance within the penis and increases arterial flow. Resulting dilation of the sinusoidal spaces then occludes the veins that pass through the tunica albuginea, dramatically reducing venous outflow. During maximal erection sinusoidal pressure at some point equilibrates with arterial inflow pressure; this value is called cavernosal artery occlusion pressure (CAOP).

During studies using fine needles inserted into the cavernous bodies, it is possible to measure CAOP with a Doppler probe. If arterial pressure is reduced by proximal occlusion, penile rigidity cannot occur. Cavernosal pressure also cannot rise when venous leakage is excessive. Such leakage can be caused by either congenital or more commonly acquired leaks through the tunica albuginea.

Techniques have been adapted from those described by Bookstein et al,[35] Goldstein,[36] and Lue et al.[37] To perform cavernosometry and cavernosography, two 21-gauge butterfly needles are placed into each corpora cavernosa for infusion of pharmacologic agents, saline solution, and pressure monitoring. Constant cavernosal pressure monitoring and an infusion pump are used. A 60 mg amount of papaverine and 1 mg of phentolamine, diluted to a total volume of 5 ml, are injected. After 15 minutes heparinized saline solution is infused at a rate of 20 ml/min. This rate is gradually increased until a rigid erection occurs. Cavernosal pressure then usually exceeds 100 mm Hg. The infusion rate is lowered to achieve steady-state cavernosal pressure at this level. The flow rate to induce erection (FIE) and FME are recorded. Infusion rate is then further increased to produce a suprasystolic cavernosal pressure of 150 mm Hg, and the infusion is stopped. The rate of fall of cavernosal pressure over the succeeding 30 seconds is recorded.

To visualize venous leaks, a diluted nonionic contrast agent is injected, and spot filming in various obliquities is performed to identify specific abnormal opacified veins. FMEs of less than 12 ml/min have been proposed as normal, whereas a rate greater than 45 ml/min exceeds the ability of even a normal arterial system to compensate for increased venous leakage. Goldstein suggests that the rate of pressure fall of greater than 1 mm Hg/sec strongly suggests cavernosal leakage.

Following these procedures, CAOP is measured. CAOP, a physiologic index of penile arterial supply, is thought to be normal when greater than 90 mm Hg. However, a cavernosal brachial gradient must be taken into consideration. In certain cases a gradient greater than 30 mm Hg suggests arterial inflow reduction even if CAOP is greater than 90 mm Hg.

ARTERIOGRAPHY

To detect arterial occlusion and to determine candidacy for vascular interventions, selective arteriographic studies are needed. Conventional aortoiliac studies are used to demonstrate large-vessel disease and should be used when PBI or lower-extremity pulses are abnormal. Highly selective internal iliac arteriography using nonionic contrast media and ICI to produce partial penile tumescence (not full erection) are needed to display pudendal and penile anatomy. As mentioned previously, DICC, CAOP, and selective arteriography are all required in potential candidates for microvascular reconstructions or venous ablation.

TREATMENT OF VASCULOGENIC IMPOTENCE

The box on p. 446 summarizes treatment options. Medical treatment is generally tried first. For all patients it is wise to recommend risk factor intervention, particularly cessation of cigarette smoking and control of hypercholes-

TREATMENT OF VASCULOGENIC IMPOTENCE

Medical
Risk factor interventions
    Smoking cessation
    Control of diabetes
    Change of blood pressure medication
Drugs
    Isoxsuprine
    Yohimbine hydrochloride
    Trazodone
Injections
    Intracorporeal papaverine*
    Phentolamine
    Prostaglandin E₁
    Vacuum constrictor devices

Surgical
Arterial dysfunction
    Aortoiliac and/or internal iliac reconstruction or dilation
    Dorsal artery bypass
    Dorsal vein arterialization
Cavernosal or neurogenic
    Prostheses
Cavernosal leakage
    Vein resection and interruption
    Transcatheter venous occlusion

*Not currently available.

terolemia. In some cases it is possible to alter antihypertensive treatment by weight control or changing drugs. After ICI using prostaglandin E₁, some men resume function. In cases of mild arteriogenic impotence, this effect can be enhanced by the addition of isoxsuprine 10 to 20 mg four times a day. In addition, yohimbine hydrochloride (Yocon) is effective in some cases. Its mechanism of action is unknown. In the author's experience 10% to 15% of patients resume satisfactory function. Self-injection programs, with proper supervision, can also be offered to carefully selected patients.

Revascularization of penile vessels and venous interruption should offer ideal options in patients failing to respond to ICI or VCD, provided an accurate diagnosis has been obtained. Presently these procedures are being reappraised.[38-40] Skepticism exists because reported results range from 33% to 100% success rates with scanty life-table data to support these claims. No uniform methods of post-operative surveillance have been agreed on. The true success rates of these procedures are currently unknown. This situation is similar to the early era of coronary revascularization. Penile artery bypass, deep dorsal vein arterialization, and venous interruption are evolving procedures. However, with accurate preoperative evaluation these procedures are of value in carefully selected patients.

Techniques of aortoiliac surgery to perfuse the internal iliac arteries and spare autonomic nerves are less controversial and more effective. In a recent report of 10 years' experience in macrovascular interventions,[8] 23 of 1145 men screened for the complaint of impotence received various aortoiliac procedures for aneurysm or occlusive disease. Among these 58% resumed continuous spontaneous erectile function in follow-ups ranging from 33 to 48 months. An additional 15% functioned using ICI or VCD.

In contrast, among 50 men undergoing penile artery bypass, deep dorsal vein arterialization, or venous interruption followed for an average of 35 to 48 months, 27% to 33% functioned spontaneously. The additional use of ICI increased function to 70% overall. All cases for these procedures should be selected on the basis of initial screening sequences,[25] failure to respond to ICI or VCD, absence of diabetes, need for hypertensive medications, and patterns of vascular disease appropriate for arterial bypass or venous ligation.

Four subsets of men with vasculogenic impotence exhibit differing and rather distinct patterns of vascular pathology; each type requires a properly selected approach. These include macrovascular aortoiliac disease, pudendal or penile artery local occlusions, diffuse penile obstructive disease, and cavernosal leakage with discrete leakage sites. About 1 in 100 impotent men may exhibit aneurysmal disease; these aneurysms might often be less than 5 cm in size. Although atheroembolism coinciding with abrupt onset of impotence can be correlated in some of these men, aneurysmectomy will not reverse this process if penile atheroembolism has been extensive. In addition, a 1% prevalence of aneurysmal disease in men in their sixth or seventh decades is not unexpected, and impotence might simply be coincidental in some of these cases.

For microvascular bypass to the dorsal penile artery using the inferior epigastric artery,[41] the best responders remain young men[42] with isolated pudendal artery involvement or those with lesions caused by trauma. Diffuse penile arterial disease not suitable for bypass, or mixed arterial and venous impotence, has been treated using deep dorsal vein arterialization.[43,44] This procedure has the disadvantage of glans hyperemia as an early or late complication. Additionally the physiologic mechanism by which this procedure influences erectile function is unclear. The direction of arterial flow appears to be mainly into the spongiosum as seen by us,[45] and documented by others using magnetic resonance imaging.[46] Similar to the author's experience[8] in arteriographically recent follow-ups, about one half to one third of these men report spontaneous function,[47,48] whereas 70% achieve erections with ICI, which was previously ineffective.

Venous interruption efficacy clearly correlates with correction of abnormally elevated FME from 80 ml/min or greater to postoperative values of 40 ml/min or less.[49] If this reduction is not obtained, there is failure to erect either spontaneously or with ICI. Although immediate postoperative function rates are high after venous ligation, there is a rapid decrement in function over the ensuing 36 months. However, 70% function overall with ICI. Studies using postoperative DICC have shown the development of sequential leakage from other sources, which accounts for this fall in function. Therefore as complete an interruption as possible is a desirable goal of the initial procedure. Anatomic factors favoring success in the author's experience are dominant leakage from the deep dorsal vein[9]; diffuse cavernous spongiosum leakage offers a poor prognosis.

SUMMARY

In summarizing treatment of vasculogenic impotence, the clinician will recognize that most men can be treated medically. Although self-injection with prostaglandin E_1 is commonly used, a search continues for locally or intraurethrally applicable vasoactive active agents.[50,51] It is now clear that orally administered drugs can induce erection and even cause priapism in the case of trazodone.[16] Investigating oral agents capable of inactivating overactive α-adrenoreceptor activity in cavernous smooth muscle is important. Prosthetic devices for diabetics with severe neurovascular dysfunction can be recommended after appropriate investigations and trials of therapy. An interesting new development is the Subrini[52,53] soft implant. This device is neither inflatable nor meant to provide rigidity. Rather the implant occupies space in the cavernous bodies; it is placed in such a manner as to minimize interference with vessels and cavernous tissue. Thus normal tumescence is enhanced in naturally erotic situations.

In a previous iteration of this chapter, the reader was provided with an algorithmic approach to diagnosis and treatment of vasculogenic impotence. It can be appreciated, however, that no single approach is currently applicable for all patients. Based on patients' goals or desires, treatment must be individualized. The author relies heavily on results of neurovascular screening and reserves invasive testing for men who fail to respond to initial therapy. It is of course imperative to rule out aneurysmal, embolic, and other life-threatening diseases sometimes signaled by the complaint of impotence.

REFERENCES

1. Leriche R: Des obliterations arterielle hautes (obliteration de la termination de l'aorte) comme cause de insufficances circulatoire des membres inferiurs, Bull Mem Soc Chir 49:1404, 1923 (abstract).
2. Leriche R and Morel A: The syndrome of thrombotic obliteration of the aortic bifurcation, Ann Surg 127:193, 1948.
3. May AG, Rob CB, and DeWeese JA: Changes in sexual function following operation on the abdominal aorta, Surgery 65:41, 1969.
4. DePalma RG, Levine SB, and Feldman S: Preservation of erectile function after aortoiliac reconstruction, Arch Surg 113:902, 1978.
5. Virag R: Intracavernous injection of papaverine for erectile failure, Lancet 2:938, 1982.
6. Brindley GS: Pilot experiments on the actions of drugs injected into the corpus cavernosum penis, Br J Psychiatry 87:495, 1986.
7. Azadzoi KM, Negra A, and Siroky MB: Effects of cavernosal hypoxia and oxygenation on penile erection, Int J Impotence Res 6(suppl I):D4, 1994 (abstract).
8. DePalma RG et al: Vascular interventions for impotence: lessons learned, J Vasc Surg 21:576, 1995.
9. DePalma RG: Mechanisms of vasculogenic impotence. In White RA and Hollier LA, eds: Vascular surgery: basic science and clinical correlations, Philadelphia, 1994, JB Lippincott.
10. Keogh ET et al: Medical management of impotence, Int J Impot Res 6(suppl I):S13, 1994 (abstract).
11. Emsellem HA et al: Pudendal evoked potentials in the evaluation of impotence, J Clin Neurophysiol 5:359, 1988.
12. DePalma RG et al: Modern management of impotence associated with aortic surgery. In Bergan JJ and Yao JST, eds: Arterial surgery: new diagnostic and operative techniques, Orlando, Fl, 1988, Grune & Stratton.
13. Sohn M et al: Histological and ultrastructural workup of cavernous tissue from impotent patients, Int J Impot Res 6(suppl I):D14, 1994 (abstract).
14. Carrier S et al: The effect of aging on erectile function in the rat, Int J Impot Res 6(suppl I):D16, 1994 (abstract).
15. Gopalakrishnakone P et al: NADPH-diaphorase and VIP positive nerve fibres in human penile erectile tissue, Int J Impotence Res 6(suppl I):A26, 1994 (abstract).
16. Adaikan PG: Physio-pharmacological basis of treatment for erectile dysfunction, Int J Impot Res 6(suppl I):PL1, 1994 (abstract).
17. Brock GB et al: Nitric oxide synthase is testosterone dependent, Int J Impot Res 6(suppl I):D42, 1994 (abstract).
18. Glina S et al: Impact of cigarette smoking on papaverine induced erection, J Urol 140:523, 1988.
19. DePalma RG et al: A screening sequence for vasculogenic impotence, J Vasc Surg 5:228, 1987.
20. DePalma RG and Michal V: Point of view; deja vu again: advantages and limitations of methods for assessing penile arterial flow, Urology 36:199, 1990.
21. DePalma RG et al: Predictive value of a screening sequence for venogenic impotence, Int J Impot Res 4:143, 1992.
22. DePalma RG and Massarin E: Occult aortoiliac disease in men with primary complaint of erectile dysfunction, Int J Impot Res 6(suppl I):A50, 1994 (abstract).
23. Lue TF: Impotence: a patients goal-directed approach to treatment, World J Urol 8:67, 1990.
24. DePalma RG: What constitutes an adequate impotence workup, World J Urol 10:157, 1992.
25. DePalma RG et al: Noninvasive assessment of impotence. In Pearce WH and Yao JST, eds: The Surgical Clinics of North America: noninvasive diagnosis of vascular diseases, Philadelphia, 1990, WB Saunders.
26. Waldhauser M and Schramek P: Efficiency and side effects of prostaglandin in the treatment of erectile dysfunction, J Urol 140:525, 1988.
27. DePalma RG, Kedia K, and Persky L: Surgical options in the correction of vasculogenic impotence, Vasc Surg 14:92, 1980.
28. Opsomer RJ et al: Pudendal cortical somatosensory evoked potentials, J Urol 135:1216, 1986.
29. Fisher-Santos BL, de Dues Viera AL, and dos Santos ES: Bulbocavernosus reflex and evoked potentials in evidentially normal males, Int J Impot Res 6(suppl I):A12, 1994 (abstract).
30. Lewis RW and King BF: Dynamic color Doppler sonography in the evaluation of penile erectile disorders, Int J Impot Res 6(suppl I):A30, 1994 (abstract).
31. Lue TF et al: Vasculogenic impotence evaluated by high-resolution ultrasonography and pulsed Doppler spectrum, Radiology 155:777, 1985.
32. Mansour MOA: Anxiety mediated impotence misdiagnosed as venogenic impotence by color duplex scanning: a comparison with nocturnal tumescence monitoring, Int J Impot Res 6(suppl I):A36, 1994 (abstract).

33. Ware JC et al, eds: Principles and practice of sleep medicine, Philadelphia, 1989, WB Saunders.

34. Udelson D et al: A new methodology of pharmacocavernosometry which enables hemodynamic analysis under conditions of known corporal smooth muscle relaxation, Int J Impot Res 6(suppl I):A17, 1994 (abstract).

35. Bookstein JJ et al: Pharmacoangiographic assessment of the corpora cavernosa, Cardiovasc Intervent Radiol 11:218, 1988.

36. Goldstein I: Overview of types and results of vascular surgical procedures for impotence, Cardiovasc Intervent Radiol 11:240, 1988.

37. Lue TF et al: Functional evaluation of penile veins by cavernosography in papaverine-induced erection, J Urol 135:476, 1986.

38. Furlow WL: Vascular surgery in the treatment of impotence, Int J Impot Res 6(suppl I):S8, 1994 (abstract).

39. Sohn M: Is there an indication for invasive diagnostic workup and vascular surgery in patients with erectile dysfunction? Int J Impot Res 6(suppl I):S7, 1994 (abstract).

40. Sharlip I: A critical evaluation of short and long-term results of penile revascularization, Int J Impot Res 6(suppl I):59, 1994 (abstract).

41. DePalma RG and Olding MJ: Surgery for vasculogenic impotence. In Greenhalgh RM, ed: Vascular and endovascular surgical techniques, ed 3, London, 1994, WB Saunders.

42. Krane RG, Goldstein I, and DeTejada IS: Impotence, N Engl J Med 321:1648, 1989.

43. DePalma RG: Surgery for sexual impotence. In Jamieson CW and Yao JST, eds: Rob and Smith's operative surgery, ed 5, London, 1994, Chapman and Hall.

44. Furlow WL, Knoll LD, and Benson RC: Deep dorsal vein arterialization in the Furlow-Fischer modification in 156 patients with vasculogenic impotence, Int J Impot Res 4(suppl 2):A133, 1992 (abstract).

45. DePalma RG and Olding MF: Surgery for vasculogenic impotence. In Greenhalgh RM, ed: Vascular surgical techniques: an atlas, London, 1989, WB Saunders.

46. Sohn MH et al: Objective follow-up after penile revascularization, Int J Impot Res 4:73, 1992.

47. Schramek P, Engelmann U, and Kaufmann F: Microsurgical arterialization in the treatment of vasculogenic impotence, J Urol 147:1028, 1992.

48. Cookson MS et al: Analysis of microsurgical penile revascularization by etiology of impotence, J Urol 149:1308, 1993.

49. Yu GW et al: Preoperative and postoperative dynamic cavernosography and cavernosography: objective assessment of venous ligation for impotence, J Urol 147:618, 1992.

50. Cavallini G: Minoxidil plus capsaicine: an association of transcutaneous drugs for erection facilitation, Int J Impot Res 6(suppl I):D71, 1994 (abstract).

51. Canning JR and Marchese KR: Prostaglandin E_1 as a topical agent for treatment of erectile dysfunction, Int J Impot Res 6(suppl I):D82, 1994 (abstract).

52. Lewis RW: Prosthesis—past, present, and future, Int J Impot Res 6(suppl I):S1, 1994.

53. Austoni E et al: Functional role of complementary erection in soft silicone prosthetic penile implant, Int J Impot Res 6(suppl I):D127, 1994 (abstract).

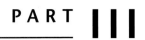

VENOUS DISEASES

CHAPTER TWENTY-SIX

DEEP VEIN THROMBOSIS

Felipe Navarro

John R. Bartholomew

Deep vein thrombosis (DVT) is a common yet often under-recognized condition, especially among hospitalized patients. Although most thrombi in the leg are small, asymptomatic, and confined to the deep calf veins, 20% of these calf vein thrombi extend into the proximal deep veins and can lead to fatal pulmonary embolism.[1]

DVT may present as a painful, swollen leg or arm or may be entirely asymptomatic. This leads to a failure to recognize and treat DVT appropriately and to a potential for significant morbidity and mortality. DVT has two major complications: pulmonary embolism (PE) and the postphlebitic syndrome. Although in this textbook DVT and PE are discussed in separate chapters, the concept that venous thromboembolism is one process is now widely accepted.[2]

Despite recent advances in the diagnosis, treatment, and prevention of venous thromboembolism, the overall incidence may have changed little in the past 30 years.[3] In the United States the actual incidence of venous thromboembolism is uncertain. An estimated 250,000 cases annually was suggested in a 1973 study published by Coon, Willis, and Keller.[4] The 1986 Consensus Conference for the Prevention of Venous Thrombosis and Pulmonary Embolism estimated that there were between 300,000 and 600,000 hospitalizations yearly in the United States for venous thromboembolism.[5] The Worcester DVT study estimated that there are 170,000 new cases of venous thromboembolism annually and another 99,000 hospitalizations for recurrent events.[6] As many as 200,000 persons die every year in the United States of venous thromboembolism, and in 1975 PE was reported to be the third most frequent cause of death in the United States.[7] More than 70% of patients who die of PE are not suspected of having it before death.[8]

HISTORICAL BACKGROUND

The earliest recorded case of DVT was highlighted by Dexter and Folch-Pi[9] in an article published in 1974. They searched the literature and found a case involving a young man in the thirteenth century presenting with a massively swollen leg and leg ulcers, whom they felt had iliofemoral thrombosis. Unilateral leg swelling following childbirth had been recognized for centuries and referred to as "milk leg." In 1769 an obstetrician named Puzo theorized that milk leg was caused by retained milk from mothers who did not nurse.[10] Others attributed this swelling to infection or lymphatic obstruction. In 1823 David D. Davis described clots in the iliac veins found at autopsy of four women who died shortly after childbirth. He is credited with the first clinical description and drawings of venous thrombosis.[10] The concept that a swollen limb could be caused by venous thrombosis was slowly accepted beginning in the latter part of the nineteenth century. Since then much has been learned.

PATHOLOGY

Venous thrombi are composed predominately of red cells, masses of platelets and leukocytes, bound together by fibrin. Venous thrombi normally have a gelatinous, moist appearance and resemble blood clotted in a test tube.[11] Most thrombi form in valve pockets of the deep veins of the calf or thigh, where there are areas of static blood flow.[12,13] Kakkar et al[1] demonstrated this by using iodine[125]–labeled fibrinogen scanning. They found that thrombi initially start in the tibial veins or soleal sinuses and later propagate to the popliteal and femoral veins. Once initiated, thrombi generally propagate in the direction of blood flow by the addition of successive layers of platelets and fibrin.[14] In larger veins thrombi are initially loosely attached to vessel walls, thus giving the potential for detachment and embolization. If embolization does not occur, thrombi resolve by canalization, organization, or lysis by the fibrinolytic system. Further formation, growth, or dissolution of venous thrombi reflects the balance between thrombogenic stimuli, direction and velocity of venous flow, and the protective mechanisms that exist in vivo.

Anatomically 90% of venous thrombi arise from the lower extremities. This has been demonstrated using radioactive fibrinogen scanning and venography.[1,15] Other sources of thrombi include the upper extremities, the right side of the heart, and the pelvic veins. Most fatal pulmonary emboli originate from the proximal veins of the legs.

PATHOGENESIS

The pathogenesis of DVT is thought to be largely due to vessel wall damage, venous stasis, and increased activation of clotting factors, also referred to as *hypercoagulability*. This concept was first described by Virchow[16] more than a century ago and still remains the fundamental basis for our understanding of thrombosis.

Venous Stasis

Static or altered blood flow in the deep veins of the lower limbs helps to initiate venous thrombi. Normally blood clearance from the lower extremities is enhanced by contractions of the calf muscles, which propel the blood from the calf toward the heart. In the immobile patient, however, the repetitive muscular massaging activity of the deep and superficial veins of the leg is removed and stasis is enhanced.[17] This contributes to venous thrombosis by preventing the activated coagulation factors from being diluted by nonactivated blood, by preventing the clearance of these factors, and by preventing their mixing with the naturally occurring inhibitors.[18,19]

The concept that venous stasis contributes to thrombosis has been demonstrated using thermal dilution techniques, in which venous blood flow is measured in the femoral and iliac veins during surgery. Blood flow decreases by as much as 50% during the induction of anesthesia, and this lower flow appears to remain constant throughout the operation.[20]

Injury to the Vessel Wall

The intact endothelium is normally thromboresistant and prevents thrombosis by eliminating contact between platelets and subendothelial collagen. If there is damage to the vessel wall, however, the exposed subendothelium leads initially to platelet adhesion, followed by platelet aggregation and platelet release.[21] Activation of components of both the intrinsic and extrinsic pathways of coagulation soon follows and further contributes to vessel wall damage.[22-26] Injury to the vessel wall has been suggested to be the strongest risk factor for venous thrombosis.[21] This may occur during any surgical procedure but is especially important in cases of trauma, knee or hip surgery, or in burn victims.

Hypercoagulability

A number of inherited and acquired disorders that can lead to a hypercoagulable state have now been identified. The classification of these disorders into primary and secondary disorders is useful to the clinician for purposes of diagnosis. Primary hypercoagulable disorders are usually inherited in an autosomal dominant manner and are discussed further in Chapter 5. The secondary hypercoagulable states, also referred to by some authors as "predisposing risk factors," are listed in the box on this page and are generally acquired. These predisposing risk factors interact

---

PREDISPOSING RISK FACTORS

Immobilization
Surgery
Trauma
Age
Malignancy
Heart failure
Previous venous thrombosis
Obesity
Pregnancy and contraceptives

---

with the components of Virchow's triad, clearly demonstrating the complexity of thrombosis.

In certain clinical situations these predisposing risk factors are known to increase the patient's susceptibility for thrombosis. Their recognition may help facilitate the early diagnosis and treatment of venous thromboembolism as well as minimize it by encouraging the use of prophylaxis.

IMMOBILIZATION. In addition to the increased risk of thrombosis during surgery, preoperative and postoperative immobility is also associated with an increased incidence of venous thrombosis.[27,28] Postoperative patients remain at risk during their entire period of immobility. This immobility may persist after discharge and must not be forgotten when trying to determine why a patient has had a thrombotic event.[29] The concept that immobilization plays an important role in thrombosis is also supported by the frequency of venous thrombosis in the paralyzed limb of stroke patients, the increased incidence of thrombosis in patients with incapacitating cardiac or pulmonary disorders, in healthy patients during long airplane rides or motor vehicle trips, or in cases of trauma and inappropriate extended bed rest. Autopsy findings have also confirmed this idea, especially in patients confined to bed for more than a week.[30]

SURGERY. The risk of venous thrombosis after surgery is related to the site and extent of the surgical procedure, the duration and nature of the operation, and the length of time that the patient remains immobilized before and after surgery. In addition, the underlying disease process and preoperative and postoperative risk factors also increase the risk for DVT. Patients undergoing orthopedic procedures involving the hip, knee, or pelvis; neurosurgery; and major pelvic or abdominal surgery for malignancy appear to be at the greatest risk. A number of well-recognized thrombogenic factors are associated with surgery and include the release of tissue thromboplastin, stasis from immobilization, and a reduction in the fibrinolytic systems activity. Intraoperative venodilation at veins distant from the operative site has also been proposed as a possible cause of postoperative thrombosis.[31] In total hip replacement operative venography shows that the femoral vein is markedly twisted and distorted. Endothelial damage likely occurs as a consequence of this distortion and is partially responsible for the unique localization of thrombi in the proximal venous segment in some patients.

TRAUMA. Patients with major trauma have a very high risk of venous thromboembolism. In a recent study predictive factors for venous thrombosis in the trauma patient included age, the need for surgery or blood transfusion, spinal cord injuries, or the presence of lower-extremity fractures.[32] Increased length of stay and reduced mobility were also associated with an increased risk for thrombosis.[32]

AGE. Increasing age is an important risk factor for venous thrombosis, but the underlying mechanism is unclear.[26,27] Age over 60 years was cited in a recent report of risk factors for DVT in outpatients.[33] Possible explanations include decreased mobility secondary to disease states and venous dilation that occurs in the elderly, which results in increased venous stasis. The fibrinolytic response may also decrease in persons above the age of 65. Other unknown mechanisms undoubtedly also contribute to the high risk of venous thrombosis that occurs with advanced age. DVT occurs in the pediatric and adolescent population; however, the incidence is not known, and the mechanisms and anatomic location for thrombosis may be different. In a study of 137 patients between the ages of 1 month and 18 years of age, the incidence of DVT/PE was 0.07 per 10,000 children with 50 of the thrombotic events located in the arm and 79 in the lower extremities. Predisposing conditions in this age group seemed related to the frequent use of central venous lines.[34]

MALIGNANCY. Patients with malignancy can develop recurrent superficial DVT, venous thrombosis in unusual anatomic sites, thrombosis resistant to anticoagulant therapy and, rarely, phlegmasia cerulea dolens.[22,26,27] The risk of venous thrombosis after surgery for malignant conditions is two to three times greater than the risk for nonmalignant conditions.

A number of factors contribute to the increased risk of venous thrombosis in patients with malignant disease. These include the elaboration of a tissue thromboplastin-like substance from the tumor, a reduced fibrinolytic activity in some patients with malignancy, compression or infiltration of the vein by the cancer, increased age of the patient, and a greater potential for surgical procedures. Patients with neoplasms of the gastrointestinal tract, lung, urogenital tract, breast, and intracranial tumors appear to be at the greatest risk for thrombosis.[35] Because of the well-known association between thrombosis and cancer, a common problem facing the physician is when to look for an underlying malignancy in patients who have no other apparent risk factors for a thrombotic event. In one study of patients presenting with an idiopathic venous thrombosis, cancer was diagnosed in 8% during a follow-up period of 2 years; however, in those individuals who had recurrent thrombosis, the incidence was 17%.[36] Other studies have also demonstrated an increased incidence of an underlying malignancy with idiopathic venous thrombosis.[35,37,38]

HEART FAILURE. Heart failure is a well-established risk factor for venous thrombosis, presumably because of the raised central venous pressure (CVP) and the immobility associated with heart failure.[18,39]

PREVIOUS VENOUS THROMBOSIS. Patients with a history of venous thrombosis have two to three times the risk of developing venous thrombi after elective abdominal surgery.[26,27] Patients with recurrent venous thrombosis also have a three to four times greater risk of developing a subsequent episode of venous thrombosis when anticoagulant therapy is discontinued 3 months instead of 6 months after the initial event.

OBESITY. Obesity is associated with venous thrombosis, probably because it impairs fibrinolytic activity and leads to greater immobility in this population.[26,27] An increased frequency of thromboembolism is noted in patients who weigh more than 20% above the standard amount for their age, sex, and frame size.

PREGNANCY AND CONTRACEPTIVES. The evidence supporting pregnancy as a risk factor is imperfect. The evidence that the low-dose estrogen pill is a risk factor for venous thrombosis is also inconclusive.[40,41]

A number of humoral and mechanical events occurring during a normal pregnancy and delivery, however, do increase the patient's risk of thrombosis. These events include a decrease in the fibrinolytic activity that occurs during the third trimester and in the early stages of labor before placental separation. In addition, the release of tissue thromboplastin at the time of placental separation, venous stasis resulting from deep venous dilation, and the mechanical pressure of the uterus on the inferior vena cava (IVC) during the third trimester and during delivery also play a role. In general, the levels of plasma fibrinogen and coagulation factors VII, VIII, and IX increase during pregnancy, but the relationship of these factors to an increased risk of venous thrombosis is unclear.

Estrogens and oral contraceptive pills produce many of the same changes that occur during pregnancy. They can produce venous dilation, and in some studies estrogens have decreased functional levels of antithrombin III, as well as a decrease in the fibrinolytic activity. Current data indicate that the use of estrogen replacement therapy in postmenopausal women, however, does not increase the risk for venous thrombosis.[42,43]

MISCELLANEOUS RISK FACTORS. Other precipitating risk factors reported to have a high association with venous thrombosis include anesthesia, chemotherapy, varicose veins, inflammatory bowel disease, thrombocytosis, polycythemia vera, systemic lupus erythematosus, and Behçet's syndrome.

DIAGNOSIS OF VENOUS THROMBI

Clinical Diagnosis

The clinical diagnosis of DVT is notoriously unreliable. Many potentially dangerous venous thrombi are clinically silent. Classic findings of pain, edema, and venous distention are not always found (Fig. 26-1). Homans' sign, which is pain in the upper calf during forced dorsiflexion of the foot, is insensitive and nonspecific. It was once considered a classic finding for DVT. The unreliability of clinical diagnosis has been demonstrated by numerous studies that

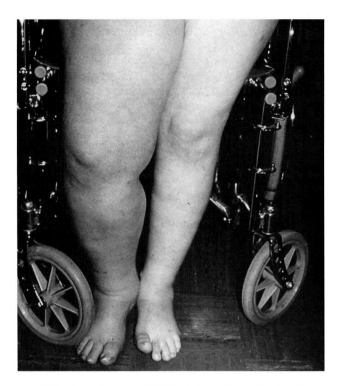

Fig. 26-1. Classic findings of DVT including edema, discoloration, and venous distention.

compare clinical findings with the results of objective testing.[26,44] Hull et al[44] evaluated more than 1000 patients by venography with clinically suspected DVT and found approximately 70% of these patients did not have this diagnosis. In this study the most common clinical findings were pain, tenderness, and swelling. Other clinical features, including night cramps, redness, cyanosis, or dilated veins, were relatively rare and occurred with approximately equal frequency in patients with and without venous thrombosis.

Patients with DVT may present with a pale, cyanotic, or reddish-purple leg. Cyanotic changes are caused by impaired venous return and stagnant anoxic blood flow in the cutaneous vessels. A pale or white leg, earlier referred to as *milk leg,* is caused by extensive iliofemoral vein thrombosis and classically seen postpartum. *Phlegmasia cerulea dolens,* an unusual presentation of DVT, is clinically recognized by pain, blue discoloration, marked swelling, and signs of arterial insufficiency (Fig. 26-2). Patients presenting with phlegmasia often have an underlying malignancy, and many of these patients will require amputation.

Although we continue to rely on the clinical examination to consider the diagnosis of DVT, it is unreliable and an objective test must be performed before continuing treatment.

Objective Diagnostic Tests
Venography has been the gold standard for diagnosing venous thrombosis. A venogram will outline the entire deep venous system of the lower extremity, including the external and common iliac veins up to the distal portion of the IVC. With the recent advances made in ultrasonogra-

phy, however, duplex scanning now rivals the venogram as the preferred diagnostic method. Duplex scanning techniques have excellent sensitivity and specificity for the diagnosis of proximal DVT.

Venography
Venography is performed by injecting a radiopaque contrast medium into a dorsal vein in the foot. The most reliable criterion for confirming an acute venous thrombosis is an intraluminal filling defect seen consistently in multiple views (Fig. 26-3). Other criteria are less reliable and include nonfilling of a segment of the deep venous system with abrupt termination of the contrast medium or nonfilling of the deep venous system above the knee despite adequate venographic technique.

Venography is invasive, and certain complications are associated with injection of the contrast medium. In addition to the pain at the site of injection, the hyperosmolar radiopaque contrast medium can damage endothelial cells and may produce a superficial phlebitis or DVT. Other less common complications include hypersensitivity reactions to the radiopaque dye, renal failure, and local skin and tissue necrosis as a result of extravasation of the contrast medium at the site of injection.

Noninvasive Methods
The advantages afforded by the development of noninvasive tests make them the method of choice for the majority of patients suspected of having a DVT. These tests include impedance plethysmography and duplex ultrasonography. In the past impedance plethysmography was considered the best noninvasive method to diagnose DVT. However, it did not detect calf thrombi, nor did it allow for exact anatomic localization of the thrombus. Duplex ultrasonography has now been proven to be the superior method. This technique often allows visualization of the thrombus. In experienced hands duplex scanning of the lower extremities has a sensitivity and specificity greater than 95% for proximal vein thrombosis. The sensitivity falls when examining the calf veins, and accuracy and reliability is generally operator dependent.

Other available methods include computed tomography (CT), magnetic resonance imaging (MRI), radionuclide venography, and the use of blood tests such as concentrations of plasma D-dimer. CT scans may be most helpful in diagnosing DVT of the abdomen and pelvis, whereas the cost and availability of MRI limit its usefulness. The possibilities of a blood test analogous to those used to exclude myocardial infarction is intriguing. This test and the noninvasive methods are discussed further in other chapters.

Differential Diagnosis
The differential diagnosis for DVT is listed in the box on p. 456. Muscle aches, muscle tears, arterial insufficiency, Baker's cyst, and neurogenic pain due to compression of a nerve can all mimic DVT. A complete history and physical examination along with objective testing is necessary to confirm the diagnosis. Other conditions such as cellulitis, lymphangitis, vasculitis, myositis, fibrositis, fibromyalgia, and panniculitis may also cause signs and symptoms

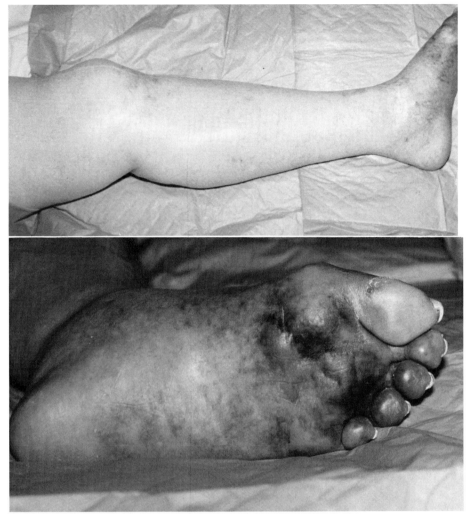

Fig. 26-2. **A** and **B,** Phlegmasia cerulea dolens, an unusual presentation of DVT. Note the marked swelling and discoloration generally seen in this setting.

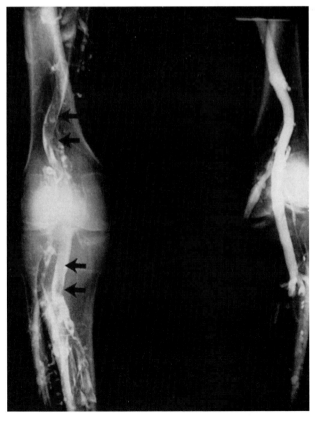

Fig. 26-3. DVT as demonstrated by an ascending venogram. The right lower extremity demonstrates an intraluminal filling defect (*arrows*) with contrast material streaming around the clot. The left leg is normal.

DIFFERENTIAL DIAGNOSIS OF DEEP VEIN THROMBOSIS

Muscle aches, muscle tears

Arterial insufficiency

Baker's cyst, arthritis

Neurogenic pain

Cellulitis

Lymphangitis

Vasculitis

Myositis

Fibrositis, fibromyalgia

Panniculitis

Superficial phlebitis, varicose veins

suggestive of a DVT. These conditions can usually be differentiated from DVT on clinical grounds. Patients with varicose veins frequently have pain and tenderness over the region of the varicosities. When superficial phlebitis (Fig. 26-4) occurs in a varicosity, it may become inflamed and tender and can produce local edema. A number of recent studies have suggested an association between DVT and superficial phlebitis and recommend noninvasive tests in all patients presenting with this condition.[45,46] Other conditions that may simulate DVT include compression of the iliac vein (Fig. 26-5) by an abscess, tumor, bladder, or other mechanical obstructing problems.

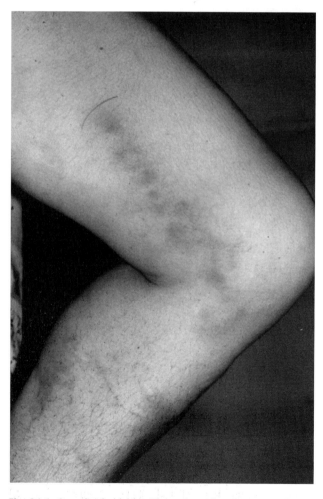

Fig. 26-4. Superficial phlebitis. The patient often presents with inflammation and erythema over the varicose vein.

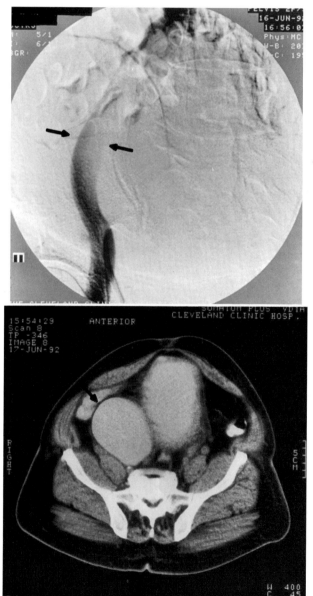

Fig. 26-5. Conditions that mimic DVT. This patient presented with a massively swollen leg. **A,** A venogram demonstrates extrinsic compression on the right iliac vein *(arrow)*. **B,** The CT scan shows a large bladder diverticulum *(arrows)* that is responsible for the compression.

TREATMENT

Anticoagulant Therapy

Treatment for DVT should be initiated as soon as the diagnosis is suspected, unless there is a contraindication to anticoagulation therapy. Traditional therapy with heparin and warfarin aims to prevent further thrombus formation and extension and minimize the potential for acute PE and the postphlebitic syndrome. Thrombolytic agents dissolve thrombi, and their use aims to restore patency of the veins and eliminate chronic venous insufficiency. In general, thrombolytic agents are adjuncts to other therapies. Their use should be monitored by clinicians experienced in the care of patients with venous or arterial thrombotic disease.

HEPARIN. Heparin remains the drug of choice for the treatment of thromboembolic disease, despite continued interest in thrombolytic therapy.

An intravenous bolus of between 5,000 and 10,000 U should be given initially, followed by a continuous infusion. The activated partial thromboplastin time (APTT) should be checked 4 to 6 hours after the initiation of therapy and then every 4 hours until the APTT is therapeutic. Clinical trials have demonstrated that the recurrence of venous thromboembolism can be prevented by maintaining the APTT at two to three times the laboratory control value, particularly during the first 24 to 48 hours after the acute event.[47-50] Unfortunately current practices for dosing heparin often result in inadequate anticoagulation, especially during the first few days of treatment.[51] A number of authors stress the advantages of using a nomogram in an attempt to minimize "underanticoagulation" and to prevent recurrent venous thromboembolism.[52,53] In these studies the nomogram enabled clinicians to obtain a therapeutic APTT more rapidly and thus decrease recurrent thrombosis.

Occasionally the APTT does not appear to be therapeutic despite large doses of heparin. Evidence from animal studies indicates that the use of a heparin assay may be helpful in these situations. Venous thrombosis can be prevented at heparin levels of 0.2 to 0.5 U/ml, measured by protamine neutralization, even when the APTT is not prolonged to twice the normal control value.[54,55]

Once a therapeutic range has been obtained, monitoring the APTT every 24 hours is sufficient. Platelet counts should be obtained every 48 to 72 hours while the patient is receiving heparin.

Although peak plasma levels can be obtained almost instantly by parenteral administration, other methods of providing heparin therapy have been tried. Intermittent, intravenous injection has been used in the past to administer heparin, but this has been demonstrated to increase the risk of bleeding.[47] The use of subcutaneous, unfractionated heparin during the acute event has also been suggested.[56-59] In one study this regimen induced an initial anticoagulant response below the therapeutic range and resulted in more recurrent venous thromboembolic events.[57] In another study it proved to be more effective and at least as safe.[59] The subcutaneous method is used in patients who fail warfarin therapy, for example patients with Trousseau's syndrome and patients with coumarin

skin necrosis. In the future this may be the method of choice for the treatment of acute uncomplicated DVT (although using low molecular weight heparins), especially if administered in the outpatient setting. Complications and other aspects of anticoagulation therapy with heparin are described in Chapter 6.

WARFARIN. Despite its acceptance and use for many decades, some aspects of therapy with warfarin (Coumadin) for the treatment of DVT (using low molecular weight heparin) remain controversial—in particular, the time at which to initiate therapy, the duration of therapy for uncomplicated or recurrent venous thromboembolism, the optimal dose for achieving adequate anticoagulation, and monitoring using the international normalized ratio (INR).

The mean half-life of a single dose of warfarin is 35 to 40 hours. In healthy volunteers the concentration of warfarin in plasma is poorly correlated with its anticoagulant effect. Its metabolism and excretion can vary greatly by individual. Some people are either fast or slow metabolizers, and therefore dosing must be individualized. The absorption of warfarin is also influenced by diet, drugs, and the underlying disease process.

Although many physicians still do not initiate warfarin therapy until the fifth day or later in the treatment of acute DVT, warfarin initiated at the same time as heparin for DVT has been shown to be effective.[60,61] Warfarin treatment should last 3 months for the patient with an initial thrombotic event, although the optimum duration for an acute DVT following surgery may be shorter.[59] Other authors have recommended periods from 1 month to 6 weeks for the treatment of acute DVT.[62,63] In patients with a recurrent event, warfarin from 6 months to 1 year is recommended, and in patients with three or more events, lifelong anticoagulation therapy is needed. These events should be of undetermined etiology, without any immediate cause, and well documented with venograms, pulmonary angiograms, lung scans, or reliable noninvasive studies, especially to prevent prolonged or unnecessary treatment as may be the case using a clinical diagnosis. Oral anticoagulants have been shown to be ineffective when used alone in the treatment of proximal DVT.[64] A loading dose of 10 mg of warfarin is generally given on days 1 and 2. Subsequent doses of warfarin are based on the INR. Warfarin and heparin should overlap for 4 to 5 days even if the INR is therapeutic sooner. In this scenario the initial rise in the INR is due to a rapid decrease in factor VII, but warfarin's peak anticoagulation effect may be delayed up until 96 hours due to the longer half-lives of factors II, IX, and X. In addition, the INR may appear "therapeutic" but if heparin is discontinued too soon, there is potential for warfarin to be thrombogenic and increase the patient's risk for extension or recurrent thrombosis.

Current recommendations are to maintain the INR between 2 and 3 for the treatment of DVT. These values are based on data that show that less intensive oral anticoagulation therapy is as efficacious as more intensive therapy.[65,66] The incidence of untoward bleeding has been greatly reduced with the newer, less intensive therapy.[65] North American patients in the past were taking higher doses of oral anticoagulants than were patients in the

United Kingdom. This difference in dose has been attributed to the source of thromboplastin used in the prothrombin time test. Rabbit brain thromboplastin has been used in North America, whereas human brain, which is more responsive to reductions in vitamin K–dependent coagulation factors, is used in the United Kingdom.

The mechanism of action, complications, and biochemical aspects of warfarin therapy are discussed in Chapter 6.

LOW-MOLECULAR-WEIGHT HEPARIN. The use of low-molecular-weight heparins (LMWHs) in the treatment of DVT provides us with a new therapeutic agent. These agents, which were developed in the 1970s, are prepared from standard unfractionated heparins by either chemical or enzymatic depolymerization.[67] These agents have an equivalent antithrombotic effect but appear to produce less bleeding than standard heparin. Their long plasma half-lives allow the LMWHs to be administered once or twice daily, dosed by a weight-adjusted regimen, and require little or no laboratory monitoring. The cost of LMWHs is more than unfractionated heparin, but since their use does not require laboratory monitoring, and since there is potential for a shorter hospital stay, their cost may be offset by these savings. The only available LMWHs approved for use in the United States are enoxaparin (Lovenox), which is available for use only in the prophylaxis of hip and knee surgery and dalteparin (Fragmin) available for prevention of DVT in abdominal surgery.

Several recent clinical studies have demonstrated that LMWHs are at least as effective and safe as unfractionated intravenous heparin in the treatment of acute DVT.[68-71] In several of these studies venographic improvement was demonstrated, whereas in others the frequency of recurrent venous thromboembolism and bleeding complications were comparable to unfractionated heparin.[68,71] These agents may make it possible to treat patients with uncomplicated acute DVT as outpatients, and the potential for cost savings is considerable.

THROMBOLYTIC THERAPY. The use of thrombolytic therapy for the treatment of DVT is a controversial issue. The goal of treatment for DVT is the prevention of PE and the postphlebitic syndrome. Although anticoagulation therapy prevents PE, its role in preventing the postphlebitic syndrome is not as clear. Thrombolytic therapy has the advantage of clot dissolution, which may lead to recanalization, restoration of normal venous hemodynamics, and the prevention of venous valvular damage (Fig. 26-6). Studies have suggested that if early recanalization can occur, it may preserve venous valve function and theoretically help prevent the postphlebitic syndrome.[72,73]

Thrombolytic therapy for DVT has been evaluated in a number of studies and has been shown to result in greater lysis of deep vein thrombi than heparin therapy.[74-86] Thirteen separate trials comparing systemic thrombolytic agents with heparin in the treatment of DVT using venographic assessment have been reported. Eleven of these compared streptokinase with heparin,[74-86] and two compared tissue plasminogen activator with heparin.[87,88] Despite the previously mentioned studies, thrombolytic therapy has not yet been definitely shown to prevent the

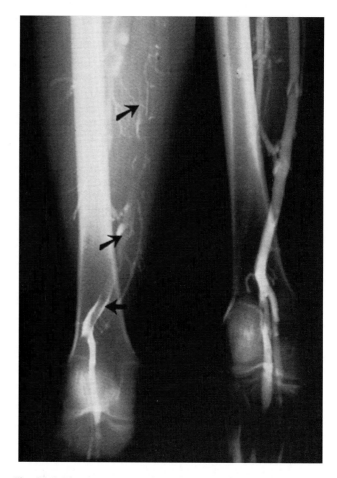

Fig. 26-6. The venogram on the right demonstrates extensive thrombosis (*arrows*). The venogram on the left was performed following 18 hours of thrombolytic therapy. Note how the clot has been dissolved, and the contrast agent flows through the venous channels.

postphlebitic syndrome. Only a few articles have reported on the long-term effects of thrombolytic therapy in the treatment of DVT.[77,89] In these studies more patients were free of postthrombotic symptoms with the use of streptokinase compared with heparin. Johansson et al[95] described a functional evaluation, using occlusion plethysmography, of the veins in patients initially treated with streptokinase for DVT. This study had a mean follow-up of 2 years and found an excellent correlation between anatomically normal venograms and normal venous outflow capacity and valvular function. Normal outcomes occurred in 42% of patients treated with streptokinase. The authors concluded that an initial complete thrombolysis provides a good opportunity for obtaining a lasting restoration of deep venous anatomy and function without developing signs and symptoms of venous insufficiency.

Other studies have not supported the use of thrombolytic therapy for the prevention of the postphlebitic syndrome. Kakkar et al,[78] in a follow-up of more than 5 years, noted that the postphlebitic syndrome was as common in patients treated with thrombolysis as in those treated with heparin. The indications for thrombolytic therapy in DVT are limited to a select group of patients.

Patients with phlegmasia cerulea dolens,[91-94] superior vena cava syndrome,[95] extensive iliofemoral DVT, and younger individuals with axillary-subclavian thrombosis should be considered candidates for thrombolysis in the appropriate setting. In phlegmasia an ipsilateral intraarterial infusion through a sheath from the contralateral femoral artery may work best. In iliofemoral DVT optimal delivery of the thrombolytic agent can be achieved through a multi-sidehole infusion catheter placed from the opposite femoral vein. An infusion catheter should also be placed directly into the thrombus in patients with axillary-subclavian vein or superior vena cava syndrome.

The usual dose of urokinase for the treatment of acute DVT is a 4400 IU/kg bolus followed by 4400 IU/kg/hr continuous infusion. For streptokinase the dose is a bolus of 250,000 IU followed by 100,000 IU/hr. For recombinant tissue plasminogen activator (rt-PA), the dose is 0.05 mg/kg/hr for up to 24 hours. The length of treatment varies with the agent used. In the past recommendations were to treat for 48 to 72 hours with streptokinase, 12 to 24 hours with urokinase, and up to 24 hours with rt-PA. Current recommendations imply that if no lysis occurs after 24 hours of treatment, the agent should be discontinued. If lysis does occur, lytic therapy should be continued until maximal clot resolution is noted. There are a number of contraindications to the use of thrombolytic therapy including recent surgery, trauma, active internal bleeding, pregnancy, a recent stroke or intracranial mass, an underlying bleeding diathesis, and recent biopsy of internal organs. In one study of 209 patients with DVT, Markel, Manzo, and Strandness[73] found that only 7% were candidates for thrombolytic therapy because of the previously listed contraindications.

The major complication associated with thrombolysis is hemorrhage. The frequency with which major bleeding occurs is difficult to assess. Straub[96] reviewed the literature to determine the frequency of bleeding in patients treated with streptokinase. His review included 549 patients treated for DVT. Fatal bleeding occurred in 0.73% of these patients, and major nonfatal bleeding occurred in 11.5%. The mean duration of treatment was extremely long (106 hours, or more than 4 days), and a uniform definition of major bleeding was not applied. This review indicates that the greatest risk for bleeding occurs when therapy is prolonged, perhaps for 3 to 4 days.

Interestingly studies on bleeding complications with heparin therapy have similar findings. Holm[97] gathered information on 280 patients treated for DVT with standard anticoagulation therapy. Fatal bleeding occurred in 0.3% of patients, and overall nonfatal major bleeding occurred in 3%, but was 8% in females and 4% in males over 70 years of age. Other complications include fever, nausea, vomiting, and an allergic reaction to the agent.

Surgical Treatment For Deep Vein Thrombosis

VENA CAVA INTERRUPTION. Some form of vena cava interruption for the prevention of PE has been used since 1893 when Bottini performed the first IVC ligation.[98] The early techniques of IVC interruption included IVC ligation, plication, or clipping—which required general anesthesia and laparotomy. These procedures were associ-

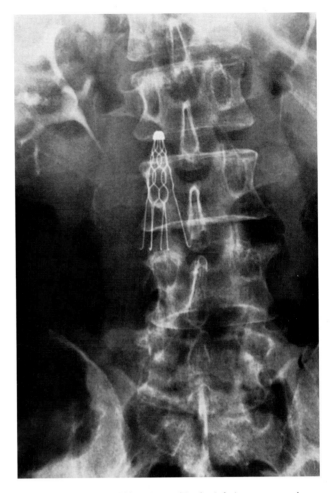

Fig. 26-7. A Greenfield filter situated in the inferior vena cava below the renal veins. The nephrogram and draining ureters can be seen on both sides of the filter.

ated with significant morbidity and mortality. Between the 1960s and 1970s several filters, balloons, and clips were introduced. However, these often resulted in IVC thrombosis, filter migration, or significant venous insufficiency. In 1973 the introduction of the Greenfield filter ushered in a new era for filters. The Greenfield filter is deployed with the base of the filter below the level of the renal veins between the second and third lumbar vertebrae (Fig. 26-7). Its cone-shaped geometry allows most of the cone to be filled with thrombus without significant reduction in caval blood flow.[99] In turn, this preservation of caval blood flow, along with renal vein blood flow, allows gradual resolution of the thrombi caught in the filter. Long-term filter patency rates are reported to be up to 98%, whereas the reported incidence of recurrent PE is 2% to 5%.[100,101] Infection or sepsis are not contraindications for placement of a Greenfield filter because its inert metal allows sterilization of the thrombus with appropriate antibiotic therapy.

The initial Greenfield filters were plagued by a high incidence of DVT at the insertion site, due to the large sheath required and the need for a femoral or internal jugular vein cutdown.[102] The newer titanium Greenfield filters can be inserted percutaneously, using a much smaller system.

Suprarenal deployment of filters is occasionally necessary in cases of thrombus propagation above a previously placed filter and to protect against thromboembolism from a gonadal source. Clinical studies have not shown renal dysfunction with this type of placement as had been a concern.[103,104] Greenfield filters have also been placed in the iliac veins of patients with very large IVCs and the superior vena cava for upper-extremity DVT.[105]

In addition to the Greenfield filters, other filters have been introduced. These filters include the bird's nest, Simon-Nitinol, VenaTech, Amplatz, and Gunther. These filters boast smaller carrier systems, but they do not share the same caval patency rates and low complication rates enjoyed by the Greenfield filters.

The indications for filter placement include a contraindication to anticoagulation therapy, recurrent PE despite adequate anticoagulation, in patients undergoing pulmonary embolectomy, and in patients with chronic recurrent PE. Other indications recommended by some authors include elderly patients at risk of falling, mentally unstable patients, a free-floating proximal thrombus, patients with low cardiopulmonary reserve or pulmonary hypertension, and patients with massive PE.[106-112]

Complications associated with caval devices include misplacement, migration, and, as noted earlier, thrombus formation above a previously placed filter (Figs. 26-8 and 26-9). In addition, procedural complications include hematoma, venous thrombosis, air embolism, perforation of the vascular wall, and filter thrombosis.

VENOUS THROMBECTOMY. The first thrombectomy of a leg vein was performed in 1938 by Lawen.[113] In the 1950s and 1960s there was considerable enthusiasm for venous thrombectomy because of initial reports of excellent patency and the absence of painful swelling and venous stasis.[114] Haller and Abrams[115] claimed an 85% patency rate in patients undergoing surgery within 10 days of the onset of the thrombus and reported normal extremities with no edema in 81% of the survivors. Soon, however, reports such as those by Lansing and Davis[116] emerged suggesting higher rates of rethrombosis and continued problems with venous stasis sequelae especially in phlegmasia cerulea dolens. In this follow-up study 94% of the patients had sufficient edema and stasis changes to require elastic support and leg elevation consistent with the classical definition of venous insufficiency. This report dampened the enthusiasm for surgical thrombectomy.

Other reports indicated that from 82% to 88% of patients could undergo a thrombectomy successfully and that postoperative anticoagulation therapy was helpful in avoiding rethrombosis.[117-119]

Venous thrombectomy can be performed, using a local or regional anesthetic, through a groin incision. This procedure is best performed within 2 or 3 days after the onset of symptoms. The venous thrombectomy is performed using a Fogarty venous catheter passed upward, ideally under fluoroscopic guidance. After the proximal thrombectomy has been completed, treatment of the distal thrombus can be undertaken. An arteriovenous fistula can then be created with a venous branch to the superficial femoral or profunda femoris artery. Systemic anticoagulation therapy with heparin is used throughout the proce-

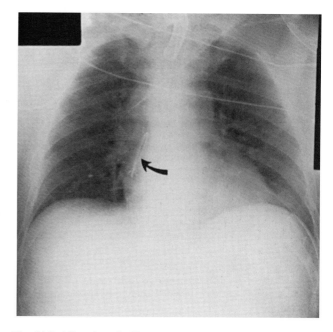

Fig. 26-8. Migration of a filter (*arrow*) into the right pulmonary artery. Although an unusual complication, migration can also occur into the retroperitoneal space or into other venous structures branching from the IVC.

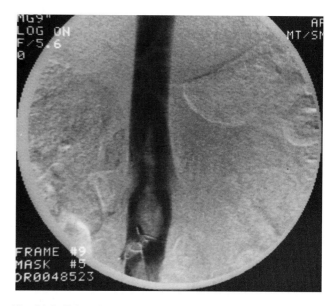

Fig. 26-9. This patient presented with signs and symptoms of a pulmonary embolism. The arrow demonstrates a large free-floating thrombus that has formed above the filter, an unusual finding.

dure. Operative mortality primarily reflects the seriousness of the underlying disease and the ability to avoid PE and to replace blood as fast as it is lost. Although the mortality in Haller and Abrams'[115] series was 9% and two of the three fatalities were related to PE, the mortality risk has dropped steadily in the past two decades. The choice of thrombectomy should be based primarily not on its risk but on its effectiveness relative to other therapies in reducing either early morbidity or the late sequelae of iliofemoral thrombosis. The patient should receive warfarin as soon as wound bleeding is eliminated as a problem and for a minimum of 6 weeks to 3 months, preferably longer if the retained thrombus remains. In selected patients venous thrombectomy has a limited but definite role in treating DVT in combination with postoperative anticoagulation therapy. Current indications for its use include phlegmasia cerulea dolens, phlegmasia alba, and extensive iliofemoral DVT, not responsive to other therapies. Venous thrombectomy is of little value in the management of patients who have recurrent thrombosis or thrombosis in the smaller vessels distal to the popliteal vein.

AXILLARY-SUBCLAVIAN VEIN THROMBOSIS

Thrombosis of the axillary and subclavian veins accounts for 1% to 2% of all DVT.[120] Recent data suggest that this incidence may be increasing, largely because of the increased use of the subclavian vein as an access site and for hemodynamic monitoring.

Although axillary-subclavian vein thrombosis is sometimes considered a benign disorder, the incidence of PE and postphlebitic syndrome suggests otherwise. The frequency of PE arising from axillary-subclavian vein thrombosis may be as high as 36%, although most authors suggest that this incidence approaches 12% to 15%.[120-124] The incidence of postphlebitic syndrome or residual disability resulting from upper-arm thrombosis varies between 7% and 74%, reflecting the various underlying causes for this syndrome.[120,124-126]

The pathogenesis of axillary-subclavian vein thrombosis is multifactorial but is generally similar to that of the lower extremity. Factors that may differ include the more common use of the subclavian vein for venous access and the use of irritating intravenous solutions or drugs, injury to the vascular endothelium directly related to venous puncture or catheter insertion, and the duration and size of catheter placement.

The causes for DVT involving the axillary-subclavian veins are diverse (see box on this page). Axillary-subclavian vein thrombosis seen in young, muscular, healthy males may be related to unusual exercise such as lifting, pulling, or hyperabduction of the arm and is referred to as *effort thrombosis* or *Paget-Schroetter's syndrome.*

Axillary-subclavian vein thrombosis also occurs with the use of CVP lines, pacemaker wires, Hickman or Broviac catheters, or intravenous drug abuse.

Signs and symptoms suggesting acute axillary-subclavian vein thrombosis include pain, local tenderness or warmth, edema, supraclavicular fullness, cyanosis, the presence of a palpable cord, or an increased venous pattern (Fig. 26-10). The diagnosis is suggested by a history and physical examination. Questions related to drug abuse, recent use of the subclavian vein for access or hemodynamic purposes, and types of physical activities should be asked. The diagnosis is established by venography or noninvasive studies. Thrombosis of the axillary-subclavian veins is treated like that of the leg: elevation, moist heat, and anticoagulants. The goal is to prevent pulmonary embolization and postphlebitic syndrome. Sympathetic ganglion blocks, conservative treatment with rest, and

---

CAUSES FOR AXILLARY-SUBCLAVIAN DEEP VEIN THROMBOSIS

Muscular effort of arms

Thoracic outlet syndrome

Trauma

Idiopathic

CVP lines

Intravenous drug abuse

Pacemaker wires

Tumor

Congenital venous malformation

---

elevation without the concomitant use of anticoagulants have no role in modern therapy. Thrombolytic agents are also successfully used to treat acute, well-documented axillary-subclavian vein thrombi.[121,126] These agents may be infused through a catheter directly into the thrombus or given systemically by a routine intravenous catheter.

Surgical approaches to axillary-subclavian vein thrombosis include the use of a superior vena caval filter, venous thrombectomy, or transaxillary first-rib resection. The use of superior vena caval filters is discussed elsewhere in this chapter. Venous thrombectomy is still advocated in many centers, although early rethrombosis is common. Transaxillary first-rib resection is probably helpful in the patient with thoracic outlet syndrome or with effort thrombosis after initial treatment with thrombolytic therapy or the more traditional use of anticoagulants.

SUPERIOR VENA CAVA SYNDROME

The superior vena cava syndrome was first recognized in 1757 by William Hunter, who reported it as a complication of a syphilitic aortic aneurysm. Infectious diseases including syphilis and tuberculosis were the most common causes for this disorder; however, the large majority of cases now recognized are related to underlying malignancy.[127-130] These include bronchogenic cancer, lymphoma, or metastatic disease arising most often from the breast or testicles. Other less commonly reported causes include fibrosing mediastinitis secondary to histoplasmosis or radiation treatment, pericardial hematoma, aortic aneurysms, polyarteritis nodosa, and iatrogenic sources resulting from the use of the axillary-subclavian vein for hemodynamic monitoring including Swan-Ganz catheters, Hickman or Broviac catheters, CVP lines, or transvenous cardiac pacemakers.

The pathogenesis of this syndrome may involve an extrinsic compression or an intrinsic process. Most commonly, extrinsic compression is the result of a slowly progressive process, such as a tumor, that eventually obstructs the vessel. This may cause only minimal clinical findings. However, direct invasion of an aggressive tumor

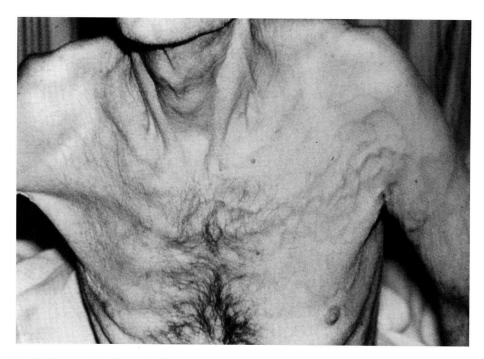

Fig. 26-10. Classic findings of axillary-subclavian DVT. Note the venous distention along the anterior portion of this patient's chest wall.

or an acute thrombosis causing acute obstruction occurs rapidly and produces a much more dramatic clinical picture.

Physical findings generally include upper-extremity and facial edema and occasionally conjunctival edema. Dilation of the superficial veins of the chest wall, neck, or arms is commonly observed. Patients may complain of cough, hoarseness, or shortness of breath and stridor due to laryngeal edema. Dysphagia secondary to esophageal edema may be present. Dizziness, headache, visual symptoms, somnolence, and changes in mental status (including stupor and coma) are reported. Symptoms are often aggravated by lying, bending, or stooping. The diagnosis of superior vena cava syndrome can be confirmed by venography. Chest x-ray studies may help in identifying an underlying malignancy or other contributing causes. CT and venous duplex scanning are effective noninvasive studies. Biopsy diagnosis can be obtained by a percutaneous needle approach or through an endovascular procedure using a biopsy device or atherectomy catheter.[131-133] Treatment has traditionally been the emergent use of radiation therapy based on the premise that the underlying disease process was cancer. This was often performed without confirming the diagnosis. Radiation therapy continues to play a major role in the treatment of this disorder; however, other modalities are now available and confirmation of the disease process is recommended before initiating treatment.

Medical measures including bed rest, diuretics, and head elevation often help. Steroids have been advocated to reduce cerebral or laryngeal edema. The use of anticoagulants is imperative if thrombotic occlusion has occurred. Thrombolytic therapy has proved to be effective.[95] Surgical therapy to remove the thrombus or bypass to replace the superior vena cava has not been highly successful and is not commonly used.

PREVENTING VENOUS THROMBOEMBOLISM

PE is the most common preventable cause of in-hospital death. In the absence of prophylaxis, the frequency of postoperative fatal PE ranges from 0.1% to 0.8% in patients undergoing elective general surgery, 0.3% to 1.7% in patients undergoing elective hip surgery, and 4% to 7% in patients undergoing emergency hip surgery.[7,134,135] Other medical illnesses such as stroke, myocardial infarction, and congestive heart failure carry a risk of developing DVT, the precursor of PE, in 25% to 60% of patients.[136] Ideally prophylaxis is most effective for preventing death and morbidity from PE. Therefore the use of prophylaxis to lower the risk of DVT and subsequent pulmonary emboli is of great importance. Effective prophylaxis is now available to most nonsurgical and surgical patients.

Despite convincing evidence that PE and DVT are largely preventable, many physicians and hospitals have no strategy for preventing venous thromboembolic disorders. This lack of strategy is explained, perhaps, by the fact that any given surgeon rarely has a patient die from PE and by the concern of physicians in all areas of practice that prophylaxis may not be as effective as some believe. This underuse of prophylaxis has been well documented. In a review of 2017 patients with multiple predisposing risk factors for DVT, only 19% of patients received appropriate prophylaxis in nonteaching hospitals and 44% in teaching hospitals.[137] Hospitals also have been reluctant to add prophylactic measures that may increase costs.[138-140] Many medical and surgical physicians rely solely on early ambulation and graded compression stockings to prevent thrombotic complications. These forms of prophylaxis are usually inadequate.

A number of predisposing risk factors for venous thromboembolism have been identified and discussed in this chapter. These risk factors were summarized in the box on p. 452.

Various prophylactic strategies have been evaluated for patients in different risk categories.[141] Selecting the most appropriate strategy for different clinical settings is an important aspect of prescribing prophylaxis.

The most commonly used strategy is a low-dose heparin regimen that prevents thrombosis by enhancing antithrombin III and by inhibiting factor Xa and thrombin. This enhancement and inhibition must occur before thrombin is activated; after thrombin is activated, low-dose heparin cannot prevent thrombosis. As a result, low-dose heparin is not effective in the treatment of acute DVTs or for prophylaxis after a clot exists. In almost all of the randomized trials with nonorthopedic patients, low-dose heparin has been found to be more effective than other treatments in preventing thrombosis.[142]

Although low-dose heparin prophylaxis is effective in the general surgical and medical populations, its use has been limited by the fear that it will induce bleeding. This fear is unsupported. The administration of 5000 U of heparin every 8 to 12 hours has not been associated with a clinically or statistically significant increase in risk of bleeding among general surgical patients.[143] Bleeding is a possibility, of course, and low-dose heparin prophylaxis should not be given to patients undergoing cerebral, eye, or spinal surgery. Heparin is also relatively ineffective in patients undergoing emergency or elective hip surgery, prostate surgery, or knee replacement surgery.[143]

Anticoagulation monitoring is not required during low-dose, subcutaneous heparin therapy. However, platelet counts should be obtained every few days to warn of the rare occurrence of heparin-associated thrombocytopenia.

A popular and effective prophylactic strategy is intermittent pneumatic leg compression, which enhances blood flow in the deep veins of the legs and prevents venous stasis.[29,144] Leg compression also stimulates fibrinolytic activity and reduces endothelial damage by the prevention of operative venodilation, both of which may help contribute to its antithrombotic properties.[31,145] It is the strategy of choice for patients in whom low-dose heparin is contraindicated or has been proven to be ineffective (i.e., patients undergoing eye, spine, prostate, or orthopedic surgery, or neurosurgery). Intermittent pneumatic leg compression is virtually free of clinically important side effects and is a valuable alternative for patients who have a high risk of bleeding. Unfortunately patient compliance is poor with these devices, and Comerota, Katz, and White[145] found that less than half of patients had properly functioning devices on their regular nursing floors.

Several other prophylactic strategies are available including low-dose oral anticoagulation therapy, dextran, aspirin, dose-adjusted subcutaneous heparin, IVC filters, and a combination of strategies. Although no prophylactic strategy has proved completely satisfactory for patients undergoing hip or knee replacement surgery, current

Table 26-1. The Common Approach to Prophylaxis in Medical and Surgical Patients

Type of Operation or Condition	Prophylaxis
Abdominal or thoracic surgery	Heparin 5000 U SQ q12h starting 2 hr preoperatively AND/OR pneumatic compression stockings
Eye surgery or neurosurgery; open prostatectomy	Pneumatic compression stockings
Orthopedic surgery; hip or knee replacement	Low molecular weight heparin 30 mg q12h OR pneumatic compression stockings OR adjusted doses of heparin SQ to prolong APTT 1-3 sec OR warfarin beginning the night of surgery
General medical patients including stroke and myocardial infarction	Heparin 5000 U SQ q12h AND/OR pneumatic compression stockings

options include LMWH, warfarin, adjusted doses of heparin, or pneumatic compression stockings. LMWH has been approved for prevention of thrombosis in elective hip and knee surgery.[146-152] In most studies to date, it has been shown to be more effective than the other current available methods for the prevention of venous thromboembolism in elective hip and knee surgery. It also has the advantage of beginning treatment postoperatively and can be administered subcutaneously. LMWH has also been used in trials in spinal injury patients, and in general medical and surgical patients and has recently been approved for prophylaxis in general abdominal surgery.[67,153,154]

The most carefully documented guidelines for selecting prophylactic strategies are those proposed by the American Heart Association for thoracic and abdominal surgery patients. Combining the American Heart Association recommendations for fixed, low-dose subcutaneous heparin therapy with early ambulation and, in some situations, pneumatic compression stockings is a reasonable strategy (Table 26-1). For patients at higher risk of thrombosis, the dose of heparin can be increased, and intermittent pneumatic leg compression can be simultaneously used. LMWH may also be an option in this type of patient.

Despite efforts at prophylaxis, DVT and PE will occur in some instances. To minimize the adverse impact of these complications, constant vigilance is required to establish an accurate diagnosis and provide effective treatment. This includes close observation following discharge. Although the incidence of thrombosis after release is unknown, an article by Huber et al[155] found about one fourth of all postoperative PE in their series occurred after hospital discharge. This is an area that has been neglected by most physicians in the past. A certain segment of patients may need prophylaxis following discharge, or at least an objective test to determine the absence or presence of thrombosis at that time.

REFERENCES

1. Kakkar VV et al: Natural history of postoperative deep vein thrombosis, Lancet 2:230, 1969.
2. Moser KM: Venous thromboembolism: state of the art, Am Rev Respir Dis 141:235, 1990.
3. Lindblad B, Sternby NH, and Bergqvist D: Incidence of venous thromboembolism verified by necropsy over 30 years, Br Med J 302:709, 1991.
4. Coon WW, Willis PW, and Keller JB: Venous thromboembolism and other venous disease in the Tecumseh community health study, Circulation 18:893, 1973.
5. Consensus Conference: Prevention of venous thrombosis and pulmonary embolism, JAMA 256:744, 1986
6. Anderson FA et al: A population based perspective of the hospital incidence and case fatality rates of deep vein thrombosis and pulmonary embolism. The Worcester DVT study, Arch Intern Med 151:933, 1991.
7. Dalen JE and Alpert JS: Natural history of pulmonary embolism, Prog Cardiovasc Dis 17:259, 1975.
8. Rosenow EC: Venous and pulmonary thromboembolism: an algorithmic approach to diagnosis and management, Mayo Clin Proc 70:45, 1995.
9. Dexter L and Folch-Pi W: Venous thrombosis. An account of the first documented case, JAMA 228:195, 1974.
10. Warren R: Behavior of venous thrombi, Arch Surg 115:1151, 1980.
11. Robbins SL: Fluid and hemodynamic derangements. In Pathologic basis of disease, Philadelphia, 1974, WB Saunders.
12. Hamer JD, Malone PC, and Silver IA: The Po_2 in venous valve pockets: its possible bearing on thrombogenesis, Br J Surg 68:166, 1981.
13. Sevitt S and Gallagher N: Venous thrombosis and pulmonary embolism: a clinico-pathological study in injured and burned patients, Br J Surg 48:475, 1961.
14. Fraser RS: Pathologic characteristics of venous thromboembolism. In Leclerc JR, ed: Venous thromboembolic disorders, Philadelphia, 1991, Lea and Febiger.
15. Browse NL and Thomas ML: Source of non-lethal pulmonary emboli, Lancet 1:258, 1974
16. Virchow RLK: Gesammelte Abhandlungen zur wissenschaftlichen Medizin, Frankfurt, 1856, AM Von Meidinger Sohn.
17. Almen T and Nylander G: Serial phlebography of the normal lower leg during muscular contraction and relaxation, Acta Radiol 57:264, 1962.
18. Hirsh J and Genton E: Thrombogenesis. In Root WS and Hoffman FG, eds: Physiological pharmacology, New York, 1974, Academic Press.
19. Wessler S and Yin ET: On the mechanism of thrombosis. In Brown EB and Moore CV, eds: Progress in hematology, New York, 1969, Grune & Stratton.
20. Cotton LT and Clark C: Anatomical localization of venous thrombosis, Ann R Coll Surg Engl 36:214, 1965.
21. Carter CJ: The pathophysiology of venous thrombosis, Prog Cardiovasc Dis 36:439, 1994.
22. Walsh PN and Griffin JH: Contributions of human platelets to the proteolytic activation of blood coagulation factors XII and XI, Blood 57:106, 1981.
23. Wilner GD, Nossel HL, and Leroy EC: Activation of Hageman factor by collagen, J Clin Invest 47:2608, 1968.
24. Zeldis SM et al: Tissue factor (thromboplastin): localization to plasma membranes by peroxidase-conjugated antibodies, Science 175:766, 1972.
25. Wiman B et al: The role of the fibrinolytic system in deep vein thrombosis, J Lab Clin Med 105:265, 1985.
26. Kakkar VV et al: Deep vein thrombosis of the leg: is there a "high-risk" group? Am J Surg 120:527, 1970.
27. Nicolaides AN and Irving D: Clinical factors and the risk of deep venous thrombosis. In Nicolaides AN, ed: Thromboembolism aetiology, advances in prevention and management, Lancaster, England, 1975, Medical and Technical Publishing.
28. Heatley RV et al: Preoperative or postoperative deep-vein thrombosis? Lancet 1:437, 1976.
29. Turpie AGG et al: Prevention of venous thrombosis in patients with intracranial disease by intermittent pneumatic compression of the calf, Neurology 27:435, 1977.
30. Gibbs NM: Venous thrombosis of the lower limbs with particular reference to bedrest, Br J Surg 45:209, 1957.
31. Comerota AJ et al: Operative venodilation: a previously unsuspected factor in the cause of postoperative deep vein thrombosis, Surgery 106:301, 1989.
32. Geerts WH et al: A prospective study of venous thromboembolism after major trauma, N Engl J Med 331:1601, 1994.
33. Cogo A et al: Acquired risk factors for deep-vein thrombosis in symptomatic outpatients, Arch Intern Med 154:164, 1994.
34. Andrew M et al: Venous thromboembolic complications (VTE) in children: first analyses of the Canadian registry of VTE, Blood 83:1251, 1994.
35. Prins MH, Lensing AWA, and Hirsh J: Idiopathic deep venous thrombosis: is a search for malignant disease justified? Arch Intern Med 154:1310, 1994.
36. Prandoni P et al: Deep vein thrombosis and the incidence of subsequent symptomatic malignant disease, N Engl J Med 327:1128, 1992.
37. Goldberg RJ et al: Occult malignant neoplasm in patients with deep venous thrombosis, Arch Intern Med 147:251, 1987.
38. Gore JM et al: Occult cancer in patients with acute pulmonary embolism, Ann Intern Med 96:556, 1982.
39. Anderson GM and Hull E: The effect of dicumarol upon the mortality and incidence of thromboembolic complications in congestive heart failure, Am Heart J 39:697, 1950.
40. Bonnar J et al: Haemostatic mechanism in the uterine circulation during placental separation, Br Med J 2:564, 1970.
41. Bonnar J, McNicol GP, and Douglas AS: Fibrinolytic enzyme system and pregnancy, Br Med J 3:387, 1969.
42. Devor M et al: Estrogen replacement therapy and the risk of venous thrombosis, Am J Med 92:275, 1992.
43. Lobo RA: Estrogen and the risk of coagulopathy, Am J Med 92:283, 1992.
44. Hull RD et al: Clinical validity of a negative venogram in patients with clinically suspected venous thrombosis, Circulation 64:622, 1981.
45. Skillman JJ et al: Simultaneous occurrence of superficial and deep thrombophlebitis in the lower extremity, J Vasc Surg 11:818, 1990.
46. Jorgensen JO et al: The incidence of deep venous thrombosis in patients with superficial thrombophlebitis of the lower limbs, J Vasc Surg 18:70, 1993.
47. Glazier RL and Crowell EB: Randomized prospective trial of continuous vs intermittent heparin therapy, JAMA 236:1365, 1976.
48. Wilson JR and Lampman J: Heparin therapy: a randomized prospective study, Am Heart J 97:155, 1979.

49. Bentley PG et al: An objective study of alternative methods of heparin administration, Thromb Res 18:177, 1980.
50. Basu D et al: A prospective study of the value of monitoring heparin treatment with the activated partial thromboplastin time, N Engl J Med 287:324, 1972.
51. Wheeler AP, Jaquiss RDB, and Newman JH: Physician practices in the treatment of pulmonary embolism and deep vein thrombosis, Arch Intern Med 148:1321, 1988.
52. Raschke RA et al: The weight-based heparin dosing nomogram compared with a "standard care" nomogram, Ann Intern Med 119:874, 1993.
53. Cruickshank MK et al: A standard heparin nomogram for the management of heparin therapy, Arch Intern Med 151:333, 1991.
54. Chiu HM, Hirsh J, and Yung WL: Relationship between the anticoagulant and antithrombotic effects of heparin in experimental venous thrombosis, Blood 49:171, 1977.
55. Levine MN et al: A randomized trial comparing activated thromboplastin time with heparin assay in patients with acute venous thromboembolism requiring large daily doses of heparin, Arch Intern Med 154:49, 1994.
56. Andersson G et al: Subcutaneous administration of heparin: a randomized comparison with intravenous administration of heparin to patients with deep-vein thrombosis, Thromb Res 27:631, 1982.
57. Hull RD et al: Continuous intravenous heparin compared with intermittent subcutaneous heparin in the initial treatment of proximal-vein thrombosis, N Engl J Med 315:1109, 1986.
58. Doyle DJ et al: Adjusted subcutaneous heparin or continuous intravenous heparin in patients with acute deep vein thrombosis, Ann Intern Med 107:441, 1987.
59. Hommes DW et al: Subcutaneous heparin compared with continuous intravenous heparin administration in the initial treatment of deep vein thrombosis, Ann Intern Med 116:279, 1992.
60. Gallus A et al: Safety and efficacy of warfarin started early after submassive venous thrombosis or pulmonary embolism, Lancet 2:1293, 1986.
61. Hull RD et al: Heparin for 5 days as compared with 10 days in the initial treatment of proximal venous thrombosis, N Engl J Med 322:1260, 1990.
62. O'Sullivan EF: Duration of anticoagulant therapy in venous thrombo-embolism, Med J Aust 2:1104, 1972.
63. Holmgren KAJ et al: One-month versus six-month therapy with oral anticoagulants after symptomatic deep vein thrombosis, Acta Med Scand 218:279, 1985.
64. Brandjes DPM et al: Acenocoumarol and heparin compared with acenocoumarol alone in the initial treatment of proximal-vein thrombosis, N Engl J Med 327:1485, 1992.
65. Hull R et al: Different intensities of oral anticoagulation therapy in the treatment of proximal vein thrombosis, N Engl J Med 307:1676, 1982.
66. Adar R and Salzman EW: Treatment of thrombosis of veins of the lower extremities, N Engl J Med 292:348, 1975.
67. Hirsh J and Levine MN: Low molecular weight heparin, Blood 79:1, 1992.
68. Prandoni P et al: Comparison of subcutaneous low-molecular-weight heparin with intravenous standard heparin in proximal deep-vein thrombosis, Lancet 339:441, 1992.
69. Simonneau G et al: Subcutaneous low-molecular-weight heparin compared with continuous intravenous unfractionated heparin in the treatment of proximal deep vein thrombosis, Arch Intern Med 153:1541, 1993.
70. Leizorovicz A et al: Comparison of efficacy and safety of low molecular weight heparins and unfractionated heparin in initial treatment of deep venous thrombosis: a meta analysis, Br Med J 309:299, 1994.
71. Hull RD et al: Subcutaneous low-molecular-weight heparin compared with continuous intravenous heparin in the treatment of proximal-vein thrombosis, N Engl J Med 326:975, 1992.
72. Strandness DE et al: Long term sequelae of acute venous thrombosis, JAMA 250:1289, 1983.
73. Markel A, Manzo RA, and Strandness DE: The potential role of thrombolytic therapy in venous thrombosis, Arch Intern Med 152:1265, 1992.
74. Arnesen H et al: A prospective study of streptokinase and heparin in the treatment of deep vein thrombosis, Acta Med Scand 203:457, 1978.
75. Browse NL, Thomas ML, and Pim HP: Streptokinase and deep vein thrombosis, Br Med J 3:717, 1968.
76. Duckert F et al: Treatment of deep vein thrombosis with streptokinase, Br Med J 1:479, 1975.
77. Elliot MS et al: A comparative randomized trial of heparin versus streptokinase in the treatment of acute proximal venous thrombosis: an interim report of a prospective trial, Br J Surg 66:838, 1979.
78. Kakkar VV et al: Treatment of deep vein thrombosis: a trial of heparin, streptokinase and Arvin, Br Med J 1:806, 1969.
79. Marder VJ, Soulen RL, and Atichartakarn V: Quantitative venographic assessment of deep vein thrombosis in the evaluation of streptokinase and heparin therapy, J Lab Clin Med 89:1018, 1977.
80. Porter JM et al: Comparison of heparin and streptokinase in the treatment of venous thrombosis, Am Surg 41:511, 1975.
81. Rosch J et al: Healing of deep venous thrombosis: venographic findings in a randomized study comparing streptokinase and heparin, AJR 127:553, 1976.
82. Seaman AJ et al: Deep vein thrombosis treated with streptokinase or heparin, Angiology 27:549, 1976.
83. Robertson BR, Nilsson IM, and Nylander G: Value of streptokinase and heparin in treatment of acute deep venous thrombosis, Acta Chir Scand 134:203, 1968.
84. Robertson BR, Nilsson IM, and Nylander G: Thrombolytic effect of streptokinase as evaluated by phlebography of deep venous thrombi of the leg, Acta Chir Scand 136:173, 1970.
85. Tsapogas MJ et al: Controlled study of thrombolytic therapy in deep vein thrombosis, Surgery 74:973, 1973.
86. Watz R and Savidge GF: Rapid thrombolysis and preservation of valvular venous function in high deep vein thrombosis: a comparative study between streptokinase and heparin therapy, Acta Med Scand 205:293, 1979.
87. Goldhaber SZ et al: Randomized controlled trial of tissue plasminogen activator in proximal deep venous thrombosis, Am J Med 88:235, 1990.
88. Turpie AG et al: Tissue plasminogen activator (rt-PA) vs heparin in deep vein thrombosis, Chest 97(suppl 4):172S, 1990.
89. Hood DB et al: Advances in the treatment of phlegmasia cerulea dolens, Am J Surg 166:206, 1993.
90. Robinson DL and Teitelbaum GP: Phlegmasia cerulea dolens: treatment by pulse-spray and infusion thrombolysis, AJR 160:1288, 1993.
91. Comerota AJ and Aldridge SC: Thrombolytic therapy for deep venous thrombosis: a clinical review, Can J Surg 36:359, 1993.
92. Wlodarczyk Z et al: Low-dose intra-arterial thrombolysis in the treatment of phlegmasia cerulea dolens, Br J Surg 81:370, 1994.
93. Gray BH et al: Safety and efficacy of thrombolytic therapy for superior vena cava syndrome, Chest 99:54, 1991.

94. Arnesen H, Hoiseth A, and Ly B: Streptokinase or heparin in the treatment of deep vein thrombosis: follow-up results of a prospective study, Acta Med Scand 211:65, 1982.

95. Johansson L et al: Comparison of streptokinase with heparin: late results in the treatment of deep vein thrombosis, Acta Med Scand 206:93, 1979.

96. Straub H: Letale komplikationen der fibrinolyse, Munch Med Wschr 124:17, 1982.

97. Holm HA et al: Heparin treatment of deep venous thrombosis in 280 patients: symptoms related to dosage, Acta Medica Scandinavica 215:47, 1984.

98. Dale WA: Ligation of the inferior vena cava for thromboembolism, Surgery 43:22, 1958.

99. Greenfield LJ et al: A new intracaval filter permitting continued flow and resolution of emboli, Surgery 73:533, 1973.

100. Greenfield LJ et al: Greenfield vena caval filter experience, Arch Surg 116:1451, 1981.

101. Greenfield LJ and Michna BA: Twelve year experience with the Greenfield vena cava filter, Surgery 104:706, 1988.

102. Kantor A, Glanz S, and Gordon DH: Percutaneous femoral insertion of the Greenfield vena cava filter: incidence of femoral vein thrombosis, AJR 149:1065, 1987.

103. Stewart JR et al: Clinical results of suprarenal placement of the Greenfield vena cava filter, Surgery 92:1, 1982.

104. Greenfield LJ et al: Late results of suprarenal Greenfield vena cava filter placement, Arch Surg 127:969, 1992.

105. Owen E Jr, Schoettle G, and Harrington OB: Placement of a Greenfield filter in the superior vena cava, Ann Thorac Surg 53:896, 1992.

106. Greenfield LJ et al: Clinical experience with the Kim-Ray Greenfield venal cava filter, Ann Surg 185:692, 1977.

107. Roehm JOF: The bird's nest inferior vena cava filter: progress report, Radiology 168:745, 1988.

108. Ricco JB et al: Percutaneous transvenous caval interruption with the "LGM" filter: early results of a multicenter trial, Ann Vasc Surg 2:242, 1988.

109. Simon M et al: Simon Nitinol inferior vena cava filter: initial clinical experience, Radiology 172:99, 1989.

110. Fobbe F et al: Gunther vena caval filter: results of long-term follow-up, AJR 151:1031, 1988.

111. Yune HY: Inferior vena cava filter: search for an ideal device, Radiology 172:15, 1989.

112. Epstein DH et al: Experience with the Amplatz retrievable vena cava filter, Radiology 172:105, 1989.

113. Lawen A: Weitere erfahrung uber operative thrombenentfehrnung bei venenthrombose, Langenbecks Arch Klin Chir 193:723, 1938.

114. Karp RB and Wylie EJ: Recurrent thrombosis after iliofemoral venous thrombectomy, Surg Forum 17:147, 1966.

115. Haller JA Jr and Abrams BL: Use of thrombectomy in the treatment of acute iliofemoral venous thrombosis in forty-five patients, Ann Surg 158:561, 1963.

116. Lansing AM and Davis WM: Five-year follow-up study of iliofemoral venous thrombectomy, Ann Surg 168:620, 1968.

117. Harris EJ and Brown WH: Patency after iliofemoral venous thrombosis, Ann Surg 167:91, 1968.

118. Lindhagen J et al: Iliofemoral venous thrombectomy, J Cardiovasc Surg 19:319, 1978.

119. Plate G et al: Thrombectomy with temporary arteriovenous fistula: the treatment of choice in acute iliofemoral venous thrombosis, J Vasc Surg 1:867, 1984.

120. Coon WW and Willis PW: Thrombosis of axillary and subclavian veins, Arch Surg 94:657, 1967.

121. Donayre CE et al: Pathogenesis determines late morbidity of axillosubclavian vein thrombosis, Am J Surg 152:179, 1986.

122. Harley DP et al: Pulmonary embolism secondary to venous thrombosis of the arm, Am J Surg 147:221, 1984.

123. Horattas MC et al: Changing concepts of deep venous thrombosis of the upper extremity—report of a series and review of the literature, Surgery 104:561, 1988.

124. Gloviczki P, Kazmier FJ, and Hollier LH: Axillary-subclavian venous occlusion: the morbidity of a nonlethal disease, J Vasc Surg 4:333, 1986.

125. Tilney NL, Griffiths HJG, and Edwards EA: Natural history of major venous thrombosis of the upper extremity, Arch Surg 101:792, 1970.

126. Demeter SL et al: Upper extremity thrombosis: etiology and prognosis, Angiology 33:743, 1982.

127. Lopez MI and Vincent RJ: Malignant superior or vena cava syndrome. In Kapoor AS, ed: Cancer and the heart, New York, 1986, Springer-Verlag.

128. Parish JM et al: Etiologic considerations in superior vena cava syndrome, Mayo Clin Proc 56:407, 1981.

129. Schraufnagel DE et al: Superior vena cava obstruction: is it a medical emergency? Am J Med 70:1169, 1981.

130. Lochridge SK, Knibbe WP, and Doty DB: Obstruction of the superior vena cava, Surgery 85:14, 1979.

131. Dake MD et al: The cause of superior vena cava syndrome: diagnosis with percutaneous atherectomy, Radiology 174:957, 1990.

132. Perez CA, Presant CA, and VanAmburg AL: Management of superior vena cava syndrome, Semin Oncol 5:123, 1978.

133. Armstrong P, Hayes DF, and Richardson PJ: Transvenous biopsy of carcinoma of bronchus causing superior vena caval obstruction, Br Med J (Clin Res) 1:662, 1975.

134. Skinner DB and Salzman EW: Anticoagulant prophylaxis in surgical patients, Surg Gynecol Obstet 125:741, 1967.

135. Kakkar VV et al: Prophylaxis for post-operative deep-vein thrombosis, JAMA 241:39, 1979.

136. Fratantoni JC and Wessler S: Prophylactic therapy of deep-vein thrombosis and pulmonary embolism, DHEW Publ No (NIH) 76-866, Washington, DC, 1977, US Government Printing Office.

137. Anderson FA et al: Physician practices in the prevention of venous thromboembolism, Ann Intern Med 115:591, 1991.

138. Salzman EW and Davies GC: Prophylaxis of venous thromboembolism: analysis of cost-effectiveness, Ann Surg 191:207, 1980.

139. Hull RD et al: Cost-effectiveness of primary and secondary prevention of fatal pulmonary embolism in high-risk surgical patients, Can Med Assoc J 127:990, 1982.

140. Carter C and Gent M: The epidemiology of venous thrombosis. In Coleman RW et al, eds: Hemostasis and thrombosis: basic principles and clinical practice, New York, 1982, JB Lippincott.

141. Salzman EW and Hirsh J: Prevention of venous thromboembolism. In Coleman RW et al, eds: Hemostasis and thrombosis: basic principles and clinical practice, New York, 1982, JB Lippincott.

142. Kakkar VV et al: Efficacy of low doses of heparin in prevention of deep-vein thrombosis after major surgery: a double-blind randomized trial, Lancet 2:101, 1972.

143. Hull RD and Hirsh J: Preventing venous thromboembolism, J Cardiovasc Med 9:63, 1984.

144. Skillman JJ et al: Prevention of deep-vein thrombosis in neurosurgical patients: a controlled, randomized trial of external pneumatic compression boots, Surgery 83:354, 1978.

145. Comerota AJ, Katz ML, and White JV: Why does prophylaxis with external pneumatic compression for deep vein thrombosis fail? Am J Surg 164:265, 1992.

146. Turpie AGG et al: A randomized controlled trial of a low-molecular-weight heparin (enoxaparin) to prevent deep-vein thrombosis in patients undergoing elective hip surgery, N Engl J Med 315:925, 1986.
147. Levine MN et al: Prevention of deep vein thrombosis after elective hip surgery, Ann Intern Med 114:545, 1991.
148. O'Brien BJ, Anderson DR, and Goeree R: Cost-effectiveness of enoxaparin versus warfarin prophylaxis against deep-vein thrombosis after total hip replacement, Can Med Assoc J 150:1083,1994.
149. Colwell CW et al: Use of enoxaparin, a low-molecular-weight heparin, and unfractionated heparin for the prevention of deep venous thrombosis after elective hip replacement, J Bone Joint Surgery 76-A:3, 1994.
150. Spiro TE et al: Efficacy and safety of enoxaparin to prevent deep venous thrombosis after hip replacement surgery, Ann Intern Med 121:81, 1994.
151. Imperiale TF and Speroff T: A meta-analysis of methods to prevent venous thromboembolism following total hip replacement, JAMA 271:1780, 1994.
152. Hull R et al: A comparison of subcutaneous low-molecular-weight heparin with warfarin sodium for prophylaxis against deep-vein thrombosis after hip or knee implantation, N Engl J Med 329:1370, 1993.
153. Green D et al: Prevention of thromboembolism after spinal cord injury using low-molecular-weight heparin, Ann Intern Med 113:571, 1990.
154. Haas S and Flosbach CW: Prevention of postoperative thromboembolism with enoxaparin in general surgery: a German multicenter trial, Thromb Hemost 19(suppl 1):164, 1993.
155. Huber O et al: Postoperative pulmonary embolism after hospital discharge, Arch Surg 127:310, 1992.

CHAPTER TWENTY-SEVEN

PULMONARY EMBOLISM

Arthur A. Sasahara
G.V.R.K. Sharma
Kevin M. McIntyre

Pulmonary embolism (PE) continues to be a common and important medical and surgical complication. Although it does not occur commonly in the practice of any individual physician, its impact globally is considerable, being responsible for some 150,000 deaths per year as the third most common cause of death in the United States, and occurring nonfatally in about 650,000 patients per year. In medical centers with active medical and surgical services, particularly with sizable numbers of orthopedic and cancer patients, the incidence of nonfatal PE approaches 15 to 20 patients per 1000 inpatients and fatal PE in approximately 4 to 5 patients per 1000[1] inpatients. Infrequently it arises de novo in patients without identifiable risk factors.

INCIDENCE OF PULMONARY EMBOLISM

The calculation of an accurate incidence of acute PE is problematic because of the inherent difficulties in distinguishing between clinically significant and incidental PE at autopsy, in coding PE on death certificates, and in correlating clinical signs and symptoms of PE with objective evidence of the diagnosis. Pathologists at autopsy do not routinely perform dissection of the leg veins to search for venous thrombi, but simply and quickly milk the blood back through the transected iliac veins and examine the effluent for gross clots. Most autopsy series attempt to differentiate between major PEs that cause or contribute to the patient's death and minor emboli that are clinically incidental. However, there is a very wide variation in the proportion of patients with major PE and those with minor PE at autopsy. In a survey of a number of these reported series, the frequency of PE ranged from 8%[2] to 64%,[3] strongly suggesting that there was a linear correlation between careful dissection of all of the vessels by the pathologist and the incidence of PE.

MORTALITY

The mortality of untreated PE is relatively high, ranging from 18% to about 38%, but once diagnosed and treated, whether heparin or thrombolytic agents are employed, mortality falls to about 8%.[4] This observation underscores the importance of early diagnosis, which leads to early treatment to reduce mortality. Early diagnosis, however, remains an important problem for the clinician. In contrast, it has been stated that overdiagnosis is a problem, particularly in hospitals where the primary care of the patient is assumed by the interns and residents. This dual status is explained by the fact that (1) the clinical picture of PE is so variable that it is often difficult to diagnose on clinical grounds; (2) there are no simple, routinely available laboratory tests that are sensitive and specific for PE, and (3) the disease, in general, is self-limiting, and if unrecognized and without recurrence, the patient will recover and be discharged from the hospital with another diagnosis.

Despite the variability of the clinical picture of PE, the history and physical examination constitute the only basis for suspecting the presence of the disease. In many patients, particularly those with recognized risk factors for venous thrombosis, the occurrence of cardiopulmonary symptoms and signs should lead the clinician to suspect the disease. At the least, a preliminary diagnosis can be made.

PREDISPOSITION

In the majority of cases PE develops while the patients are hospitalized because of other disease processes. A number of risk factors have now been recognized that predispose patients to venous thromboembolism. These include prolonged immobilization[5] (especially of patients more than 40 to 45 years of age),[6,7] trauma[8] (especially lower-leg trauma),[5] hip fractures,[9] surgery and the postoperative period[5,6] (especially in patients with malignant disease[6,9] and those undergoing orthopedic procedures),[9] paralysis,[10] and air travel.[11]

Other predisposing conditions are obesity,[9] oral contraceptive use,[12] pregnancy and the puerperium,[13] varicose veins,[6] prior venous thromboembolism,[6] heart disease (especially with congestive heart failure),[9] group A blood type,[14] inflammatory bowel disease,[15] the nephrotic syndrome,[16] phospholipid antibodies,[17] proteins C and S and antithrombin III deficiency.[18]

In some instances the presence of a risk factor may alert the physician to the possibility of PE—for example, an operative procedure in a patient with malignant disease or previous PE. Other factors, such as heart disease, may simply complicate the diagnostic process because of overlapping symptoms and signs. It is also useful from a therapeutic viewpoint to categorize a risk factor as either acute and self-limited (e.g., immobilization following trauma, surgery, or obstetric delivery) or chronic (e.g., chronic congestive heart failure or venous insufficiency). Chronic factors with continued risk for recurrent thromboembolism require careful management on a long-term basis.

CLINICAL SYNDROMES

Most patients who suffer PE have nonspecific symptoms and signs. Any number of cardiopulmonary abnormalities could evoke and mimic the clinical picture. However, it is possible to group the clinical picture into three syndromes: (1) acute cor pulmonale, (2) pulmonary infarction, and (3) PE.

Patients with acute cor pulmonale usually have sudden and dramatic development of dyspnea, cyanosis, right ventricular failure, and/or systemic hypotension. Patients with pulmonary infarction usually complain of dyspnea, pleuritic pain, and hemoptysis and may have a pleural friction rub. Patients with PE may complain only of sudden dyspnea or of not feeling well and have only tachycardia, tachypnea, or low-grade fever. Which of these "clinical syndromes" is seen is usually determined by the massiveness of the embolic process and the presence or absence of underlying cardiopulmonary disease.

CLINICAL PICTURE

Symptoms and Signs

When PE occurs, a number of nonspecific symptoms and signs occur. When they occur in patients without prior cardiopulmonary disease, they are clues to the diagnosis, whereas when they occur in patients with prior heart or lung disease, they may be mistaken for manifestations of the underlying disease. The following analysis was made from data obtained from the National Institutes of Health (NIH)-sponsored Urokinase Pulmonary Embolism Trial (UPET)[4] (Table 27-1).

1. *Dyspnea* was the most common symptom, occur-

Table 27-1. Presenting Symptoms with Pulmonary Embolism

Symptoms	Incidence (%)		
	All	**Massive**	**Submassive**
Dyspnea	81	79	83
Pleural pain	72	62	84*
Apprehension	59	61	56
Cough	54	50	60
Hemoptysis	34	27	44
Sweats	26	27	24
Syncope	14	22*	4

(Adapted from Sasahara AA et al: The urokinase pulmonary embolism trial: a national cooperative study, Circulation 47[suppl II]:66, 1973.)
*Differences in last two columns are significant.

ring in 81% of patients with angiographically proved PE. Characteristically the severity of this complaint appears to be out of proportion to the degree of objective abnormal findings.
2. *Chest pain,* frequently pleuritic, occurred in 72% of patients. It is usually associated more often with submassive PE than with massive PE (massive defined as the obstruction of two or more lobar arteries).
3. *Apprehension,* though very nonspecific, occurred in 59% of patients. In massive embolism patients feel a sense of impending catastrophe, whereas in lesser obstruction anxiety appears out of proportion to the physical findings noted.
4. *Cough* occurred in 54% of patients. It is usually nonproductive unless the patient has underlying chronic obstructive pulmonary disease.
5. *Hemoptysis,* although at one time requisite for considering PE in the differential diagnosis, occurred in only 34% of patients. It is characteristically blood-streaking, in contrast to diseases such as mitral stenosis, in which pure blood is expectorated. Serious blood loss is uncommon.
6. *Sweats,* also a very nonspecific finding, occurred about equally in both the massive and submassive groups.
7. *Syncope* occurred in 14% of patients, usually associated with massive PE. When it occurred in patients with submassive PE, significant underlying cardiopulmonary disease was present. (Physical examination findings tabulated from the UPET study[4] were relatively nonspecific and could also be associated with other cardiopulmonary disorders [Table 27-2].)
8. *Tachypnea* (respiratory rate greater than 16 breaths/min) was the most frequent sign, occurring in 87% of patients. It is generally characterized as "fast and shallow" respiration.
9. *Tachycardia* (heart rate greater than 100 beats/min) occurred in 44% of patients. In general, there tends

Table 27-2. UPET Presenting Signs of Pulmonary Embolism

Signs	Incidence (%)		
	All	**Massive**	**Submassive**
Rales	53	50	57
Increased P₂ second heart sound	53	60*	44
Phlebitis	33	42	21
S₃, S₄ gallop heart sounds	34	47*	17
Sweating	34	41	24
Cyanosis	18	28*	6
Respiratory rate >16 breaths/min	87	–	–
Pulse >100/min	44	–	–
Fever >37.8° C	42	–	–

(Adapted from Sasahara AA et al: The urokinase pulmonary embolism trial: a national cooperative study, Circulation 47[suppl II]:66, 1973.)
*Differences are significant; $P < 0.005$.

to be a direct relation between size of the embolic process and the increase in heart rate. When tachycardia ceases suddenly in a patient with massive PE, it is an ominous sign and may herald a cardiac arrest.

10. *Accentuation of the pulmonary closure sound* occurred in 53% of patients. Because it is usually a manifestation of large PE and the development of sudden pulmonary hypertension, its detection generally denotes significant embolic obstruction.
11. *Rales,* which occurred in 53% of patients, were a manifestation of congestive heart failure and occurred more often in patients with underlying cardiopulmonary disease.
12. *Fever* was found in 42% of patients. It was generally greater than 37.8° C and lacked the "spiking" nature of systemic infectious processes.
13. *Sweating* occurred in 34% of patients. It results from sympathetic discharge occurring in patients with anxiety and cardiopulmonary distress. Hence, it is more often found in patients with massive PE.
14. *Thrombophlebitis* was uncommon in these patients, although asymptomatic deep vein thrombosis (DVT) was not. This latter observation is of clinical importance because most PEs arise from thrombi in the deep venous system of the legs. Only by use of objective diagnostic studies can deep vein thrombi be detected with any degree of sensitivity.
15. *Gallop heart sounds,* S₃ and/or S₄ were detected in 34% of patients, usually with massive obstruction. The occurrence pathophysiologically is related to abnormal right ventricular hemodynamics, which result from sudden elevation of pulmonary arterial pressure. The right ventricular origin can occasionally be confirmed by its phasic variation with respiration.

16. *Cyanosis,* noted in 18% of patients, represented a more severe degree of the very frequent hypoxemia and desaturation that occur in patients with PE. Hence, it is a finding of massive PE.

It is quite evident from this analysis that the majority of patients with PE have signs and symptoms that could be part of other heart and lung disorders. The physician must be prepared to accept a clinical presentation short of the classic hemoptysis, pleural pain, and thrombophlebitis and initiate as expeditiously as possible a diagnostic evaluation.

HEMODYNAMIC RESPONSES TO PULMONARY EMBOLISM

Hemodynamic responses to PE have been the subject of discussion and speculation for many years. Hemodynamic measurements made during diagnostic pulmonary angiography often have been said to represent the "response" to the embolism.[19,20] Patients with a prior hemodynamic abnormality such as pulmonary hypertension or congestive heart failure will have hemodynamic abnormalities after PE that are merely the result of their underlying cardiac or pulmonary disease. It is often difficult to determine how much of the abnormality is due to embolism and how much is due to the primary cardiopulmonary disturbance. Accordingly the term hemodynamic "response" to PE perhaps should be restricted to those circumstances in which no other process that could independently disturb the hemodynamics is present—that is, the postembolic hemodynamic status in patients with no preembolic cardiopulmonary disease. Similarly the term hemodynamic "status" after PE would more accurately apply to patients with preembolic cardiopulmonary disease.

It appears that the hemodynamic status after PE is primarily determined by the magnitude of the embolic event and the preexisting cardiopulmonary status. Because the preembolic condition of the heart and lungs plays such an important role in the postembolic hemodynamic status, it is worthwhile to consider separately patients with and without prior heart and lung disease.

Hemodynamic Responses in Patients Without Underlying Cardiopulmonary Disease
SYSTEMIC ARTERIAL HYPOXEMIA. The most frequently observed hemodynamic abnormality in patients with PE and a previously normal cardiopulmonary system (Fig. 27-1) has been shown to be systemic arterial hypoxemia.[19,20] Hypoxemia is usually the only manifestation of embolism when obstruction is 25% or less; it has been observed with as little as 13% angiographic obstruction. The arterial oxygen tension (Pao₂) may provide useful information when other disease states that depress Pao₂ are absent, although Pao₂ has been found to be normal in about 6% to 10% of patients after embolism.[4,21] It appears therefore that PE is unlikely when Pao₂ is normal. The extent to which Pao₂ may be depressed after PE in normal patients is worth noting; values as low as 32 mm Hg were observed. A reduction of this magnitude could induce a sympathetic response that may play an important part in

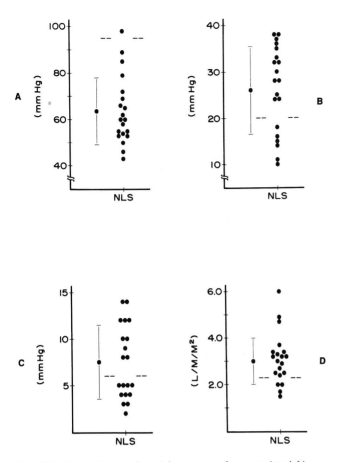

Fig. 27-1. Systemic arterial partial pressures of oxygen *(top left)* mean pulmonary arterial pressure *(top right)*, mean right atrial pressure *(bottom left)*, and cardiac index *(bottom right)* are plotted for each of 20 patients. The mean and one standard deviation are shown for each index. Horizontal broken lines indicate normal values. *(From McIntyre KM and Sasahara AA: Pulmonary angiography, scanning, and hemodynamics in pulmonary embolism: critical review and correlations, CRC Crit Rev Radiol Sci 3:489, 1972. Used by permission.)*

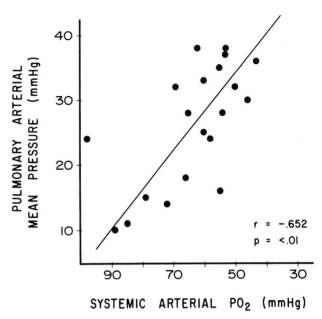

Fig. 27-2. The relation between pulmonary arterial mean pressure and systemic arterial hypoxemia after pulmonary embolism. *(From McIntyre KM and Sasahara AA: Pulmonary angiography, scanning, and hemodynamics in pulmonary embolism: critical review and correlations, CRC Crit Rev Radiol Sci 3:489, 1972. Used by permission.)*

the total cardiovascular status after PE in humans.[22] Some correlation between the degree of Pao_2 depression and the extent of pulmonary vascular obstruction was observed, which indicates that in previously normal patients this measurement could roughly quantify the extent of embolus (Fig. 27-2). Mechanisms for this hypoxemia have been shown to include venous admixture, diminished diffusion, and/or ventilation-perfusion ($\dot{V}/\dot{Q}$) imbalance.[23]

PULMONARY HYPERTENSION. The next most frequent hemodynamic derangement after PE in patients free of prior cardiopulmonary disease was pulmonary hypertension (Fig. 27-1). The angiographic observation that PE obstruction of 25% to 30% of the pulmonary vasculature is associated with pulmonary hypertension is not inconsistent with results of animal and human studies following unilateral balloon occlusion of the pulmonary artery and pneumonectomy,[24] which showed that pulmonary hypertension does not usually occur until about 50% of the pulmonary vasculature is occluded. In addition to mechanical obstruction, other factors have been shown to be

important in the production of pulmonary hypertension. These include hypoxia, localization of emboli in the small pulmonary vasculature,[25] and probably release of serotonin from platelet-rich thromboemboli, all of which can induce pulmonary artery vasoconstriction.[26,27] Angiography is not capable of quantitating vasoconstriction. Whatever the roles of these factors, there nonetheless appears to be a definite relation between the extent of angiographically demonstrated embolic obstruction and severity of pulmonary hypertension (Fig. 27-3).

It is of particular interest to note that no patient developed a pulmonary artery mean pressure in excess of 40 mm Hg, even though obstruction was massive in some. It was concluded that this pressure approximates the maximum that a previously normal right ventricle can generate. This conclusion is consistent with observations of other investigators.[28] Accordingly we believe that a pulmonary arterial mean pressure of 30 to 40 mm Hg represents severe pulmonary hypertension in a patient with no prior cardiopulmonary disease. As a corollary it may be stated that a mean pulmonary arterial pressure level over 40 mm Hg after PE should suggest either chronic recurrent embolization or prior nonembolic causes of pulmonary hypertension.

RIGHT VENTRICULAR FILLING PRESSURE. Elevation of right atrial mean pressure was less frequent than pulmonary hypertension in patients with previously normal cardiopulmonary status; it occurred in only half the patients (Fig. 27-1). An elevation of filling pressure was a reliable indication of encroachment on right ventricular reserve. It appears to bear a direct relation to the degree of pulmonary hypertension, as shown in Fig. 27-4. The right

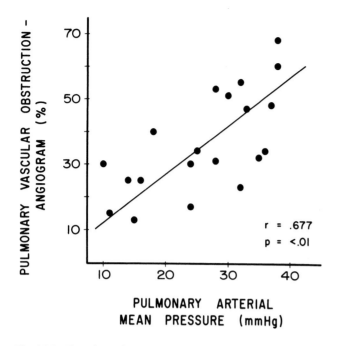

Fig. 27-3. The relation between estimated angiographic obstruction and pulmonary arterial mean pressure following PE. *(From McIntyre KM and Sasahara AA: Pulmonary angiography, scanning, and hemodynamics in pulmonary embolism: critical review and correlations, CRC Crit Rev Radiol Sci 3:489, 1972. Used by permission.)*

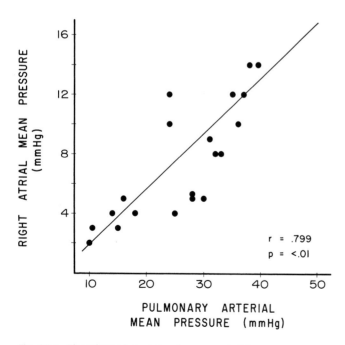

Fig. 27-4. The relation between pulmonary arterial mean pressure and right atrial mean pressure following PE. *(From McIntyre KM and Sasahara AA: Pulmonary angiography, scanning, and hemodynamics in pulmonary embolism: critical review and correlations, CRC Crit Rev Radiol Sci 3:489, 1972. Used by permission.)*

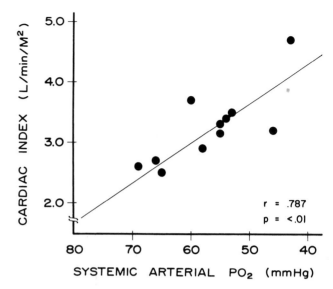

Fig. 27-5. The relation between cardiac index and systemic arterial hypoxemia following PE. *(From McIntyre KM and Sasahara AA: Pulmonary angiography, scanning, and hemodynamics in pulmonary embolism: critical review and correlations, CRC Crit Rev Radiol Sci 3:489, 1972. Used by permission.)*

atrial mean pressure was occasionally elevated when pulmonary arterial mean pressure was less than 30 mm Hg, but usually it was not. When pulmonary arterial mean pressure exceeded 30 mm Hg, however, right atrial mean pressure was consistently elevated. Therefore severe pulmonary hypertension (pulmonary arterial mean pressure of 30 to 40 mm Hg for patients free of prior cardiopulmonary disease) could be diagnosed after PE if neck vein distention was prominent or if central venous pressure was elevated. However, more than 30% embolic obstruction could be present without any signs of venous pressure elevation.

CARDIAC INDEX. The cardiac index was rarely depressed after PE (Fig. 27-1). In most patients it was normal or increased. Previous studies suggested that an increase in cardiac index may be a characteristic response to embolization in the absence of cardiac failure.[4,23] One factor that may be responsible is systemic arterial hypoxemia. Observations in the unanesthetized dog indicate that an increase in cardiac output in response to hypoxia is not observed until Pa_{O_2} is less than 30 mm Hg. In humans Kontos, Levasseur, and Richardson[29] showed that acute depression of Pa_{O_2} below 40 mm Hg was consistently followed by increased cardiac output. Their study also suggested that less striking increases in cardiac index may be expected when the Pa_{O_2} drops acutely to a range of 50 to 60 mm Hg. Nine of eleven patients in our study in whom this relation was examined had Pa_{O_2} values below 60 mm Hg, which made hypoxemia a tenable explanation for the increase in cardiac output observed (Fig. 27-5). Experimental evidence further suggests that the high-flow response to hypoxemia may be mediated by a marked increase in cardiac sympathetic discharge both in animals and in humans.[30] Another explanation may be that the hypoxic stimulus to systemic vasoconstriction may result in an increase in venous return with a resultant increase in stroke output.[31] This explanation is consistent with the observation that increases in cardiac index in our study were mediated primarily by increases in stroke volume rather than in heart rate.[19] It is likely that enhancement of both cardiosympathetic tone and venous return are involved as compensatory phenomena after PE in previously normal patients. Failure of these mechanisms to sustain stroke output may ultimately result in a low cardiac index, a high right atrial mean pressure, and a predominantly chronotropic response to cardiosympathetic influences. This appeared to be the condition of three of the four patients in our series in whom the cardiac index was depressed (Fig. 27-1).

When the cardiac index dropped, it was virtually always associated with massive obstruction and what we previously defined as severe pulmonary hypertension for patients with a normal preembolic cardiopulmonary status—that is, a pulmonary arterial mean pressure between 30 and 40 mm Hg. It is interesting that right atrial mean pressure may be elevated without a depression in cardiac index, which again suggests that the Frank-Starling mechanism plays some role, however limited, as a compensatory mechanism after PE. Observations that a mild elevation of right atrial mean pressure improves right ventricular performance in the course of acute myocardial infarction support this position. It may be said as a corollary, however, that when the cardiac index is depressed in the absence of an elevated right atrial mean pressure or central venous pressure, PE is not the sole cause, and an additional cardiovascular disturbance should be sought.

In summarizing the hemodynamic status after PE in patients free of prior heart and lung disease, we conclude that clinically detectable PE usually does not occur without a low Pa_{O_2}; this may be the only abnormality. Once angiographically demonstrable obstruction exceeds 25% to 30%, pulmonary arterial mean pressure is likely to be elevated. Right atrial mean pressure is less frequently elevated and usually requires embolic obstruction of 30% to 35% and a pulmonary arterial mean pressure of 30 mm Hg or more before it is consistently observed. Reduced cardiac index is less common and, when caused by PE, should be associated with pulmonary vascular obstruction greater than 40% to 50% and with elevated right ventricular filling pressure.

Dalen, Banas, and Brooks[28] reported similar hemodynamic data in patients free of cardiopulmonary disease before PE. Pulmonary arterial mean pressure was usually but not always increased. It never exceeded 40 mm Hg despite extensive obstruction in some patients. Right atrial pressure was normal more frequently than pulmonary arterial mean pressure. The cardiac index was often increased even though right atrial mean pressure was elevated. Although depressions of the cardiac index were infrequent (approximately 15%), when present they were usually associated with substantial increases in right atrial mean pressure and systemic hypotension. Miller et al[25] reported on the clinical and hemodynamic findings in 23 patients who had massive PE proved by angiographic evidence of involvement of at least half of the major

pulmonary artery branches. All but 2 patients were free of prior cardiopulmonary disease. Pulmonary embolectomy was performed in 12 of these cases, and the extent of embolic obstruction was confirmed at that time. There were no deaths. Hemodynamic findings were similar to those in our patients, although depression of the cardiac index and hypotension were more frequent among their patients, possibly because all had massive embolism. Furthermore, pulmonary arterial mean pressure was lower, suggesting that inability of the previously normal right ventricle to maintain output may be associated with a failure of pressure generation. Hirsh, Hale, and McDonald[32] reported hemodynamic observations that were comparable to ours, although (as in the study of Miller et al) all of their patients had major emboli.

Hemodynamic Responses in Patients With Prior Cardiopulmonary Disease

A comparison of patients free of prior cardiopulmonary disease with 30 patients with preembolic cardiopulmonary disease was very instructive.[33] Patients with prior heart and lung disease had significantly less angiographic obstruction (Fig. 27-6). Mean obstruction (23%) in this group was less than that required to produce pulmonary hypertension in previously normal patients. Massive obstruction was quite infrequent; as shown by angiography no patient with prior cardiopulmonary disease had more than 50% obstruction. The degree of pulmonary hypertension, however, was significantly greater. The apparent upper limit of pulmonary hypertension for the previously normal subjects, a pulmonary arterial mean pressure of approximately 40 mm Hg, was the average for patients with prior cardiopulmonary disease, and normal pulmonary arterial pressures were unusual (Fig. 27-6). The relation of angiographically demonstrated obstruction to the severity of pulmonary hypertension is shown for each group in Fig. 27-7. When judged by the responses observed in normal patients, patients with prior cardiopulmonary disease clearly showed a level of pulmonary hypertension that was disproportionate to the degree of embolic obstruction. Furthermore, the fact that the mean value for pulmonary arterial pressure in patients with prior cardiopulmonary disease exceeded the highest values observed in patients free of prior cardiopulmonary disease indicated that the pressure-generating capability of the right ventricle in those cases was greater than normal—that is, that right ventricular hypertrophy had likely occurred.

Although embolic obstruction shown by angiography was significantly greater in patients with previously normal hearts and lungs, the decrease in Pa_{O_2} was not significantly different in the two groups. The depression of Pa_{O_2} in previously normal patients could be attributed to the embolic event per se, whereas in patients with preembolic heart and lung disease, such depressions could be caused by lung disease, heart disease, or PE, alone or in combination. Accordingly the roughly quantitative value of Pa_{O_2} depression in predicting the extent of vascular involvement in previously normal patients is invalid in those with prior cardiopulmonary disease. Furthermore, because the Pa_{O_2} may already be depressed because of preexisting heart

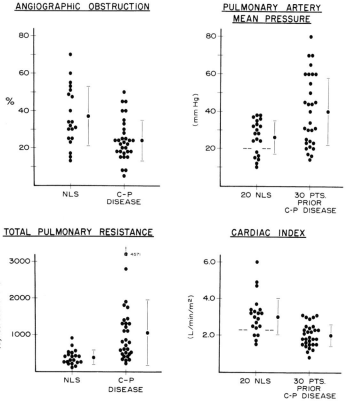

ANGIOGRAPHIC OBSTRUCTION

PULMONARY ARTERY MEAN PRESSURE

TOTAL PULMONARY RESISTANCE

CARDIAC INDEX

Fig. 27-6. The extent of angiographic obstruction in percent *(top left)*, pulmonary arterial mean pressure *(top right)*, total pulmonary resistance *(bottom left)*, and cardiac index *(bottom right)* are shown for 20 patients free of prior cardiopulmonary disease *(NLS)* and 30 patients with prior cardiopulmonary disease *(C-P disease)*. The mean and 1 SD are shown for each group. *(From McIntyre KM and Sasahara AA: Pulmonary angiography, scanning, and hemodynamics in pulmonary embolism: critical review and correlations, CRC Crit Rev Radiol Sci 3:489, 1972. Used by permission.)*

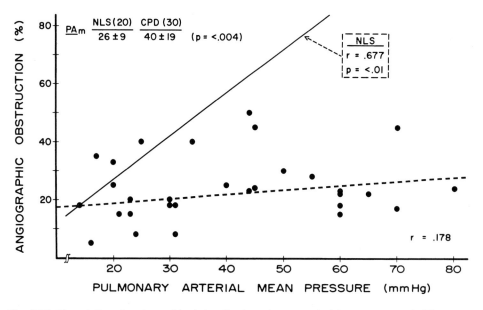

Fig. 27-7. The relation of angiographic obstruction to pulmonary arterial mean pressure in 30 patients with prior cardiopulmonary disease *(CPD)*. No predictable relation was found *(dotted line)*. The regression line for the two values in 20 patients free of prior cardiopulmonary disease *(NLS)* is superimposed. The mean and 1 SD for both groups are shown in the upper left. *(PAm, Pulmonary arterial mean [pressure].) (From McIntyre KM and Sasahara AA: Pulmonary angiography, scanning, and hemodynamics in pulmonary embolism: critical review and correlations, CRC Crit Rev Radiol Sci 3:489, 1972. Used by permission.)*

or lung disease in these patients, a depression of Pa_{O_2} cannot be used to support the diagnosis of PE in this group.

Right atrial mean pressure was also an unreliable indicator of the severity of PE in patients with prior cardiopulmonary disease. When elevated, it could often be attributed to underlying cardiopulmonary disease rather than PE. The value of elevated central venous pressure or jugular venous distention as a sign of life-threatening pulmonary vascular obstruction by embolism may be lost in this group of patients.

Decreased cardiac index was usually seen only after extensive embolic obstruction (40% to 50% or more) in patients free of prior cardiopulmonary disease, but among those with prior heart and lung disease, it was the rule after PE, despite less obstruction (Fig. 27-6). The difference in the cardiac index after embolism therefore appeared to be determined more by the preembolic hemodynamic status than by the impact of the embolism itself. A depressed cardiac index was usually associated with massive angiographically demonstrable obstruction (greater than 40%) and with "severe" pulmonary hypertension (30 to 40 mm Hg) in patients with no preembolic cardiopulmonary disease, whereas depressions of the cardiac index appeared to be independent of both the magnitude of obstruction and the pulmonary arterial pressure in patients with preexisting cardiopulmonary disease. Previously normal patients usually had a normal or increased cardiac index when pulmonary arterial mean pressure was normal or mildly elevated (20 to 30 mm Hg), whereas the cardiac index in the other group was often depressed at this level. The cardiac index was depressed in patients free of preembolic cardiopulmonary disease when pulmonary arterial mean pressure was 30 to 40 mm Hg. Pressures in excess of 40 mm Hg were observed only in patients with underlying cardiopulmonary disease, all but one of whom had a depressed cardiac index. The extent to which depression of the cardiac index resulted from PE alone or from previous cardiopulmonary abnormalities was not clearly determinable in this group.

Comparing the relation between the postembolic hemodynamic status and the extent of angiographic obstruction in previously normal patients with that in patients with preembolic heart and lung disease was useful, however, in determining the extent to which prior cardiopulmonary disease altered the relatively predictable relation seen in previously normal patients. Such a comparison may have prognostic and therapeutic importance when the cardiac index is depressed in patients who have had prior cardiopulmonary disease. It appears that when the cardiac index is depressed after PE in previously normal patients, PE is life-threatening but potentially reversible. In patients with preembolic cardiopulmonary disease, the same may be true, but less extensive embolic obstruction may result in depression of a previously normal cardiac index because of preexisting alterations in the pulmonary vasculature and the heart. It is equally possible that an angiographically detectable clot may be totally incidental to impairment of cardiac output in patients with preembolic cardiac failure.

A comparison between total pulmonary vascular resistance and the extent of angiographically shown obstruction provided additional insight into the mechanism involved in determining the postembolic hemodynamic status. This relation suggests that for previously normal patients, total pulmonary resistance is proportional to the extent of embolic obstruction. It appears that a total pulmonary resistance of 800 dynes/sec/cm^{-5} approximates the highest level likely to be seen acutely, because this was the maximum seen in patients with massive obstruction. The average total pulmonary resistance was similar to that observed by Dalen, Banas, and Brooks[28] in a group of patients free of prior cardiopulmonary disease. When pulmonary vascular obstruction reached 40%, total pulmonary resistance was in the range of 200 to 400 dynes/sec/cm^{-5}. When obstruction exceeded 40%, total pulmonary resistance was higher. The difference between total pulmonary resistance in patients with and without prior cardiopulmonary disease makes clear the extent to which the preembolic pulmonary vascular status affected the postembolic status.

DIAGNOSTIC EVALUATION

The objective of a diagnostic evaluation for acute PE should be to confirm the presumptive diagnosis, to begin therapy promptly, or to exclude its presence and seek other diagnoses. Because PE is complex, can recur and be fatal, a simple, unqualified algorithmic approach to diagnosis should not be carried out, in contrast to many other major diseases that do not have serious consequences if a diagnosis is delayed or hindered for a few days. Hence, the diagnostic evaluation should be tailored to the clinical urgency and the facilities that are readily available to the physician.

Clinical Laboratory Tests

Although a number of biochemical abnormalities may occur in PE, the routine laboratory tests available are nonspecific. The white blood cell count is frequently normal in patients with PE/pulmonary infarction. Particularly with infarction, where the presence of a pulmonary infiltrate on the chest x-ray may suggest pneumonia, a normal white blood cell count should raise the suspicion of pulmonary infarction rather than pneumonia. In our own series the white blood cell count was less than 15,000/mm^3 in over 90% of patients with PE and was within normal limits in approximately 80%.[34] Similarly lacking in sensitivity and specificity was the biochemical triad of the elevated levels of serum bilirubin and lactic dehydrogenase and normal levels of glutamic oxaloacetic transaminase.[34,35] In fact, a raised level of serum bilirubin in patients with PE correlated better with the presence of right ventricular failure.[34]

Other investigations have reported the usefulness of measuring the byproducts of thrombosis and to a lesser degree, fibrinolysis: fibrin degradation products, fibrinopeptide A, urinary thromboxane B2, soluble fibrin complexes, and the platelet protein β-thromboglobulin.[36-39] Unfortunately these tests lacked the sensitivity and specificity to become an accepted part of the diagnostic evaluation and were not available on a routine basis.

In recent years considerable interest has been focused

on the diagnostic use of D-dimer (DD) in patients with suspected PE.[40] DD is an epitope produced from the plasmin degradation of a cross-linked fibrin clot. It can be measured accurately by a monoclonal antibody assay in plasma. Although the test is very sensitive (about 96%), it lacked specificity in a metaanalysis of over 400 patients with suspected PE. In another recent study[41] the enzyme-linked immunosorbent assay (ELISA) DD with a cutoff value of 300 ng/ml was compared with a latex agglutination assay with a cutoff value of 500 ng/ml in patients with suspected PE. The ELISA DD showed a sensitivity and negative predictive value of 100% in all patients and patients with non–high-probability $\dot{V}/\dot{Q}$ scans, but the corresponding specificities were only 26% and 13%, respectively. The latex agglutination assay showed a sensitivity of 84% in all patients and 90% in patients with non–high-probability $\dot{V}/\dot{Q}$ scans, negative predictive values of 93% in all patients and 98% in patients with non–high-probability scans, and specificities of 56% in all patients and 55% in patients with non–high-probability scans. This study showed that an ELISA DD value of less than 300 ng/ml excludes PE but occurs in a small proportion of patients with clinically suspected PE. The latex agglutination assay with a cutoff of 500 ng/ml has clinical use in excluding PE in the subgroup of patients with non–high-probability lung scans. However, the 95% confidence interval on the observed sensitivity in this group is wide.

In addition, levels of DD are raised in patients with DVT[42] and also acute myocardial infarction.[43] A technical problem with the ELISA measuring DD is the relatively long time required to complete the test, precluding its use in the urgent situation. It seems more useful to proceed directly with the more diagnostic imaging procedures.

Chest Radiograph

The plain film of the chest continues to be a standard tool by which all disorders of the lung are evaluated. It is readily obtained and aside from the radiation exposure, which is small, it is a harmless, noninvasive procedure. Although a number of findings have been described over the years, a useful combination was described by the radiologists in the NIH-sponsored UPET: the combination of a pulmonary infiltrate and an elevated hemidiaphragm on the same side, found in 41% of the patients (Table 27-3). The pulmonary infiltrate often was thought to represent pneumonia initially. The elevated hemidiaphragm on the involved side represented the decreased lung volume that resulted from atelectasis occurring in PE. The combination therefore of a pulmonary infiltrate and an elevated hemidiaphragm on the same side should suggest PE infarction rather than pneumonia.

Electrocardiogram

Although a number of electrocardiogram (ECG) findings have been described in PE, few are specific enough to raise suspicion of the disease. Aside from the previously described pattern of acute cor pulmonale, or the $S_1Q_3T_3$ pattern, other findings are nonspecific and can be encountered in many other cardiopulmonary disorders: arrhythmias, QRS abnormalities, and ST-T wave changes (Table 27-4).

Table 27-3. UPET Frequency of Chest X-Ray Abnormalities in Pulmonary Embolism

Abnormality	Patients (%)
Consolidation	41
High diaphragm	41
Pleural effusion	28
Plump pulmonary arteries	23
Atelectasis	20
Enlarged left ventricle	16
Focal oligemia	15
Enlarged right ventricle	5

(Adapted from Sasahara AA et al: The urokinase pulmonary embolism trial: a national cooperative study, Circulation 47[suppl II]:66, 1973.)

Table 27-4. Frequency of Electrocardiogram Abnormalities Among Patients in UPET

Abnormality	(%)	Patients
Rhythm disturbances	–	11
Atrial ectopic beats	3	–
Ventricular ectopic beats	9	–
Atrial fibrillation	3	–
P pulmonale	–	4
QRS changes	–	65
Right axis deviation	5	–
Left axis deviation	12	–
Incomplete RBB block	5*	–
Complete RBB block	11*	–
$S_1Q_3T_3$	11*	–
ST-segment changes	–	44
T wave inversion	–	40

*Findings of massive PE.

The most frequent arrhythmias are ventricular and atrial ectopy, whereas the most common sustained arrhythmia is paroxysmal atrial fibrillation. Although paroxysmal atrial flutter may occur in PE with a high degree of specificity, it is not common. QRS abnormalities are frequent, having been noted in 65% of patients in the NIH-sponsored UPET.[4] A number of other abnormalities were also observed, including right and left axis deviation; right bundle branch (RBB) block, incomplete and complete; and the $S_1Q_3T_3$ pattern. Nonspecific and common were ST-T wave changes, which were found in 40% to 44% of patients in the trial. Aside from the $S_1Q_3T_3$ pattern, RBB block, and the T wave inversions over the right precordial leads, which generally occur only with significant PE, the other findings had no apparent relation to the size of the embolus. In essence, ECG is quite sensitive in patients with PE, although many of the changes are nonspecific. Nonetheless, it remains an important part of the workup for cardiopulmonary disorders and should always be obtained. It can be particularly useful in patients who suffer syncope or have extensive chest discomfort when one must consider acute myocardial infarction in the differential diagnoses.

Arterial Oxygen Tension

One of the most commonly used laboratory tests in suspected PE is measurement of Pa_{O_2}. Its usefulness derives from the fact that the vast majority of patients with PE have some degree of hypoxemia. In fact, in patients with PE, but without underlying cardiopulmonary disease, there is an inverse relation between the size of the emboli and the Pa_{O_2}.[19] Approximately 6% of patients with confirmed PE will have a Pa_{O_2} of 90 mm Hg or more, despite the size of the emboli.[4] As a general rule therefore it can be stated that in patients suspected of PE, if the Pa_{O_2} is 90 mm Hg or more, the likelihood that PE is present is only about 6%. It is most useful in patients without underlying cardiopulmonary disease in whom a normal Pa_{O_2} may help exclude PE with a relatively high degree of probability.

More recently the alveolar-arterial oxygen gradient has been evaluated as a diagnostic aid in the diagnosis of PE. Considered a more sensitive measure of the alteration in oxygenation than the Pa_{O_2},[44] a retrospective analysis of the relationship of the alveolar-arterial oxygen gradient to the diagnosis of PE was carried out in 109 patients discharged with the diagnosis of PE.[45] Of these, only 1 of 57 patients (1.8%) without a history of PE or DVT and with a normal alveolar-arterial oxygen gradient had PE. Thus from this small study, a normal alveolar-arterial oxygen gradient among patients without a history of PE or DVT makes the diagnosis of PE unlikely. However, in the Prospective Investigation of Pulmonary Embolism Diagnosis (PIOPED) study,[46-48] a normal alveolar-arterial oxygen gradient (up to 20 mm Hg) was noted in almost 15% of patients with PE, and the mean oxygen gradients of those with PE and without PE were virtually identical.[46]

Lung Scanning

Central to the adequate evaluation of patients with suspected PE is the perfusion lung scan, with or without a ventilation scan. Vagaries of the clinical presentation preclude making a solid clinical decision on the basis of clinical findings. The perfusion lung scan is an extremely useful aid in helping confirm the clinical impression or in excluding the diagnosis. If multiple-view scans are normal, clinical PE is extremely unlikely, and therefore the diagnostic evaluation can be directed toward other disorders. If the scans are abnormal, other procedures should be performed to arrive at a firmer basis for diagnosis. The modern, more realistic approach to the interpretation of lung scans considers the limitations of scanning. It recognizes the fact that lung scanning is a procedure that characterizes only the regional distribution of pulmonary arterial blood flow. Because it is now known that a number of abnormalities may alter the distribution of flow, the interpretation of abnormal lung scans should state the probability of PE as the causative disease. Lesions on perfusion scans are now categorized as having high, intermediate, or low probability of having been caused by PE (Fig. 27-8).

High-probability lung scans are those in which the lesions or scan defects are (1) multiple (in one or both lungs) and (2) have configurations compatible with vascular lesions. These include lesions that occur as concave defects on the lateral edges of the lung or along a pleural surface, or wedge-shaped or segmental lesions that conform to a vascular pattern. Intermediate- or low-probability lung scans are those in which the lesions may be either single or multiple, generally corresponding with some other abnormality on the plain chest film. The lesions are not clearly definable as segmental or vascular in origin. They tend to be round or elongated, crossing lung segments. They are most commonly noted in those with chronic obstructive airways disease. It should be noted, however, that patients with obstructive airways disease may also show segmental or other types of lesions that have a vascular configuration. The only difference is that these vascular lesions occur much more frequently in patients with PE. The simultaneous performance of ventilation scanning (before or shortly after perfusion scanning) will add specificity to lung scanning ($\dot{V}/\dot{Q}$ scanning). Characteristically a normal ventilation scan over an area that shows a perfusion defect(s) is said to be highly specific for PE. Such "mismatched" defects are generally seen only in patients with PE. Lesions that are "matched" (poor ventilation and poor perfusion) are indicative of other diseases such as chronic obstructive airways disease. However, it is in this category of patients that the specificity of combined ventilation and perfusion scanning is less secure. If PE occurred in an area of lung that already had poor perfusion and ventilation, the lung scan would not change significantly and the resulting "matched" lesion would be interpreted as being consistent with chronic lung disease. In addition, an infiltrate on the plain chest film because of pulmonary infarction or pneumonia will also produce a $\dot{V}/\dot{Q}$ scan of poor perfusion and ventilation. Hence, it is important that $\dot{V}/\dot{Q}$ lesions be interpreted in areas of lung that appear normal in the plain chest x-ray. In these clinical situations other diagnostic procedures such as selective pulmonary angiography should be performed. If not available, objective assessment of the deep venous system of the legs for DVT may be helpful. In general, however, a compatible history for PE in a young patient without underlying heart or lung disease, plus an abnormal lung scan with high-probability segmental or lobar lesions, may be adequate documentation to begin therapy.[47]

To determine the sensitivities and specificities of $\dot{V}/\dot{Q}$ lung scans for acute PE, a random sample of 933 of 1493 patients was studied prospectively in the PIOPED study.[48] Nine hundred thirty-three patients underwent scintigraphy and seven hundred fifty-five patients underwent pulmonary angiography. A total of 251 patients (33%) of the 755 demonstrated PE. Almost all patients with PE had abnormal scans of high, intermediate, or low probability, but so did most without PE (sensitivity of 98%, specificity of 10%). Of 116 patients with high-probability scans and definitive angiograms, 102 (88%) had PE, but only a minority with PE had high-probability scans (sensitivity of 41%, specificity of 97%). Of 322 with intermediate-probability scans and definitive angiograms, 105 (33%) had pulmonary embolism. Follow-up and angiography together showed that PE occurred in 12% of patients with low-probability scans. Clinical assessment combined with the $\dot{V}/\dot{Q}$ scan established the diagnosis or exclusion of PE for only a minority of patients—those with clear and concordant clinical and $\dot{V}/\dot{Q}$ scan findings.

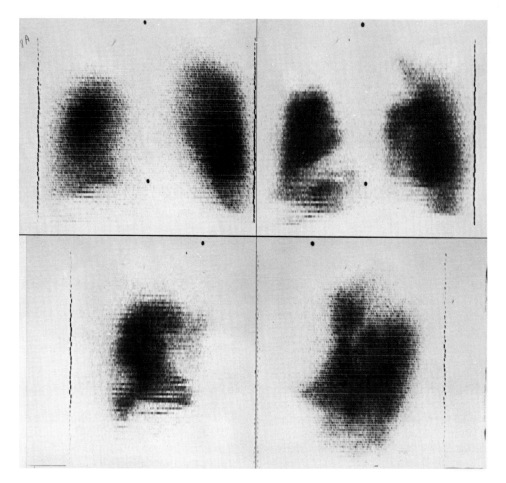

Fig. 27-8. Four-view perfusion lung scan of patient with massive pulmonary embolism: anterior *(upper left)*, posterior *(upper right)*, right lateral *(lower left)*, and left lateral *(lower right)* views. Striking are multiple lesions and substantial perfusion deficits in both the right and left lungs.

The PIOPED Central Scan Interpretation Categories and Criteria used in assessing scans are reproduced in the box on p. 479 because of their usefulness in providing uniformity of interpretation.[48]

Selective Pulmonary Angiography

Since selective pulmonary angiography was introduced in 1964,[49] it has become the standard by which PE can be diagnosed with assurance during life. Although a number of angiographic findings have been reported, only two have been accepted as confirmatory for PE: (1) an intravascular filling defect and (2) an arterial vessel cutoff (Fig. 27-9). Other findings that have been described in PE but are not diagnostic of the disease when present alone are (1) focal flow retardation or asymmetry of filling with contrast material, (2) pruning of vessels or the "winter tree" effect, and (3) nonfilling of vessels.[50,51]

Pulmonary angiography is most helpful in demonstrating thromboembolism in patients with underlying heart or lung disease, where the clinical presentation may be nonspecific and compatible with an exacerbation of the underlying disease and where the V̇/Q̇ scan may be less specific. Visualization of the impacted emboli would secure the diagnosis and obviate the need for other studies.

Pulmonary angiography is also very useful in other patients without previous heart or lung disease who are suspected of having PE. In addition to confirming the diagnosis, the measurement of pressures in the pulmonary circulation and right side of the heart provides an index of the degree of competency of the heart in coping with the embolic obstruction. Because there is a direct relation between size of the emboli and right ventricular pressures, these measurements can provide valuable diagnostic and therapeutic information.[19]

Recurrence of PE is also best confirmed by pulmonary angiography. At the bedside it is virtually impossible to differentiate true recurrence from fragmentation of the original emboli with distal migration.[52] Performing a repeat pulmonary angiogram may be the only reliable method for making this distinction. If a repeat angiogram showed the disappearance of a previous proximal embolus, and with poor or no visualization of the distal vessels subserved by the larger, originally occluded vessel, one could conclude that the original embolus fragmented with resulting distal migration or embolization of the smaller fragments. In contrast to true recurrence, fragmentation and distal migration are not considered a failure of treatment requiring a change in therapy.

PIOPED CENTRAL SCAN INTERPRETATION CATEGORIES AND CRITERIA

High Probability
≥2 Large (>75% of a segment) segmental perfusion defects without corresponding ventilation or roentgenographic abnormalities or substantially larger than either matching ventilation or chest roentgenogram abnormalities

≥2 Moderate segmental (≥25% and ≤75% of a segment) perfusion defects without matching ventilation or chest roentgenogram abnormalities and 1 large mismatched segmental defect

≥4 Moderate segmental perfusion defects without ventilation or chest roentgenogram abnormalities

Intermediate Probability (Indeterminate)
Not falling into normal, very low, low, or high-probability categories

Borderline high or borderline low

Difficult to categorize as low or high

Low Probability
Nonsegmental perfusion defects (e.g., very small effusion causing blunting of the costophrenic angle, cardiomegaly, enlarged aorta, hila, and mediastinum, and elevated diaphragm)

Single moderate mismatched segmental perfusion defect with normal chest roentgenogram

Any perfusion defect with a substantially larger chest roentgenogram abnormality

Low Probability
Large or moderate segmental perfusion defects involving no more than four segments in one lung and no more than three segments in one lung region with matching ventilation defects either equal to or larger in size and chest roentgenogram either normal or with abnormalities substantially smaller than perfusion defects

>3 Small segmental perfusion defects (<25% of a segment) with a normal chest roentgenogram

Very Low Probability
≤3 Small segmental perfusion defects with a normal chest roentgenogram

Normal
No perfusion defects present

Perfusion outlines exactly the shape of the lungs as seen on the chest roentgenogram (hilar and aortic impressions may be seen, chest roentgenogram and/or ventilation study may be abnormal)

(The PIOPED Investigators: Value of the ventilation/perfusion scan in acute pulmonary embolism, JAMA 263:2753, 1990.)

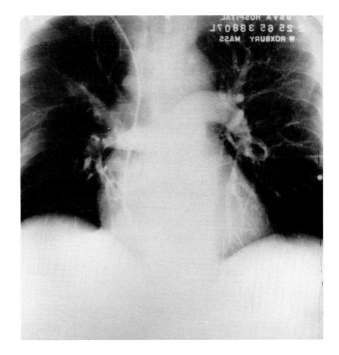

Fig. 27-9. Pulmonary angiogram shows massive embolism. Large filling defect (saddle embolus) at junction of right upper, intermediate, and lower lobar arteries with multiple filling defects obstructing almost all of the blood flow to the right lung.

Pulmonary angiography, however, is an invasive procedure that has some morbidity and mortality, albeit very small. It is one of the more difficult angiographic procedures to perform well and requires expensive equipment and a trained team to perform safely and expertly. Because of its invasive nature, it does not lend itself to serial performance. Hence, other diagnostic measures have been sought. One such test is electrical impedance plethysmography.

Electrical Impedance Plethysmography
Assessment of the deep venous system of the legs as a diagnostic aid stems from observations made by Sevitt and Gallagher[53] some years ago when they reported that on postmortem examination the great majority of their patients who died of massive PE embolized from the deep venous system of the legs. Some years later Kakkar, Howe, and Flanc[54] noted a similar correlation in a radioactive fibrinogen leg scan survey of patients undergoing elective abdominal or thoracic operation. Because radioactive fibrinogen was not available for leg scans at that time, we chose to assess impedance plethysmography as the noninvasive diagnostic aid in PE, a technique originally described by Wheeler et al.[55] The procedure is a physiologic test that detects and measures venous outflow obstruction in the deep veins, as well as the capability of the venous system to expand and constrict, as it would do in the normal state. It does this very effectively and has a sensitivity reported to average 97% and a specificity of 93%[56] in detecting deep vein thrombi. It does not, however, detect thrombi in the calf veins as efficiently as it does in the deep system. However, because of its noninvasive

nature, serial observations can be made in a patient who is in a high-risk clinical situation for developing thromboembolism.

In our validating study 95% of patients who had PE confirmed by angiography showed an abnormal impedance tracing indicative of deep venous obstruction. None of these patients had history or evidence of major pelvic disease, pelvic operation, or pelvic manipulation that might predispose to thrombosis of the pelvic veins. It was also shown that in patients with suspected PE, if an assessment of the deep veins was positive, the probability of pulmonary angiographic confirmation was 90%, whereas if the impedance assessment was normal bilaterally, the probability of a negative pulmonary angiogram was 90%.[47,56] However, in studies assessing impedance plethysmography in other patient populations with PE, its usefulness was less apparent, being positive for DVT in only 57%.[57]

The results in our own patients, however, were very encouraging and prompted its routine clinical use in our institution, because the procedure again established a strong relation between PE and the deep veins of the legs as the source of the emboli. Other techniques to detect DVT include contrast venography, which is the current standard against which all other methods to detect DVT must be compared. However, as a procedure used for diagnosing PE by detecting the surrogate marker of DVT, contrast venography is probably not ideal because of its inability to visualize clearly the pelvic veins in all patients. Moreover, it is expensive, requires specialized equipment, as well as experience and some degree of expertise on the part of the radiologist. Patient discomfort is prominent.

Color-flow venous duplex scanning (CFVDS), present in most vascular laboratories now, has also been examined as an aid to the diagnosis of PE.[58] In a study of 51 patients with suspected PE, CFVDS was carried out before pulmonary angiography. Forty-one patients also had $\dot{V}/\dot{Q}$ scanning plus CFVDS before angiography. The results unfortunately showed that the combination of $\dot{V}/\dot{Q}$ lung scanning and CFVDS was positive in only 62% of patients with angiographically proven PE.

Another test, radionuclide venography, is a simple diagnostic technique using a radioactive bolus of technetium-99m injected into pedal dorsal veins. The venographic images are visualized by a computerized gamma camera, which permits sequential imaging. The accuracy of radionuclide venography in assessing the venous system of the leg is high, and it is enhanced by observing the transit of the bolus and comparing each leg to the other. However, it has had no validation in this diagnostic situation.

Other newer techniques including imaging with radioisotopes (labeled platelets, monoclonal antibodies), high-resolution computed tomography (CT), or magnetic resonance imaging (MRI) look promising but will require extensive testing for validating its usefulness in the diagnosis of DVT and PE.

Echocardiography

The recent application of echocardiography, including Doppler echocardiography, has provided an excellent, objective assessment of the complex hemodynamic impact on the cardiopulmonary system. Initially reported in identifying intracardiac clots,[59] it was found to be of greater value in assessing the right ventricular pressure and volume overload of PE.[60,61] Other echocardiographic parameters reported to be of value in patients with PE are the ratio of right ventricular and left ventricular end-diastolic size, the abnormal pattern of septal wall motion, hypokinesis of the dilated thin right ventricle, compression of the left ventricle, assessment of the degree of tricuspid regurgitation, estimation of the right ventricular and pulmonary arterial pressures, and an estimate of the size of the right pulmonary artery.[62,63] Having suddenly occurred with the lodgment of emboli in the pulmonary vasculature, these changes remain transient depending on the fate of the obstructing emboli. As noted by several investigators, these changes can revert rapidly to normal, following successful thrombolysis of the emboli.[64,65] These studies are impressive in demonstrating the qualitative and quantitative usefulness of echocardiography in both the diagnostic and therapeutic aspects of PE.

Differential Diagnosis

The clinical diagnosis of PE, as previously pointed out, is not a simple diagnostic exercise in the majority of patients. Because the disease may present in an atypical fashion, a number of disease entities must initially be considered. Moreover, the diagnostic difficulties often are compounded by the association of these other diseases with PE: chronic obstructive airways disease, congestive heart failure, pneumonia, acute myocardial infarction, angina pectoris, carcinoma of the lung, viral pleuritis, and postoperative atelectasis. Many of these diseases share clinical features with PE and hence cannot be excluded purely on a clinical basis.

Diagnostic Recommendations (Fig. 27-10)

When PE is initially suspected, heparin coverage is recommended, especially when the various diagnostic studies and the $\dot{V}/\dot{Q}$ lung scan may require some hours to complete. Key to the diagnosis and decision-making process is the lung scan. PE can be excluded if the multiple views of the scan are normal, unless the history is so compelling that pulmonary angiography is necessary (albeit a rare event). When the lung scan is abnormal, different factors enter into the decision tree. If the lung scan is of high probability of having been caused by PE, and if the history is highly suggestive of PE, especially in patients with risk factors, therapy can begin. If the lung scan is interpreted as low or intermediate probability, pulmonary angiography may be performed for a definitive answer. However, in the absence of angiography, objective assessment for DVT, a surrogate marker for PE, may be carried out. Ninety percent of PEs have their source of emboli in the deep venous system of the legs. Whether impedance plethysmography, color duplex scanning, or contrast venography is used, a positive result warrants treatment. If negative, however, pulmonary angiography should be performed, or if still not available, continued clinical observation, supported by repeated testing over the next several days should be carried out. It should be stressed that in the very urgent

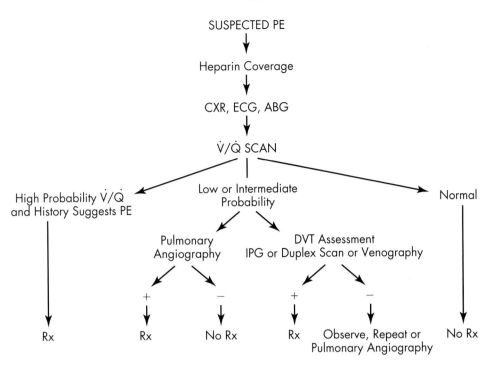

Fig. 27-10. Flow diagram outlining our recommended approach to PE diagnosis (see text).

situation of massive PE, pulmonary angiography, as the only definitive diagnostic study, should be performed as soon as possible.

TREATMENT OF PULMONARY EMBOLISM

The treatment of PE begins when the diagnosis is first suspected. Unless all of the diagnostic studies can be completed within a few hours of suspecting PE, heparin bolus injections of 5000 U are recommended. If the diagnosis is established, the treatment can be continued or changed to thrombolytic agents. If not confirmed, heparin can be terminated.

Heparin

Heparin is a glycosaminoglycan with powerful anticoagulant activity. Its action is mediated by binding to a serine protease inhibitor, antithrombin III, and enhancing its inhibitory effect. It is isolated for commercial preparations from intestinal mucosa of hogs and beef lung.

Heparin administration has been the mainstay of therapy for venous thromboembolism for many years and probably will be for some years to come. Despite the long history of effective use, there has not been, until recently, a consensus concerning the mode of administration and the requirements for laboratory monitoring. Following the demonstration of the relation between the frequency of bleeding complications and the level of heparin activity in the blood,[4] and the subsequent clinical demonstration of reduced bleeding complications, the intravenous administration of heparin by continuous pump infusion appears to be the optimal method of administering the anticoagulant.[21,66]

Heparinization regimens are many and increase as new and novel approaches are investigated. However, until other regimens are shown to be more effective and safer, the following are recommended: a loading dose of 5,000 to 10,000 U intravenously, followed immediately by a continuous pump infusion regulated to deliver approximately 1,200 U/hr. After several half-lives (several hours) any of several clotting tests (activated partial thromboplastin time or thrombin time) should be obtained to maintain the level of anticoagulation at approximately two to three times the control value. Following each adjustment, several hours should elapse before another monitoring sample is obtained. Generally, most patients will require between 1,200 to 1,800 U/hr to maintain the blood clotting test values within the recommended therapeutic range. Once stabilized, clotting tests can be obtained daily. Administered in this fashion, Salzman et al[66] observed only a 1% major bleeding complication, contrasted to the 8% to 10% complication when heparin was administered intravenously on an intermittent basis every 4 hours. In recent years the subcutaneous route of administering heparin has become more popular, particularly in clinical situations where an intravenous line is difficult to place or where constant surveillance of an intravenous setup is difficult. It is also more convenient to administer and is more comfortable for the less symptomatic patient.[67] Though heparin activity control is more difficult because of the vagaries of subcutaneous absorption of heparin, effective anticoagulation can usually be carried out by administering the projected total daily dose in divided doses every 12 hours. In most patients 15,000 to 20,000 U subcutaneously every 12 hours suffices. The initial subcutaneous dose should be given with 5,000 U of heparin intravenously. Blood clotting tests should be performed at the midpoint (sixth hour) after beginning therapy. Appropriate adjustment should be made based on the value of the clotting test.

The duration of heparin administration depends on the subsidence of the acute embolic process, which can be assessed by clinical improvement such as the diminishing of symptoms and signs. However, it has been shown in the experimental animal that 7 to 12 days are required before a thrombus stabilizes, becomes firmly cross-linked, shows cellular infiltration, and becomes firmly attached to the vein wall,[68] which is particularly important in preventing recurrence of PE. More recently it has been shown that a 5-day course of heparin compared with 10 days was equally effective in the treatment of patients with proximal venous thrombosis.[69]

Oral Anticoagulation

Oral anticoagulation therapy is necessary to maintain the antithrombotic state for a period depending on the duration of the high-risk state for recurrent thromboembolism. Unlike heparin, which has a direct antithrombotic effect the instant it is administered, the oral anticoagulants require a prolonged period to be effective. Their action is based on their antagonism with vitamin K, which reduces the activity of the vitamin K–dependent clotting factors (II, VII, IX, and X). Sodium warfarin is the most widely used agent.

In patients with massive PE who have complicating congestive failure, hypotension, or other comorbid conditions, it is recommended that only heparin be administered to simplify management during the period of complete bed rest when venous stasis is maximal. When clinical improvement is sufficient to consider ambulation, warfarin should be begun concurrently with heparin, realizing that 3 to 5 days will be necessary before all of the vitamin K–dependent clotting factors will be sufficiently depleted to achieve effective anticoagulation. Because of the short half-life of 6 hours for factor VII, which most influences the prothrombin time, it is possible to prolong the prothrombin time within 24 to 48 hours to therapeutic levels without achieving an antithrombotic state. Because factor II has a half-life of some 60 hours, a minimum of 3 or more days will be required to achieve an effective antithrombotic state. At this point heparin can be discontinued.

If the patient is not critically ill, oral drugs may be initiated simultaneously with heparin, providing a longer time in which to achieve the desired therapeutic range. When heparin is discontinued, only minor adjustments of dosage are generally required.

There is no unanimity concerning the optimal duration of chronic oral anticoagulant therapy. Coon, Willis, and Symous[70] showed that after 4 to 6 months of outpatient therapy, there was no significant difference between the recurrence rates of thromboembolism in the anticoagulated group and the nonanticoagulated group. Up to 4 to 6 months the frequency of recurrences was strikingly higher in the nonanticoagulated group. Others have recommended that patients receive anticoagulation therapy for 3 months.[71] After this, if the patient is well and fully ambulatory, the oral agent can be stopped.

Thrombolytic Therapy

The investigational use of thrombolytic agents for venous thromboembolism has a long history, but it was not until the late 1970s that the two major activators of the fibrinolytic system, streptokinase (SK) and urokinase (UK), became available to the professional community. SK is a bacterial catabolite with a single chain that indirectly activates plasminogen through an SK-plasminogen complex, whereas UK, produced by the parenchymal cells of the kidney, directly converts plasminogen to plasmin.

Clinical Efficacy

Although many investigations have demonstrated the clinical efficacy of both SK and UK, the major studies that most clearly established the usefulness of fibrinolytic agents in acute venous thromboembolism were the Phase 1 and Phase 2 trials sponsored by the National Heart, Lung and Blood Institute.[4,72]

The multicenter Phase 1 UPET compared the effect of 12 hours of UK therapy followed by heparin therapy with the effects of heparin therapy alone in patients with acute PE. Resolution of pulmonary thromboemboli during the first 24 hours of therapy was greater and more rapid in patients treated with both UK and heparin than in patients treated with heparin alone, according to the results of pretherapy and posttherapy pulmonary angiography (to assess clot resolution), perfusion lung scanning (to evaluate lung reperfusion), and measurements of right ventricular and pulmonary hemodynamics.

The phase 2 Urokinase-Streptokinase Pulmonary Embolism Trial (USPET) compared the efficacy of 12- and 24-hour UK therapy and 24-hour SK therapy in three treatment groups randomized out of 167 patients with acute PE. All three fibrinolytic regimens proved essentially identical in the degree to which they produced clot resolution (Fig. 27-11), lung reperfusion (Fig. 27-12), and hemodynamic improvement (Fig. 27-13). However, the fibrinolytic-treated patients experienced significantly greater improvement than did the heparin-treated patients in the Phase 1 trial. For example, the mean angiographic improvement was significantly better. Similarly, the percentage of overall perfusion scan defect resolution in the three groups of fibrinolytic-treated patients was 23% (range, 18% to 29%), compared with 7% in the heparin group, and finally, the fibrinolytic-treated groups showed considerably greater decrease in right atrial, right ventricular systolic and diastolic, and pulmonary arterial pressures, and considerably greater increases in Pa_{O_2}.

In the subgroup of patients with massive PE, there was a significant difference in the degree of lung reperfusion (Fig. 27-14) and lowering of pulmonary hypertension (Fig. 27-15) favoring the 24-hour UK regimen over the 24-hour SK regimen. Although the trials were not designed to test mortality differences because of the huge number of patients that would have been required, other studies show benefits of thrombolytic therapy not associated with heparin therapy. These include the much higher frequency of preserving venous valve cusps and valve function in the deep veins of the legs, which may have long-term implications in preventing chronic venous hypertension and venous insufficiency.[73,74] In addition, it has been shown that thrombolytic therapy may prevent permanent damage to the pulmonary vasculature by lysing thromboem-

PHASE I AND II RESULTS: ANGIOGRAPHIC CHANGE

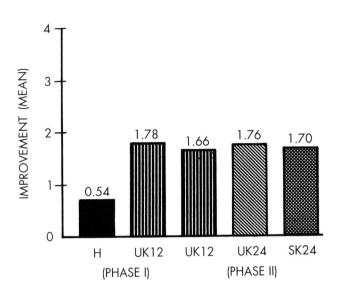

Fig. 27-11. Angiographic assessment of the mean changes following therapy in the five groups of patients in the UPET and USPET trials (see text). Note the virtually identical degrees of improvement in the lytic groups, all of which are superior to the heparin group. *(Reproduced from Sasahara AA et al: Thromb Diathes Haemorrh 33:464, 1975.)*

PHASE II: SCAN DEFECT CHANGES

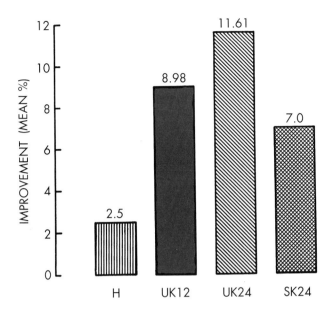

Fig. 27-12. Lung scan assessments of the mean percent improvement in perfusion in the thrombolytic and heparin groups (Phase II) at approximately 24 hours. Note the minimal improvement of the heparin group, compared with the significant return of perfusion in the thrombolytic groups. *(Reproduced from Sasahara AA et al: Thromb Diathes Haemorrh 33:464, 1975.)*

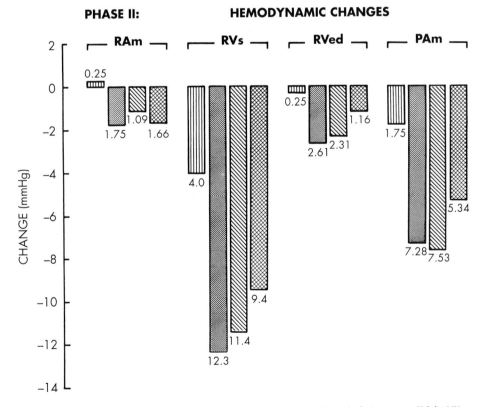

Fig. 27-13. Mean hemodynamic changes in the heparin and three thrombolytic groups (12-hr UK, 24-hr UK, 24-hr SK). The grouping of the four treatment groups for each pressure measurement (right atrial mean, right ventricular systolic, and end-diastolic and pulmonary arterial mean pressures) are as follows, left to right: heparin, 12-hr UK, 24-hr UK and 24-hr SK. Though minimal reductions in the abnormal pressures were noted in the heparin group, significant improvements occurred in the lytic groups. *(Reproduced from Sasahara AA et al: Thromb Diathes Haemorrh 33:464, 1975.)*

PHASE II: SCAN CHANGE: MASSIVE PE

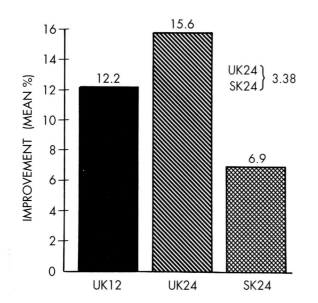

Fig. 27-14. Perfusion lung scan change in massive PE. The degree of reperfusion at 24 hours in the 24-hr UK group was significantly greater than the reperfusion in the 24-hr SK group. The 12- and 24-hr UK groups were not significantly different, though there was a strong trend. *(Reproduced from Sasahara AA et al: Thromb Diathes Haemorrh 33:464, 1975.)*

PHASE II: PAm CHANGE: MASSIVE PE

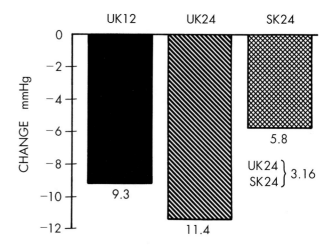

Fig. 27-15. Pulmonary arterial mean *(PAm)* pressure change in massive PE. The degree of lowering of PAm pressure was significantly greater in the 24-hr UK group compared with the 24-hr SK group. The two UK groups were not significantly different. *(Reproduced from Sasahara AA et al: Thromb Diathes Haemorrh 33:464, 1975.)*

boli and restoring the capacity of the pulmonary microcirculation to normal.[75]

RESOLUTION OF EMBOLI IN THE PULMONARY MICROCIRCULATION

Most patients without underlying cardiopulmonary disease recover from PE without apparent sequelae. The perfusion lung scans and pulmonary angiograms return to normal. In the UPET abnormal lung scans of 86% of the patients followed for 1 year returned to normal or had only a minimal (10% or less) residual defect. However, neither the pulmonary angiogram nor the lung scan is a sensitive measure of the state of the pulmonary microcirculation. When properly performed, the pulmonary angiogram may visualize only down to third-order segmental vessels of the 25 to 26 divisions of the pulmonary vasculature before the capillaries. The lung scan is also grossly handicapped by the limits of resolution of the detector-collimator system, which is now about 0.5 cm or slightly less.

We therefore chose to measure the pulmonary capillary blood volume as a sensitive index of the pulmonary microcirculation. Forty patients without prior clinical cardiopulmonary disease were selected for this study so that any abnormality of this measurement could be reasonably attributed to PE and not to any other underlying disorder. When determined 2 weeks following therapy (Fig. 27-16), the mean pulmonary capillary blood volume was 30 ml/m² (normal = 47 ± 5 ml/m² body surface area) in the heparin-treated group and 44 ml/m² in the lytic therapy groups (*P* < 0.001; not shown in Fig. 27-16). At

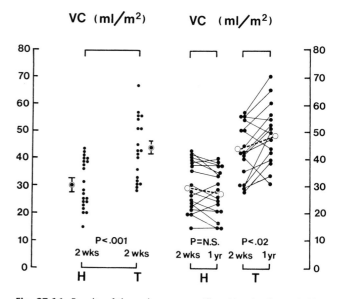

Fig. 27-16. Results of the pulmonary capillary blood volume *(VC)* measured in the heparin *(H)* and thrombolytic *(T)* treated groups, expressed as milliliters per square meter of body surface area. The left panel shows the results at 2 weeks and the right compares the 1-year results with the 2-week results in each group. The open circles represent mean values. There were significant differences in the normal pulmonary capillary blood volumes of the thrombolytic group compared with the abnormally reduced volumes in the heparin group at 2 weeks and at 1 year. *(Reproduced from Sharma GVRK, Burleson VA, and Sasahara AA: Effect of thrombolytic therapy on pulmonary capillary blood volume in patients with pulmonary embolism, N Engl J Med 303:842, 1980.)*

1-year follow-up the mean capillary blood volume was 28 ml/m^2 in the heparin group (no significant difference compared with the 2-week value) and 49 ml/m^2 (significant when compared with the 2-week value) in the lytic group.[75]

Our use of pulmonary capillary blood volume was intended to be a sensitive index of the status of the pulmonary microcirculation. The restoration of the capillary blood volume to normal in the lytic therapy group, in contrast to the abnormally low volume in patients treated with heparin, indicated that residual thromboemboli were present in the heparin-treated patients, whereas there was complete or near-complete clearing of emboli from the microcirculation in the lytic therapy group. The importance of these observations may affect the long-term morbidity from PE.

Therefore 20 of the 40 patients who had angiographically proven PE and who had initially been randomized to an intravenous infusion of heparin ($n = 11$) or a thrombolytic agent (UK or SK, $n = 12$) were restudied after a mean follow-up of 7.4 years to measure the right-sided pressures and to evaluate their response to exercise during supine bicycle ergometry.[76] Results showed that, at rest, the pulmonary arterial mean pressure and the pulmonary vascular resistance were significantly higher in the heparin group compared with the thrombolytic group (22 vs. 17 mm Hg, $P < 0.05$, and 351 vs. 171 dynes/sec/cm^{-5}, $P < 0.02$, respectively). During exercise both the parameters rose to a significantly higher level in the heparin group (from rest to exercise, pulmonary arterial mean pressure: 22 to 32 mm Hg, $P < 0.01$, and pulmonary vascular resistance: 351 to 437 dynes/sec/cm^{-5}, $P < 0.01$, respectively), but not in the thrombolytic group (rest to exercise, pulmonary arterial mean pressure: 17 to 19 mm Hg, $P = $ ns, and pulmonary vascular resistance: 171 to 179 dynes/sec/cm^{-5}, $P = $ ns).

Interim clinical course during the follow-up period as assessed by the occurrence of death, recurrent DVT and PE, inferior vena caval interruption procedures, and functional status was more favorable in the thrombolytic group compared with the heparin group (cumulative event rate: 15.3% vs. 38.3%, respectively, $P < 0.02$). It was concluded that thrombolytic therapy, by virtue of its superior initial resolution of thromboemboli, preserves the normal hemodynamic response to exercise. It may also prevent recurrences of venous thromboembolism and the development of pulmonary hypertension.

New Thrombolytic Regimens

More recently there has been a renewed interest in thrombolysis of PE by employing new and novel regimens of high-dose/short-duration therapy of several plasminogen activators. Since one of the major factors involved in the bleeding from thrombolytic therapy is duration of therapy, investigators have sought to design regimens that employed high doses over a short period to maximize efficacy and safety.[77-80] In a comparative study of recombinant tissue plasminogen activator (rt-PA) (100 mg) and UK (3,000,000 U) regimens administered over 2 hours, it was shown that 67% of patients randomized to UK showed angiographic improvement (9% marked, 33% moderate,

25% mild), compared with 79% of patients randomized to rt-PA (12% marked, 22% moderate, and 45% slight improvements).[79] The changes in lung scan improvement obtained at 24 hours were similar for both treatment regimens. Despite the shortened course some significant bleeding did occur, requiring transfusions in 11% of the UK patients and 14% of the rt-PA patients. Two patients randomized to rt-PA and one to UK sustained intracranial bleeds. This trial did demonstrate that a shortened course of UK or rt-PA administered over 2 hours resulted in significant angiographic improvement with an improved safety profile.

In another study[81] 58 patients with PE (33 patients randomized to rt-PA, 25 patients to saline placebo) received intravenous heparin plus rt-PA 0.6 mg/kg or placebo as a single bolus. The mean relative improvement of the scan defect was 37% in the rt-PA group compared with 19% in the placebo group. No major bleeds occurred. The investigators suggested this regimen as an alternative and convenient approach to thrombolytic therapy in patients with PE. In the plasminogen activator Italian multicenter study 2 (PAIMS-2) trial,[82] 100 mg of rt-PA was administered over 2 hours and compared with heparin therapy in 36 patients with PE. Clot lysis at the posttreatment angiogram and the reduction in pulmonary arterial pressure were noted only in the thrombolytic group. Two patients in the rt-PA group and one in the heparin group died—one from renal failure and one from intracranial hemorrhage in the rt-PA group and one from recurrent PE in the heparin group.

Another novel approach that seems to bridge the conventional and approved 24-hour regimen of UK and the abbreviated and bolus regimens of rt-PA and UK is the bolus plus 12-hour low-dose intrapulmonary infusion of UK.[83] In 16 patients with PE, UK therapy was administered with a bolus dose of 500,000 IU followed by a right atrial catheter infusion of 1,000,000 IU over 12 hours (83,333 IU/hr). There was a mean improvement of the angiographic score of 57% when repeat angiography at 48 hours was compared with the control series and significant improvement (over 30%) in all of the hemodynamic parameters measured. All patients improved, and only one patient sustained a significant bleed at the catheter insertion site. The investigators concluded that this new and novel regimen was useful in the safe and efficacious administration of urokinase. Another trial of importance was the UKEP study that compared two dosages of UK in patients with massive PE: the standard 4400 IU/kg/hr and a reduced dosage of 2000 IU/kg/hr plus heparin.[84] Equal efficacy was achieved with improved safety in both groups and bleeding complications were severe in only 4.5% and 3% respectively.

Our belief currently is that thrombolytic therapy has significant benefits to offer patients with PE. The selection of an agent, at this time, is probably less important than making the decision to employ thrombolytic therapy in patients with "significant" PE. The recent studies offering different regimens are important in that the designs incorporate the principle of high-dose/short-duration therapy to achieve efficacy with maximal safety. Significant emboli previously indicated the involvement of several segmental defects on lung scan or three segmental pulmonary arteries on angiography, indicating that approximately 20% to 25% of the lung vascular volume was compromised by the PE. A more recent procedure to assess the overall hemodynamic impact of PE is echocardiography. As the size of the embolic process increases, the more alterations in normal right ventricular hemodynamics take place—for example, right ventricular enlargement, left ventricular compression, right ventricular wall hypokinesis in the absence of right ventricular hypertrophy and varying degrees of tricuspid regurgitation. Because of the correlation between right ventricular hemodynamics and echocardiographic changes, the echo is capable of detecting the patient with hemodynamically significant PE. These patients, in the absence of any contraindication to thrombolytic therapy, may be the optimal candidates for thrombolytic therapy.[85]

SURGICAL THERAPY

Aside from pulmonary embolectomy, the surgical techniques employed in PE are for the purpose of preventing recurrent episodes. Because more than 90% of thrombi originate in the lower extremities, surgical maneuvers have been directed toward interruption of the inferior vena cava. As such, the following indications can be recommended for interruption: (1) contraindications to anticoagulation therapy, (2) recurrence during adequate anticoagulation therapy, (3) septic pelvic thrombophlebitis with emboli, (4) recurrent pulmonary emboli, and (5) pulmonary embolectomy.

The majority of patients requiring surgical venous interruption are those in whom some contraindication to anticoagulation therapy exists. These include severe systemic hypertension associated with grade III or IV hypertensive retinopathy; presence of an actively bleeding lesion in the gastrointestinal or genitourinary tract (symptomatic lesions without active bleeding are considered relative contraindications); craniotomy or cerebrovascular accident within the prior 2 months or evidence of a lesion known or suspected to be associated with intracranial hemorrhage including cerebral neoplasms; presence of an uncontrolled hypocoagulable state including coagulation factor deficiencies, platelet abnormalities, or other spontaneous hemorrhagic or purpuric phenomena; and severe renal or hepatic insufficiency. Relative contraindications to anticoagulation therapy must be considered on an individual patient basis, weighing the risk and impact of bleeding against the morbidity of surgical venous interruptions.

The recognition of true recurrence during the acute phase of PE is a difficult clinical problem that cannot be resolved without the aid of lung scanning or pulmonary angiography. Only by angiography can the distinction between recurrent PE and fragmentation and distal migration of the original clot be answered with any assurance.[1,4] The importance of this distinction lies in the therapy. Adequate anticoagulation implies the intravenous administration of heparin in adequate doses to achieve and maintain therapeutic levels. Should true recurrence occur during this period, the patient may be considered a "heparin failure" and caval interruption can be subsequently performed. The fragmentation and migration

process, on the other hand, requires only continuation of the heparin.

If recurrence develops during well-controlled orally administered anticoagulation therapy, during the recovery period, or during long-term anticoagulation, reanticoagulation with heparin is recommended. Subsequently several courses are available depending on a number of factors: cardiopulmonary status of the patient, magnitude of reembolism, assessment of deep veins in the legs, and nature of the predisposing event. If the underlying cardiopulmonary status is satisfactory, the embolic episode submassive (less than 35% to 40% of total pulmonary vasculature affected), the deep veins minimally abnormal, and the predisposing event temporary (e.g., leg trauma), retreatment with intravenously administered heparin following the same time-course sequence as in the initial event may be carried out. However, if the underlying cardiopulmonary status is unstable, or the reembolic episode massive, or the deep veins grossly abnormal, or the predisposing condition chronic (e.g., recurrent heart failure), caval interruption is recommended. Assessment of patency of deep veins in the legs is best performed by ascending phlebography or alternatively by one of the noninvasive methods (e.g., electrical impedance color-flow venous duplex scanning)[34,55] and is extremely helpful in this decision process. If a sizable clot in the deep vein is seen, with the proximal end "free floating," or if the noninvasive study indicates deep venous obstruction, it can be assumed that the patient is still at risk of sustaining recurrent PE.

Although interrupting the inferior vena cava will prevent further embolization in the acute period, recurrences can occur.[86] One of the earliest nonsurgical interruptions of the cava was carried out by insertion of an umbrella filter.[87] Many thousands had been inserted with a 1% complication rate and a 3% recurrent embolism rate. However, the majority of umbrella filters eventually became occluded, converting a partial obstruction to a total obstruction. The Greenfield filter, in contrast, is characterized by a high patency rate (96%), low recurrence rate of PE (4%), low complication rate (4.1%), and low operative mortality rate (0.5%).[88] The complications of the Greenfield filter occur early, during placement or late, after satisfactory placement. Misplacement of the filter is related to technique of insertion (2% to 7%).[89,90] Tilting and angulation occur without seemingly compromising the function of the filter, but they do not provide optimal protection. Distal migration of the filter is common and is thought to be due to failure of firm attachment to the caval wall, a large cava, thrombus formation around the filter during insertion, trauma, and increased abdominal pressure.[91] As originally introduced, its large carrier size made percutaneous introduction difficult and therefore it was better suited for operative placement, avoiding the high incidence of venous thrombosis induced by the larger carrier. This led to the development of other filters, as well as a downsizing of the Greenfield filter. This modified filter was reported to be 97% effective in preventing recurrent PE, with no occlusion of the inferior vena cava.

The Gianturco-Roehm bird's nest filter was designed to correct some of the problems associated with the Greenfield filter, particularly the relatively high incidence of

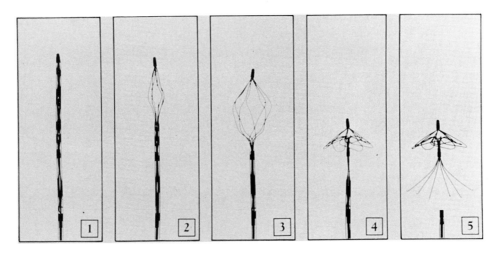

Fig. 27-17. The five panels of this figure show the different steps and configurations of the Simon-Nitinol filter. Panel 1 shows the straight, pliable form maintained within the introducer by cold saline solution. The subsequent panels demonstrate the progressive extrusion of the filter from the introducer and the assumption of the clot-trapping configuration upon warming to body temperature.

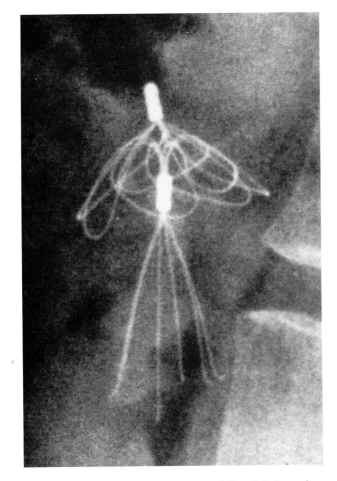

Fig. 27-18. Lateral view of the Simon-Nitinol filter, fully formed within the inferior vena cava.

filter angulation. The bird's nest filter, in 440 patients, has been effective in preventing recurrent PE in 97.3% of the patients, with an inferior vena cava rate of occlusion of 2.9% at 6 months.[92]

The latest filter that appears effective is the Simon-Nitinol filter, an ingenious device using a thermal shape-memory nitinol alloy that is introduced percutaneously with a small 7 Fr introducer within which the filter is straight in shape but assumes its complex clot-trapping shape upon being extruded and exposed to body temperature (Figs. 27-17 and 27-18). In a multicenter trial of 238 patients, recurrent PE occurred in only 1.3% and filter occlusion occurred in 7% of the patients.[93] The authors report that the great majority of patients did not receive anticoagulation therapy after filter placement. Current data from slightly over 10,000 implants show a patency rate of 93.5%, a 1.1% incidence of recurrent PE, and five filter migrations.[93a] No venous thrombosis was reported at the entry site, probably as a result of the very small introducer (7 Fr).

Other devices include the LGM-France,[94] the Gunther basket filter,[95] and the Hunter-Sessions balloon device.[96] Each was designed with specific features, presumably to correct defects associated with the Greenfield filter.

Pulmonary embolectomy, a dramatic and heroic procedure, is now being performed in fewer patients with PE.[97] The procedure should be performed with cardiopulmonary bypass in patients with angiographically confirmed massive embolism with shock who do not respond to vigorous medical therapy and who, without mechanical removal of the emboli, would probably die.[98,99] The mortality ranges between 40% and 100% in different series, but in the infrequent appropriate clinical situation, it may be lifesaving.[99,100]

ADJUNCTIVE THERAPY

Since most patients with clinically detectable PE will have some degree of hypoxemia, oxygen therapy is an important adjunct. Though cyanosis may be noted only in the very ill, Pa_{O_2} will invariably be reduced. Regardless of the mechanism of hypoxemia in the individual patient (venous admixture, $\dot{V}/\dot{Q}$ reduction, or diffusion defect), the administration of oxygen will relieve or diminish the symptoms of hypoxemia in many patients.[34] Since hypoventilation is rarely a cause of hypoxemia in PE, oxygen may be administered comfortably by nasal catheter without fear of suppressing ventilation.

In patients who sustain major to massive PE, cardiac failure is frequently observed particularly when there is preexisting cardiopulmonary disease. The cardiac index may fall below 2.0 L/min/m^2.[33] In such circumstances the administration of an isoproterenol hydrochloride drip of 2 to 4 mg/500 ml of 5% dextrose in water is helpful as a cardiotonic agent; it increases cardiac output and decreases pulmonary arterial pressure. In the event that hypotension is present and persists after isoproterenol administration, levarterenol bitartrate 2 to 6 ml of 0.2% in 500 ml of 5% dextrose in water should be administered. Occasionally, when the central venous pressure is low, administration of intravenous fluids may be helpful in restoring near-normal hemodynamics. Digitalis glycosides, intravenously administered diuretics, and various antiarrhythmic agents should be used in the appropriate clinical situation in the usual dosages.

In patients who complain of severe pleuritic pain or who exhibit apprehension, morphine sulfate slowly administered intravenously 1 mg at a time (up to 5 to 10 mg) may be very useful. Apprehension is lessened and ventilation is frequently improved. Codeine sulfate 30 to 60 mg may be given for lesser pain.

Since the great majority of patients who suffer acute PE have their site of thromboemboli in the deep veins of the legs, appropriate measures, such as leg elevation, are useful. One cannot rely on clinical symptoms of thrombophlebitis since nearly 50% to 60% of those with DVT are without symptoms or signs.[6]

REFERENCES

1. Sasahara AA: Current problems in pulmonary embolism: introduction. In Sasahara AA, Sonnenblick EH, and Lesch M, eds: Pulmonary embolism, New York, 1975, Grune & Stratton.
2. Roe BB and Goldthwait JC: Pulmonary embolism: a statistical study of postmortem material at the Massachusetts General Hospital, N Engl J Med 241:679, 1949.
3. Freiman DG, Suyemoto J, and Wessler S: Frequency of pulmonary thromboembolism in man, N Engl J Med 272:1278, 1965.
4. Sasahara AA et al: The urokinase pulmonary embolism trial: a national cooperative study, Circulation 47(suppl II):66, 1973.
5. Plate G, Einarsson E, and Eklof B: Etiologic spectrum in acute iliofemoral venous thrombosis, Internat Angio 2:59, 1986.
6. Kakkar VV et al: Deep vein thrombosis of the leg, Am J Surg 120:527, 1970.
7. Coon WW, Willis PW, and Keller JB: Venous thromboembolism and other venous disease in the Tecumseh Community Health Study, Circulation 158:839, 1973.
8. Shackford SR et al: Venous thromboembolism in patients with major trauma, Am J Surg 159:365, 1990.
9. Coon WW: Risk factors in pulmonary embolism, Surg Gynecol Obstet 143:385, 1976.
10. Frisbie JH and Sasahara AA: Low dose heparin prophylaxis for deep venous thrombosis in acute spinal cord injury patients: a controlled study, Paraplegia 19:343, 1981.
11. Sasahara AA: Vacation emboli, Med World News 9:22, 1968.
12. Inman WHW et al: Thromboembolic disease and the steroidal content of oral contraceptives: a report to the committee on safety of drugs, Br Med J 2:203, 1970.
13. Sipes SL and Weiner CP: Venous thromboembolic disease in pregnancy, Semin Perinatol 2:103, 1990.
14. Jick H et al: Venous thromboembolic disease and ABO blood type, Lancet 1:539, 1969.
15. Koenigs KP, McPhedran P, and Spiro HM: Thrombosis in inflammatory bowel disease, J Clin Gastroenterol 9:627, 1987.
16. Panicucci F et al: Comprehensive study of haemostasis in nephrotic syndrome, Nephron 33:9, 1983.
17. Ginsburg KS et al: Anticardiolipin antibodies and the risk for ischemic stroke and venous thrombosis, Ann Int Med 117:997, 1992.
18. Nachman RL and Silverstein R: Hypercoagulable states, Ann Int Med 119:819, 1993.
19. McIntyre KM and Sasahara AA: The hemodynamic response to pulmonary embolism in patients without prior cardiopulmonary disease, Am J Cardiol 28:288, 1971.
20. Sasahara AA, Sidd JJ, and Tremblay G: Cardiopulmonary consequences of acute pulmonary embolism, Prog Cardiovasc Dis 9:259, 1966.
21. Szucs MM Jr, Brooks HL, and Grossman W: Diagnostic sensitivity of laboratory findings in acute pulmonary embolism, Ann Intern Med 74:161, 1971.
22. Richardson DW, Kontos HA, and Raper AJ: Modification by beta-adrenergic blockade of the circulatory responses to acute hypoxia in man, J Clin Invest 46:77, 1967.
23. Sasahara AA: Pulmonary vascular response to thromboembolism, Mod Concepts Cardiovasc Dis 36:55, 1967.
24. Brandfonbrener M, Turino GM, and Himmelstein A: Effects of occlusion of one pulmonary artery on pulmonary circulation in man, Fed Proc 7:19, 1958 (abstract).
25. Miller GAH et al: Comparison of streptokinase and heparin in treatment of isolated acute massive pulmonary embolism, Br Med J 2:681, 1971.
26. Comroe JH Jr, Van Lingen B, and Stroud RC: Reflex and direct cardiopulmonary effects of 5-OH-tryptamine (serotonin): their possible role in pulmonary embolism and coronary thrombosis, Am J Physiol 173:379, 1966.
27. Thomas DP, Gurewich V, and Ashford TP: Platelet adherence to thromboemboli in relation to the pathogenesis and treatment of pulmonary embolism, N Engl J Med 274:953, 1966.
28. Dalen JE, Banas JS, and Brooks HL: Resolution rate of acute pulmonary embolism in man, N Engl J Med 280:1194, 1969.
29. Kontos HA, Levasseur E, and Richardson DW: Comparative circulatory responses to systemic hypoxia in man and in unanesthetized dog, J Appl Physiol 23:381, 1967.
30. Downing SE and Siegel JH: Some factors concerned with the regulation of sympathetic discharge to the heart, Clin Res 10:171, 1962 (abstract).
31. Eckstein JW and Harsley AW: Effects of hypoxia on peripheral venous tone in man, J Lab Clin Med 56:847, 1960.
32. Hirsh J, Hale GS, and McDonald IG: Streptokinase therapy in acute major pulmonary embolism: effectiveness and problems, Br Med J 4:729, 1968.
33. McIntyre KM and Sasahara AA: Pulmonary angiography, scanning, and hemodynamics in pulmonary embolism:

critical review and correlations, CRC Crit Rev Radiol Sci 3:489, 1972.

34. Sasahara AA et al: Clinical and physiologic studies in pulmonary thromboembolism, Am J Cardiol 20:10, 1967.

35. Wacker WEC et al: Diagnosis of pulmonary embolism and infarction, JAMA 178:8, 1961.

36. Bynum LJ, Crotty CM, and Wilson JE: Use of fibrinogen/fibrin degradation products and soluble fibrin complexes for differentiating pulmonary embolism from nonthromboembolic lung disease, Am Rev Respir Dis 114:285, 1976.

37. Yudelman IM et al: Plasma fibrinopeptide A levels in symptomatic venous thromboembolism, Blood 51:1189, 1978.

38. Klotz TA, Cohn LS, and Zipser RD: Urinary excretion of thromboxane B2 in patients with venous thromboembolic disease, Chest 8:329, 1984.

39. Van Hulstein H et al: Diagnostic value of fibrinopeptide A and beta-thromboglobulin in acute deep venous thrombosis and pulmonary embolism, Acta Med Scand 211:323, 1982.

40. Bounameaux H et al: Measurement of D-dimer in plasma as diagnostic aid in suspected pulmonary embolism, Lancet 337:196, 1991.

41. Ginsburg JS et al: D-dimer in patients with clinically suspected pulmonary embolism, Chest 104:1679, 1993.

42. Heaton DC, Billings JD, and Hickton CM: Assessment of D-dimer assays for the diagnosis of deep vein thrombosis, J Lab Clin Med 110:588, 1987

43. Francis CW et al: Increased plasma concentration of cross-linked fibrin polymers in acute myocardial infarction, Circulation 75:1170, 1987.

44. Hockberger RS and Rothstein: Pulmonary embolism, Emerg Med Clin North Am I:393, 1983.

45. McFarlane MJ and Imperiale TF: Use of alveolar-arterial oxygen gradient in the diagnosis of pulmonary embolism, Am J Med 96:57, 1994.

46. Stein PD et al: Clinical laboratory, roentgenographic and electrocardiographic findings in patients with acute pulmonary embolism and no pre-existing cardiac or pulmonary disease, Chest 100:598, 1991.

47. Sasahara AA et al: Methodology in diagnosis of pulmonary embolization. In Bergan JJ and Yao JST, eds: Venous problems, Chicago, 1978, Year Book Medical Publishers.

48. The PIOPED Investigators: Value of the ventilation/perfusion scan in acute pulmonary embolism, JAMA 263: 2753, 1990.

49. Sasahara AA et al: Pulmonary angiography in the diagnosis of thromboembolic disease, N Engl J Med 270:1075, 1964.

50. Stein PD et al: Angiographic diagnosis of acute pulmonary embolism: evaluation of criteria, Am Heart J 73:730, 1967.

51. Ferris EL et al: Pulmonary angiography in pulmonary embolic disease, Am J Roentgenol 100:355, 1967.

52. Walsh PW et al: An angiographic severity index for pulmonary embolism, Circulation 47(suppl 11):101, 1973.

53. Sevitt S and Gallagher NG: Venous thrombosis and pulmonary embolism: a clinicopathological study in injured and burned patients, Br J Surg 48:475, 1961.

54. Kakkar VV et al: Natural history of deep vein thrombosis, Lancet 2:230, 1969.

55. Wheeler HB et al: Diagnosis of occult deep vein thrombosis by a noninvasive bedside technique, Surgery 70:20, 1971.

56. Sasahara AA, Sharma GVRK, and Parisi AR: New developments in the detection and prevention of venous thromboembolism, Am J Cardiol 43:1214, 1979.

57. Hull RD et al: Pulmonary angiography, ventilation lung scanning and venography for clinically suspected pulmonary embolism with abnormal perfusion lung scan, Ann Int Med 98:891, 1983.

58. Killelewich LA, Nunnelee JD, and Auer AI: Value of lower extremity venous duplex examination in the diagnosis of pulmonary embolism, J Vasc Surg 17:934, 1993.

59. Covarrubias EA, Sheikh MU, and Fox LM: Echocardiography and pulmonary embolism, Ann Int Med 87:720, 1977.

60. Steckley R, Smith CW, and Robertson RM: Acute right ventricular overload: an echocardiographic clue to pulmonary thromboembolism, Johns Hopkins Med J 143:122, 1978.

61. Shiina A et al: Echocardiographic manifestations of acute pulmonary thromboembolism: a case report, Jpn Heart J 22:853, 1980.

62. Kasper W et al: Echocardiographic findings in patients with proved pulmonary embolism, Am Heart J 112:1284, 1981.

63. Come PC: Echocardiographic recognition of pulmonary arterial disease and determination of its cause, Am J Med 84:384, 1988.

64. Come PC et al: Early reversal of right ventricular dysfunction in patients with acute pulmonary embolism after treatment with intravenous tissue plasminogen activator, Am Coll Cardiol 10:971, 1987.

65. Okuba S et al: Role of echocardiography in acute pulmonary embolism, Jpn Heart J 30:655, 1989.

66. Salzman EW et al: Management of heparin therapy: controlled prospective trial, N Engl J Med 292:1046, 1975.

67. Hommes DW et al: Subcutaneous heparin compared with continuous intravenous heparin administration in the initial treatment of deep vein thrombosis—meta-analysis, Ann Int Med 116:279, 1992.

68. Wessler S et al: Experimental pulmonary embolism with serum induced thrombi, Am J Pathol 38:89, 1961.

69. Hull RD et al: Heparin for 5 days as compared with 10 days in the initial treatment of proximal venous thrombosis, N Engl J Med 322:1260, 1990.

70. Coon WW, Willis PW, and Symous MJ: Assessment of anticoagulant treatment of venous thromboembolism, Ann Surg 170:559, 1969.

71. Research Committee of the British Thoracic Society: Optimum duration of anticoagulation for deep-vein thrombosis and pulmonary embolism, Lancet 340:873, 1992.

72. Urokinase streptokinase pulmonary embolism trial: Phase II results, JAMA 229:1606, 1974.

73. Kakkar VV: Results of streptokinase therapy in deep vein thrombosis, Postgrad Med J 49(suppl):60, 1973.

74. Common HH, Seaman AJ, and Rosch J: Deep vein thrombosis treated with streptokinase or heparin: follow-up of a randomized study, Angiology 27:645, 1976.

75. Sharma GVRK, Burleson VA, and Sasahara AA: Effect of thrombolytic therapy on pulmonary capillary blood volume in patients with pulmonary embolism, N Engl J Med 303:842, 1980.

76. Sharma GVRK et al: Long-term benefits of thrombolytic therapy in pulmonary embolic disease, J Am Coll Cardiol 15:65A, 1990.

77. Dickie KJ et al: Hemodynamic effects of bolus infusion of urokinase in pulmonary thromboembolism, Am Rev Resp Dis 109:48, 1974.

78. Pettipretz P et al: Effects of a single bolus of urokinase in patients with life-threatening pulmonary emboli: a descriptive trial, Circulation 70:861, 1984.

79. Goldhaber SZ et al: Recombinant tissue-type plasminogen activator versus a novel dosing regimen of urokinase in acute pulmonary embolism: a randomized controlled multicenter trial, J Am Coll Cardiol 10:24, 1992.

80. Diehl JL et al: Effectiveness and safety of bolus administration of alteplase in massive pulmonary embolism, Am J Cardiol 70:1477, 1992.
81. Levine MN et al: A randomized trial of a single bolus regimen of recombinant tissue plasminogen activator in patients with acute pulmonary embolism, Chest 98:1473, 1990.
82. Dalla-Volta S et al: PAIMS-2: alteplase combined with heparin versus heparin in the treatment of acute pulmonary embolism: Plasminogen Activator Italian Multicenter Study 2, J Am Coll Cardiol 20:520, 1992.
83. Gonzalez-Juanatey JR et al: Treatment of massive pulmonary thromboembolism with low intrapulmonary dosages of urokinase, Chest 102:341, 1992.
84. The UKEP Study Research Group: The UKEP study: multicentre clinical trial on two local regimens of urokinase in massive pulmonary embolism, Eur Heart J 8:2, 1987.
85. Goldhaber S: Contemporary pulmonary embolism thrombolysis, Chest 107:455, 1995.
86. Gurewich V, Thomas DP, and Rabinov KR: Pulmonary embolism after ligation of the inferior vena cava. N Engl J Med 274:1350, 1966.
87. Mobin-Uddin K et al: Caval interruption for prevention of pulmonary embolism: long-term results of a new method, Arch Surg 99:711, 1969.
88. Greenfield LJ and Michna BA: Twelve year clinical experience with the Greenfield vena cava filter, Surgery 104:706, 1988.
89. Berland LL, Maddison FE, and Bernhard VM: Radiology follow-up of vena cava filter devices, AJR 134:1047, 1980.
90. Castenada F et al: Migration of a Kimray-Greenfield filter into the right ventricle, Radiology 149:690, 1983.
91. Taheri SA et al: A complication of the Greenfield filter: fracture and distal migration of two struts—a case report, J Vasc Surg 16:96, 1992
92. Roehm JOF et al: The bird's nest inferior vena cava filter: progress report, Radiology 168:745, 1988.
93. Simon M et al: Simon-Nitinol inferior vena cava filter: initial clinical experience: work in progress, Radiology 172:99, 1989.
93a. Simon M: Personal communication.
94. Ricco JB et al: Percutaneous transvenous caval interruption with the LGM filter: early results of a multicenter trial, Ann Vasc Surg 3:242, 1988.
95. Gunther RW and Schild H: Basket filter for prevention of pulmonary embolism, Semin Intervent Radiol 3:220, 1986.
96. Hunter JA et al: Inferior vena cava interruption with the Hunter-Sessions balloon: eighteen years' experience in 191 cases, J Vasc Surg 10:450, 1989.
97. Sautter RD, Myers WO, and Wenzel FJ: Implications of the urokinase study concerning the surgical treatment of pulmonary embolism, J Thorac Cardiovasc Surg 63:54, 1972.
98. Sautter RD et al: Pulmonary embolectomy: review and current status. In Sasahara A, Sonnenblick EH, and Lesch M, eds: Pulmonary emboli, New York, 1975, Grune & Stratton.
99. Cross FS and Mowlem A: A survey of the current status of pulmonary embolectomy for massive pulmonary embolism, Circulation 35(suppl 1):1967.
100. Sasahara AA and Barsamian EM: Another look at pulmonary embolectomy, Ann Thorac Surg 16:317, 1973.

CHAPTER TWENTY-EIGHT

CHRONIC VENOUS INSUFFICIENCY AND VARICOSE VEINS

Thomas F. O'Donnell, Jr.
Harold J. Welch

Although arterial occlusive disease receives more attention than chronic venous insufficiency (CVI), CVI is a significant problem in the United States affecting as much as a quarter of the population. Venous disease afflicts a younger segment of the population and the morbidity of edema, leg pain, and ulceration may result in life-style alterations, loss of work, and frequent hospitalizations. In the following sections we review the pathophysiology, clinical findings, classification, diagnosis, and treatment of CVI.

In a discussion of the prevalence of venous disease in the population, simple varicose veins must be distinguished from advanced CVI with venous ulcer. Browse, Burnand, and Lea[1] have reviewed this subject and summarized the results of the following four national surveys on the prevalence of varicose veins: the U.S. National Survey of 1935-1936,[2] The Survey of Sickness conducted in the United Kingdom in 1950,[3] The Sickness Survey of Denmark, 1952-1953,[4] and The Canadian Sickness Survey, 1950-1951.[5] These summaries revealed a prevalence that ranged from 1.53% of the population in the Canadian study to 2.25% in the U.S. and U.K. studies (Table 28-1). These national surveys, however, probably underestimate the true prevalence of varicose veins in the population because the data were gathered from questionnaires and the surveys were conducted by nonmedical personnel. Therefore local or regional studies may provide a truer definition of varicose vein prevalence. Widmer's[7] survey typifies the true prevalence in an industrialized society. He conducted a clinical study that included physical examinations and photographs of the extremities of over 4000 chemical workers. Varicose veins affected men (5.27%) more frequently than women (3.2%). The incidence of varicose veins increased with age, so that patients under

the age of 35 had a 10% incidence, whereas 50% of those over the age of 65 were affected. In any event, if 2% of the population is affected by varicose veins, it represents a substantial health problem.

The prevalence of venous ulceration is more difficult to determine than the prevalence of varicose veins. The earliest studies on this subject by Dickson-Wright[8] and Linton[9] appear to be extrapolations. Linton estimated that 300,000 to 400,000 patients in the United States had venous ulcers. A Swedish study demonstrated a prevalence of less than 0.1%.[11] Specific studies of a defined population perhaps provide the best data on venous ulcer. Widmer's[7] study of chemical workers uncovered a 1.3% incidence of venous ulcer. The Callam et al[12] West Lothian leg ulceration survey, which was conducted in the form of mailed questionnaires to nurses, physicians, and hospital outpatient facilities, demonstrated an incidence of 0.15%—quite similar to that described by Hellgren[11] in his Swedish study. A compilation of these studies suggests that nearly 1% of the population has experienced or currently has an active leg ulceration.[1] Like varicose veins the incidence of venous ulcer increases with age, but unlike varicose veins, appears to be more common in females.

NORMAL VENOUS ANATOMY

Superficial Veins

To understand the anatomic classification of CVI, one must appreciate the anatomy of a normal venous system. The long, or greater, saphenous vein is the main superficial vein in the lower extremity and begins anterior to the medial malleolus, rising obliquely and posteriorly to this bony prominence as it crosses the anteromedial surface of

Table 28-1. Prevalence of Chronic Venous Insufficiency

Study	Location	Type	Years	Prevalence (%)
Varicose Veins				
U.S. National Survey[2]	US	Interview	1935-1936	2.25
U.K. Survey of Sickness[3]	UK	Interview	1950	2.25
Denmark Sickness Survey[4]	Denmark	Hospital	1953	–
Canadian Sickness Survey[5]	Canada	Interview	1951	1.53
Bobeck (regional)[6]	Czechoslovakia	Medical examination	>15	
Widmer[7]	Switzerland	Medical examination	1974	4.2
Venous Ulcer				
Dickson-Wright[8]	UK	?	1931	0.5
Linton[9]	US	? Extrapolation	1948	300-400K*
Lockhart-Mummery[10]	UK	Derivation	1951	0.2-0.5
Hellgren[11]	Sweden	Survey	1967	0.1
Widmer[7]	Switzerland	Medical examination	1974	1.3
Callam[12]	UK	Survey district hospital	1985	0.15

*An estimation of the total number of people in the United States with venous ulcers.

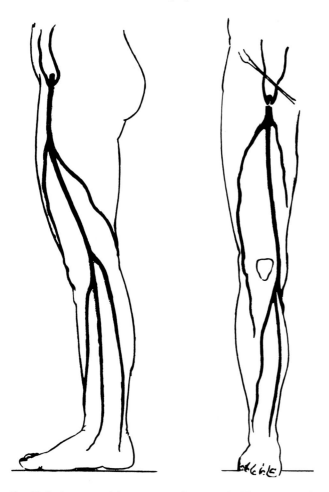

Fig. 28-1. Anatomy of the greater saphenous vein. The major trunk of the greater saphenous vein lies superficial to the deep fascia. At the thigh level the greater saphenous has an anterior and a posterior branch that run in a more superficial plane, while at the knee, the saphenous trifurcates with both anterior and posterior branches. Varicosities usually occur in the branches and lie more superficial in the loose areolar subcutaneous tissue.

the tibia (Fig. 28-1). Below the knee joint the saphenous vein is joined by the posterior arch vein. This significant tributary drains the mediodorsal lower leg and communicates with the deep system by medial perforating veins. Other important tributaries include the superficial anterior vein in the lower leg, and the anterolateral and posteromedial veins in the thigh. These latter branches usually join the saphenous vein near the inguinal ligament and are frequently responsible for recurrent varicosities if not properly identified and ligated during initial surgical procedures. The long saphenous vein usually lies on top of the deep fascia and joins the common femoral vein at the fossa ovale. In a large series using duplex ultrasound mapping of the greater saphenous vein, a dominant single system was seen in only 67% of patients, whereas 25% had branching double systems and 8% had complete double systems.[13]

The short, or lesser, saphenous vein lies posterior to the lateral malleolus and courses upward, lateral to the Achilles tendon (Fig. 28-2). It is typically joined by a perforating vein in its lower portion. As the lesser saphenous vein reaches the lower and middle third of the calf, it becomes midline and lies on the deep fascia. The vein then penetrates the deep fascia of the calf at the upper third so that it enters the popliteal space between the heads of the gastrocnemius muscles. The saphenopopliteal junction is usually found within 3 to 7 cm above the knee fold. In up to one third of cases, however, the lesser saphenous vein may drain directly into the greater saphenous vein or deep femoral vein.[14]

Perforating (Communicating) Veins

The perforating, or communicating, veins provide the bridges between the superficial and deep system. Blood flows through one-way valves from the superficial to the deep system (Fig. 28-3). Perforating veins are classified as either *direct*, when they permit the superficial venous systems to communicate directly with the main veins, or *indirect*, when the perforating veins connect with the deep

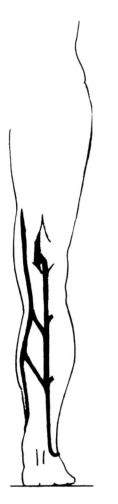

Fig. 28-2. Anatomy of the lesser saphenous vein. This posterior view of the lower extremity shows the lesser saphenous vein with its intercommunication to the greater saphenous (located medially). The lesser saphenous vein originates posterior to the lateral malleolus and courses proximally to enter the popliteal vein, above the popliteal crease.

veins by way of a muscular vein. The direct perforating veins are most important, lying on the medial aspect connecting the posterior tibial vein to the posterior arch vein and are often called the Linton or Cockett perforators. These direct perforators are generally constant in anatomic location. The greatest number are located posterior to the medial malleolus in an area overlying the posterior tibial vein—the lower perforating vein.[15] By contrast, the middle perforating vein is found approximately 7 to 10 cm above the medial malleolus and posterior to the tibia. This perforating vein communicates directly with the posterior tibial vein. Finally, the most superior of the three medial perforating veins is located in the upper third of the calf, posterior to the tibia. Although this vein usually connects with the long saphenous vein by means of a tributary, it drains directly into the posterior tibial vein. The thigh perforating vein is usually located within Hunter's canal, from which it derives its name. This vein communicates with a superficial vein and enters either the long saphenous vein directly or indirectly through one of its branches.

Deep Veins

In the calf the deep veins are paired and usually accompany the named arteries with venous tributaries intertwining over the surface of the artery. At the knee joint the veins usually join to form the popliteal vein, which may be a single trunk, a dual system, or even a plexus. The deep veins transport blood from the muscles of the limb and provide an important carrier function for the calf muscle pump. The soleal sinusoids and the calf muscle veins are encased within a tight muscle-fascial envelope, similar to an elastic support stocking. This may prevent dilation of the deep veins in contrast to the superficial veins, which are contained within loose nonsupportive areolar tissue.[14] The soleal sinuses and calf muscle veins communicate in a latticework manner with the posterior tibial and peroneal veins. The superficial femoral vein is a continuation of the popliteal vein and may commonly be duplicated or bifid. Although the term "superficial femoral vein" is well understood by vascular surgeons, that segment of vein is commonly known as the "femoral vein" by nonsurgeons.[16] In about 10% of cases the profunda femoris vein communicates directly with the popliteal vein. The classic textbook description is present in less than 20% of cases, and symmetry between right and left legs is unusual with both normal and "variant" anatomy.

NORMAL VENOUS PHYSIOLOGY

To understand the altered physiology of CVI, normal venous physiology should first be reviewed. The calf muscles and deep veins of the calf act like the cardiac ventricles so that the phasic changes in the calf veins, which occur with walking, can be compared with systole and diastole of the cardiac cycle.[17] During the *systolic phase* of the ambulatory venous calf muscle pump cycle, contraction of the calf muscles compresses the blood contained within the venous sinuses and deep calf veins, thereby pumping the blood toward the heart. Valves in the communicating (perforating) veins, which link the deep with the superficial system, are closed to prevent retrograde flow of venous blood from the deep veins to the superficial system (Fig. 28-3). The pressure within the deep system at this point may reach 120 mm Hg during peak systolic contraction (Fig. 28-4). During the *diastolic phase* of the venous calf muscle pump, the relaxation of the calf muscle allows the soleal sinuses and deep calf veins to refill, thus recharging the pump and allowing blood to flow from the superficial to the deep venous system through the perforating veins whose valves are now open. At this point, the higher pressure in the superficial venous system favors flow to the deep system.

CHRONIC VENOUS INSUFFICIENCY

Pathophysiology

In the limb with CVI the systolic phase of the calf muscle pump is altered, whereas the diastolic phase is similar to that of the normal limb. The basic underlying pathophysiologic mechanism in CVI is venous hypertension, especially that created during the systolic phase. The

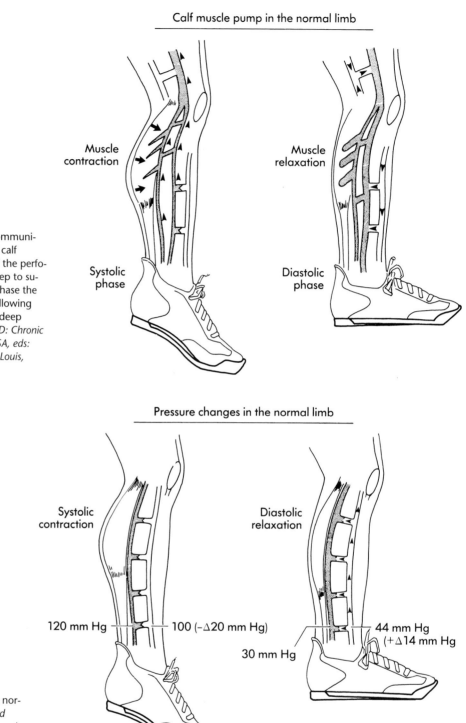

Calf muscle pump in the normal limb

Muscle contraction

Muscle relaxation

Systolic phase

Diastolic phase

Fig. 28-3. Anatomy of the perforating (communicating) veins. During the systolic phase of calf muscle contraction, the one-way valves of the perforating veins are closed, which prevents deep to superficial blood flow. During the diastolic phase the valves of the perforating veins are open, allowing superficial to deep blood flow to refill the deep veins. *(From O'Donnell TF Jr and Shepard AD: Chronic venous insufficiency. In Jarrett F and Hirsch SA, eds: Vascular surgery of the lower extremities, St Louis, 1985, The CV Mosby Co.)*

Pressure changes in the normal limb

Systolic contraction

Diastolic relaxation

120 mm Hg — 100 (−Δ20 mm Hg)

44 mm Hg (+Δ14 mm Hg

30 mm Hg

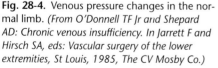

Fig. 28-4. Venous pressure changes in the normal limb. *(From O'Donnell TF Jr and Shepard AD: Chronic venous insufficiency. In Jarrett F and Hirsch SA, eds: Vascular surgery of the lower extremities, St Louis, 1985, The CV Mosby Co.)*

venous hypertension is created either by blocking the outflow (obstruction), inefficient or insufficient outflow or backflow (reflux), or a combination of both. Obstruction is most often due to thrombosis but may result from congenital abnormalities, extraluminal compression (e.g., tumors, ascites, bandages), and intraluminal obstructions (e.g., webs, tumors). Segmental occlusion in the deep system creates resistance to venous outflow and concomi-

tantly elevates distal venous pressure. Reflux is the result of valvular dysfunction: valves scarred or destroyed by thrombi, or floppy, incompetent valves seen in primary valvular insufficiency. Incompetence of the valves in the perforating veins permits the higher pressures generated in the deep system during the systolic phase to be transmitted to the superficial veins, subcutaneous tissue, and skin. Incompetent valves permit an uninterrupted column of

Direction of blood flow
in limb with chronic venous insuffiency

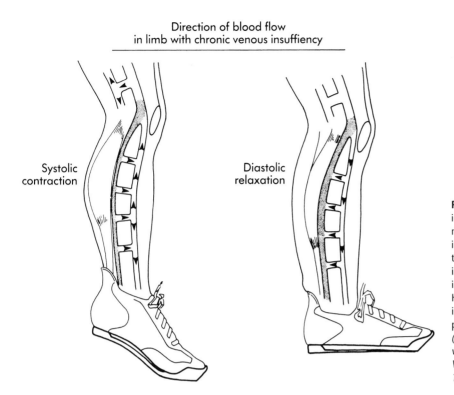

Systolic
contraction

Diastolic
relaxation

Fig. 28-5. Venous blood flow in chronic venous insufficiency. In contrast to flow direction in the normal limb (Fig. 28-3), with chronic venous insufficiency, blood flows paradoxically from the deep to the superficial system across the incompetent valves of the perforating veins during the systolic phase of the calf muscle pump. High pressure, as shown in Fig. 28-4, is therefore introduced from the deep system into the superficial system during this phase of the cycle. *(From O'Donnell TF Jr and Shepard AD: Chronic venous insufficiency. In Jarrett F and Hirsch SA, eds: Vascular surgery of the lower extremities, St Louis, 1985, The CV Mosby Co.)*

blood under the influence of gravity in the upright position to exert additional hydrostatic pressure on the deep venous system. These two mechanisms, obstruction and reflux, may further increase superficial venous system pressure. Thus the increased venous pressure within the superficial venous system during the systolic phase of the calf muscle pump plays a major role in the development of CVI[18] (Fig. 28-5).

Although the venous hypertension seen in CVI is a macrocirculatory change, it ultimately exerts its influence on the microcirculation of the subdermal and dermal tissues. Although several theories have been proposed, more recent developments have increased focus on white blood cells (WBCs) as a major contributor to ulcer formation.

Older theories speculated on tissue hypoxia as the cause for ulcer formation. The possibility of small arteriovenous (AV) fistulas shunting blood away from the skin was discounted by experiments using microspheres that showed an increase in AV shunting in CVI.[19,20] Tissue hypoxia was also proposed as a result of a "fibrin cuff" seen histologically around capillaries in the skin of patients with CVI.[21] The venous hypertension results in a leakage of proteins, most significantly fibrinogen, through the capillary walls. Decreased fibrinolytic activity in patients with venous disease may explain the formation of the fibrin cuffs. The fibrin cuff theory rested on the premise that there was decreased oxygen in the skin because the fibrin blocked oxygen diffusion. Unfortunately there has been no evidence supporting significant resistance to diffusion of oxygen, nor has anyone shown decreased oxygen levels in patients with venous ulcerations.

The white cell theory has been championed by Coleridge-Smith and Scurr,[22] and is essentially a two-component theory. Because WBCs are much larger than red blood cells, they significantly affect blood rheology and peripheral vascular resistance in the microcirculation.[23] Moyses, Cederholm-Williams, and Michel[24] examined the effect of increased venous pressure by measuring ankle greater saphenous vein WBC concentrations before and after 40 minutes of limb dependency and found a 25% decrease in WBCs after dependency. Thomas, Nash, and Dormandy[25] compared normal limbs with those with CVI in a similar study and found normal limbs "trapped" 7% of WBCs after 60 minutes, whereas CVI limbs "trapped" 30%. Coleridge-Smith and Scurr[22] examined the microcirculation in patients with normal limbs, varicose veins, and lipodermatosclerosis, focusing on the number of capillary loops per unit area. They found marked decrease in the number of capillary loops only in those patients with lipodermatosclerosis and attributed it to white cell trapping.

White cell trapping alone would not explain ulcer formation, and thus the second component of the white cell theory is the activation of the cells. Activated white cells release a variety of agents such as superoxide radicals, cytokines, proteolytic enzymes, and chemotactic agents. Coleridge-Smith and Scurr[22] studied skin biopsies in patients with varicose veins, liposclerotic skin, and healed ulcers and found progressively more white cells in the skin with progression of venous disease. Those with healed ulcers had 40 times the number of WBCs than those with varicose veins and normal skin, with most of the cells identified as macrophages, with some T lymphocytes.[22]

Limb swelling, a characteristic early finding in the limb with CVI, develops through a disturbance in at least one of three mechanisms.[17] First, hydrostatic pressure on the venous side of the capillary is increased because of the

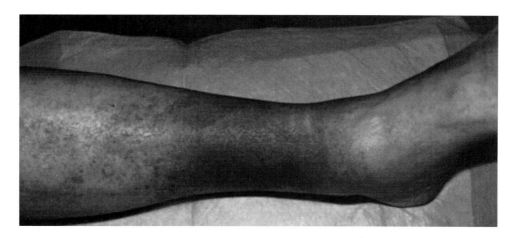

Fig. 28-6. Clinical findings in longstanding and advanced chronic venous insufficiency. Edema to the supramalleolar level and pronounced pigmentary changes are observed, which are indicative of stage II disease. *(From O'Donnell TF Jr: Clinical diagnosis and classification of chronic venous insufficiency. In Rutherford RB, ed: Vascular surgery, ed 3, Philadelphia, 1989, WB Saunders Co.)*

mechanisms previously discussed, and this favors transfer of fluid out of the capillary into the interstitial space. Second, the lymphatics in many patients have been damaged and fibrosed by recurrent skin infections, thereby preventing the normal transport of water and protein by the lymphatics out of the interstitial space. Third, edema formation in the limb with CVI is favored by the increased protein content within the interstitial space, which develops because of leaky capillary walls. These mechanisms are associated with the transfer of osmotically active particles from the intravascular to the interstitial space and produce a phenomenon called "water-trapping."

Clinical Findings

The chief clinical manifestations of CVI are dilated veins, leg pain, edema, and cutaneous changes, and their frequency is related to both the site of anatomic involvement (superficial or deep system) and to the severity of disease.

Before the clinical classification is discussed, the individual symptoms and physical findings are discussed separately. It is somewhat artificial to discuss each one of these clinical manifestations individually because they usually occur together.

EDEMA. Edema may be the first manifestation of early CVI. The patient usually notes that the swelling is mild and limited to the area just above the shoe line around the malleoli. The edema usually resolves with bed rest, particularly if the legs are elevated during sleep. In the early phases of CVI the distribution of the edema is limited to the perimalleolar area, but with longstanding CVI the edema may progress to involve the midcalf (Fig. 28-6). As opposed to limb swelling associated with lymphedema (Fig. 28-7), the metatarsal area usually is not involved in the early phases of CVI. Initially the edema may be pitting, but with chronic edema formation subcutaneous fibrosis occurs so that the edema may fail to pit. This fibrosis is probably related to deposition of protein within the subcutaneous tissue and the subsequent inflammatory process. Although

it has been taught that only lymphedema fails to pit, the critical factor that determines pitting is the degree of subcutaneous fibrosis, irrespective of a venous or lymphatic cause.

VENOUS DILATION. With involvement of the superficial venous system, the most common initial sign, in addition to mild edema, may be cosmetically displeasing dilated superficial veins. Initially the venous dilation may be most apparent in the dependent portion of the limb, particularly on the medial aspect of the lower calf. The patient may observe dilation of small veins underneath the medial malleolus, the so-called "ankle flare" sign, pathognomonic of CVI. As with edema formation, the veins may become most prominent following prolonged standing or in women at the time of menses. With progression of CVI the veins become more tortuous and larger, and the patient will note their appearance in the proximal portion of the limb (Fig. 28-8). Although some mild varicosities may develop in women during adolescence, they usually progress rapidly in size and number during pregnancy. With each successive pregnancy, the number and width of these varicosities usually increase. In the postpartum period, or with cessation of oral contraceptives, there may be improvement in the varicose veins.

LEG PAIN. Although not all patients with CVI experience pain, several distinct types of pain are commonly associated with CVI. The most frequent type is limb heaviness or ache, which occurs after prolonged standing. The pain is usually experienced in the calf area, and as opposed to the calf pain associated with arterial insufficiency, this ache may be eased by walking. Lying down, particularly with elevation of the limb, relieves limb heaviness within a short period. The aching sensation may be worse in warm, humid weather or for women during their menses, because both conditions are associated with greater salt and water retention, which worsens the edema. Edema presumably produces the pain by increasing both intracompartmental and subcutaneous tissue volume and pressure. Mild calf pain or ache after prolonged standing is

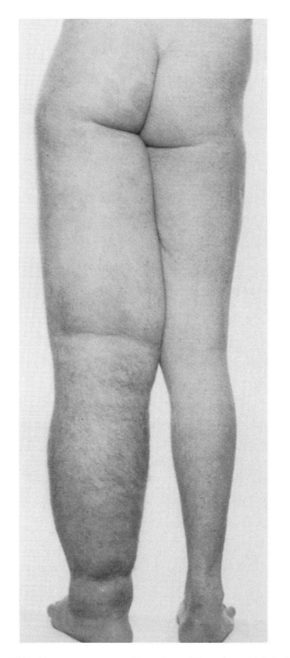

Fig. 28-7. Nonvenous causes of leg edema. The enlarged left limb of this patient with lymphedema has no significant pigmentary changes or prominent varices, which is in striking contrast to the patients with chronic venous insufficiency shown in Figs. 28-8 to 28-10.

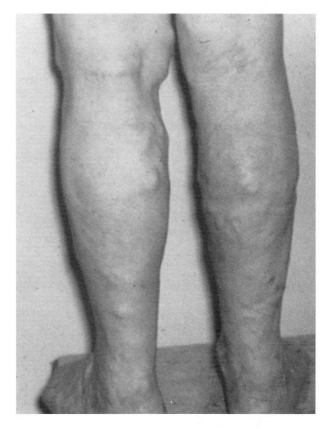

Fig. 28-8. Early stage II venous disease. Posterior view of patient with stage II chronic venous insufficiency—characteristically prominent bilateral varicosities involving both calves and the right thigh. Mild bilateral edema is present.

usually characteristic of CVI involving the superficial system. In addition, patients may experience pain along the course of dilated varicose veins after prolonged standing, which is probably a result of venous stasis within the varicosity and distention of the vein wall.

The pain associated with deep venous insufficiency is related to the cause of deep system disease. Patients with obstruction of the deep venous system may experience "venous claudication." Although mild aching sensation is experienced at rest, ambulation produces an intense burst-ing cramping sensation in the calf. As with the patient with arterial insufficiency, the patient with venous claudication may have to stop and allow the venous congestion to resolve. Studies by Negus and Cocket[26] and recent investigations by Killewitch et al[27] have shown that venous claudication is caused by a rapid increase in both superficial and deep venous pressure. The increased resistance to venous blood flow out of the limb, which is usually related to iliofemoral occlusion, sharply elevates venous pressure. Patients with inadequate venous collateral flow around an iliofemoral occlusion usually experience venous claudication. The second type of pain experienced by a patient with chronic deep venous insufficiency is related to valvular incompetence. On standing, the patient may note the sudden development of leg heaviness. Patients have described it as similar to the sensation of water being poured into the leg to fill it up. After standing for a while, this sensation may be followed by a bursting type of heaviness in the calf, which can be quite incapacitating.

Cutaneous infection, secondary to dermatitis or, alternatively, an open ulcer, can produce pain in the limb with CVI, but this pain is related to the primary process rather than to actual venous involvement (Fig. 28-9).

CUTANEOUS MANIFESTATIONS. Finally, the patient may observe skin pigmentary changes, usually characterized by brownish hemosiderin deposits in the skin

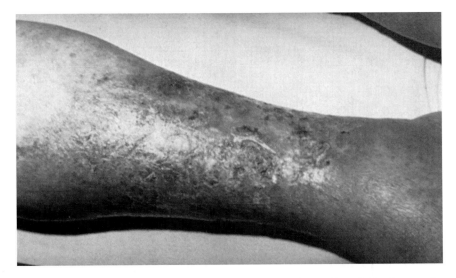

Fig. 28-9. Advanced stage II venous disease. Scaling eczematous dermatitis and skin changes characteristic of longstanding disease. *(From O'Donnell TF Jr: Clinical diagnosis and classification of chronic venous insufficiency. In Rutherford RB, ed: Vascular surgery, ed 3, Philadelphia, 1989, WB Saunders Co.)*

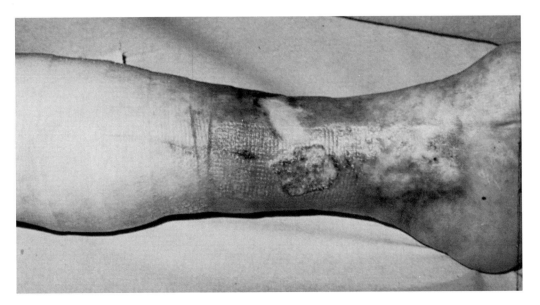

Fig. 28-10. Stage III venous disease. The medial view of a limb with end stages of venous disease as characterized by a chronic venous ulcer *(above the medial malleolus)* and marked cutaneous pigmentary changes. *(From O'Donnell TF Jr: Clinical diagnosis and classification of chronic venous insufficiency. In Rutherford RB, ed: Vascular surgery, ed 3, Philadelphia, 1989, WB Saunders Co.)*

(Fig. 28-6). Frequently the eczematous dermatitis associated with advanced CVI may prompt referral to a skin specialist for treatment (Fig. 28-10). In general, such skin changes are manifestations of longstanding venous insufficiency.

Classification

CVI is classified broadly into three areas (see the box, p. 499). The first is *anatomic*—where the system(s) involved are described (superficial and deep levels) or segments involved are defined (proximal-iliofemoral or distal popliteal and calf veins). The second is *clinical*—where the severity of the disease is estimated. The third is *hemo-*

dynamic—where the extent and severity of the disease is determined objectively by noninvasive vascular laboratory testing.

ANATOMIC. The anatomic classification of CVI is important because it relates directly to the causes of the clinical manifestations of CVI, and it influences the type of therapy. CVI can involve the superficial venous system alone (greater and lesser saphenous veins) or can combine with involvement of the deep venous system as is usual in more advanced cases. The perforating veins are included with the superficial venous system in the classification system used in this chapter (see the box, p. 499). Finally, deep venous system involvement alone, without involve-

CLASSIFICATIONS OF CHRONIC VENOUS INSUFFICIENCY

I. Anatomic
 A. System(s) involved: superficial or deep
 B. Segment(s) involved: proximal or distal

II. Clinical
 A. Severity: stage I (mild) to stage III (severe)

III. Hemodynamic
 A. Extent
 B. Severity

ANATOMIC CLASSIFICATION

I. System(s) Involved
 A. Superficial
  1. Saphenous (greater or lesser)
  2. Perforating (communicating) veins
 B. Deep
 C. Combination of A and B

II. Segment(s) Involved
 A. Deep veins
  1. Calf veins
  2. Femoral veins: iliofemoral
  3. Iliac veins: iliofemoral
  4. Cava
 B. Superficial veins
  1. Greater
  2. Lesser
  3. Perforating

III. Morphology
 A. Obstruction
 B. Valve incompetence

ment of the perforating (communicating) veins or segments of the superficial venous system, is unusual.

Figure 28-11 illustrates schematically the major anatomic components of the superficial and deep venous systems of the lower extremity in the normal limb. CVI of the superficial venous system includes the most frequently encountered form of CVI, varicose veins. In a clinical, phlebographic, and Doppler study of nearly 600 consecutive patients who went to a venous clinic, Darke[28] demonstrated that 78% were related to varicose veins and therefore involved predominantly the superficial venous system. Traditionally involvement of the superficial venous system alone has been termed *primary varicose veins,* which implies a congenital or inherited cause rather than an acquired one. The congenital cause of varicose veins is strengthened by the strong family history of varicose veins in over 75% of the patients who have them.[17,29]

The deep system may be involved in approximately one quarter of all patients with CVI[28] (Fig. 28-12). Although deep venous insufficiency is usually attributed to the sequelae of acute deep venous thrombosis, a history of documented deep venous thrombosis may be elicited in only 40% to 50% of patients.[30,31] Bauer[32] demonstrated nonthrombotic valvular incompetence in 30 of 55 limbs with typical postthrombotic clinical changes. Subsequently Kistner[33] described primary valvular incompetence in approximately 50% of "postthrombotic" limbs examined by phlebography, because none of these 22 limbs had typical phlebographic evidence of previous deep venous thrombosis.

Recently Darke[28] performed descending phlebographic studies in a series of patients with characteristic clinical changes of the postthrombotic limb. The venograms showed anatomic alterations typical of the postthrombotic limb in only 15 out of 65 limbs (23%) with grade II reflux and in 7 out of 32 limbs (21%) with grade III or IV reflux. As in Kistner's study, these data imply that a congenital cause or acquired weakness in the vein from causes other than an episode of deep venous thrombosis may be more common than the postthrombotic state as a cause of deep venous insufficiency.[34]

We have observed that patients with typical postthrom-

botic changes on phlebography in their calf or popliteal veins distally may have floppy and redundant valve leaflets in the femoral vein at a more proximal level. Thus the dual cause may confound simple ascription to either post–deep venous thrombosis or primary valvular incompetence.

The anatomic distribution of CVI is further subdivided by the specific location within the superficial or deep venous systems (see the box on this page). In the superficial system varicose veins may involve the greater or lesser saphenous veins or perforating veins (Figs. 28-11 and 28-12). In chronic deep venous insufficiency the iliac, superficial femoral, profunda femoris, popliteal, and calf veins may be affected. Chronic deep venous insufficiency can be further classified anatomically as to whether obstruction, valvular incompetence, or a combination of both is present. The anatomic finding has important clinical implications for the subsequent pathophysiology, as discussed previously in this chapter. Traditionally authors have divided the anatomic involvement of the deep system into central (iliofemoral) or peripheral (popliteal-tibial) disease (see the box on this page). This distinction is somewhat artificial, and it is perhaps better to specify the actual site involved and whether the process is caused by obstruction or valvular incompetence.

CLINICAL. The Subcommittee for Standards in Vascular Surgery formulated a classification of CVI that could be based on the clinical evaluation of the patient.[35]

There are three clinical categories that are related to the severity of the disease. The various symptoms and physical findings previously described help classify the disease. Table 28-2 shows the three grades of CVI.

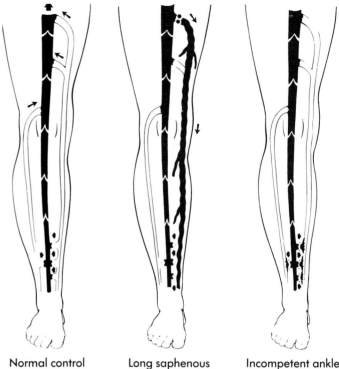

Fig. 28-11. Blood flow alterations in superficial venous insufficiency. Normal limb *(left)* is contrasted to limb with long saphenous incompetence *(middle)*, where valvular damage in the superficial system alters flow. Similar changes are observed in the limb with incompetent ankle perforators alone *(right)*. *(From O'Donnell TF Jr: Clinical diagnosis and classification of chronic venous insufficiency. In Rutherford RB, ed: Vascular surgery, ed 3, Philadelphia, 1989, WB Saunders Co.)*

Normal control

Long saphenous incompetence (SFI)

Incompetent ankle perforators alone (ICPV)

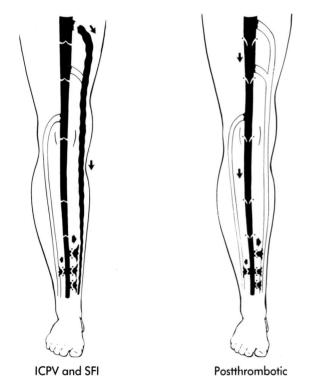

ICPV and SFI

Postthrombotic

Fig. 28-12. Blood flow alterations in combined saphenous and perforating vein incompetence *(left)* are contrasted to patient with deep venous valvular incompetence and obstruction *(right)*. *(From O'Donnell TF Jr: Clinical diagnosis and classification of chronic venous insufficiency. In Rutherford RB, ed: Vascular surgery, ed 3, Philadelphia, 1989, WB Saunders Co.)*

Table 28-2. Clinical Classification of Chronic Venous Insufficiency

Grade	Symptoms	Physical Findings
I	Mild swelling Heaviness Vein dilation	Ankle edema <1 cm Dilated superficial veins Normal skin and subcutaneous tissue
II	Moderate to severe swelling Heaviness Varicosities Skin changes	Edema >1 cm Multiple dilated veins Incompetent perforating veins (mild) Pigmentation (mild) Liposclerosis (mild)
III	Severe swelling Calf pain with or without claudication	Edema >2 cm Multiple dilated veins Incompetent perforating veins (severe) Multiple vein varicosities Marked skin pigmentation Severe liposclerosis Ulcer

Grade I CVI is characterized by symptoms of mild swelling, limb heaviness after prolonged standing, and dilation of the superficial veins, particularly underneath the medial malleolus. On physical examination the ankle girth is usually increased by less than 1 cm when compared with the contralateral limb. Superficial venous dilation usually involves the greater saphenous system, particularly at the lower thigh and calf areas. Incompetent perforating veins are unusual. The skin has normal pigmentation and the subcutaneous tissue lacks fibrosis.

By contrast, grade II CVI indicates a more extensive anatomic process. The greater saphenous system is extensively involved with varicosities and the perforating (communicating) veins are usually incompetent. Varicosities are quite numerous and easily observable. The patient complains of moderate to severe swelling and limb heaviness and observes mild skin pigmentary changes. On physical examination the edema is usually greater than 1 cm in girth. There are multiple dilated tributaries of the greater saphenous vein in the calf and thigh. Incompetent perforating veins are palpated. Cutaneous changes are limited to mild pigmentary deposition—brownish-red streaks, particularly in the gaiter or supramalleolar area. The subcutaneous tissue is slightly indurated secondary to liposclerosis.

Finally, with grade III CVI the swelling is severe and extends up from the ankle area to involve the calf. The patient complains of calf ache and heaviness, which occur earlier in the day or after short periods of standing. If iliofemoral involvement is present, venous claudication may occur. An active ulcer is observed or it may have recently healed. Physical findings include more significant edema of greater than 2 cm in girth at the ankle level, multiple dilated superficial veins, and evidence of incompetent perforating veins. There is marked dark brown–black skin pigmentation with brawny edema. Eczematous changes of the skin are observed. Severe induration of the subcutaneous fat is palpated, which reflects more advanced liposclerosis.

Diagnosis

The physician diagnosing CVI relies on a thorough history and physical examination, the use of bedside maneuvers, and the assistance of the noninvasive vascular laboratory.

PHYSICAL EXAMINATION. The physical examination of the limb with CVI may play a more important role in guiding therapy than it does for the limb with arterial insufficiency. The patient should be examined in the upright position, preferably standing on a stool or bench. The use of a nonfluorescent lamp is quite helpful to allow the varicosities, if present, to cast shadows. The four traditional stages of the physical examination—inspection, palpation, percussion, and auscultation—are followed in succession with particular emphasis on the first two. The patient's limb is inspected in a standing position from the front, side, and rear. Specially prepared anatomic diagrams of the lower extremity for CVI are helpful for making clinical notations. We usually examine the limb from the ankle up to the abdomen in a standard fashion. The presence of the ankle venous flare underneath the medial malleolus is sought and is usually found as one of the first signs of CVI. Next, the degree of edema formation and its extent are assessed at the foot, ankle, and lower calf levels. Limb girths should be measured at specified anatomic points to document objectively the extent of edema. The presence of skin pigmentary changes, particularly in the

supramalleolar area, should be observed (Fig. 28-6). An associated scaling dermatitis may be present (Fig. 28-9).

The location of a venous ulcer is charted. The size and depth of the ulcer as well as the degree of granulation tissue should be described (Fig. 28-10). Venous ulcers usually occur over the gaiter area (medial supramalleolar area), the site of the lower three major perforating veins, and also the area that is under the maximum influence of hydrostatic pressure. As opposed to arterial ulcers, venous ulcers are superficial and do not frequently penetrate through the fascia. The location of incisions from previous venous surgery should be sought for anterior to the medial malleolus, in the inguinal area, or over the perforating vein area. Finally, the distribution of dilated superficial veins should be charted.

Next the limb is palpated. The compliance of the subcutaneous tissue edema is assessed. Does the edema pit easily? And at what level? What is the extent of subcutaneous fibrosis? The limb with more advanced CVI will feel woody and resilient to palpation. The skin temperature is assessed, and an increased temperature may indicate underlying cellulitis. The saphenofemoral junction should be palpated for valvular incompetence. The fingers are placed over the foramen ovale and the patient is instructed to cough or to perform Valsalva's maneuver. In the limb with saphenofemoral incompetence a definite expansile impulse will be felt at the origin of the greater saphenous vein, which is caused by reflux of blood in a retrograde direction. Since some veins will not be readily visible in patients with moderate obesity, palpation may be the best method to locate dilated superficial varicosities of the thigh and calf. In the calf region, palpation of circular defects in the subcutaneous tissue usually reveals the site of incompetent dilated perforating veins.[15] These sites should be marked on the skin before surgery or noted on the diagram what their distance is from the malleoli.

The physical examination is not complete without auscultation. Although it is an unusual occurrence, arteriovenous fistulas can be associated with the development of prominent lower-extremity varicosities. Auscultation over the varicosities will usually reveal a continuous murmur. A pulsatile arterial component will be heard if a Doppler probe is placed over the varicose veins. In addition, there will be increased skin temperature.

Tourniquet Tests. Although tourniquet tests, originally developed by Brody and subsequently by Trendelenburg, have confused generations of medical students, their purpose is twofold: to determine the level of valvular incompetence in the superficial system and to ascertain whether deep venous system involvement is present. We prefer a multilevel tourniquet test. The patient should be in a supine position with the limb elevated for at least a minute before the examination is begun. This latter maneuver empties the veins by reducing venous congestion in the superficial venous system. Tourniquets (½-inch Penrose drains) are then placed at several levels: (1) at the upper thigh just below the origin of the greater saphenous vein, (2) at the lower thigh below the adductor canal, (3) at the upper calf below the level of the lesser saphenous vein, and (4) at the upper ankle level above the malleoli (Fig. 28-13). The patient is then instructed to stand. If the

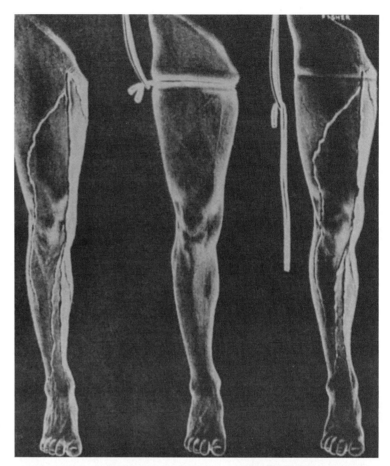

Fig. 28-13. Sequence of findings in tourniquet test shows incompetence of the greater saphenous vein. *(From O'Donnell TF Jr: Clinical diagnosis and classification of chronic venous insufficiency. In Rutherford RB, ed: Vascular surgery, ed 3, Philadelphia, 1989, WB Saunders Co.)*

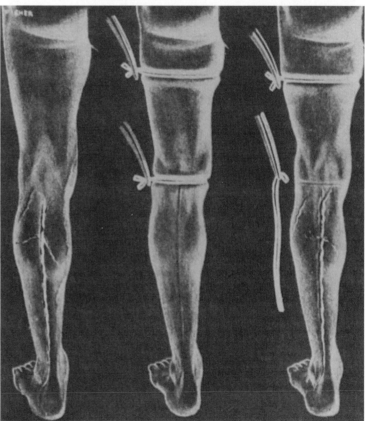

Fig. 28-14. Tourniquet test demonstrates lesser saphenous incompetence. *(From O'Donnell TF Jr: Clinical diagnosis and classification of chronic venous insufficiency. In Rutherford RB, ed: Vascular surgery, ed 3, Philadelphia, 1989, WB Saunders Co.)*

superficial veins of the calf segment fill, perforating vein incompetence is usually present. The tourniquets are usually removed from the bottom upward (Fig. 28-14). As previously stated, if removing the ankle tourniquet fills the superficial venous system, perforating vein incompetence is suspected. If, after removal of the below-knee tourniquet, the lesser saphenous system fills, lesser saphenous incompetence is most likely. Next the above-knee tourniquet is removed to assess the competence of the Hunter's canal perforator. Finally, if the superficial venous system remains empty, the high thigh tourniquet is removed to detect whether saphenofemoral incompetence is present (Fig. 28-13).

Different sequences of tourniquet removal will help to define the level of valvular incompetence. The tourniquet test is used similarly with quantitative photoplethysmography by light reflection rheography (LRR) to document the level of incompetence.[36]

In addition to observation and direct palpation of incompetent perforating veins, a tourniquet test with exercise is helpful in establishing the condition of perforating veins. The patient should exercise in place by elevating the heels, and the extent of superficial venous congestion should be observed. Next a tourniquet is applied to the upper calf to compress the superficial venous system. This tourniquet prevents filling of the greater and lesser saphenous system from above. The patient then reexercises to activate the calf muscle pump. Various responses may be observed. If the superficial calf veins become less congested with exercise, the perforating veins are usually competent, because of the normal direction of venous flow from the superficial to deep venous systems. Alternatively, if the calf veins fail to decompress or if congestion increases, this is indicative of incompetent perforating veins. In addition to the tourniquet tests for perforator incompetence, digital control of the perforating veins can be carried out. The physician's fingers are placed over the sites of the perforating veins, and the limb is elevated to decompress the superficial venous system. The patient is then instructed to stand and the physician's fingers are removed from the perforating veins individually as if he or she were playing notes on a piano keyboard. Veins will bulge at the sites of incompetent perforators when the fingertip is removed.

NONINVASIVE ASSESSMENT. The purpose of the noninvasive assessment of CVI is to answer three questions:

1. What *systems* are involved—deep, communicating veins or superficial venous system?
2. What is the *pathologic process*—valvular incompetence, obstruction, or a combination of both?
3. What *anatomic level* is involved by the pathologic changes?

Like the noninvasive assessment of arterial occlusive disease, the present methods for evaluation of CVI can be divided into those that provide hemodynamic or functional information and those that provide anatomy. The various noninvasive tests are described as they are used in our diagnostic evaluation of the patient with CVI.

Photoplethysmography. Quantitative photoplethysmography (light reflection rheography [LRR]) is a useful screening tool in the assessment of patients with and without venous disease. Photoplethysmographic technique uses a probe attached to the supramalleolar skin which emits light through the skin into the subdermal plexus and records light reflected back to the probe (Fig. 28-15). A tracing of the amount of reflected light is produced, thus giving a measurement of dermal venous blood flow. In the normal limb the blood content of the skin, which is predominantly in the subdermal plexus, decreases in response to calf muscle exercise (ankle dorsiflexion or manual calf compression) and returns to baseline after 25 seconds. Most healthy patients have venous refill times (VRTs) of 35 to 45 seconds. If the VRT is less than 25 seconds, tourniquets are placed above and below the knee and the test repeated with sequential removal of these tourniquets. This helps determine the amount of reflux contributed by the superficial venous system. Total normalization of an abnormal VRT with the addition of tourniquets is diagnostic of superficial venous insufficiency alone, whereas partial correction of the VRT indicates superficial and deep venous insufficiency. Other studies have shown decreased venous emptying with photoplethysmography to be useful in the diagnosis of deep venous thrombosis.[37] LRR is an excellent tool to exclude venous disease in those patients with limb swelling and no physical findings of CVI. Although LRR will also identify significant obstruction and reflux, there may be variability or overlap of VRT values with varying degrees of reflux. Additionally, it does not localize the pathology as well as duplex scanning does. For these reasons, in addition to economy of test use, we now order LRR less than in the past.

Bidirectional Doppler Velocity Probe. With the advent of duplex scanning, bidirectional Doppler examination should be relegated to a bedside test by an experienced examiner. This test can detect valvular incompetence or obstruction of the superficial and deep venous systems[38,39] but is less reliable for detecting incompetence or obstruction below the knee. Although incompetent perforating veins can be identified in approximately 60% to 70% of patients with CVI,[40] many investigators, including the senior author,[15] consider such findings at times confusing, inconclusive, and difficult to interpret. Since only a relatively short segment of vein can be studied at a time, incompetence of an entire vein should not be based on retrograde flow through a single venous segment.[41] The Doppler examination is simple in methodology and extremely portable; however, this technique requires significant examiner experience. This test is subjective and highly operator dependent. Furthermore, it may be insensitive to minor venous anatomic abnormalities that do not influence overall venous flow patterns.

Air Plethysmography. Air plethysmography (APG) was described as a diagnostic modality in 1987 by Christopoulos et al,[42] and is a technique that measures several parameters of venous physiology. APG measures venous volume of the calf, the rate at which the volume is achieved (which is related to reflux), the pumping capacity

PPG   LRR

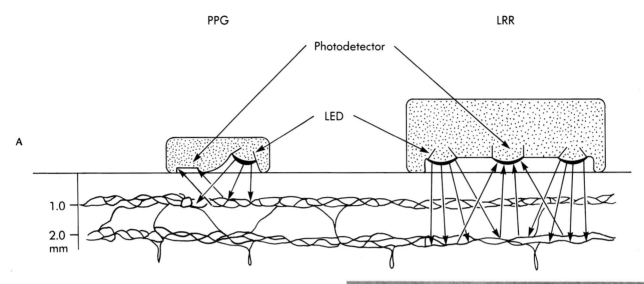

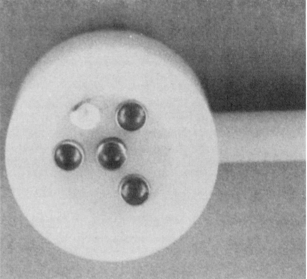

B

Fig. 28-15. Schematic of photoplethysmographic determination of venous refill time. **A,** Comparison of photoplethysmography *(PPG)* to light reflection rheography *(LRR)*. The latter has greater skin depth penetration and three light emitting sources. *(From O'Donnell TF Jr and Shephard AD: Chronic venous insufficiency. In Jarrett F and Hirsch S, eds: Vascular surgery of the lower extremity, St Louis, 1985, CV Mosby Co.)* **B,** Actual LRR probe demonstrates central photodetector. *(From O'Donnell TF Jr, McEnroe CS, and Heggenick P: Chronic venous insufficiency, Surg Clin North Am 70:159, 1990.)*

of the calf muscle, and indirectly measures ambulatory venous pressure. APG uses an air-filled polyvinyl cuff surrounding the calf, which is connected to a pressure transducer that has been calibrated with known quantities of air. A standard protocol is then carried out as follows (Fig. 28-16). The air-filled cuff is applied to the calf and the leg is elevated to 45 degrees, emptying the leg. Volume changes within the calf are reflected by pressure alterations in the sensing cuff. After a steady state has been acheived, which indicates emptying of the leg, the patient quickly stands while holding on to a walker so that the body weight is supported by the contralateral leg. Venous filling of the leg is then recorded continuously until a plateau is reached, which signifies that the *functional venous volume* (VV) is reached. By convention, 90% of the VV (90%VV) is used in calculating the *venous filling index* (VFI). The time to reach 90%VV is defined as *venous filling time 90%* (90% VFT). The VFI, a measure of reflux, is calculated from 90%VV/90%VFT, which is expressed as milliliters per second. The patient then performs one tiptoe maneuver to activate the calf muscle pump. The decrease in calf volume associated with one calf muscle exercise represents the

ejection volume (EV). The *ejection fraction* (EF) can be calculated based on the VV and is expressed as EV/VV × 100. EF represents the capability of the calf muscle pump. When a steady volume plateau is again achieved, the patient performs 10 rapid tiptoe maneuvers to thoroughly empty the calf venous reservoir. The volume is recorded at the end of the exercise and the *residual volume* (RV) is the difference between that volume and the baseline volume. The *residual volume fraction* (RVF) is calculated as RV/VV × 100 and has been shown to correlate with ambulatory venous pressure.[42] In summary, APG determines the degree of reflux, the capability of the calf muscle pump, and ambulatory venous pressure.

Duplex Imaging. Duplex scanning is the test of choice in the evaluation of venous disease. It is highly sensitive, noninvasive, and readily available. Its major disadvantage is the fact it is highly operator and interpreter dependent, so considerable experience is necessary for high accuracy. Duplex scanning permits evaluation of superficial, deep, and perforator veins, although visualization of the iliac veins is sometimes difficult. It also provides both anatomic and hemodynamic information as well as

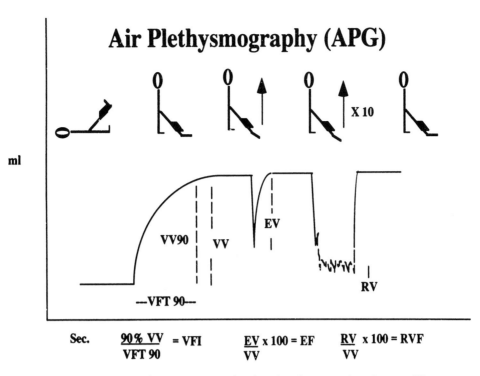

Fig. 28-16. Air plethysmography patient protocol and tracings for generation of venous filling index, ejection fraction, residual volume fraction (see text). *(From Christopoulos DG et al: Air-plethysmography and the effects of elastic compression on venous hemodynamics of the leg, J Vasc Surg 5:148, 1987.)*

detecting other pathology such as venous aneurysm, Baker's cyst, or hematoma. Importantly, it allows for determination of obstruction or thrombosis, and reflux.

In the evaluation of venous thrombosis several parameters are examined. Doppler insonation is used to identify spontaneity of flow and phasicity of flow with respiration. Squeezing the extremity distal to the probe will produce augmentation of venous flow through a nonobstructed system. Perhaps the most important parameter is B-mode visualization of the vein and its ability to collapse or compress with external pressure. A fresh thrombus is not echogenic but will not allow the vein walls to coapt with pressure. As the thrombus ages and becomes more organized with increased collagen content, it becomes more echogenic (Fig. 28-17). Thus duplex scanning is also able to determine the age of the thrombus. Other changes can also be identified including thickened, irregular vein walls and recanalization. Color-flow duplex scanning is especially useful in the latter (Fig. 28-18).

Other tests may determine the functional severity of venous outlet obstruction. These include strain-gauge plethysmography, maximum outflow fraction measured by APG, arm-foot pressure differential, and ambulatory venous pressure.

Valvular incompetence attributed to postthrombotic changes is indicated morphologically by B-mode imaging by thickening of the valve leaflets or their absence. On dynamic scanning no motion of the leaflets is observed, and they also fail to coapt. Primary valvular incompetence appears as redundant or multifolded valve structures.

Improvements in duplex scanning have allowed for

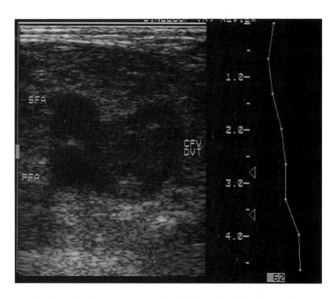

Fig. 28-17. Duplex scan of organized thrombus in the common femoral vein. Chronicity of thrombus is evident by the echogenicity of the fibrin clot within the thrombus.

quantitation of venous reflux. A variety of techniques have been used to produce reflux, with the patient either supine or standing. The Valsalva maneuver, manual compression, and cuff deflation have all been used to elicit reflux with various results. Although van Bemmelen et al[43] showed Valsalva's maneuver to be insufficient in a significant number of patients in producing reflux, especially distally,

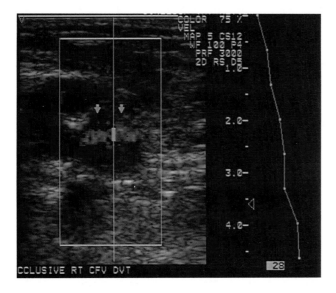

Fig. 28-18. Color-flow duplex scan illustrates nonocclusive thrombus in the common femoral vein.

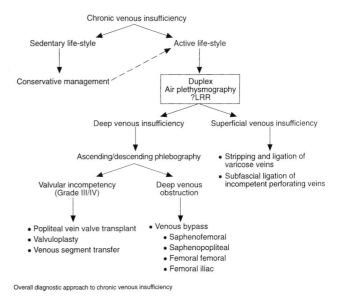

Overall diagnostic approach to chronic venous insufficiency

Fig. 28-19. Overall diagnostic approach to chronic venous insufficiency.

Masuda, Kistner, and Eklof[44] found no difference in the techniques. We believe that reflux is a physiologic response most pronounced when standing so the patient should be examined in the upright position. In addition, the intensity of the Valsalva maneuver varies by patient, so the patient-independent cuff deflation technique described by van Bemmelen et al[45] is our test of choice for venous reflux. By using Doppler spectral analysis, the duration of venous reflux is recorded objectively, what we have termed the valve closure time (VCT).[46] van Bemmelen et al[45] determined the normal VCT to be less than 0.5 seconds. With a thigh cuff, the common, superficial, and profunda femoral veins, as well as the saphenofemoral junction and midsaphenous vein are studied. A calf cuff is used to evaluate the popliteal and lesser saphenous veins and the tibial veins are tested using a foot cuff. Our laboratory has demonstrated that a sum of the superficial femoral and popliteal vein VCTs of 4 seconds or more is highly accurate in predicting severe venous reflux when compared with descending phlebography.[46] Other measurements using duplex scanning to quantify reflux include peak reflux velocity[47] and venous reflux flow.[48] Additional noninvasive tests to evaluate reflux include foot volumetry[49] and strain-gauge plethysmography.[50]

Overall Diagnostic Approach (Fig. 28-19)

After a thorough history and physical examination in the clinic, patients are referred to the vascular laboratory. Although we occasionally obtain an LRR, primarily to objectively exclude those without venous insufficiency, most patients will undergo duplex ultrasound examination, including VCTs, which accurately assesses both the superficial and deep veins. Additionally, duplex scanning is used to identify and locate incompetent perforating veins (ICPVs). If there is significant deep venous insufficiency, an APG evaluation of the limb is performed. The use of tourniquets with APG in our laboratory has not been consistently helpful in distinguishing the degree of super-

Table 28-3. Phlebographic Classification of Reflux (Kistner)

Grade	Symptom
0	No evidence of reflux
1	Reflux to proximal thigh
2	Reflux to above the knee
3	Reflux to below the knee
4	Reflux to the ankle

ficial reflux. Based on the anatomic and functional characterization of the patient's CVI, and of course the clinical symptoms and their response to nonoperative management, certain patients would be considered potential candidates for operative intervention. Such patients would undergo ascending phlebography, wherein tourniquets are used to prevent filling of the superficial system. Visualization of contrast material in the superficial venous system usually indicates flow from the deep system via incompetent perforating veins. Specific anatomic details (recanalization, obstruction, or avalvular segments) of the deep venous system are sought. If the deep system shows no major (bypassable) obstruction, the patient will undergo descending phlebography. With the patient on the tilt table, either the ipsilateral or contralateral common femoral vein can be cannulated. The patient is positioned at 70 to 90 degrees and contrast material is injected while the patient performs Valsalva's maneuver. The rate and level of descent within the deep venous system permits categorization of the degree of deep venous incompetence according to the Kistner grade (Table 28-3). Surgery for valvular incompetence is usually reserved for those in whom dye refluxes to below the knee popliteal or tibial vein segments (Fig. 28-20). This overall method (Fig. 28-19)

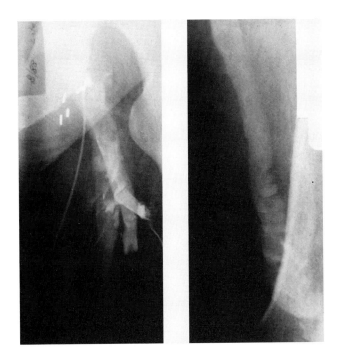

Fig. 28-20. Descending phlebogram shows competent profunda femoris vein valves and reflux in the superficial femoral vein to the level of the knee.

of evaluation allows more definitive selection of the patient for superficial venous surgery such as ligation, stripping, and interruption of incompetent perforating veins, or deep venous reconstructive surgery to correct valvular incompetence or to bypass obstruction.

Epidemiology

INCIDENCE OF SUPERFICIAL VERSUS DEEP VENOUS SYSTEM DISEASE. The relative proportion of limbs with involvement of the superficial venous system alone is important, because this incidence reflects the number of patients who may benefit from relatively straightforward surgery. Several biases, however, enter into the assessment of the relative proportion of superficial and deep venous system involvement. Many reports originate in large teaching hospitals, where patients with more severe forms of CVI may be referred. On the other hand, other reports are based only on candidates for surgery and therefore may be biased toward a greater proportion of limbs with more severe disease, or alternatively concern only those limbs that would benefit from surgery. Allowing for these limitations, Table 28-4 summarizes the relative proportion of limbs with superficial or deep CVI in several series. Our own review of nearly 720 limbs[51] showed that the proportion of limbs with deep venous involvement was three times greater than those with superficial venous insufficiency (21%). Another 14% had combined superficial and deep venous disease. The incidence of deep venous involvement (65%) in our study was three times greater than that reported by Darke[28] in his series of a comparable size. Like Darke we studied a full range of patients with CVI, in contrast to Raju,[52] who examined only limbs with the classic clinical changes of the postthrombotic syndrome.

The relatively high incidence of deep venous insufficiency in our study is probably related to the increased proportion of limbs with advanced CVI (stage III disease). In our series 142 limbs had stage III disease. Two other studies[53,54] focused on candidates for venous surgery and reported a much lower incidence of deep venous involvement. This finding may be related not only to the surgical character of these series but also to the type of surgery under consideration, namely ligation and stripping of the saphenous vein or subfascial ligation of incompetent perforating veins. This would bias toward a greater proportion of superficial venous involvement. As can be seen from Table 28-5, obstruction of the deep system is an infrequent cause of deep venous disease. In our series only 5% of patients with deep venous disease had outflow obstruction. Although Shanzer and Peirce's[55] smaller series had an incidence of venous obstruction comparable to ours, Moore, Himmel, and Sumner[56] and Raju[52] reported double our frequency of obstructive venous disease. However, the majority of limbs (85%) had valvular insufficiency as the cause of their CVI.

Several studies have used descending phlebography to determine the anatomic location of deep venous valvular incompetence. They indicate that the popliteal vein segment was incompetent in over 80% of the 300 limbs examined (Table 28-5). Alternatively, other studies that used a bidirectional Doppler instrument for assessment of deep venous valvular function demonstrated a comparable proportion of limbs (80%) with popliteal vein valve incompetence. From this, one would conclude that (1) valvular incompetence is the chief cause of chronic venous insufficiency and (2) the popliteal vein valve is usually incompetent in significantly symptomatic patients.

SPECTRUM. There are few studies that have correlated the clinical stages of CVI in a large unselected population. Our study showed that 40% of limbs had advanced stage III disease,[51] which is twice the proportion observed by Darke.[28] In his study only 20% of limbs had venous ulceration. These patients with an open or recently healed venous ulcer represent the most challenging management problem in CVI. Since the major proportion of patients with venous ulcer have valvular incompetence of the deep venous system as the cause of their CVI, there exists a relatively large population of potential candidates for deep venous reconstruction. Of additional interest, however, is the 13% to 15% of patients with venous ulcers who have involvement solely of the superficial venous system.[57] By contrast, these patients may benefit from ligation and stripping with or without ligation of perforating veins.

Treatment

The choice of nonsurgical versus surgical treatment is usually dictated by the severity of symptoms and the anatomic system(s) affected by the disease process. Our approach has been to define the severity of CVI by clinical examination, aided by noninvasive objective measurements that also suggest what systems are involved. Patients with stage I disease are usually treated by nonsurgical means unless involvement of the superficial venous system has produced moderate symptoms or the superficial varicosities are cosmetically displeasing to the patient. A

Table 28-4. Incidence of Deep Venous Disease

Study	No. of Limbs	Criteria for Entry	Methods of Diagnosis				System Involved (%)	
			Clin	Dop	AVP	Phleb	Superficial	Deep
Darke[28]	594	CVI	+	+		+	78	22
NEMCH[51]	346	CVI	+	+	+		35	65
Moore et al[56]	174	PT	+	+			65	38
Raju and Fredericks[53]	147	PT	+		+	+	27*	73
St. Thomas Hospital[54]	119	Surg	+		+	+	66	37
Schanzer and Peirce[55]	52	Surg	+		+	+	65	35

*Combined with superficial.

Clin, Clinical; *Dop,* bidirectional Doppler; *AVP,* venous pressure; *Phleb,* ascending or descending phlebogram; *CVI,* chronic venous insufficiency; *PT,* postthrombotic syndrome; *Surg,* candidate for surgery.

Table 28-5. Type and Location of Deep Venous Insufficiency

Study	No. of Limbs	Criteria for Entry	Methods of Diagnosis				Obstruction (%)	Valvular Incompetence	
			Clin	Dop	AVP	Phleb		Proximal	Distal (Popliteal)
Darke[28]	100	Ulcer	+	+		+	0	19	88
NEMCH[51]	346	CVI	+	+	+		5	11	80
Moore et al[56]	113	PT	+	+			12	22	78
Raju and Fredericks[53]	100	PT	+		+	+	13		
Schanzer and Peirce[55]	17	Surg	+		+	+	7		
Pearce et al[109]	48	PT	+		+	+	0	47	14
Bruns-Slot et al	194	PT	+	+			0	14	86
Gooley and Sumner[108]	74	PT	+	+	+		0	54	46

CVI, Chronic venous insufficiency; *Surg,* candidate for surgery; *Clin,* clinical; *Dop,* bidirectional Doppler; *AVP,* venous pressure; *Phleb,* Ascending or descending phlebogram; *PT,* postthrombotic syndrome.

similar approach is used for early stage II disease. For advanced stage II and stage III CVI (venous ulcer), a full workup including phlebography is undertaken. The patient's age, medical risks, and preferences for therapy dictate the form of treatment. If isolated superficial venous insufficiency is defined, surgery is the preferred option. If both superficial and deep systems are affected, usually surgery is directed initially at the superficial system, with deep venous reconstruction performed later if necessary for control of symptoms. Occasionally, for primary valvular incompetence, a superficial femoral vein valvuloplasty is performed concomitantly with superficial ligation and stripping. By contrast, depending on the patient's medical condition and the severity of the venous ulceration, conservative nonsurgical methods are the first line of therapy.

NONSURGICAL THERAPY. The goals of nonsurgical therapy are reduction of ambulatory superficial venous hypertension by external compression and improvement of skin nutrition.[17] Wound healing is obviously a focus in the treatment of stage III disease.

External Compression. The benefits of external compression were recognized by the Romans. A compression linen bandage was recommended by Celsus[58] to treat venous ulcers, and Wiseman[59] developed a forerunner of today's elastic stocking—a laced leather stocking. This garment was contoured to fit the lower extremity—a remarkable feature in 1676.

Three forms of external compression presently are available: compression wraps, elastic stockings, and intermittent pneumatic compression devices. The theoretic advantage of external compression is that it blocks transcapillary fluid flow during the ambulatory venous pressure cycle. The pressure required to achieve this effect at the ankle varies with the clinical state of the limb. Starling[60] has shown that approximately 40 to 50 torr are required at the ankle in patients with stage III disease to reduce transcapillary fluid flow. External compression has also been shown not only to increase the fibrinolytic activity of veins[61] but also to improve deep venous blood flow.

Compression Bandages. Compression bandages are the simplest and least expensive form of external compression. Unfortunately they are associated with poor patient compliance because of difficulty in consistently applying the correct pressure, loss of elasticity with repeated washing, and problems in maintaining the wrap in the correct position. Many have commented that the wrapping of a leg is an art form, and great variability has been noted from physician to physician or nurse to nurse.

Despite these disadvantages the Ace wrap bandage is helpful for the elderly patient who cannot pull on an elastic stocking, or it is useful in instances where there is a weeping wound and bulky dressings that require frequent dressing changes. Finally, Ace wraps are useful in abnormally contoured limbs. We generally avoid an elastic stocking when there is an ulcer requiring treatment so that an Ace wrap is used. Before wrapping the leg, an ABD pad or gauze or foam pad can be placed over an area requiring special compression, such as large varices or incompetent perforating veins. The wrap is started at the malleoli for the first turn and then continued distally to the forefoot from ankle to forefoot. The wrap is continued back up over the leg in a medial to lateral direction, with the outside of the roll applied to the leg.

Elastic Stockings. Specially, custom-fitted elastic compression stockings are the standard for treatment of CVI. Like compression bandages, elastic stockings should employ graduated pressure with the highest pressure placed at the ankle level and the lowest pressure at the calf level. Below-knee stockings are usually prescribed, whereas thigh-high or other forms of above-knee stockings are to be avoided because they bind in the popliteal fossa—and theoretically, high pressures are really not needed above the knee but rather at the ankle area. The graduated elastic compression stocking reduces superficial venous volume and prevents transcapillary leakage of fluid into the interstitium. In a study assessing the effects of elastic stockings on ambulatory venous pressure measurements in the postthrombotic limb, we showed that the major hemodynamic effect of these stockings was to reduce the peak systolic pressure achieved during the ambulatory walking cycle (Fig. 28-21).[62] All patients had ascending phlebography that showed extensive postthrombotic involvement of the deep venous system. All patients had advanced stage II or stage III disease. Neither venous refill time nor percent reduction in ambulatory venous pressure was altered by elastic compression. A study by Noyes et al[63] demonstrated a reduction in VRT, as measured by photoplethysmography. This benefit appeared to be present even without application of the elastic stocking. The reason for this improvement without external compression is difficult to explain. Unfortunately, in contrast to our study, Noyes et al[63] did not have any anatomic definition of the extent of involvement of either the superficial or the deep venous system. In addition, no clinical classification was mentioned.

Assessment of the tension produced by an elastic stocking is beyond the scope of this chapter, but the British Standards Commission has tested various elastic stockings

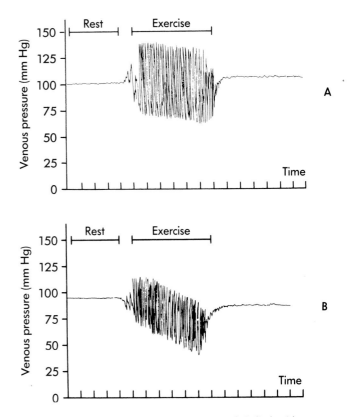

Fig. 28-21. A, Ambulatory venous pressure study in limb with postthrombotic syndrome without elastic compression. Note the high peak systolic pressure, which rises to nearly 150 mm Hg, mostly with exercise and rapid refilling. **B,** Ambulatory venous pressure study in limb **(A)** with elastic compression. The effect of elastic compression is to lower the peak systolic pressure. Venous emptying and refill time are unaffected. *(From O'Donnell TF Jr and Shephard AD: Chronic venous insufficiency. In Jarrett F and Hirsch S, eds: Vascular surgery of the lower extremity, St Louis, 1985, CV Mosby Co.)*

and measured the pressure at contact points underneath the elastic stocking.[64] Certainly the choice of the brand of stocking is up to the physician, who should be guided by the reliability of fit, durability, comfort, and finally, patient acceptance, which usually arises from the previous factors. Stockings come in several varieties of compression, 20 to 30 torr, 30 to 40 torr, and 40 to 50 torr. For mild venous disease, stage I, a 20- to 30-torr seamless, double-weave stocking is prescribed, whereas for patients with stage II or stage III (healed ulcer) we prefer the 40- to 50-torr stocking. The life of a pair of elastic stockings is from 4 to 6 months, depending on the brand. Generally four stockings per limb per year will be required. The patient is instructed to put the stocking on before arising from bed, because presumably this is the time of maximal edema reduction. The tension of the elastic stockings is checked on office visits, and when the stocking feels easy to apply it has obviously lost its elasticity.

The major disadvantage to elastic compression stockings is the difficulty of putting them on and taking them off, and several aids are commercially available to help patients. The use of standard rubber kitchen gloves also greatly helps patients put on the stockings, and zippered stockings are also available.

Circ-Aid. An alternative approach to elastic compression stockings is the Circ-Aid. This is a custom-fitted device composed of a series of Velcro straps from the ankle to below the knee. This allows the patient to adjust the tension of each strip and to fit the compression device to an abnormally contoured leg. Circ-Aid also allows dressing changes to be carried out more easily. Recent trials have shown improved hemodynamic and healing benefits with the use of this device.[65]

Intermittent Pneumatic Compression. Intermittent pneumatic compression devices have been used extensively for the prevention of deep vein thrombosis.[66] These devices have been shown by controlled trials to prevent deep vein thrombosis by promoting increased deep venous blood flow. In addition, the fibrinolytic activity of veins has been enhanced.[67] These devices come as single-unit cells, two- or three-cell units, or multicell sequential units. A significant number of patients with CVI also have lymphatic involvement complicating the edema and its treatment. Intermittent compression devices have been shown to improve ulcer healing and improve the microcirculatory changes seen in CVI and should be considered for those patients with stage III ulcers or marked edema. In our experience the devices should have sequential inflation of at least three chambers to "milk" the fluid up the leg.

Skin Care. Patients with stage I and early stage II disease should be encouraged to use skin cream to improve skin nutrition. A water-based, soluble cream or lotion is preferred. Since Polysorb Hydrate is not oil-based, it does not act on the overlying elastic compression stocking. Its lack of greasy feeling improves patient compliance. Patients with advanced stage II disease and eczematous skin changes complain bitterly of pruritus. Topical steroid cream is helpful in reducing this symptom and therefore preventing scratching. Excoriations may convert a stage II limb to a stage III limb. The addition of an oral antihistamine supplements the topical application of the steroid in such patients. Patients with acute infection should be treated vigorously to prevent damage to the lymphatics. Lymphatic obliteration compounds the edema of CVI. In general, the cellulitic infection is related to group B streptococci, and therefore penicillin or erythromycin is appropriate treatment. Fungal infection should not be overlooked in patients with scaling dermatitis. If fungal infection is suspected, a skin scraping should be obtained for microscopic examination and oral antifungal agents prescribed.

Ulcer Care. Venous ulcer represents the end stage of CVI. Unfortunately most studies gauge the effect of any treatment modality for venous ulcer by the incidence of ulcer healing, but few provide follow-up data on ulcer *recurrence.* It is important to focus on ulcer recurrence as the gold standard rather than on the initial healing of the venous ulcer, because as Browse has stated, "Almost all venous ulcers can be healed with good medical treatment, but universal prevention of recurrence cannot yet be achieved."[1] Therefore the true measure of success for any treatment method should be determined by its prevention of ulcer recurrence rather than ulcer healing alone. Implicit in the assessment of ulcer recurrence is a long-term follow-up program similar to the reporting of arterial reconstructive procedures or survival with antineoplastic

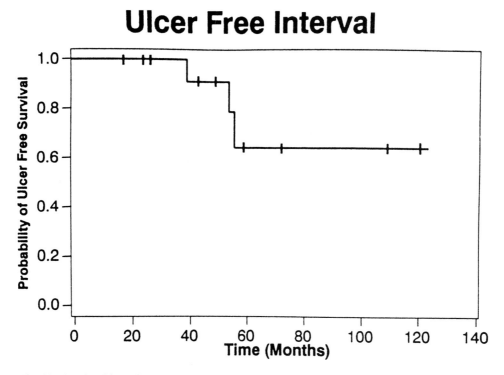

Fig. 28-22. Life-table analysis of 15 patients treated by popliteal vein valve transplant for recurrent venous ulcer. The curve shows the ulcer-free interval following surgery. *(From Bry JDL et al: The clinical and hemodynamic results after axillary-to-popliteal vein valve transplantation, J Vasc Surg 21:110, 1995.)*

medicines. We have used a life-table method for assessing the results of ulcer healing. This method is similar to that used for determining the graft patency of arterial grafts. This measure of ulcer recurrence has been termed *the ulcer-free interval rate* (Fig. 28-22).

External compression is essential to promote ulcer healing. We prefer a frequently changed, high-tension elastic compression bandage or the Circ-Aid device to complement wound care. Occasionally patients will be able to wear an elastic compression stocking over the dressing, but this is difficult to apply over bulkier dressings. These external compression methods may be supplemented by the nightly use of an external pneumatic compression device. Although considered a form of external compression, the Unna boot is addressed subsequently as a form of wound care.

The goal of ulcer treatment is to prevent recurrence and frequent hospitalizations with lost time from work, which has a significant socioeconomic impact.

Ulcer care should reduce the bacterial population of the ulcer, arrest periulcer infection, and promote epithelialization of the ulcer. Three types of dressings are currently available to treat venous ulcers: (1) absorbent dressings, (2) occlusive dressings, and (3) impregnated bandages. We do not use dressings impregnated with antibiotic cream, another form of wound care, because of the danger of sensitization.

Absorbent dressings, such as gauze sponges, should "blot" or "sponge up" the ulcer exudate. In ulcers with exudate several options exist. Calcium alginate dressings are very absorbent but need to be changed when saturated, which may occur in hours or days. Betadine-soaked gauze sponges thoroughly wrung out can be used in a wet-to-dry fashion initially changed every 6 hours. Once the ulcer is no longer purulent and granulation tissue is observed, a variety of wound options are available. These include saline wet-to-dry gauze dressings, occlusive dressings such as DuoDerm, polyurethane sheets, or foam dressings.

Impregnated bandages, such as the Unna boot, are widely used in the management of venous ulcers. The term *Unna boot* is used in a generic sense, because the medication, developed by a dermatologist, is a mixture of gelatin, zinc oxide, sorbitol, gelatin magnesium, aluminum silicate, and calamine. Unna boots represent a popular form of bandage and are used in many large outpatient clinics in urban hospital settings. The advantages of an Unna boot are that both wound care and external compression are contained in one unit; the boot can be changed on a twice- or once-weekly basis depending on the amount of exudate, and the boot prevents the patient from doing damage to the skin by scratching. The disadvantages of this treatment are the obvious personal hygiene problem, sensitization to the paste, and exudate forming underneath the boot, which could further macerate the skin.

Results of Treatment. Cranley[68] has shown that 86% of 18,055 ulcerated extremities, monitored from 1952 to 1987, could be healed by a combination of pressure bandage applications and wound care alone. Similarly, Browse, Burnand, and Lea[1] found that over 80% of leg ulcers would heal within the first year after treatment in a special venous clinic when treated by a combination of paste bandages and elastic compression. Recently, occlusive hydrocolloid dressings, such as DuoDerm,[69] have been used in conjunction with external compression. A randomized, prospective, comparative study by Kikta et al[70] showed superiority of the Unna boot regimen (70% healing rate) (Table 28-6) over that of the hydrocolloid dressing treatment (38% healing rate). Although the hydrocolloid dressing was more acceptable to the patient with respect to comfort and convenience, 10 patients in the hydrocolloid dressing group required cessation of therapy because of complications. Eriksson[71] showed diametrically opposite results in a comparative study (Table 28-6). The incidence of healing was comparable between the hydrocolloid dressing group and the Unna boot group. Rubin et al[73] recently reported a comparative trial of Unna boot versus polyurethane foam dressings (PFDs). During a 12-month period 36 consecutive ambulatory patients with lower-extremity chronic venous ulcer were randomized into the two treatment programs. Of the patients treated with PFDs, 52% withdrew from the study because of wound odor, while conversely there was 100% compliance in the Unna boot group. In addition, the overall wound-healing rate was better in the Unna boot group (95% vs. 41% of the PFD group). Finally, the healing rate was superior in the Unna boot group (0.5 cm^2/day) than in the PFD group (0.07 cm^2/day). This most recent study suggests that the Unna boot should not be abandoned as a form of therapy. Unfortunately, little data are available on subsequent ulcer recurrence. In the most extensive series reported on conservative therapy, Cranley[68] observed a 21% incidence of recurrent ulcers with documented deep venous disease in patients treated in his clinic. This rate is similar to the 18% recurrence rate noted

Table 28-6. Results of Ulcer Healing with Nonsurgical Treatment

Study	No. of Cases	Method	Ulcers Healed (%)
Cranley[68]	18,055	Pressure bandage and wound care	86
Browse[1]	>100	Elastic compression Paste bandage	80
Kikta[70]	30	Unna boot	70
	39	Hydrocolloid dressing	38
Eriksson[71]	17	Hydrocolloid and elastic compression	53
van Rijswijk[72]	152	Hydrocolloid	62

MEDICAL THERAPY FOR CHRONIC VENOUS INSUFFICIENCY

I. External Compression
A. Elastic stockings: custom fitted
B. Ace wrap or variant
C. Circ-Aid
D. Intermittent external pneumatic compression

II. Skin Care
A. Lanolin
B. Water-based lotion: Polysorb Hydrate
C. Topical antifungal agent

III. Ulcer Care
A. Absorbent
  1. Wide-mesh gauze
    a. Purulent: half-strength Betadine
    b. Nonpurulent: saline wet to dry
B. Occlusive dressing
  1. Hydrogels: Synthaderm
  2. Hydrocolloids: DuoDerm
  3. Polyurethane: Op-Site
  4. Foam: LYOfoam
C. Impregnated compression bandages
  1. Unna boot

Table 28-7. Results with Sclerotherapy

Study	No. of Patients	Years of Follow-Up Care	Recurrence (%)
Fegan[74]	760	6	15
Hobbs*[75]		1	18
		5	93
Strother[103]	348	1-3	11
		>4	32
Dejode[104]	146	1-5	17
Reid[105]	1080	1	10
Chant[106]	155	3	22

*Greater saphenous vein.

in patients with superficial venous disease who were treated with wound care and compression bandages. For a review of medical therapy see the box on this page.

Sclerotherapy. Sclerotherapy is an important adjunct to the treatment of CVI (Table 28-7). There is some debate as to the proper role of sclerotherapy, but most physicians use this method in selected circumstances. Sclerotherapy depends on producing a limited inflammatory response in a segment of vein. Subsequent external compression of that vein segment produces adherence of the vein walls. Fibrosis and possible reabsorption eventually ensue. Fegan[74] demonstrated that only a small amount of sclerosing solution entered the deep venous system and was rapidly diluted if the patient exercised.

As stated previously, patient selection is critical. Hobbs'[75] prospective study, which compared sclerotherapy with surgery, showed that sclerotherapy was most useful for the treatment of incompetent perforating veins and for recurrent veins after surgery. Long saphenous incompetence was associated with a high incidence of recurrence in the sclerotherapy-treated group. Saphenopopliteal and saphenous vein high thigh incompetence had poor results with sclerotherapy, usually caused by the difficulty in obtaining compression and the large volume of sclerosant required. Hobbs suggested surgery for these groups to avoid such problems. With sclerotherapy, however, some physicians use high ligation of the vein with

sclerotherapy or with stripping to the knee. Sclerotherapy of the calf varices is also carried out.

In many cases cosmetic improvement is an important factor leading one to decide on treatment for varicosities. Although surgical and injection treatment options are available for varicose veins, spider telangiectasias respond only to injection therapy, and the response may be quite variable. Surgical removal is inappropriate and nearly impossible.

Sclerotherapy for venous telangiectasia is best accomplished using 23% saline and a 30-gauge needle to enter the vein (Fig. 28-23). Complete filling of the telangiectatic area should be easily accomplished with the injection, and extravasation should be avoided. Resolution of the veins following adequate injection should occur within 2 to 6 weeks. This technique is ideal for cosmetic management of venous telangiectasias.

Various sclerosing solutions are available for larger veins. Sodium tetradecyl 3% is FDA approved and widely used. Alternatively, hypertonic saline solution can be used but may be painful to the patient. Some of the discomfort of hypertonic saline solution can be avoided by mixing a local anesthetic agent, such as lidocaine (Xylocaine) or bupivacaine (Marcaine), with the solution. The concentration of the sclerosant depends on the size of the vein sclerosed. For smaller veins sodium tetradecyl 3% can be diluted in half or in quarter with saline solution. While the patient is standing the veins are marked and a 25- or 30-gauge needle can be inserted attached to the end of a tuberculin syringe and taped into place. Five to six syringes may be required. Alternatively the vein may be entered with the patient in the horizontal position. If carried out with the patient lying down, a 25- or 30-gauge scalp vein can be used. The leg is elevated to empty the vein. A small amount of air is injected first to be sure that the needle is in the vein and to prevent extravasation of the sclerosant solution. Next, 0.1 to 0.75 ml of the sclerosing solution is injected. The physician's index and ring fingers are placed a few centimeters above and below the site of injection to maintain the sclerosing solution in the proper location. A gauze or foam pad provides compression over the vein segment. Care should be taken to avoid tension on the skin with the tape holding the pads, because the tape may cause

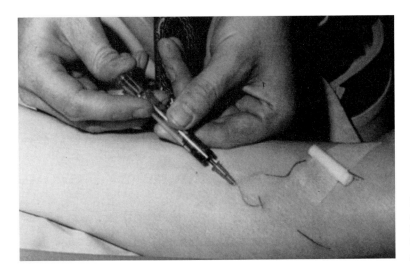

Fig. 28-23. Sclerotherapy for superficial calf varicosities. A 25+-gauge needle has aspirated blood before injection of sclerosant. A dental roll is placed over the vein for direct compression of the leg. Elastic stockings or Ace wraps are then worn.

traction burns. The patient is instructed to walk at least a mile or two a day following sclerotherapy to dilute the sclerosing solution in the deep venous system. There is argument over how long the Ace wrap should stay in place. Personal hygiene demands a shorter period than the usual 4 to 6 weeks originally recommended. European specialists suggest a period of at least 3 weeks, although shorter periods may be used with good results. We generally advise sclerotherapy to be done in the cooler months so that the patient is more comfortable wearing the Ace wraps. After a week of compression the patient may remove the Ace bandage and take a bath, or alternatively the Ace wrap limb may be placed in a large garbage bag to allow showering. The patient should be seen 10 to 14 days after injection. If thrombus is present in a vein segment, it can be evacuated with a No. 11 blade and compression. This decreases unsightly pigmentation.

Complications such as extravasation may lead to skin sloughing in a small percentage of patients. This can be avoided by absolute assurance that the needle is in the vein and by the use of dilute sclerosing solution for small veins. Thrombophlebitis is unusual with this technique. Pigmentation along the vein will usually fade by 4 to 6 months if present.

SURGICAL TREATMENT. Until recently the patient with advanced CVI was treated according to the regimen outlined by John Hunter in 1642: "The sores of poor people are often mended by rest in the horizontal position, fresh provisions, and warmth in hospitals."[76] Now, however, as an alternative to medical therapy, direct reconstruction of the deep venous system may be offered to selected patients with advanced chronic venous disease. The candidates for such surgery are few, as Darke's study[28] implied, numbering less than one quarter of patients with chronic venous disease. To determine the site and degree of valvular dysfunction or obstruction in potential candidates, a thorough diagnostic evaluation is performed preoperatively (as summarized previously). Surgical options for CVI are listed in the box on this page.

Ligation and Stripping. Burnand et al[54] have previously shown that ligation and stripping of the greater saphenous system restores hemodynamics to normal

---

SURGICAL OPTIONS FOR CHRONIC VENOUS INSUFFICIENCY

Superficial Venous Insufficiency
Ligation and stripping of varicose veins
  Greater saphenous vein
  Lesser saphenous vein
Subfascial ligation of incompetent perforators

Chronic Deep Venous Obstruction
Iliofemoral
  Crossover saphenofemoral vein graft
SFV
  In situ saphenopopliteal bypass

Deep Valvular Incompetence
Primary
  Valvuloplasty
Secondary
  Vein valve transplant
  Venous segment transfer

---

where ambulatory pressure and VRT are normalized. When physical examination and noninvasive tests show the greater saphenous vein to be incompetent, it is ligated flush with the femoral vein and stripped. Stripping is usually performed to the level of the knee to reduce the chance of injury to the saphenous nerve. If the greater saphenous vein is competent and not dilated, it may be preserved for possible future use as an arterial conduit. Reports have shown greater saphenous vein preservation has recurrence rates of varicose veins comparable to greater saphenous vein stripping.[77] Tributary varicosities are avulsed through small 3-mm incisions. Obvious incompetent perforators can also be approached through small

Table 28-8. Surgical Results with Varicose Veins

Study	No. of Patients	Length of Follow-Up Care (Yrs)	Recurrence (%)
Lofgren[107]	1000	10	15
Haeger[29]	578	5	8
Rivlin[108]	2000	>6	7
Hobbs[75]	170	10	29
Chant[106]	100	3	14

incisions and ligated. Table 28-8 summarizes the results with superficial venous surgery.

Subfascial Ligation. There are several options in the surgical treatment of incompetent perforating veins (ICPVs). If only one or two obvious ICPVs are identified, they can be approached directly and ligated. More extensive ICPVs can be approached through the standard (Linton) medial calf incision (Fig. 28-24) or conversely through a posterior stocking seam incision, which avoids the often liposclerotic or ulcerated medial gaiter area. Because of wound complications and prolonged recovery time with a long calf incision, video-assisted subfascial vein ligation

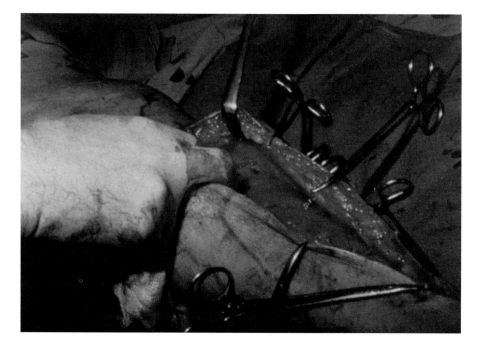

Fig. 28-24. Subfascial vein ligation. Incompetent perforating veins are exposed through the medial or posterior subfascial approach. They are then ligated and interrupted. Perforating veins are seen at the top of the scissors and underneath the retractor *(right)*.

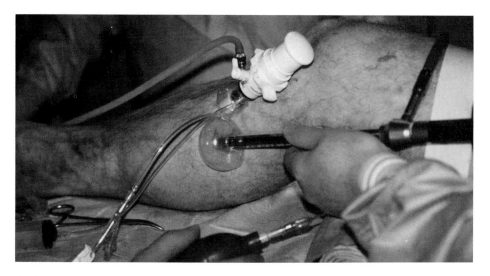

Fig. 28-25. Video-assisted subfascial ligation uses small incisions placed proximally in the lower leg to avoid incisions in chronic skin changes in the gaiter area. Carbon dioxide insufflation is used for dissection in this illustration; gasless techniques with retractors are also used.

has become an attractive option. After preoperative localization of the ICPVs by duplex ultrasound, small incisions for the camera and instruments are placed on the upper medial calf away from liposclerotic skin (Fig. 28-25). This technique has been successful in effectively treating ICPVs and decreasing hospital length of stay.

Venous Reconstructive Surgery. Burnand et al[79] showed that recurrence of venous ulcer was common following ligation of ICPVs in patients with concomitant deep venous disease, as demonstrated by phlebography. By contrast, recurrence of ulcer was unusual if the perforating veins and the superficial system were involved, but there was no evidence of deep venous disease, and hemodynamics improved. Direct venous reconstruction is designed to either bypass isolated obstruction within the deep system

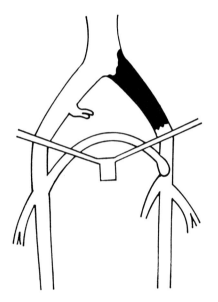

Fig. 28-26. Saphenofemoral bypass (Palma procedure). This procedure uses the contralateral saphenous vein, which is anastomosed to the ipsilateral femoral vein to bypass an iliac obstruction. *(From O'Donnell TF Jr and Shephard AD: Chronic venous insufficiency. In Jarrett F and Hirsch S, eds: Vascular surgery of the lower extremity, St Louis, 1985, CV Mosby Co.)*

or to interpose a functioning valvular segment in a patent but incompetent deep venous system.

Crossover-Saphenofemoral Venous Bypass. The natural history of deep venous thrombosis is recanalization of the involved vein with destruction of valves. If the recanalization process is incomplete and collateral vessel formation is inadequate, functional venous obstruction may result. When anatomic obstruction is limited to a short segment of vein, such as the iliac, and severe symptoms of edema or venous claudication are present, the patient may be a candidate for a venous bypass procedure. The number of postthrombotic patients who fall into this category appears limited and has been estimated to be between 2% and 4%.[80] In the crossover-saphenofemoral bypass, initially described by Palma and Esperson in 1960,[78] the saphenous vein from the nonaffected limb is mobilized to the level of the distal thigh, ligated distally and tunneled suprapubically to the inguinal region of the obstructed side. The saphenous vein is anastomosed to either the common femoral or superficial femoral vein to bypass the obstructed ipsilateral iliac vein (Fig. 28-26). Methods to increase venous blood flow in the transposed saphenous segment appear important to prevent graft thrombosis. An AV fistula may be created distal to the anastomosis, or intermittent pneumatic compression devices may be applied postoperatively. In addition, we generally employ carefully monitored heparin therapy with conversion to warfarin in these patients. Table 28-9 summarizes the results of several series. Although clinical criteria have been used to judge the success, only two series report follow-up care with anatomic and functional studies.[30,78] Our smaller series has used B-mode ultrasound as a method for demonstrating late anatomic and functional patency of the bypass.[30] Long-term follow-up study has shown adequate patency.

Saphenous Bypass. The greater saphenous vein has been used to bypass an isolated obstruction of the superficial femoral vein as popularized by Husni.[86] The early experience of Linton[9] showed few sequelae to ligation of the superficial femoral vein. Indeed, this vein has even been used as a conduit for arterial bypass without any deleterious consequences. It is unusual to find a patient in this

Table 28-9. Crossover-Saphenofemoral Venous Bypass for Postthrombotic Syndrome

Study	No. of Patients	Clinical Results (Percent of Patients)		
		Excellent	**Good**	**Unimproved**
Palma (1960)[78]	7	57	29	14
Dale (1969)[85]	23	43	43	14
May (1981)[81]	66	73	0	27
Husni (1981)[86]	82	61	15	24
Halliday (1985)[80]	50*	76	0	24
O'Donnell et al (1986)[30]	6†	83	17	0

*Patent by phlebography.
†Patent by late B-mode ultrasound.

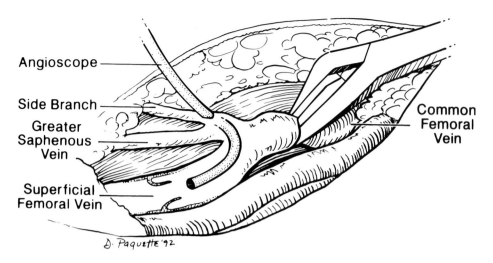

Fig. 28-27. Angioscope is inserted through tributary or stump of previously ligated greater saphenous vein into superficial femoral vein. Diagnosis of valvular incompetence is made, the valve repaired under direct vision, and competency of the repair is assessed through an angioscope. *(From Welch HJ, McLaughlin RL, and O'Donnell TF: Femoral vein valvuloplasty: intraoperative angioscopic evaluation and hemodynamic improvement, J Vasc Surg 16:694, 1992.)*

Table 28-10. Valvuloplasty: Surgical Results

Author	No. of Limbs	Ulcers (%)	Follow-Up (Mo)	Patent (%)	Hemodynamic Improvement (%)
Masuda and Kistner[87]	51	57	48-252	67	60
Cheatle Perrin[99]	52	40	NA	69	NA
Eriksson[100]	22	NA	6-84	100	62
Raju[53]	107	71	24-96	NA	63
Simkin[101]	7	100	NA	NA	50
Sottiurai[102]	20	100	10-73	NA	80
O'Donnell[83]	9	100	2-51	100	100

situation who has not undergone a previous saphenectomy or whose saphenous vein is unaffected by the same disease process. Therefore this procedure is rarely used.

Venous Valvuloplasty. Repair of an incompetent valve can be performed in those patients with primary valvular incompetence. The typical vein valve seen in these patients is elongated, redundant, and floppy. The excess valve leaflet can be reefed up with fine sutures by a number of techniques. First described by Kistner,[82] the valvuloplasty is most commonly performed on the highest valve within the superficial femoral vein. Previously described techniques have used either a transverse or longitudinal venotomy to visualize the incompetent valve. Repair is then performed using interrupted sutures to reef up or "tighten" the floppy valve. We have adopted the use of the angioscope[83] in vein valvuloplasty, as first described by Gloviczki.[84] Insertion of the angioscope through the saphenous vein stump or side branches eliminates the need for femoral venotomy (Fig. 28-27). Visualization from within the lumen allows the surgeon to make the proper diagnosis and also guides precise placement of the externally placed sutures through the edges of the valve leaflets.

The competency of the repair can be visually checked with gentle instillation of saline solution through the scope. We have shown significant improvement in venous hemodynamics after angioscopically guided valvuloplasty, which allows for improved ulcer healing.[83] Kistner's series of venous reconstruction was recently reviewed[87] and vein valvuloplasty has shown to be a durable procedure with long-term ulcer healing of 72% at 10 years. Although this procedure is not applicable to the majority of patients with deep venous insufficiency whose valve leaflets are scarred and destroyed by thrombosis, in those patients who are eligible for valve repair, it should be the first procedure attempted because of its results, durability, and restriction to one venous segment without transplantation (Table 28-10).

Venous Segment Transfer (Table 28-11). This procedure is used for patients in whom the valves of the superficial and common femoral venous system have been destroyed. A competent valve-bearing venous segment is transposed into the main deep venous system at the groin level (Fig. 28-28). Several varieties of transposition have been used, either the ipsilateral saphenous vein or competent pro-

Table 28-11. Venous Segment Transfer: Clinical, Hemodynamic, and Phlebographic Results

Study	No. of Limbs	Preoperative Ulcer (%)	Ulcer Healing		Pain Relief		VRT Improved		AVP Improved		Patent and Functioning Segment by Phlebography	
			Short-term (%)	Long-term (%)	Short-term (%)	Long-term (%)	Short-term (%)	Long-term (%)	Short-term (%)	Long-term (%)	Short-term (%)	Long-term (%)
Masuda and Kistner[87]	14	?	80	–	64	–	–	–	92	–	100	57
Queral[90]	12	33	100	–	75	–	92	–	50	–	75	–
Johnson[88]	12	33	0	0	–	25	–	25	0	0	–	–

VRT, Venous refill time; *AVP,* ambulatory venous pressure.

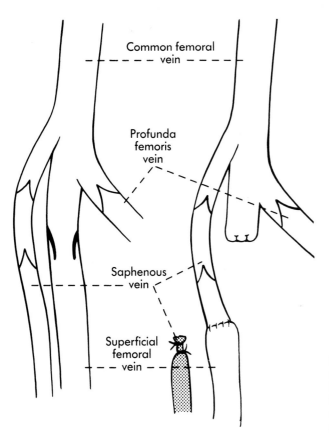

Fig. 28-28. Venous segment transposition. This procedure interposes a normal valve from saphenous or preferably profunda femoris vein into the deep venous circuit to correct incompetence of a superficial femoral vein valve. *(From O'Donnell TF Jr: The clinical management of deep venous valvular incompetence. In Rutherford RB, ed: Vascular surgery, ed 3, Philadelphia, 1989, WB Saunders Co.)*

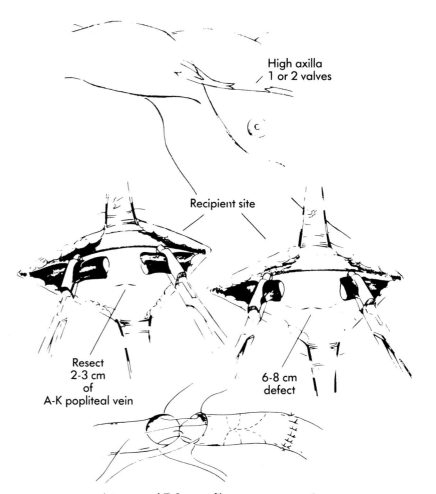

Fig. 28-29. Popliteal vein valve transplant. Axillary vein valve whose competence has previously been confirmed by B-mode ultrasound is transplanted to the above-knee popliteal vein as an interposition graft.

Table 28-12. Vein Valve Transplant, Surgical Results

Author	Taheri[95]	Nash[96]	Raju[53]	Eriksson[97]	Sottiurai[98]	Cheatle[99]	Bry[94]
Year published	1985	1988	1988	1988	1991	1993	1995
Number	66	23	18	35	8	26	15
Ulcers (%)	27	74	42	–	100	74	93
Procedure	B to F	B to P	A to F	A to F (26%) A to P (74%)	B to F	A to F	A to P
Follow-up results							
Mean (years)	–	1.5	>2	2.3	2.8	4	5.3
Symptomatic relief	78	–	50	–	–	48	92
Ulcer recurrence (%)	6	18	54	–	25	31	21
VVT thrombosis (%)	3	0	–	–	0	48	0

B, Brachial; *F,* femoral; *P,* popliteal; *A,* axillary.

funda femoris vein. Although Ferris and Kistner's studies showed excellent results,[89] the work of the Northwestern group showed degeneration of both clinical and functional state by 1 year.[88,90] In contrast to Ferris and Kistner's patients, the Northwestern group did not treat incompetent perforating veins and found that patients with the most significant clinical and hemodynamic recurrence following venous segment transfer had concomitant perforator vein disease.[88]

Vein Valve Transplantation. Until the development of heterologous valve grafts or durable autologous "neovalve" reconstructions, vein valve segment transplantation will remain a viable and necessary option in the treatment of CVI. Taheri et al[91] deserve the credit for introducing and popularizing the use of vein valve transplantation (VVT) for severe venous reflux. Taheri et al's concept is similar to Ferris and Kistner's venous segment transposition—namely, to ameliorate deep system reflux by placing a competent valve in the main deep system at the level of the thigh. Initially Taheri et al used a short segment of superficial femoral vein just below the femoral bifurcation and replaced that segment with a 2- to 2.5-cm valve-bearing segment of the brachial vein. Raju and Fredericks[53] have used the superficial femoral vein level, but they used the large-caliber axillary vein as the valve-containing segment.

Our approach to VVT differs from others by using the larger-caliber axillary vein and transplanting it to the above-knee popliteal vein (Fig. 28-29). The larger-caliber axillary vein is a better size match for the popliteal vein, which theoretically may avoid late dilation of the transplanted segment and secondary valvular incompetence. A second benefit to placing the valve at the popliteal vein level is suggested in the work of Bauer,[32] Shull et al,[92] and Moore et al,[93] which showed that the function of the popliteal vein valve is important in avoiding ulceration. The New England Medical Center (NEMC) experience with VVT was recently reviewed.[94] With an average follow-up of 5.3 years, the late ulcer-free probability was 62%. Despite variable improvements in venous hemodynamics measured postoperatively, clinically there was marked improvement in pain levels, edema, and ulcer healing (Table 28-12). Two patients in the series with recurrent ulceration

were found to have a competent VVT, but ICPVs, wherein subfascial ligation of these produced lasting ulcer healing. We believe, in addition to correcting venous valvular insufficiency, ICPVs should be ligated before, or concomitant with, deep venous reconstruction.

REFERENCES

1. Browse NL, Burnand KG, and Lea TM, eds: Diseases of the veins: pathology, diagnosis and treatment. London, 1988, Edward Arnold.
2. US Department of Health, Education, and Welfare: National health survey 1935-1936, Washington, DC, 1938.
3. General Register Office: Studies on medical and population subjects, #12. The survey of sickness 1943-52, Logan WPD and Brooke EM, London, 1957, HM Stationery Office.
4. The Sickness Survey of Denmark: The committee on the Danish national morbidity survey, Copenhagen, 1960.
5. Illness and Health Care in Canada: Canadian Sickness Survey 1950-1951. The Department of National Health and Welfare and the Dominion Bureau of Statistics, Ottawa, 1960.
6. Bobek K et al: The study of the frequency of venous disorders and the influence of several etiologic factors, Phlebologie 19:217, 1966.
7. Widmer LK: Peripheral venous disorders: prevalence and sociomedical importance—observations in 4529 apparently healthy persons, Basle III Study, Bern Hans Huber, 1978.
8. Dickson-Wright A: The treatment of indolent ulcer of the leg, Lancet 1:457, 1931.
9. Linton RR: The communicating veins of the lower leg and the operating techniques for their ligation, Ann Surg 107:582, 1938.
10. Lockhart-Mummery HE and Smithan JH: Varicose ulcer: a study of the deep veins with special references to retrograde venography, Br J Surg 38:284, 1951.
11. Hellgren L: An epidemiology survey of skin diseases, tatooing and rheumatic diseases, Ups Linquist Wiksel, 1967.
12. Callam MJ et al: Chronic ulceration of the leg: extent of the problem and provision of care, Br Med J 290:1855, 1985.
13. Darling RC and Kupinski AM: Preoperative evaluations of veins, Semin Vasc Surg 6:155, 1993.
14. Kosinski C: Variations of the external saphenous vein, J Anat 60:131, 1926.

15. O'Donnell TF et al: Doppler examination versus clinical and phlebographic detection of the location of incompetent perforating veins, Arch Surg 112:31, 1977.

16. Bundens WP et al: Deep venous anatomy of the thigh: clinical implications of nomenclature in thrombotic disease. Presented at the American Venous Forum, Seventh Annual Meeting, Ft Lauderdale, Fla, February 23, 1995.

17. O'Donnell TF and Shepard AD: Chronic venous insufficiency. In Jarrett F and Hirsh J, eds: Vascular surgery of the lower extremity, St. Louis, 1985, The CV Mosby Co.

18. Haeger K: Leg ulcers. In Hobbs JT, ed: The treatment of venous disorders, Lancaster, England, 1977, MPT.

19. Hehne HJ et al: Zur Bedentung arteriovenoeser anastosen bei dem primaeren varicosis und der chronischvenoesen insuffizienz, Vasa 3:396, 1974.

20. Lindmayr W et al: Arteriovenous shunts in primary varicosis: a critical essay, Vasc Surg 6:9, 1972.

21. Browse NL and Burnand KG: The cause of venous ulceration, Lancet 2:243, 1982.

22. Coleridge-Smith PD and Scurr JH. Current views on the pathogenesis of venous ulceration. In Bergan JJ and Yao JST, eds: Venous disorders, Philadelphia, 1991, WB Saunders.

23. Braide M et al: Quantitative studies of leukocytes on the vascular resistance in a skeletal muscle preparation, Microvasc Res 27:331, 1984.

24. Moyses C, Cederholm-Williams SA, and Michel CC: Haemoconcentration and the accumulation of white cells in the feet during venous stasis, Int J Microcirc Clin Exp 5:311, 1987.

25. Thomas PRS, Nash GB, and Dormandy JA: White cell accumulation in the dependent legs of patients with venous hypertension: a possible mechanism for trophic changes in the skin, Br Med J 296:1693, 1988.

26. Negus D and Cocket FB: Femoral vein pressures in post-phlebitic iliac vein obstruction, Br J Surg 54:522, 1967.

27. Killewitch LA et al: Pathophysiology of venous claudication, J Vasc Surg 1:502, 1984.

28. Darke SG: Reconstructive surgery for chronic venous insufficiency in the lower limbs. In Greehalgh RA, Jamieson CW, and Nicolaides AN, eds: Vascular surgery issues in current practice, London, 1986, Grune & Stratton.

29. Haeger K: Five-year results of radical surgery for superficial varices with or without coexisting perforator insufficiency, Acta Chir Scand 131:38, 1966.

30. O'Donnell TF et al: Clinical, hemodynamic, and anatomic follow-up of direct venous reconstruction, Arch Surg 122:474, 1987.

31. Negus D and Friedgood A: The effective management of venous ulceration, Br J Surg 70:623, 1983.

32. Bauer G: The etiology of leg ulcers and their treatment by resection of popliteal vein, J Int Chir 8:937, 1948.

33. Kistner RL: Primary venous valve incompetence of the leg, Am J Surg 140:218, 1982.

34. Lodin A and Lindvall N: Congenital absence of valves of the deep veins of the leg: a factor in venous insufficiency, Arch Derm Venereol 41(suppl 45):1, 1961.

35. Porter JM et al: Reporting standards in venous disease—venous subcommittee, J Vasc Surg 8:172, 1988.

36. Shepard AD et al: Light reflection rheography: a new non-invasive test of venous function, Bruit 8:266, 1984.

37. Arora S et al: Light reflection rheography: a simple noninvasive screening test for deep vein thrombosis, J Vasc Surg 18:767, 1993.

38. Barnes RW: Noninvasive tests for chronic venous insufficiency. In Bergan JJ and Yao JST, eds: Surgery of the veins, New York, 1985, Grune & Stratton.

39. Sigel B et al: A Doppler ultrasound method for diagnosing lower extremity venous disease, Surg Gynecol Obstet 127:339, 1986.

40. Miller SS and Foote AV: The ultrasonic detection of incompetent perforating veins, Br J Surg 61:653, 1974.

41. Folse R and Alexander RH: Directional flow detection for localizing venous valvular incompetence, Surgery 67:114, 1970.

42. Christopoulos DG et al: Air-plethysmography and the effects of elastic compression on venous hemodynamics of the leg, J Vasc Surg 5:148, 1987.

43. van Bemmelen PS et al: The mechanism of venous valve closure. Its relationship to the velocity of reverse flow, Arch Surg 125:617, 1990.

44. Masuda EM, Kistner RL, and Eklof B: Prospective study of duplex scanning for venous reflux: correlation of Valsalva and pneumatic cuff techniques in the reverse Trendelenburg and standing positions, J Vasc Surg 20:711, 1994.

45. van Bemmelen PS et al: Quantitative segmental evaluation of venous valvular reflux with duplex ultrasound scanning, J Vasc Surg 10:425, 1989.

46. Welch HJ et al: Comparison of descending phlebography with quantitative photoplethysmography, air plethysmography, and duplex quantitative valve closure time in assessing deep venous reflux, J Vasc Surg 16:913, 1992.

47. Araki CT et al: Refinements in the ultrasonic detection of popliteal vein reflux, J Vasc Surg 18:742, 1993.

48. Vasdekis SN, Clarke GH, and Nicolaides AN: Quantification of venous reflux by means of duplex scanning, J Vasc Surg 10:670, 1989.

49. Bradbury AW et al: Foot volumetry and duplex ultrasonography in patients with recurrent venous ulceration after superficial and perforator vein ligation, Br J Surg 80:845, 1993

50. Barnes RW et al: Noninvasive quantitation of venous hemodynamics in the post-phlebitic syndrome, Arch Surg 107:807, 1973.

51. McEnroe CS, O'Donnell TF, and Mackey WC: Correlation of clinical findings with venous hemodynamics in 396 patients with chronic venous insufficiency, Am J Surg 156:148, 1988.

52. Raju S: Venous insufficiency of the lower limb and stasis ulceration: changing concepts and management, Ann Surg 197:688, 1983.

53. Raju S and Fredericks R: Valve reconstruction procedures for nonobstructive venous insufficiency: rationale, techniques and results in 107 procedures, J Vasc Surg, 7:301, 1988.

54. Burnand KG et al: The relative importance of incompetent communicating veins in the production of varicose veins in venous ulcer, Surgery 82:9, 1977.

55. Schanzer H and Peirce EC: A rational approach to surgery: the chronic venous stasis syndrome, Ann Surg 195:25, 1982.

56. Moore EJ, Himmel PD, and Sumner DS: Distribution of venous valvular incompetency in patients with the post-phlebitic syndrome, J Vasc Surg 3:49, 1986.

57. Abramowitz HB, Queral LA, and Flinn WR: Use of photoplethysmography in the assessment of chronic venous insufficiency: a comparison to venous pressure measurements, Surgery 86:434, 1979.

58. Celsus AC: Of medicine in eight books, London, 1756, Wilson (translated by J Grieve).

59. Wiseman R: Eight surgical treatises, London, 1676, Meridon.

60. Starling EH: On the absorption of fluid from the connective tissue spaces, J Physiol (Lond) 19:312, 1986.

61. Clark RL, Orandi A, and Clifton EE: Tourniquet induction of fibrinolysis, Angiology 11:367, 1960.

62. O'Donnell TF et al: Effect of elastic compression on venous hemodynamics in the postphlebitic limb, JAMA 242:2766, 1979.

63. Noyes LD, Rice JC, Kerstein M: Hemodynamic assessment of high compression hosiery in chronic venous disease, Surgery 102:813, 1987.

64. Burnand KG and Layer G: Graduated elastic stockings, Br Med J 293:224, 1986.

65. Vilavicencio JL et al: Leg ulcers of venous origin. In Cameron JL, ed: Current surgical therapy-three, Toronto, 1989, BC Decker.

66. Hills NH et al: Prevention of deep vein thrombosis by intermittent compression of calf, Br Med J 1:131, 1972.

67. Clark RL, Orandi A, and Clifton EE: Tourniquet induction of fibrinolysis, Angiology 11:367, 1960.

68. Cranley J: The management of venous disorders. In Rutherford R, ed: Vascular surgery, Philadelphia, 1989, WB Saunders.

69. Friedman SJ and Su WDD: Management of leg ulcers with hydrocolloid occlusive dressings, Arch Dermatol 120:1329, 1984.

70. Kikta MJ et al: A prospective randomized trial of Unna's boots versus hydroactive dressing in the treatment of venous stasis ulcers, J Vasc Surg 7:478, 1988.

71. Ericksson G: Comparison of two occlusive bandages in the treatment of leg ulcers, Br J Dermatol 114:227, 1986.

72. van Rijswijk L, Brown D, and Friedman S: Multicenter clinical evaluation of a hydrocolloid dressing for leg ulcers, Cutis 35:173, 1985.

73. Rubin JR et al: Unna's boots and polyurethane foam dressing for the treatment of venous ulceration, Arch Surg 125:489, 1990.

74. Fegan WG: Continuous compression treatment for injecting varicose veins, Lancet 2:109, 1963.

75. Hobbs JT: Surgery and sclerotherapy in the treatment of varicose veins: a randomized trial, Arch Surg 109:793, 1974.

76. Hunter J: Of specific diseases, tumours, hydatids, etc. In Palmer JF, ed: The works of John Hunter, London, 1837, Longman, Reese, Orme, Brown, Green and Longman.

77. Large J: Surgical treatment of saphenous varices with preservation of the main great trunk, J Vasc Surg 2:886, 1985.

78. Palma ED and Esperson R: Vein transplants and grafts in the surgical treatment of the post-phlebitic syndrome, J Cardiovasc Surg 1:94, 1960.

79. Burnand KG et al: Relationship between post-phlebitic changes in the deep veins and results of surgical treatment of venous ulcers, Lancet 1:936, 1976.

80. Halliday P, Harris J, and May J: Femoral-femoral cross-over grafts (Palma operation): a long-term follow-up study. In Bergan JJ and Yao JST, eds: Surgery of the veins, New York, 1985, Grune & Stratton.

81. May R: Späkergebnissr nach venosom femoralis bypass, Vasa 8:67, 1974.

82. Kistner RL: Surgical repair of the incompetent femoral vein valve, Arch Surg 110:1336, 1975.

83. Welch HJ, McLaughlin RL, and O'Donnell TF: Femoral vein valvuloplasty: intraoperative angioscopic evaluation and hemodynamic improvement, J Vasc Surg 16:694, 1992.

84. Gloviczki P, Merrell SW, and Bower TC: Femoral vein valve repair under direct vision without venotomy: a modified technique with use of angioscopy, J Vasc Surg 14:645, 1991.

85. Dale WA: Crossover vein grafts for relief of iliofemoral block, Surgery 57:608, 1965.

86. Husni EA: Issues in venous reconstruction, Vasc Diagn Ther 2:37, 1981.

87. Masuda EM and Kistner RL: Long-term results of venous valve reconstruction: a four to twenty-one year follow-up, J Vasc Surg 19:391, 1994.

88. Johnson ND et al: Late objective assessment of venous valve surgery, Arch Surg 116:1461, 1981.

89. Ferris ED and Kistner RL: Femoral vein reconstruction and the management of chronic venous insufficiency: a 14-year experience, Arch Surg 117:1571, 1982.

90. Queral LA et al: Surgical correction of chronic deep venous insufficiency by valvular transposition, Surgery 87:685, 1980.

91. Taheri SA et al: Surgical treatment of post-phlebitic syndrome with vein valve transplant, Am J Surg 144:221, 1982.

92. Shull KS et al: Significance of popliteal reflux in relationship to ambulatory venous pressure and ulceration, Arch Surg 114:1304, 1979.

93. Moore EJ, Himmel PD, and Sumner DS: Distribution of venous valvular incompetency in patients with the postphlebitic syndrome, J Vasc Surg 3:49, 1986

94. Bry JDL et al: The clinical and hemodynamic results after axillary-to-popliteal vein valve transplantation, J Vasc Surg 21:110, 1995.

95. Taheri SA, Pendergast DR, and Lazar E: Vein valve transplantation, Am J Surg 150:201, 1985.

96. Nash T: Long term results of vein valve transplants placed in the popliteal vein for intractable postphlebitic ulcers in pre-ulcer skin changes, J Cardiovasc Surg 29:712, 1988.

97. Eriksson JI and Almgren B: Surgical reconstruction of incompetent deep vein valves, Uppsala J Med Sci 93:139, 1988.

98. Sottiurai VS: Surgical correction of recurrent venous ulcer, J Cardiovasc Surg 32:104, 1991.

99. Cheatle TR and Perrin M: Surgical options in the post-thrombotic syndrome, Phlebology 8:50, 1993.

100. Eriksson JI and Almgrem B: Surgical reconstruction of deep vein valves, Uppsala J Med Sci 93:139, 1988.

101. Simkin R, Estembam JC, and Bulloj R: Bypass veno-venosos y valvuloplastias en el tratamiento quirugico del sindrome post-trombotico, Angiologia 30:4, 1988.

102. Sottiurai VS: Surgical correction of recurrent venous ulcer, J Cardiovasc Surg 32:104, 1991.

103. Strother IG, Bryson H, and Alexander S: Treatment of varicose veins by compression sclerotherapy, Br J Surg 61:387, 1974.

104. Dejode LR: Injection compression treatment of varicose veins, Br J Surg 57:285, 1970.

105. Reid RG and Rothne NG: Treatment of varicose veins by compression sclerotherapy, Br J Surg 55:889, 1968.

106. Chant ADB, Jones HO, and Weddel JM: Varicose veins: a comparison of surgery and injection/compression sclerotherapy, Lancet 2:1188, 1972.

107. Lofgren KA: Post phlebitic syndrome (chronic deep venous insufficiency). In Haimovici H, ed: Vascular surgery principles and techniques, ed 1, New York, 1971, McGraw-Hill.

108. Rivlin S: The surgical care of primary varicose veins, Br J Surg 62:613, 1975.

109. Gooley NA and Summer DS: Relationship of venous reflux to the sight of venous valvular incompetence: implications for venous reconstructive surgery, J Vasc Surg 7:50, 1988.

110. Pearce WH, Ricco JB, Quertl LA et al: Hemodynamic assessment of venous problems, Surgery 93:715, 1983.

PART IV

LYMPHEDEMA

CHAPTER TWENTY-NINE

LYMPHEDEMA

Alexander Schirger

Peter Gloviczki

The term *lymphedema* describes accumulation of fluid in a part of the body—most commonly in the extremities but also in the lower part of the abdomen, the scrotum, the external genitalia, and the face. Lymphedema is caused by the inability of the lymphatic system to carry lymph, which causes stasis of the lymph. Lymphedema must be distinguished from other forms of edema of systemic, venous, or allergic origin.

Lymphatic vessels develop from mesenchymal cells. Their existence was first recognized by Gasparo Aselli (1581-1626), an Italian anatomist and surgeon at the University of Pavia.[1] During an operation on a dog, designed to study the action and innervation of the diaphragm, Aselli discovered enlarged lymphatic vessels in the dog's mesentery. When he incised one of these structures, a whitish fluid was released. In a similar experiment on a second animal no such vessels were noted. Aselli realized that the difference between the two experiments was that the second animal had not been fed before the operation, and he concluded that the structures observed in the first experiment represented channels in which some substance was carried from the intestine.

Although the clinical entity of lymphedema has been recognized since ancient times, and the similarity of the grossly disfigured human extremities to the legs of an elephant has led to the term *elephantiasis*, the correlation of these disfiguring conditions with Aselli's discovery of the lymphatic system some three centuries earlier did not occur until Milroy[2] in 1928 and Allen[3] in 1934 described lymphatic malfunction. Both of these clinicians published accurate descriptions of the clinical entities of idiopathic lymphedema. The introduction of lymphangiography into clinical medicine by Kinmonth et al[4] has aided in establishing the link between the areas of knowledge for which Aselli laid the foundation 300 years earlier and the conclusions derived from the astute clinical observations and vast bedside experience of eminent clinicians such as Milroy and Allen.

ANATOMY AND PATHOPHYSIOLOGY

Lymph is collected from the interstitial space by the initial or terminal lymphatic capillaries and then transported through major collecting lymph channels. In the lower extremity, major collecting channels are located both in the deep compartments and subcutaneously. The deep lymphatic system of the lower extremities follows the tibial, popliteal, and femoral vessels. The more significant superficial lymphatic system carries 80% of the lower-extremity lymph fluid. This system consists of 10 to 15 large lymphatic channels that are located mostly along the greater saphenous vein. The two systems join in the inguinal nodes, and the lymph then is transported through iliac and paraaortic lymph channels and nodes into the thoracic duct. The duct, which also carries chyle from the mesenteric lymph vessels, has an average output of 1.5 L daily, which is emptied into the venous system at the left jugulosubclavian junction. The lymphatic system of the left upper extremity and the left side of the neck and head drains into the thoracic duct, but that of the right upper extremity and the right side of the head and neck drains through the right cervical trunk directly into the right subclavian vein.

Unidirectional flow in the collecting lymphatic channels is ensured by the presence of fine valves. Congenital or acquired obstruction of lymphatic flow results in accumulation of protein-rich fluid in the subcutaneous space. Because lymphatic capillaries of the dermis do not contain valves, in lymphatic obstruction the lymph refluxes through these dermal lymphatics, a phenomenon called *dermal reflux*. This can be demonstrated in patients with lymphedema by intradermal injection of blue dye. If collateral lymphatic circulation is not satisfactory and the function of the tissue macrophages is exhausted, lymphedema develops. The mechanism of the development of acute and chronic lymphedema after surgical excision of lymph vessels and lymph nodes is outlined in Fig. 29-1. It is not unusual for chronic lymphedema to develop several

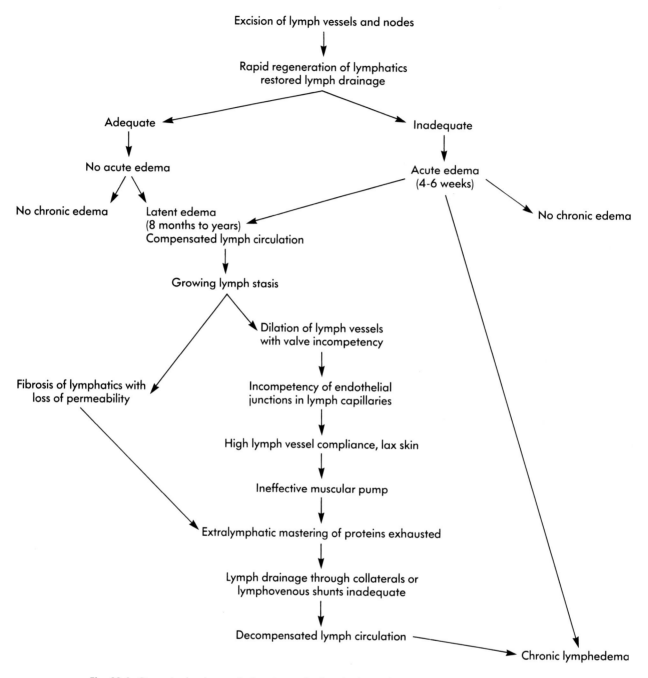

Fig. 29-1. Stages in development of postoperative lymphedema. *(From Gloviczki P and Schirger A: Lymphedema. In Spittell JA Jr, ed: Clinical medicine, Philadelphia, 1985, Harper & Row.*

months or even years after interruption of the lymphatic transport system.

CLASSIFICATION

Lymphedema can be classified as primary (idiopathic) or secondary. Primary lymphedema may be present at birth or make its appearance later in life. When present at birth, it may occur in a single patient or cluster in a family. It is to this form of congenital familial lymphedema that the eponym "Milroy's disease" is properly applied because it corresponds to the description by Milroy[2] in 1928. When primary lymphedema makes its appearance later in life, it

is usually at the time of menarche or in the late teens or early twenties. It was because of this temporal relationship that Allen[3] assigned the term *lymphedema praecox* to the noncongenital type of primary lymphedema.

Experience has taught clinicians that when lymphedema does make its appearance later in life, most commonly it is because of an identifiable cause and is therefore secondary in nature. Nevertheless, one occasionally may see an older patient with truly primary lymphedema. To this group of cases Kinmonth et al[4] applied the term *lymphedema tarda.*

Secondary lymphedema may result from obstruction of, interruption in, or replacement of lymphatic channels and nodes. The etiology can be a mechanical process such as trauma, surgical intervention, invasion by tumor, or a fibrosing process including radiation fibrosis. The other form of secondary lymphedema is caused by an inflammatory process in which lymphatic channels are obstructed by acute or recurrent lymphangitis and cellulitis. In the Western world the most common cause of inflammatory lymphedema is streptococcal infection, usually via a portal of entry caused by trichophytosis, but in many other parts of the world, Bancroft's filariasis and other parasitic infections account for this form of lymphedema.

CLINICAL PICTURE

Primary Lymphedema

The clinical picture of *congenital lymphedema,* that of a child born with lymphedema, whether familial or nonfamilial, is identical. There is a visible enlargement of the extremity or extremities or affected parts of the body. The swelling is painless and is more resistant to pitting than venous edema; the extremity color is normal. There are no signs of venous insufficiency or venous malformations. Although congenital lymphedema may involve only one extremity, we have seen it in both lower extremities and in the hands and arms as well. External genitalia and parts of the face also may be affected. During the first year of life, when the child is supine most of the time, gravity does not play a significant role, and the swelling may not become apparent until the child is fully ambulatory.

Association of congenital lymphedema with other congenital abnormalities—such as Turner's syndrome,[5,6] congenital absence of the nails,[7] bilateral pleural effusion, and the presence of yellow nails (referred to as "the yellow nail syndrome")—has been described.[8] In rare instances children with the congenital familial type of lymphedema have been noted to have an extra row of eyelashes.[9]

Lymphedema praecox is the form of lymphedema that makes its appearance around puberty (during the mid or late teens) or, rarely, at the beginning of the third decade. In his description of 300 such patients, Allen et al[3,10] coined the term "lymphedema praecox." Data from Allen's series and from a later series[11] at the Mayo Clinic revealed a preponderance of cases in women with a female-to-male ratio of approximately 10:1. In congenital lymphedema, by definition, the swelling is detected by family members or attendant physicians or nurses. In lymphedema praecox it is the patient who most commonly calls the condition to the attention of the physician. The first thing that may be noted is a painless, spontaneously occurring swelling, usually on the dorsum of the foot and gradually involving the ankle and lower leg and the remainder of the forefoot and toes, which are often squared (Figs. 29-2 and 29-3).

Characteristically ulceration is absent, and there are none of the hallmarks of deep venous insufficiency such as increased pigmentation, evidence of enlarged collateral veins, or ulceration. The swelling is painless and is more resistant to pitting than venous edema. In a Mayo Clinic series[11] in about one third of the cases there was an antedating traumatic event such as a contusion. At first the

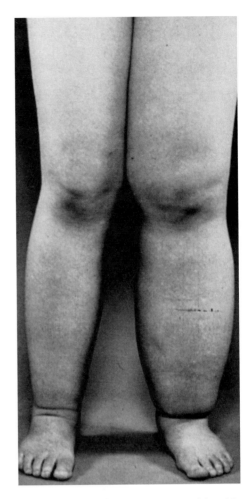

Fig. 29-2. Idiopathic lymphedema (praecox type) in a 19-year-old woman.

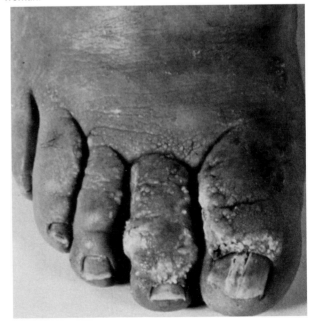

Fig. 29-3. Squaring of toes in a 47-year-old man with secondary lymphedema (obstructive type). *(From Gloviczki P and Schirger A: Lymphedema. In Spittell JA Jr, ed: Clinical medicine, Philadelphia, 1985, Harper & Row.)*

swelling in the extremity will disappear after a night's rest in the horizontal position, but if allowed to persist, only prolonged periods of bed rest (often with mechanical attempts to resolve the swelling) will result in its disappearance. In Allen's original series 13% of the patients had a history of complicating lymphangitis and cellulitis. The swelling may be unilateral or bilateral and, as in primary lymphedema of the congenital type, may be associated with other congenital abnormalities such as yellow nails[12] or with pleural effusions,[13] primary pulmonary hypertension, unequal breasts, bronchiectasis,[14] and pes cavus.[15] A rare cause of secondary lymphedema has been reported in human immunodeficiency virus type 1 (HIV-1) seropositive patients with Kaposi's sarcoma.[16] In children the lymphedema of the extremities may be associated with intestinal lymphangiectasia and accompanying gastrointestinal symptoms, resulting in failure to grow.[17] In rare instances hereditary intermittent cholestasis may be associated with lymphedema praecox.[18] Hereditary intrahepatic cholestasis with lymphedema is an autosomal recessive inherited syndrome. Seventy-five percent of the known cases came from Norway, mostly in the southwest. Cholestasis is postulated to be due to lymphatic drainage.[19] The association of yellow nail syndrome in lymphedema with rhinosinusitis has recently been reported.[20]

In the series of cases of primary and secondary lymphedema reported from the Mayo Clinic, the majority of patients with primary lymphedema had onset of swelling before the age of 39. However, there are genuine cases of primary lymphedema in which onset of swelling occurs later in life, and no cause can be identified. Thus the appearance of lymphedema before age 39, in the absence of signs and symptoms of acute lymphangitis and cellulitis, indicates an idiopathic process in all likelihood.

Secondary Lymphedema

Secondary lymphedema may be caused by obstruction of the lymphatic pathways by trauma, surgery, irradiation, or replacement of lymph channels or lymph nodes by metastatic tumor, or it may be caused by inflammatory changes (Fig. 29-4). The hallmark of obstructive lymphedema is the fairly abrupt onset, usually the unilateral nature of the swelling initially, and the absence of inflammatory changes. Onset after age 39 distinctly points to this possibility. In a Mayo Clinic series[21] in men, carcinoma of the prostate was the most common cause of secondary obstructive lymphedema; in women, carcinoma of the ovary was high on the list of the cancerous tumors, but lymphoma appeared to be more common. Lymphedema of an upper extremity after radical or modified radical mastectomy is a distinct form of secondary obstructive lymphedema. The swelling may appear at variable intervals postoperatively (Fig. 29-5).

The signs of inflammatory lymphedema are recurrent lymphangitis and cellulitis, characterized by acute onset, shaking chills, a temperature up to 40.6° C, and either de novo onset of swelling or intensification of swelling already present. There usually are red streaks on the feet, lower extremities, and thighs along the course of lymphatic channels and palpable, enlarged, tender lymph

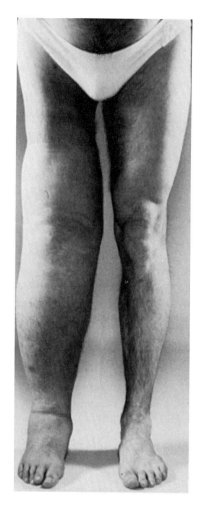

Fig. 29-4. Secondary lymphedema of lower extremities in a 55-year-old man. *(From Gloviczki P et al: Microsurgical lymphovenous anastomosis for treatment of lymphedema: a critical review, J Vasc Surg 7:647, 1988, by permission of the Society for Vascular Surgery and the North American chapter of the International Society for Cardiovascular Surgery.)*

nodes in the retropopliteal space and groin. There also may be a diffuse cellulitis involving the entire leg. Frequently the portal of entry for the offending organism, most commonly a streptococcus, can be detected as dermal fissures in the web spaces between the toes, indicating trichophytosis. The systemic symptoms of fever and chills may be accompanied by an intense malaise, headaches, nausea, vomiting, and diffuse sweats. Although acute thrombophlebitis may be accompanied by an increase in body temperature, the degree of increase seen in acute lymphangitis and cellulitis is seldom seen in thrombophlebitis, with the exception of pelvic septic thrombophlebitis. In Third-World countries filariasis is a frequent and important cause of secondary inflammatory lymphedema. Nodular lymphangitis is a special form of lymphangitis caused by *Sporothrix schenckii, Nocardia brasiliensis, Mycobacterium marinum, Leishmania braziliensis,* and *Francisella tularensis.* Diagnosis is made on skin biopsy.[22,23] Lymphedema is a rare complication of rheumatoid arthritis and seems to be unaffected by treatment of the primary underlying condition.

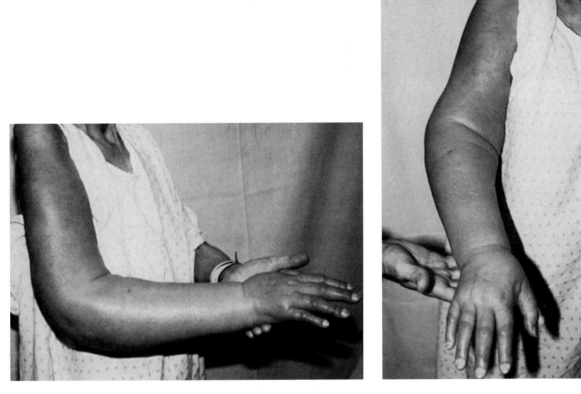

Fig. 29-5. Lymphedema of right upper extremity after mastectomy.

DIAGNOSIS

Diagnosis of lymphedema is based on the history, the characteristic appearance of the involved extremity, and the absence of symptoms and signs indicating a systemic cause for the swelling or arterial or deep venous insufficiency. Arterial pulses characteristically are normal unless the swelling is excessive when they may be difficult to feel. The venous pattern is not prominent, and there is no tenderness along the course of the deep veins of the calf and thigh.

The age of onset is of great aid in the differential diagnosis of primary or secondary lymphedema, even though an idiopathic swelling may develop late in life. Of the tests found helpful in confirming the diagnostic impression of either primary or secondary lymphedema, the ultrasonographic examination of the pelvis and prostate is valuable, as is computed tomographic examination of the abdomen and pelvis.

Lymphoscintigraphy uses technetium-99m as a radioactive label and antimony trisulfide for labeling particles. We inject 400 to 500 μCi of ^{99m}Tc-labeled antimony trisulfide colloid (Cadema Medical Products, Inc., Middletown, N.Y.) subcutaneously into the second interdigital space in the foot or the hand (0.3 to 0.6 ml). We ask the patient to squeeze a rubber ball or to perform toe stands for 3 minutes after the injection. In the first hour 12-minute images are obtained with the gamma camera. At 1 and 3 hours additional 5-minute images are made (Figs. 29-6 and 29-7). In selected cases images are recorded at 6 and 24 hours (Fig. 29-8).

Semiquantitative evaluation of the lymphatic drainage and visual interpretation of the different image patterns in 190 lymphoscintigraphic examinations at The Mayo Clinic showed a sensitivity of 92% and a specificity of 100% for distinguishing lymphedema from edemas of other origin.[24] We could not distinguish primary from secondary lymphedema consistently by using this method. Because lymphoscintigraphy is a reliable and safe method and has no side effects, it has replaced contrast lymphangiography in our institution for the routine evaluation of a swollen extremity. In a more recent report, Cambria et al[25] confirmed the effectiveness of lymphoscintigraphy in the noninvasive diagnosis of lymphedema.[26] Magnetic resonance imaging has been reported to be useful in diagnosing lymphedema through a specific honeycomb pattern in the subcutaneous tissues (Fig. 29-9, B and C).[27] Contrast lymphangiography is used frequently, however, in the evaluation of patients with lymphangiectasia (Fig. 29-10). For a differential diagnosis of the swollen limb see Chapter 38.

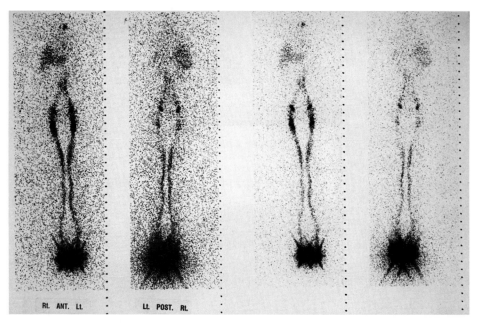

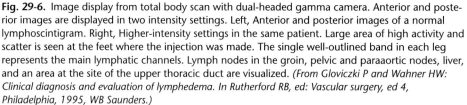

RI. ANT. LI.   LI. POST. RI.

Fig. 29-6. Image display from total body scan with dual-headed gamma camera. Anterior and posterior images are displayed in two intensity settings. Left, Anterior and posterior images of a normal lymphoscintigram. Right, Higher-intensity settings in the same patient. Large area of high activity and scatter is seen at the feet where the injection was made. The single well-outlined band in each leg represents the main lymphatic channels. Lymph nodes in the groin, pelvic and paraaortic nodes, liver, and an area at the site of the upper thoracic duct are visualized. *(From Gloviczki P and Wahner HW: Clinical diagnosis and evaluation of lymphedema. In Rutherford RB, ed: Vascular surgery, ed 4, Philadelphia, 1995, WB Saunders.)*

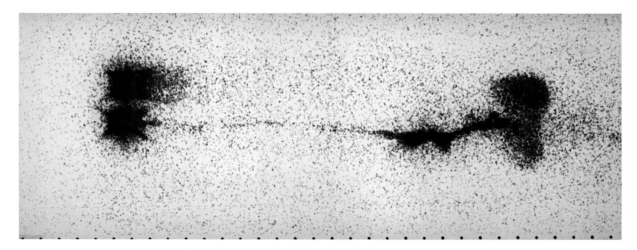

Fig. 29-7. Lymphoscintigram of a 65-year-old woman with primary lymphedema tarda of the right lower extremity. There is minimal dermal backflow above the right ankle 3 hours after injection, and no lymph vessels or lymph nodes are visualized. Normal pattern in the left leg. *(From Gloviczki P and Wahner HW: Clinical diagnosis and evaluation of lymphedema. In Rutherford RB, ed: Vascular surgery, ed 4, Philadelphia, 1995, WB Saunders.)*

Fig. 29-8. Lymphoscintigram of a 25-year-old woman with congenital familial lymphedema of both lower extremities. Note the absence of lymph vessels and lymph nodes at 6 hours, with only minimal dermal backflow visible in the distal calves. This patient also had recurrent familial cholestasis due to absence of intrahepatic bile ducts (Aagenaes syndrome). *(From Gloviczki P and Wahner HW: Clinical diagnosis and evaluation of lymphedema. In Rutherford RB, ed: Vascular surgery, ed 4, Philadelphia, 1995, WB Saunders.)*

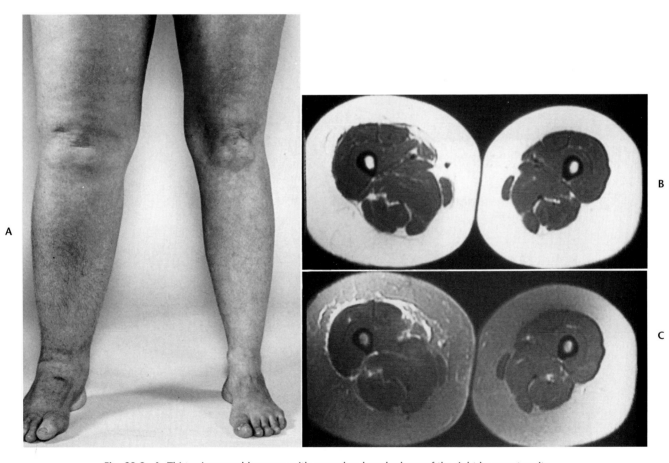

Fig. 29-9. A, Thirty-six-year-old woman with secondary lymphedema of the right lower extremity. **B,** Magnetic resonance imaging of the legs reveals enlargement of the subcutaneous tissues and the deep compartment on the right with considerable stranding within the subcutaneous tissues, predominantly anteriorly and medially. **C,** T2-weighted image reveals the region of soft tissue stranding that is now of high signal intensity in the deep layers of the subcutaneous tissue. *(From Gloviczki P and Wahner HW: Clinical diagnosis and evaluation of lymphedema. In Rutherford RB, ed: Vascular surgery, ed 4, Philadelphia, 1995, WB Saunders.)*

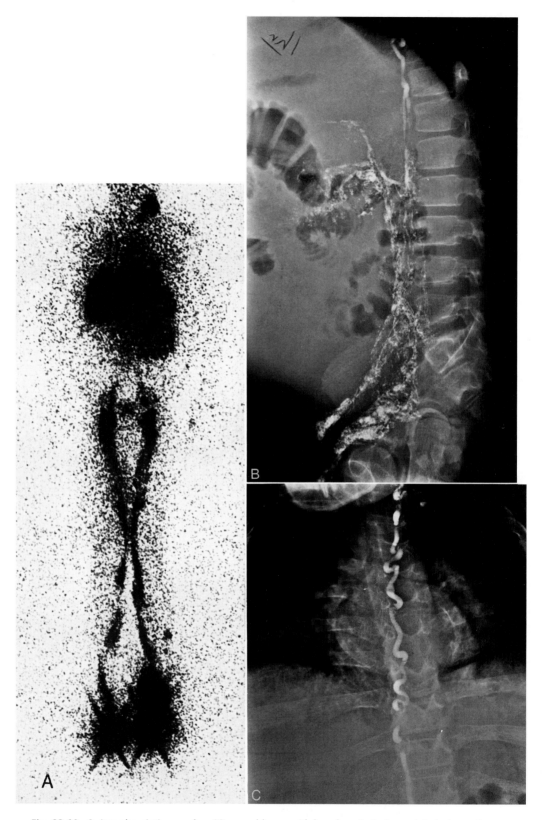

Fig. 29-10. A, Lymphoscintigram of an 18-year-old man with lymphangiectasia, protein-losing enteropathy, and chylous ascites. Note large leg lymphatics and reflux of colloid into the mesenteric lymph vessels, filling almost the entire abdominal cavity. **B,** Lymphangiogram of the same patient reveals reflux of dye into the dilated mesenteric lymphatics. **C,** Note extremely dilated and tortuous but patent thoracic duct. *(From Gloviczki P and Wahner HW: Clinical diagnosis and evaluation of lymphedema. In Rutherford RB, ed: Vascular surgery, ed 4, Philadelphia, 1995, WB Saunders.)*

TREATMENT

Medical Therapy

There is no known cure for lymphedema once the swelling appears. At present, with few exceptions, we have no way of completely restoring normal lymphatic flow. The aim of treatment thus should be to remove as much fluid as possible from the affected extremity and to maintain an edema-free state. Currently used modalities of edema reduction include bed rest with elevation of the leg in a lymphedema sling, the use of intermittent compression pumps, and physical therapy in the form of manual lymph massage.

In the most advanced cases the removal of fluid is best done in the hospital. The extremity is elevated in a lymphedema sling. A diuretic, such as furosemide, is administered while the patient is being protected from the hazards of venous thromboembolism by subcutaneous injection of heparin in doses of 5,000 to 10,000 U twice daily. Because a vigorous diuresis may ensue, attention needs to be focused on potassium losses and, if necessary, on potassium replacement. This becomes more imperative in patients who are prone to cardiac arrhythmias or who are taking digitalis. However, diuresis does not change the protein content of the subcutaneous space, and its effect on edema of lymphatic origin is temporary.

The drainage of the fluid from the affected extremity is aided by the use of the lymphedema sling, which allows the patient to keep the extremity elevated without flexing the back. It also affords periods of rest, which provide comfort and will not jeopardize the gains already made by having the extremity elevated for several hours. In some patients maximal fluid drainage can be obtained in 24 to 48 hours; in others several days of in-hospital treatment is necessary. We have been very impressed by the effectiveness of this simple method, when strict bed rest was reinforced in our patients.

Once all the fluid that can be removed has been removed, the patient is measured for an elastic stocking. If the lymphedema involves only the leg, a knee-length stocking (30 to 40 or 40 to 50 mm Hg of compression) suffices. If it involves the thigh, thigh-length stockings or a pantyhose type of support may be necessary.

Edema can also be removed from lymphedematous limbs by mechanically pumping the limbs for 2 to 8 hours to make them edema-free. This intensive treatment is continued at home daily for 1 or 2 hours. Of the different intermittent pneumatic compression devices available, we prefer those that have several cells for sequential compression. The effectiveness of these was reported by Pappas and O'Donnell.[28] Many patients find it helpful to have a period of rest at midday with their extremities elevated. Others use an intermittent pneumatic compression device during the night to massage the fluid out of the affected extremity. The use of manual lymphatic massage has been popularized by Földi.[29] This technique of manual lymph drainage used together with compressive bandaging, and specific physical therapy exercises is used with increasing frequency to treat lymphedema not only in Europe and Australia, but in the United States as well.[30,31] Alteration of the morphology of the lymphatics after manual massage in patients with lymphedema was recently reported.[31]

The hope is that early drainage of the fluid and use of an elastic stocking will prevent accumulation of lymphedematous fluid and avoid overgrowth of tissue, induration, fibrosis, and eventual disfiguring distortion of the extremity. The intermittent use of a thiazide diuretic 3 days a week will aid in maintaining the decrease in fluid accumulation in some patients with a lymphedematous extremity. Benzopyrones have been reported by Casley-Smith, Morgan, and Piller[32] to reduce the volume of high-protein edema fluid by stimulating proteolysis. They are felt to provide a method for removing excess protein and its consequence. A slow but safe reduction of the lymphedema of the extremities could be achieved. In addition, 5,6-benzo-alpha-pyrone has also been found to be efficacious in reducing lymphedema in filariasis and elephantiasis.[33]

If more than one episode of lymphangitis and cellulitis occurs, the intermittent use of antibiotic prophylaxis is indicated. We prescribe penicillin VK 500 mg orally four times daily for 7 to 10 days or in patients allergic to penicillin, erythromycin 250 mg four times daily for 7 to 10 days each month for a minimum of 12 months. Good skin and nail care, and especially the early treatment of tinea pedis, are important to prevent portals of entry for bacterial invasion.

Liu and Olszewski[34] studied the influence of microwave and hot water immersion hyperthermia on lymphedema and lymphedematous skin of the leg in 12 patients. They noted decreased volume of the leg but no improvement in the lymph flow. Dermal inflammation decreased, and the authors postulated that subsidence of local inflammation in the lymphedematous limb with alteration in the extracellular protein matrix after regional heating accounted for the reduction in peripheral edema. Another treatment of lymphedema has recently been reported in the form of elimination or drastic reduction of long-chain dietary triglycerides.[35] The reduction in the lymphedematous limb occurred despite no weight reduction in one patient. A recent case of yellow nail syndrome responded favorably to zinc supplementation for 2 years.[36] The lymphedema likewise was reported to have resolved.

The goal of treatment of lymphedema is the achievement and maintenance of as normal-appearing an extremity as possible. This is particularly important for children during their period of physical, social, and emotional growth. We try not to interdict in young patients those activities that clearly will not aggravate the lymphedema. All forms of exercise involving the legs, other then contact sports, are encouraged. Swimming seems to be ideally suited as a disciplined, regular, repetitive activity because the water exerts pressure on the extremity during the time that the muscle pump is being used. The need for psychologic support in all age groups, particularly in teenagers afflicted with lymphedema is most important.[37]

Surgery

Despite the best efforts medical therapy will fail in some patients. Then surgical consultation needs to be obtained to determine whether an operation might help to control the swelling. In general, there are two types of operations: excisional or debulking operations and the so-called physiologic operations, which include microvascular reconstruction of the lymph drainage with lymphovenous anastomosis or lymph vessel transplantation. No procedure currently available is going to cure the disease.

In the excisional or debulking operations, first introduced by Sir Havelok Charles, some or most of the edematous subcutaneous tissue and the underlying fascia are resected.[38] The skin of the extremity may be so diseased that it cannot be used for coverage, and skin grafting to the entire excised area has to be performed. Wound healing can be a significant problem, and additional skin grafting frequently is needed. There may remain a difference in circumference between the edematous and excised areas, at the ankle or at the knee, creating a cosmetic deformity. Joint stiffness, secondary skin changes, hypesthesia or burning sensation, or hyperesthesia at and distal to the operated area may occur. For us, the only indication for excisional operation is disabling severe lymphedema—that is, elephantiasis. We favor the staged excisional procedure[39] originally described by Homans[40] and modified by Kinmonth[41] and, in the United States, by Miller.[42] We make every attempt to use local skin flaps for coverage after excision.

Thompson's buried dermal flap operation is partly excisional and partly a physiologic operation. Thompson[43] claimed to improve lymphatic drainage of the superficial tissue to the deep compartments by suturing one of the skin flaps down to the muscles. Although the improvement probably is only the result of excision of some of the edematous tissue,[44] we have had patients who were pleased with the outcome many years afterward. Because of persisting lymphedema, these patients need continuous, conservative treatment, but problems with healing the incision are less than with other excisional operations.

The enteromesenteric bridge operation was suggested by Kinmonth.[41] He reported decreased edema in several patients with primary lymphedema who had proximal pelvic lymphatic obstruction. Postoperative lymphangiography in three patients confirmed good lymphatic drainage from the inguinal lymph nodes to the mesenteric lymphatic circulation. Experience with this operation has been very limited.

Perfection of microsurgical techniques has made direct reconstructions of the lymph vessels possible. Lymph node–to-vein and lymph vessel–to-vein anastomoses have been performed for more than 25 years now, but long-term effectiveness and patency have yet to be demonstrated with objective tests. O'Brien and Shafiroff[45] reported an improvement in two thirds of their patients treated surgically; however, in many cases an additional excisional operation also was performed.

In our laboratory we found patency of lymphovenous anastomoses in dogs up to 8 months after the operation by using contrast cine lymphangiography.[46] Our experience with 18 patients treated surgically has been reported[47]; 14 underwent successful lymph vessel–to-vein anastomosis. Decrease in limb circumference, frequency of postopera-

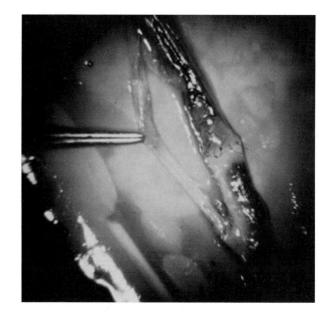

Fig. 29-11. Lymphaticovenous anastomosis in a patient with secondary lymphedema.

tive cellulitis, patient satisfaction, and lymphoscintigraphic findings were used to assess the results. Only one of seven patients with primary lymphedema and four of seven with secondary lymphedema showed improvement at a mean of 36 months after the operation (Figs. 29-11 and 29-12). Lymphoscintigraphy provided only indirect evidence of patency. We continue to perform this operation only in carefully selected patients with secondary lymphedema who have no history of cellulitis. Preoperative evaluation includes lymphoscintigraphy, which in ideal cases demonstrates distended lymphatics of the thigh distal to a pelvic lymphatic obstruction (Fig. 29-13). We admit that contrast lymphangiography could be the only test that proves late patency. However, this procedure is invasive and is uncomfortable for the patient, and we are reluctant to advise it unless it has definite therapeutic consequences. Worsening of lymphedema has been described after lymphangiography.[45]

Baumeister, Frick, and Hofmann[48] performed lymphatic grafting to bypass obstruction in 55 patients. Lymph vessel transplantation from the thigh to the arm was done to treat patients with postmastectomy lymphedema. With a follow-up of more than 3 years, objective improvement was found in 80% of the patients. The same group performed suprapubic lymph vessel transplantation to treat unilateral secondary lower-extremity lymphedema with improvement in 8 of 12 patients. At this time the effectiveness of this operation has not yet been proven by other centers.

Results of surgical interventions for chronic lymphedema are far from satisfactory at this time. Because the number of patients needing surgical attention is not large, it should be performed only by those who have special interest and expertise in this field.

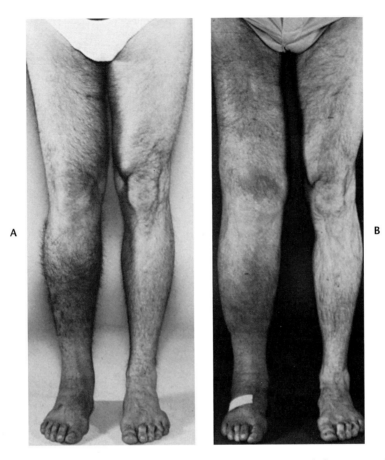

Fig. 29-12. At 3 **(A)** and 12 **(B)** months after lymphaticovenous anastomosis (same case as in Fig. 29-4). *(A: From Gloviczki P et al: Microsurgical lymphovenous anastomosis for treatment of lymphedema: a critical review, J Vasc Surg 7:647, 1988, by permission of the Society for Vascular Surgery and the North American chapter of the International Society for Cardiovascular Surgery.)*

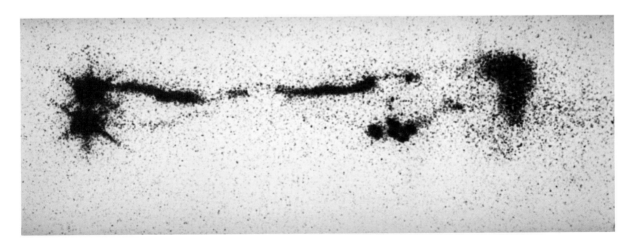

Fig. 29-13. Bilateral lower-extremity lymphoscintigraphy in a patient with right lower-extremity lymphedema secondary to obstruction of the right iliac nodes. Note the dilated lymph vessels in the right thigh distal to the obstruction suitable for direct lymphatic reconstruction. *(From Gloviczki P: Lymphatic reconstructions. In Rutherford RB, ed: Vascular surgery, ed 4, Philadelphia, 1995, WB Saunders.)*

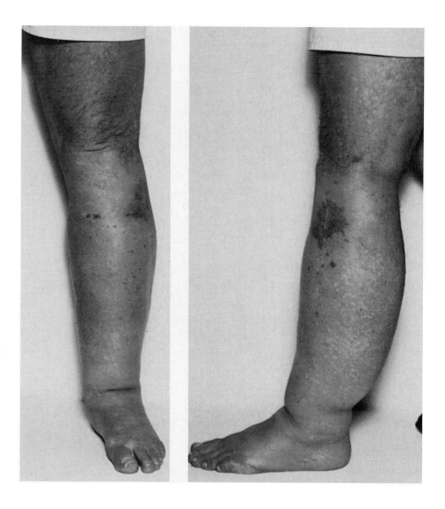

Fig. 29-14. Idiopathic lymphedema of 25 years' duration and early appearance of lymphangiosarcoma in a 52-year-old man. *(From Schirger A and Peterson LFA: Lymphedema. In Juergens JL, Spittell JA Jr, and Fairbairn JF II, eds: Allen-Barker-Hines peripheral vascular diseases, ed 5, Philadelphia, 1980, WB Saunders, by permission of the Mayo Foundation.)*

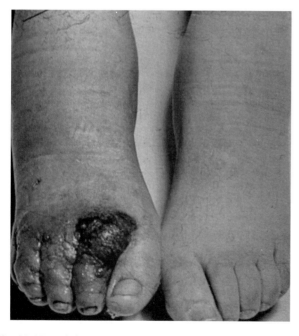

Fig. 29-15. Early lymphangiosarcoma in a 24-year-old man with idiopathic lymphedema. *(From Schirger A: Lymphedema, Cardiovasc Clin 13:293, 1983, by permission of FA Davis Co.)*

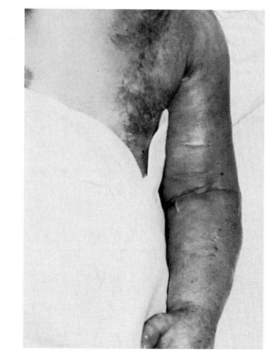

Fig. 29-16. Postmastectomy lymphedema of 9 years' duration in an 82-year-old woman, complicated by lymphangiosarcoma.

LATE COMPLICATIONS

In lymphedema the deleterious sequelae generally are only esthetic and emotional. In some cases there may be loss of working time because of acute increases in swelling such as when acute lymphangitis and cellulitis develop. Occasionally a late and serious life-threatening complication may occur: the appearance of a malignant lymphangiosarcoma originating from the distorted, enlarged lymphatic channels. This was first described in postmastectomy lymphedema by Stewart and Treves.[49] It also may be seen, although rarely, in patients with idiopathic lymphedema of long duration. The clinical picture is that of a new lesion appearing in the skin of the affected extremity (Figs. 29-14, 29-15, and 29-16). The patient at first identifies the bluish flat lesion as a bruise, even though being unable to recall a trauma. The bruise subsequently enlarges and satellite lesions appear. The central portion of the lesion may ulcerate. Such a sequence of events should lead the clinician to suspect lymphangiosarcoma and mandates immediate biopsy and appropriate therapy.[50] Unfortunately this therapy involves fairly radical surgery, because wide excision is insufficient and blood-borne metastases occur early. Because of this, an appropriate high amputation, sometimes followed by radiation therapy, usually is favored. At the present time there is no proven method of chemotherapy. We have observed one patient for over 20 years who was cured by a high amputation of a lymphangiosarcoma of many years' duration that occurred in a lymphedematous extremity. Recurrent lymphangitis in chronic lymphedema has recently been reported as a milieu for the development of multiple basal cell carcinomas of the leg.[51]

REFERENCES

1. Asellius G: De Lactibus sive Lacteis Venis Quarto Vasorum Mesaraicorum Genere Novo Inuento, Mediolani, 1627, JB Biddellium.
2. Milroy WF: Chronic hereditary edema: Milroy's disease, JAMA 91:1172, 1928.
3. Allen EV: Lymphedema of the extremities: classification, etiology and differential diagnosis; a study of three hundred cases, Arch Intern Med 54:606, 1934.
4. Kinmonth JB et al: Primary lymphoedema: clinical and lymphangiographic studies of a series of 107 patients in which the lower limbs were affected, Br J Surg 45:1, 1957.
5. Benson PF, Gough MH, and Polani PE: Lymphangiography and chromosome studies in females with lymphoedema and possible ovarian dysgenesis, Arch Dis Child 40:27, 1965.
6. Courtecuisse V et al: Lymphedema tarda in Turner syndrome (in French), Arch Fr Pediatr 35:988, 1978.
7. Maisels DO: Anonychia in association with lymphoedema, Br J Plast Surg 19:37, 1966.
8. Siegelman SS, Heckman BH, and Hasson J: Lymphedema, pleural effusions and yellow nails: associated immunologic deficiency, Dis Chest 56:114, 1969.
9. Robinow M, Johnson GF, and Verhagen AD: Distichiasis-lymphedema: a hereditary syndrome of multiple congenital defects, Am J Dis Child 119:343, 1970.
10. Allen EV and Ghormley RK: Lymphedema of the extremities: etiology, classification and treatment; report of 300 cases, Ann Intern Med 9:516, 1935.
11. Schirger A, Harrison EG Jr, and Janes JM: Idiopathic lymphedema: review of 131 cases, JAMA 182:14, 1962.
12. Anonymous: Yellow nails and oedema, Br Med J 4:130, 1972.
13. Runyon BA, Forker EL, and Sopko JA: Pleural-fluid kinetics in a patient with primary lymphedema, pleural effusions, and yellow nails, Am Rev Respir Dis 119:821, 1979.
14. Bowers D: Unequal breasts, yellow nails, bronchiectasis and lymphedema, Can Med Assoc J 100:437, 1969.
15. Jackson BT and Kinmonth JB: Pes cavus and lymphoedema: an unusual familial syndrome, J Bone Joint Surg 52B:518, 1970.
16. Frans E et al: Kaposi's sarcoma presenting as generalized lymphedema, Acta Clinica Belgica 49:19, 1994.
17. Vardy PA, Lebenthal E, and Schwachman H: Intestinal lymphangiectasia: a reappraisal, Pediatrics 55:842, 1975.
18. Aagenaes TO: Hereditary recurrent cholestasis with lymphoedema—two new families, Acta Paediatr Scand 63:465, 1974.
19. Aagenaes O and Medbo S: Hereditary intrahepatic cholestasis with lymphedema—Aagenaes syndrome, Tidsskr Nor Laegeforen 113:3673, 1993.
20. Varney VA et al: Rhinitis, sinusitis and the yellow nail syndrome—a review of symptoms and response to treatment in 17 patients, Clin Otolaryngol 19:237, 1994.
21. Smith RD, Spittell JA Jr, and Schirger A: Secondary lymphedema of the leg: its characteristics and diagnostic implications, JAMA 185:80, 1963.
22. Lymphatic filariasis—tropical medicine's origin will not go away, Lancet 1:1409, 1987 (editorial).
23. Mak JW: Epidemiology of lymphatic filariasis, Ciba Found Symp 127:5, 1987.
24. Gloviczki P et al: Noninvasive evaluation of the swollen extremity: experiences with 190 lymphoscintigraphic examinations, J Vasc Surg 9:683, 1989.
25. Cambria RA et al: Noninvasive evaluation of the lymphatic system with lymphoscintigraphy: a prospective, semiquantitative analysis in 386 extremities, J Vasc Surg 18:773, 1993.
26. Case TC et al: Magnetic resonance imaging in human lymphedema: comparison with lymphoscintigraphy, J Magn Reson Imag 10:549, 1992.
27. Kinmonth JB: Lymphangiography in man: a method of outlining lymphatic trunks at operation, Clin Sci 11:13, 1952.
28. Pappas CJ and O'Donnell TF: Long-term results of compression treatment for lymphedema, J Vasc Surg 16:555, 1992.
29. Földi E, Földi M, and Weissleder H: Conservative treatment of lymphoedema of the limbs, Angiology 36:171, 1985.
30. Boris M et al: Lymphedema reduction by noninvasive complex lymphedema therapy, Oncology 8:95, 1994.
31. Eliska O and Eliskova M: Lymphedema—morphology of the lymphatics after manual massage, Lymphology 27:132, 1994.
32. Casley-Smith JR, Morgan RG, and Piller NB: Treatment of lymphedema of the arms and legs with 5,6-benzo-[alpha]-pyrone, N Engl J Med 329:1158, 1993.
33. Casley-Smith JR, Wang CT, and Zi-hai C: Treatment of filarial lymphedema and elephantiasis with 5,6-benzo-alpha-pyrone (coumarin), Br Med J 307:1037, 1993.
34. Liu NF and Olszewski W: The influence of local hypothermia on lymphedema and lymphedematous skin of the human leg, Lymphology 26:28, 1993.
35. Soria P et al: Dietary treatment of lymphedema by restriction of long-chain triglycerides, Angiology 45:703, 1994.
36. Arroyo JF and Cohen ML: Improvement of yellow nail syndrome with oral zinc supplementation, Clin Exp Dermatol 18:62, 1993.
37. Gold R et al: Lymphedema in Pickwickian syndrome, Eur J Dermatol 4:663, 1994.

38. Charles RH: Elephantiasis scroti. In Latham A, ed: A system of treatment, vol 3, London, 1912, Churchill.

39. Sakulsky SB et al: Lymphedema: results of surgical treatment in 64 patients (1936-1964), Lymphology 10:15, 1977.

40. Homans J: The treatment of elephantiasis of the legs: a preliminary report, N Engl J Med 215:1099, 1936.

41. Kinmonth JB: The lymphatics: surgery, lymphography and diseases of the chyle and lymph systems, London, 1982, Edward Arnold.

42. Abdou MS, Ashby ER, and Miller TA: Excisional operations for chronic lymphedema. In Rutherford RB, ed: Vascular surgery, ed 4, Philadelphia, 1995, WB Saunders.

43. Thompson N: Buried dermal flap operation for chronic lymphedema of the extremities: ten-year survey of results in 79 cases, Plast Reconstr Surg 45:541, 1970.

44. Sawhney CP: Evaluation of Thompson's buried dermal flap operation for lymphoedema of the limbs: a clinical and radioisotopic study, Br J Plast Surg 27:278, 1974.

45. O'Brien BM and Shafiroff BB: Microlymphaticovenous and resectional surgery in obstructive lymphedema, World J Surg 3:3, 1979.

46. Gloviczki P et al: The natural history of microsurgical lymphovenous anastomoses: an experimental study, J Vasc Surg 4:148, 1986.

47. Gloviczki P et al: Microsurgical lymphovenous anastomosis for treatment of lymphedema: a critical review, J Vasc Surg 7:647, 1988.

48. Baumeister RGH, Frick A, and Hofmann T: 10 years experience with autogenous microsurgical lymph vessel-transplantation, Eur J Lymphol 6:62, 1991.

49. Stewart FW and Treves N: Lymphangiosarcoma in postmastectomy lymphedema: a report of six cases in elephantiasis chirurgica, Cancer 1:64, 1948.

50. Taswell HF, Soule EH, and Coventry MB: Lymphangiosarcoma arising in chronic lymphedematous extremities: report of thirteen cases and review of literature, J Bone Joint Surg 44A:277, 1962.

51. Lotem M et al: Multiple basal cell carcinomas of the leg after recurrent erysipelas and chronic lymphedema, J Am Acad Dermatol 31:812, 1994.

PART V

VASCULAR DISEASES OF DIVERSE ORIGIN

CHAPTER THIRTY

PERIPHERAL VASCULAR DISEASE IN CHILDREN

Douglas S. Moodie
David Driscoll
Dawn Salvatore

With the aging of the U.S. population, we are seeing more adult patients with peripheral vascular disease. The number of physicians trained specifically to deal with peripheral vascular disease is very limited. Even more limited is the expertise in pediatrics about the unusual peripheral vascular problems that present in infancy, childhood, and young adulthood. No one center is able to accumulate enough patients to define the broad scope of peripheral vascular disease in children, and so one must look to what is collectively presented in the literature. This chapter deals with peripheral vascular disease in children and attempts to present information as it relates to specific disease entities, their clinical manifestations, diagnosis, and treatment.

KLIPPEL-TRENAUNAY SYNDROME

Klippel-Trenaunay syndrome (KTS) consists of a triad of cutaneous capillary hemangioma, bone and soft tissue hypertrophy, and venous varicosities.[1] The etiology of KTS is unknown, but some authors have suggested that it results from a mesodermal abnormality that occurs during fetal development, leading to the maintenance of microscopic arteriovenous communications in the limb bud.[2] Most commonly it is a sporadic event. Although a few cases have been reported in which more than one family member had the syndrome, other authors suggest that this may have not been the case.[3,4] It has been suggested that KTS could result from the action of a mosaic gene abnormality that is lethal to the gamete when present in all cells of the embryo.[5] We have seen two patients with intriguing associations. One patient has prolonged QT interval syndrome and the other a translocation of chromosomes 8 and 14. Whether these are coincidental abnormalities or provide a clue to the location of a causative gene is unknown.

KTS should be distinguished from Parks-Weber syndrome. In Parks-Weber syndrome there are clinically apparent and important arteriovenous fistulas, whereas in KTS any arteriovenous fistulas that exist are microscopic in size and unassociated with the typical clinical findings of arteriovenous fistulas. The natural history of these syndromes is different. For example, because patients with KTS do not have arteriovenous fistulas, high-output cardiac failure does not occur.

The manifestations of KTS are variable (Figs. 30-1, 30-2, and 30-3). In a study of 144 patients evaluated at The Mayo Clinic,[6] 132 had lower-extremity involvement, 37 had upper-extremity involvement, 21 had pelvic and abdominal involvement, 25 had involvement of the thorax, and 7 had head and neck involvement.

With occasional exceptions the appearance of the baby shortly after birth will define the ultimate appearance of the child and young adult. The exceptions to this include (1) the cutaneous capillary hemangioma (port-wine stain) may become lighter or darker; (2) dark small nodular excrescence may develop on the skin; (3) as growth occurs, the limb length discrepancy may increase; (4) some of the apparent increased mass may regress as baby fat regresses; (5) subcutaneous masses may appear; and (6) venous varicosities and, possibly, dependent lymphedema will become more prominent with time. Parents should be reassured, however, that unaffected extremities and organs will not become affected in the future.

Clinical Manifestations

VENOUS VARICOSITIES AND MALFORMATIONS. The venous involvement in KTS can range from subtle abnormalities to massive varicosities and absence of important deep venous structures. The venous abnormalities usually involve the affected extremity and are apparent as superficial varicose veins. Dilation of superficial varicose

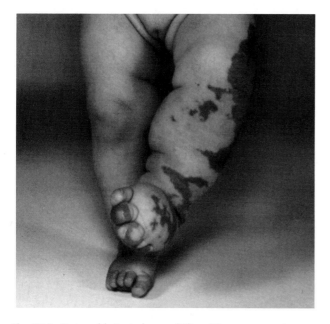

Fig. 30-1. Reasonably typical case of Klippel-Trenaunay syndrome. Note the foot and toe enlargement.

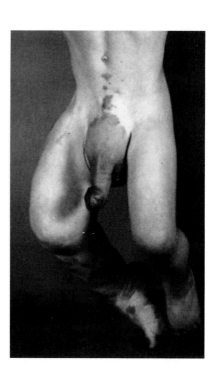

Fig. 30-3. Klippel-Trenaunay syndrome involving the right leg and genitalia.

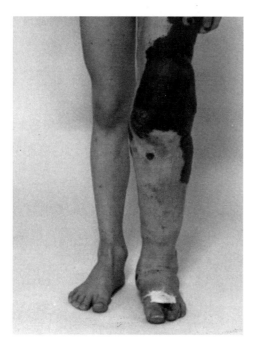

Fig. 30-2. Relatively severe involvement of the leg. Note the verrucous appearance of the cutaneous hemangioma. A bandage covers a lesion on the dorsal aspect of the left foot that chronically drains.

veins may be unapparent in infancy but become apparent with increasing age. Not all patients with KTS have superficial venous varicosities.

In addition to superficial varicosities many patients have abnormalities of the deep venous system of the extremity. The deep venous abnormalities can include dilation of the deep veins, absent venous valves, hypopla-

sia of the veins, and complete absence of the deep venous system. It is critically important to ascertain the status of the deep venous system if one is considering removal of superficial varicosities since the superficial venous system cannot be removed if the deep venous system is inadequate to provide venous drainage of the extremity. Because of the venous malformations some patients with KTS can develop thrombophlebitis.

Venous varicosities also can involve intraabdominal and intrapelvic organs. In Gloviczki's series 10% of the patients manifested rectal bleeding and 3% had hematuria.[6] Others have reported that 20% of their patients have had rectal bleeding, 10% had hematuria, and 33% had evidence of abnormal intrapelvic veins.[7] Venous or arteriovenous malformations have been described in other locations in rare patients with KTS. These include bone, spinal, and intracranial locations.

In addition to the complete absence of the deep venous system of an extremity, absence of the inferior vena cava has been reported,[8] and we have observed absence of the internal jugular veins.

LYMPHATIC ABNORMALITIES. Many patients with KTS have abnormalities of the lymphatic system. Since in no series of patients have these abnormalities been looked for in a systematic fashion, the incidence of lymphatic abnormalities is unknown. In one series it was reported that 20% of patients have cutaneous vesicles that leak lymph. However, in our experience, exudation of lymph is less common. It frequently is unclear if the edema of an affected dependent extremity is a result of venous insufficiency, abnormal lymphatic drainage, or a combination of the two. Some patients do develop soft tissue masses that are reminiscent of cystic hygromas. These masses can occur on an affected extremity or over the trunk, head, or neck.

CAPILLARY HEMANGIOMAS AND OTHER CUTANEOUS LESIONS. There is a broad spectrum of cutaneous manifestations of KTS. Most commonly there is a port-wine stain that can be very light in color to deep maroon. This lesion can be flat or elevated. The integrity of the skin over the hemangioma may be excellent or poor. In some cases the capillary hemangioma is raised considerably from the surface and may be verrucous in nature. Some areas of the malformation may be prone to skin breakdown, bleeding, and infection. In general, the intensity of the color of the hemangioma lessens as the child ages. However, some patients develop dark (deep blue to black) 1- to 2-mm nodules on the top of the hemangioma or at times over seemingly unaffected portions of skin. These can be quite friable and prone to spontaneous bleeding or bleeding after minor trauma. Cutaneous or subcutaneous cavernous hemangiomas occur in 40% of patients.[1] These can produce a spongy feel to the skin and frequently are associated with lymphangiomas.

Other cutaneous manifestations of KTS include phlebectasia, hyperhidrosis, hyperthermia, and hypertrichosis. Patients with KTS are prone to cellulitis. It is unclear if these episodes are always secondary to bacterial infection or to a local inflammatory response in response to pockets of lymph accumulation.

BONE AND SOFT TISSUE HYPERTROPHY. In Gloviczki's series 95 of 144 patients had one extremity longer than the other, and 100 of 144 patients had a swollen or circumferentially enlarged extremity.[6] Most commonly a lower extremity is affected, but in a fourth of the patients an upper extremity is involved. Usually the longer, bigger extremity is also the extremity that exhibits the skin and vascular changes, but occasionally the extremity with skin and vascular involvement is the shorter or smaller extremity. The bony hypertrophy may affect all the bones in an extremity or be limited to one or two bones. Some patients may have macrodactyly.

In addition to bony hypertrophy many patients have soft tissue hypertrophy. This can be quite limited, for example, to a localized mass on the back or the chest, or can be quite widespread, for example, involving an entire arm or leg. The soft tissue hypertrophy is usually fatty and contains variable amounts of venous structures.

Other limb findings that have been described in KTS include syndactyly, clinodactyly, polydactyly, split hand deformity, metatarsal and phalangeal agenesis, osteolysis, congenital dislocation of the hip, and peripheral neuropathy.[1]

HEAD, CENTRAL NERVOUS SYSTEM, AND EYE INVOLVEMENT. Patients with KTS can have macrocephaly and less frequently, microcephaly. Intracranial angiomas, arteriovenous malformations, and intraspinal angiomas have been described. More than 40 cases of KTS have been described in association with Sturge-Weber syndrome.[9]

Ophthalmologic findings reported in association with KTS include conjunctival telangiectasia, retinal varicosities, choroidal angioma, glaucoma, coloboma iridis, heterochromia iridis, intraorbital varix, and enophthalmos.[1,10]

ADDITIONAL FINDINGS AND PROBLEMS

Coagulopathy. Some patients with KTS exhibit evidence of an intravascular coagulopathy. This usually is mild but in some patients can be relatively severe and result in bleeding after minor trauma or major bleeding associated with surgical procedures. This coagulopathy probably represents a form of Kasabach-Merritt syndrome and may be manifested by thrombocytopenia, reduced fibrinogen, and the presence of fibrin-split products.[11] It is prudent to assess patients' coagulation status before planned surgical procedures.

Pulmonary Emboli. There have been several instances of fatal and nonfatal pulmonary emboli in patients with KTS. It is unclear at this point which patients with KTS are at risk for this complication. Some episodes have been associated with bed rest following a surgical procedure. One author has recommended that patients with KTS receive anticoagulation therapy when admitted to a hospital or long-term anticoagulation therapy for those who have had a documented thrombotic event.[7]

Syncope. Patients with large venous capacitance in the legs can be prone to light-headedness and syncope when standing.

MANAGEMENT ISSUES

Compression Therapy. Most patients with lower-extremity involvement experience some degree of lower-extremity edema. This usually is not manifested until after the child begins walking and gravitational forces become a factor. It is important to remember that an extremity may be enlarged because of increased bony and soft tissue mass as well as edema. Compression of the extremity with elastic support will acutely lessen the edema *but there are no data that chronic compressive therapy will result ultimately in less bony or soft tissue mass.* Also, compression will not affect the ultimate length of the leg. Patients with a major component of lymphedema and those with severe venous insufficiency seem to derive the most benefit from chronic compressive therapy. Compressive therapy also should be used for patients with edema and recurrent cellulitis. It may reduce the frequency of episodes of cellulitis. Compression may or may not be useful for patients with friable skin lesions that tend to bleed. In some cases the compression garment will protect the sites and lessen the bleeding, but in other cases the garment may irritate the skin and increase the bleeding episodes. Compression therapy may slow the progression of lower-extremity varicose veins, and is useful for patients with upper-extremity involvement who have problems with edema.

We do not favor compression therapy for young children. In general, young children will not tolerate wearing a compression garment. They will rapidly outgrow the garment and the parents will become frustrated.

In general, a compression garment should extend from the tip of the toes to well above the involved site.

Removal of Varicose Veins. Unsightly or painful superficial varicose veins can be removed in selected patients. It is critical that the status and integrity of the deep venous system be established before superficial veins are removed. If the deep venous system is inadequate, the superficial veins should not be removed.

Epiphysiodesis. Epiphysiodeses are done to assure relatively equal leg lengths at full maturation. This procedure is necessary only if the projected limb-length discrepancy exceeds 2.0 cm. It is important that this operation be done at the appropriate time. Parents need to be reassured that the operation need not be done during early childhood. Most epiphysiodeses are done between 10 and 14 years of age. For limb-length discrepancies less than 2.0 cm, shoe lifts can be used.

Intentional destruction of growth plates also can be done to control excessive growth of digits.

Amputation and Ray Resection. Amputation of digits and portions of an extremity should be undertaken only to improve function of the extremity and to manage otherwise uncontrollable infection or bleeding. Many of these children manage to obtain excellent function from an extremity that is enlarged and malformed. An important dictum in managing these patients is to operate to improve function rather than for cosmesis and never to sacrifice function to obtain improved cosmesis.

Patients with discordant foot size may have difficulty fitting the foot into a shoe. We have found that ray resection is a very satisfactory procedure to reduce excessive foot width.

Debulking Procedures. The potential complications of debulking procedures should be considered carefully before undertaking this type of treatment. The potential drawbacks of debulking procedures include (1) the bulk can return, (2) the bulk is traded for a scar, (3) the debulking procedure may interrupt the venous and lymphatic drainage in an extremity with compromised drainage to begin with, (4) wound infection, and (5) poor skin healing with resultant chronic lymphatic ooze. In general, the more proximal on a extremity a debulking procedure is considered, the greater are the risks for interfering with venous and lymphatic drainage. Conversely, debulking procedures on digits, the hands, and feet are tolerated better than those on more proximal locations. As noted above, one must always consider function above form when contemplating surgical procedures for patients with KTS.

Laser Therapy. Laser therapy can be used to reduce the discoloration of capillary hemangiomas. Before embarking on this treatment, it must be remembered that the procedure is painful. Also, frequently it is the parent who opts to have the lesion treated, but it is the child who must undergo the discomfort. It may be preferable to wait until the child is old enough to participate in the decision.

Antibiotics. Antibiotics are used to treat cellulitis. For patients who have recurrent cellulitis, maintaining the patient on prophylactic antibiotics may be helpful.

Gastrointestinal Bleeding. Gastrointestinal bleeding can occur in patients with perirectal or pericolonic varicose veins. Bleeding can range from minimal to life-threatening. As with all cases of gastrointestinal bleeding, the source of bleeding needs to be defined. If the bleeding is secondary to varicose veins and is not life-threatening, treatment should consist of stool softeners and iron re-

placement. Surgery may be necessary to deal with massive recurrent bleeding.

KASABACH-MERRITT SYNDROME

Hemangiomas are the most frequently encountered tumors in childhood.[12,13] Typical progression of these tumors is one of rapid growth initially followed by slow, gradual involution.[14] In many instances the tumor, if small, recedes completely. In approximately 20% of cases the tumor may cause serious complications—for example, congestive heart failure secondary to arteriovenous shunting, vital organ impingement, and the Kasabach-Merritt syndrome. This syndrome is characterized by thrombocytopenia and localized consumptive coagulopathies associated with the hemangioma.[15] Giant angiomatous nevi may affect the lower extremities of children. Although the natural history of these giant angiomas is of spontaneous regression with thrombosis and subsequent fibrosis, the mortality in untreated cases may be 30%, coagulopathy being the major cause.[16,17] Simultaneous samples from the angioma and peripheral blood have indicated intense coagulopathy localized to the angioma involving both coagulation and fibrinolysis.[16] It is believed that endothelial abnormalities within the lesion cause thrombosis, with consumption of platelets and clotting factors.

Numerous pediatric cases have been described involving the soft tissues of the upper extremity, retroperitoneum, chest wall, scalp, neck, and scapula.[18,19] A 6-week-old girl with a large subcutaneous angiomatous nevus involving the left leg from midthigh to midcalf has been reported.[20]

As the Kasabach-Merritt syndrome is very rare and many forms of treatment have been used, assessment of efficacy of various treatments has been difficult. Surgery of the extremity is frequently complicated by uncontrolled bleeding.[21] Embolization has also involved numerous additional complications.[21] Systemic corticosteroids have been successful in reducing the size of angiomatous nevi and suppressing the coagulopathy. However, a prolonged course may be required.[17] In a recent review of 153 cases, radiation therapy in combination with steroids or surgery gave the best outcome.[16] Inhibitors of fibrinolysis, such as aminocaproic acid, often given with cryoprecipitate, have reduced the size of the angiomatous nevi and improved thrombocytopenia.[20] Aylett et al[20] have described the use of pneumatic compression in a 6-month-old infant with leg angiomatosis. Two blood pressure cuffs sewn together encircled the angiomatous nevus, held in place with a lightweight bandage. They were attached to a compression device, which provided intermittent pneumatic compression. This treatment can obviously be carried over a long period and has had some dramatic results. A recent report has described the use of α interferon in a full-term baby with a large flank hemangioma and life-threatening coagulopathy.[22]

TAKAYASU'S DISEASE

Takayasu's arteritis is a chronic inflammatory disease of unknown etiology that usually affects young Asian women, involving the aortic arch and the proximal portion of its major branches as well as the pulmonary arteries. Histologic changes consist of granulomatous inflammatory infiltrates involving the adventitia and the media of the artery and its branches with a picture of necrotizing arteritis. Inflammation usually leads to wall thickening and lumen stenosis or occlusion of the arteries involved.[23] Since Takayasu first described a case of pulseless disease with retinal changes in 1908, many series and cases have been reported in adults. There are few large series of cases in children. Although the most common presentations are in Asian females between ages 20 and 30 years, Hong et al[24] have reported on 70 cases seen in Korea between 1962 and 1980 in children. In this study[24] the youngest patient was a 3-year-old female; 81% of the patients were female, and the male-to-female ratio was 1:4.4. Six females presented at ages 4 years and under, twenty-five between 5 and 9 years, and twenty-six between 10 and 15 years. Six males presented between ages 5 and 9 years, and seven males between ages 10 and 15 years.[24]

The most common complaints were dyspnea, headache, palpitation, edema or puffy face, and generalized weakness. Five patients presented with intermittent claudication, four with abdominal pain, one with lower-extremity pain, and one with paralysis of the lower extremities.[24]

Compared with adults, where Takayasu's arteritis frequently involves the aortic arch and its vessels, the abdominal aorta with or without renal involvement was the most commonly involved site in pediatric patients[24] (Figs.

30-4 and 30-5). Because of these lesions, 93% of the pediatric patients had hypertension. Two cases of Takayasu's arteritis have been associated with nephrotic syndrome.[24]

Tuberculin skin testing was positive in 90% of the patients. The high frequency of tuberculin-positive hypersensitivity in children with Takayasu's arteritis has been noted previously.[24] The mechanism of the high association of a positive skin test in Takayasu's arteritis has not been elucidated. Coronary artery involvement[23,25] has been described, usually with narrowing of the coronary ostia, and the development of myocardial infarction and congestive heart failure.[23,25,26]

Morales et al[27] described 26 children from Mexico City with Takayasu's arteritis under 16 years of age. Arterial hypertension was found in 22 of the 26 cases. Interestingly, two thirds of the patients presented with congestive heart failure, and one third of the patients had limb claudication.

Children with Takayasu's arteritis may suffer an aggressive, often lethal illness, and a mortality rate of 35% to 40% has been described.[27,28] Gronemeyer and deMello[29] described Takayasu's disease in a 7-month-old infant with aneurysm of the right common iliac artery and an iliocaval fistula.

Sharma et al[30] described the sites of arterial involvement in 32 consecutive children studied with digital subtraction angiography. The mean age of 21 females and 11 males was 10.8 years. Aneurysms were uncommon (16% of the patients) and were usually small and saccular. Twenty-four had involvement of the abdominal aorta and

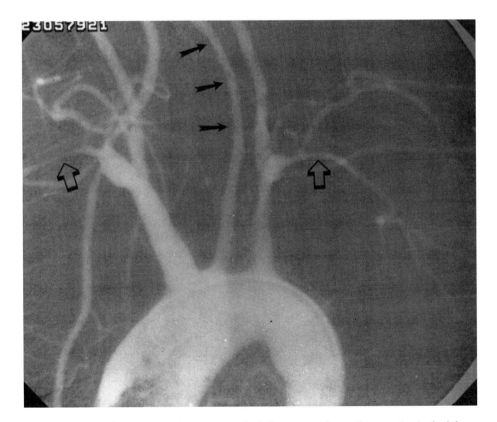

Fig. 30-4. Aortic arch angiogram demonstrates classic long areas of smooth narrowing in the left common carotid artery *(closed arrow)* and subclavian arteries *(open arrows).*

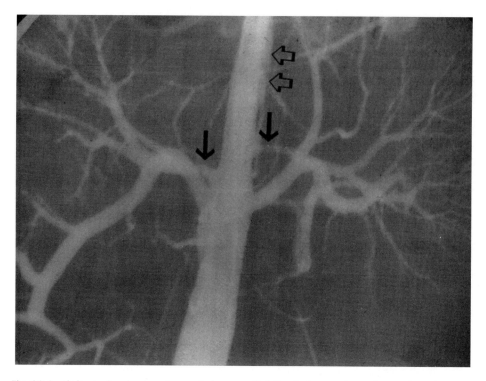

Fig. 30-5. Abdominal aortogram demonstrates a small abdominal aorta above the renal arteries *(open arrows)* with hypoplasia of the renal arteries *(closed arrows)*. The abdominal aorta with renal involvement is the most commonly involved site in pediatric patients.

four had involvement of the femoral artery. There was one aneurysm of the abdominal aorta, one in the left common iliac, and one in the right renal artery.[30]

Transluminal angioplasty was performed in eight patients, seven with proximally located renal artery stenosis and abdominal aortic stenosis in one patient. The initial success rate was 80%.

The management of these patients can be difficult. Steroids are still controversial; surgery (bypass operations) has shown good results in the majority of patients.[24] Percutaneous intertransluminal angioplasty as management of the arterial stenosis in Takayasu's arteritis has been effective in 65% to 80% of cases.[24,29] Its place in the management of this condition is yet to be established with short-term and long-term follow-up of these patients.

PERIPHERAL ARTERIAL VENOUS FISTULAS

Congenital arterial venous fistulas are abnormal vascular communications between high-pressure arterial and low-pressure venous channels. The clinical presentation in children is frequently associated with pain when the lesions occur on weight-bearing surfaces. Increased blood flow through an extremity fistula may improve oxygen delivery to the tissues, resulting in growth discrepancy between the normal and affected limbs, and cardiac output may be increased with subsequent congestive heart failure.[31] Ford et al[31] reviewed 26 patients, 11 males and 15 females with a mean age of 7.2 years, who had congenital peripheral arteriovenous malformations (AVMs). Lower-extremity lesions were most common (12), followed by upper extremity (8), shoulder girdle (3), and thorax and

neck (3). Seventeen of the twenty-six patients had lesions in more than one location. All patients presenting under 1 year of age had upper-extremity lesions. All patients between 5 and 10 years old had lower-extremity lesions.

The authors[31] concluded that neither surgery nor embolization alone offers cure to patients with congenital AVM. Fluoroscopic-directed transcatheter embolic techniques offered good tumor control and good cosmetic results with a minimum complication rate. Although all the patients undergoing embolization alone had residual disease, they were all functioning well.[31]

KAWASAKI SYNDROME (MUCOCUTANEOUS LYMPH NODE SYNDROME)

Kawasaki syndrome was first described by Thomas Saku Kawasaki in the Japanese medical literature in 1967, when he reported his experience from 1961 to 1967 with 50 children who manifested a distinctive clinical illness.[32] More than 105,000 cases of Kawasaki syndrome have now been recognized in Japan, and approximately 5,000 cases have been reported to the Centers for Disease Control and Prevention in Atlanta since 1976 in the United States.[33] Kawasaki syndrome appears now to have replaced acute rheumatic fever as the leading cause of acquired heart disease in children in the United States.[33] The incidence of the syndrome appears to be increasing in both Japan and the United States.[34]

Coronary artery involvement with its serious myocardial complications is a regular finding of Kawasaki syndrome.[35] Inflammation and resulting aneurysm formation in other medium-sized muscular arteries throughout the body occur in about 1% to 2% of patients in Japanese studies.[36,37] Complications seen in infants less than 7 months old, which appear to be more common in non-Asian than Asian children, are the development of peripheral ischemia of the hands and feet leading to dry gangrene and autoamputation.[38-44] Prostaglandin E[44] or repeated sympathetic blocks[39] have been reported as treatments of this complication, which may be due to vascular spasm, thrombosis and/or arteritis.

VENOUS THROMBOEMBOLIC COMPLICATIONS IN CHILDREN AND PULMONARY EMBOLISM

Deep venous thrombosis and pulmonary embolism are rare in children. From 1975 to 1991 a total of 308 children were reported to have deep venous thrombosis of the extremities or pulmonary embolism, or both, from Montreal, Quebec, and Hamilton, Ontario.[45] The children ranged in age from 2 months to 18 years, and essentially all of the patients with deep venous thrombosis (98%) had a serious underlying disorder or predisposing factor (Table 30-1). Twenty-six percent of the cases were secondary to the use of central venous catheters.

The authors identified 231 cases in the literature,[45] excluding reviews of autopsy series, that had deep venous thrombosis in the lower extremities. The clinical manifestations almost universally included pain and swelling in the affected extremity, occasionally fever, and abdominal or inguinal pain less frequently.[45] The cardinal signs and symptoms of pulmonary embolism in children are similar to those in adults; however, there may be less dyspnea and tachypnea in adolescents or young adults with pulmonary embolism and a higher incidence of signs and symptoms of deep venous thrombosis than in adult patients.[46,47] Ages of the patients with deep venous thrombosis in the leg or with pulmonary artery embolism ranged from 3 months to 18 years with a mean age of 13 years and an equal number of male and female patients.[45] The incidence appeared to increase during adolescence, and the cause was unknown. In one retrospective review of clinically diagnosed deep venous thrombosis in children, an incidence of 1.2 cases per 10,000 hospital admissions was reported.[48] Another study reported an incidence of pulmonary embolism of 7.8 cases per 10,000 hospital admissions in adolescents and young adults.[46]

The authors recommend treating pediatric patients with deep venous thrombosis and pulmonary embolism as aggressively as adults with heparin therapy followed by anticoagulant therapy, and in some patients thrombolytic therapy followed by anticoagulant therapy.[46] The authors recommend that streptokinase not be used[46] to reestablish catheter patency because of the possibility of allergic reactions with repeated doses. One common protocol is to instill 2 to 3 ml/hr of urokinase (5000 U/ml) for 2 to 4 hours. Another approach is to infuse urokinase at 150 U/kg/hr for 8 hours and reassess.

The risk factors for pulmonary embolism in children were recently described by Evans and Wilmott.[49] Risk factors in decreasing order of importance were (1) presence of a central venous catheter, (2) immobility, (3) congenital heart disease, (4) ventricular atrial shunt, (5) trauma, (6)

Table 30-1. Underlying Disorders or Other Predisposing Factors in Children and Adolescents with Venous Thrombosis in the Extremities or Pulmonary Embolism or Both (n = 308)

Disorder or Other Factor	Subjects	
	No.	%
Indwelling catheter	65	21.1
Surgery	40	13.0
Trauma	27	8.8
Systemic lupus erythematosus	23	7.5
Infection	19	6.2
Tumor	18	5.8
None or unknown	17	5.5
Total parenteral nutrition	17	5.5
Disorder of hemostasis causing predisposition to thrombosis	12	3.9
Athletic activity	11	3.6
Leukemia	9	2.9
Nephrotic syndrome	9	2.9
Estrogen use	7	2.3
Obesity	6	2.0
Ulcerative colitis; other enteropathy	6	2.0
Paralysis	5	1.6
Immobilization	4	1.3
Abortion	2	0.7
Homocystinuria	2	0.7
Pregnancy	2	0.7
Ventriculoatrial shunt	2	0.7
Hemolytic anemia	1	0.3
Hughes-Stovin syndrome	1	0.3
Hydrocephalus	1	0.3
Sickle cell anemia	1	0.3
Vascular malformation	1	0.3

neoplasm, (7) operation, (8) infection, (9) medical illness, (10) dehydration, (11) shock, and (12) obesity.

MOYAMOYA DISEASE

Moyamoya disease is a rare chronic occlusive cerebrovascular disorder characterized by progressive stenosis of the arteries of the circle of Willis. Initially this stenosis involves the intracranial carotid arteries bilaterally. It may progress to involve both the middle cerebral and posterior cerebral arteries. An abnormal capillary network develops at the base of the brain, which the Japanese first characterized in 1969 as "moyamoya disease" because the word "moyamoya" describes the "hazy puff of smoke" appearance of the abnormal capillary vessels at the base of the skull[50,51] (Fig. 30-6). The cause of moyamoya disease is unknown. The formation of the abnormal small moyamoya vessels distal to the narrowing of the carotid arteries is now considered a secondary process in the development of collateral circulation.[52,53]

In children the usual manifestations are transient ischemic attacks, strokes, and seizures.[51] The mortality rate

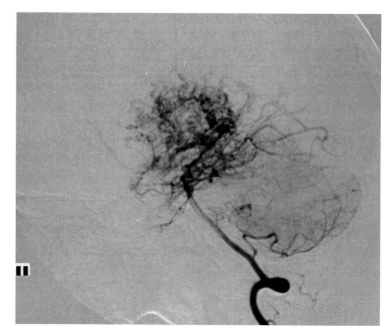

Fig. 30-6. Cerebral angiogram demonstrates the abnormal capillary vessels at the base of the skull, giving the appearance of a puff of smoke.

described for children is 4.3%.[51] The cause of death was intracranial bleeding in five of nine children (55.5%).[51] AVMs are rarely associated with moyamoya disease.[51]

Three major surgical techniques are employed in the treatment of this condition. Direct anastomosis, such as a superficial temporal artery to middle cerebral artery bypass can be effective for revascularization of the brain.[51] Encephaloduroarteriosynangiosis (EDAS) is a procedure in which the superficial temporal artery is sutured along the longitudinal dural defect to approximate the artery to the brain surface. Encephalomyosynangiosis (EMS) is a surgical technique where the temporal muscle is sutured, approximating the muscle to the surface of the brain.[51] Both EMS and EDAS are indirect anastomotic procedures; the goal is to develop neovascularization from the extracranial arterial and soft tissue system to the ischemic brain.[51] These procedures are easier and safer than the superficial temporal artery to middle cerebral artery anastomosis, especially in small children.

In 1992 Karasawa, Touho, and Ohnishi[54] reported a series of 104 children with moyamoya disease treated with superficial temporal artery to middle cerebral artery anastomosis, or EMS, or both, with a follow-up of almost 10 years. Surgical results were excellent[54] with the incidence of transient ischemic attacks and major strokes substantially reduced and intellectual function maintained. Kinugasa et al[55] recently described a combined procedure of EDAS and EMS with good surgical results.

STROKE

Cerebrovascular disease, although a rare entity in the pediatric population, has been well documented in infants and children since the seventeenth century. Initially all cases of pediatric stroke, regardless of presentation or etiology, were grouped together and reported.[56-61] In 1927 Ford and Schaffer published the first study that analyzed the etiology of each case of stroke in a pediatric population.

Table 30-2. Age Distribution of 61 Patients, Age 21 Years or Less, with Stroke

Age (Yr)	Male	Female	Total
0-4	8	5	13
4-10	6	5	11
10-16	11	4	15
17-21	7	15	22
			61

During the next decade postmortem reports describing pediatric cerebral infarcts were available.[57-61] By the 1950s extensive investigations were being conducted evaluating specific variables (i.e., clinical presentation, age, autopsy findings).[57-61]

Although not a common pediatric problem—the average incidence rate being 2.52 cases per 100,000 per year[57-61]—given the tremendous potential for disability and the need to identify risk factors as early as possible, pediatric stroke warrants investigation and discussion.

Demographics

Between 1973 and 1989 61 patients ranging in age from 3 days to 21 years (mean, 20.9 years) presented to the Cleveland Clinic Foundation with evidence of a stroke (Table 30-2). Fifty-two percent (32 of 61) were males and forty-eight percent (29 of 61) were females. This is comparable to a 1983 Swedish study[57] extending over a decade in which 27 pediatric stroke victims were evaluated with 52% (14 of 27) being male and 48% (13 of 27) being female, ranging in age from 6 months to 15 years. Racial distribution in our series was as follows: 88% (54 of 61) white and 12% (7 of 61) black. Gender distribution in each racial group was as follows: 54% white male (29 of 54) and 48%

white female (25 of 54); 46% black male (3 of 7) and 57% black female (4 of 7).

Age distribution (Table 30-2) revealed a preponderance in males 10 to 16 years (11 of 32) and in females 17 to 21 years (15 of 29). Over 50% of females in our population were over the age of 17 years, which may be a reflection of tobacco use, substance abuse, or use of birth control pills. In the Bogousslavsky and Regli[62] study on ischemic stroke in adults less than 30 years of age, up to two thirds of females were using birth control pills. Two of our female patients were known to be taking birth control pills at the time of stroke.

Presentation

As in the adult population, cerebrovascular disease in children can be manifested as various neurologic changes, depending on the site of the central nervous system involved. But unlike adults, atherosclerosis and hypertension are not commonly present in the pediatric population. In addition, no data are available indicating these risk factors are antecedents of childhood stroke.[59]

Clinical signs and symptoms occurred either as isolated findings or more commonly in combination. In Table 30-3 one or more of the clinical findings were present in any given patient.

In our study the most common presentation, seen in 80% of patients, was hemiparesis (left in 43% and right in 57%). In contrast, in the Eeg-Olofsson study[57] 67% (18 of 27) presented with hemiplegia, and disturbance of consciousness occurred in 70% (19 of 27).

Other common signs included cranial nerve palsy 51% (with facial nerve affected in 18 patients), aphasia 38%, paresthesia 31%, and visual changes 23% (most commonly as visual field cuts with two patients experiencing complete loss of vision). Seizures were part of the presentation in seven patients. Headache, coma, dysarthria, and ataxia were less common findings.

Head computed tomography (CT) was the most frequently performed study (59 of 61 patients) with a yield of 78% (46 of 59); radiographic findings correlated with clinical findings in all cases (Table 30-4). Head magnetic resonance imaging (MRI) gave a higher yield of 84% but was performed on only 25 patients. In 7 patients with a normal head CT scan, MRI was positive. An electroencephalogram was abnormal in 58% (26 of 45) of cases, but in general the results were nonspecific.

Etiology

Stroke in adults is most commonly related to underlying disease such as hypertension or arteriosclerosis. In children these are rare disorders, therefore the focus of predisposing factors shifts. Nine etiologic categories were defined in our study group: (1) preexisting cardiac disease, (2) vascular abnormalities, (3) underlying malignancy, (4) complicated migraine, (5) history of trauma, (6) hematologic abnormality, (7) substance abuse, (8) infection, and (9) idiopathic (Table 30-5).

Congenital Heart Disease

Congenital heart disease occurs in 8 to 10 per 1000 live births. In previously reported studies cerebrovascular dis-

Table 30-3. Clinical Presentation of Stroke in 61 Patients Age 21 Years or Less

Clinical Presentation	No.
Hemiparesis	49
Left	21
Right	28
Cranial nerve palsy	31
VII	18
III	4
VI, IX, and/or XII	6
V, X, and/or XI	3
Aphasia	23
Paresthesias	19
Visual changes	14
Right VF cut	6
Left VF cut	4
Loss of vision	2
Blurred vision	1
Diplopia	1
Seizure	7
GTC	3
Focal	4
Headache	6
Coma	6
Dysarthria	3
Ataxia	5

VF, Visual field; *GTC*, Generalized tonic clonic.

Table 30-4. Diagnostic Studies Performed in 61 Patients, Age 21 Years or Less, with Stroke

Diagnostic Study	No. Performed	No. Positive/ Abnormal
Head CT	59	46
ECHO	46	8
EEG	45	26
Cerebral angiogram	40	28
Brain MRI	25	21
Cardiac catheterization	3	2

CT, computed tomography; *ECHO*, echocardiography; *EEG*, electroencephalogram.

ease associated with congenital heart disease may result from several different processes—that is, embolism, thrombosis (arterial or venous), polycythemia (secondary to decreased Pao_2), dehydration, congestive heart failure, and intracerebral hemorrhage, which is usually related to hemostasis defects, telangiectasias, or aneurysm.[59] In addition, open heart surgery to correct congenital heart disease may result in stroke perioperatively due to air, calcium, fibrin, or fat emboli, hypotension and/or hypocarbia (secondary to decreased cerebrovascular blood flow during surgery).[59]

In the Mayo Clinic experience, early in life the risk of stroke in children with congenital heart disease is 5% if a

Table 30-5. Possible Etiology for Stroke in 61 Patients Age 21 Years or Less

Etiology	No.	%
Cardiac—congenital heart disease*	10	16
Vascular abnormalities*	8	13
Underlying malignancy	6	10
Complicated migraine	5	8
Trauma	6	10
Blood dyscrasias	2	3
Substance abuse*	2	3
Infection	1	2
Idiopathic	23	38

*Two patients repeated in these categories.

right-to-left shunt is present and 2% if no shunt is present.[59] In patients with patent foramen ovale or atrial septal defect, a left-to-right shunt may change to a right-to-left shunt with the Valsalva maneuver, with the potential for a paradoxic embolus to the brain. In such patients pulmonary emboli or venous thrombosis may precede the event.[63,64]

Vascular Abnormalities

Structural abnormalities of the internal carotid artery system and intracranial vessels may predispose to stroke in children. Among these are agenesis or hypoplasia of the internal carotid artery, kinks and coils of the internal carotid artery, aneurysm, AVM, and vein of Galen aneurysm.[59] Aneurysms may be either venous or arterial. In general, arterial intracranial aneurysms are less common in children than adults. Their association with polycystic kidney disease and coarctation of the aorta is well documented.[59] In our study three patients presented with intracranial aneurysms.

As in aneurysms, AVMs may present as intracranial hemorrhage. The heralding feature may be seizure or neurologic deficit. The vein of Galen aneurysm, a misnomer, is actually an enlarged vein from a deep midline AVM. Typically one or more branches of the carotid or vertebral circulation—most commonly the posterior communicating artery—communicates directly with this vein. A vein of Galen aneurysm may present in any age group but commonly presents in the newborn with high-output congestive heart failure.

Underlying Malignancy

Malignancy may result in or present as a stroke via various mechanisms including hypercoagulability. Intracranial hemorrhage occurs in up to 10% of patients with leukemia,[65] either from severe thrombocytopenia caused by chemotherapy or drug-resistant disease, or from increased blood viscosity associated with extreme leukocytosis in the acute stage of the disease. Primary brain tumors or metastatic lesions may result in secondary hemorrhage, increased intracranial pressure secondary to mass effect, or subdural hematoma.

Complicated Migraine

More than 40 years ago Wolff formulated his classic theory of migraine consisting of a prodrome due to intracranial vasoconstriction followed by headache due to extracranial vasodilatation. Both of the preceding events can be associated with severe head pain secondary to muscle tension.[66] Migraine is a common disease with stroke being the most frequent serious complication of the prodrome phase. It has been suggested that 15% to 30% of patients with stroke have a history of migraine headaches.[67,68] A neurologic deficit may be the result of cerebral ischemia or infarction secondary to vasospasm of cerebral arteries during the migraine crisis. In a paper on migraine stroke, Bogousslavsky[69] points out that patients with migraine also frequently have mitral valve prolapse (MVP). Since stroke in young patients may be due to emboli originating from MVP, strokes in migraine patients may also be embolic from the heart.[70] Patients frequently have recurring episodes.[71]

In our series three out of five patients were female. Three of these five patients had a positive family history of migraine; it is unknown whether there was a similar history of stroke in family members. In all cases there was eventual resolution of the neurologic deficits.

Trauma

Head trauma or injury to the carotid artery secondary to a fall may result in cerebral ischemia or internal carotid artery thrombosis. Typically trauma to the carotid artery produces an intimal tear, leading to dissection with subsequent vessel thrombosis. Because of this scenario onset of neurologic signs tends to be delayed, usually 2 to 24 hours.[65] Most commonly this occurs from falling on a stick held in the mouth, producing intraoral trauma.[65] A basilar skull fracture can be complicated by laceration of the carotid artery.[65] Of note, fat emboli only infrequently cause neurologic symptoms; such emboli tend to pass through the brain and become lodged in the pulmonary vasculature by unclear mechanisms.[59]

Blood Dyscrasias

Sickle cell anemia, hemophilia, idiopathic thrombocytopenic purpura, thrombotic thrombocytopenic purpura, hemolytic uremic syndrome,[72] thrombocytosis, and infections (vasculitis, disseminated intravascular coagulation, emboli, hemorrhages) are among the hematologic abnormalities that may predispose to the development of stroke.[59] In our study only two patients were in this category. Acute hemiplegia in children has also been associated with thrombocytosis following an acute infectious process.[59]

Substance Abuse

The relationship of drug use to the development of neurologic sequelae remains controversial. The four types of vascular problems found to occur are thrombosis, vasculitis, embolism, and hemorrhage. Thrombosis has been shown to occur in patients using lysergic acid diethylamide (LSD) or heroin by vasoconstriction or vascular hypersensitivity, respectively.[59] Necrotizing angiitis has been demonstrated in patients with a history of amphetamine use alone or in combination with LSD or heroin.[59] Cerebral emboli occur, though rarely, in subacute bacterial endocarditis associated with intravenous drug abuse.[59] In addition, intracerebral and subarachnoid hemorrhages have been identified in intravenous drug abusers.

Infection

Either local or systemic infectious processes may result in pediatric stroke. Vasculitis, resulting in ischemia or vessel thrombosis, disseminated intravascular coagulation, emboli, and hemorrhage, as occurs with rupture of a mycotic aneurysm, are possible mechanisms.[59] Arteritis secondary to meningitis may cause thrombosis of intracranial arteries. Also, thrombophlebitis of cerebral veins or dural sinuses may occur in purulent meningitis or following otitis media, mastoiditis, sinusitis, and local scalp and face infections.[65] Only one patient fell into this category in our study group.

Idiopathic

There were 10 patients in the idiopathic group, ranging in age from 3 days to 10 years with a mean of 4.3 years. There were six males and four females. Six of the patients had been known to have a seizure disorder, but there was no family history of stroke and no history of peripheral vascular disease, syncope, or hypertension. Diagnostic studies were negative for an etiologic cause for a stroke.

Because of the previous reported relationship of hyperlipidemia and unexplained stroke,[73-75] we measured lipid levels in 9 of the 10 patients. Total cholesterol was measured in 8 patients in this group and was found to be elevated in 6. Total triglycerides were measured in 7 patients and were found to be elevated in 6 (85%). High-density lipoprotein (HDL) cholesterol was measured in 6 patients and was low in 4 (67%).

Lipid studies were also done on all the family members of 5 of these patients. A total of 17 members were studied. Total cholesterol was found to be elevated in 5 of 17 or 30%. Triglyceride levels were elevated in 4 of 17 (23%). Total HDL cholesterol was normal in all 17 family members; however, HDL-2 was low in 8 of 17 family members (47%). This subfraction has been shown to be associated with early and severe coronary atherosclerosis in patients in our institution.

In most pediatric stroke patients an etiology can be identified using standard testing. In one third of our series the etiology was unknown. Hyperlipidemia may represent a risk factor for stroke in childhood. Low HDL cholesterol levels and elevated triglyceride and cholesterol appear to be the most common lipid abnormalities. Whether early identification and treatment of families at risk for developing stroke would decrease the incidence of this disabling disorder in children remains uncertain. Whether abnormal lipid values are markers for stroke or are secondary events is unclear, but the question demands further study.

REFERENCES

1. Stickler G: Klippel-Trenaunay syndrome. In Gomez M, ed: Neurocutaneous diseases, a practical approach, Boston, 1987, Butterworths.
2. Baskerville P, Ackroyd J, and Browse N: The etiology of the Klippel-Trenaunay syndrome, Ann Surg 202:624, 1985.
3. Aelvoet G, Jorens P, and Roelen L: Genetic aspects of the Klippel-Trenaunay syndrome, Br J Dermatol 126:603, 1992.
4. Jorgenson R et al: Prenatal diagnosis of the Klippel-Trenaunay-Weber syndrome, Prenat Diagn 14:989, 1994.
5. Happle R: Lethal Henes surviving by mosaicism: a possible explanation for sporadic birth defects involving the skin, J Am Acad Dermatol 16:899, 1987.
6. Gloviczki P et al: Klippel-Trenaunay syndrome: the risks and benefits of vascular interventions, Surgery 110:469, 1991.
7. Browse N et al: Klippel-Trenaunay syndrome. In Browse N et al: Diseases of the veins, pathology, diagnosis and treatment, Baltimore, Williams & Wilkins, 1988.
8. Stewart G and Farmer G: Sturge-Weber and Klippel-Trenaunay syndromes with absence of inferior vena cava, Arch Dis Child 65:546, 1990.
9. Deutsch J et al: Combination of the syndrome of Sturge-Weber and the syndrome of Klippel-Trenaunay, Klin Paediatr 188:464, 1976.
10. Brod R et al: Unusual retinal and renal vascular lesions in the Klippel-Trenaunay-Weber syndrome, Retina 12:355, 1992.
11. D'Amico J et al: Klippel-Trenaunay coagulation and massive osteolysis, Cleve Clin Q 44:181, 1977.
12. Brown SH, Neerhou RC, and Fonkalsrude: Prednisone therapy in the management of large hemangiomas in infants and children, Surgery 71:168, 1972.
13. Enjolras O et al: Management of alarming hemangiomas in infancy: a review of 25 cases, Pediatrics 85:494, 1990.
14. Hurvitz CH et al: Cyclophosphamide therapy in life-threatening vascular tumors, J Pediatr 109:360, 1986.
15. Kasabach HH and Merritt KK: Capillary hemangioma with extensive purpura (report of a case), Am J Dis Child 59:1063, 1940.
16. El-Dessouky M et al: Kasabach-Merritt syndrome, J Pediatr Surg 23:109, 1988.
17. Neidhert JA and Roach RW: Successful treatment of skeletal hemangioma and Kasabach-Merritt syndrome with amino-caproic acid, Am J Med 73:434, 1982.
18. Henley JD et al: Kasabach-Merritt syndrome with profound platelet support, Am J Clin Pathol 99:628, 1993.
19. Zukerberg LR, Nickoloff BJ, and Weiss SW: Kaposiform hemangioendothelioma of infancy and childhood, Am J Surg Pathol 17:321, 1993.
20. Aylett SE et al: The Kasabach-Merritt syndrome: treatment with intermittent pneumatic compression, Arch Dis Child 65:790, 1990.
21. Varsenialar SEN et al: Kasabach-Merritt syndrome: therapeutic consideration, Pediatrics 79:971, 1987.
22. Hatley RM et al: Successful management of an infant with a giant hemangioma of the retroperitoneum and Kasabach-Merritt syndrome with alpha-interferon, J Pediatr Surg 28:1356, 1993.
23. Basso C et al: Sudden cardiac arrest in a teenager as first manifestation of Takayasu's disease, Int J Cardiol 43:87, 1994.
24. Hong CY et al: Takayasu arteritis in Korean children: clinical report of seventy cases, Heart Vessels 7(suppl):91, 1992.
25. Chiasson DA et al: Acute heart failure in an 8-year-old diabetic girl, J Pediatr 116:472, 1993.
26. Seguchi M et al: Ostial stenosis of the left coronary artery as a sole clinical manifestation of Takayasu's arteritis: a possible cause of unexpected sudden death, Heart Vessels 5:188, 1990.
27. Morales E et al: Takayasu's arteritis in children, J Rheumatol 18:1081, 1991.

28. Lee S, Young S, and Yee H: Primary arteritis pulseless disease in Korean children, Acta Pediatr Scand 56:526, 1967.

29. Gronemeyer PS and deMello DE: Takayasu's disease with aneurysm of right common iliac artery and iliocaval fistula in a young infant: case report and review of the literature, Pediatrics 69:626, 1982.

30. Sharma S et al: Non-specific aorto-arteritis (Takayasu's disease) in children, Br J Radiol 64:690, 1991.

31. Ford EG et al: Peripheral congenital arterial venous fistulae: observe, operate, or obturate, J Pediatr Surg 27:714, 1992.

32. Kawasaki T: Acute febrile mucocutaneous syndrome with lymphoid involvement with specific desquamation of the fingers and toes in children (in Japanese), Jpn J Allergy 16:178, 1967.

33. Taubert KA et al: A U.S. nationwide hospital survey of Kawasaki's disease in acute rheumatic fever 1984-1987, Presented at the 29th Interscience Conference on Antimicrobial Agents of Chemotherapy, Houston, Tex, September 1989.

34. Nakamura Y, Fujita Y, and Nagai M: Epidemiology of Kawasaki's disease in Japan (1988), Presented at the Third International Kawasaki's Disease Symposium, Tokyo, Japan, December, 1988.

35. Tanaka N, Sekimoto K, and Naoe S: Kawasaki's disease: relationship with infantile periarteritis nodosa, Arch Pathol Lab Med 100:81, 1976.

36. Suzuki A et al: Coronary artery lesions of Kawasaki's disease. Cardiac catheterization findings of 100 cases, Pediatr Cardiol 7:3, 1986.

37. Tako H, Inoue O, and Akaji T: Kawasaki disease: cardiac problems and management, Pediatr Rev 9:209, 1988.

38. Ames EL et al: Bilateral hand necrosis in Kawasaki's syndrome, J Hand Surg 10A:391, 1985.

39. Edwards W and Burney RG: Use of repeated nerve blocks in management of an infant with Kawasaki's disease, Anesth Analog 67:1008, 1988.

40. Fukushige J, Nihill MR, and McNamara DG: Spectrum of cardiovascular lesion in mucocutaneous lymph node syndrome: analysis of eight cases, Am J Cardiol 45:98, 1980.

41. Kainou Y et al: Case of Kawasaki's disease with gangrene on the left fourth and fifth fingers (in Japanese), J Jpn Pediatr Soc 88:1184, 1984.

42. Teixeira O, Pong AH, and Blad P: Amputating gangrene in Kawasaki's disease, Can Med Assn J 127:132, 1982.

43. Trumble T and Fitch RD: Kawasaki's disease: a cause of vasculitis in children, J Pediatr Orthop 6:92, 1986.

44. Westphalen MA et al: Kawasaki disease with severe peripheral ischemia: treatment with prostaglandin E$_1$ infusion, J Pediatr 112:431, 1988.

45. David M and Andrew M: Venous thromboembolic complications in children, J Pediatr 123:337, 1993.

46. Bernstein D, Coupey S, and Schonberg SK: Pulmonary embolism in adolescents, Am J Dis Child 140:667, 1986.

47. Green RM et al: Pulmonary embolism in younger patients, Chest 101:1507, 1992.

48. Wise RC and Todd JK: Spontaneous lower extremity venous thrombosis in children, Am J Dis Child 126:766, 1973.

49. Evans DA and Wilmott RW: Laboratory medicine II, Pediatr Clin North Am 41:569, 1994.

50. Suzuki J and Takaku A: Cerebral vascular "Moya Moya disease": disease showing abnormal net-like vessels in base of brain, Arch Neurol 20:288, 1969.

51. Ueki K, Meyer FB, and Mellinger JS: Moya Moya disease: the disorder in surgical treatment, Mayo Clin Proc 69:749, 1994.

52. Kudo T: Spontaneous occlusion of the circle of Willis. A disease apparently confined to Japanese, Neurology 18:485, 1968.

53. Suzuki J: Moya Moya disease, Berlin, 1986, Springer-Verlag.

54. Karasawa J, Touho H, and Ohnishi H: Long-term follow-up study after extracranial intercranial bypass surgery for anterior circulation ischemia in childhood Moya Moya disease, J Neurosurg 77:84, 1992.

55. Kinugasa K et al: Surgical treatment of Moya Moya disease: operative technique for encephalo-duro-arterio-myosynangiosis, its follow-up, clinical results, and angiograms, Neurosurgery 32:527, 1993.

56. Adams HP, Butler MJ, and Biller J: Non-hemorrhagic cerebral infarction in young adults, Arch Neurol 43:793, 1986.

57. Eeg-Olofsson O and Ringheim Y: Stroke in children. Clinical characteristics and prognosis, Acta Paediatr Scand 72:1982.

58. Hilton-Jones D and Warlow CP: The causes of stroke in the young, J Neurol 232:137, 1985.

59. Saha AL et al: Report of the Joint Committee for Stroke Facilities. IX. Strokes in children (Part I), Washington, DC, 1973, US Department of Health, Education, and Welfare, Health Resources Administration.

60. Saha AL, Huber WV, and Greenhouse AH: Report of the Joint Committee for Stroke Facilities. IX. Strokes in children (Part II), Washington, DC, 1973, U.S. Department of Health, Education, and Welfare, Health Resources Administration.

61. Schoenberg BS, Mellinger JF, and Schoenberg DG: Cerebrovascular disease in infants and children: a study of incidence, clinical features, and survival, Neurology 28:763, 1978.

62. Bogousslavsky J and Regli F: Ischemic stroke in adults younger than 30 years of age, Arch Neurol 44:479, 1987.

63. Jones HR et al: Cerebral emboli of paradoxical origin, Ann Neurol 13:314, 1983.

64. Alexander J et al: A 'functional murmur' and stroke in a young adult, Arch Intern Med 143:519, 1983.

65. Swaiman KF: Pediatric neurology principles and practice, St Louis, 1989, CV Mosby.

66. Plum F, ed: Hemiplegic migraine and focal ischemia, Neurol Alert 6:19, 1988.

67. Henrich JB: The association between migraine and cerebral vascular events: an analytical review, J Chron Dis 40:329, 1987.

68. Pereira P et al: Migraine and cerebral infarction: three case studies, Headache 429, 1985.

69. Bogousslavsky J et al: Migraine stroke, Neurology 38:223, 1988.

70. Boughner DR et al: Incidence of mitral valve prolapse in patients with stroke, Abstracts of the 51st Scientific Sessions II-57:213, 1970.

71. Rothrock JF et al: Mitral valve prolapse and ischemic stroke in the young, Abstracts of the 61st Scientific Sessions II-601:2398, 1988.

72. Trevathan E and Dooling EC: Large thrombotic strokes in hemolytic-uremic syndrome, J Pediatr 111:863, 1987.

73. Glueck CJ, Daniels SR, and Bates S: Pediatric victims of unexplained stroke and their families: familial lipid and lipoprotein abnormalities, Pediatrics 69:308, 1982.

74. Kannel WB, Gordon T, and Bawber TR: Role of lipids in the development of brain infarction: the Framingham Study in stroke, Stroke 5:679, 1974.

75. Mathew NT et al: Hyperlipoproteinemia in occlusive cerebrovascular disease, JAMA 232:262, 1975.

CHAPTER THIRTY-ONE

THORACIC OUTLET SYNDROMES

Edwin G. Beven

The thoracic outlet syndromes are a group of disorders that produce symptoms affecting the neck, shoulder, and upper extremity by compression or mechanical irritation of the brachial plexus, subclavian artery, or subclavian vein as these structures pass through the thoracic outlet (Fig. 31-1). The syndromes are divided into three types—neurologic, arterial, and venous—based on the predominant structure compromised. The neurologic type is the most common type, accounting for 95% of all thoracic outlet patients, and results from compression of elements of the brachial plexus. It occurs mainly in young to middle-aged adults from their second to fifth decade with a 3:1 predominance in women. The arterial type is the least common, accounting for 1% to 2% of all thoracic outlet patients, but it is the most serious. It can produce arterial lesions with thromboembolic complications that can jeopardize the viability of the upper extremity. The venous type is caused by compression of the subclavian vein and accounts for about 3% to 4% of all thoracic outlet patients. It is most commonly observed from the third to the fourth decade and is more prevalent in men. A small number of patients have symptoms of compression of more than one of these structures, exhibiting a combination of symptoms.

The thoracic outlet syndrome has been surrounded by confusion, misconceptions, and controversy regarding etiology, diagnosis, and methods of treatment.[1-6] Thus depending on the (attributed) offending structure or the provocative maneuver thought to cause compression of the neurovascular structures in the cervical-axillary canal, the thoracic outlet syndrome has been known in the past as *cervical rib syndrome*[7]; *scalenus anticus syndrome, Naffziger's syndrome*[8,9]; *first thoracic rib syndrome*[10]; *costoclavicular syndrome*[11-13]; and *hyperabduction syndrome*.[14] Peet et al, in 1956, recommended that all of these clinical entities be grouped together as the *thoracic outlet syndrome*.[15] Two years later Rob and Standeven referred to it as the *thoracic outlet compression syndrome* in describing arterial complications of the syndrome.[16] During the last three decades the term *thoracic outlet syndrome* has become the accepted name, but its plural, *thoracic outlet syndromes*, is

probably a better term because it denotes more than one group or subdivision.[4]

Paralleling the historic development of the differently named syndromes that describe the cause of the compression of the neurovascular bundle, surgical treatment was directed at the presumed corresponding offending anatomic structure by excision of the cervical rib,[17] first thoracic rib,[18] or by division of the anterior scalene muscle[19] or the pectoralis minor tendon.[20]

Although there has been general agreement regarding the etiology, diagnosis, and treatment of the arterial and venous thoracic outlet syndromes—the least common—much of the controversy surrounding the subject of thoracic outlet syndrome has centered around the diagnosis and treatment of the neurologic type, which paradoxically is most commonly diagnosed. The vague and diffuse pattern of pain that lacks accepted neuroanatomic basis, the absence of objective findings or diagnostic confirmatory tests, and the lack of agreement as to its management form the basis of this continued controversy. The neurologic thoracic outlet syndrome is accepted as a definite syndrome by those who treat it surgically,[21-26] but is seriously questioned by many neurologists and others who label it "disputed" thoracic outlet syndrome,[2,27] and still others deny its existence.[28]

NEUROLOGIC TYPE

Etiology

The anatomic abnormalities in the thoracic outlet that can cause neurologic symptoms are various skeletal or soft tissue abnormalities that compress, displace, or irritate the brachial plexus as it exits between the anterior and middle scalene muscles (Fig. 31-1). Although the most obvious and easily detected of these are diverse osseous abnormalities (i.e., cervical ribs, elongated transverse process of C7 vertebra with its fibrous band that functionally acts as a cervical rib, hypoplasia or anomalies of the first thoracic rib, and abnormal callous formation or angulation from

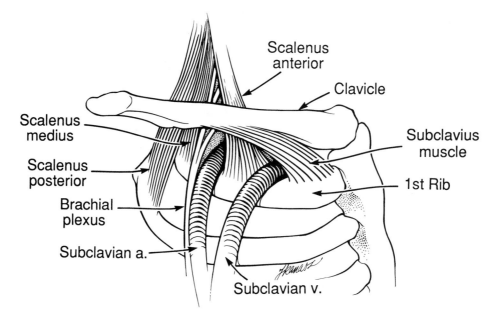

Fig. 31-1. Schematic drawing of the right thoracic outlet. The subclavian artery and brachial plexus exit through the scalene triangle, bordered by the anterior and middle scalene muscles and the first rib. The subclavian vein crosses the first rib between the anterior scalene and subclavius muscles anteriorly.

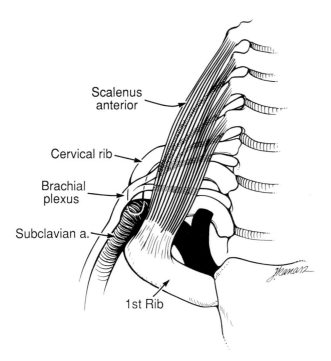

Fig. 31-2. Schematic drawing of the right cervicoaxillary region, demonstrating the usual anatomic position of a cervical rib coursing underneath the lower trunks of the brachial plexus and compressing the subclavian artery against the anterior scalene muscles. Note the presence of poststenotic dilation of the subclavian artery.

clavicular or first rib fractures), these congenital and acquired abnormalities account for only 10% of all causes of thoracic outlet syndrome[28] (Fig. 31-2). In contrast, the more common soft tissue structural changes in the thoracic outlet, such as various congenital myofascial bands or anomalies of the scalene muscles[21,22,28] that compress the brachial plexus, are more elusive because their contribution to the clinical syndrome can be inferred only from the symptoms they produce and can be recognized only by the surgeon at operation.

Roos[30] has identified 10 different congenital fibromuscular bands that compress the brachial plexus at its lower C8 and T1 nerves and 7 other anomalies of the anterior scalene muscle that encroach on the brachial plexus at its upper C5, C6, and C7 nerves. Undoubtedly there are factors other than congenital anomalies that trigger the symptoms of thoracic outlet syndrome, in order to explain why the onset of symptoms often occurs during a patient's third and fourth decades. Postural changes, such as drooping shoulders and those associated with activities involving arm elevation above the shoulders, are probably important. The fact that a significant number of patients develop symptoms of thoracic outlet syndrome following hyperextension injuries of the neck may be attributed to stretch injury of the scalene muscles, with resultant edema, hemorrhage, and spasm. Eventually muscle fibrosis may occur, which in turn can entrap the brachial plexus and cause symptoms of thoracic outlet syndrome.[8,23] Using histochemical stains, histologic abnormalities of the scalene muscles in these patients have been observed.[31-32] The significance of these findings remains unclear.

Clinical Manifestations

Pain and paresthesias of the neck and upper limb are the most prominent symptoms. The pain is variously described as aching or throbbing, but rarely as burning. It is of variable intensity and commonly insidious in onset, with various degrees of progression and severity. The pain is frequently aggravated by activity, especially that involving arm elevation above the shoulders. It may last for hours after the physical activity has ceased.

Roos has described two separate patterns of distribution of pain.[33] The more common pattern is that associated with compression of the *lower* nerves of the brachial plexus (C8 and T1) that eventually form the ulnar nerve. The pain is described in the infraclavicular and supraclavicular areas; in the posterior aspect of the neck, down the upper back medial to the scapula and down the medial aspect of the arm; and in the forearm and hand to the fourth and fifth fingers. The intensity of the pain may vary in different areas. Paresthesias along the ulnar nerve distribution to the hand and medial two fingers are frequently associated with this neurologic type. The paresthesias at times can affect all the fingers. Weakness of the arm and hand can also accompany this pattern. These symptoms are commonly aggravated by arm activity and especially with activity above the head. Nocturnal exacerbation of pain or numbness is common.

The second pattern of pain distribution is that attributed to compression or irritation of the *upper* nerves of the brachial plexus (C5, C6, and C7). The pain is commonly described in the anterolateral aspect of the neck, extending at times from the upper anterior chest to the mandible, face, and temporal and occipital areas of the head. It can also extend to the scapular and deltoid regions and down the lateral aspect of the arm and forearm to the dorsal surface of the hand between the thumb and index fingers. A third pattern of pain distribution involves a combination of the *upper and lower* brachial plexus involvement. From a therapeutic point of view it is important to identify each of these patterns so that appropriate surgical treatment can be tailored specifically to each group.[24-25,33]

In more than half the patients with thoracic outlet syndome, the symptoms appear to follow an injury to the neck or upper back, commonly of the hyperextension type.[24-26,30] Pain and neck stiffness, often accompanied by headache, become severe. After a variable period of days to weeks, pain and paresthesia of the upper limb appear with all the features of thoracic outlet syndrome. An asymptomatic interval between injury and symptoms is frequently described. Many patients are involved in litigation for work-related accidents or motor vehicle "whiplash" injuries, which may lead the physician to label the patient a "malingerer." Headache is not an unusual symptom of thoracic outlet syndrome and can be severe enough to incapacitate the patient. It is commonly occipital, radiating from the posterior part of the neck, and may extend to affect the ipsilateral hemicranium. It is not unusual for the diagnosis of thoracic outlet syndrome to be seriously questioned for patients in whom headache is a prominent part of the symptom complex, especially in nervous and tense patients prone to psychosomatic complaints. Generally, most patients with thoracic outlet syndrome have had symptoms for months or even years and have sought repeated medical attention with little relief because of misdiagnosis.

Physical examination should include a careful evaluation of the neck, supraclavicular area, shoulder, and the entire upper extremity, and a complete neurologic examination, to exclude other causes of pain. Palpation of the supraclavicular fossa and neck may demonstrate the presence of a cervical rib or prominent C7 transverse process. Tenderness of the upper nerves of the brachial plexus or the anterior scalene muscle is a common finding. Spasm and tenderness of the trapezius and paraspinal muscles are frequently observed in patients with a history of trauma. Radicular pain may be elicited by rotation and extension of the head or by axial cervical spine compression, indicating cervical disk disease. Pain and tenderness of the shoulder joint may be caused by rotator cuff injury or tendonitis.

All muscle groups should be tested for strength. Patients with upper brachial plexus involvement may exhibit objective weakness of the deltoid and trapezius muscles, demonstrated by the patient's inability to keep the arms extended in the abduction position, especially against mild resistance.[30] Other compression syndromes, such as entrapment of the ulnar nerve at the elbow (cubital tunnel syndrome) or median nerve at the wrist (carpal tunnel syndrome), can coexist with thoracic outlet syndrome and should be excluded by percussion at the elbow and over the volar carpal ligaments (Tinel's sign), respectively. Hand weakness, associated with wasting of the intrinsic muscles of the hand and the presence of an ipsilateral cervical rib or its analog, is seen in the extremely rare form of "true" or "classic" thoracic outlet syndrome.[34-35]

Sensation in all dermatomes is usually intact in thoracic outlet syndrome, although a mild decrease in pinprick sensation can be observed over the ulnar nerve distribution in patients with lower brachial nerve involvement. However, major sensory changes with decreased deep tendon reflexes may be caused by nerve root compression from a herniated cervical disk, spinal cord tumor, or superior pulmonary sulcus tumor.

The thoracic outlet maneuvers initially described for testing for what was mistakenly attributed to the arterial type of thoracic outlet syndrome contribute little to the diagnosis of neurologic thoracic outlet syndrome. These tests simply indicate arterial compression, a common finding in over 50% of normal individuals[14] and in 30% to 50% in the asymptomatic, contralateral arm of patients with unilateral thoracic outlet syndrome.[36,37] The thoracic outlet maneuvers include Adson's maneuver,[19] performed by rotation and extension of the head of the seated patient with the arms resting on his or her lap; the costoclavicular maneuver (exaggerated military position)[11]; and the hyperabduction maneuver.[14] These are considered positive when reduction or obliteration of the radial pulse is obtained and therefore reflect only compression of the subclavian or axillary artery in these extreme positions.

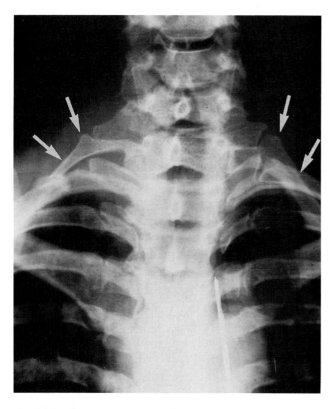

Fig. 31-3. Chest roentgenogram demonstrates well-formed and ossified bilateral cervical ribs *(arrows)*. The patient had severe bilateral neurologic type of thoracic outlet syndrome.

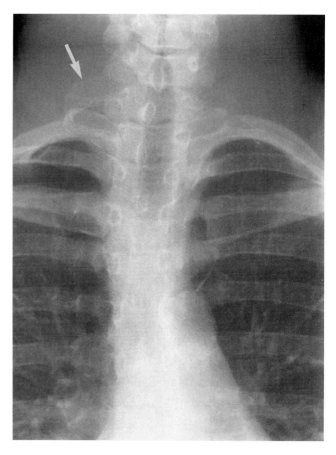

Fig. 31-4. Chest roentgenogram of a patient with elongated C7 transverse process *(arrow)* and symptoms of thoracic outlet syndrome on the right. An operation revealed a tight fibrous band stretched from the tip of the C7 transverse process to the inner aspect of the first rib, elevating the T1 nerve and inferior trunk of the brachial plexus.

They do not necessarily identify the patient with thoracic outlet syndrome.

Roos described the Elevated Arm Stress Test (EAST) as reliable for diagnosing neurologic thoracic outlet syndrome.[30] It is performed by holding the arms at 90-degree abduction and external rotation while the patient opens and closes the hands for 3 minutes. The test is considered positive when the symptoms of thoracic outlet syndrome are reproduced. Vascular examination should be complete with evaluation of all pulses and blood pressure determination in both arms to exclude arterial stenoses, obstructions, or aneurysms. Roentgenograms of the chest and cervical spine should be performed routinely. These may demonstrate skeletal abnormalities such as a cervical rib, elongated C7 transverse process, anomalous first rib, or remote fractures of the clavicle that could be the cause of thoracic outlet symptoms (Figs. 31-3 and 31-4). If significant degenerative cervical spine disease is present, and if clinically indicated, further evaluation can be done with oblique views of the cervical spine, myelography, computed tomography (CT) scan, or magnetic resonance imaging (MRI).

After an initial enthusiasm for electrodiagnostic testing such as electromyograms (EMG), nerve conduction velocity, and somatosensory evoked potentials (SSEP)[38-40] these tests have been found to be nonspecific, and they add little to the evaluation of patients with thoracic outlet syndrome, except for those patients with suspected nerve entrapment syndromes.[41-45] Similarly, arteriography and phlebography have no role in the routine evaluation of patients with neurologic symptoms but are indispensable for patients with vascular complications of thoracic outlet syndrome. Arteriography should also be considered for patients with a supraclavicular bruit, diminished upper limb pulses, or a blood pressure differential in the arms. Noninvasive vascular studies such as pulse-volume recordings (segmental pressures) and Doppler ultrasound examination (duplex scan) should likewise be confined to patients with obvious vascular symptoms, because these tests add little to the diagnosis of neurologic thoracic outlet syndrome.

Management

Conservative treatment in the form of occupational and physical therapy should be the initial management for all patients with neurologic thoracic outlet syndrome. There is no risk involved in this treatment, and most patients with mild to moderate symptoms show enough improvement that no further treatment is necessary. Physical therapy is directed at strengthening the suspensory muscles of the shoulder girdle by specific exercises for the trapezius, levator scapulae, and rhomboid muscles. These should be supplemented with stretching exercises and correction of any abnormal posture. Patients with severe associated muscle spasm of the back and neck may need initial management with a variety of treatments including heat; massage; ultrasound; and the administration of muscle relaxants, analgesics, and antiinflammatory drugs. After initial improvement patients are instructed to avoid prolonged periods with the arm elevated or in positions that reproduce symptoms.[46-47] This program should be tried for a minimum of 3 months to properly evaluate its effectiveness. A small number of patients, especially those with severe symptoms, are either unaffected by this treatment or cannot tolerate it because their symptoms are aggravated by the exercises.

Surgical treatment for neurologic thoracic outlet syndrome should be restricted to those patients with severe, intolerable symptoms unchanged by conservative therapy or for those who consider their symptoms unacceptable because they interfere with their occupation or normal daily activities. Mere failure of conservative treatment does not warrant surgical treatment as long as the symptoms are tolerable to the patient. It is estimated that 15% to 30% of patients require surgical treatment.[21,24,48] Treatment is based on the concept that excision or division of the structure or structures causing the neurovascular compression will result in the relief of the neurologic symptoms. Thus historically the procedures described have been excision of a cervical rib, the first operation for thoracic outlet syndrome, performed by Coote in 1861[17]; excision of a normal, first thoracic rib via the supraclavicular approach, performed by Murphy in 1910[18]; division of the anterior scalene muscle or "scalenotomy," performed by Adson and Coffey in 1927[19]; excision of the clavicle, performed by Rosati and Lord in 1968[49]; excision of the pectoralis minor tendon, performed by Lord in 1953[20]; and excision of the scalene muscles or "scalenectomy," performed by Sanders, Monsour, and Gerber in 1979.[24]

Although the early reports of first rib resection effectively decompressed the thoracic outlet, the operation never became popular. The scalenotomy became the preferred operation for over 3 decades because of its simplicity, lack of complications, and immediate favorable results. In 1962 Clagett,[50] because of the disappointing long-term results of scalenotomy with a 50% to 60% recurrence of symptoms,[50-51] revived interest in first rib resection for thoracic outlet syndrome. The common denominator in the compression mechanism is the first rib, and Clagett advocated its excision through a posterior parascapular approach, an operation that never gained much popularity because of the morbidity associated with this incision.

In 1966 Roos revolutionized the surgical treatment of thoracic outlet syndrome when he described a new technique for first rib resection through the transaxillary approach. This method presumably was less traumatic, safer, and easier to perform.[52] Although other approaches to first rib resection (for example, the supraclavicular,[13] the posterior,[50] and the anterior subclavicular[53]) had been described, Roos's transaxillary approach was the one that became widely adopted.[33,54-56] This approach allows for wide decompression of the thoracic outlet because it permits complete excision of the first rib, and the cervical rib when present, as well as division and partial excision of

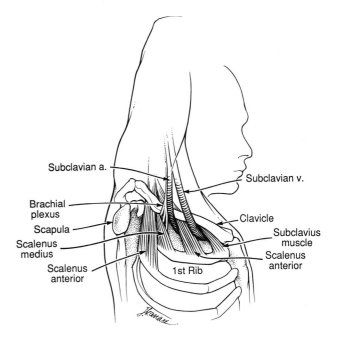

Fig. 31-5. Schematic drawing of the right thoracic outlet as viewed from the axillary approach. Note that excision of the first rib and division of the scalene and subclavius muscles would amply decompress the thoracic outlet.

the scalene muscles and congenital fibromuscular bands (Fig. 31-5). This technique was a major factor in the improved results of surgical management with 72% to 92% "good" results reported in large representative series.[25,33,54-58]

From 1984 to 1996, for various reasons, there has been a trend by many surgeons toward performing supraclavicular operations. There have been concerns regarding the safety of the transaxillary route for first rib resection because of the incidence of brachial plexus traction injuries.[59] In addition, recurrence of symptoms has been reported by some in up to 15% of patients following first rib resection.[24,25] Others have found that most patients are relieved of symptoms by excision of supraclavicular soft tissue structures, without the need for first rib resection,[60] whereas still others have found the supraclavicular approach to first rib resection technically easier to perform.[36] Roos prefers transaxillary first rib resection for patients with lower brachial plexus involvement (the majority of patients) and anterior scalenectomy for those with upper brachial plexus compression. In his experience this latter group accounts for only 2% of all primary operations for thoracic outlet syndrome.[33] Sanders, Monsour, and Gerber prefer anterior and middle scalenectomy without rib resection for both groups of patients because of their observed lower incidence of complications with this technique.[24] Presently there is still no agreement among surgeons with respect to the choice of operation for thoracic outlet syndrome.

Serious complications associated with all thoracic outlet operations include injuries to the subclavian artery or vein, brachial plexus, phrenic nerve, or long thoracic nerve.[61] Fortunately these occur infrequently. Pneumothorax, although observed more commonly, is easily managed with needle aspiration or occasionally with a chest tube. Sensory disturbance in the inner aspect of the arm caused by injury to the intercostal brachial nerve occurs in 35% of patients who undergo transaxillary surgery.[24] Following transaxillary first rib resection, recurrence of symptoms within 2 years after an initial successful result occurs in 15% to 20% of operations.[24,25,33,62] Recurrent symptoms of thoracic outlet syndrome can be caused by scalene muscle reattachment to the bed of the first rib and dense scar formation, which can entrap the brachial plexus.[63] At times retained periosteal cells can regenerate another rib, which, when associated with scar tissue, can again result in brachial plexus compression with recurrence of symptoms. Technical failure with incomplete rib resection during the original operation accounts for some of the reported recurrences.[63] Reoperation for recurrent symptoms is recommended for those patients who had an initial good result following transaxillary first rib resection and whose recurrent symptoms are severe. The operation of choice is scalenectomy with neurolysis of the brachial plexus through the supraclavicular approach.[24,26,33,63] Although the initial success rate for reoperations is similar to that of primary operations,[62] the incidence of brachial plexus injury is greater.[63]

Patients whose symptoms are unchanged following operations for thoracic outlet syndrome may have been misdiagnosed and therefore should be completely reevaluated so that the true cause of their symptoms can be established.

ARTERIAL TYPE

Arterial complications of thoracic outlet syndrome are the least common, but have the most serious implications because they frequently result in severe ischemia of the upper extremity.[64-67] They usually occur in adults from the third to the sixth decade with equal incidence in men and women. In contrast to the more common neurologic thoracic outlet syndrome, these patients almost always have a congenital bony abnormality in the thoracic outlet.

Etiology

The basic pathophysiologic mechanism is chronic compression of the subclavian artery with resultant arterial wall changes, leading to intimal injury and thickening, mural thrombus formation, and eventually peripheral embolization. The compression site is usually at the scalene triangle where a cervical rib compresses and angulates the subclavian artery from behind, against the anterior scalene muscle and first rib (Fig. 31-2). A fully developed cervical rib appears to be the most common mechanism for arterial compression, being present in 50% of cases.[4,64] Congenital anomalies of the first rib, exostosis of the first rib, and, less commonly, malunion following fracture of the clavicle are other causes of arterial compression. Although soft tissue structures, such as congenital fibromuscular bands or abnormalities of the anterior scalene muscle, commonly produce neurologic symptoms, they rarely lead to arterial complications, accounting for only 12% of this group.[21,65,66]

The arterial compression eventually causes thickening of the arterial wall, with inflammation and periarterial fibrosis. Poststenotic dilation then follows, secondary to blood flow turbulence just beyond the constricted segment.[68] In time a true aneurysm may form from the longstanding effects of flow disturbance.

Thromboembolic events can result from either an intimal lesion formed at the site of compression or from mural thrombus layered in the subclavian aneurysm. Platelet aggregates tend to deposit on intimal lesions and can dislodge, resulting in microembolization of the hand and fingers. Embolization from mural thrombus usually causes occlusion of larger, more proximal arteries. Thrombosis of the subclavian artery is an infrequent event.[69] Retrograde subclavian artery thrombosis with cerebral embolization is extremely rare.[70,71]

The severity of the ischemic symptoms depends on the site and extent of the arterial occlusion. Microembolization of the fingers and hand can result in Raynaud's phenomenon as the only initial symptom. Repeated embolization may eventually obliterate the distal arterial bed, resulting in severe ischemia, which can progress to irreversible changes and gangrene. Larger emboli that lodge in the proximal arteries tend to result in milder ischemic symptoms because of the rich collateral vessels available around the shoulder girdle.

Clinical Manifestations

The earliest clinical manifestation of arterial thoracic outlet syndrome is most frequently an ischemic episode of the affected upper extremity resulting from an embolic event. Depending on the size and number of emboli, and on the site of occlusion, this may appear as Raynaud's phenomenon, secondary to microemboli of the digital arteries and palmar arch. It can also appear as distinct ischemia of one or more digits, as a single event, or in "showers," with repeated and varied episodes of ischemia of the hand and forearm or even of the entire arm.

The diagnosis of arterial thoracic outlet syndrome is rarely made before thromboembolic events occur. On occasion, early diagnosis is possible in patients examined for asymptomatic subclavian aneurysm or in patients with neurologic symptoms associated with a cervical rib or other bony abnormality.[72] The diagnosis can be made easily if all patients with upper limb ischemia are investigated for possible sources of emboli. The diagnosis should be suspected in young patients with unilateral arm, hand, or finger ischemia. A history of the presence of a cervical rib or previous trauma with healed fractures of the clavicle or upper ribs should alert the physician to the possibility of thoracic outlet syndrome.

Physical examination will reveal the usual characteristics of tissue ischemia with pallor, cyanosis, and coldness, depending on the severity and level of the arterial occlusion. A complete vascular examination should be performed to search for a proximal source of emboli. Examination may reveal a palpable subclavian aneurysm, or a prominent subclavian artery that has been displaced anteriorly and superiorly by a cervical rib. A supraclavicular bruit is frequently audible with the arm in the neutral

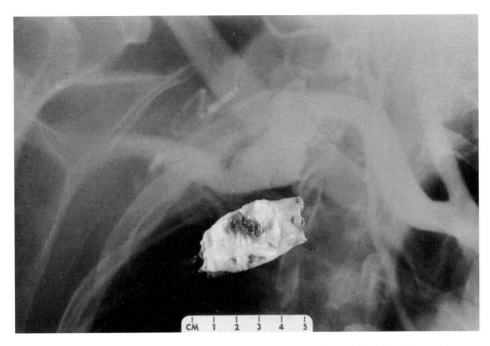

Fig. 31-6. Right subclavian arteriogram shows an aneurysm secondary to thoracic outlet syndrome. Superimposed is the surgical specimen demonstrating the intimal thrombus that was the source of distal emboli.

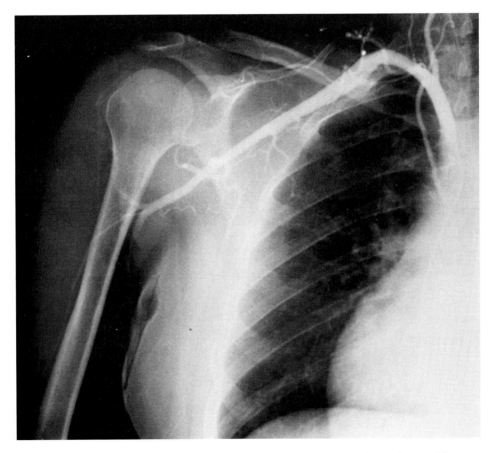

Fig. 31-7. Right subclavian arteriogram in a patient with thoracic outlet syndrome shows mild post-stenotic dilation.

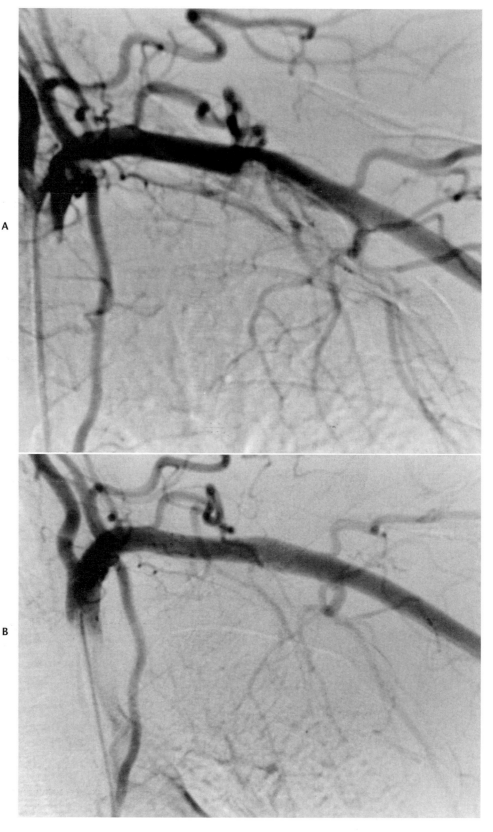

Fig. 31-8. A, Left subclavian arteriogram demonstrates a partially occluding thrombus at the thoracic outlet. **B,** Normal appearing subclavian artery after intraarterial thrombolytic treatment.

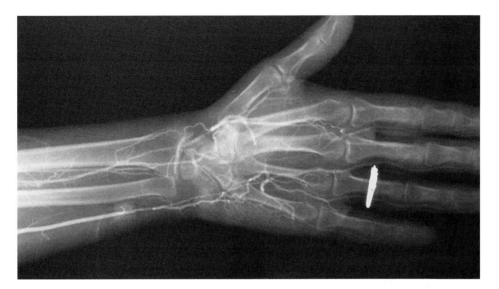

Fig. 31-9. Arteriogram of the left forearm and hand shows embolic occlusion of the proximal radial and distal ulnar arteries from a subclavian intimal thrombus caused by thoracic outlet syndrome secondary to cervical rib.

position, indicating a subclavian stenosis at the point of compression. Examination of the contralateral arm and lower extremities should be carefully performed to exclude evidence of other embolic occlusions from a cardiac source. Upper thoracic and cervical roentgenograms are critical, because a bony abnormality is almost always present. Noninvasive vascular studies with pulse-volume recordings are important in the evaluation to determine the level of the arterial occlusion, the severity of the ischemia, and the degree of collateral circulation present. Duplex scanning of the subclavian and axillary arteries may reveal the presence of a subclavian aneurysm or poststenotic dilation with the presence of mural thrombus.

Arteriography is the most specific diagnostic test and should be obtained routinely in any patient with ischemic symptoms of the upper extremity. It should include the entire arm from the aortic arch to the digital arteries. In most cases the arteriographic changes are obvious, demonstrating severe angulation of the subclavian artery with poststenotic dilation or a subclavian artery aneurysm (Fig. 31-6). Careful examination of the films is necessary for patients in whom the subclavian artery shows only subtle findings such as minor intimal changes or small intravascular filling defects (Figs. 31-7 and 31-8, A and B). Evaluation of the distal arteries is crucial in patients with severe ischemia in order to plan appropriate surgical treatment, which may include embolectomy, thrombolytic therapy, or arterial bypass to improve perfusion (Fig. 31-9).

Management

Surgery is the treatment for arterial complications of thoracic outlet syndrome. It is frequently performed as an emergency because of the common clinical presentation as an acute embolic event with resultant severe ischemia. Surgical management consists of three steps: (1) excision of the anatomic abnormality responsible for the arterial compression, (2) removal of the source of emboli by arterial reconstruction, and (3) improvement in distal perfusion by appropriate thromboembolectomy.

Thoracic outlet decompression is performed through the supraclavicular approach, which allows for adequate access to the cervical rib or other anomalies that may be present and for control of the subclavian artery for subsequent arterial reconstruction. The thoracic outlet should be fully decompressed with excision of the first rib and all anomalous osseous and soft tissue elements.[72] After decompression of the thoracic outlet, the subclavian-axillary artery becomes more accessible and mobile, and thus the arterial component of the operation can be performed through the same incision. For extensive aneurysms, however, an infraclavicular counterincision will improve the surgical exposure for arterial reconstruction. This may entail excision of the subclavian aneurysm with end-to-end anastomosis when this is feasible, or replacement of the aneurysm with a saphenous vein or prosthetic graft for more extensive involvement. For lesser intimal lesions, an endarterectomy or intimectomy may be all that is required.[72,73] Intraoperative use of the duplex scan is helpful in determining the presence and extent of the intimal lesion when the subclavian artery appears normal on external inspection.

For most patients with mild chronic ischemia, removal of the source of emboli is all that is necessary. For patients with recent thromboembolic episodes to the forearm and hand, or for patients with recent subclavian artery thrombosis, catheter-directed thrombolytic treatment can be an effective method to restore arterial perfusion.[74] For severe distal ischemia caused by *remote* digital artery and palmar arch embolization not amenable to embolectomy or thrombolytic treatment, dorsal sympathectomy may improve perfusion. Patients with repeated embolization and obliteration of the distal arterial tree of longstanding duration may be candidates for revascularization with vein bypass graft to any available patent target artery in the forearm or wrist. Some patients are not candidates for these reconstructions and require a major amputation for rehabilitation.[64,66,73]

The results of surgery for arterial complications of thoracic outlet syndrome are excellent when early diagnosis is made and treatment is instituted before multiple emboli occlude the distal arterial run-off, with resultant irreversible ischemia. In an excellent collective review, Sanders and Haug reported good results in 84% of 137 patients reported since 1970.[75]

VENOUS TYPE

Extrinsic compression of the subclavian vein in the thoracic outlet has been implicated as one of the common causes of spontaneous axillosubclavian vein thrombosis. It is known as *Paget–von Schröetter syndrome* from the first two authors who described it independently.[76,77] It is also commonly referred to as "effort" thrombosis because of its temporal relationship between vigorous physical activity of the arm and shoulder and the development of symptoms. It is prevalent in men in their third and fourth decades. The right side is affected in two thirds of the patients, probably because the physical activity or "effort" is generally related to the dominant arm.[78,79] Sanders and Haug postulate that the acute angle at the junction between the right subclavian vein and innominate vein may be another factor in the higher incidence of right-sided symptoms compared with the left side.[80]

Etiology

The most accepted etiologic factor in primary thrombosis of the axillosubclavian vein is external compression resulting from anatomic structures in the anterior portion of the thoracic outlet (Fig. 31-1). These include a large costoclavicular ligament or subclavius muscle, a more anterior insertion of the anterior scalene muscle, or congenital fibromuscular bands.[21] The pectoralis minor muscle tendon can also compress the axillary vein more laterally.[81] Repetitive arm and shoulder movements then lead to chronic intermittent compression of the vein, with eventual traumatic inflammation and fibrosis that finally culminates in thrombosis. Other factors that have been incriminated are intrinsic abnormalities such as malformation or hypertrophy of the subclavian vein valves.[82,83]

Clinical Manifestations

The symptoms of axillosubclavian vein thrombosis are pain, swelling, and cyanosis of the upper extremity. The onset is usually sudden and dramatic. Some patients, however, develop slowly progressive or intermittent symptoms over a period of days or even weeks. The severity of the symptoms depends on the extent of the thrombotic process and the degree of collateralization that develops. Pulmonary embolism is an uncommon complication.[84] Physical examination reveals a swollen, cyanotic arm with distended superficial veins around the shoulder and anterior chest. Depending on the severity of the symptoms, the arm may be tender to palpation. A tender thickened cord is sometimes palpable in the axilla.[85] The diagnosis is confirmed with upper-extremity venography. The study dem-

onstrates occlusion of the axillosubclavian vein (Fig. 31-10). In patients with intermittent symptoms, venograms should be obtained with the arm in the neutral position and also with the arm abducted to 90 degrees to demonstrate extrinsic subclavian vein compression (Fig. 31-11, *A* and *B*). The contralateral arm also should be studied with positional venograms because extrinsic vein compression is found in a significant number of patients, some of whom might be at risk for subclavian vein thrombosis and therefore may be candidates for prophylactic thoracic outlet decompressive surgery.[81,86]

Duplex scanning is helpful, but adequate visualization of the vein is limited by the clavicle and can be misleading because collateral veins may be erroneously mistaken for the axillary vein.[80] Therefore it should complement, but not exclude, venography. Intravascular ultrasound (IVUS) can be used at the time of the diagnostic venogram, and it supplements diagnostic information because in addition to the intraluminal findings, it can identify changes in the vein wall thickness as well as surrounding extraluminal anatomy. The site of venous compression can be accurately identified and assessed.[87]

Management of Acute Obstruction

Considerable changes have occurred in the management of acute axillosubclavian vein thrombosis during the 1980s. Before the 1980s there were essentially two approaches for the management of this syndrome: the most commonly used, conservative treatment with anticoagulation therapy or the infrequently performed surgical thrombectomy.[79] The poor results of anticoagulation,[84,88] the high rate of recurrent thrombosis following thrombectomy coupled with the improvement in thrombolytic techniques, have dramatically changed the treatment of Paget-Schröeter syndrome. The development of a multidisciplinary approach, using pharmacologic and interventional catheter-based techniques combined with surgical decompressive procedures have resulted in more consistent relief of symptoms and in the prevention of recurrent thrombosis.[89-92]

Treatment begins with the diagnostic venogram. Once the diagnosis of axillosubclavian vein thrombosis is confirmed, the catheter is introduced into the thrombus for the local delivery of urokinase, the most commonly used thrombolytic agent. Heparin is also used to prevent thrombus formation around the catheter. After 12 to 24 hours a completion venogram is performed to determine the efficacy of the treatment. If there is no residual thrombus, a positional venogram is obtained to determine the presence of extrinsic compression of the subclavian vein (Fig. 31-10). If extrinsic compression is noted, decompressive thoracic outlet surgery, usually transaxillary first rib resection, should be planned to prevent rethrombosis. The surgery can be performed shortly after completion of the thrombolytic therapy,[93] or else it can be staged 2 to 3 months later.[92] Anticoagulation therapy with warfarin should be instituted during the interval between the diagnosis and the operation to prevent recurrent thrombosis of the subclavian vein.

Although most surgeons prefer transaxillary first rib resection with division of the costoclavicular ligament,

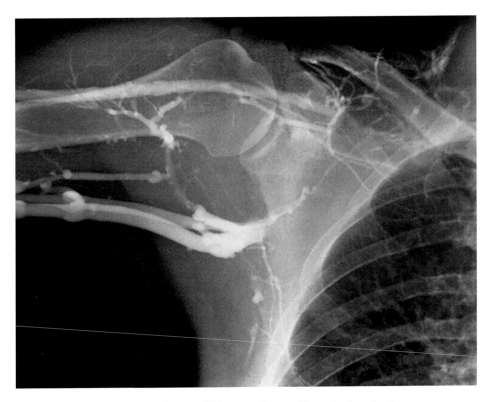

Fig. 31-10. Right arm phlebogram shows axillary vein thrombosis.

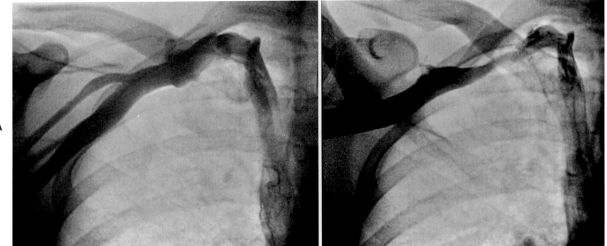

Fig. 31-11. The patient presented with intermittent symptoms of venous obstruction of the right arm. **A,** Normal left arm venogram with the arm in the neutral position. **B,** Extrinsic compression of the vein as it crosses the first rib, when the arm is abducted.

and subclavius and anterior scalene muscles to decompress the subclavian vein, some opt for other approaches such as supraclavicular or "paraclavicular" approaches.[94] When the compression site is at the pectoralis minor tendon, its division without first rib resection is all that is needed.[20,60]

For those instances where significant residual vein stenosis is seen on the venogram, "venolysis" can be performed at the time of the first rib resection,[94] or percutaneous balloon angioplasty can be used *after* first rib resection to correct the stenosis.[90,95]

Surgical thrombectomy either alone or combined with a thoracic outlet decompressive procedure is now rarely performed because of the popularity and effectiveness of the multidisciplinary approach as described.[96] The only patients that should be considered for operation are those in whom thrombolytic therapy is contraindicated. The onset of the acute axillary vein thrombosis should be no longer than a few days to obtain a favorable outcome. The operation can be performed through the infraclavicular, supraclavicular, or transclavicular approach.[58-59] After removal of the thrombus and closure of the venotomy, with or without a patch, decompression of the thoracic outlet should follow. This is accomplished by excision of the first rib and division of the costoclavicular ligament and subclavius and anterior scalene muscles. If the transclavicular approach is used, claviculectomy amply decompresses the thoracic outlet with relatively minimal deformity.[81,92,96] Patients with symptoms of intermittent obstruction of the subclavian vein, who demonstrate extrinsic compression on positional venography and no thrombosis, should be considered for elective decompression to prevent subclavian vein thrombosis.[78,86]

Conservative therapy is indicated for patients with mild symptoms, in whom the thrombosed segment is limited in extent so that collateral pathways are expected to be ample and effective. It is also indicated for patients with contraindications for thrombolytic treatment and for those who are poor surgical candidates. The treatment consists of arm elevation and anticoagulation therapy. The upper extremity should be elevated in a forward position, thus avoiding any possible venous compression in the thoracic outlet by some degree of abduction, which invariably occurs when the arm is elevated to the patient's side. Anticoagulation is instituted by administering heparin by the continuous intravenous route and is continued with warfarin therapy for 3 to 6 months.

The results of conservative treatment vary widely in reported series. Sanders and Haug, in their collective review, found that disabling arm swelling occurred in 49% of 185 patients who received anticoagulant therapy alone.[80]

Management of Chronic Obstruction

Patients who delay seeking medical treatment after the onset of symptoms of axillosubclavian vein occlusion, or those patients in whom thrombectomy has failed, may reach a chronic stage in their clinical course when the collateral development is not adequate enough to keep their symptoms at an acceptable level. Some patients may report only mild symptoms at rest but develop severe pain and swelling with moderate physical activity. Because most of these patients are young and active, other treatment options must be considered.

Thoracic outlet decompression by transaxillary first rib resection has been reported to result in symptomatic improvement in patients with chronic axillosubclavian occlusion.[73] The authors theorize that first rib resection decompresses the functioning venous collateral vessels with resultant improvement in symptoms. Subclavian vein reconstruction by endovenectomy[88] or venous bypass[97-99] is probably the only effective method available for correction of the resultant venous hypertension in patients with poor collateral vessels. Because of the relatively high incidence of thrombosis following venous reconstructions, the operation should be combined with the construction of a temporary arteriovenous fistula to increase flow and improve patency.[100]

Early recognition of acute axillosubclavian vein thrombosis and aggressive treatment using a multidisciplinary approach, hopefully will reduce the number of patients with severe symptoms resulting from chronic subclavian vein thrombosis.

REFERENCES

1. Barker WF: An historical look at the thoracic outlet compression syndrome, Ann Vasc Surg 3:293, 1989.
2. Wilbourn AJ and Porter JM: Thoracic outlet syndromes, Spine 2:597, 1988.
3. Gilliatt RW: Thoracic outlet syndromes. In Dyck PJ et al, eds: Peripheral neurology, ed 2, Philadelphia, 1984, WB Saunders Co.
4. Lord JW: Thoracic outlet syndromes: real or imaginary? N Y State J Med 81:1488, 1981.
5. Porter JM et al: Thoracic outlet syndrome: a conservative approach, Vasc Diagn Ther 3:35, 1982.
6. Dale A: Thoracic outlet compression syndrome. In Management of vascular surgical problems, New York, 1985, McGraw-Hill, Inc.
7. Todd TW: Posture and the cervical rib syndrome, Ann Surg 75:105, 1922.
8. Ochsner A, Gage M, and DeBakey M: Scalenus anticus (Naffziger) syndrome, Am J Surg 28:669, 1935.
9. Naffziger HC and Grant WT: Neuritis of the brachial plexus mechanical in origin: Scalenus syndrome, Surg Gynecol Obstet 67:722, 1938.
10. Hvoslef J: Abnormal first thoracic rib simulating cervical rib, J Minn State Med Assoc and NW Lancet 31:251, 1911.
11. Keen WW: The symptomatology, diagnosis and surgical treatment of cervical ribs, Am J Med Sci 133:173, 1907.
12. LeVay AD: Costoclavicular compression of brachial plexus and subclavian vessels, Lancet 2:164, 1945.
13. Falconer MA and Li FW: Resection of first rib in costoclavicular compression of brachial plexus, Lancet 1:59, 1962.
14. Wright IS: The neurovascular syndrome produced by hyperabduction of the arms, Am Heart J 29:1, 1945.
15. Peet PM et al: Thoracic outlet syndrome: evaluation of a therapeutic exercise program, Mayo Clin Proc 31:281, 1956.
16. Rob CG and Standeven A: Arterial occlusion complicating thoracic outlet compression syndrome, Br Med J 2:709, 1958.
17. Coote H: Exostosis of the left transverse process of the seventh cervical vertebra, surrounded by blood vessels and nerves: successful removal, Lancet 1:360, 1861.
18. Murphy T: Brachial neuritis caused by pressure of first rib, Aust Med J 15:582, 1910.
19. Adson AW and Coffey JR: Cervical rib: a method of anterior approach for relief of symptoms by division of the scalenus anticus, Ann Surg 85:839, 1927.
20. Lord JW: Surgical management of shoulder girdle syndromes, Arch Surg 66:69, 1953.
21. Roos DB: Congenital anomalies associated with thoracic outlet syndrome: anatomy, symptoms, diagnosis and treatment, Am J Surg 132:771, 1976.
22. Thomas GI et al: The middle scalene muscle and its contribution to the thoracic outlet, Am J Surg 145:589, 1983.
23. Urschel H and Razzuk MA: Thoracic outlet syndrome. In Sabiston DC and Spencer FC, eds: Gibbon's surgery of the chest, Philadelphia, 1989, WB Saunders Co.
24. Sanders RJ, Monsour JW, and Gerber WF: Scalenectomy versus first rib resection for treatment of thoracic outlet syndrome, Surgery 85:109, 1979.
25. Qvarfordt PG, Ehrenfeld WK, and Stoney RJ: Supraclavicular radical scalenectomy and transaxillary first rib resection for the thoracic outlet syndrome: a combined approach, Am J Surg 148:111, 1984.

26. Reilly LM and Stoney RJ: Supraclavicular approach for thoracic outlet decompression, J Vasc Surg 8:329, 1988.

27. Wilbourn AJ: The thoracic outlet syndrome is overdiagnosed, Arch Neurol 47:328, 1990.

28. Cherington M: Thoracic outlet syndrome: rise of the conservative viewpoint, Am Fam Physician 43:1998, 1991 (editorial).

29. Reference deleted in proofs.

30. Roos DB: Thoracic outlet nerve compression. In Rutherford RB, ed: Vascular surgery, Philadelphia, 1989, WB Saunders Co.

31. Machleder HJ, Moll F, and Verity A: The anterior scalene muscle in thoracic outlet compression syndrome: histochemical and morphometric studies, Arch Surg 121:1141, 1986.

32. Sanders RJ et al: Scalene muscle abnormalities in traumatic thoracic outlet syndrome, Am J Surg 159:231, 1990.

33. Roos DB: The place for scalenectomy and first rib resection in thoracic outlet syndrome, Surgery 92:1077, 1982.

34. Gilliatt RW et al: Wasting of the hand associated with a cervical rib or band, J Neurol Neurosurg Psychiatry 33: 615, 1970.

35. Wilbourn AJ: Case report no. 7: true neurogenic thoracic outlet syndrome, Rochester, Minn, 1982, American Association of Electromyography and Electrodiagnosis.

36. Hempel GK et al: Supraclavicular resection of the first rib for thoracic outlet syndrome, Am J Surg 14:213, 1981.

37. Sallstrom J and Gjores JE: Surgical treatment of thoracic outlet syndrome, Acta Chir Scand 149:555, 1983.

38. Urschel HC and Razzuk MA: Thoracic outlet syndrome, N Engl J Med 286:1140, 1972.

39. Glover JL et al: Evoked responses in the diagnosis of thoracic outlet syndrome, Surgery 89:86, 1981.

40. Machleder HJ et al: Somatosensory evoked potentials in the assessment of thoracic outlet compression syndrome, J Vasc Surg 6:177, 1987.

41. Jerrett SA, Cuzzone LJ, and Pasternak BM: Thoracic outlet syndrome: electrophysiological reappraisal, Arch Neurol 41:960, 1984.

42. Cherington M: Ulnar conduction velocity in thoracic outlet syndrome, N Engl J Med 294:1185, 1976.

43. Raskin NH, Howard MN, and Ehrenfeld WK: Headache as the leading symptom of thoracic outlet syndrome, Headache 25:208, 1985.

44. Wilbourn AJ and Lederman RJ: Evidence for conduction delay in thoracic outlet syndrome is challenged, N Engl J Med 310:1052, 1984.

45. Veilleux M, Stevens JC, and Campbell JK: Somatosensory evoked potentials: lack of value for diagnosis of thoracic outlet syndrome, Muscle Nerve 11:571, 1988.

46. Walsh MT: Therapist management of thoracic outlet syndrome, J Hand Ther 7:131, 1994 (review).

47. Aligne C and Barral X: Rehabilitation of patients with thoracic outlet syndrome, Ann Vasc Surg 6:381, 1992 (review).

48. Pretre R, Spiliopoulos A, and Megevand R: Transthoracic approach in the thoracic outlet syndrome: an alternative operative route for removal of the first rib, Surgery 106: 856, 1989.

49. Rosati LM and Lord JW: Neurovascular compression syndromes of the shoulder girdle. In Modern surgical monographs, New York, 1968, Grune & Stratton, Inc.

50. Clagett OT: Presidential address: research and prosearch, J Thorac Cardiovasc Surg 44:153, 1962.

51. Raaf J: Surgery for cervical rib and scalenus anticus syndrome, JAMA 157:219, 1955.

52. Roos DB: Transaxillary approach for first rib resection to relieve thoracic outlet obstruction, Ann Surg 163:354, 1966.

53. Nelson RM and Davis RW: Thoracic outlet compression syndrome: collective review, Ann Thorac Surg 8:437, 1969.

54. Urschel HC and Razzuk MA: Thoracic outlet syndrome, N Engl J Med 286:1140, 1972.

55. Dale WA and Lewis MR: Management of thoracic outlet syndrome, Ann Surg 181:575, 1975.

56. Kelly TR: Thoracic outlet syndrome: current concepts of treatment, Ann Surg 190:657, 1979.

57. Green R, McNamara J, and Ouriel K: Long-term follow-up after thoracic outlet decompression: an analysis of factors determining outcome, J Vasc Surg 14:739, 1991.

58. Sellke FW and Kelly TR: Thoracic outlet syndrome, Am J Surg 154:56, 1988.

59. Dale WA: Thoracic outlet compression syndrome: critique in 1982, Arch Surg 117:1437, 1982.

60. Stallworth JM, Quinn GJ, and Aiken AF: Is rib resection necessary for relief of thoracic outlet syndrome? Ann Surg 185:581, 1977.

61. Melliere D et al: Severe injuries resulting from operation for thoracic outlet syndrome: can they be avoided? J Cardiovasc Surg 32:599, 1991.

62. Sanders RJ, Haug CE, and Pearch WH: Recurrent thoracic outlet syndome, J Vasc Surg 12:390, 1990.

63. Cheng SW and Stoney RJ: Supraclavicular reoperation for neurogenic thoracic outlet syndrome, J Vasc Surg 19:565, 1994.

64. Judy KL and Heymann RL: Vascular complications of thoracic outlet syndrome, Am J Surg 123:536, 1974.

65. Dorazio RA and Ezzet F: Arterial complications of the thoracic outlet syndrome, Am J Surg 138:246, 1979.

66. Short DW: The subclavian artery in 16 patients with complete cervical ribs, J Cardiovasc Surg 16:135, 1975.

67. Cormier JM et al: Arterial complications of the thoracic outlet syndrome: fifty-five operative cases, J Vasc Surg 9:778, 1989.

68. Pairolero PC et al: Subclavian axillary artery aneurysms, Surgery 90:757, 1981.

69. Bouhoutsos J, Morris T, and Martin P: Unilateral Raynaud's phenomenon in the hand and its significance, Surgery 82:547, 1977.

70. DeVillers JC: A brachiocephalic vascular syndrome associated with cervical rib, Br Med J 2:140, 1966.

71. Al-Hassan HK, Sattar MA, and Eklof B: Embolic brain infarction: a rare complication of thoracic outlet syndrome. A report of two cases, J Cardiovasc Surg 29:322, 1988.

72. Kieffer E and Ruotolo C: Arterial complications of thoracic outlet compression. In Rutherford RB, ed: Vascular surgery, Philadelphia, 1989, WB Saunders Co.

73. Etheredge S, Wilbur B, and Stoney RJ: Thoracic outlet syndrome, Am J Surg 138:175, 1979.

74. Sullivan KL, Minken SK, and White RI: Treatment of a case of thromboembolism resulting from thoracic outlet syndrome with intra-arterial urokinase infusion, J Vasc Surg 7:568, 1988.

75. Sanders RJ and Haug C: Review of arterial thoracic outlet syndrome with a report of five new instances, Surg Gynecol Obstet 173:415, 1991 (review).

76. Paget J: Clinical lectures and essays, London, 1875, Longmans, Green & Co.

77. von Schröetter L: Erkrankungen der Gefossl. In Nathnogel, Handbuch der Pathologie und Therapie, Wein, 1884, Holder.

78. Adams JT et al: Intermittent subclavian vein obstruction without thrombosis, Surgery 63:147, 1968.

79. DeWeese JA, Adams JT, and Gaiser DL: Subclavian venous thrombectomy, Circulation 16(suppl 2):158, 1970.

80. Sanders RJ and Haug C: Subclavian vein obstruction and thoracic outlet syndrome: a review of etiology and management, Ann Vasc Surg 4:397, 1990.

81. Daskalakis E and Bouhoutsos J: Subclavian and axillary compression of musculoskeletal origin, Br J Surg 67:573, 1980.

82. Cucci CE, Bottino CG, and Ciampa V: Venous obstruction of the upper extremity caused by a malformed valve of the subclavian vein, Circulation 27:275, 1963.

83. Wilder JR, Haberman ET, and Nach RL: Subclavian vein obstruction secondary to hypertrophy of the terminal valve, Surgery 55:214, 1964.

84. Tilney NL, Griffiths HJG, and Edwards EA: Natural history of major venous thrombosis of the upper extremity, Arch Surg 101:792, 1970.

85. Hughes ESR: Venous obstruction in the upper extremity, Br J Surg 36:155, 1948.

86. Machleder HI: Evaluation of a new treatment strategy for Paget-Schroetter's syndrome: spontaneous thrombosis of the axillary-subclavian vein, J Vasc Surg 17:305, 1993.

87. Chengelis DL et al: The use of intravascular ultrasound in the management of thoracic outlet syndrome, Am Surg 60:592, 1994.

88. Gloviczki P, Kazmier FJ, and Hollier LH: Axillary subclavian venous occlusion: the morbidity of a nonlethal disease, J Vasc Surg 4:333, 1986.

89. Taylor LM et al: Thrombolytic therapy followed by first rib resection for spontaneous ("effort") subclavian vein thrombosis, Am J Surg 149:644, 1985.

90. Perler BA and Mitchell SE: Percutaneous transluminal angioplasty and transaxillary first rib resection: a multi-disciplinary approach to the thoracic outlet compression syndrome, Am Surg 52:485, 1986.

91. Kunkel JM and Machleder HI: Treatment of Paget-Schroetter syndrome: a staged, multi-disciplinary approach, Arch Surg 124:1153, 1989.

92. Machleder HI: Evaluation of a new treatment strategy for Paget-Schroetter's syndrome: spontaneous thrombosis of the axillary-subclavian vein, J Vasc Surg 17:305, 1993.

93. Urschel HC Jr and Razzuk MA: Improved management of the Paget-Schroetter syndrome secondary to thoracic outlet compression, Ann Thorac Surg 52:1217, 1991.

94. Thompson RW et al: Circumferential venolysis and paraclavicular thoracic outlet decompression for "effort thrombosis" of the subclavian vein, J Vasc Surg 16:723, 1992.

95. Baron B, Kiproff PM, and Khoury MB: Local thrombolysis and percutaneous transluminal venoplasty for the venous complications of thoracic outlet syndrome: case report, Angiology 43:957, 1992.

96. Lord JW Jr and Wright IS: Total claviculectomy for neurovascular compression in the thoracic outlet, Surg Gynecol Obstet 176:609, 1993.

97. Rabinowitz R and Goldfarb D: Surgical treatment of axillosubclavian venous thrombosis: a case report, Surgery 70:703, 1971.

98. Hashmonai M, Schramek A, and Farbstein J: Cephalic vein crossover bypass for subclavian vein thrombosis: a case report, Surgery 80:563, 1976.

99. Jacobson JH and Haimov M: Venous revascularization of the arm: report of three cases, Surgery 81:599, 1977.

100. Sanders RJ, Rosales C, and Pearce WH: Creation and closure of temporary arteriovenous fistulas for venous reconstruction or thrombectomy: description of technique, J Vasc Surg 6:504, 1987.

CHAPTER THIRTY-TWO

REFLEX SYMPATHETIC DYSTROPHY AND CAUSALGIA

Alvin J. Mathe
Jess R. Young

REFLEX SYMPATHETIC DYSTROPHIES

Reflex sympathetic dystrophy (RSD) and causalgia represent a family of overlapping disorders, and a number of terms have been used to describe them (see the box on this page). Although many of these terms are descriptive, their use has confused clinicians and has obscured the clinical features of these disorders. Confusion is not surprising since RSD occurs in different forms at different times during its course. The various names given in the past have mainly been used to describe separate clinical aspects of this syndrome.

The subcommittee on taxonomy of the International Association for the Study of Pain (IASP) 1986[1] defined *RSD* as "continuous pain in a portion of an extremity after trauma, which may include fracture but does not involve a major nerve, associated with sympathetic hyperactivity."

Causalgia is a type of RSD associated with major nerve injury. The IASP defines *causalgia* as "burning pain, allodynia, and hyperpathia usually in the hand or foot after partial injury of a nerve or one of its major branches" (see the box, p. 568, for definitions of terms used).

Most authorities list causalgia as a type of RSD. This is logical since there is evidence of sympathetic overactivity associated with this condition, and the pain can be stopped by sympathetic blocks or sympathectomy. RSDs can therefore be divided into two major types, one associated with major nerve injury (causalgia) and the other not associated with major nerve injury (RSD).

Causes of the RSD syndromes can be grouped under three categories: traumatic (after an injury), nontraumatic (after a noninjurious condition), and idiopathic (see the box, p. 568).

In the past patients with causalgia and RSD were often misdiagnosed and mistreated by physicians because confusing and conflicting descriptions made diagnosis and treatment difficult. With a better understanding of these conditions, physicians no longer need to be confused and

TERMS USED TO DESCRIBE RSD SYNDROMES

Algodystrophy

Algoneurodystrophy

Disuse phenomenon

Posttraumatic dystrophy

Reflex neurovascular dystrophy

Causalgia

Mimocausalgia

Minor causalgia

Major causalgia

Sudeck's osteodystrophy

Osteoporosis with disability

Painful osteoporosis

Posttraumatic osteoporosis

Posttraumatic fibrosis

Shoulder-hand syndrome

Posttraumatic sympathalgia

Postinfarctional sclerodactyly

Acute atrophy of bone

Traumatic angiospasm

Traumatic vasospasm

Posttraumatic pain syndrome

Posttraumatic neurovascular pain syndrome

Posttraumatic spreading neuralgia

Peripheral trophoneurosis

Disability after real or alleged venous thrombosis

Posttraumatic neurovascular pain syndrome

DEFINITIONS OF TERMS USED IN PAIN

Allodynia: pain resulting from a non-noxious stimulus to normal skin

Dysesthesia: an unpleasant abnormal sensation produced by normal stimuli

Hyperesthesia: increased sensitivity to stimulation

Hyperpathia: abnormally exaggerated subjective response to painful stimuli

---

DISORDERS ASSOCIATED WITH RSD SYNDROMES

Traumatic (60%)
Fractures

Sprains

Contusions

Muscle strains

Crush injuries

Peripheral nerve injuries

Burns

Iatrogenic injuries

Dislocations

Lacerations

Nontraumatic (25%)
Cerebrovascular accident with hemiplegia

Myocardial infarction

Thrombophlebitis

Prolonged bed rest

Neoplasm

Metabolic bone disease

Cervical osteoarthritis

Herpes zoster

Idiopathic (15%)

---

frustrated. Increased awareness of the clinical pictures, knowledge of the wide array of predisposing events, and prompt initiation of proper therapy will prevent protracted cases with persistent limitation of function of the extremity.

Reflex Sympathetic Dystrophy

The term *reflex sympathetic dystrophy* in this discussion will be applied to patients with a persistent pain syndrome in an extremity, usually after an injury or an insult to the extremity. It is not associated with major nerve injuries, and there may be clinical evidence of sympathetic overac-

tivity. RSD is a common, frequently misdiagnosed condition characterized by pain, tenderness, limitation of motion, and a favoring of one limb. It is the result of a failure of a patient to become rehabilitated normally.

Although RSD has been known for a long time, knowledge of it is still quite limited. Mitchell, Morehouse, and Keen[2] wrote the first clinical description of causalgia based on cases of gunshot wounds to the nerves and blood vessels during the Civil War. Sudeck[3] described cases of painful joint involvement giving rise to the term *Sudeck's syndrome* after injury. Leriche[4] called attention to the role of the sympathetic nervous system in these disorders. Evans[5] coined the term RSD to describe posttraumatic pain syndromes that were not related to major nerve damage.

ETIOLOGY. As mentioned, the precipitating causes for RSD can be discussed under three headings: traumatic, nontraumatic, and idiopathic (see the box on this page). An illustrative review is provided by Patman,[6] who described 113 patients, 25 with causalgia, 88 with "mimocausalgia," or RSD by current terminology. Of these 88 patients the precipitating factor in 30 was fracture; 31 patients had minor trauma such as cuts, sprains, or falls; 6 had major trauma such as a crush injury; 6 had miscellaneous injuries not otherwise specified; there were 4 shoulder-hand syndromes and 5 of unknown cause.

In 1983 Linson[7] described 29 patients with RSD of the arm. The precipitating cause in 15 of these patients was fracture; 11 of these were of the distal radius. In an overall review of the literature, about 60% of the cases of RSD are posttraumatic, about 25% are associated with nontraumatic conditions such as failure to rehabilitate after a stroke, myocardial infarction, or thrombophlebitis, and the other 15% are idiopathic.

The trauma or injury that precipitates RSD can also be iatrogenic (e.g., after surgical procedures on the hand including carpal tunnel release or palmar fasciotomy). Transaxillary resection of the first rib for thoracic outlet syndrome has also been complicated by RSD. Five of the twenty-nine patients from Linson's[7] group were status post–carpal tunnel release. RSD has also been associated with metabolic bone disease, neoplasm, cervical osteoarthritis, and herpes zoster.

In a comprehensive review by Kozin[8] RSD was found to occur most frequently after fractures. In 25% to 30% of the cases, no specific precipitating event could be identified. In a review by Pak[9] of 140 cases, the precipitating cause was not recognized in 15%.

The syndrome can be aggravated and prolonged by incorrect diagnosis on the part of the physician. The physician may keep the patient in bed or immobilized for an unreasonably long time. When the patient finally does become active, the tender, painful limb is often misdiagnosed as thrombophlebitis, and an additional period of bed rest and immobilization is prescribed. This furthers the development of RSD.

EPIDEMIOLOGY. It is difficult to determine how common RSD is in the general population because most studies of RSD patients are from pain treatment centers. Therefore the sample population is skewed. For example, Stiltz[10] reported 133 patients with RSD among 1463 patients at the University of Virginia Pain Clinic over 2 years.

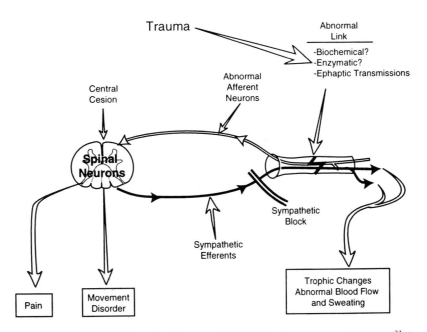

Fig. 32-1. A theory of pathophysiology of reflex sympathetic dystrophy as proposed by Janig.[31] See text for description.

Plewes[11] estimated that RSD occurred in 0.05% of patients seen in a trauma unit. Others suggest that it may be up to 5% of patients with injuries. Chan and Chow[12] reported 3000 patients with hand injuries admitted to an orthopedic unit in Hong Kong. Twenty developed persistent pain, tenderness, swelling, and stiffness of the hand despite at least 1 month of treatment.

PATHOPHYSIOLOGY. The exact mechanism by which the initial trauma and tissue damage result in a chronic irritation of the peripheral sensory nerves is unknown. It may be enzymatic, biochemical, or bioelectric in nature. Regardless of the mechanism, the result is a prolonged stimulation of pain impulses.

Most theories of pathophysiology involve a vicious circle. Janig[31] proposed a hypothesis (Fig. 32-1) briefly described as follows: Afferent neurons with small-diameter fibers in the affected territory become sensitized by trauma or some other inciting event. The sympathetic efferent fibers traveling in the same nerve bundle are coupled in some way to the abnormal afferent neuron, possibly by chemical factors or ephaptic transmission of impulses across the nerves. This leads to abnormal afferent impulses back to the spinal cord. Neurons in the spinal cord are barraged by the abnormal afferent activity. There may be a central lesion that also provides abnormal input to the spinal neurons (dorsal horn area). The result of this spinal neuron activity is the clinical manifestations of RSD. Thalamic and higher centers interpret the abnormal spinal activity as pain. The abnormal milieu around the spinal neurons may lead to stimulation of adjacent motor neurons, leading to the movement disorder of RSD. The abnormal milieu also stimulates sympathetic efferents, which completes the circle and leads to trophic changes and abnormal regulation of blood flow and sweating. Since

sympathetic activity is one arc of the circle, it explains why sympathetic block stops the cycle. Components of this theory are supported by studies by Livingston,[32] Janig,[33] Blumberg and Janig,[34] Bond et al,[35] and Willis.[36]

The abnormal sympathetic activity leads to spasm in the arteriolar and venule ends of the capillary loops, thus raising filtration pressure. Edema and swelling result. Cyanosis and anoxemia increase capillary permeability, further worsening the edema. Edema stimulates the afferent neurons, perpetuating the vicious circle.

CLINICAL PICTURE. RSD is a dynamic process that has just one common denominator to all forms and all stages: pain. Changes in bones, blood vessels, muscles, tendons, connective tissue, and skin may occur.

The pain of RSD is usually described as an aching or throbbing discomfort that is aggravated by weight bearing or by use of the extremity. Pain at rest, if present, is usually mild. It is usually worse when the extremity is dependent. Because of the pain with weight bearing, limping and the use of a cane, crutch, or wheelchair are common. If an arm is involved, it is often carried in a sling. RSD is found twice as often in the lower extremities, and a dominant extremity is most often affected.

Steinbrocker and Argyros[37] suggested dividing RSD into three stages. This classification has proven to be of great help to us clinically and is illustrated in Table 32-1. These stages appear sequentially but with great variability. The groupings should be used only as a rough clinical classification since there is considerable overlap between the various stages. This may cause difficulty in diagnosis and classification.

It is important to recognize that there is a stage of RSD after an injury or insult to the extremity, stage 1, that is not associated with any clinical evidence of sympathetic over-

Table 32-1. Clinical Features of Reflex Sympathetic Dystrophy

Stage	Pain	Sympathetic Activity	Function	Trophic Changes	Color	Edema
Stage 1 (acute) From injury to 3-6 mo	Out of proportion to original injury; increased with dependency	*No evidence of overactivity*	Minimal impairment	Increased hair and nail growth; bony changes may be present on x-ray films	Erythematous	++
Stage 2 (dystrophic) Another 3-6 mo	Burning, throbbing, may increase over stage 1	Increased; skin is cool, hyperhydrotic with color changes	Restricted	Nails are ridged, cracked, brittle; hair loss; diffuse osteopenia	Livedo reticularis, cyanosis	+++
Stage 3 (atrophic) May last years	Burning, throbbing; may decrease; may spread proximally	Less, as compared with stage 2	Severely restricted, contractures may occur; *irreversible impairments*	Atrophy of skin and subcutaneous tissues; marked demineralization on x-ray films	Cyanotic	++

activity. Because of this lack of evidence of sympathetic dysfunction, clinicians often miss the diagnosis. They think that there must be evidence of sympathetic overactivity to qualify for the diagnosis of RSD. There are more patients with RSD who do not have evidence of sympathetic dysfunction than those who do.

RSD can occur in any age group. It was originally thought that RSD was rare in children, but there have been increasing numbers of reports of children with this disorder.[38-42] RSD in children appears to differ somewhat from that in adults. The children do not appear to be as disabled; there usually are few or no roentgenographic or bone scan changes, vasomotor disturbances are mild, and the children usually respond well to conservative therapy. Breuhl and Carlson[43] reported that children with RSD tend to have a history significant for life stressors such as abuse or separation of parents, and that psychologic factors play a larger role in children than in adults.

Osteoporosis can develop in any of the stages of RSD and is termed *Sudeck's atrophy*. It is a later development and should never be considered an antecedent to RSD or a cause of RSD. Osteoporosis developed in 31% of the patients described by Drucker et al.[44]

Although Lexer, Kuliga, and Turk[45] described four types of osteoporosis, most workers simply describe the bone changes as acute or chronic. In the acute form there are numerous small, round lucent areas in the juxtaarticular bone. In the chronic form the trabeculas are very fine and difficult to see, and patchy areas of rarification are seen. In severe cases the next stage is marked with diffuse demineralization.

Patients with RSD often appear to be emotionally unstable and anxious. Chronic invalidism, drug addiction, psychiatric commitment, and suicide can occur. Disparity between the degree of pain reported by the patient and the physical examination findings, combined with the patient's anxiety, leads many physicians to think that the pain is psychogenic. Some observers believe that emotional instability is a result of chronic pain and report that emotional disturbances are usually resolved with successful treatment of the condition.[46] However, Pak's[9] review of 140 patients with RSD revealed that emotional disturbances and psychiatric problems were thought to be present before the onset of RSD. Julsrud[47] and Owens[48] believe that patients with RSD are "sympathetic reactors" with a background of emotional and vasomotor instability that makes them more prone to develop the syndrome.

A classic case history demonstrating the three stages of RSD would be a patient with disability after deep venous thrombosis. Typically this involves an anxious patient with a low pain threshold who is treated for deep thrombophlebitis with abnormally prolonged bed rest for weeks or even months. When ambulation is attempted, the leg becomes swollen, feels tight and stiff, and hurts on weight bearing. The patient limps, producing more discomfort because of abnormal weight bearing. The muscles become increasingly sore and tender, and a wrong diagnosis of recurrent phlebitis is made. Additional bed rest and immobilization only worsens the condition. The leg continues to ache and throb constantly. The patient cannot bear much

weight on the extremity and resorts to a cane or crutches. On examination, a full-blown picture of RSD is seen with mild to moderate swelling, generalized tenderness in the muscle and bones, and limitation of motion of the toes and ankles. In this first stage there may be increased skin blood flow with increased warmth and rubor. After 2 or 3 months the skin becomes cool, sweaty, and frequently cyanotic. X-ray films show osteoporosis. These are typical signs and symptoms of sympathetic overactivity found in the second stage. In the third stage symptoms include increased stiffness, muscle atrophy, tight skin, diffuse osteoporosis, and rigid joints.

DIAGNOSIS. The diagnosis of RSD is primarily clinical. A history of persistent pain, usually after an injury or insult to an extremity, is of primary importance in making an accurate diagnosis. If pain is out of proportion to that expected from the initial incident, a diagnosis of RSD must be seriously entertained. RSD is initially misdiagnosed in approximately 70% of all cases.[49]

The criteria used to identify RSD vary widely. Some authors require only the presence of the typical pain syndrome, whereas others insist that evidence of sympathetic overactivity be present. Evidence of sympathetic overactivity is usually absent in stage 1 RSD.

Kozin[50] has proposed criteria for a diagnosis of definite, probable, possible, and doubtful RSD. Patients would be considered to have definite RSD when pain, tenderness, swelling, and vasomotor and sudomotor changes are present. Probable RSD would be present if pain, tenderness, and vasomotor and sudomotor changes are present, but swelling is absent. Possible RSD would be diagnosed if only vasomotor or sudomotor changes are present and doubtful RSD if only unexplained pain and tenderness are present. These criteria may be of some help in evaluating the patient with persistent pain.

Many believe that the failure of a lumbar sympathetic nerve block to relieve pain excludes the diagnosis of RSD, providing that the block was properly done. Although relief is usually obtained, this is not invariably seen.

Laboratory tests are generally helpful only to exclude other causes of painful limbs (e.g., collagen vascular diseases or bone or soft tissue infections). Radiologic features are important in the diagnoses of RSD. Standard roentgenograms may show some other cause for the persistent pain in the extremity such as a stress fracture. With the use of fine-detail roentgenography, osteoporosis can be found in 90% of patients with definite RSD.[51] It may take 4 to 8 weeks to develop. The acute form is characterized by an irregular mottled appearance, usually marked most in the tarsal bones and heads of the metatarsals. In the chronic form of osteoporosis the trabeculas of the bones are very fine and sometimes difficult to recognize, and a diffuse osteopenia may be present.

Abnormal bone scans using technetium-99m are present in over 80% of patients with RSD.[52] Asymmetric blood flow is typically present. In most patients increased flow and uptake are noted, but diminished flow and uptake can also be seen. The delayed images generally show increased uptake in periarticular tissues, although a few patients have reduced uptake in the entire affected extremity. Holder and Mackinnon[53] have suggested specific criteria for judging the bone scan in patients suspected of having RSD.

Kozin et al[52] compared the sensitivity and specificity of roentgenography and bone scan in patients with RSD. The sensitivity was found to be 69% in roentgenography and 60% in bone scans, whereas the specificities were 71% and 86%, respectively. Bone scans may also be helpful in predicting prognosis in RSD. Kozin et al[52] reported that 90% of the patients identified by positive bone scan had a good response to corticosteroid treatment.

DIFFERENTIAL DIAGNOSIS. The differential diagnosis of RSD depends on the major clinical features at the time of presentation. The list of conditions that can cause pain, tenderness, swelling, and heat or coldness of an extremity is long. This list would include tendinitis, myositis, tenosynovitis, septic or inflammatory arthritis, collagen vascular disorders, metabolic arthropathy, chondromalacia, digital sheath infections or abscesses, muscle strains, sprains, senile or postmenopausal osteoporosis, unrecognized fracture (e.g., stress fractures), thrombophlebitis, arterial insufficiency, osteomyelitis, compartment syndrome, fascial hernias, overstretched sensory nerves, severe fibromyalgia (fibrositis), peripheral neuropathy, radiculitis, and hysterical conversion reaction. The clinician must also consider false presentation by a patient who is thereby anticipating compensation, disability, or physician attention. In stage 3, the atrophic stage of RSD, the tight skin and joint contractures may suggest scleroderma.

Erythermalgia, also called erythromelalgia, is an uncommon condition with a typical triad of symptoms: erythema, heat, and burning pain of the involved part. Symptoms are intermittent and are related to increases in environmental temperature or to exercise. Relief can be obtained by administering aspirin or by cooling the environment. These features should make the condition easy to distinguish from RSD.

A careful check of the pulses should be made to exclude the possibility of arterial ischemia in the patient with a painful, tender, cool extremity. If the pulses are not easily felt, assessment of the arterial status by Doppler pressure determination or by referring the patient to a noninvasive vascular laboratory will be helpful.

If nerve involvement is suspected as a cause of a painful extremity, electromyogram with nerve conduction studies may be helpful. Laboratory tests should help exclude other conditions such as infections of bone or soft tissue and collagen vascular diseases.

The changes seen on bone scan are similar to any disease that causes a chronically inflamed joint such as synovitis, gout, or osteomyelitis. The changes seen on roentgenography are similar to any disease that causes increased bone turnover such as prolonged immobilization, hyperparathyroidism, degenerative joint disease, Wilson's disease, thyrotoxicosis, Cushing's syndrome, Paget's disease, metastatic cancer, or multiple myeloma.

Since osteoporosis is a component of the later stages of RSD, patients who have been successfully treated may present later with a stress fracture mimicking a recurrence of RSD. If malingering is suspected, the physician may test the affected extremity while distracting the patient to see if symptoms occur when the patient is not focused. Malingering should also be suspected if the patient is noncompliant to a treatment program.

TREATMENT. The most effective treatment for RSD is prevention. The importance of early mobilization of an injured extremity, after even minor trauma, must be emphasized. Early mobilization is essential for patients known to be predisposed to RSD such as those with hemiplegia, myocardial infarction, fracture, or trauma. This is especially true if these conditions occur in a patient with a severe anxiety state or a low pain threshold.

Once RSD is established, the most important factor in successful treatment is early diagnosis and treatment. The goal is to restore the normal use of the disabled extremity. This may be accomplished in the early stages of RSD by a careful explanation of the disorder, along with copious reassurance and encouragement. An attempt should be made to convince a patient that it is not a serious disease and that a full recovery is expected. A patient should be instructed to walk without aid and to make a real effort to avoid limping. The use of crutches or canes is strictly avoided. The patient should be cautioned that there may be increased discomfort in the limb for the first days or even weeks of rehabilitation.

If the patient is not responding adequately and rapidly to these simple measures, an intensive physical therapy program should be started. The role of physical therapy in the treatment of patients with RSD is well established and should be tried before proceeding to more complicated forms of treatment. Trudel et al[54] reported good to excellent results in 44 of 50 RSD patients treated with physical therapy.

The physical therapy program should include full range-of-motion exercises, stretching of taut muscles and tendons, gait training for normal weight bearing, and exercises in a whirlpool bath. Active exercises are encouraged. Desensitization massage may help some patients. Contrast baths of the affected extremity often help, alternating four minutes at 40.6° C (105° F) with 4 minutes of melting ice water at 0° C (32° F) until hot and cold baths total 32 minutes. The final bath should be hot water, immediately followed by range-of-motion exercises. Intensive physical therapy may be sufficient, especially early in the course of the disease (i.e., stage 1 or stage 2). Patients with too much pain to participate in physical therapy should initially be treated with pain medications or sympathetic blocks.

Transcutaneous electrical nerve stimulation (TENS) can be useful in some patients with RSD.[55] The TENS unit is postulated to relieve pain by the electrically generated barrage of nerve impulses in large axons. Although there have been mixed results reported in the use of this form of therapy, recent experiences with TENS have been encouraging. Since this method is rapid and safe, it should be tried before more invasive treatments are used. It was reported effective as the only treatment in a child with RSD.[56] TENS may be a useful adjunct to sympathetic blockade, providing analgesia between intermittent blocks. It may also help control pain in chronic cases that do not respond to other modes of therapy.

For the patient who is not responding to reassurance,

physical therapy, and TENS, the next step should be a trial of high-dose corticosteroids. Several reports have indicated that this treatment may be of benefit to RSD patients. Fair to excellent responses have been reported in 63% to 67% of patients.[52,57,58] Most patients were started on 60 to 200 mg of prednisone daily, with gradual tapering over 2 to 6 weeks. A typical regimen would start with a daily dose of 60 mg of prednisone or equivalent doses of related preparations. This is tapered every 3 days by 5 mg, for a total therapy duration of about 5 weeks. Few side effects are noted with this regimen. If the symptoms increase too much during tapering, therapy may have to be extended.

In the past, paravertebral sympathetic ganglion blockade has been one of the most widely recommended treatments for RSD.[59-62] Good to excellent results have been reported in 50% to 80% of patients, though improvement may not be permanent. When the sympathetic block is indicated, the sooner the treatment is initiated, the better the prognosis. A block performed within the first 4 weeks of symptoms may give long-term or permanent relief. When symptoms have been present longer than 6 to 8 weeks, a series of blocks over several days or weeks may be needed. If no significant improvement has appeared after three to five sympathetic blocks given daily or every other day, this approach should be abandoned. Loh and Nathan[59] stressed the importance of hyperpathia in predicting the response to sympathetic blocks. Most patients with hyperpathia responded well to blocks, and only a small percentage without that symptom responded.

Paravertebral ganglionectomy should be considered for patients whose relief with sympathetic blocks is only temporary and whose overall course shows little improvement. In elderly or poor-risk patients, chemical sympathectomy using an injection of phenol or alcohol into the sympathetic chain is an alternative to surgery. This approach cannot be used in the upper extremity because of the proximity of the brachial plexus to the cervical sympathetic chain.

Several authors have reported the results of paravertebral ganglionectomy in patients with RSD.[62-66] Complete relief of symptoms was obtained in 58% to 100% of patients during a follow-up period of 6 months to 17 years. Results were better when surgery was done within 6 months of the onset of symptoms. Failures of treatment were seen most often in patients with severe, longstanding disease or in those with incomplete sympathetic denervation.

Bier blocks have been successfully used in RSD patients. A Bier block is a method used for regional anesthesia. The limb is elevated, a tourniquet applied, and an anesthetic or other substance is injected into the limb intravenously for up to 15 minutes. The tourniquet is then removed. Success has been reported[67-69] using Bier blocks with 10 to 20 mg of guanethidine sulfate, with pain relief lasting from hours up to 6 months. This treatment seemed to be most effective in patients with hyperesthesia or hyperpathia. Poplawski, Wiley, and Murray[70] used Bier blocks with lidocaine hydrochloride (Xylocaine) and methylprednisolone sodium succinate (Solu-Medrol) for 28 patients with RSD. Excellent results were obtained in 16 patients, 5 had some improvement, and 7 had no response. All patients had been symptomatic for more than 9 months. The exact role of Bier blocks in the treatment of RSD is not clear. This method of treatment should be considered when symptoms recur after ganglionectomy or when the patient refuses ganglionectomy.

RSD has been treated by direct infusion of reserpine (Serpasil)[71,72] or guanethidine monosulfate (Ismelin)[73] into the affected limb followed by physical therapy. Neither of these agents has been approved by the Food and Drug Administration for intravenous use, and intravenous reserpine is no longer commercially available. Both deplete the peripheral nerves of noradrenaline, the primary agent for vasoconstriction, thus producing a chemical sympathectomy that may last 4 to 5 days or longer.

Steinberg[74] found that the use of periarterial blocks with any anesthetic agent was effective in the treatment of RSD. Severe cases were treated with daily blocks. An average of 3 to 12 treatments were required to resolve the condition.

Antiinflammatory agents may help patients with RSD. Other agents, including oral vasodilating agents such as guanethidine,[75] reserpine, and hydralazine, have been reported to be effective. Beta blockers such as propranolol have also been used.[76] Other agents include griseofulvin 3 g orally per day[77] and calcitonin 100 to 160 IU intramuscularly daily.[78]

Portwood, Lieberman, and Taylor[79] reported on three patients with lower-extremity RSD who responded dramatically to daily, low-dose ultrasound therapy to the tarsal tunnel and plantar nerve distribution of the foot and the use of a shoe insert. Several weeks of daily treatments were required to bring about significant improvement. Another measure employed in the treatment of RSD is acupuncture.[14]

In the past, one frequent suggestion was to immobilize the affected part with a cast or splint. Casting or immobilization is not recommended since this not only exacerbates the problem[38,80] but also can cause the problem. Other treatment modalities that have been reported with varied success are nifedipine,[13] topical clonidine,[81] clonidine Bier blocks,[30] and topical capsaicin.[82]

It is difficult to compare studies dealing with RSD because each investigator may use his own diagnostic criteria. The evaluation of pain and pain relief is subjective, and methods to quantify pain vary from study to study. It has been reported that chronic pain patients' memory for pain is unreliable.[83] Finally, there are few controlled trials and placebo effects are often great.

Treatment of patients with chronic, stage 3, atrophic RSD, with symptoms enduring a year or more, is difficult, and the recovery rate is small. High-dose corticosteroids, sympathetic blocks, and sympathectomy should be considered, but most patients do not respond well. The use of vasocoolant spray, followed by stretching of the restricted myofascial tissues may help. Manipulation of the joints with the patient anesthetized may be necessary for severe contractions. Therapy should also include reducing drug dependency by psychiatric pain therapy units when available and the use of psychotrophic agents such as tricyclic antidepressants. Amitriptyline is one of the more potent tricyclics. Vocational guidance and rehabilitation may also be helpful.

SUGGESTED TREATMENT PROGRAMS FOR RSD SYNDROMES

RSD Stage I (Acute Stage)
Education and reassurance of patient

Intensive physical therapy

Transcutaneous electrical nerve stimulation (TENS)

If not responding in reasonable amount of time, proceed to modalities outlined for stage 2

RSD Stage 2 (Dystrophic Stage)
Try steps outlined for stage 1 (usually not effective)

If not responding, try oral corticosteroid course of therapy

If not responding, try sympathetic blocks and sympathectomy

RSD Stage 3 (Atrophic Stage)
Try steps outlined for stages 1 and 2 (usually not effective)

Free adhesions under general anesthesia

Tricyclic antidepressants

Referral to pain therapy unit

Vocational rehabilitation

Causalgia
Trial course of phenoxybenzamine

If not responding, try sympathetic blocks and sympathectomy

This great variety of treatment modalities proposed in the literature attests to the fact that the management of RSD is controversial. The main point regarding therapy is that the degree of disability and response to treatment depend greatly on the time between the onset of the problem and initiation of proper treatment. Problems arise because of difficulties in diagnosis and great variability of the disease expression and course.

Based on a review of the literature and experience with this condition, the following broad guidelines for treatment are suggested (see the box on this page):

1. *Stage 1 RSD* (acute stage). Early recognition and initiation of early physical therapy is important. Recognize that there is no clinical evidence of sympathetic overactivity in this stage. Success is often achieved by education and reassurance of the patient and a vigorous physical therapy program (the TENS unit may also be useful at this stage). A local nerve block or sympathetic block may be necessary to facilitate these exercises. For patients unresponsive to these measures, a course of corticosteroid therapy should be given.
2. *Stage 2 RSD* (dystrophic stage). Education, reassurance, and physical therapy should be combined with corticosteroid therapy in this patient with clinical evidence of sympathetic overactivity. Steroid therapy should not be delayed. For patients unresponsive to this course of therapy, sympathetic blocks and sympathectomy should be considered.
3. *Stage 3 RSD* (atrophic stage). Corticosteroid therapy should be tried but may be unsuccessful. Sympathetic blocks and sympathectomy should also be considered but likewise may not be greatly successful. Manipulation of the joints under general anesthesia may be necessary for severe contractures. Pain therapy units, antidepressants, and vocational guidance may be helpful.

PROGNOSIS. RSD may follow a benign course, causing moderately severe symptoms and resolving with minimal therapy, or it may be severe, lasting years with chronic pain and disability. In general, the earlier the treatment, the more effective the result.

The majority of patients with RSD respond dramatically to nonsurgical therapy. In a series of 75 patients reported by Trudel et al,[54] 44 had good to excellent results with encouragement, reassurance, and physical therapy. An additional 16 had good to excellent results with lumbar sympathetic blocks and physical therapy. Another 8 patients had good results with physical therapy, sympathetic blocks, and sympathectomy. Only 7 of 75 patients had poor results after all forms of therapy.

Pak,[9] in his review of 140 patients, reported that, of those receiving physical therapy for more than 3 days, 80% showed subjective or objective improvement. In a follow-up of 68 patients, 92% showed continued improvement.

Bonica,[84] reviewing his and other data, reported that over 80% of patients achieved lasting benefits from sympathetic blocks. Wang, Johnson, and Ilstrup[85] found that 40% of their patients obtained good to excellent results from sympathetic blocks, 22% had partial relief, and 38% had a poor outcome. Lower success rates occur if treatment has been postponed for several months.

Although high-dose corticosteroid therapy has been used only in recent years, there are several series of patients with fair to excellent responses in 63% to 76% of cases.[52,57,58] Patients with RSD whose symptoms have been present for a year or more are much less likely to respond to corticosteroid therapy, nerve blocks, or sympathectomy. Irreversible muscle, tendon, and joint dysfunction develop making rehabilitation difficult.

Secondary-gain motives or negative feedback from family members aggravate the situation in a patient with RSD. If litigation is pending, drawn-out legal proceedings may markedly slow rehabilitation efforts. The use of tranquilizers, hypnotics, and narcotics further complicates the situation. The recovery rate in this group of chronic patients is small.

Causalgia

Although causalgia is a form of RSD, it seems advantageous to separate it from the other clinical states already described (i.e., stages 1, 2, and 3 of RSD). Causalgia has sufficiently different diagnostic criteria to be separated from these other conditions. In addition, patients with causalgia fail to respond to physical therapy, whereas practically 100% respond to sympathectomy.

In 1813 Denmark[86] described an agonizing pain in the arm of a soldier after a battle injury. In 1838 Hamilton[87] reported on patients with painful extremities after nerve injuries. In 1864 Mitchell, Morehouse, and Keen[2] described a painful syndrome in soldiers suffering from gunshot wounds during the Civil War. Mitchell[88] later introduced the term *causalgia* to describe the most striking feature of this condition: a persistent, severe, burning pain. His vivid description remains unsurpassed in describing the clinical picture of causalgia.

Causalgia has a place in the history of vascular surgery. Leriche noticed a warming of the extremities in his patients after sympathectomy. He then successfully used sympathectomy to treat ischemic legs. He established his "school for vascular surgoens" based on his techniques of sympathectomy. Some of Leriche's students who went on to greater things were Dos Santos, Kunlin, and DeBakey.[89]

Causalgia is a strictly defined syndrome and represents a subcategory of RSD itself. Terms such as causalgia-like states, mimocausalgia, major causalgia, and minor causalgia are inaccurate and should not be used.

ETIOLOGY. Causalgia may occur after a wide spectrum of injuries in both military and civilian populations. It is most frequently seen in wartime after penetration of the body by a high-velocity projectile, usually a bullet or shell fragment, that causes an incomplete lesion of the peripheral nerve. Other nerve injuries can occur from knife wounds, motor vehicle accidents, falls, athletic accidents, and iatrogenic injuries. Although most injuries are partial nerve injuries, causalgia occasionally is associated with total transection. Shumacker[90] found complete transection lesions in 10% of patients that he saw with causalgia. There appears to be no clinical correlation between the severity of the nerve injury and the intensity of the symptoms.

Richards[91] concluded from a review of nine papers about causalgia from 1945 to 1949, including 9781 nerve injuries, that causalgia occurs in less than 5% of wounds of major nerves. It almost always occurs with high-velocity missile injuries, and the most frequent nerves involved are the median and sciatic.

Causalgia is a disease of war. Mitchell[2] made his classic observations with Civil War soldiers. Leriche[4] used sympathectomy to treat World War I soldiers. Richards[91] and others observed World War II soldiers. Rothberg[92] studied the epidemiology of causalgia during the Vietnam War.

PATHOGENESIS. The exact neurophysiologic explanation of causalgia remains uncertain. Theories proposed to explain this syndrome are the same outlined in the pathogenesis section of RSD. Three theories are commonly proposed. The first is that artificial synapses are produced by the nerve injury so that sensory afferent fibers are activated by efferent sympathetic fiber impulses. The second theory is that nerve impulses from the site of injury alter the vasomotor status of the skin in the painful areas, thus increasing afferent nociceptor activity. The third

CLINICAL FEATURES OF CAUSALGIA

Severe sustained burning pain in distribution of injured nerve or distal to it

Often associated with hyperalgesia (increased sensitivity to noxious stimuli)

Often associated with allodynia (increased sensitivity to nonnoxious stimuli)

Sympathetic overactivity usually present with coolness, hyperhidrosis, cyanosis

theory is that increased spinal cord neuronal activity occurs secondary to changes in the peripheral nervous system. There is little available evidence to fully support any of these theories.

CLINICAL MANIFESTATIONS. The discomfort of causalgia is usually so severe that the clinical presentation is characteristic (see the box on this page). The patient keeps the extremity constantly protected and immobile. In addition the patient is tense, nervous, and apprehensive and devises all sorts of measures to lessen the pain, including moist towels to protect the extremity from drafts of air.

The discomfort of causalgia is usually described as an intense, agonizing burning or aching. It is usually present along the distribution of a major peripheral nerve (e.g., the median, ulnar, femoral, or sciatic nerve) distal to the site of injury. The pain can be diffuse and spread to the proximal and distal portions of the limb without following specific dermatome patterns.

The pain usually begins soon after the injury and reaches peak intensity within a few days to weeks. Onset can be delayed as long as 3 weeks. The pain is usually spontaneous and persistent but subject to exacerbations by various sensory or emotional stimuli. The slightest sensory stimulus, whether tactile, auditory, visual, or emotional, may greatly increase the severity of the pain. Examples include moving or touching the involved part, touching slick objects, touching dry objects, feeling the slightest breeze, hearing certain words, feeling vibrations, experiencing upsetting emotional situations, or just gazing upward or downward. Bandages, towels, stockings, or gloves are often worn by the patient to limit sensory stimuli. Causalgia frequently is associated with hyperalgesia and allodynia in the painful area, but these characteristics are not essential for the diagnosis.

Because of the unrelenting burning pain and frequent hyperesthesia, most patients cannot continue working or carry out regular daily activities. They tend to become extremely irritable and withdrawn and may even exhibit psychotic behavior. Severe depression, drug addiction, and suicide have been reported.[91,93,94] Because of these reactions, patients suffering from causalgia may be thought to be malingering or hysterical. However, these personality disorders are a result of the condition and not the cause of it. The personality disorders usually clear after pain relief with suitable treatment. Psychologic studies done after successful treatment have failed to show any predisposing personality disturbances.[95,96]

The distribution of the pain is a point of controversy. Some authors state that the pain should be restricted to the skin distribution of the involved nerve. Others state that the pain is not restricted to this segment and is usually distal in the hand or foot. Mitchell[88] wrote that "the seat of burning is very various, but it never attacks the trunk, rarely the arm or thigh, and not often the forearm or leg. Its favorite site is the foot or hand." All 20 patients reported by Jebara and Saade[97] had pain distally in the hand or foot. Patients with causalgia may have such severe pain that they have difficulty describing the exact distribution, and this may account for the discrepancies in reported series. In a report by Kirklin, Chenoweth, and Murphey[98] pain was not limited to the exact distribution of one nerve in 43% of patients.

Altered sympathetic activity is usually present in causalgia. Shumacker, Spiegel, and Upjohn,[99] in a study of 54 patients, found a cooler than normal limb in 10 patients and a warmer than normal limb in 25. Other signs of altered sympathetic activity may be present including edema, increased or decreased sweating, and erythema or cyanosis. If the syndrome has been persistent for months to years, dystrophic changes can occur such as skin or muscle atrophy, muscle fibrosis, demineralization of bone, flexion contractures, and joint ankylosis.

Most patients with causalgia have nerve injuries proximal to the knee or elbow.[91] The tibial division of the sciatic nerve, the median nerve, and the medial cord of the brachial plexus are frequent sites of involvement. Upper limbs are more frequently involved than lower limbs with a 5:4 ratio.[2]

DIAGNOSIS. Physicians, especially those dealing with acute trauma patients, should recognize the possibility that a nerve injury, usually a penetrating nerve injury, can be followed by causalgia. Early diagnosis and treatment are important for a favorable outcome. Without proper treatment, long-suffering neurotic tendencies and narcotic dependency can develop in many patients.

Since causalgia is most often seen in wartime, it is unfamiliar to most physicians whose training and experience are limited to civilian practice. As a result, when it is seen in a non–wartime setting, the diagnosis is frequently missed, causing needless protracted suffering and disability.

Although not in agreement, most authorities believe that the criteria for diagnosis of causalgia should include the presence of a continuous burning pain distal to the site of an injury, hyperalgesia and allodynia in the painful area, a traumatic event occurring proximal to the painful area (either immediately or within a few weeks before the onset of pain), and the relief of symptoms with a sympathetic nerve block (see the box on this page). Clinical evidence of nerve injury, sympathetic dysfunction, and trophic changes are not required for the diagnosis.

DIFFERENTIAL DIAGNOSIS. The clinical picture is so striking and unique that causalgia should not be confused with other clinical conditions. It should easily be differentiated from the three stages of classical RSD, Sudeck's atrophy, painful osteoporosis, and a painful amputated stump (with or without neuroma).

PROPOSED CRITERIA FOR DIAGNOSIS OF CAUSALGIA

Traumatic event, often a penetrating wound, occurring proximal to the painful area, either immediately or within a few weeks before onset of pain

Continuous burning pain distal to site of injury

Hyperalgesia and allodynia often present

Relief with a sympathetic block

TREATMENT. Spontaneous remission of causalgia is rare. Treatment should be started as early as possible to prevent contractures, atrophy, and psychologic disturbances. Although physical therapy is the cornerstone of treatment for other forms of RSD, it is ineffective in causalgia. Manipulations and other modalities of therapy only serve to aggravate the suffering.

Narcotic analgesics may relieve causalgia pain, especially when given in large doses, but the danger of addiction is great. Oral medications, including sympatholytic agents and β-adrenergic blocking agents, have been sporadically reported to be useful in causalgia, but medications usually do not adequately control symptoms. TENS has occasionally been reported to be effective,[55] but it is usually not helpful and can aggravate symptoms.

Sympathetic blocks will relieve the pain of causalgia only temporarily, and the pain will return to the preinjection levels within hours. Some authors[91,100,101] have advocated neurolysis or resection of the damaged section of nerve with suture sealing of the proximal and distal stumps, but others[95,98] have reported failures of this treatment. Another procedure that has been attempted but abandoned is periarterial sympathectomy.

In the past the best method of treatment has been paravertebral ganglion sympathectomy. The first documented cure of a patient with causalgia was reported in 1930 by Spurling,[102] a neurosurgeon who performed a successful cervical thoracic sympathectomy. Although some surgical series may confuse causalgia with other forms of RSD, the success rate for complete relief from symptoms of causalgia after surgical sympathectomy range from 84% to 91%, and only 4% to 5% fail to improve.[103,104] The failure of some patients to improve may be related to incomplete sympathectomy or to severe dystrophic changes in muscles and joints in prolonged causalgia.

Jebara and Saade[97] described 20 patients with causalgia resulting from war injuries by high-velocity missiles. All patients were treated with sympathectomy and had complete dramatic relief in the immediate postoperative period. The follow-up period ranged from 4 months to 10 years, with a mean of 5.3 years. No return of symptoms was found.

Chemical sympathectomy using an injection of phenol or alcohol into the sympathetic chain is an alternative to surgical sympathectomy, especially in elderly or poor-risk patients with lower-extremity causalgia. It is not applicable in the upper extremity because of the proximity of the cervical sympathetic chain to the brachial plexus.

In 1984 Ghostine et al[19] reported a method of treatment that should be seriously considered before sympathetic blocks or sympathectomy. They treated a series of 40 causalgia patients with a postsynaptic α_1-blocker and presynaptic α_2-blocker, phenoxybenzamine (Dibenzyline). Although none of the patients had a sympathetic block to test the diagnosis of causalgia, all fulfilled the criteria of a deep burning pain that was exacerbated by physical or emotional stimuli, was associated with partial nerve injury to a major peripheral nerve, and often followed the cutaneous innervation of the injured nerve. Phenoxybenzamine was given in a daily dose of 40 to 120 mg for 6 to 8 weeks. Total resolution of pain was achieved in all patients, with a follow-up period from 6 months to 6 years. Thus this regimen appears to be highly successful and should be tried as the initial treatment in patients with causalgia.

PROGNOSIS. Left untreated, the pain of causalgia may gradually subside in a number of patients. According to Echlin, Owens, and Wells[105] there was a gradual improvement of discomfort within 2.5 months in 38% of patients and within 6 months in an additional 20%. Other workers report patients whose pain persisted for many years.[65,106] With phenoxybenzamine treatment or sympathectomy the prognosis is excellent.

REFERENCES

1. International Association for the Study of Pain: Classification of chronic pain, descriptions of chronic pain syndromes and definitions of terms, Pain 6(suppl 3):529, 1986.
2. Mitchell SW, Morehouse CR, and Keen WW: Gunshot wounds and other injuries of nerves, Philadelphia, 1864, JB Lippincott.
3. Sudeck P: Über die akute (reflecktorische) Knochenatrophie nach Entzündungin und Verletzungin an den Extremitäten und ihre Klinichen Erscheinungen, Fortschr Geb Rontgenstra 5:277, 1901-1902.
4. Leriche R: The surgery of pain, Baltimore, 1939, Williams & Wilkins (Translated and edited by A. Young).
5. Evans J: Reflex sympathetic dystrophy: report on 57 cases, Ann Intern Med 26:417, 1947.
6. Patman RD: Management of post traumatic pain syndromes, Ann Surg 177:780, 1975.
7. Linson MA: The treatment of upper extremity reflex sympathetic dystrophy with prolonged continuous stellate ganglion blockade, J Hand Surg 8:153, 1983.
8. Kozin F: The painful shoulder and reflex sympathetic dystrophy syndrome. In McCarty DJ, ed: Arthritis and allied conditions, ed 10, Philadelphia, 1985, Lea & Febiger.
9. Pak TJ: Reflex sympathetic dystrophy: a review of 140 cases, Minn Med 53:507, 1970.
10. Stiltz RJ: Reflex sympathetic dystrophy in a 6 year old: successful treatment by transcutaneous nerve stimulation, Anesth Analg 56:438, 1977.
11. Plewes LW: Sudeck's atrophy in the hands, J Bone Joint Surg [Br] 38:195, 1956.
12. Chan CS and Chow SP: Electroacupuncture in the treatment of post-traumatic dystrophy (Sudeck's atrophy), Br J Anesth 53:899, 1981.
13. Prough DS: Efficacy of oral nifedipine in the treatment of reflex sympathetic dystrophy, Anesthesiology 62:796, 1985.
14. Reiestad F: Intrapleural analgesia in treatment of upper extremity reflex sympathetic dystrophy, Anesth Analg 69:671, 1989.
15. Arner S: Intravenous phentolamine test: diagnostic and prognostic use in reflex sympathetic dystrophy, Pain 46:17, 1991.
16. Mockus MB: Sympathectomy for causalgia, Arch Surg 122:668, 1987.
17. Olcott C: Reflex sympathetic dystrophy—the surgeon's role in management, J Vasc Surg 14:488, 1991.
18. Christensen K: The reflex dystrophy syndrome—response to treatment with corticosteroids, Acta Chir Scand 148:653, 1982.
19. Ghostine SY et al: Phenoxybenzamine in the treatment of causalgia—report of 40 cases, J Neurosurg 60:1263, 1984.
20. Schwartzman RJ: The movement disorder of reflex sympathetic dystrophy, Neurology 40:57, 1990.
21. Kozin F: The reflex sympathetic dystrophy syndrome, Am J Med 60:321, 1976.
22. Carron H: The treatment of post-traumatic dystrophy, Adv Neurol 4:485, 1974.
23. Gellman H: Reflex sympathetic dystrophy in brain injured patients, Pain 51:307, 1992.
24. Goblet C: The effect of adding calcitonin to physical treatment on reflex sympathetic dystrophy, Pain 48:171, 1991.
25. Glick EN: Reflex dystrophy (algoneurodystrophy)—results of treatment by corticosteroids, Rheumatol Rehabil 12:84, 1973.
26. Glynn CJ: The role of peripheral sudomotor blockade in the treatment of patients with sympathetically maintained pain, Pain 53:39, 1993.
27. Genant HK: The reflex sympathetic dystrophy syndrome, Radiology 117:21, 1975.
28. Demangeat JL: Three phase bone scanning in reflex sympathetic dystrophy of the hand, J Nucl Med 29:26, 1988.
29. Rocco AG: A comparison of regional guanethidine and reserpine in reflex sympathetic dystrophy, a controlled, randomized, double blind crossover study, Clin J Pain 5:205, 1989.
30. Glynn CJ: An investigation of the role of clonidine in the treatment of reflex sympathetic dystrophy. In Stanton-Hicks M et al, eds: Reflex sympathetic dystrophy, Norwell, Mass, 1990, Kluwer Academic.
31. Janig W: Pathobiology of reflex sympathetic dystrophy: some general considerations. In Stanton-Hicks M et al, eds: Reflex sympathetic dystrophy, Norwell, Mass, 1990, Kluwer Academic.
32. Livingston WK: Pain mechanisms, New York, 1943, Macmillan.
33. Janig W: Pathophysiology of nerves following mechanical injury. In Dubner R, Gebhart GF, and Bond MR, eds: Pain research and clinical management, Amsterdam, 1988, Elsevier.
34. Blumberg H and Janig W: Reflex patterns and post ganglionic vasoconstrictor neurons following chronic nerve lesions, J Auton Nerv Syst 14:157, 1985.
35. Bond MR et al: Proceedings of the 6th World Congress on Pain, Amsterdam, 1991, Elsevier.
36. Willis WD: Hyperalgesia and allodynia, New York, 1992, Raven Press.
37. Steinbrocker O and Argyros TG: The shoulder-hand syndrome: present status as a diagnostic and therapeutic entity, Med Clin North Am 42:1538, 1958.
38. Bernstein BH et al: Reflex neurovascular dystrophy in childhood, J Pediatr 93:211, 1978.
39. Bermaglich DR: Reflex sympathetic dystrophy in children, Pediatrics 60:881, 1977.

40. Ruggeri SB et al: Reflex sympathetic dystrophy in children, Clin Orthop 163:225, 1982.
41. Silber TJ and Majd M: Reflex sympathetic dystrophy syndrome in children and adolescents: report of 18 cases and review of the literature, Am J Dis Child 142:1325, 1988.
42. Kesler RW et al: Reflex sympathetic dystrophy in children: treatment with transcutaneous electric nerve stimulation, Pediatrics 82:728, 1988.
43. Breuhl S and Carlson CR: Predisposing psychological factors in the development of reflex sympathetic dystrophy, Clin J Pain 8:287, 1992.
44. Drucker WR et al: Pathogenesis of post-traumatic sympathetic dystrophy, Am J Surg 97:454, 1959.
45. Lexer E, Kuliga R, and Turk W: Untersuchgen über Knochenarterien, Berlin, 1904, Hirschwald.
46. Echlin F, Owens FM, and Wells WL: Observations on "major" and "minor" causalgia, Arch Neurol 62:183, 1945.
47. Julsrud ME: A review of reflex sympathetic dystrophy, J Am Podiatr Med Assoc 70:512, 1980.
48. Owens JC: Causalgia, Am Surg 23:636, 1957.
49. DeTakats G: Sympathetic reflex dystrophy, Med Clin North Am 49:117, 1965.
50. Kozin F: Reflex sympathetic dystrophy syndrome, Bull Rheum Dis 36:1, 1986.
51. Kozin R et al: The reflex sympathetic dystrophy syndrome. II. Roentgenographic and scintigraphic evidence of bilaterality and of periarticular accentuation, Am J Med 60:332, 1976.
52. Kozin F et al: The reflex sympathetic dystrophy syndrome. III. Scintigraphic studies, further evidence for the therapeutic efficacy of systemic corticosteroids and proposed diagnostic criteria, Am J Med 70:23, 1981.
53. Holder LE and Mackinnon SE: Reflex sympathetic dystrophy in the hands: clinical and scintigraphic criteria, Radiology 152:517, 1984.
54. Trudel J et al: Disuse phenomenon of the lower extremity: diagnosis and treatment, JAMA 186:1129, 1963.
55. Meyer GA and Fields HL: Causalgia treated by selective large fibre stimulation of peripheral nerve, Brain 95:163, 1972.
56. Kesler RW et al: Reflex sympathetic dystrophy in children, Clin Orthop 163:225, 1982.
57. Glick EN: Reflex dystrophy (algoneurodystrophy): results of treatment by corticosteroids, Rheumatol Rehabil 12:84, 1973.
58. Rosen PS and Graham W: The shoulder-hand syndrome: historical review with observations on 73 patients, Can Med Assoc J 77:86, 1957.
59. Loh L and Nathan PW: Painful peripheral states and sympathetic blocks, J Neurol Neurosurg Psychiatry 41:664, 1978.
60. Subbarao J and Stillwell GK: Reflex sympathetic dystrophy syndrome of the upper extremity: analysis of total outcome of management of 125 cases, Arch Phys Med Rehabil 62:549, 1981.
61. Betcher AM, Bean G, and Casten DF: Continuous procaine block of paravertebral sympathetic ganglions, JAMA 154:288, 1953.
62. Shumacker HB and Abramson DI: Posttraumatic vasomotor disorders: with particular reference to late manifestations and treatment, Surg Gynecol Obstet 88:417, 1949.
63. Patman RD, Thompson JE, and Persson AV: Management of post-traumatic pain syndrome: report of 113 cases, Ann Surg 177:780, 1973.
64. Holden WD: Sympathetic dystrophy, Arch Surg 57:373, 1948.
65. Barnes R: The role of sympathectomy in the treatment of causalgia, J Bone Joint Surg [Br] 35b:172, 1953.
66. Evans JA: Sympathectomy for reflex sympathetic dystrophy: report of 29 cases, JAMA 172, 1946.
67. Glynn CJ, Basedow RW, and Walsh JA: Pain relief following postganglionic sympathetic blockade with IV guanethidine, Br J Anaesth 53:1297, 1981.
68. Tabira T, Shibasaki H, and Kuroiwa Y: Reflex sympathetic dystrophy (causalgia) treatment with guanethidine, Arch Neurol 40:430, 1983.
69. Loh L et al: Effects of guanethidine infusion in certain painful states, J Neurol Neurosurg Psychiatry 43:446, 1980.
70. Poplawski ZJ, Wiley AM, and Murray JF: Post-traumatic dystrophy of the extremities, J Bone Joint Surg [Am] 65:642, 1983.
71. Chuinard RG et al: Intravenous reserpine for treatment of reflex sympathetic dystrophy, South Med J 74:1481, 1981.
72. Benzon HT, Chomka CM, and Brunner EA: Treatment of reflex sympathetic dystrophy with regional intravenous reserpine, Anesth Analg 59:500, 1980.
73. Bonnelli S et al: Regional intravenous guanethidine vs stellate ganglion block in reflex sympathetic dystrophies: a randomized trial, Pain 16:297, 1983.
74. Steinberg MD: Gout and Sudeck's atrophy: a simplified office approach to treatment, J Am Podiatr Med Assoc 65:379, 1975.
75. Headley B: Historical perspective of causalgia: management of sympathetically maintained pain, Phys Ther 67:1370, 1987.
76. Visitsunthorn U and Prete P: Reflex sympathetic dystrophy of the lower extremity—a complication of herpes zoster with dramatic response to propranolol, West J Med 135:62, 1981.
77. Doury P: Reflex sympathetic dystrophy (algodystrophy), Int Med Specialist 6:67, 1985.
78. Doury P and Pattin S: Treatment of algodystrophy with calcitonin, Rheumatology 32:111, 1980.
79. Portwood MM, Lieberman JS, and Taylor RG: Ultrasound treatment of reflex sympathetic dystrophy, Arch Phys Med Rehabil 68:116, 1987.
80. Kim HJ et al: Reflex sympathetic dystrophy syndrome of the knee following meniscectomy, Arthritis Rheum 22:177, 1979.
81. Davis KD et al: Topical application of clonidine relieves hyperalgesia in patients with sympathetically maintained pain, Pain 47:309, 1991.
82. Cheshire WP and Snyder CR: Treatment of reflex sympathetic dystrophy with topical capsaicin—case report, Pain 42:307, 1990.
83. Engel GL: "Psychogenic pain" and the pain prone patient, Am J Med 26:899, 1959.
84. Bonica JJ: Causalgia and other reflex sympathetic dystrophies, Postgrad Med 53:143, 1973.
85. Wang JK, Johnson KA, and Ilstrup DM: Sympathetic blocks for reflex sympathetic dystrophy, Pain 23:13, 1985.
86. Denmark A: An example of symptoms resembling tic douloureux produced by a wound in the radial nerve, Med Chir Trans 4:48, 1813.
87. Hamilton J: On some effects resulting from wounds of nerves, Dublin J Med Sci 13:38, 1838.
88. Mitchell SW: Injuries of nerves and their consequences, Philadelphia, 1872, JB Lippincott.
89. Barker WF: comment with Olcott C et al: Reflex sympathetic dystrophy—the surgeon's role in management, J Vasc Surg 14:488, 1991.

90. Shumacker HB Jr: Causalgia. III. A general discussion, Surgery 24:485, 1948.

91. Richards RL: Causalgia: a centennial review, Arch Neurol 16:339, 1967.

92. Rothberg JM: The epidemiology of causalgia among soldiers wounded in Vietnam, Mil Med 148:347, 1983.

93. Horowitz SH: Brachial plexus injuries with causalgia resulting from transaxillary rib resection, Arch Surg 120:1189, 1985.

94. Shumacker HB Jr: A personal overview of causalgia and other reflex dystrophies, Ann Surg 201:278, 1985.

95. Mayfield FH and Devine JW: Causalgia, Surg Gynecol Obstet 80:631, 1945.

96. DeTakats G: Causalgic states in peace and war, JAMA 128:699, 1945.

97. Jebara VA and Saade B: Causalgia: a wartime experience—report of twenty treated cases, J Trauma 27:519, 1987.

98. Kirklin JW, Chenoweth AI, and Murphey F: Causalgia: a review of its characteristics, diagnosis, and treatment, Surgery 21:321, 1947.

99. Shumacker HB, Spiegel LL, and Upjohn RH: Causalgia, Surg Gynecol Obstet 86:76, 1948.

100. Allbritten FF Jr and Maltby GL: Causalgia secondary to injury of the major peripheral nerves, Surgery 19:407, 1946.

101. Paget J: Effects from a wound to the radial nerves, Med Times 612:1, 1864.

102. Spurling RG: Causalgia of the upper extremity: treatment by dorsal sympathetic ganglionectomy, Arch Neurol Psychiatr 23:784, 1930.

103. Bonica JJ: Causalgia and reflex sympathetic dystrophies. In Bonica JJ and Albe Fessard D, eds: Advances in pain research and therapy, vol 3, New York, 1979, Raven Press.

104. Mayfield FH: Causalgia, Springfield, Ill, 1951, Charles C Thomas.

105. Echlin F, Owens FM Jr, and Wells WL: Observations on major and minor causalgia, Arch Neurol Psychiatr 62:183, 1949.

106. Abram SE and Lightfoot R: Treatment of long-standing causalgia with prazosin, Reg Anesth 6:79, 1981.

CHAPTER THIRTY-THREE

VASCULAR ANOMALIES

Earl Z. Browne, Jr.

In no area of peripheral vascular disease is there more confusion than in the etiology and pathophysiology of vascular anomalies. A bewildering classification exists, contrasting numerous eponyms and lengthy Latin descriptions with the tendency to describe all types of vascular malformations as hemangiomas.[1-3] This has been especially true in the British literature, where the term *cavernous hemangioma* is applied to a wide variety of pathologic variants.[4] The use of syndromes often adds to the confusion. Although there are some syndromes associated with relatively uniform manifestations (see the box on this page), others are not so clear. For example, Ollier's disease, that of multiple congenital enchondromatosis, is referred to as Maffucci's syndrome when vascular malformations are present, and the actual malformations have been described in many different ways.[5]

GENERAL CONSIDERATIONS

Classification

As with all diseases, it is best to minimize the use of long Latin names and base classification on pathophysiology. Common to all vascular lesions is the presence of endothelial cells. Studies of the characteristics of these cells in various vascular lesions indicate that the lesions fall into two major categories. These include lesions with proliferative endothelium and lesions with static endothelium (or vascular malformations) (see the box on this page).

LESIONS WITH PROLIFERATIVE ENDOTHELIUM. The normal process of healing is a form of vascular proliferation. Angiogenesis is one of the earliest histologic activities in healing, leading to granulation tissue formation in the open wound. Proliferative vascular masses, primarily the true hemangiomas, are vascular tumors with increased endothelial cell turnover during an early phase of proliferation.[6] Although not true neoplasms, capillary hemangiomas demonstrate increased mast cell activity, angiogenesis, and capillary migration.[7] Immunohistochemical analysis of these lesions during the prolifera-

---

CLASSIFICATION OF VASCULAR ANOMALIES

I. Lesions with Proliferative Endothelium
A. True hemangiomas (strawberry nevus)

B. Pyogenic granulomas

C. Neoplasms (hemangiopericytoma, angiosarcoma)

II. Lesions with Static Endothelium (Vascular Malformations)
A. Capillary malformations (port-wine stains)

B. Lymphatic malformations (cystic hygromas and lymphangiomas)

C. Venous malformations (cavernous hemangiomas)

D. Arteriovenous malformations
1. Congenital
2. Acquired
   a. Trauma (penetrating injuries, fractures)
   b. Iatrogenic (surgery)
   c. Spontaneous

SYNDROMES IN WHICH VASCULAR LESIONS ARE PRESENT

Sturge-Weber syndrome (port-wine stain)

Klippel-Trenaunay syndrome (port-wine stain)

Kasabach-Merritt syndrome (true hemangiomas, venous malformations)

Maffucci's syndrome (Ollier's disease)

tion stage demonstrates high levels of cytokines found during angiogenesis such as vascular endothelial growth factor and basic fibroblast growth factor. These lesions characteristically enlarge rapidly in the initial stage, then stabilize, and usually regress. Other lesions with proliferative endothelium include pyogenic granuloma and neoplasms of vascular origin.

LESIONS WITH STATIC ENDOTHELIUM. Lesions with static endothelium are most appropriately called *vascular malformations*. Depending on the structures that are present, vascular malformations may be arterial, venous, lymphatic, capillary, or any combination of those forms. Since they do not have increased endothelial cell turnover, nor do they express cytokine markers of endothelial proliferation, their increased size represents enlargement of previously existing vascular channels.[7,8] A misnomer in the group is the cavernous hemangioma. This is not a proliferative lesion like the capillary, or true hemangioma, although it usually enlarges with time because of hemodynamic changes.[9] Vascular malformations are generally congenital lesions but can be caused by penetrating trauma such as a stab wound.

A study of the embryology of the vascular system provides insight into how these abnormalities, and the various combinations, might occur.[10] The vascular system in the early embryo initially consists of blood spaces forming a diffuse network in the mesenchyme. There is then a coalescence of these spaces into a primitive capillary network. At that stage there is no differentiation of the type of vessel. In the second so-called "retiform" phase there is a coalescence of this primitive capillary network into large plexiform structures, which appear to be separate from one another. It appears that the collateral vessel system is established during this phase, especially in the extremities, and regions of the body develop their own autonomous microcirculation. In the third stage large blood vessels grow out from the great vessels, and communications develop between these vessels and the preexisting retiform plexuses. Arterial, venous, and lymphatic systems are thus established. Depending on the phase in which an embryologic insult occurs, any of these systems may fail to evolve or to involute, causing excessive or faulty development of one or more elements during that time of the embryologic differentiation. Therefore there can be nests of capillaries, veins, or arteries, persistence of arteriovenous connections from the retiform stage, lymphatic accumulations, or any combination of these. Common to all of these malformations, however, is the presence of mature endothelial cells, which do not proliferate to a greater extent than normal cells.[9] Enlargement to "cavernous" structures is a manifestation of blood inherently following the path of least resistance and dilating existing structures.

The classification of these lesions is therefore best done by naming them all vascular malformations and then subclassifying them according to the most predominant element present.[6] Thus the term *malformation* is more descriptive than cavernous hemangioma, and a capillary malformation might be considered to be venous, lymphatic, or mixed. Only if it can be demonstrated that definite shunting is present should a structure be called an arteriovenous malformation. It is also convenient from a clinical standpoint to subcategorize lesions as high flow or low flow.[11] No matter what type of lesion is present, those that have high flow are more apt to enlarge and to require consideration for treatment.

Diagnosis

Although sophisticated tests may sometimes be necessary to determine the extent of a vascular lesion, the diagnosis can almost always be made on physical examination. Lesions characterized by proliferation of endothelium will grow and increase in size over a period of time out of proportion to the surrounding part of the body. Lesions that are static may slowly increase in size but will do so by becoming more engorged with blood and will not truly grow. In addition to obtaining this history, it is possible to determine whether there is a high or low degree of blood flow in the lesion on physical examination. High-flow lesions are characterized by warmth and evidence of increased metabolic activity in the area of the lesion. There may be obvious overgrowth in the area. If there is an arterial component, a thrill may be felt on palpation, a bruit heard when listening to the lesion with a stethoscope, and characteristic sounds of either arterial or venous flow can be heard with the Doppler. Plain radiographs can be helpful in determining the presence of localized increased metabolic activity, and in lesions with large venous spaces phleboliths can also be seen. Arteriography and computerized imaging can sometimes be of value and are discussed in relation to the individual lesions.

Treatment

In general, large vascular lesions are diffuse and are not often symptomatic. Many times the patient or family members are primarily concerned about the appearance of the lesion and its potential for worsening. The physician must first be very accurate in establishing the pathophysiology of the lesion, and then he or she must consider which is worse, the treatment or the disease. For the most part symptomatic treatment and psychologic reassurance are the best approaches for diffuse lesions. Only if it can be determined that a small localized lesion can be easily treated, or that a large lesion has a significant potential for threatening life or limb, should specific treatment measures be considered for relatively asymptomatic lesions.

LESIONS WITH PROLIFERATIVE ENDOTHELIUM

True Hemangioma

The true hemangioma is the so-called "strawberry nevus" of infancy. This classically appears during the second to fourth week of life, having sometimes been noted at birth as a small red cutaneous spot.[10] By 1 year of age approximately 12% of children will have developed a hemangioma, and it is more commonly found in white female infants.[12] The hemangioma characteristically grows very rapidly and is most commonly found in the head and neck region. There is an initial bright red swelling that becomes raised and rapidly shows signs of involution on the surface[13] (Fig. 33-1). After growing rapidly for the first 8 to 10 months of the infant's life, significant involu-

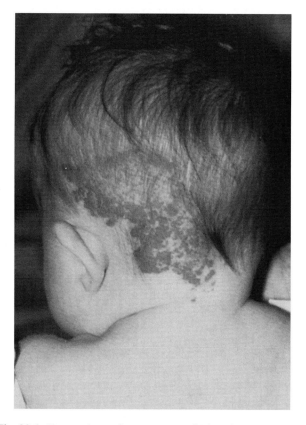

Fig. 33-1. Hemangioma of recent onset, which is already undergoing involution in scattered areas.

tion occurs, and a large number of the lesions have completely involuted by 2 years of age. Studies of the immunohistochemical markers during this stage show a difference from the proliferation stage, and there is found to be an elevation of the tissue inhibitor of metalloproteinase, TIMP 1, an inhibitor of new blood vessel formation.[7] Many studies have indicated that complete resolution occurs in at least 50% of patients by the age of 5 years and in 90% by 7 years.[14,15] The involution, which occurs on the surface, generally starting at the center, causes lighter areas of scarring, which gives this lesion its characteristic appearance of a strawberry. Although they are usually small, occasionally the lesion will proliferate to an enormous size and can cause problems by encroachment on important structures such as the eyelid (Fig. 33-2). They may also ulcerate and bleed. The syndrome of disseminated intravascular coagulation (DIC) in association with extensive, rapidly growing hemangioma in the young infant has been named Kasabach-Merritt syndrome.[16] Although this is rare, it can be associated with a profound bleeding diathesis, and there is a high mortality rate in untreated cases.[17,18]

In general, these lesions are best left alone, since they will typically involute with time.[13,14] The results of treatment are often worse in terms of scarring than the subsequent results of the involution. Occasionally the lesion will not completely involute and surgical excision is warranted, but this is generally reserved for those circumstances where involution of very large lesions has left redundancy of the skin and subcutaneous tissue. The results of cryotherapy, sclerotherapy, and laser ablation are fraught with excessive scarring, so in general they are less desirable than complete surgical excision. These mea-

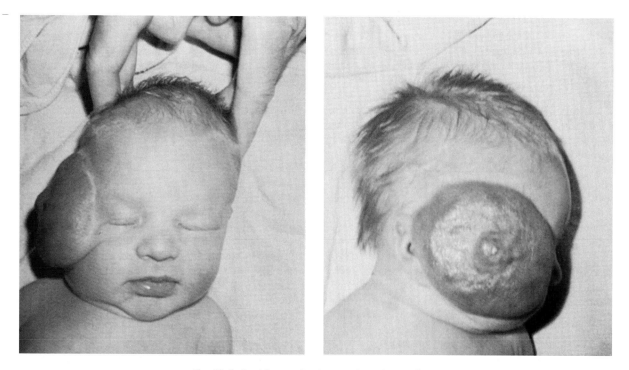

Fig. 33-2. Rapidly growing hemangioma in an infant.

sures, however, may be of value in helping to reduce the size of massive lesions.[9,11] Sometimes because of excessively rapid growth, airway obstruction can develop, which may require treatment. One specific problem requiring intervention is extensive involvement of the eyelid. Amblyopia will develop if obstructed vision is left untreated. Early surgical excision in these circumstances has resulted in encouraging reports.

Systemic steroid therapy is used to treat infants with large hemangiomas, especially if there is significant bleeding or ulceration, encroachment on an important structure such as the eye, or such widespread involvement that there is concern about cardiac failure.[17] Hemorrhage associated with the coagulopathy of the Kasabach-Merritt syndrome usually responds to steroids, but it is important that treatment begin at a very early age. If the lesion is sensitive, a response will occur within a few weeks with a dosage of 2 to 3 mg/kg/day.[18]

Because as many as 40% of severe life-threatening hemangiomas do not respond to steroids, treatment with interferon alpha may be useful. Since interferons are known to inhibit endothelial cell proliferation, experimental protocols using alpha interferon for infants with life-threatening or sight-threatening hemangiomas are being developed, and promising case reports have been published.[19]

Intramuscular Hemangioma

Intramuscular hemangioma is a very unusual form of hemangioma that typically develops in the muscles in young adults. There are no visible signs of vascular change, but a tender area can be palpated and there is typically pain with exercise of the affected muscle. Intramuscular hemangiomas can be identified clearly on magnetic resonance imaging (MRI) studies, as shown in the pectoralis minor muscle in Fig. 33-3. A close association of abnormal blood vessels and nerve fibers is found histologically, as well as the presence of vasoactive neuropeptides.[20] Although histologically indistinguishable from cutaneous hemangiomas, these lesions proliferate and enlarge within the muscle much like a benign tumor (Fig 33-4). The lesion shown in Fig 33-4 was found to contain vascular endothelial growth factor, as well as substance P, accounting for the severe muscle pain encountered with physical activity.

Pyogenic Granuloma

An interesting proliferative vascular lesion is the pyogenic granuloma. It is a localized tumorous growth appearing in small wounds that often have been chronically infected.

Histologically similar to the capillary hemangioma, the pyogenic granuloma is a small polypoid growth that generally develops in the area of trauma (Fig. 33-5). Often there is a small laceration that becomes chronically infected, although these lesions may arise de novo and in apparently well-healed wounds. Although an infectious cause is indicated by its name, seldom is there bacterial growth present unless the lesion ulcerates and becomes secondarily infected.[9] These lesions may spontaneously regress, though many of them have a history of repeated episodes of ulceration and bleeding. They are generally

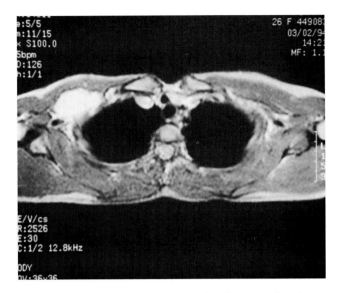
Fig. 33-3. MRI showing hemangioma within the pectoralis minor muscle.

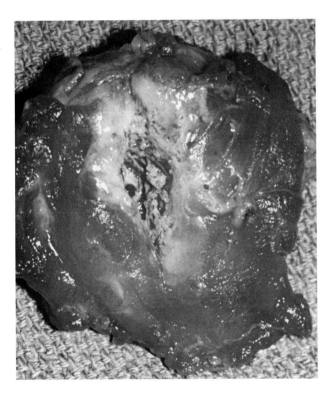
Fig. 33-4. Intramuscular hemangioma in resected pectoralis minor.

treated either by excision or electrodesiccation and seldom have the opportunity to proliferate to a very large size.

Vascular Neoplasms

Although quite rare, there are true neoplasms of vascular origin such as hemangiopericytoma or angiosarcoma, which also have cells that proliferate to a greater than normal extent. These are discussed in Chapter 36.

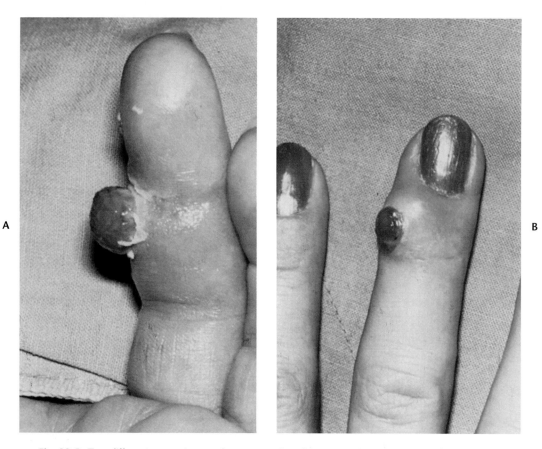

Fig. 33-5. Two different pyogenic granulomas occurring after penetrating injury. **A** is polypoid, resembling granulation tissue. **B** is tumorous, involving adjacent normal tissue, resembling a hemangioma.

LESIONS WITH STATIC ENDOTHELIUM

Capillary Malformations (Port-Wine Stains)

The most common lesion is the purplish cutaneous staining, commonly seen on the face along the distribution of one of the trigeminal nerves (Fig. 33-6). These are always low-flow lesions that characteristically thicken over the years, developing a raised nodular surface.[21] Histologically there are numerous dilated capillary- or venule-size structures present in the dermis. They are always present at birth, although they never appear to be as extensive as the network eventually becomes. Especially in the lower extremities, not only does the surface of the skin become much thicker and involved with dilated vessels, but also more and more of these vessels open in the collateral bed with time, so that the lesion has the appearance of spreading centripetally (Fig. 33-7). However, there is no evidence at all of endothelial proliferation in these lesions.[6-7]

There are two fairly characteristic syndromes associated with port-wine stains. The presence of a stain in the trigeminal nerve distribution may be associated with an underlying venous or arteriovenous malformation of the leptomeninges. This is referred to as the Sturge-Weber syndrome.[22] The Klippel-Trenaunay syndrome is a port-wine stain of the trunk and/or extremities, associated with muscular hypertrophy and varicose veins.[23] Congenital

venous malformations may be present. Often very large tortuous vascular channels develop in the leg (Fig. 33-8). There is characteristically increased warmth of the extremity and often overgrowth, especially if it involves the lower extremity.

Port-wine stains are always permanent defects; the color usually darkens with age, and in adults the surface becomes raised and irregular. One should always keep in mind the possibility of an underlying vascular malformation such as the Sturge-Weber syndrome with a facial stain or the Klippel-Trenaunay syndrome when a stain is present on an extremity.

Most of the concerns for treatment of these lesions have to do with appearance, since they can be quite psychologically disturbing. Over the years there have been many techniques used, including electrical desiccation, cryotherapy, tattooing, serial excision, and skin grafting, but although helpful in extreme cases, most of these result in such excessive scarring that the appearance is worse than the lesion itself.[24] There are several very good camouflage makeups that can be used, and skillful application of one of these is probably the best form of therapy available.

There is considerable interest in the use of lasers to treat port-wine stains.[24,25] The principle of this is the absorption by hemoglobin of energy in a relatively narrow wavelength. Theoretically, if the lesion is purely capillary, it would be possible to deliver enough localized energy in a

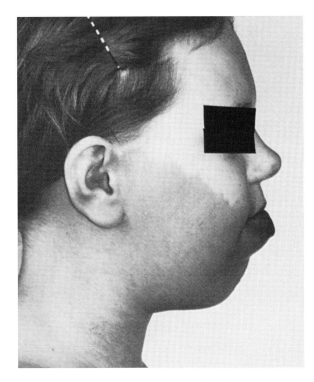

Fig. 33-6. Port-wine stain of the face.

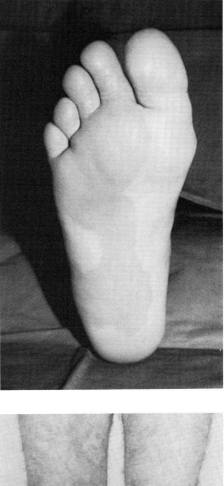

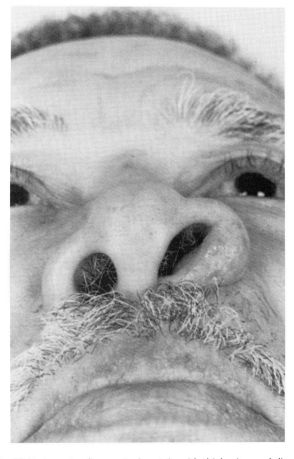

Fig. 33-7. Longstanding port-wine stain with thickening and distortion of the nasal skin.

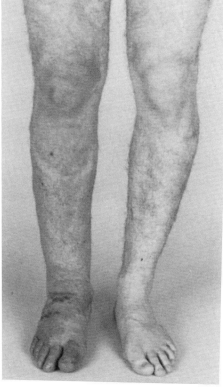

Fig. 33-8. Features of Klippel-Trenaunay syndrome, showing portwine stain, tortuous venous channels, and hypertrophy of the extremity.

small focused beam that the treated area could be vaporized, not harming adjacent tissue. This is only applicable to very small vessels and not dilated channels. By the use of multiple treatments, using a grid pattern, which is changed for each successive treatment, the lesion can be obliterated over a period of time. The argon laser has been used for this purpose in many instances, but unfortunately there is a tendency toward hypertrophic scarring, especially in very young children.[24] Scarring is caused by absorption of energy into the surrounding dermis as well as the vessels. Theoretically it is advisable to use the lowest energy level possible and concentrate the absorption in the vessels by selecting the most desirable wavelength. Many modifications have been tried, and improved results have been achieved, both in eradication of the stain and reduced scarring, with use of other lasers. Flashlamp-pumped dye lasers tuned to wavelengths of 577 nm with low intensity have been reported to be especially effective.[25] Increasing blood flow within the stain improves the result of laser therapy, and simultaneous administration of calcitonin gene-related peptide, the most potent vasodilator known, has been reported to be very effective.[26] Depending on the skin color and texture, light of a color other than red may be effective, and use of the copper vapor laser, which emits rapidly pulsed yellow and green light, appears to be very effective when the skin is hypertrophic or cobblestoned.[27] It appears that successful laser therapy will depend on the ability to select the proper modality for each individual patient; at the present time this is by far the best method of treatment available.

Lymphatic Malformations

Lymphatic malformations are almost always low-flow vascular lesions, although they may become quite large because of increased resistance. Two characteristic forms are lymphangioma and cystic hygroma. A lymphangioma most commonly involves the extremity. It might involve only superficial vessels in the skin, which characteristically become nodular over a period of years. It may also develop into quite large diffuse cystic channels, causing extensive swelling of the entire extremity. Cystic hygromas are always much larger and more diffuse than they appear. They usually appear as spongy-feeling swellings in the neck, which may enlarge with straining or crying. These lesions consist of large dilated cystic spaces filled with lymphatic fluid. If located in areas that are frequently traumatized, they may increase and become chronically inflamed and scarred (Fig. 33-9).

Lymphatic malformations are all low-flow lesions and are best treated only if complications develop. Often surface irregularities develop, leading to cracking and scaling, and over a period of years cutaneous infections may develop. This, just as in the case with lymphedema, can become a significant problem with recurrent bouts of cellulitis and lymphangitis. Because of this, excision and skin grafting may sometimes be necessary for cutaneous lesions (Fig. 33-10). Although well-localized deeper lesions can be totally excised, these lesions typically are much more extensive than they appear, and recurrence after excision is the rule rather than the exception. This is especially true in the cervical cystic hygroma. Prevention

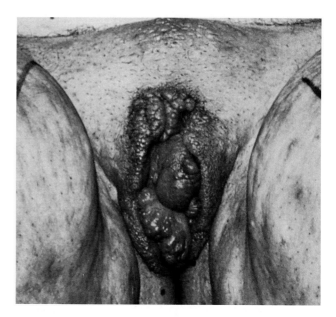

Fig. 33-9. Chronically inflamed, painful, lymphatic malformation of vulva.

of infection with good skin care and compression with elastic garments to help prevent subsequent lymphedema are the primary methods of treatment. Bouts of cellulitis should be treated vigorously with antibiotics to help prevent scarring and progressive lymphatic obliteration in adjacent areas.

Venous Malformations

CLINICAL PICTURE. Venous malformations are lesions that have been commonly called cavernous hemangiomas. They may be low flow, relatively localized, and appear only as a cystic dilated nest of blood vessels (Fig. 33-11). Venous malformations may also be quite diffuse and involve a very large portion of the body as in the Klippel-Trenaunay syndrome. These lesions may expand with trauma and frequently enlarge around the time of puberty or hormonal change. Thrombosis often occurs within these channels because of sluggish flow and may lead to intermittent localized pain and tenderness. Phleboliths can be palpated as lumps in the affected areas and are always seen on radiographic evaluation. There can also be a low-grade DIC present, a form of the Kasabach-Merritt syndrome.[16]

Small, localized lesions are generally asymptomatic. Large diffuse lesions involving the extremities may slowly enlarge to the point where significant problems can occur because of the size of the dilated vessels. Skin changes of stasis, ulceration, and hemorrhage can occur and may become quite painful. Pain may also be produced by pressure on deep structures, especially nerves passing through confined spaces. Nerve deficit may be present because of direct involvement of the nerve by the malformation, but symptoms of nerve entrapment may develop as well. One frequent manifestation is carpal tunnel syndrome caused by compression of the median nerve either in the carpal tunnel or the distal forearm. If allowed to

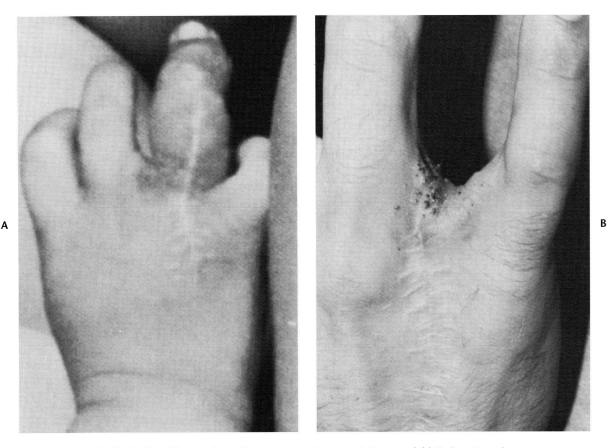

Fig. 33-10. A, Digital lymphatic malformation requiring amputation in a child. **B,** Symptomatic ulceration of residual lesion in a teenager, which was subsequently excised and skin grafted.

persist for a long time, permanent nerve deficit may result from degeneration caused by localized pressure (Fig. 33-12).

DIAGNOSIS. On physical examination there may be very few findings except for a soft compressible mass. Since there is no arterial component, there are no thrills or bruits present, although there is generally a diffuse continuous nondirectional venous sound heard over the involved area when listening with the Doppler. Larger lesions imply not only a more diffuse network of vessels, but also a higher flow causing increased resistance and opening up of more channels. In this circumstance the involved area is often warmer than the rest of the body, and there may be evidence of hypertrophy (Fig. 33-8). Skeletal overgrowth of the involved extremity is a classic finding in the Klippel-Trenaunay syndrome.[9,28] Hypertrophy can be seen on radiographic examination as well as on physical examination (Fig. 33-13).

Plain radiographs almost always demonstrate phleboliths present in the involved area (Fig. 33-14). This is generally a sign of stasis and subsequent thrombosis within the lesion, connoting that it is a relatively stable lesion.[28] With higher flow, especially in arteriovenous malformations, phleboliths seldom develop. Arteriography is not especially useful in purely venous malformations. The arterial phase is characteristically normal, demonstrating normal-caliber arteries and no evidence of shunting.[29]

Small puddles of contrast medium can be seen on late-phase follow-up films during the venous phase but are seldom valuable in determining the entire extent of the lesion (Fig. 33-15). Venograms can sometimes outline the lesion reasonably well, but depend on being able to inject relatively directly into a vein traversing the lesion (Fig. 33-16). Computed tomographic (CT) scans and MRI studies are of much greater value in helping to determine the size and extent of involvement (Fig. 33-17).

TREATMENT. Venous malformations, like the deeper lymphatic lesions, are more diffuse than they appear and are best treated symptomatically with elastic compression. Although occasionally DIC can develop as part of the Kasabach-Merritt syndrome, it is unusual for these purely venous conditions to require specific therapy. Small lesions may respond to injection of thrombosing agents. The obvious limitation of this technique is the ability to confine the agent only to the lesion. Although in the past Klippel-Trenaunay syndrome was treated by excision of varicosities, this form of therapy has not been especially successful.[30] Surgical excision is best done for lesions in which ulcerations or bleeding develop. This does happen occasionally in chronically traumatized areas, such as the foot, and may require excision of the involved area and skin grafting (Fig. 33-18). No attempts should be made to excise the entire involved area unless it is small and localized.

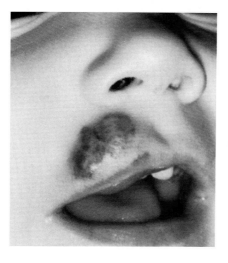

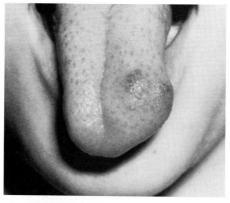

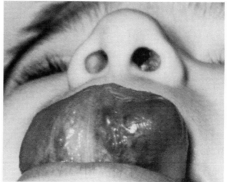

Fig. 33-11. Localized venous malformations. Although erroneously referred to as "cavernous hemangiomas," these are not proliferative lesions.

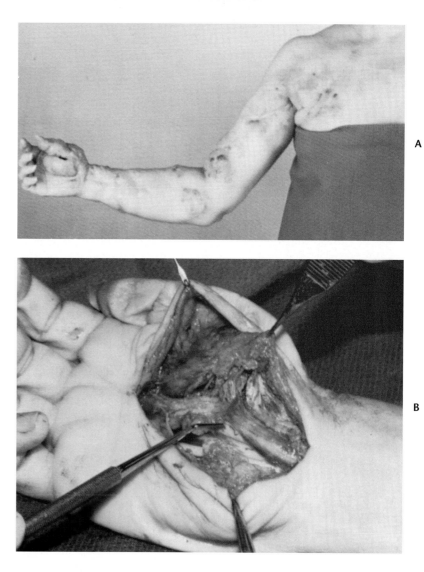

A

B

Fig. 33-12. A, Diffuse venous malformation of the upper extremity causing severe compression of the median nerve in the carpal tunnel **(B).**

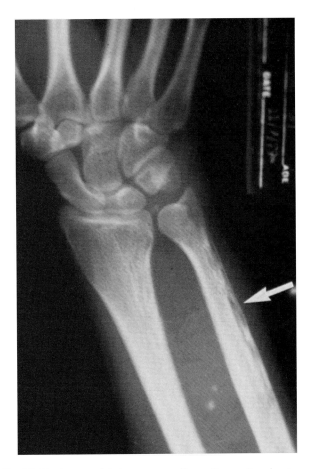

Fig. 33-13. Arrow points to venous malformation centered over ulna in forearm with bony overgrowth seen on radiograph.

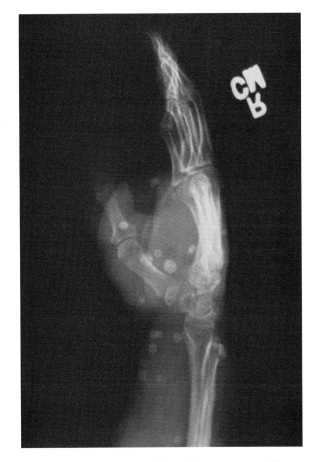

Fig. 33-14. Phleboliths scattered throughout a venous malformation of upper extremity.

A   B   C

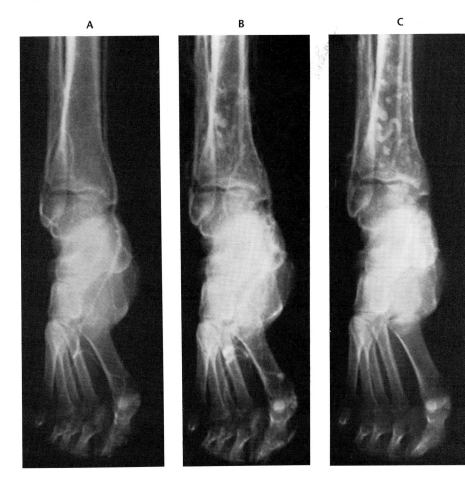

Fig. 33-15. **A,** Normal arteriogram of venous malformation of the lower extremity. **B,** Shows "puddling" of contrast medium in the early venous phase. **C,** Residual tortuous venous channels seen in the later phase.

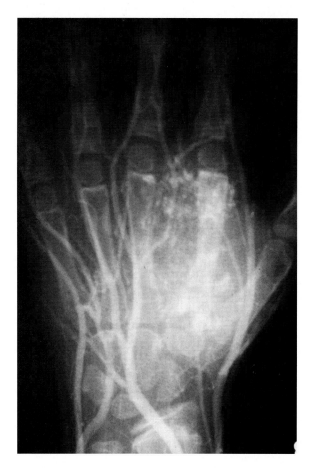

Fig. 33-16. Venous study showing veins and dilated malformation channels over the second metacarpal.

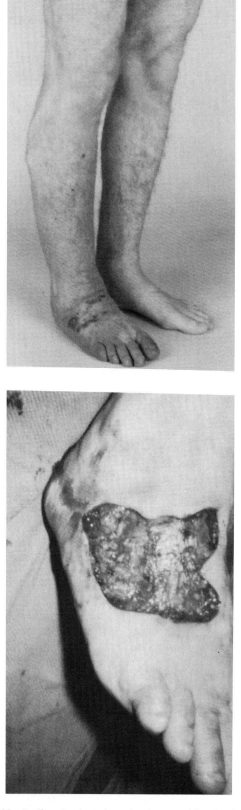

Fig. 33-18. A, Chronic ulceration over dorsum of foot in Klippel-Trenaunay syndrome. **B,** Extent of excision and skin grafting.

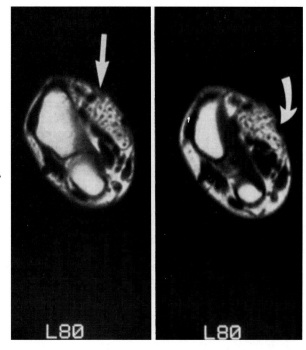

Fig. 33-17. A and **B,** Two sections of an MRI study of a venous malformation at the level of the distal forearm, showing that the lesion is confined to skin and subcutaneous tissue *(arrows).*

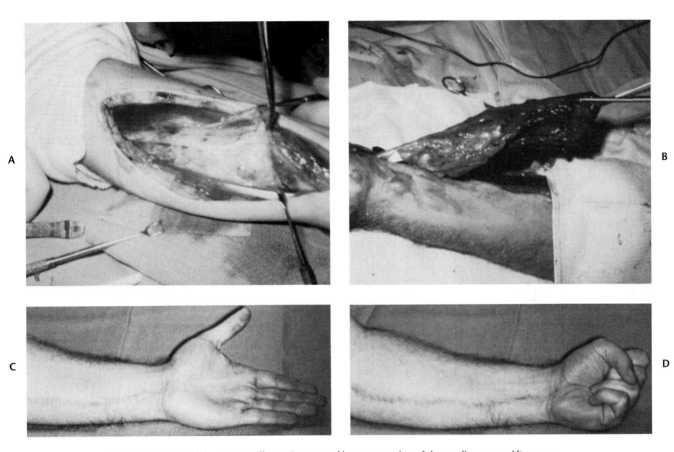

Fig. 33-19. A, Painful venous malformation caused by compression of the median nerve. After complete resection of involved muscle **(B)** and tendon transfer, complete function is preserved **(C** and **D).**

One specific indication for consideration of surgical treatment of venous malformations is the presence of pain. This in itself should raise the possibility of an arterial component, but pain caused by compression by the enlarging malformation can occur. This is most common in the upper extremity, and partial excision of the lesion or decompression may be necessary for pain relief. Compression of nerves can occur, especially in the forearm and in the carpal tunnel. These nerve entrapments are slow in onset, and the symptoms can be subtle. It is easy to overlook these symptoms, blaming the pain on vascular engorgement. It is very important for the physician to make the distinction between entrapment and engorgement. Simple decompression of the nerve, while leaving the malformation alone, can afford marked symptomatic relief of entrapment. Complete resection of the lesion can sometimes be done, providing it will not compromise function (Fig. 33-19).

Arteriovenous Malformations

PATHOPHYSIOLOGY. Arteriovenous malformations can be congenital or acquired. Acquired arteriovenous fistulas are usually caused by penetrating injuries or fractures. They have also been reported after many types of surgical procedures and may occur spontaneously as a result of arteriosclerotic or mycotic aneurysms.[22]

The pathophysiologic changes occurring in congenital lesions are the same as those in acquired fistulas. The basic principle is that blood follows the path of least resistance.[31] The arteriovenous malformation is an abnormal connection between a high-pressure arterial system and a low-pressure venous system with high capacity. Because of the difference in resistance, blood flows preferentially through the fistula rather than continuing along the artery into the normal capillary bed. This causes decreased flow in the artery distal to the fistula and increased flow in the venous system. In addition to causing a steal of blood from the distal bed, the hemodynamic changes that are present lead to the development of increased collateral circulation around the fistula.

CLINICAL PICTURE. Many small congenital arteriovenous malformations are relatively asymptomatic, but acquired lesions often cause such significant shunting that they can become a danger to life or limb. Blood volume, heart rate, and stroke volume can increase, progressing to pulmonary hypertension and even cardiac failure in extreme conditions.[31] This almost never happens in congenital arteriovenous malformations of the extremities, but it is not uncommon for them to become painful, and for ulceration and bleeding to take place (Fig. 33-20). As is the case with large venous malformations, vascular engorgement of an extremity can be a cause of nerve entrapment such as carpal tunnel syndrome.

Acquired arteriovenous malformations often appear as

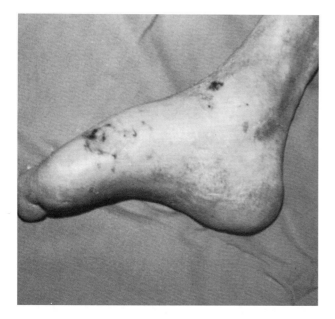

Fig. 33-20. Vascular insufficiency and ulceration of the foot distal to an arteriovenous malformation.

emergent problems. They characteristically tend to worsen fairly rapidly and cause problems because of distal ischemia as well as proximal overload. Even vascular access in the forearm for dialysis can cause significant ischemia of the hand, which can be painful and threaten the survival of the digits.

With an early lesion it is often difficult to determine on physical examination whether a malformation is venous or if there is an arterial component. As changes progress, however, visible signs of shunting will become apparent.[29] Characteristically the area of the malformation will be enlarged and warm, and there will be a palpable thrill present over the fistula. Veins may appear pulsatile, and there will be signs of atrophic changes in the extremity distal to the lesion (Fig. 33-21). Decreased growth occurs distal to the shunt.[32] A bruit is heard with the stethoscope, and marked prominence of both arterial and venous sounds is heard diffusely over the area with the Doppler. It is usually possible to identify several unidirectional feeding arteries with this instrument. The classic sign on physical examination is the Nicoladoni-Branham sign. In this the heart rate slows with compression of the arterial venous communication.[33] This is a reliable sign in acquired fistulas, but if there are many diffuse feeding vessels present in congenital malformations, this sign is not always present.

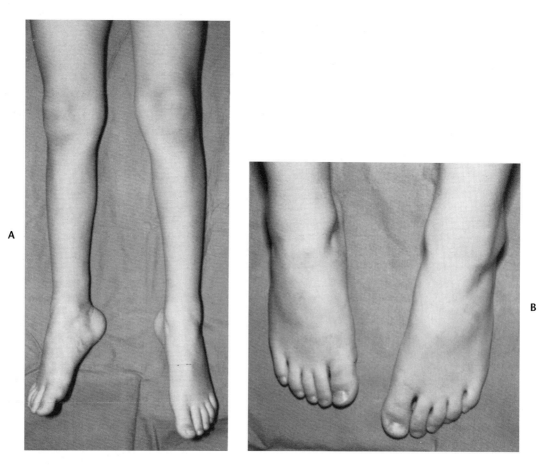

Fig. 33-21. A and **B,** Decreased growth of foot distal to arteriovenous malformation at level of the ankle.

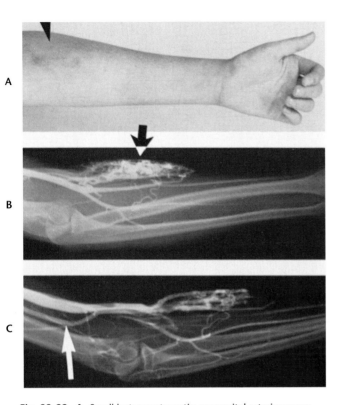

Fig. 33-22. **A,** Small but symptomatic congenital arteriovenous malformation of proximal volar forearm *(arrow).* **B,** Rapid filling of lesion through multiple feeders from radial and ulnar arteries *(arrow).* **C,** Prominent venous return seen before contrast agent has reached the hand *(arrow).*

DIAGNOSIS. The most important consideration in evaluation of a vascular malformation is whether the lesion is a true arteriovenous malformation. If it can be determined that this is not the case, treatment is generally only supportive. True arteriovenous malformations are considered to be unstable lesions because of their tendency to progressively enlarge and because of their potential life- or limb-threatening nature.[22,31] If the diagnosis is very plausible on a clinical basis, it is probably wise to confirm by selective arteriography even though no specific therapy is indicated at that time. An angiogram serves not only to confirm the diagnosis but also to indicate the extent of involvement. In addition, it serves as a baseline for comparison should subsequent deterioration take place in the future.

Although plain radiographs may show skeletal changes of decreased growth and even atrophy, the most important imaging technique is angiography.[29] Selective angiograms show almost immediate shunting with blood present in veins before the contrast medium has progressed any appreciable distance past the fistula (Fig. 33-22). In addition, many tortuous channels are demonstrated, and the largest of the feeding vessels are identified. In congenital lesions, however, there are usually multiple feeding channels, and only the largest ones can be identified angiographically. A very good estimation of the size of the malformation can be gained with angiography, but some-

times CT or MRI studies can also be of value in determining the extent of the lesion, especially if there is concern that bony involvement may be present[34] (Fig. 33-23).

TREATMENT OF CONGENITAL LESIONS

General Remarks. Congenital arteriovenous malformations are usually slowly progressive but may enlarge rapidly following trauma, during growth spurts, or during periods of hormonal or vascular changes such as adolescence or pregnancy. In the absence of life- or limb-threatening problems, treatment must be determined on the basis of whether it is possible to completely eradicate the lesion. Any form of treatment other than complete eradication is doomed to failure because of the presence of multiple feeding vessels.[9,22,31]

If the lesion is threatening life or limb, there is no choice and the lesion must be treated. On the other hand, if it is small and relatively asymptomatic, especially a congenital lesion, then probably no treatment is indicated. As most cases will fall somewhere in between, consideration must be given not only for the problem that the patient has at the time but also for the potential of it becoming worse. For example, even though a small localized lesion may not be terribly symptomatic, it might be that the potential for complete eradication would be quite good. In that circumstance, treatment might be justified on the basis that if the lesion significantly enlarged, the consequences would be much worse—either in terms of the extent of treatment necessary for eradication, or the problems that the lesion itself might cause. An example of this could be decreased growth in a hand or foot distal to an arteriovenous malfunction. If it would be possible to remove the lesion without sacrificing function, then this seemingly more radical approach would end up more conservative in the long run. In general, however, consideration of treatment in marginal cases depends on the presence of complications such as ulceration, bleeding, and pain.

Embolization. Once the decision is made to treat a congenital arteriovenous malformation, embolization with superselective angiography has become an increasingly important form of therapy.[35-37] Theoretically it should be possible to inject material into the feeding vessels, which would then cause occlusion at the capillary level. Small particles of many materials such as absorbable Gelfoam sponge or various nonabsorbable polymers have been used for this purpose. These particles are small enough to pass into minute feeding vessels but too large to pass through the capillary bed.[36-38] The obvious drawback with this technique is not only the ability to successfully do this but also to prevent systemic spread of the embolizing material. Especially in the case of congenital lesions, it also means being able to identify all of the feeding vessels so that the entire structure can be brought under control. This requires very careful planning and an extremely high level of competence in very selective catheterization.[39]

Two obvious problems exist with this technique. The first is the significant incidence of recurrence of arteriovenous malformation, especially congenital malformations. The second is the potential for severity of complications, such as stroke, if the embolizing material cannot be confined to the lesion. Consequently this technique pres-

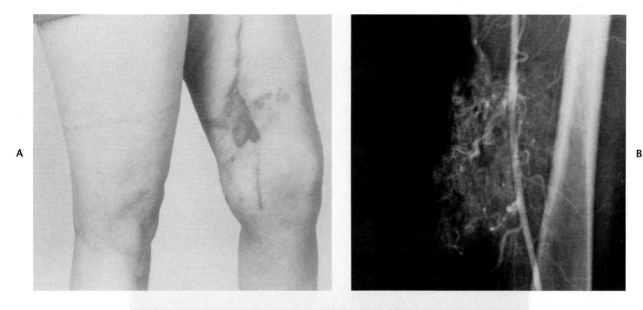

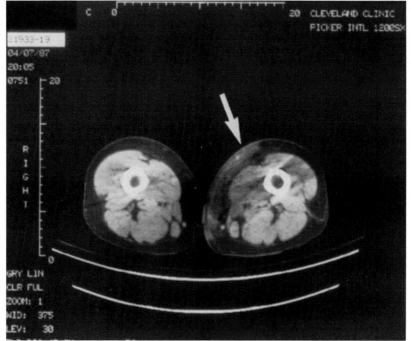

Fig. 33-23. A, Recurrent arteriovenous malformation of the inner thigh. **B,** Arteriogram shows lesion with multiple feeders and early venous phase. **C,** Section of CT scan shows extent of involvement of subcutaneous tissue onto surface of muscle *(arrow.)*

ently is seldom used as the only mode of therapy except in those instances where surgical eradication of the lesion would not be considered feasible, and yet the condition is deemed life-threatening.[38,40] So far, the most valuable use for this technique is in combination with surgical excision. By preoperatively embolizing the main trunks with a substance such as a gelatin sponge or collagen, the mass of the arteriovenous malformation can be temporarily reduced so that the operative blood loss can be markedly reduced.[41]

Surgical Treatment. Two problems are encountered in attempting to eradicate only the feeding vessels of an arteriovenous malformation. Because the fistula results in reduced peripheral blood flow, ligation of proximal inflow serves only to decrease the perfusion in the distal extremity. It has been known for years that gangrene is a common result of ligation of proximal vessels for acquired fistula.[22] The second problem is that ligation of only some of the feeders, by causing anoxia in the peripheral bed, will serve as a potent stimulus for opening up of collaterals. This establishes many more feeders for the fistula, which results in the arteriovenous malformation growing larger and larger.

In addition to opening existing collateral channels,

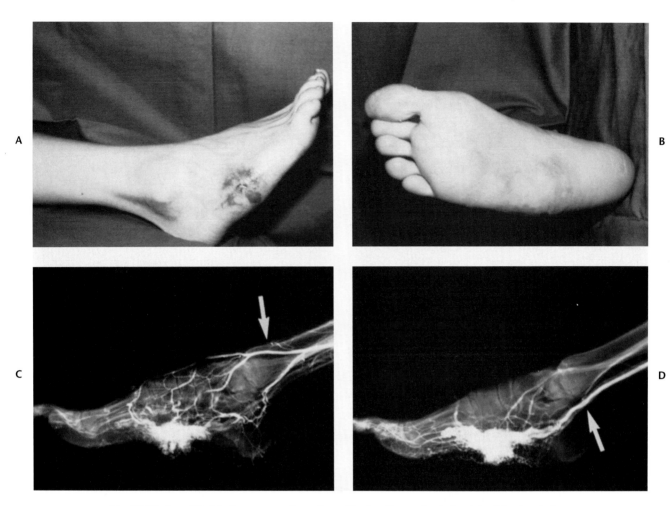

Fig. 33-24. **A** and **B,** Arteriovenous malformation with ulceration and pain involving lateral and plantar surface of the foot. **C** and **D,** Angiograms show multiple feeders from both anterior *(arrow)* and posterior *(arrow)* tibial systems. Resection will create a significant functional defect.

anoxia itself is a potent stimulus of angiogenesis. Anoxic endothelial cells liberate vascular endothelial growth factor (VEGF), which is a potent mediator of vascular permeability and neovascularization.[42] In experimental investigation of ischemic rabbit hindlimbs, administration of VEGF has been shown to significantly augment revascularization. This has been documented by noting increased vessels on angiograms and increased capillaries histologically.[43]

Ligation of vessels is not usually feasible in congenital lesions, since they represent a mass of collaterals with multiple malformed vessels in the given area. When it is feasible to remove this entire mass and still preserve function, then total excision is carried out. When combined with preoperative embolization 2 or 3 days before the operation, blood loss is minimized. It has been difficult in the past to excise some of these lesions even though they were relatively localized because of the subsequent tissue defect (Fig. 33-24). With the advent of free tissue transfer by microsurgical means, however, it is now possible to replace these defects with tissue that can be spared from another part of the body. One of the most common of these procedures is the use of part or all of a relatively

expendable muscle such as the latissimus dorsi or rectus abdominus. The muscle is removed as a free graft with its vascular pedicle and placed into the surgical defect, then circulation is reestablished by microvascular anastomosis (Fig. 33-25). This accomplishes two functions. The first is to resurface the defect and make appearance and function better. The second is to make this microsurgically revascularized tissue healthy with good blood supply. One of the most potent stimuli to angiogenesis is local tissue ischemia. Radical excision of large amounts of tissue, combined with poor wound coverage such as skin grafting, results in scarred, locally anoxic wound beds (Fig. 33-26). In these wound beds collaterals open up and new arterial feeders develop, resulting in recurrent arteriovenous malformations. In addition to the vascular problem, resulting scar contracture may markedly limit function. If the arteriovenous malformation is excised and replaced by healthy, well-vascularized tissue, minimal stimulus for collateralization will be present. This provides the best chance of all for reducing the possibility of recurrence as well as preservation of function[44] (Fig. 33-27). Therefore when treatment is necessary, the combination of preoperative embolization to reduce blood loss and complete

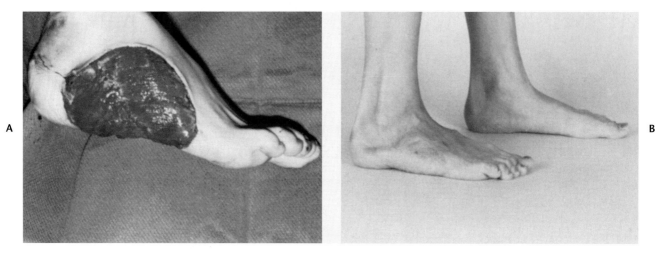

Fig. 33-25. A, The patient in Fig. 33-24 has had total resection of lesion and defect replaced with latissimus dorsi microvascular flap and skin graft. **B,** Function is normal with no pain or ulceration 3 years later.

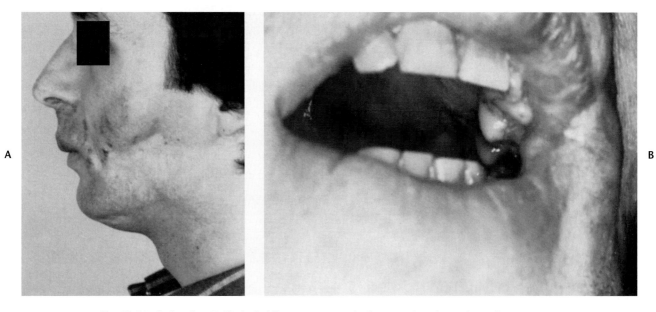

Fig. 33-26. A, Scarring. **B,** Limited ability to open mouth after resection of vascular malformation.

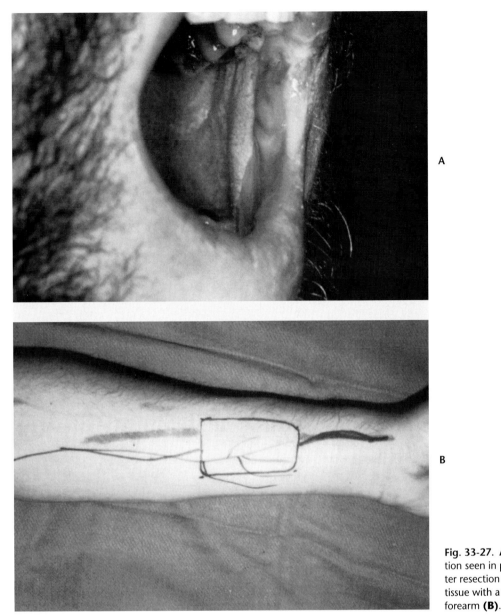

Fig. 33-27. A, Marked improvement in function seen in patient shown in Fig. 33-26 after resection and replacement of intraoral tissue with a free microvascular flap from the forearm **(B)**.

excision of the lesion, combined with replacement of the tissue with a well-vascularized free tissue transfer, is recommended as the treatment of choice.[45]

TREATMENT OF THE ACQUIRED LESION. In the acquired fistula the so-called quadruple ligation method can be effective, especially in the distal extremity.[31] In this procedure ligation of both artery and vein above and below the fistula, along with ligation of any significant collateral, is employed. A more effective method, however, is eradication of the fistula itself with reconstruction of flow in both artery and vein.

REFERENCES

1. South DA and Jacobs AH: Cutis marmorata telangiectatica (congenital generalized phlebectasia), J Pediatr 93:944, 1978.
2. Malan E and Puglionisi A: Congenital angiodysplasia of the extremities. I: Generalities and classification: venous dysplasia, J Cardiovasc Surg 5:87, 1964.
3. Malan E and Puglionisi A: Congenital angiodysplasia of the extremities. II: Arterial, arterial and venous, and haemolymphatic dysplasis, J Cardiovasc Surg 6:255, 1965.
4. Simpson JR: The natural history of cavernous hemangiomata, Lancet 2:1057, 1959.
5. Loewinger RJ et al: Maffucci's syndrome: a mesenchymal dysplasia and multiple tumour syndrome, Br J Dermatol 96:317, 1977.
6. Mulliken JB and Glowacki J: Hemangiomas and vascular malformations in infants and children: a classification based on endothelial characteristics, Plast Reconstr Surg 69:412, 1982.
7. Takahashi K et al: Cellular markers that distinguish the phases of hemangioma during infancy and childhood, J Clin Invest 93:2357, 1994.

8. Mulliken JR, Zetter BR, and Folkman J: In vitro characteristics of endothelium from hemangiomas and vascular malformations, Surgery 92:348, 1982.

9. Mulliken JB: Cutaneous vascular lesions of children. In Serafin D and Georgiade NG, eds: Pediatric plastic surgery, St Louis, 1984, The CV Mosby Co.

10. Woollard HH: The development of the principal arterial stems in the forelimb of the pig, Cont Embryol 14:65, 1922.

11. Jackson IT et al: Hemangiomas, vascular malformations, and lymphovenous malformations: classification and methods of treatment, Plast Reconstr Surg 91:1216, 1993.

12. Holmdahl K: Cutaneous hemangiomas in premature and mature infants, Acta Paediatr 44:370, 1955.

13. Hidano A and Nakajima S: Earliest features of the strawberry mark in the newborn, Br J Dermatol 87:138, 1972.

14. Bowers RE, Graham EA, and Tomlinson KM: The natural history of the strawberry nevus, Arch Dermatol 82:667, 1960.

15. Lister WA: The natural history of the strawberry naevi, Lancet 1:1429, 1938.

16. Kasabach HH and Merritt KK: Capillary hemangioma with extensive purpura: report of a case, Am J Dis Child 59:1063, 1940.

17. Zarem HA and Edgerton MT: Induced resolution of cavernous hemangiomas following prednisolone therapy, Plast Reconstr Surg 39:76, 1967.

18. El-Dessouky AF et al: Kasabach-Merritt syndrome, J Pediatr Surg 23:109, 1988.

19. Ezekowitz A, Mulliken J, and Folkman J: Interferon alpha therapy of hemangiomas in newborns and infants, Br J Haematol 79(suppl 1):67, 1991.

20. Robinson D et al: Neuropeptidergic innervation of intramuscular hemangiomas, Exp Molec Pathol 56:186, 1992.

21. Mulliken JB and Murray JE: Natural history of vascular birthmarks. In Williams HB, ed: Symposium on vascular malformations and melanotic lesions, St Louis, 1982, The CV Mosby Co.

22. Gloviczki P and Hollier LH: Arteriovenous fistulas. In Haimovici H, ed: Vascular surgery: principles and techniques, ed 3, New York, 1989, Appleton & Lange.

23. Klippel M and Trenaunay P: Du naevus variqueux osteohypertrophique, Arch Gen Med (Paris) 3:641, 1900.

24. Noe JM et al: Port wine stains and the response to argon laser therapy: successful treatment and the predictive role of color, age, and biopsy, Plast Reconst Surg 65:130, 1980.

25. Reid WH et al: Treatment of portwine stains using the pulsed dye laser, Br J Plast Surg 45:565, 1992.

26. Jernbeck J and Malm M: Calcitonin gene-related peptide increases the blood flow of port-wine stains and improves continuous-wave dye laser treatment, Plast Reconstr Surg 91:245, 1993.

27. Dinehart SM, Waner M, and Flock S: The copper vapor laser for treatment of cutaneous vascular and pigmented lesions, J Dermatol Surg Oncol 19:370, 1993.

28. Rosen RJ, Riles TS, and Berenstein A: Congenital vascular malformations. In Rutherford RB, ed: Vascular surgery, ed 3, Philadelphia, 1989, WB Saunders Co.

29. Sumner DS and Rutherford RB: Diagnostic evaluation of arteriovenous fistulas. In Rutherford RB, ed: Vascular surgery, ed 3, Philadelphia, 1989, WB Saunders Co.

30. Gloviczki P et al: Surgical implications of Klippel-Trenaunay syndrome, Ann Surg 197:353, 1983.

31. Sumner DS: Hemodynamics and pathophysiology of arteriovenous fistulas. In Rutherford RB, ed: Vascular surgery, ed 3, Philadelphia, 1989, WB Saunders Co.

32. Boyd JB et al: Skeletal changes associated with vascular malformations, Plast Reconstr Surg 74:789, 1984.

33. Branham HH: Aneurysmal varix of the femoral artery and vein following a gunshot wound, Int J Surg 3:250, 1890.

34. Berquist TH: Bone and soft tissue tumors. In Berquist TH, ed: Magnetic resonance of the musculoskeletal system, New York, 1987, Raven Press.

35. Merland JJ et al: Les malformations vasculaires cervico-cephaliques protocole actuel de tratement. Á propos de 230 cas, Phlebologie 33:95, 1980.

36. Rosen RJ: Embolization in the treatment of arteriovenous malformations. In Goldberg HI, Higgins CB, and Ring EJ, eds: Contemporary imaging, San Francisco, 1985, University of California Press.

37. Gomes AS, Mali WP, and Oppenheim WL: Embolization therapy in the management of congenital arteriovenous malformations, Radiology 144:41, 1982.

38. Forbes G et al: Therapeutic embolization angiography for extra-axial lesions in the head, Mayo Clin Proc 61:427, 1986.

39. Coldwell DM, Stokes KR, and Yakes WF: Embolotherapy: agents, clinical applications and techniques, Radiographics 14:623, 1994 (review).

40. Stanley P et al: Therapeutic embolization of infantile hepatic hemangioma with polyvinyl alcohol, Am J Roentgenol 141:1047, 1983.

41. Loose DA: Combined treatment of congenital vascular defects: indications and tactics, Semin Vasc Surg 6:260, 1993 (review).

42. Miller JW et al: Vascular endothelial growth factor/vascular permeability factor is temporally and spatially correlated with ocular angiogenesis in a primate model, Am J Pathol 145:574, 1994.

43. Takeshita S et al: Therapeutic angiogenesis, J Clin Invest 93:662, 1994.

44. Hurwitz DJ and Kerber CW: Hemodynamic considerations in the treatment of arteriovenous malformations of the face and scalp, Plast Reconstr Surg 67:421, 1981.

45. Yamamoto Y et al: Experience with arteriovenous malformations treated with flap coverage, Plast Reconstr Surg 94:476, 1994.

CHAPTER THIRTY-FOUR

TRAUMA AND PERIPHERAL VASCULAR DISEASE

Malcolm O. Perry

Trauma ranks overall as the fourth leading cause of death in the United States, but in the first four decades of life, it is first.[1] Over 140,000 people die each year from accidents, and injuries lead to more than 140,000,000 bed days of annual disability.

Most major arterial injuries are the result of aggressive acts of violence, and although few communities are spared, these events are more likely to occur in urban areas, where violence is endemic and drug abuse is common. In fact, recent government studies indicate that most violent crimes now are drug related.[2,3]

ETIOLOGY

Penetrating wounds caused by bullets and knives are usually seen, but accidental stab wounds resulting from motor vehicle accidents or industrial mishaps also may be encountered[4,5] (see the accompanying box). Stab wounds are seen more frequently than gunshot wounds; many of them are not serious, and vital organs may be spared. Gunshot wounds usually penetrate deeply and often involve the trunk as well as the extremities. Many of the patients with bullet wounds of the abdomen and chest do not survive long enough to reach the hospital. Multiple vascular wounds are often encountered in these patients, and although any major vascular wound can lead to lethal bleeding, death is more common with injuries of major vessels in the chest or abdomen, where early detection and rapid control of hemorrhage are more difficult (see the accompanying box).

Those injuries that are the result of substance abuse present particularly difficult problems.[6,7] The patients generally do not seek medical aid until complications of the arterial punctures have occurred, usually false aneurysms, infection, and occasionally sepsis. In many of these people thromboembolism has already supervened, and viability of the extremities is in doubt at the time they are first seen. Moreover, a major threat at any time is rupture of an infected artery.[8]

With the increasing use of transarterial procedures for various studies, and balloon dilation of stenotic arteries, there are more iatrogenic injuries of major vessels.[9] The incidence of complications varies a great deal depending on the indication for the arterial procedure.[10,11] Trans-

DISTRIBUTION OF ARTERIAL INJURIES IN 665 PATIENTS

Extremity	501
Aorta	31
Visceral	37
Cervical	96
TOTAL	665

From Perry MO: The management of acute vascular injuries, Baltimore, 1981, Williams & Wilkins.

ASSOCIATED INJURIES (%) IN 665 PATIENTS WITH ARTERIAL INJURIES

Large vein	34
Major nerve	18
Separate artery	7
Lung, abdominal viscera	39

From Perry MO: The management of acute vascular injuries, Baltimore, 1981, Williams & Wilkins.

femoral catheter studies are often uncomplicated, even in patients with atherosclerosis. One study reported an overall complication rate of only 1%.[12] If the common femoral artery is used for balloon dilation of stenotic arteries, the problems are more numerous, probably related to the length and complexity of the procedures.[13] Intraaortic assist procedures and transfemoral cardiac valve operations, such as valvuloplasty, are even more risky; complications are seen in 5% to 11% of patients.[12]

Most angiographers and cardiologists try to use the femoral artery rather than the brachial or axillary arteries. These routes also carry a higher risk, not only of arterial damage, but also of major nerve problems. Although these problems can be severe, the complications usually are identified early since the patient is under direct observation in the hospital.[14] An accurate diagnosis and expedient repair is usually feasible, and therefore the results generally are satisfactory. If initial arterial repairs are not undertaken, delayed complications can occur, even after months or years.[15]

PATHOPHYSIOLOGY

Penetrating injuries, producing direct vascular wounds, are usually caused by knives or bullets traveling at a low velocity, and most of the damage is confined to the wound tract. Lacerations of the artery are the most common finding, but contusions, punctures, and transections are also encountered. High-velocity bullets can produce severe damage to the structures in their path, and the blast effect can cause more remote injuries. Contusion or even vessel transection can follow the cavitation effect associated with bullets traveling at velocities of 2000 to 3000 ft/sec. Even if immediate arterial disruption does not occur, mural contusions can result in delayed thrombosis or wall necrosis, late hemorrhage, and false aneurysm formation.

Although unusual in the civilian environment, a high-velocity bullet or metal fragment can produce a great deal of damage because of its high energy. Secondary missiles consisting of bullet or shell fragments or bone splinters also may be created, and they in turn produce other wounds. There is a powerful suction effect as the blast cavity collapses, and surface structures such as clothing and dirt can be drawn into the wound. Such widespread destruction may not be suspected from inspection of the skin surface where, in some cases, rather small entrance and exit wounds are seen, despite the extent of the interior damage.

Motor vehicle accidents also result in vascular trauma, and usually the victims have multiple injuries. Direct injury to the arteries can occur, but often vascular wounds are the result of fractures. This is especially likely to occur to vessels located near the joints; there they are relatively fixed and more vulnerable to shear forces.

The break of large, heavy bones such as the femur or the tibia releases tremendous amounts of energy. The damage to the soft tissues in the area can be extensive, and the effects are similar to those produced by high-velocity bullets. After the bones fall back to a near-normal position, the magnitude of the injuring forces may not be appreciated, and the severity of the damage is easily underestimated.

DIAGNOSIS

Clinical Diagnosis

Injuries of large arteries usually can be identified readily because of severe hemorrhage, large hematomas, and pulse deficits[5] (see the box on this page). Less extensive injuries may not be as obvious. Ischemia distal to the area of the arterial injury may not be present, especially when intervening collateral vessels are adequate and hypotension is absent. The assessment of the adequacy of blood flow based on the detection of distal extremity pulses is limited by specific hemodynamic features. The pulse wave is a pressure wave that attains velocities of up to 10 m/sec, while the flow wave of blood has a velocity of 40 cm/sec. The physical examination must take this fact into account because the pulse wave can be transmitted past intimal flaps, through collateral arteries, or even beyond limited areas of fresh soft clot. Moreover, if the injuries are limited only to damage of the vessel wall, then distal pulses usually will be unimpaired (Fig. 34-1). One series reported that up to 18% of patients with operatively proven major arterial injuries in the extremities had normal distal pulses at the time of the initial examination.[5,16] Such a combination of findings is especially likely to be seen in patients who have penetrating wounds near the hip or shoulder where the collateral circulation is abundant.

Most major arterial injuries caused by penetrating trauma to the extremities can be detected by obtaining a detailed history and performing a careful physical examination.[17] Although small, occult vascular wounds can be missed, studies have shown that these rarely cause significant problems.[18] A careful, long-term follow-up of these patients is required because missed injuries of major arteries are capable of causing serious delayed complications.[19]

Injuries of the great vessels in the chest and abdomen present special problems in diagnosis since they are inaccessible for direct evaluation. A hemopneumothorax or mediastinal bleeding is common with penetrating injuries to the chest even in patients who do not have major vascular wounds. These patients may initially be stable and are thought only to have parenchymal lung damage or minor arterial injuries, and sudden hemodynamic collapse may be the first sign of more severe problems. In such patients a wide mediastinum, cardiac arrest, persistent shock, cardiac tamponade, and recurring hemothorax strongly suggest the presence of major vascular injuries.[5,16]

CLINICAL FEATURES OF ARTERIAL INJURIES

Diminished or absent pulse

Enlarging hematoma

Pulsatile arterial bleeding

Symptoms of ischemia

Injury of anatomically related nerves

Major hemorrhage with hypotension

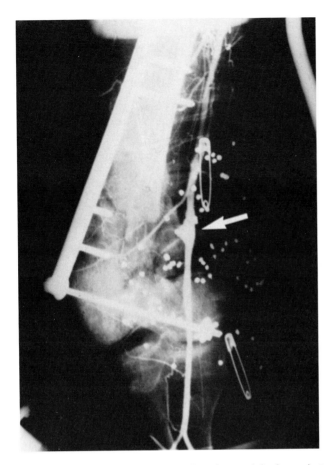

Fig. 34-1. This injury from shotgun pellets shattered the femur, but the patient had palpable pedal pulses, despite the injury to the superficial femoral artery *(arrow)*.

Patients with penetrating or blunt trauma to the abdomen also are vulnerable to vascular injuries although not with as great a frequency as in the extremities. The diagnosis of a vascular wound in these patients rests primarily on the detection of continued bleeding.[20]

Adjunctive Diagnostic Methods

Although ordinary radiographs rarely establish the diagnosis of an arterial injury, they are of value in evaluating these patients since such studies may disclose the presence of subcutaneous or mediastinal air, collections of fluid or blood, and displacement of viscera. The wound tract of a bullet is not usually a straight line, but x-ray film studies may offer some assistance in determining the nature and the extent of the wound, and thus suggest a need for other studies. An assessment of the vulnerable structures between the entry site and exit site (or final resting place) of the bullet should be undertaken.

Computerized tomography (CT) is of benefit in the examination of injured patients, and even without the administration of contrast medium, soft tissue distortion, hematomas, and some injuries of solid organs can be detected.[16] Magnetic resonance imaging (MRI) promises to be of even greater value in the evaluation of trauma patients. Specialized adjustments, which change the resonance frequency, can generate images of the blood vessels even without radiopaque contrast material. Although these methods are not sufficiently refined so as to permit them to be used exclusive of other techniques, they do offer valuable data in the evaluation of vascular injuries.

Doppler techniques may be helpful in detecting vascular injury, and also in assessing the adequacy of arterial blood flow in the extremities. The measurement of distal arterial systolic blood pressure is helpful, but specificity of these methods suffers from hemodynamic limitations, which also govern arterial pulses. Subtle abnormalities in the Doppler-derived measurements are common, but relatively normal values are also seen. This may be a particular problem in the patient with multiple injuries who is hypotensive. These techniques are of considerable value as an extension of the physical examination in the initial evaluation of the patient, and they offer a great deal of assistance postoperatively, but none can be relied on to exclude an arterial injury.[5]

ARTERIOGRAPHY. In the management of trauma patients preoperative arteriography is used for three main reasons: (1) to exclude the presence of a vascular injury in a patient who otherwise has no indications for operative exploration, (2) to detect a lesion that was not exposed by other diagnostic techniques, and (3) to plan the operative management of a patient with a major vascular injury.

In patients who have penetrating trauma to the lower extremity a simple needle puncture of the common femoral artery and single plane arteriograms may be quite useful in excluding the need for operation when other indications for exploration do not exist (Fig. 34-2). Feliciano et al have clearly demonstrated that this is a safe and reliable technique, and although their follow-up series was relatively short, no serious immediate complications were seen.[4] Snyder et al have emphasized that high-grade biplane arteriography is reliable, although not infallible, in detecting arterial injuries.[21] In a prospective study of 183 patients with penetrating trauma of the extremity, biplane arteriography was evaluated. All of the patients had arteriograms and then were operated on for the listed indications regardless of the arteriographic findings. There were 28 false-positive studies, 32 true-positive studies, one false-negative examination, and the rest were true negatives in this series, thus confirming the usefulness of this technique in establishing the diagnosis of major vascular injuries in the extremities. Studies have suggested that in those patients who have no firm indications for operation, if arteriography is performed solely because of the proximity of the injury to a vessel, it is likely to have a positive yield of less than 10%.[22] In such situations a careful selection of patients must be undertaken to avoid performing unnecessary studies, keeping in mind that an abbreviated arterial procedure can be of considerable assistance at times in excluding the need for operation in such patients.

Although direct punctures are possible, more often than not transfemoral Seldinger catheter techniques have been used for these studies. They enable the angiographer to examine many portions of the arterial tree via a single arterial entry. In the unstable patient it is best not to undertake these prolonged procedures but to go directly to the operating room. In such situations sudden hemody-

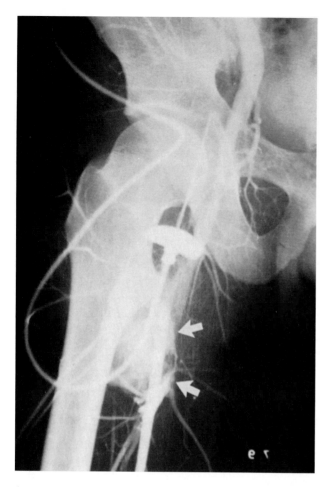

Fig. 34-2. A stab wound of the profunda femoris artery caused this false aneurysm *(arrows)*. The patient had normal pedal pulses.

namic collapse may occur; it often will have a lethal outcome if the patient is not in a position where bleeding can be controlled immediately. Diagnostic studies in a hemodynamically unstable patient should be performed in the operating room so the surgical team may intervene immediately if necessary.

Special problems are presented when drug abuse patients with arterial wounds are seen.[6] Since these wounds are invariably infected, arteriography may be particularly valuable in planning the operative procedure. Remote bypass techniques using subcutaneous grafts may be required to maintain viability of the extremities in such patients, since direct repairs in the grossly contaminated field are not safe.[23] A careful and complete evaluation of the vascular system in the involved area must be undertaken in these patients, and that usually means biplane arteriography as well as CT or MRI scans.

For people in whom injuries to the internal carotid artery at the base of the skull or at the root of the neck are suspected, preoperative arteriography is of considerable value in planning the operation (Fig. 34-3). Moreover, if the patient has a neurologic deficit, biplane intracranial films should be obtained at the same time to determine if distal thromboembolism has already supervened. Specialized surgical procedures for exposure and vascular repair may be required in these patients, and it is best to have this knowledge before beginning the operation.[5]

A special situation also exists in the evaluation of patients who are thought to have renal artery or kidney injury.[16] In a patient with hematuria an intravenous pyelogram (IVP) is performed, and if there was a prior disturbance in renal function, this is followed by an arteriogram. In such a patient if the major vascular architecture to the kidney is intact, and if there is no disruption of the collecting system, observation rather than exploration is preferred. In such people injuries to the kidney

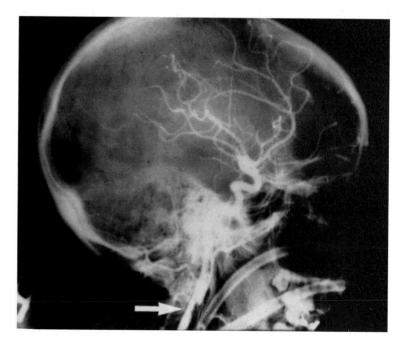

Fig. 34-3. Injuries to the internal carotid artery can be difficult to diagnose. This mural damage and intraluminal clot resulted from blunt trauma *(arrow)*.

cortex can be expected to heal if Gerota's fascia is left intact. On the other hand, if major arterial injury or collecting system disruption is identified, then surgical repair is required.

Arteriography also may be of use when patients are suspected of having injuries to other major visceral arteries, again primarily to identify the area of injury and to accurately plan the operation. If these patients are unstable, however, abbreviated arteriographic studies can be performed in the operating room during the course of the procedure; this offers considerable assistance both in identifying other lesions and in planning the repairs. The intraoperative method is not as satisfactory as the more sophisticated studies available in the radiology suite, but it is the preferred solution for an unstable patient.

MANAGEMENT

General Principles

A patient with a major vascular injury usually has dramatic symptoms—bleeding, pallor, shortness of breath, and often hypotension. Successful resuscitation requires that certain priorities be established and specific plans for treatment be formulated. In all of these people initial attention to the airway and stopping the bleeding is first. Once control of the airway has been obtained and the vital signs assessed, an overall evaluation can be completed and proper priorities assigned. If external bleeding is present, it is usually controlled with direct finger pressure, pressure dressings, or pressure on proximal vascular structures. Blind attempts to clamp bleeding vessels located deep in the wound are ineffective and often dangerous, and should not be done. Tourniquets are rarely necessary.

After control of the airway is secured and respiratory assistance initiated, ventilation and pulmonary function are evaluated. Chest trauma is not uncommon in these patients and a hemothorax or pneumothorax must be treated initially. If chest tubes are needed, these should be inserted early during the resuscitation before pressure-assisted ventilation causes more severe mechanical problems by increasing the air leak and perhaps producing a tension pneumothorax.

Since these patients often require large amounts of fluid and blood, large catheters are placed into uninjured upper and lower extremity veins and carefully secured. One line is committed only for fluid replacement and is not used for drug administration or anesthetic manipulations.

In most cases these patients require a combination of a balanced electrolyte solution and whole blood to replace losses. As described by Shires and Shires, trauma and shock cause internal shifts of interstitial fluid that are best treated with appropriate infusions of electrolyte solutions and blood. It is wise not to overtransfuse, especially if cardio-pulmonary disease is present, since this may lead to cardiac overload. It appears that a whole blood hematocrit of approximately 30% is optimum; further increases in hemoglobin are unneeded and may increase blood viscosity unnecessarily. There are little convincing data showing that the infusion of a colloid solution such as albumin or dextran is of any additional value, and some studies suggest that colloid solutions may be harmful.[1]

During the initial examination if there is a need for special monitoring techniques, this is usually obvious. Hemodynamically stable patients with minor wounds of the extremities require only routine procedures, especially if they are young and free of intercurrent illnesses. In contrast, the patient who has multiple injuries or shock, or someone with preexisting cardiopulmonary problems, is almost certain to need continuous monitoring of vital signs, pulmonary mechanics, and cardiac function. Some estimate of cardiac filling and output is needed in these patients. A venous catheter to measure central venous pressure is helpful, but most of these people will benefit from a Swan-Ganz balloon catheter for direct evaluation of pulmonary artery pressure and cardiac function.

Control of Bleeding

Most bleeding wounds can be controlled with direct digital pressure. In the majority of instances brisk hemorrhage has stopped in patients who have survived to reach the emergency room, but often large hematomas are present, and some bleeding may persist. If the wound is not bleeding it is best not to disturb it during the initial resuscitation; no attempt should be made to remove foreign bodies, or to evacuate clots until a general assessment has been completed and measures for obtaining proximal control are under way. Penetrating objects that are in the wound must be protected during transportation because they are capable of causing further damage, and it is best not to extract these foreign bodies until the patient reaches the operating room.

If fatal hemorrhage appears likely to occur in the emergency room, the wound can be extended and vascular clamps applied under direct vision. In large trauma centers even thoracotomy can be performed rapidly and safely in the emergency room, and in some hospitals patients have been placed on cardiopulmonary bypass in the emergency pavilion before being transported to the operating room.[24] These are unusual requirements, and they should be approached with caution, especially by those who are not experienced in such operations. A separate indication for emergency thoracotomy may exist when patients are admitted in profound hypovolemic shock from penetrating trauma. In such people open cardiac massage can be lifesaving, and an aggressive approach is needed.

Operative Management

The patients are usually placed supine in the anatomic position and prepared to allow access to the thorax and abdomen as well as the involved extremities. Vertical incisions are preferred since they parallel the neurovascular structures and can be extended in either direction if required. Generous incisions are made to permit proximal and distal control of major vessels above and below the area suspected of being injured. Once the wound has been exposed and the clot carefully evacuated, the extent of the damage is ascertained. Every effort is made to avoid fragmenting and dislodging intraluminal clots which can result in thromboembolism. In patients with atherosclerosis the arteries are often fragile, and it is easy to extend the damage by a hasty and rough exposure. Specific arterial repairs are not begun until hemorrhage has been arrested, all the injuries are identified, and priorities set.

Methods of Repair

Lacerations of large vessels are easily repaired with lateral suture techniques if wide debridement is not required, but in patients who have sustained wounds as a result of medium- or high-velocity bullets, or have associated blunt trauma, it is often necessary to resect the damaged area and perform an end-to-end anastomosis if sufficient mobility can be obtained[16] (Fig. 34-4). If it is not possible to restore vascular continuity directly, then interposition grafts are chosen, usually using the saphenous vein if it is an appropriate size, although in some cases the hypogastric artery or other grafts may be used. In injuries involving the aortoiliac system autogenous grafts of suitable size are not available, and it will be necessary to employ plastic grafts.

Although autogenous tissue is preferred in the repair of vessels, both for patch-graft angioplasty and interposition grafts, in large arteries such as the aorta or iliac vessels plastic prostheses are needed. Special problems exist if the patient has associated injuries of the colon that have resulted in widespread bacterial contamination. In these patients, rather than insert a plastic prosthesis into a severely contaminated field, the surgeon can oversew the ends of the arteries, cover them with viable tissue, and construct remote subcutaneous bypass grafts (axillary-femoral, femoral-femoral, obturator).[4,16] When the threat of infection has passed, a direct reconstruction can be considered.

Special Problems

Although most arterial injuries can be repaired directly, once identified, particular difficulties are encountered in patients who have arterial damage as a result of substance abuse and repeated arterial punctures.[6] The usual complications of untreated vascular injuries such as thrombosis, delayed bleeding, arteriovenous fistulas, and false aneurysms are more likely to be seen in these people than in the normal trauma patient. Moreover, these arterial lesions are invariably associated with infection, both local and remote, and, in many patients, inanition and other illnesses as well.

A false aneurysm is the result of an incomplete injury of an artery, usually tangential, that permits continued bleeding. Transection of an artery is customarily followed by retraction and clotting, and in the case of small vessels, cessation of bleeding. The tangential laceration of an artery permits the blood to escape into the surrounding tissues, and sometimes to form a tamponading clot. In other cases it continues to bleed, resulting initially in what is called a "pulsating hematoma," and then subsequently a false aneurysm. If there is a contiguous tangential wound of an artery and vein an arteriovenous (AV) fistula can accompany the false aneurysm.

These lesions are easily diagnosed; there is a pulsatile mass, commonly in the groin, following a penetrating wound. There may be a bruit over the mass as a result of the blood escaping into the cavity of the false aneurysm, or if there is an AV fistula, there can be a continuous "machinery-like" murmur at and proximal to the area of injury.

False aneurysms and AV fistulas can heal only by thrombosis. In many patients thrombosis of a major artery

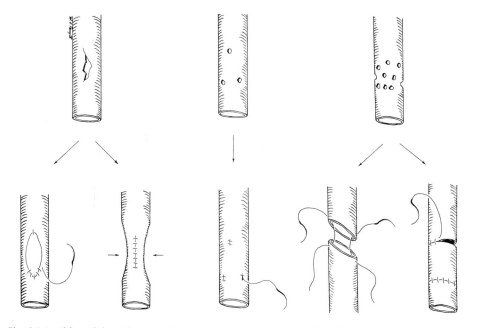

Fig. 34-4. Although lateral repair of injuries of large arteries is possible without narrowing, smaller ones require either patch-graft angioplasty or perhaps an interposition graft after resection of the damaged artery.

will not be tolerated without severe distal ischemia. Previous studies by Shumacker and Wayson demonstrated that spontaneous cure is unlikely, occurring in only 3% of posttraumatic AV fistulas and less than 6% of posttraumatic false aneurysms.[25] The incidence of spontaneous cure in infected aneurysms following substance abuse is likely to be even lower. Many of these patients are first seen when there is threatened or overt erosion of the skin as a result of expansion of the aneurysm and invasive infection. Thus a patient may require an emergency operation to control bleeding (Fig. 34-5).

Although the diagnosis of false aneurysms and AV fistulas can be made on physical examination, a B-mode ultrasonic scan or CT scan is of assistance in determining the exact size and extent of the lesions. Preoperative arteriography is recommended in the hemodynamically stable patient to plan the operative repair.

There is no unanimity of opinion about how these

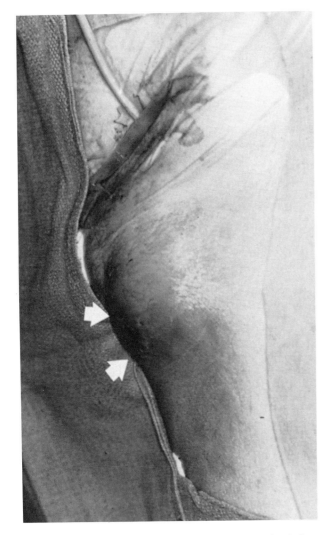

Fig. 34-5. This large, infected false aneurysm of the profunda femoris artery is eroding through the skin of the thigh *(arrows)*. The Rummel tourniquet is around the distal external iliac artery, placed there to obtain proximal control of bleeding.

lesions should be handled when infection is present. Studies suggest that even when the common femoral artery is involved, repair may be possible by using techniques of remote revascularization, bringing the graft through the obturator foramen, or perhaps via a lateral approach to reach uninvolved vessels distal to the area of infection.[26] A study by Johnson, Ledgerwood, and Lucas and a study by Reddy suggest that in many patients the extent of arterial infection is such that a direct repair is not safe.[23,27] In some patients it may be feasible to control the bleeding by direct suture of the artery, then follow-up on extremity viability carefully, perhaps with the patient receiving heparin. If the limb is not viable, the patient is returned to the operating room for a remote bypass graft. Other surgeons have suggested that an initial direct repair can be performed if properly staged, with an amputation rate no higher than 15%.[26] All of these series contain relatively small numbers of patients, and the types of cases that have been studied, although similar, vary somewhat. It is not possible to state with finality which procedure usually is safer. It is clear that direct reconstruction in the infected field is not likely to be successful. If some type of vascular repair is required, it must be remote, and placed in uninfected tissues.

Even if the initial repair is successful and the infection is controlled, recidivism is high, and many of the patients return. If the newly placed graft is accessible, it is often used for the injection of additional drugs by the addict. Clearly there is no single answer to the management of these serious problems, and a variety of reconstructive techniques will be required.

Operative Evaluation

In most situations the success of the operation is easily validated by the restoration of distal pulses and the return of function. In patients with multiple injuries the adequacy of the repair can be difficult to ascertain, and intraoperative Doppler techniques may confirm the return of arterial blood flow. In other people completion arteriography may be required, and in many trauma centers this is considered almost a routine, especially in patients who have had repairs of carotid or lower extremity arteries.[16] If there is any question as to the adequacy of the repair, completion arteriography is indicated.

Postoperative Care

If the vascular repair has been successful, only routine care is needed during the patient's recovery. The adequacy of the vascular repair is evaluated by repeated evaluations of neuromuscular function. The sine qua non for continued viability of the extremities includes the normal perception of light touch and the maintenance of intrinsic motor function. If there are disturbances in these neuromuscular modalities, then repeat arteriography is usually required, regardless of limb blood pressures, distal pulses, skin temperature, or appearance.

In the evaluation of patients who have had repairs of the visceral or splanchnic vessels repeated assessment of organ function is necessary. Disturbances in the function of the kidney, for example, suggest the need for repeat arteriography, and perhaps retrograde urography.

RESULTS

The overall results of repairing major vascular wounds are quite good, as shown in the accompanying box. If the initial repair is successful, and viability of the extremity has been gained, postoperative disability is usually a result of nerve injury, fractures, or soft tissue problems.

When evaluating the results of treating injuries of specific arteries, there is clearly a difference depending on the vessel involved. Injuries of the abdominal aorta, for example, particularly at the diaphragm, are often lethal; over half of these patients die.[20] In contrast, it is unusual for a patient with a penetrating wound distal to the knee or to the elbow to die. As seen in Table 34-1 the results of repairing penetrating wounds of the carotid artery are good if the patient does not have a neurologic deficit before surgery. It is unusual for complications to occur postoperatively if a successful repair has been performed. Most neurologic disability associated with these injuries is present before the operation. Although any vascular repair can clot, it is rare. Many trauma patients are young and have relatively normal arteries. Once the initial recovery is completed, the majority of patients have no further problems related to the vascular injury.

ARTERIAL INJURIES: RESULTS OF REPAIR IN 665 PATIENTS (%)

Failure of repair	5.2
Bleeding	2.0
Infection	3.1
Amputation	1.8
Death	10.4

From Perry MO: The management of acute vascular injuries, Baltimore, 1981, Williams & Wilkins.

Table 34-1. Penetrating Carotid Artery Injuries: Results of Repair

Preoperative Status	Number	Mortality
Group 1—no neurologic deficit	61	0
Group 2—mild neurologic deficit	9	1
Group 3—severe neurologic deficit	15	5
TOTALS	85	6 (7%)

(From Perry MO: The management of acute vascular injuries, Baltimore, 1981, Williams & Wilkins.)

REFERENCES

1. Shires GT III and Shires GT: Trauma. In Schwartz SI, Shires GT, and Spencer FC, eds: Principles of surgery, ed 5, New York, 1989, McGraw-Hill.
2. The New York Times, January 6, 1986.
3. The Tennessean, January 1, 1989.
4. Feliciano DV et al: Civilian trauma in the 1980's, Ann Surg 199:717, 1984.
5. Perry MO: The management of acute vascular injuries, Baltimore, 1981, Williams & Wilkins.
6. Carey JP and Penn I: Cardiovascular complications of parenteral drug abuse, Contemp Surg 27:59, 1985.
7. Wright CB, Hobson RW, and Hollis HW: Acute vascular insufficiency due to drug abuse. In Rutherford RB, ed: Vascular surgery, ed 3, Philadelphia, 1989, WB Saunders Co.
8. Maxwell TM, Olcott C, and Blaisdell FW: Vascular complications of drug abuse, Arch Surg 105:875, 1972.
9. Natali J and Benhamou AC: Iatrogenic vascular injuries, J Cardiovasc Surg 20:169, 1979.
10. McFadden PM, Ochsner JL, and Mills N: Management of thrombotic complications of invasive arterial monitoring of the upper extremity, J Cardiovasc Surg 24:35, 1983.
11. Shield CF et al: Pseudoaneurysm of the brachiocephalic arteries: a complication of percutaneous internal jugular vein catheterization, Surgery 78:190, 1975.
12. Skillman JJ, Kim D, and Baim DS: Vascular complications of percutaneous femoral cardiac interventions: incidence and operative repair, Arch Surg 123:1207, 1988.
13. Orcutt MB et al: Iatrogenic vascular injury, Arch Surg 120:384, 1985.
14. Soderstrom CA et al: Infected false femoral artery aneurysm secondary to monitoring catheters, J Cardiovasc Surg 24:63, 1983.
15. Mills JL et al: Minimizing mortality and morbidity from iatrogenic arterial injuries: the need for early recognition and prompt repair, J Vasc Surg 4:22, 1986.
16. Snyder WH, Thal ER, and Perry MO: Peripheral and abdominal injuries. In Rutherford RB, ed: Vascular surgery, Philadelphia, 1984, WB Saunders Co.
17. Schwartz MR et al: Refining the indications for arteriography in penetrating extremity trauma: a prospective analysis, J Vasc Surg 17:116, 1993.
18. Frykberg ER et al: Nonoperative observation of clinically occult arterial injuries: a prospective evaluation, Surgery 109:85, 1991.
19. Perry MO: Complications of missed arterial injuries, J Vasc Surg 17:399, 1993.
20. Lim RC, Trunkey DD, and Blaisdell FW: Acute abdominal aortic injury, Arch Surg 109:706, 1974.
21. Snyder WH et al: The validity of normal arteriography in penetrating trauma, Arch Surg 113:424, 1978.
22. Reid JDS et al: Assessment of proximity of a wound to major vascular structures as an indication for arteriography, Arch Surg 123:943, 1988.
23. Johnson JR, Ledgerwood AM, and Lucas CE: Mycotic aneurysm, Arch Surg 118:557, 1983.
24. Baker CC, Thomas AN, and Trunkey DD: The role of emergency room thoracotomy and trauma, J Trauma 20:848, 1980.
25. Shumacker HB and Wayson EE: Traumatic arteriovenous fistulas and false aneurysms, Am J Surg 79:532, 1950.
26. Patel KR, Semel L, and Clauss RH: Routing revascularization with resection of infected femoral pseudoaneurysms from substance abuse, J Vasc Surg 8:321, 1988.
27. Reddy DJ: Treatment of drug related infected false aneurysm of the femoral artery: is routine revascularization justified? J Vasc Surg 8:344, 1988.

CHAPTER THIRTY-FIVE

VASCULAR DISEASES RELATED TO EXTREMES IN ENVIRONMENTAL TEMPERATURE

Jeffrey W. Olin
Walid Arrabi

The vast majority of cold injuries in the past have been encountered in the military population. However, with the spread of winter sports (e.g., skiing, hiking, and mountain climbing), prevalence of alcoholism, and the increasing age of the U.S. population, cold-induced injuries are more commonly encountered among the civilian population. In addition, there are various abnormal sensitivities to heat that may occur. A useful classification for vascular diseases related to extremes in environmental temperature is as follows:

1. Freezing injuries (frostbite)
2. Nonfreezing injuries (acute and chronic pernio, immersion foot, and trench foot)
3. Erythromelalgia
4. Nonspecific sensitivities to cold and heat
5. Generalized hypothermia and hyperthermia

This chapter focuses on the first four categories since their pathogenesis is related to alterations in peripheral circulation. Raynaud's phenomenon and disease, which are vasospastic disorders usually precipitated by cold, have been discussed in detail in Chapter 23.

Some patients are bothered by a persistent coldness in the extremities, which they attribute to circulatory problems. Often the circulation is normal and this cold sensation is caused by neural factors, vasoconstriction, or what is often called *vasomotor instability*. This is a "grab bag" term that illustrates the scientific community's lack of understanding as to why some people have cold, erythematous, or cyanotic extremities.

FROSTBITE

Frostbite is defined as a state of actual freezing of tissues resulting from exposure to cold. Frostbite is usually caused by below-freezing temperatures but may occur at above-freezing temperatures under certain circumstances (wetness, strong wind, or high altitude).[1] Although frostbite implies injury of varying degrees to superficial and deep tissues, frostnip is an injury to superficial tissues and is completely reversed with rewarming (i.e., placing hand in axilla). It has been shown experimentally that slow freezing begins in mammalian tissues when the temperature in the deeper parts reaches 10° C, and cells rarely survive when the temperature is less than 5° C.[2,3] Freezing may involve the skin, subcutaneous fat, musculoskeletal components, blood vessels, and nerves. The damage done to these tissues is directly related to the depth of the temperature and the length of exposure. The two most important environmental factors that modify the effects of frostbite are wind velocity and humidity. Wind accelerates heat loss from the victim by convection and by increasing the evaporation of sweat. The effect of wind velocity is expressed as the wind chill factor.[4,5] Moisture, as a good heat conductor, also accelerates heat loss from the skin. Wet skin cools faster than dry skin and freezes at a higher ambient temperature.[5] A number of environmental, social, and host factors have been shown to predispose tissue to cold injury either by enhancing heat loss or by decreasing body heat production. These factors include tobacco, alcohol, inappropriate clothing, underlying vascular disease, previous cold injury, fatigue, anxiety,[6] high altitude, and race (blacks may be more susceptible to cold injury than whites).[7,8]

Those at greatest risk for developing frostbite fall into one of several categories.[9] Those with altered mental status due to psychiatric disorders, alcohol abuse, or head trauma may experience prolonged exposure to the cold and not recognize the early warning signs of frostbite or hypothermia. Likewise, the homeless, elderly, and debilitated individuals are predisposed to frostbite. It has been recognized for years that frostbite is seen in military personnel or other individuals who work in cold environments. Ervasti et al[10] sent questionnaires to 2081 male reindeer herders in Finland asking about the prevalence and predisposing factors of frostbite in this high-risk population. Twenty-two percent of the respondents reported frostbite during the previous 12 months, the most common areas being the face, fingers, and toes. Snowmobiling was a major predisposing factor to the development of frostbite in this series. In those individuals who have vibration-induced white finger syndrome,[11] the prevalence of frostbite increased significantly in the hands.

There is an increased prevalence of frostbite in individuals participating in outdoor sports such as skiing, running, mountain climbing, and snowmobiling.

A person's response to cold is aimed at conserving the core (internal body) temperature and the extremity viability. Assuming intact thermoregulatory mechanisms, the body reacts to cold exposure by reducing heat loss and/or augmenting heat production. Heat loss is reduced by peripheral vasoconstriction caused by sympathetic stimulation and catecholamine release. At the same time maintenance or augmentation of body heat production is accomplished by muscular activities such as shivering.[12] However, the heat production from shivering cannot be sustained for more than a few hours because of glycogen depletion, which is the source of heat energy during the shivering process. The extremities are protected by the "hunting reaction," which consists of alternating periods of vasoconstriction and vasodilation.[13,14] These cycles are irregular and last for 5 to 10 minutes. During vasodilation there is rewarming of the extremities. This recurrent rewarming is known as "cold-induced dilation" or "temperature hunting response." This serves to protect the extremities against excessive sustained vasoconstriction at minimal loss of internal body temperature.[1] However, when the body is exposed to cold of such magnitude or duration so as to threaten the internal body temperature, this mechanism fails. Since the disruption of core temperature is much more deleterious to the body than peripheral vasoconstriction, conservation of core temperatures takes precedence over rewarming of the extremities, and the hunting response is replaced by continuous and more intense vasoconstriction, thus placing the extremities at a higher risk for developing frostbite.

Pathogenesis

The exact mechanism by which freezing causes cold tissue injury is not known but three pathogenetic factors are recognized: ice crystal formation, cellular dehydration, and thrombosis of the microvasculature. Cold may directly freeze the tissues, resulting in the formation of ice crystals.[15] Ice crystals may form both intracellularly and extracellularly if freezing is rapid. The formation of intracellular crystals, as seen in rapid freezing, will disrupt cellular structures in an irreversible manner. However, in most clinical situations, freezing occurs slowly and ice crystals are formed extracellularly and, as such, cause only moderate cellular derangement.[16,17] Cellular dehydration

and tissue destruction occur by a shift of water from intracellular to extracellular compartments.[18,19]

Another mechanism of tissue necrosis is related to reactive vascular changes.[20-22] After exposure to cold, local and reflex arterial and venous constriction ensue, with resultant reduced perfusion to the affected area. Cold directly increases blood viscosity and thus causes sludging.

One of the earliest pathologic changes is endothelial cell damage with increased capillary membrane permeability (thus explaining edema formation in early frostbite). In the early thawing period vessels in the affected tissue dilate, and circulation is restored. Platelets start to aggregate and may occlude the vessels.[21] The stimulus for platelet aggregation may be prior endothelial injury. Platelet aggregation is followed by red cell aggregation, which occurs first in the venules and then in the capillaries and arterioles of the injured tissue. Because of the increased capillary permeability from endothelial injury, fluid and plasma proteins leak into the interstitial space. This resulting increase in intravascular viscosity leads to stasis and promotes further sludging. Simultaneously, rising levels of fibrinogen and lipid levels augment red cell aggregation. The net result is stasis with occlusion of the microvasculature by thrombi.

Tissues manifest variable susceptibility to frostbite. Skin, muscles, blood vessels, and nerves are highly sensitive. Connective tissue, tendons, and bones exhibit more resistance.[23] Recent studies implicate the release of prostaglandins and thromboxane (both metabolites of arachidonic acid) in the pathogenesis of frostbite.[24] The vasoconstrictor prostaglandins (prostaglandin F_2 [PGF_2] and thromboxane B_2 [TXB_2]) have been found to be present in high levels in frostbite blister fluid. Raine et al,[25] using an experimental frostbite model, showed that antiprostaglandin agents and thromboxane inhibitors significantly improve survival of injured tissues.

Clinical Features

Shortly after exposure to cold the patient senses pain in the affected part, which gradually progresses to numbness. Soon all sensation is lost. The frozen part looks white because of intense vasospasm. With thawing, circulation is restored to the affected parts, which then become hyperemic. Edema can develop within the first hour of thawing and may remain for days or weeks. Blisters appear within the first 24 hours and are resorbed within 1 or 2 weeks with little or no tissue loss. With mild frostbite blisters are usually large, filled with clear fluid, and extend to the tips of the digits[26] (Fig. 35-1, *A*). In severe frostbite blisters are small, dark colored (hemorrhagic), and do not involve the tips.[12,26] The blisters may look similar to those seen in patients who have reperfusion bullae. After resorption blisters are replaced by black eschar, which can give the false impression of a deep gangrene. However, after several weeks the eschar often sloughs, and the tissues heal. An initially fragile skin covering eventually develops into a normal healthy skin. In severe and deep frostbite demarcation between viable and mummified dead tissue takes place. Amputation can be spontaneous or surgical (Fig. 35-1, *B*). A few days after thawing a throbbing pain caused

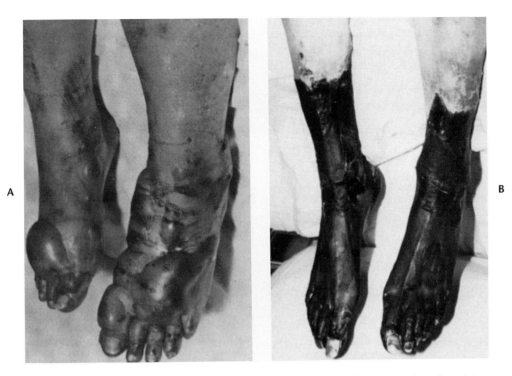

Fig. 35-1. A, Severe frostbite 24 hours after cold injury. Note extensive blister formation. *(From Spittell JA Jr: Vascular syndromes related to environmental temperature. In Juergens JL, Spittell JA, and Fairbairn JF, eds: Peripheral vascular diseases, Philadelphia, 1980, WB Saunders Co. By permission of the Mayo Foundation.)* **B,** Bilateral deep frostbite resulting in bilateral gangrene. This patient required bilateral below-knee amputations.

by inflammation develops and may last for weeks.[12] A persistent prickly pain may be present or shooting electric current–like sensations resembling tabes dorsalis may occur, especially at night, both reflecting ischemic neuritis.[27] Hyperhidrosis and a burning sensation in the feet can occur and have been ascribed to overactivity of the sympathetic nervous system. These may respond well to sympathectomy. All patients develop some loss of touch, pain, and temperature that may later resolve or may persist indefinitely.[12]

Chronic Sequelae

After frostbite up to 70% of victims develop symptoms including cold sensitivity, pain, and sensory disturbances. These symptoms may remain for years, and their presence has been reported 30 years after frostbite.[28] Color changes, hyperhidrosis, and swelling, as well as wound formation with scarring, are common. Many symptoms in postfrostbite victims resemble those seen in patients with reflex sympathetic dystrophy. Frostbite arthritis is also occasionally seen after cold injury. In children, frostbite injury is due in large part to epiphyseal damage. Fragmentation or absence of the epiphysis in premature fusion may occur. This may lead to brachydactyly, clinodactyly, and malalignment of the articular surfaces. Eventually, premature osteoarthritis may occur.[26,29,30] In adults clinical and radiologic features of osteoarthritis may be seen.[31,32] A rare complication of frostbite is the late development of squamous cell carcinoma at the site of injury.[33]

Diagnostic Considerations

The diagnosis of frostbite is easily made, given a history of cold exposure associated with typical clinical manifestations. However, two diagnostic problems exist when evaluating a frostbite victim. These include establishing the depth of frostbite and determining tissue viability. There are two methods of classifying frostbite according to the depth of injury (Table 35-1). The first divides frostbite into four degrees and is analogous to a burn classification.[9] The major difficulty with this classification is that it is based on the outcome of frostbitten tissue after thawing but cannot assess the depth of frostbite on appearance. The second classification may be more convenient. Superficial frostbite is differentiated from deep frostbite by palpation. In superficial frostbite deep tissues are soft, whereas in deep frostbite the whole part is stony hard. However, even this classification is often unreliable. Early classification has little clinical use in terms of management decisions since all frostbite victims, except for the ones with injuries that are obviously superficial, are treated along the same lines.[5]

Early in the course of frostbite, clinical signs and symptoms do not provide a reliable way to assess tissue viability. Tissue viability is usually determined weeks or months after cold injury when the demarcation zone and sloughing of dead tissue takes place. Investigators have attempted to use thermography or technetium-99m HDP scintigraphy to assess the tissue viability in experimentally produced frostbite in the rabbit ear.[34,35] Triple-phase bone scanning has been used in seven patients and was found to

Table 35-1. Classification of Cold Injury According to Severity

Depth of Involvement	Symptoms
Superficial	
First degree: partial skin freezing	Transient stinging and burning
Erythema, edema, hyperemia	Throbbing and aching possible
No blisters or necrosis	May have hyperhidrosis
Occasional skin desquamation (5-10 days later)	
Second degree: full-thickness skin freezing	Numbness; vasomotor disturbance in severe cases
Erythema, substantial edema	
Vesicles with clear fluid	
Blisters that desquamate and form blackened eschar	
Deep	
Third degree: full-thickness skin and subcutaneous tissue freezing	Initially no sensation
Violaceous/hemorrhagic blisters	Involved tissue feels like "block of wood"
Skin necrosis	Later, shooting pains, burning, throbbing, aching
Blue-gray discoloration	
Fourth degree: full-thickness skin, subcutaneous tissue, muscle, tendon, and bone freezing	Possible joint discomfort
Little edema	
Initially mottled, deep red, or cyanotic	
Eventually dry, black, mummified	

(From Britt LD, Dascombe WH, and Rodriguez A: New horizons in management of hypothermia and frostbite injury, Surg Clin North Am 71:345, 1991.)

be useful in predicting tissue viability as early as 2 days after cold injury.[36] More experience with these techniques will be necessary to recommend their routine use in frostbite victims.

Treatment

Initially all patients with frostbite should be admitted to the hospital to evaluate the degree of injury. In mild cases the use of daily whirlpool baths with bed rest is sufficient. Treatment of deep frostbite should be considered a medical emergency since early institution of medical therapy may substantially reduce the amount of tissue loss. It is equally important to remember that thawing, which is the mainstay of therapy, should not be implemented if the patient may be reexposed to the cold. Refreezing thawed tissue promotes further tissue damage,[12] but walking on frozen limbs produces substantially less damage than walking on thawed ones.[23]

After transporting the victim to an adequate medical facility and removing any constricting garments, further treatment of frostbite depends on whether the tissue is still frozen or whether complete thawing has occurred. If the affected tissue is still frozen, the most important therapeutic step is rapid rewarming of the frozen tissue. The affected part is immersed in a waterbath at 40° C to 42° C (104° F to 108° F) for 15 to 30 minutes until complete thawing has occurred.[37] This is manifested by reappearance of normal color to the frozen part signifying reestablishment of blood flow. If gangrene is already present, one can hope to preserve tissue around the area of gangrene by rapid rewarming and thus limit the amount of amputation required. Rapid rewarming restores perfusion more rapidly than slow thawing at lower temperatures. Rewarming at

temperatures above 42° C may increase tissue loss and is not recommended. Tissue should not be thawed by an open flame or dry heat since this may cause a burn injury. Putting ice on a frostbitten extremity will worsen the amount of injury and should never be done. When thawing is complete, the tissue should be kept dry and exposed. The thawing process is often very painful and may require the administration of narcotics for adequate pain relief. If the feet are involved, the patient should be permitted no weight bearing until healing ensues. The extremities should be elevated to minimize the amount of edema, and smoking should not be allowed under any condition.

The extremity with necrotic tissue should be cleansed for 20 minutes twice daily in a whirlpool bath with an aseptic solution at 35° C to 37° C (95° F to 99° F). Meticulous care should be taken to prevent secondary infections. Although some clinicians advocate prophylactic antibiotics in every case of frostbite, we believe that it is best to administer antibiotics only when infection occurs. Tetanus prophylaxis should be administered. Early reports suggested that vesicles should be left intact until they resorb spontaneously (usually 1 to 2 weeks) to minimize the chance of infection. However, Heggers et al[38] treated 56 patients with their frostbite protocol and compared the results in a retrospective fashion to 98 patients treated with warm saline solution, sulfadiazine silver (Silvadene), or mafenide acetate (Sulfamylon). Their frostbite protocol consisted of debridement of clear blisters with topical application of aloe vera, oral ibuprofen at a dose of 12 mg/kg/day, intramuscular penicillin, and daily hydrotherapy. Those patients treated with their new protocol had less tissue loss and amputations as well as a shorter hospital stay compared with patients treated in the standard fashion. Active exercise of the muscles, joints, and tendons is very important to prevent contractures.[39]

There has been an enormous amount of research on the role of neutrophil-endothelial cell adhesion in various inflammatory conditions.[40] Mileski et al[41] tested the hypothesis that blocking neutrophil adherence and/or aggregation reduces tissue injury in frostbitten hind limbs of the New Zealand white rabbit. The left hind limbs of three groups of rabbits were immersed in a −15° C salt water bath for 30 minutes to freeze the foot. The foot was rewarmed in a 39° C waterbath. Neutrophil adherence and aggregation were blocked with a monoclonal antibody (MAb) 60.3 in two of the groups of rabbits, whereas the third group was treated with saline solution. Those rabbits treated with a MAb had significantly less tissue loss, suggesting that at least some component of the cold injury was mediated by neutrophil adhesion and aggregation. It will be interesting to see if these studies can be corroborated in humans. Sirr et al[42] published an abstract reporting on 14 patients with third-degree frostbite who received recombinant tissue plasminogen activator (r-tPA) and compared that with 10 patients treated with supportive therapy only. All patients treated with supportive therapy had amputation. Those treated with r-tPA salvaged much more tissue. Further study will be required before this form of therapy can be recommended for patients with frostbite.

Since it is difficult and sometimes impossible to assess tissue viability early in the course of treatment, and since the eventual amount of tissue loss is often much less than initially expected, an important principle in the management of frostbite injury is to avoid early debridement or amputation. Definitive debridement should be delayed until either autoamputation occurs or tissue demarcation is obvious. This may take weeks or months but is the only way now available to ensure maximum tissue preservation. It is important to appreciate that the gangrene of frostbite is often superficial.[23] Early amputation or debridement is indicated only when infected gangrene or generalized sepsis occurs.

In the literature there are conflicting reports regarding the efficacy of sympathectomy in the treatment of acute frostbite. Proponents believe it prevents ischemic tissue loss resulting from vasospasm in the area adjacent to the injured tissue. Some studies suggest that sympathectomy in the acute therapy of frostbite enhances resolution of edema and decreases tissue loss, with faster healing of the wound and fewer late sequelae.[43-46] We do not advocate early sympathectomy. Although sympathectomy is controversial in the acute phase of frostbite, there is general agreement that sympathectomy is effective for the treatment of some chronic frostbite sequelae.

Low-molecular-weight dextran has been effective in treating animals with frostbite when they are treated early, but it has not been effective in treating humans.[47]

Prevention of Frostbite

Most cases of frostbite are preventable if appropriate measures are followed. Several thin layers of loose clothing should be worn with a first layer of water-resistant clothing (i.e., polypropylene) and an outer layer of waterproof material. Warm, loose footwear should be worn. Careful inspection and care of the feet are important, and the skin of the feet should be kept well oiled since this greatly protects the skin from low temperatures.[5] Mittens should be worn on the hands. Facial hair growth increases the likelihood of frostbite on the face because of moisture collecting on the mustache or beard.

Sato and Shimada[48] recently studied peripheral skin temperatures in the Muztagata expedition of 1992 (Himalayan Association of Japan). Peripheral skin temperature was measured at rest and then after a cold water challenge test at 4300 m and 5300 m. One group received placebo, one group received 5 μg of the oral prostaglandin E_1 analog limaprost and one group received 10 μg of limaprost. The prostaglandin E_1 analog helped to improve peripheral tissue perfusion at high altitude. Further studies will be necessary to see if, in fact, it will be a useful prophylactic measure for cold injuries at high altitudes.

PERNIO (CHILBLAINS)

Pernio* is a term used to denote localized inflammatory lesions of the skin as a result of an abnormal response to the cold. In the past pernio has been viewed as a skin disease, but now it is recognized as a cold-induced vascular disorder that is associated with skin manifestations.[49]

The prevalence of pernio varies considerably according to the geographic location. It is more common now in the temperate, humid climates of northwestern Europe than in the United States.[50] Winner and Cooper-Willis[51] suggested that up to 50% of women during wartime conditions developed chilblains by the time they were 40. It has been suggested that pernio is much less common than it used to be because of the availability of appropriate clothing in colder climates and because of the improvement in home and office heating.

During exposure to cold there is increased blood viscosity, resulting in a sluggish circulation in the superficial vessels accompanied by redistribution of flow to the deeper vascular network.[52] Humidity is an important predisposing factor for pernio since moisture promotes heat loss from the skin. Pernio develops only in susceptible subjects who are exposed to nonfreezing cold. Lynn has suggested that susceptibility seems to be related to a defective cutaneous circulation consisting of intense and prolonged vasospasm of parts of the skin during cold exposure.[5,53] This is consistent with the observation that in the same environment, subjects likely to develop pernio have cooler hands and feet than do those who are not.[5,53,54] Pernio is frequent in conditions with deficient limb circulation such as poliomyelitis, syringomyelia, and disuse phenomenon.

Pathology and Pathophysiology

The vasospasm, which is induced by cold, is supplemented by structural changes in the skin that present characteristic, though not pathognomonic, histologic features. The most prominent changes are found in the dermis and subcutaneous fat and include (1) edema of the papil-

---

*Pernio is a Latin word that literally means frostbite. Its synonym, chilblain, is an Anglo-Saxon term that means cold sore.

lodermis, (2) vasculitis characterized by perivascular infiltration of the arterioles and venules of the dermis and subcutaneous fat by mononuclear and lymphocytic cells, (3) thickening and edema of the blood vessel walls, (4) fat necrosis, and (5) chronic inflammatory reaction with giant cell formation.

Not all of these changes are necessarily present, and fat necrosis and giant cell formation may be frequently absent.[55] The most consistent feature is perivascular lymphocytic or mononuclear infiltrates. In a recent study eight of nine women with pernio demonstrated histologic evidence of a lymphocytic infiltration of the blood vessel walls. Although fibrinoid necrosis was not seen, some have suggested that this disease is a vasculitis.[56] The vascular changes seen on histology may also be caused by repeated episodes of vasospasm or prolonged vasospasm leading to tissue anoxia.[49]

Why one patient exposed to cold develops Raynaud's phenomenon and another develops pernio is not clear, but these diseases appear to be a continuum with Raynaud's phenomenon representing acute and readily reversible vasospasm and pernio representing more prolonged vasospasm with more chronic changes.

Clinical Features

Pernio occurs most commonly in young women between the ages of 15 and 30 but may occur in children[57] or adults of any age. The reason for this female predominance is not clear. It has been suggested that women have an increased responsiveness of the cutaneous circulation to cold, and the pattern of female fat distribution reduces cutaneous blood flow in some areas.[58] It has also been suggested that women who wear skirts are more exposed to the effect of cold.

Acute pernio may develop 12 to 24 hours after exposure to cold. Single and multiple erythematous, purplish edematous lesions appear accompanied by intense itching and burning. Their size varies from a few millimeters to several centimeters. The lesions tend to affect the toes and dorsa of the proximal phalanges. The fingers, nose, ears, and thighs have also been involved. Milkers' chilblains has been reported and at times is disabling to the point that the patients had to give up milking cows.[59] Often this acute phase of pernio is bilateral and symmetric.[5] Ulcerations may occur and are usually shallow, vary in shape and size, and may have a hemorrhagic base. The acute lesions usually disappear in 1 to 3 weeks and may not recur unless there is reexposure to cold. Acute pernio is a self-limited condition, although it may be recurrent. The legs may be slightly swollen, cool to touch, and may demonstrate varying degrees of cyanosis. Characteristically the peripheral pulses, pulse-volume recordings, and arterial pressures are normal. Chronic pernio occurs when repeated exposure to cold results in the persistence of lesions with subsequent scarring and atrophy. Characteristically the lesions begin in winter or fall and disappear as the warm season begins. These lesions, like those of acute pernio, often itch and burn. The natural history of pernio differs slightly depending on the age of the patient.[50] Children often have recurrences each winter for several years, and then complete recovery is the rule. In adults there is a

tendency toward worsening of the pernio over the years, and this may lead to chronic occlusive vascular disease.[58] In advanced cases the seasonal variation may disappear. Pernio has been described in association with poliomyelitis,[53] monocytic leukemia,[60,61] and with cutaneous lupus erythematosus.[62] The question arises whether lupus pernio or chilblain lupus erythematosus represents genuine chilblains in the course of lupus erythematosus or a lupuslike lesion resembling chilblains.[63] There is a clear female preponderance of lupus pernio, and although the lesions of banal pernio have a clear-cut preponderance of distribution on the lower extremities, most cases of lupus pernio occur on the hands. There have also been reports of pernio occurring in women with anorexia nervosa.[64] Erythrocyanosis[5,65] represents the nodular chronic form of pernio. Some investigators consider it a distinct though closely related condition.[50] Clinically nodular lesions with swelling and fibrosis appear on deeply cyanotic skin after cold exposure. These lesions occur in the lower extremities and thighs. Adolescent girls are most commonly affected.

Diagnosis

In its classic form pernio is usually not difficult to diagnose. The patient develops violet or yellow blisters, brown plaques, and shallow ulcers on the toes, which burn and itch (Fig. 35-2). These lesions first appear at the onset of winter and disappear each spring. However, in some chronic cases in which the lesions do not disappear in the warm weather or in which the lesions cause severe pigmentation and disfiguration of the lower part of the leg, the diagnosis may be more difficult.

It is beneficial to view the differential diagnosis of pernio under two main categories of diseases. The first category consists of recurrent erythematous, nodular, and ulcerative lesions that are of primary interest to the dermatologist and include four conditions: erythema induratum, nodular vasculitis, erythema nodosum, and cold panniculitis. The second category, atheromatous emboli, is of major concern to the vascular physician (see Chapter 14).

Erythema induratum (Bazin's disease) is usually, but not always, a cutaneous form of tuberculosis, which usually affects adolescent girls who develop nodular ulcerating lesions of the calves.[53,65] In biopsies from the skin, caseating granulomas are present in some cases. However, *Mycobacterium* is rarely cultured from the skin lesions. Tuberculin skin tests are usually positive. Nontuberculous forms of recurrent painful nodules are called nodular vasculitis.[65] No apparent cause is known. Women over the age of 30 years are usually affected. The two features that differentiate this condition from either pernio or erythema induratum are that the nodules of nodular vasculitis are extremely painful and rarely ulcerate.

Erythema nodosum can be differentiated from pernio in that it may be associated with fever, arthralgias and malaise, and a secondary underlying disease. The lesions are painful and generally do not ulcerate.

Cold panniculitis is characterized by painful nodules that appear on the skin after cold exposure. These lesions can be reproduced by the application of an ice cube. The histology of the lesion reveals fat necrosis.[66]

The palpable purpuric lesion that is sometimes present

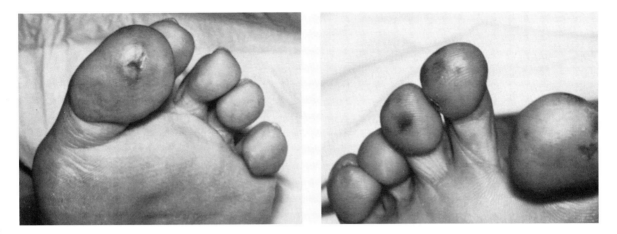

Fig. 35-2. These patients have the typical yellow-brown discoloration with shallow ulcers on the toes. This represents chronic pernio. (The photograph on the right is reproduced in color before p. 1.)

in pernio must be differentiated from other types of vasculitis, especially leukocytoclastic vasculitis. The lack of systemic manifestations and laboratory abnormalities and the relation of the lesions to cold exposure serve to separate these two conditions. Rarely a skin biopsy may be needed to make a definitive diagnosis. The other important entity that must be differentiated from pernio is atheromatous emboli. This presents a significant diagnostic problem in older patients because lesions produced by atheromatous emboli may appear identical to those of pernio. When a history of cold exposure is uncertain, arteriographic studies are often warranted in an attempt to demonstrate atheroma in the aorta or iliac vessels. A biopsy of these lesions establishes a definitive diagnosis in that the characteristic cholesterol clefts are present in atheromatous emboli (see Chapter 14).

Treatment

As in all cold-induced vascular disorders, prevention is the best form of treatment, and this consists of avoiding or minimizing cold exposure. When this is not feasible, adequate protection by suitable clothing forms the cornerstone of therapy. When lesions have already appeared, symptomatic therapy should be initiated. Many remedies have been used for treating pernio. They include calcium, nicotinic acid, phenoxybenzamine, and other vasodilators. The beneficial effects of these drugs are inconsistent. Ultraviolet light treatment was used 25 years ago and found to be beneficial to some patients.[67] Three doses of ultraviolet light were administered weekly at the beginning of winter. However, a recently performed randomized double-blind prospective trial in 9 female patients showed that there was no benefit between ultraviolet light administration and sham ultraviolet light treatment on the course of pernio.[68]

Nifedipine was recently found to be beneficial in 10 patients with severe pernio.[69] When given at a daily dose of 60 mg, shortly after the appearance of lesions, nifedipine was shown to significantly reduce the severity of symptoms and shorten their duration in the majority of patients. In a double-blind, placebo-controlled, randomized study followed by a long-term open trial, Rustin et al[70]

have shown that nifedipine in a dose of 20 to 60 mg daily reduced the time to clearance of existing perniotic lesions and prevented the development of new lesions. Nifedipine reduced the pain and soreness associated with these lesions. There was less dermal edema and perivascular infiltration on the skin biopsy after the treatment with nifedipine compared with before treatment. Therefore it seems reasonable to treat patients who have chronic pernio with nifedipine or another dihydropyridine calcium channel blocking agent. The severe itching may be treated with a local application of antipruritic agents.

In a letter to the editor[71] Ganor has reported on treating "hundreds of patients" with 0.025% fluocinolone acetonide cream under an occlusive dressing. The itch disappeared in a few days and the lesions in 1 to 2 weeks. Others have reported adverse effects with topical steroids.[72] Fitzgerald[73] has suggested that calcium and vitamin K administered intramuscularly will cure pernio. Until these dramatic results are confirmed, more conventional forms of therapy are recommended.

In severe chronic cases of pernio, sympathectomy has been used.[5,50] Although it enhances the resolution of the active lesions, it does not prevent the recurrence of new lesions, and this form of therapy is usually not necessary.

TRENCH FOOT AND IMMERSION FOOT

Trench foot is a nonfreezing cold injury resulting from exposure to cool, wet surroundings for a period of 24 hours to several days. The temperature is usually between 15° C and 0° C. Coldness alone generally will not cause trench foot. Two very important components are moisture (e.g., wet socks) and immobility. As its name indicates, this condition occurred in soldiers who were immobilized in trenches for a long period. Immersion foot is a more recent variety of nonfreezing cold injury, which was first reported during World War II in shipwreck survivors.[74] In fact, immersion foot accounted for significant morbidity and mortality in World War I, World War II, the Korean War, and the Vietnam War.[75] Prolonged immersion of the feet in cold or cool water is the usual initiating event. These two entities are probably different spectra of the same disease.

Both conditions are primarily military injuries. However, civilian cases do occur occasionally, especially in alcoholics and in the neglected elderly.[76] One recent report described several cases of immersion foot occurring in the homeless who were exposed to persistent, damp, cool environments.[77]

The pathophysiology of these conditions is related to cold-induced vasospasm, which results in hypoxia, endothelial injury, and capillary stasis.[78,79] Vascular occlusion and gangrene may occasionally occur.[5,78] Factors predisposing to these conditions, in addition to moisture and immobility, include dependency and fatigue.[16,74,79] Constricting footwear aggravates this condition by causing pressure necrosis on already ischemic areas. In World War I the British recommended wearing boots that were at least one size too large in an attempt to prevent trench foot and frostbite.[77]

Clinical Features

There are three clinical phases in the development of these conditions.[5,74] In the initial ischemic phase (also called vasospastic or prehyperemic phase), the feet are edematous, cold to touch, and pale with patchy cyanosis. Patients note heaviness and numbness of their extremities. The pulses are often reduced or absent because of intense vasospasm. The second phase (hyperemic phase) occurs within a few hours after removal of the extremity from cold exposure and is characterized by an increase in blood flow in the extremity as a result of extreme vasodilation. This phase may persist for weeks and is characterized by the presence of red, hot extremities with marked edema. The pulses are bounding. Initially the feet are numb, but this is replaced by an intense burning pain 8 to 10 days later. Vesicles, ulcers, and ecchymoses may develop, and in severe cases gangrene ensues. The hyperemic phase may resolve without sequelae or in severe cases may be followed by a late ischemic (posthyperemic) phase, which is characterized by cold sensitivity, numbness, and hyperhidrosis and may persist for years. Persistent pain may occur and has been attributed to either ischemic neuropathy, irritation of sensory nerve endings by scar tissue, or reflex sympathetic dystrophy.[16]

Treatment

Prophylaxis is the most important aspect in the management of immersion foot and trench foot because they are largely preventable conditions. Treatment of established cases consists of removing the wet, cold footwear and providing a warm environment for the victim. Affected extremities should be elevated to reduce edema. Nonsteroidal antiinflammatory agents as well as narcotics may be required for pain relief. Antibiotics should be reserved for cases of clear-cut bacterial infection. As in prevention of frostbite, silicone grease applied to the feet may delay the onset and decrease the severity of immersion foot.[80]

The hyperemic stage should not be left untreated. If this phase is allowed to persist, large bullae, or blebs, rapidly develop followed by massive swelling. This is a reperfusion injury and can be prevented by placing the patient in a cooler environment and elevating the legs. Since the gangrene of nonfreezing cold injuries is superficial,[78] surgery should be delayed until complete demarcation and sloughing of nonviable tissues takes place. Long-term sequelae, which are related to vasospasm and sympathetic overactivity, respond well to medical and surgical sympathectomy.[5]

WARM WATER IMMERSION INJURIES

Warm water immersion injuries are primarily military injuries that are caused by protracted exposure (greater than 72 hours) to water at temperatures of 22° C to 32° C (72° F to 90° F).[81] Two distinct forms of warm water immersion injury are now recognized: warm water immersion foot and tropical immersion foot. Warm water immersion foot occurs within 3 days of contact with water and is clinically characterized by painful, white, wrinkled soles accompanied by burning sensations in the affected extremities.[81,82] Tropical immersion foot represents an extension of the injury into the ankle and dorsum of the foot and requires 3 to 7 days of continuous exposure to water to occur.[82]

Treatment consists of cessation of water exposure and elevation of the extremities when edema is present. Complete recovery from warm water immersion foot occurs in 2 to 3 days, whereas complete recovery from tropical immersion foot may take 7 to 10 days. Prophylaxis is of paramount importance. Silicone preparations are effective in the prevention of these conditions.[80]

ERYTHROMELALGIA (ERYTHERMALGIA)

The term *erythromelalgia* was introduced by Mitchell in 1878[83] and is a combination of three Greek words: *erythros,* meaning red; *melos,* meaning extremity; and *algos,* meaning pain. It literally means red, painful extremities.

Erythermalgia is another term suggested by Smith and Allen.[84] This term was suggested because it emphasized the fact that increased temperature of the affected part is integral to this syndrome.

Erythromelalgia is uncommon. Brown[85] from The Mayo Clinic reported that its incidence was 1 in 40,000 patients seen in the 1930s. It is much less common at institutions that are not major referral centers.

A useful classification of patients with erythromelalgia is shown in the box on p. 15.[5] The primary, or idiopathic, variety may occur in a simple nonfamilial form or in a familial form that has various patterns of inheritance.[86,87] Secondary erythromelalgia is associated with a variety of underlying conditions. Myeloproliferative disorders, primarily polycythemia vera, occur in the majority of cases.[88] In a review of 51 cases of erythromelalgia at The Mayo Clinic, 30 (59%) had a primary erythromelalgia, and in 21 (41%) the erythromelalgia was secondary to another underlying disease, mainly myeloproliferative disorders.[89] Kurzrock and Cohen[88,90] reviewed erythromelalgia in detail and specifically the association of erythromelalgia and myeloproliferative disorders. As of 1993 there were 76 cases of erythromelalgia associated with a myeloproliferative syndrome reported in the literature.[91] The two most common conditions associated with erythromelalgia were

CLASSIFICATION OF ERYTHROMELALGIA

I. Primary (idiopathic)
  A. Simple nonfamilial
  B. Familial (autosomal dominant, recessive, and sex-linked)

II. Secondary
  A. Associated with myeloproliferative disorders (polycythemia vera and essential thrombocythemia)
  B. Associated with other diseases
    1. Hypertension
    2. Diabetes
    3. Rheumatoid arthritis
    4. Gout
    5. Spinal cord disease
    6. Multiple sclerosis
    7. Systemic lupus erythematosus
    8. Cutaneous vasculitis
    9. Viral infection
  C. Drug induced
    1. Nifedipine, nicardipine, verapamil
    2. Bromocriptine
    3. Pergolide

polycythemia vera and essential thrombocythemia. Agnogenic myelometaplasia and chronic myelogenous leukemia have been reported in 1 patient each. This predisposition toward patients with myeloproliferative disorders has led Kurzrock and Cohen[91] to term this paraneoplastic erythromelalgia. Itin[92] reported on the cutaneous manifestations in patients with essential thrombocythemia. In 268 patients studied retrospectively, 15 patients (22%) manifested features of erythromelalgia. These features were the initial complaint in 11 patients.[92,93]

Erythromelalgia-like eruptions have been described with the use of certain drugs, notably bromocriptine and nifedipine, nicardipine, and verapamil.[94-98]

Drenth and Michiels[99] have recently proposed a new classification for erythromelalgia. This consists of three forms: (1) erythromelalgia that is linked tightly to thrombocythemia or polycythemia vera, (2) secondary *erythermalgia* associated with other disease entities, and (3) primary *erythermalgia* that begins in childhood. The reason Drenth and Michiels separate erythromelalgia associated with thrombocythemia and polycythemia vera is that they believe the myeloproliferative disorder is important in the pathogenetic features of the disease and that this subgroup of patients receives prompt relief of pain with a single dose of aspirin.

Histopathology

Because of the rarity of this condition, few histologic studies are available, and most are based on individual case reports. The histologic findings represent a spectrum that varies from completely normal histology to arteriolar occlusion with thrombus formation. This disparity may reflect a difference in histology between mild and severe cases as well as primary and secondary forms of erythromelalgia. A biopsy of two cases of primary erythromelalgia revealed normal histology with no vascular changes.[100,101] In a third case dilated and proliferating capillaries were found.[101] In patients with erythromelalgia associated with polycythemia vera and thrombocythemia, skin biopsies revealed arteriolar inflammation with sparing of the venules and capillaries.[102,103] Arteriolar occlusion by thrombi was a common finding, especially in cases associated with gangrene. These lesions were partially reversed with aspirin. In a single case report of a patient with primary erythromelalgia, there was a decreased number of nerve terminals containing acetylcholinesterase and catecholamines, compared with normal skin,[104] suggesting that a disorder of peripheral vasomotor tone exists in these patients. Similar findings were found in a diabetic patient on skin punch biopsy.[105] Two patients with systemic lupus erythematosus and erythromelalgia have been reported with histopathologic evidence of lymphocytic vasculitis.[106]

Pathogenesis

The exact pathogenesis of erythromelalgia is not known. However, there have been advances in the understanding of this condition, and several newer theories have been advocated. As with histopathology, different pathogenetic mechanisms may be operating, depending on the type of erythromelalgia present. One proposed mechanism is temperature-triggered release of vasoactive substances such as histamine, serotonin, kinins, and prostaglandins. Methysergide, a serotonin agonist, was found to be effective in treating some cases of erythromelalgia, implying that serotonin may have a role in the pathogenesis of erythromelalgia in some patients.[107] Recently a poxvirus was isolated from the throats of school students with epidemic erythromelalgia in China, suggesting a possible etiologic role of viral infection.[108,109]

In a study involving two patients with primary erythromelalgia, increased concentrations of prostaglandins PGE_1, PGE_2, and $PGF_{1\alpha}$ were demonstrated in skin profusates.[110] PGE is a vasodilator known to cause erythema and pain in the skin. Jorgensen and Sondergaard[110] postulate that an increased rate of synthesis of prostaglandins may be an important pathogenetic mechanism to explain some clinical features of this entity. Platelet activation with the release of various mediators including prostaglandins, especially thromboxane, may cause secondary platelet aggregation and thrombus formation in secondary forms of erythromelalgia.[103] It is noteworthy that after a single dose of aspirin, the symptoms may be relieved for 2 to 4 days, which is the duration of inhibition of the rate-limiting enzyme cyclooxygenase within the platelets. Increased limb blood flow has been demonstrated in patients with erythromelalgia. However, skin oxygenation as measured by transcutaneous oxygen diffusion was extremely reduced, indicating ischemia to the microvasculature.

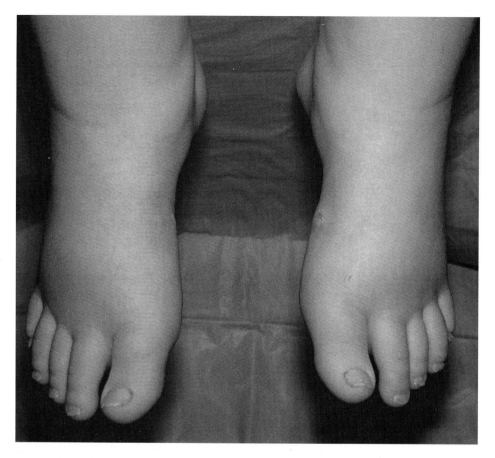

Fig. 35-3. Erythematous swollen feet of a young woman with primary erythromelalgia. (This figure is reproduced in color before p. 1.)

Clinical Features and Differential Diagnosis

Erythromelalgia is characterized by the clinical triad of erythema, burning pain, and increased temperature, usually of the extremities (Fig. 35-3). In both the idiopathic and the secondary forms, middle-aged persons are affected. Rarely the primary type may occur in children, whereas secondary erythromelalgia usually occurs after the age of 40. The feet, especially the soles, are more commonly involved than the hands, and involvement is usually bilateral in the idiopathic variety. Asymmetric or even unilateral involvement is more common in the secondary type.[88] Gangrene is not a feature of the idiopathic variety, whereas acryocyanosis progressing to gangrene may occur in the secondary variety.[88,103] The peripheral pulses are generally normal in the primary type and variable in secondary erythromelalgia. Usually the symptoms occur in "attacks" that last from minutes to hours and occasionally for days. The "attacks" are characteristically induced by a warm environment or exposure of an extremity to it. Exercise and dependency tend to exacerbate the symptoms. There is an individual critical skin temperature above which symptoms are induced.[111] The range of this critical temperature is 32° C to 36° C (90° F to 97° F). When the temperature is lower than the critical value, the symptoms disappear.

Erythromelalgia has been regarded as the antithesis of Raynaud's phenomenon since its symptoms are induced by warmth and relieved by exposure to the cold.[112]

However, others have described patients with coexistent Raynaud's phenomenon and erythromelalgia.[113] Patients often seek relief by exposing the affected extremity to a cooler environment (i.e., placing their extremity in cold water, walking on a cold floor barefoot, or running the air conditioning at all times). Patients usually continue to suffer "attacks" with variable severity. Spontaneous remissions have been described.

The diagnosis of erythromelalgia is based on (1) erythema, (2) severe burning pain, (3) increased temperature, (4) precipitation by a warm environment, (5) relief by a cool environment, and (6) exclusion of other diseases that may mimic erythromelalgia.

Other causes of painful erythematous extremities include reflex sympathetic dystrophy, arteriosclerosis obliterans (ASO), and thromboangiitis obliterans (Buerger's disease). In ASO and Buerger's disease, although the extremities may be red and painful, they are often cool to touch, and arterial pulsations are diminished. Reflex sympathetic dystrophy (see Chapter 32) is often characterized by burning pain with swelling of the affected extremity. Usually the affected part is cyanotic and cool but sometimes may be red and warm. There is no relationship to the temperature of the environment. Peripheral neuropathy may cause burning painful extremities, but they should not be erythematous or warm and the symptoms likewise are not temperature related. Rarely a peripheral neuropathy may be associated with erythromelalgia. The association of peripheral neuropathy and erythromelalgia may respond well to tricyclic antidepressants.[114] In children erythromelalgia has to be differentiated from Fabry's disease.[88]

In the majority of patients with myeloproliferative disorders, erythromelalgia preceded the clinical appearance of these disorders by several years.[88] Thus patients with erythromelalgia who are over 30 to 40 years of age should be observed by periodic blood counts.

The treatment of erythromelalgia is often difficult. In cases of secondary erythromelalgia, treatment of the underlying disease (i.e., phlebotomy of polycythemia vera and normalization of platelet count in thrombocythemia) often relieves the symptoms of erythromelalgia.[103] However, symptoms do not always correlate with the level of the hematocrit or platelet count.[88] It is important to instruct patients to avoid all potential situations that may increase peripheral vasodilation. They should try to avoid any exposure of their extremities to increased warmth and may need to avoid exercise and alcohol because of the resultant effects on vasodilation.

Aspirin is probably the most effective modality available. Patients often demonstrate rapid and prolonged relief after a single dose of aspirin therapy. Aspirin may be effective in both the primary and secondary forms of erythromelalgia.[5] Other drugs that have been used, with variable results, include methysergide,[107] ephedrine, propranolol,[115] phenoxybenzamine, nitroglycerin, and sodium nitroprusside.[101,116] Corticosteroids have been effective in patients with systemic lupus erythematosus and erythromelalgia.[117] Since the response to any of these drugs is unpredictable for the individual patient, trial with individual drugs for 2 to 3 weeks is warranted. In some cases a combination of drugs may be successful where monotherapy has failed. Nonsteroidal antiinflammatory drugs such as indomethacin may be effective even when aspirin is not. Biofeedback and hypnotherapy may be successful in some patients.[118,119]

Surgical sympathectomy has been tried with a few patients and has produced variable results. It cannot be recommended as a form of routine therapy in these patients.

The prognosis of a secondary erythromelalgia is that of the underlying disease. In severe refractory forms of idiopathic erythromelalgia, the symptoms may be continuously debilitating but are generally not life-threatening.

COLD AND HEAT URTICARIA

Cold and heat urticaria are two forms of urticaria occurring within a larger class of urticarias induced by a variety of physical agents.

Cold Urticaria (Cold Sensitivity)

Cold urticaria develops in response to cold exposure such as exposure to wind, drinking cold water, or eating cold food. Patients with this disorder who swim in cold water may develop severe hypotension and could die.[50] Two forms of cold urticaria are recognized: a rare familial form transmitted as an autosomal dominant condition and a more common acquired form.

In the hereditary or familial form symptoms develop during infancy, and urticaria is accompanied by fever, headache, arthralgias, and leukocytosis. The urticaria lesions are characteristically burning rather than pruritic.[5] Symptoms may occur immediately after cold exposure, or there may be a delay of 9 to 18 hours between symptoms and exposure. Familial urticaria is not immunologically mediated since it cannot be passively transferred. Biopsy specimens do not show degranulation of mast cells, and histamine release often does not occur.[120]

In the acquired form of cold urticaria, symptoms develop in childhood or during adult life. The vast majority of cases are idiopathic. However, cryoglobulins, cryofibrinogens, cold hemolysins, and cold agglutinins have been demonstrated especially in association with infectious mononucleosis.[121] Symptoms of pruritus and swelling appear within minutes of cold exposure and vary in severity from mild to incapacitating. In some patients symptoms resolve within weeks or months, whereas in others they tend to remain indefinitely with exacerbations and remissions related to cold challenge. Angioedema may occasionally occur. In contrast to hereditary urticaria, acquired cold urticaria is immunologically mediated. This condition can be passively transferred by a serum factor or IgE to normal skin.[122] Degranulation of mast cells and histamine release has been demonstrated. Other released mediators included neutrophil and eosinophil chemotactic factors.[120,123,124]

The diagnosis is made on a clinical basis, for example, by the appearance of symptoms after cold exposure. Champion has suggested that the disease can be provoked by placing an ice cube wrapped in a plastic bag on the skin of the patient. If weals form on rewarming, it may be diagnostic of cold urticaria.[50]

The treatment for cold urticaria is uniformly disappointing. Therefore it is essential that the patient take preventive measures to avoid exposure to swimming and cold water or other cold exposure. Antihistamines have been used with partial relief of symptoms in some patients. Success has been claimed in some cases with intramuscular penicillin. Oral penicillin has not been found to be helpful. Desensitization may help in some instances and consists of immersing the extremity in water at 15° C, initially for a few minutes every hour with a gradual increase in immersion periods and decrease in water temperature. Once tolerance is achieved, daily immersion is necessary to avoid relapse.

Heat Urticaria (Heat Sensitivity)

Heat urticaria may be of two types: a generalized type also known as cholinergic urticaria and an extremely rare localized type. Cholinergic urticaria is characterized by the development of characteristic small (1 to 3 mm) pruritic urticarial lesions that persist for minutes or hours in response to an increase in core body temperature. This may be brought about by fever, exercise, exposure to hot water, or at times by eating spicy food. Associated symptoms may include asthma, flushing, and syncope. Release of histamine as well as neutrophil and eosinophil chemotactic factors have been demonstrated. Patients may suffer from this disorder for months or years and then suddenly improve for no apparent reason.[125] Treatment consists of using antihistamines during or before attacks.

A localized form of heat urticaria has been described in a few patients. Itching and swelling are localized to the exposed part. Therapy consists of administration of antihistamines and/or desensitization.

REFERENCES

1. Purdue GF and Hunt JL: Cold injury: a collective review, J Burn Care Rehabil 7:331, 1986.
2. Merryman HT: Mechanics of freezing in living cells and tissue, Science 124:515, 1956.
3. Kulka JP: Histopathologic studies in frostbitten rabbits. In Ferrer MI, ed: Cold injury, New York, 1956, Josiah Macey Jr Foundation.
4. Washburn B: Frostbite: what it is and how to prevent it—emergency treatment, N Engl J Med 266:974, 1962.
5. Spittell JA Jr: Vascular syndromes related to environmental temperature. In Juergens JL, Spittell JA, and Fairbairn JF, eds: Peripheral vascular diseases, Philadelphia, 1980, WB Saunders Co.
6. Sampson JB: Anxiety as a factor in the incidence of combat cold injury: a review, Mil Med 149:89, 1984.
7. Post PW, Daniels F, and Binford RT: Cold injury and the evolution of "white" skin, Hum Biol 47:65, 1975.
8. Sumner DS, Criblez TL, and Doolittle WH: Host factors in human frostbite, Mil Med 41:454, 1965.
9. Britt LD, Dascombe WH, and Rodriguez A: New horizons in management of hypothermia and frostbite injury, Surg Clin North Am 71:345, 1991.
10. Ervasti O et al: Frostbite in reindeer herders, Arctic Med Res 50(suppl 6):89, 1991.
11. Virokannas H and Anttonen H: Risk of frostbite in vibration-induced white finger cases, Arctic Med Res 52:69, 1993.
12. Bangs CC: Hypothermia and frostbite, Emerg Med Clin North Am 2:475, 1984.
13. Lewis T: Observations upon the reactions of the vessels of the human skin to cold, Heart 15:177, 1930.
14. Dana AS, Rex IH, and Samitz MH: The hunting reaction, Arch Dermatol 99:441, 1969.
15. Lewis RB: Local cold injury: frostbite, Mil Surg 110:25, 1952.
16. Eubanks RG: Heat and cold injuries, J Arkansas Med Soc 71:53, 1974.
17. Merryman HT: Mechanics of freezing in living cells and tissue, Science 124:515, 1956.
18. Merryman HT: Osmotic stress as a mechanism of freezing injury, Cryobiology 8:489, 1971.
19. Merryman HT: Tissue freezing and local cold injury, Physiol Rev 37:233, 1957.
20. Cummings R and Lykke AWJ: Increased vascular permeability evoked by cold injury, Pathology 5:107, 1973.
21. Sumner DS et al: Peripheral blood flow in experimental frostbite, Ann Surg 171:116, 1970.
22. Weatherley-White RCA et al: Experimental studies in cold injury: circulatory hemodynamics, Surgery 66:208, 1969.
23. Ward M: Frostbite, Br Med J 1:67, 1974.
24. Robson MC and Heggers JP: Evaluation of hand frostbite blister fluid as a clue to pathogenesis, J Hand Surg 6:43, 1981.
25. Raine TJ et al: Antiprostaglandins and anti-thromboxanes for the treatment of frostbite, Surg Forum 31:557, 1980.
26. Mills WJ: Frostbite: a discussion of the problem and a review of an Alaskan experience, Alaska Med 15:27, 1973.
27. Suri ML et al: Neurological manifestations of frostbite, Indian J Med Res 67:292, 1978.
28. Ervasti E: Frostbite of the extremities and their sequelae: a clinical study, Acta Chir Scand Suppl 299:1, 1962.
29. Carrera GF et al: Radiologic changes in the hands following childhood frostbite injury, Skeletal Radiol 6:33, 1981.
30. Galloway H et al: Frostbite, Orthopedics 14:198, 1991.
31. Glick R and Parhami N: Frostbite arthritis, J Rheumatol 6:456, 1979.
32. Dreyfuss JR and Glemcher MJ: Epiphyseal injury following frostbite, N Engl J Med 253:1065, 1955.
33. Eun HC, Kim JA, and Lee US: Squamous cell carcinoma in a frost-bite scar, Clin Exp Dermatol 11:517, 1986.
34. Junila J et al: Assessment of tissue viability by thermography after experimentally produced frostbite of the rabbit ear, Acta Radiol 34:622, 1993.
35. Junila J et al: Assessment of tissue viability in frostbite by $^{99}TC^m$-HDP scintigraphy: an experimental study in New Zealand white rabbits, Nucl Med Commun 13:542, 1992.
36. Mehta RC and Wilson MA: Frostbite injury: prediction of tissue viability with triple-phase bone scanning, Radiology 170:511, 1989.
37. Fuhrman FA and Fuhrman GJ: The treatment of experimental frostbite by rapid thawing: a review and new experimental data, Medicine 36:465, 1957.
38. Heggers JP et al: Experimental and clinical observations on frostbite, Ann Emerg Med 16:1056, 1987.
39. McCauley RL et al: Frostbite injuries: a rational approach based on the pathophysiology, J Trauma 23:143, 1983.
40. Korthuis RJ, Anderson DC, and Granger DN: Role of neutrophil-endothelial cell adhesion in inflammatory disorders, J Crit Care Med 9:47, 1994.
41. Mileski WJ et al: Inhibition of leukocyte adherence and aggregation for treatment of severe cold injuries in rabbits, J Appl Phys 74:1432, 1993.
42. Sirr SA et al: Recombinant tissue plasminogen activator therapy of third-degree frostbite: role of scintigraphy, Radiology 118:222, 1991.
43. Mills WJ: Frostbite: summary of treatment of the cold injured patient, Alaska Med 25:33, 1983.
44. Golding MR et al: On settling the controversy on the benefit of sympathectomy for frostbite, Surgery 56:221, 1961.
45. DeJong P et al: The role of regional sympathectomy in the early management of cold injury, Surg Gynecol Obstet 115:45, 1962.
46. Kyosola K: Clinical experience in the management of cold injuries: a study of 110 cases, J Trauma 14:32, 1974.
47. Kapur BML, Gulati SM, and Talwar JR: Low molecular weight dextran in the management of frostbite in monkeys, Indian J Med Res 56:1675, 1968.
48. Saito S and Shimada H: Effect of prostaglandin E_1. Analog administration on peripheral skin temperature at high altitude, Angiology 45:455, 1994.
49. McGovern T, Wright IS, and Kruger E: Pernio: a vascular disease, Am Heart J 22:583, 1941.
50. Champion RH: Reactions to cold. In Rook DS et al, eds: Textbook of dermatology, ed 5, Oxford, 1992, Blackwell Scientific Publications.
51. Winner A and Cooper-Willis ES: Chilblains in service women, Lancet 1:663, 1946.
52. Zolar GL and Harber LC: Reactions to physical agents. In Moschella SL and Hurley HJ, eds: Dermatology, Philadelphia, 1985, WB Saunders Co.
53. Lynn RB: Chilblains, Surg Gynecol Obstet 99:720, 1954.
54. Lewis ST: Observations on some normal and injurious effects of cold upon the skin and underlying tissues: chilblains and allied conditions, Br Med J 2:837, 1941.

55. Wall LM and Smith NP: Perniosis: a histopathological review, Clin Exp Dermatol 6:263, 1981.
56. Herman EW, Kezis JS, and Silver DN: A distinctive variant of pernio: clinical and histopathologic study in 9 cases, Arch Dermatol 117:26, 1981.
57. Lucky AW and Prendiville JS: Painful digital vesicles and acrocyanosis in a toddler, Pediatr Dermatol 9:77, 1992.
58. Jacob JR et al: Chronic pernio: a historical perspective of cold-induced vascular disease, Arch Intern Med 146:1589, 1986.
59. Duffill MB: Milkers chilblains, N Z Med J 106:101, 1993.
60. Mark R, Lim CC, and Borrie PF: A perniotic syndrome with monocytosis and neutropenia: a possible association with a preleukemic state, Br J Dermatol 81:327, 1969.
61. Kelly JW and Dowling JP: Pernio: a possible association with chronic myelomonocytic leukemia, Arch Dermatol 121:1048, 1985.
62. Millard LG and Rowell NR: Chilblain lupus erythematosus (Hutchinson), Br J Dermatol 98:497, 1978.
63. Doutre MS et al: Chilblain lupus erythematosus. Report of 15 cases, Dermatology 184:26, 1992.
64. White KP et al: Perniosis in association with anorexia nervosa, Pediatr Dermatol 11:1, 1994.
65. Montgomery H, O'Leary PA, and Barker NW: Nodular vascular diseases of the legs, JAMA 128:335, 1945.
66. Solomon LM and Beerman H: Cold panniculitis, Arch Dermatol 88:897, 1961.
67. Holti G and Ingram JT: Physiotherapy in dermatology, Lancet 1:141, 1963.
68. Langtry JAA and Diffey BL: A double-blind study of ultraviolet phototherapy in the prophylaxis of chilblains, Acta Derm Venereol (Stockh) 69:320, 1989.
69. Dowd PM, Rustin MHA, and Lanigan S: Nifedipine in the treatment of chilblains, Br Med J 293:923, 1986.
70. Rustin MH et al: The treatment of chilblains with nifedipine: the results of a pilot study, a double-blind placebo-controlled, randomized study and long-term open trial, Br J Dermatol 120:267, 1989.
71. Ganor S: Corticosteroid therapy for pernio, J Am Acad Dermatol 8:136, 1983.
72. Burry JN: Adverse effects of topical fluorinated corticosteroid agents on chilblains, Med J Aust 146:451, 1987.
73. Fitzgerald KJ: Cure for chilblains, Med J Aust 1:676, 1980.
74. Francis TJR: Non-freezing cold injury: a historical review, J R Nav Med Serv 70:134, 1984.
75. Haller JS: Trench foot—a study in military-medical responsiveness in the great war, 1914-1918, West J Med 152:729, 1990.
76. Ramstead KD, Hughes RG, and Webb AJ: Recent cases of trench foot, Postgrad Med J 56:579, 1980.
77. Wrenn K: Immersion foot. A problem of the homeless in the 1990's, Arch Intern Med 151:785, 1991.
78. Pruitt BA and Goodwin CW: Burns: including cold, chemical and electrical injuries. In Sabiston DC, ed: Textbook of surgery, Philadelphia, 1986, WB Saunders Co.
79. Dembert M: Medical problems from cold exposure, Am Fam Physician 25:99, 1982.
80. Douglas JS and Eby CS: Silicone for immersion foot prophylaxis: where and how much to use? Mil Med 137:386, 1972.
81. Allen AM and Taplin D: Tropical immersion foot, Lancet 2:1185, 1973.
82. Catterall MD: Warm water immersion injuries of the feet: a review, J R Nav Med Serv 61:22, 1975.
83. Mitchell SW: On a rare vasomotor neurosis of the extremities, and on the maladies with which it may be confounded, Am J Med Sci 76:17, 1878.
84. Smith LA and Allen EV: Erythermalgia (erythromelalgia) of the extremities: a syndrome characterized by redness, heat and pain, Am Heart J 16:175, 1938.
85. Brown GE: Erythromelalgia and other disturbances of the extremities accompanied by vasodilation and burning, Am J Med Sci 183:468, 1932.
86. Cohen IJK and Samorodin CS: Familial erythromelalgia, Arch Dermatol 118:953, 1982.
87. Finley WH et al: Autosomal dominant erythromelalgia, Am J Med Genet 42:310, 1992.
88. Kuzrock R and Cohen PR: Erythromelalgia and myeloproliferative disorders, Arch Intern Med 149:105, 1989.
89. Babb RR, Alarcon-Segovia D, and Fairbairn JF II: Erythromelalgia: review of 51 cases, Circulation 29:136, 1964.
90. Kuzrock R and Cohen PR: Erythromelalgia: review of clinical characteristics and pathophysiology, Am J Med 91:416, 1991.
91. Kuzrock R and Cohen PR: Paraneoplastic erythromelalgia, Clin Dermatol 11:73, 1993.
92. Itin PH and Winkelmann RK: Cutaneous manifestations with essential thrombocythemia, J Am Acad Dermatol 24:59, 1991.
93. Michiels JJ and ten Kate FJW: Erythromelalgia in thrombocythemia of various myeloproliferative disorders, Am J Dermatol 39:131, 1992.
94. Eisler T et al: Erythromelalgia-like eruption in Parkinsonian patients treated with bromocriptine, Neurology 31:1368, 1981.
95. Alcalay J, David M, and Sandbank M: Cutaneous reactions to nifedipine, Dermatologica 175:191, 1987.
96. Fisher JR, Padnick MB, and Olstein S: Nifedipine and erythromelalgia, Ann Intern Med 98:671, 1983.
97. Drenth JPH: Erythromelalgia induced by nicardipine, Br Med J 298:1582, 1989.
98. Drenth JPH et al: Verapamil-induced secondary erythermalgia, Br J Dermatol 127:292, 1992.
99. Drenth JPH and Michiels JJ: Erythromelalgia and erythermalgia: diagnostic differentiation, Int J Dermatol 33:393, 1994.
100. Priollet P et al: Erythromelalgia without arteriolar changes, Ann Intern Med 103:639, 1985.
101. Kvernebo K and Seem E: Erythromelalgia-pathophysiological and therapeutic aspects: a preliminary report, J Oslo City Hosp 37:9, 1987.
102. Michiels JJ et al: Histopathology of erythromelalgia in thrombocythemia, Histopathology 8:669, 1984.
103. Michiels JJ et al: Erythromelalgia caused by platelet-mediated arteriolar inflammation and thrombosis in thrombocythemia, Ann Intern Med 102:466, 1985.
104. Uno H and Parker F: Autonomic innervation of the skin in primary erythromelalgia, Arch Dermatol 119:65, 1983.
105. Taub DB et al: Erythromelalgia as a form of neuropathy, Arch Dermatol 128:1654, 1992.
106. Drenth JPH and Michiels JJ: Erythermalgia secondary to vasculitis, Am J Med 94:549, 1993.
107. Pepper H: Primary erythromelalgia: report of a patient treated with methysergide maleate, JAMA 203:162, 1968.
108. Zheng ZM et al: Poxviruses isolated from epidemic erythromelalgia in China, Lancet i:96, 1988.
109. Zheng ZM et al: Further characterization of the biologic and pathogenic properties of the erythromelalgia-related pox viruses, J Gen Virol 73:2011, 1992.
110. Jorgensen HP and Sondergaard J: Pathogenesis of erythromelalgia, Arch Dermatol 114:112, 1978.
111. Lewis T: Clinical observations and experiments related to burning pain in the extremities and to so-called "erythromelalgia" in particular, Clin Sci 1:175, 1933.

112. Mandell F, Folkman J, and Matsumoto S: Erythromelalgia, Pediatrics 59:45, 1977.

113. Lazareth I and Priollet P: Coexistence of Raynaud's syndrome and erythromelalgia, Lancet i:1286, 1990.

114. Herskovitz S et al: Erythromelalgia: association with hereditary sensory neuropathy in response to amitriptyline, Neurology 43:621, 1993.

115. Bada JI: Treatment of erythromelalgia with propranolol, Lancet 2:412, 1977.

116. Ozsoylu S, Caner H, and Gokalp A: Successful treatment of erythromelalgia with sodium nitroprusside, J Pediatr 94: 619, 1979.

117. Alarcon-Segovia D and Diaz-Jouanen E: Erythromelalgia in systemic lupus erythematosus, Am J Med Sci 266:149, 1973.

118. Putt A: Erythromelalgia: a case for biofeedback, Nurs Clin North Am 13:625, 1978.

119. Chakravarty K et al: Erythromelalgia—the role of hypnotherapy, Postgrad Med J 68:44, 1992.

120. Soter NA and Wasserman SI: Cutaneous changes in disorders of altered reactivity. In Fitzpatrick TB et al, eds: Dermatology in general medicine, New York, 1987, McGraw-Hill.

121. Lemanske RF and Bush RK: Cold urticarias in infectious mononucleosis, JAMA 247:1604, 1982.

122. Sherman WB and Seebohm PM: Passive transfer of cold urticaria, J Allergy 21:41, 1950.

123. Kaplan A et al: In vivo studies of mediator release in cold urticaria and cholinergic urticaria, J Allergy Clin Immunol 55:394, 1975.

124. Soter NA, Wasserman SI, and Austen KF: Cold urticaria: release into the circulation of histamine and eosinophil chemotactic factor of anaphylaxis during cold challenge, N Engl J Med 294:687, 1976.

125. Soter NA et al: Mast cell mediator release and alterations in lung function in individuals with cholinergic urticaria, N Engl J Med 302:604, 1980.

CHAPTER THIRTY-SIX

VASCULAR TUMORS

Kandice Kottke-Marchant
John R. Bartholomew

Vascular tumors can lead to significant morbidity and mortality, and an understanding of their pathophysiology, clinical manifestations, diagnosis, and treatment is important to physicians caring for patients with vascular disease. We have elected to discuss vascular tumors under three headings: those that involve major blood vessels; those that involve blood vessels but may present as thrombi; and those presenting as soft tissue masses. It is by no means a complete review. The reader is also referred to Chapter 33 for additional information on some of the benign vascular tumors.

Vascular tumors are rare and are an unanticipated finding during physical examination. They also may be found unexpectedly while the patient is undergoing a diagnostic procedure such as arteriography, venography, computerized tomography (CT), magnetic resonance imaging (MRI), ultrasonography, or radiography. Frequently these tumors are found at autopsy. Vascular tumors may present as a soft tissue mass, as an intracardiac body, as an obstruction to a major blood vessel, or as thrombi or emboli. The clinical manifestations may be varied. Headache, pulsatile tinnitus, vertigo, conductive hearing loss, hoarseness, and dysphagia have all been described. In addition, symptoms of a systemic illness including fever, weakness, anorexia, and weight loss are reported. Chest pain, palpitations, dyspnea and syncope—all suggesting a cardiac or pulmonary problem—are also noted. Abdominal pain, bleeding manifestations, renal insufficiency, and claudication can be seen. On physical examination, hypertension, a mass in the neck, a carotid bruit, Horner's syndrome, or a heart murmur may be present. The patient may have arm or leg edema or ascites. Jaundice, cyanosis, or skin findings including ulcerations, papules, and blue or purple discoloration may be present.

TUMORS INVOLVING MAJOR BLOOD VESSELS

Sarcomas

Sarcomas involving the major blood vessels are generally further classified as leiomyosarcomas, angiosarcomas, and intimal sarcomas based on their histologic presentation. These are rare tumors that are accompanied by diverse symptoms, which usually are related to the size of the tumor and the degree of obstruction of the involved vessel, as in the case of involvement of the pulmonary artery and great veins. They may also be accompanied by nonspecific findings, including fever, weakness, and anorexia.[1] Symptoms also reflect the different growth patterns of these sarcomas. Although angiosarcomas can involve the major blood vessels, they most often present as soft tissue masses. Angiosarcomas are discussed in the section entitled "Vascular tumors appearing as soft tissue masses."

Leiomyosarcomas of the vena cava and pulmonary artery grow into the lumen, obstructing the vessel, whereas the intimal sarcomas grow in an infiltrating pattern along the vessel wall.[1,2] In thin-walled veins, leiomyosarcomas extend through the wall into adjacent structures relatively early in their course, while in arteries, with their elastic lamina, the tumor tends to remain confined to the artery much longer (Fig. 36-1). Fewer than 200 cases of leiomyosarcomas have been reported; however, the incidence may be underestimated.[1,3] Leiomyosarcomas found in the retroperitoneum and other deep soft tissue sites may arise from blood vessels, but by the time the tumor is discovered, the vascular origin may be obscure.[1,3] The most common site of origin for leiomyosarcomas is the inferior vena cava, followed by the iliac, femoral, and saphenous veins.[1-3] The superior vena cava has rarely been reported to be involved.[4] When the arterial circulation is involved, the pulmonary artery is the most common site.[5]

Intimal sarcomas are rare pleomorphic sarcomas that originate in major arteries and spread in a fashion similar to that of leiomyosarcomas of the pulmonary artery.[1,2] This pleomorphic sarcoma may contain areas suggestive of leiomyosarcoma, malignant fibrous histiocytoma, rhabdomyosarcoma, osteogenic sarcoma, and chondrosarcoma. The pleomorphic appearance is attested to by a plethora of synonyms including osteogenic sarcoma, intimal sarcoma, pleomorphic chondrosarcoma, and malignant mesenchymoma. The distinctive feature of the intimal sarcomas is their growth, both within the lumen and

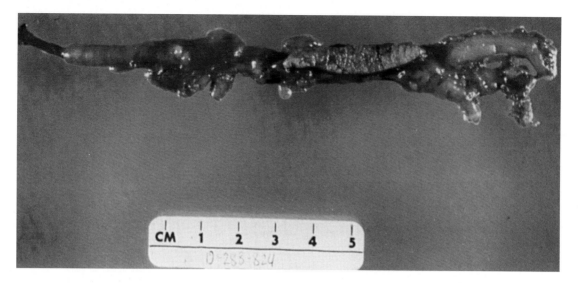

Fig. 36-1. Gross photograph of a leiomyosarcoma arising in a brachial artery. Note the apparent intravascular nature of the mass.

along the surface of the blood vessel.[6] They closely resemble thrombi when they are predominately luminal. Intimal sarcomas can cause thinning and aneurysmal dilatation of the vessel wall. In this setting they can be mistaken for an atherosclerotic aneurysm.[7]

INFERIOR VENA CAVA. Leiomyosarcomas of the inferior vena cava are often large, fleshy masses that obliterate the vascular lumen and erode through the vascular wall (Fig. 36-2, *A*). Despite the slow growth of these tumors, they have usually reached considerable size by the time of diagnosis, with extensive local invasion (Fig. 36-2, *B*). They can metastasize to the hepatic or renal veins, right atrium or ventricle, liver, lymph nodes, kidneys, adrenal glands, ribs, and skin.[8] Of the patients with this tumor, 80% to 90% are women, with an average age of 50 years.[1] In one series the female-to-male ratio was 6:1 with male patients significantly older than their female counterparts.[9] These leiomyosarcomas are difficult to diagnose because the symptoms are generally nonspecific.

Leiomyosarcomas of the inferior vena cava may be divided into superior, middle, or inferior types by their location within the inferior vena cava. This division may be helpful in classification, clinical presentation, and treatment. Leiomyosarcomas of the middle type are found in the middle third of the cava between the hepatic and renal veins, typically causing right upper quadrant pain. This pain is a nonspecific finding and can mimic cholecystitis or cholelithiasis. The tumor may extend into the renal veins, resulting in renal insufficiency or renal vein thrombosis. Extension into the right atrium and right ventricle has also been reported. Right ventricular failure, cardiac arrhythmias, and cardiac arrest have also been reported.[10-12] Tumors that arise in the superior or suprahepatic region typically develop a picture similar to Budd-Chiari syndrome because of hepatic vein obstruction or thrombosis.[13] These symptoms include jaundice, ascites, edema, and hepatomegaly. Tumors that arise in the lower third of the inferior vena cava below the renal veins often cause lower-extremity edema. This may be minimal if the

tumor is small or nonobstructive but can be massive if inferior vena cava obstruction is extensive or accompanied by secondary thrombosis.[13] In the past the diagnosis of leiomyosarcomas of the inferior vena cava was often made at autopsy or unexpectedly during surgical exploration. An ultrasound, CT scan, or MRI study may now contribute to the diagnosis earlier, either expectantly based on the patient's symptoms or as an unexpected finding. Venacavography is still one of the best methods to detect these rare tumors (Fig. 36-3). It will help to visualize the extent of the tumor and to assess the venous circulation before any planned surgery. In addition, the successful use of a transvenous biopsy to confirm the diagnosis has been reported.[12]

Treatment for leiomyosarcomas is wide local surgical excision when the middle third and lower third of the inferior vena cava are involved. Tumors that arise in the superior aspect of the inferior vena cava are usually unresectable, and the effectiveness of chemotherapy or radiation therapy has not been adequately studied.[14] Prognosis is poor and, although in one series patients who received a combination of surgery, radiation therapy, and chemotherapy remained free of disease for longer periods, the disease is generally lethal.[9]

OTHER VEINS. Leiomyosarcomas arise in veins other than the inferior vena cava. They also are found in the iliac, femoral, or saphenous veins and usually appear as a mass. Ankle swelling and lower-leg edema are the most common clinical findings, although numbness may be a complaint if the tumor produces pressure on nerves adjacent to the vessel involved. Leiomyosarcomas of the ovarian and renal veins have also been reported.[15] In contrast to leiomyosarcomas of the vena cava, the sex distribution of these tumors is almost equal. They should be treated as other leiomyosarcomas.

PULMONARY ARTERY. Sarcomas involving the pulmonary arteries are rare, and both intimal sarcomas and leiomyosarcomas have been reported.[1-4] Most of these tumors originate at the trunk of the pulmonary artery and

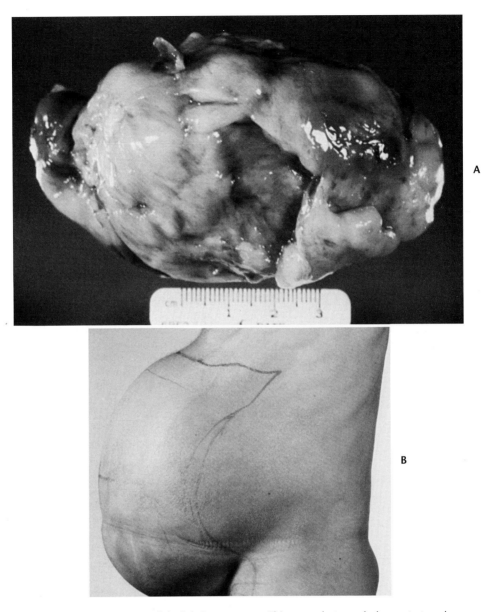

Fig. 36-2. A, Leiomyosarcoma of the inferior vena cava. This gross photograph demonstrates a large, lobulated tumor mass with no preservation of the vessel wall. **B,** This patient demonstrates the potential for the very large size of leiomyosarcomas. He presented with a large, swollen abdomen.

spread in the direction of the blood flow to the left and right pulmonary arteries and to the distal pulmonary branches. They arise during adulthood usually in the fourth or fifth decade and have no predilection for either sex. Symptoms are related to pulmonary artery obstruction and include syncope, palpitations, dyspnea, chest pain, and overt right ventricular failure. In addition, intractable cough and hemoptysis have been reported.[16] Physical findings may include cyanosis, jugular venous distention, and a systolic murmur.[16] Chest x-ray films demonstrate a large cardiac silhouette, enlarged pulmonary trunk, or solitary or multiple pulmonary nodules. Ventilation-perfusion lung scans demonstrate multiple perfusion defects indistinguishable from pulmonary embolism. Large filling defects near the pulmonary trunk may be seen on

pulmonary angiography. Contrast-enhanced MRI and CT scanning have been reported to assist in the diagnosis of the leiomyosarcomas.[17] The definitive diagnosis is made by either thoracotomy, thoracostomy with biopsy, or percutaneous CT-guided needle biopsy. Leiomyosarcomas are so unusual that the diagnosis is seldom considered until the tumor is found during surgery or autopsy. Patients are usually incorrectly treated for pulmonary embolism. The prognosis for patients with these tumors is poor. Treatment is local surgical resection, although the use of heart-lung transplantation has been reported.[17,18] This treatment is potentially curative. Chemotherapy and radiation therapy are of little benefit.[19]

AORTA. Most sarcomas of the aorta occur in the abdominal aorta and the descending thoracic aorta and are

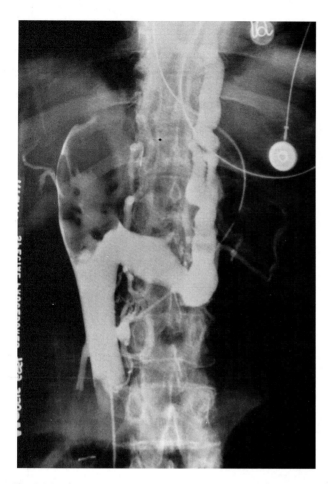

Fig. 36-3. This cavagram demonstrates a large intravascular filling defect that may easily be mistaken for a thrombus. Biopsy demonstrated a leiomyosarcoma.

usually intimal sarcomas or leiomyosarcomas. Aortic sarcomas may have different growth patterns. They may be found entirely in the lumen, in which case they resemble thrombi. Their growth pattern may also be predominately luminal with extension into the surrounding adventitia. A third growth pattern is along the vessel wall with aneurysmal dilatation of the aorta. This last type of sarcoma may be mistaken for an aneurysm and diagnosis may be made only on histologic examination of the "aneurysm." Symptoms are related to embolic phenomena or obstruction and have been reported to include claudication, back and abdominal pains, and occasionally shock from rupture.[4,7] Most patients are in their sixth decade and there is generally no sex predilection.[4] Aortic sarcomas also have been reported to occur after aortic graft placement, although what relationship this has to the surgery or the prosthesis is unknown.[4] Metastases to the kidney, thyroid, pancreas, and brain have been reported.[6] The prognosis is grim, although surgical repair and chemotherapy and radiation have been tried.

OTHER ARTERIES. Sarcomas of other arteries are quite unusual. Leiomyosarcomas of the internal mammary artery, brachial artery, inferior mesenteric artery, splenic artery, common iliac artery, and popliteal arteries have been reported.[15,20] Symptoms usually arise from vascular

obstruction. Treatment for these rare tumors is surgical, although case reports have been cited in which radiation and chemotherapy have been tried in combination with surgical intervention.[15]

Paragangliomas

Paragangliomas arise in association with major blood vessels and include carotid body paragangliomas, jugulotympanic paragangliomas, and mediastinal paragangliomas, also known as aortic body tumors.[1,21] Some confusion persists in the classification of these tumors. Those originating from the ear and jugular vein are commonly referred to as glomus jugulare or glomus tympanicum tumors. The reader is referred to other appropriate texts for discussion of this paraganglioma. Paragangliomas in the mediastinum are referred to as aortic body tumors, whereas those found in the carotid body are referred to as carotid body tumors or chemodectomas. In spite of these names, which are firmly embedded in the literature, these are all paragangliomas and not true glomus tumors. A true glomus tumor originates in association with the glomus body, a specialized form of arterial venous anastomosis, important to thermal regulation.[22] True glomus tumors do not occur in association with large vessels and are characteristically found in subungual or subcutaneous sites on the extremities.[23]

Paragangliomas arise in association with autonomic ganglia and are often classified as chromaffin or nonchromaffin tumors. The nonchromaffin tumors are concentrated in the head and neck or mediastinum, whereas the chromaffin tumors are generally found in the retroperitoneum. The autonomic ganglia systems, which give rise to the paragangliomas, include adrenal medulla, thoracic, intraabdominal, retroperitoneal ganglia, the vagal body, and chemoreceptors. The common histologic finding, which links the paraganglion system, is the presence of neurosecretory granules containing catecholamines. Since the paragangliomas may be functional, it is advisable to assess the status of the tumor before surgery in those individuals demonstrating certain clinical manifestations such as palpitations, headache, hypertension or arrhythmias.

CAROTID BODY PARAGANGLIOMA (CHEMODECTOMA, NONCHROMAFFIN PARAGANGLIOMA, OR GLOMUS CAROTICA). Carotid body paraganglioma arises in association with the carotid body, which is found on the posterior aspect of the bifurcation of the common carotid artery. It usually is incorporated into the adventitia of the vessel.[21,24,25] Carotid body paragangliomas are the most common of the extraadrenal paragangliomas and are frequently seen in patients living at altitudes greater than 6000 ft.[25,26] In addition, they are seen in patients with cyanotic heart disease and with chronic obstructive pulmonary disease. It appears that this relationship is caused in part by continued exposure to hypoxic conditions. Males and females are about equally affected, although there are some reports indicating that females are more commonly affected at higher altitudes.[26] Carotid body tumors have been reported in children but are more frequently found in patients between 40 and 60 years of age. There may be a familial predilection, suggest-

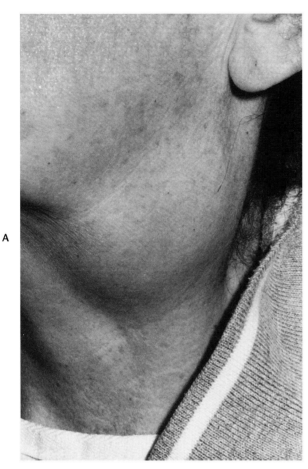

Fig. 36-4. A, Carotid body paraganglioma. This patient presented with a mass in his neck that later was found to be a carotid body tumor. **B,** This gross photograph of a large carotid body tumor demonstrates the homogeneous consistency of the tumor and its encapsulation and lack of necrosis. Despite the apparent encapsulation, these tumors may metastasize.

ing an autosomal dominant inheritance,[24,25] and when this occurs, the incidence of bilateral tumor increases dramatically.[1] Paragangliomas of all types tend to be multifocal, and a percentage of carotid body tumors are bilateral.[24]

Although carotid body tumors may have some worrisome histologic features, they rarely demonstrate unequivocal microscopic features of malignancy. As with all neuroendocrine tumors, it is difficult to predict the biologic behavior from the microscopic appearance, and carotid body paragangliomas with no obvious malignant features may still metastasize. However, multicentric paragangliomas must be considered before concluding that a given tumor has metastasized.

Carotid body tumors usually appear as a slowly enlarging mass in the neck (Fig. 36-4, *A*) and are found by the patient or discovered during routine physical examination. They may be pulsatile, and a carotid bruit may be heard. These tumors are associated with symptoms resulting from their involvement of local nerves, from pressure on the hypopharynx, or invasion of the skull. These symptoms include neck or ear pain, dysphagia, tongue weakness, hoarseness, tinnitus, headache, and syncope. Vocal cord paralysis and Horner's syndrome have also been described, and hypertensive crises can occur. Carotid body tumors may be functional, and elevated levels of urinary catecholamines can be demonstrated.[27,28]

The diagnosis is often initially made by ultrasonography. It is generally confirmed with selective arteriography,

which classically reveals a tumor sitting in the crotch of the carotid bifurcation. Arteriography may also demonstrate a characteristic tumor blush, caused by its rich vasculature. Bilateral angiographic studies should be performed to evaluate collateral flow, to look for other paragangliomas or carotid body tumors, and to assess the extent of atherosclerosis. CT and MRI may help make the diagnosis and differentiate other disease processes involving the neck. The differential diagnosis of a mass in the neck includes carotid body tumors, tuberculous lymphadenitis, branchial cleft cyst, carotid artery aneurysm, schwannoma, metastatic carcinoma, and lymphoma.

The majority of carotid body tumors are clinically benign, slow growing, and are cured by total surgical excision (Fig. 36-4, *B*). A very small number behave in a malignant manner and spread to the lungs and lymph nodes, or they invade locally.[29,30] The difficulty of surgical resection is related to the degree of involvement of the carotid artery.[31] Shamblin et al[32] classified carotid body tumors as I, II, or III, depending on their attachment to the carotid artery. Group I carotid body tumors have only minimal carotid artery involvement and are easily removed surgically. Groups II and III demonstrate more involvement of the carotid artery and are more difficult to remove. In addition to the degree of carotid involvement, surgery is also affected by the patient's age and underlying medical condition.[33] Complications of surgery include hemorrhage, stroke, and cranial and sympathetic nerve dysfunctions. Larger tumors are more apt to lead to cranial nerve complications, which may involve nerves VII, IX, X, and XII. The recurrent laryngeal nerve may also be affected.

Another approach to treatment involves selective intravascular embolization of the external carotid artery. This technique, using gelatin sponge emboli or particles of polyvinyl alcohol, reduces the size of the tumor by decreasing its blood supply and makes the tumor more accessible to surgery.[34,35] It may also be used in the poor surgical candidate, although it is not without some risks, including stroke. Radiation therapy has also been used in those patients who are not acceptable surgical candidates. Recurrences, although uncommon, are more apt to happen when there is a family history of carotid body tumors or in patients with multiple paragangliomas.[31] The prognosis is excellent following surgery.

AORTIC BODY TUMORS (MEDIASTINAL PARAGANGLIOMAS). Paragangliomas that arise from the mediastinum are associated with the pulmonary artery, aortic arch, or the sympathetic chain.[36,37] Those that originate in the pulmonary artery and aortic arch are termed *aortic body tumors* and are located in the anterior mediastinum. These aortic body tumors can be found wherever aortic body chemoreceptors are present,[1] and sites include the following: adjacent to the main pulmonary artery on its upper right border, in the angle between the ligamentum arteriosum and the descending thoracic aorta, and lateral to the innominate artery.

Aortic body tumors often present as an asymptomatic mass detected as an incidental finding on chest x-ray films. Symptoms such as pressure and hoarseness have been reported.[36,38] As with carotid body tumors, the majority of the aortic body tumors occur in people over 40, and the sex incidence is approximately equal. As with all paragangliomas, there may be an association with similar tumors at other sites.

Angiography reveals a highly vascular tumor supplied by arteries from both the aortic arch and the intercostal system with drainage into the superior vena cava.[39] Angiography should be performed in all patients who are undergoing surgical treatment. Although these tumors are histologically identical to the paragangliomas of the carotid body, aortic arch paragangliomas are more locally aggressive in their behavior.[1] Only 6% of these tumors metastasize, although up to 40% of patients may die from local invasion.[36] Complete surgical excision is the preferred treatment.

Intravascular Papillary Endothelial Hyperplasia

Also known as Masson's pseudoangiosarcoma, vegetant intravascular hemangioendothelioma, or intravascular angiomatosis, this peculiar lesion is one that is more likely to confuse the pathologist than the surgeon. Although the cause is unknown, the evidence suggests that it is no more than an unusually prolific organizing thrombus. It is not an angiosarcoma, the lesion with which it is most often confused.[40]

Papillary endothelial hyperplasia is generally an intravascular lesion that may develop in any vessel, including the vascular channels of a hemangioma, vascular malformations, or pyogenic granuloma. It rarely has been reported to occur extravascularly including the thyroid gland, intracranially, in association with an adrenal cyst, as a mass in the shoulder and cutaneously.[41] It generally presents as a mass, most commonly in veins on the head, neck, fingers, and trunk.[1] There may be a slight female preponderance. There have been case reports noting an association with trauma, hormonal influence (pregnancy or oral contraceptives), and the use of exogenous steroids.[41] Grossly the lesion is typically intravascular, about 2 cm in diameter, cystic and reddish-purple, and contains clotted blood. Occasionally the vessel will have ruptured, allowing the lesion to extend into the surrounding tissue. The histologic appearance may be confused with an angiosarcoma, but the lack of significant endothelial pleomorphism and mitotic activity, and the intravascular location, do not indicate angiosarcoma. The lesion is cured by excision, unless it is superimposed on an underlying vascular lesion.

NEOPLASMS THAT MAY PRESENT AS THROMBI

This category is composed of neoplasms that present as thrombi or emboli clinically and one variant form of thrombosis that may be misinterpreted as a neoplasm.

Low-grade Endometrial Stromal Sarcoma

Endometrial stromal sarcomas are tumors of the stromal cells of proliferating endometrium. In the older literature this neoplasm was known as "endolymphatic stromal myosis."[42,43] This neoplasm characteristically invades the myometrium, but may invade lymphatic and vascular channels. It grows and permeates along those channels, thus the older name. It usually presents as a uterine mass, but may present as an occlusive or stenotic lesion of pelvic veins extending into the inferior vena cava before there is any indication of a uterine neoplasm. Swelling of the lower extremities may be the only clinical manifestation, other than abnormal vaginal bleeding. Intracardiac invasion has also been reported.[44,45] In this setting cardiac symptoms may be minimal. Fatigue, palpitations, dizziness, arrhythmias, conduction defects, and sudden cardiac death can occur.[44] Transthoracic or transesophageal echocardiography and MRI will demonstrate a tumor or a mass. This tumor may be confused with thrombus (Fig. 36-5). The clinical progression of the lesion is quite unlike a thrombus, so recognition of the entity via frozen section is not ordinarily difficult if the operating surgeon thinks of the possibility and does a biopsy. Treatment is surgical resection if the patient is a good medical candidate.

Intravenous Leiomyomatosis of the Uterus

Leiomyoma of the uterus is a common benign tumor that involves the myometrium. Rarely this tumor may extend outside the uterus growing into the pelvic veins, the inferior vena cava, hepatic veins, the right side of the heart, and even the pulmonary vasculature.[46,47] In this setting some authors prefer the term *intravenous leiomyomatosis.*[48] Intravenous leiomyomatosis consists of a proliferation of benign uterine smooth muscle cells, analogous to the common uterine leiomyoma but with a propensity to grow within vascular channels (Fig. 36-6). Most patients with

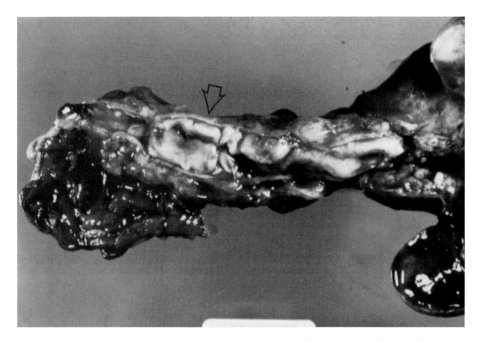

Fig. 36-5. Endometrial stromal sarcoma. This gross photograph of an endometrial stromal sarcoma shows tumor extension into an ovarian vein *(arrow)*. These tumors may often grow into and occlude pelvic veins.

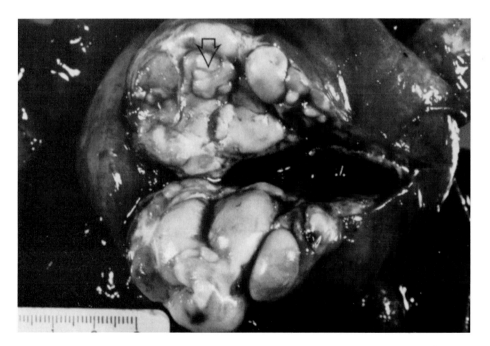

Fig. 36-6. Gross photograph of ovarian veins filled with a lobulated, bulging tumor mass *(arrow)*. This is one way in which intravenous leiomyomatosis can develop.

leiomyomas present with a pelvic mass and vaginal bleeding or pelvic pain. When vascular involvement occurs, symptoms of venous obstruction and even heart failure may be present. Dyspnea, generalized weakness, syncope from cardiac obstruction, and death have been reported. Clinical findings may include systolic and diastolic murmurs, and a gallop or pericardial rub. Atrial fibrillation and atrial flutter have also been reported.[49] Lower-extremity

swelling, ascites, and the Budd-Chiari syndrome have been noted.[48] Most patients presenting with this tumor are in their fifth decade and/or are postmenopausal. The diagnosis is usually made during surgery. However, CT, MRI, and ultrasound may demonstrate a mass, leading to further investigational studies. Venacavography remains the gold standard. When there is cardiac involvement, the diagnosis is best made by transesophageal echocardiography.

Unless the tumor is in a surgically inaccessible location, excision should be curative. Patients should also receive a total abdominal hysterectomy and bilateral oophorectomy at some point. Estrogen antagonists have also been reported to play a therapeutic role.[50]

Renal Cell Carcinoma

The propensity of this neoplasm to invade blood vessels is well known. As many as 10% of renal cell carcinomas will exhibit invasion of veins in the renal pelvis at the time they are discovered.[51] The presenting clinical manifestations may include gross hematuria, flank pain, fullness, lower-extremity swelling, and pulmonary embolism.[51] This tumor may quickly reach the renal veins and inferior vena cava and develop as an obstructive lesion, mimicking a thrombus[52] (Fig. 36-7). This presence in the vena cava potentially carries the threat of pulmonary tumor embolism. In this setting a suprarenal Greenfield filter has been recommended by some to protect the patient.[53]

Renal cell carcinoma generally affects patients older than 40 years of age.[1] Evaluation of the extent of the tumor may be accomplished by the use of CT, MRI, venacavography, or echocardiography. Treatment is surgical removal of the tumor, as vena cava extension has not been shown to be as prohibitive an indicator as previously believed.[54] Extension into the atrium, however, has a worse prognosis.[55]

Embryonal or Undifferentiated Sarcoma of the Liver

This rare neoplasm occurs predominantly in people under 20 years of age and usually involves the liver,[56] but we have seen one case in a middle-aged individual in which the neoplasm appeared as a lesion in the right atrium and inferior vena cava with a preoperative diagnosis of cardiac myxoma and thrombus. These tumors are also known as malignant mesenchymoma, fibromyxosarcoma, or simply sarcomas. Patients often remain asymptomatic until the tumors are quite large. Right upper quadrant pain, weight loss, or low-grade temperature may be the only abnormal clinical finding.[57] Liver function tests may be abnormal. The diagnosis is usually made by ultrasound or CT. However if initial symptoms are cardiac, transesophageal or M-mode echocardiogram may be used to confirm the diagnosis.

Cardiac Myxomas

Cardiac myxomas are the most common intracardiac tumors. They occur in people of all ages, may be familial, and are found equally in both males and females, generally between the third and fifth decades. The myxomas are most commonly located in the left atrium at the fossa ovalis, followed by the right atrium, and either ventricle.[58] They are usually 4 to 8 cm in diameter, globular, and may be pedunculated. Other less common primary intracardiac tumors such as papillary fibroelastoma, angiosarcoma, and malignant fibrous histiocytoma (MFH), may also be pedunculated masses and give rise to systemic or pulmonary emboli.[59-61]

The classic clinical manifestations include obstructive, embolization, and constitutional symptoms. Obstructive

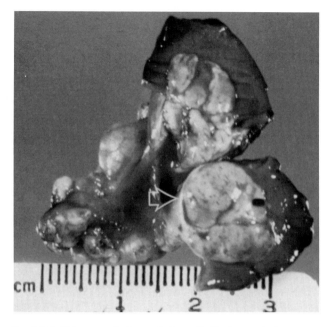

Fig. 36-7. This gross photograph dramatically demonstrates a nephrectomy specimen with renal cell carcinoma filling and distending the renal vein *(arrow)*. These tumors may grow intravascularly to fill the entire inferior vena cava and may reach the right atrium.

symptoms are due to mitral valve involvement and include shortness of breath, weakness, fatigue, and rarely syncope. Systemic embolization is generally directed toward the central nervous system and may present as a stroke, seizure, headache, vertigo, aphasia, ataxia, or visual disturbance.[62] Embolization also can occur to any other artery or organ[63] (Fig. 36-8). Embolic events to the coronary arteries have also been reported.[64] Constitutional symptoms including fever, arthralgias, myalgias, anorexia, or weight loss may also be reported. Abnormal laboratory findings reported include anemia and rarely polycythemia, elevated erythrocyte sedimentation rate, thrombocytopenia or thrombocytosis, hypergammaglobulinemia, and hypocomplementemia.[58]

The diagnosis of myxoma must be considered in cases of systemic embolization and can be easily overlooked because of the wide variety of clinical findings and abnormal laboratory studies found. A systemic illness such as a collagen vascular disease, malignancy, endocarditis, or the antiphospholipid antibody syndrome[65] is often suspected. Two-dimensional echocardiogram or transesophageal echocardiography are invaluable in identifying the intracardiac mass and confirming the diagnosis. Cardiac catheterization, used more frequently in the past, is no longer essential given the reliability of the noninvasive procedures. It is still used when the status of the coronary arteries is in question. Surgical excision is the treatment of choice.

An unusual form of myxoma, referred to as Carney's complex or Carney's syndrome, is characterized by cardiac myxomas, cutaneous myxomas, mammary myxoid fibroadenomas, spotty mucocutaneous pigmentation, primary pigmented adrenal cortical disease, large cell calcifying Sertoli cell tumors of the testes, growth hormone–secreting pituitary adenomas, and psammomatous mel-

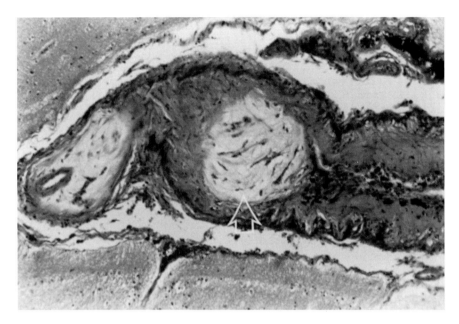

Fig. 36-8. Photomicrograph of a cerebral vessel containing an embolus *(arrow)* from a cardiac myxoma. Note the partial recanalization of the tumor embolus. (Hematoxylin-eosin stain; x300).

anotic schwannomas. Systemic embolization is especially true of myxomas, which are part of this syndrome.[66,67] The complex is familial and probably autosomal dominant. It occurs primarily in young people. Individual patients usually do not manifest all of the components of the complex. In contrast to the typical cardiac myxoma, those associated with Carney's complex tend to be multicentric or multifocal and do exhibit more aggressive behavior than does the typical isolated cardiac myxoma.

VASCULAR TUMORS PRESENTING AS SOFT TISSUE MASSES

Benign Tumors

CAVERNOUS HEMANGIOMAS. Cavernous hemangiomas may be deep seated. They are composed of large vascular channels that may exert pressure on adjacent structures and become locally destructive. The Kasabach-Merritt syndrome is a syndrome of thrombocytopenic purpura and consumptive coagulopathy associated with hemangiomas. It presents a difficult therapeutic problem because of the high risk of bleeding and infection associated with it.[1] The reader is referred to Chapter 33 for more information on this tumor.

ARTERIAL VENOUS HEMANGIOMAS. These lesions may also be in a deep location and may be associated with significant degrees of arterial venous shunting. In a deep location it is not clear whether these are truly neoplasms, as is implied by the term *hemangioma,* or whether they are really arterial venous malformations. They most commonly affect the head, neck, and lower extremities, and the larger shunts may visibly pulsate. Synonyms for this lesion include "racemose hemangioma" and "cirsoid aneurysm."[1] In addition to problems caused by the shunting, these lesions may be very painful because of pressure on adjacent nerves. The arterial venous communications are usually numerous, so ligation is not curative. Surgical excision of the lesion is often required.

Deep-seated cavernous and arteriovenous hemangiomas are the two hemangiomas that are most likely to come to the attention of the vascular physician and surgeon. The vascularity of the lesions, multiple feeding vessels, and associated bleeding problems may result in a therapeutic challenge even though they are benign.

Malignant Tumors

ANGIOSARCOMA. Angiosarcomas are rare, malignant vascular tumors of endothelial cells.[68] In contrast to other sarcomas, they have a predilection to involve skin and superficial subcutaneous tissue rather than deep soft tissue.[69] They vary from tumors resembling benign hemangiomas to very anaplastic, highly undifferentiated neoplasms, which are difficult to distinguish from carcinoma or melanoma. Angiosarcomas that arise in the setting of chronic lymphedema have been called *lymphangiosarcomas*[70] but are histologically indistinguishable from other angiosarcomas. However, since these lymphangiosarcomas have a distinct clinical presentation, they are considered here as a separate entity.

Angiosarcomas can arise at any age, but are most often seen in the sixth and seventh decades.[68] The most common sites are the skin, especially the scalp and subcutaneous tissue,[69,71] but they also have been described in the breast, bone, and liver.[72,73] Angiosarcomas of the liver have been found to be associated with vinyl chloride and thorotrast exposure.[73,74] Radiation-induced angiosarcomas have also been reported.[71]

Even though angiosarcomas are tumors of endothelial cells, tumors arising in the heart and major blood vessels are rare, comprising only 3% of all angiosarcomas.[3,75,76] Those that do arise in the major blood vessels have most often been associated with the aorta[75] but may rarely involve veins such as the superior vena cava or axillary vein.[77,78] These rare tumors can cause vascular obstruction or develop as a pulsatile mass lesion.

Cutaneous angiosarcomas usually present as a bruise-like, firm, or ulcerated lesion on the scalp of an elderly person.[79] Angiosarcomas of the breast usually occur in reproductive-age women as rapidly growing masses that cause diffuse breast enlargement with a blue or purple discoloration of the overlying skin.[72] Symptoms of hepatic angiosarcomas are more nonspecific including fatigue, weight loss, and abdominal pain.[73]

Grossly angiosarcomas, regardless of location, are ill-defined hemorrhagic masses with areas of spongelike cystic spaces.[69,72] In angiosarcomas involving the skin, the overlying skin surface may be ulcerated.[69,79] Histologically these tumors range from deceptively benign-looking neoplasms with large dilated vessels resembling hemangiomas to very high grade tumors composed of sheets of anaplastic cells.[72] The characteristic pattern consists of an interanastomosing network of vessellike structures lined by large cells with malignant features. Positive identification of the cell type as endothelial is not always possible, since many angiosarcomas fail to react with immunohistochemical stains for endothelial cells, such as factor VIII–related antigen.[68,80]

The prognosis in most types of angiosarcoma, whether located in the skin, breast, or liver, is relatively poor.[72,79] In a series of 72 patients with angiosarcoma of the face and scalp, Holden, Spittle, and Jones[79] found only a 12% 5-year survival rate. Angiosarcomas of the breast are among the most malignant of breast tumors, with 90% of patients dead of disease within 2 years.[72] Metastasis is usually early and is primarily hematogenous, with most of the spread occurring to the lungs, skin, and bone. However, lymph node metastasis has also been described, especially in angiosarcomas of the head and neck.[69] In cutaneous angiosarcoma, tumors less than 5 cm have a better prognosis than larger lesions.[71] The prognosis also is better if the primary tumor can be completely excised.[71] The value of adjunct radiation or chemotherapy is minimal, since little seems to halt the progression of this highly malignant neoplasm.

LYMPHANGIOSARCOMA. Lymphangiosarcomas are highly aggressive tumors that generally arise in the setting of chronic lymphedema. Most cases are reported following the development of postmastectomy lymphedema for breast cancer and are referred to as *Stewart-Treves syndrome*[81] (Fig. 36-9). These rare tumors are found in less than 1% of all patients with breast cancer.[82]

Although generally found in the upper extremity, lymphangiosarcomas are also found in the lower extremity; in areas without lymphedema; and in congenital, late-onset hereditary, idiopathic, or traumatic lymphedema.[83-90]

Lymphangiosarcomas are actually angiosarcomas that arise from vascular endothelial cells and are histologically identical to angiosarcomas arising without lymphedema. They usually occur in the fifth to seventh decade of life, approximately 10 years after the original mastectomy. In the congenital, late-onset hereditary, traumatic, or idio-

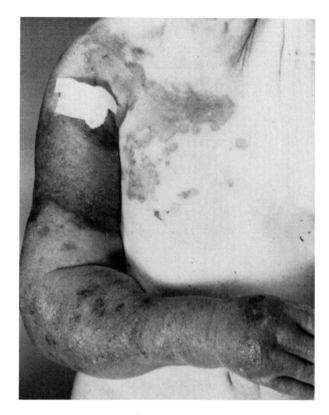

Fig. 36-9. Gross photograph of a lymphangiosarcoma arising in the right arm following mastectomy for breast carcinoma. Note the presence of lymphedema in the affected limb.

pathic setting, they may occur at a much younger age but at later intervals from the onset of lymphedema.[86]

The etiology of lymphangiosarcomas may be multifactorial and includes persistent lymphedema following radical mastectomy, radiation therapy, and local defects in cellular immunity.[83,87,88,91] Greater than 90% of all cases reported in one series were associated with a chronic lymphedematous extremity after mastectomy.[83]

Clinically lymphangiosarcomas appear either as solitary or multiple lesions, purplish-red to bluish-red, and as macular lesions or palpable purpura and nodules. They may progress to ulcerations or become necrotic. Lymphangiosarcomas may be initially confused with an ecchymosis or cellulitis, often delaying their correct diagnosis. They frequently recur locally, following wide local excision. They spread proximally and distally and eventually metastasize to the lungs, pleura, chest wall, shoulder, liver, or bone.[1]

Current treatment methods include surgery, chemotherapy, or irradiation. Overall, all three have a poor prognosis, although amputation, including shoulder disarticulation and hindquarter or forequarter amputation, offers the best option.[83,91,92] Wide local excision is not as effective. Radiotherapy and chemotherapy have not been proven as effective, although some success has been reported by Yap et al[92] with the use of multiple chemotherapeutic agents. Despite aggressive surgical intervention including amputation, median survival time is only 19 months in those patients who develop lymphangiosarcoma following mastectomy and 34 months following the development of these tumors in the nonmastectomy patient.[83] Exceptions do occur and two patients survived longer in one recent report (13 and 19 years) in which they received actinomycin D, surgery, and radiation therapy.[93] Early recognition and prompt biopsy followed by aggressive surgical intervention afford the best treatment.[94] Several authors have speculated that the current trend toward the use of less radical surgical procedures involving breast cancer and the prompt treatment of cellulitis may help decrease the incidence of this condition.[90]

KAPOSI'S SARCOMA. Kaposi's sarcoma was first described by Moritz Kaposi in 1872 and initially termed *idiopathic multiple pigmented hemorrhagic sarcoma*.[95] This tumor has been largely found in the central equatorial regions of Africa where it is endemic and represents as many as 9% of all reported malignancies.[96] Kaposi's sarcoma was considered an uncommon tumor in the United States and Europe, found mainly in the lower extremities of older men, until the epidemic emergence in association with the acquired immunodeficiency syndrome (AIDS).

There are four epidemiologic classifications of Kaposi's sarcoma, which include classic, or sporadic; endemic; epidemic; and that associated with immunosuppressive therapy.[97] Classic or sporadic Kaposi's sarcoma is a disease of elderly men found between the fifth and seventh decade of life, with a predilection for Ashkenazi Jews and southern Europeans. It is usually located on the lower extremities and generally has a relatively benign course. Endemic Kaposi's sarcoma is found in central Africa, often in younger patients. It may affect the lower extremities but can also be found in the gastrointestinal tract, lymph nodes, or bones. Four subtypes have been described including florid, infiltrative, nodular, and lymphadenopathic.[97,98] Epidemic Kaposi's sarcoma is associated with AIDS and is seen most often in homosexual and bisexual men. The incidence is lower in the other AIDS risk groups—heterosexual drug addicts, blood transfusion recipients, and hemophiliacs.[99-101] This is an aggressive disease involving visceral dissemination and multiple skin lesions. The immunosuppressive form of Kaposi's sarcoma is found in renal transplant recipients or in patients who have received immunosuppressive agents for other diseases.[102]

The etiology of Kaposi's sarcoma is multifactorial. Genetic, geographic, and viral factors all play a role as well as the immunocompetence of the host.[1] Its association with AIDS is highly suggestive of a viral cause, given the high transmission rate of hepatitis B and cytomegalovirus (CMV) in this group. The immunocompetence of the host is suggested by the presence of Kaposi's sarcoma in patients receiving immunosuppressive agents and in AIDS. Genetic and geographic roles are suggested because of the striking incidence in the indigenous black population of Africa and the increase in certain other population groups including the Ashkenazi Jews and southern Europeans.

Kaposi's sarcoma is a vascular tumor of endothelial origin. Grossly it appears on the skin or viscera as a multicentric, red-blue, purple, or reddish-brown nodule or plaque. Histologically there are two important features: the spindle cell and the presence of vascular proliferation. Initially an inflammatory pattern is seen with large numbers of lymphocytes, plasma cells, and large mononuclear

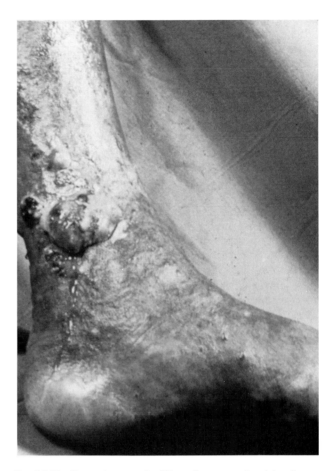

Fig. 36-10. Gross photograph of Kaposi's sarcoma involving the medial aspect of the left leg.

cells. This may resemble granulation tissue. As the lesions evolve, proliferating vascular channels or capillaries are seen, and the inflammatory response diminishes. Later the spindle cell, the first neoplastic element, becomes recognizable. These cells often form interlacing bundles and consist of round or oval nuclei with elongated cytoplasms.

Clinically Kaposi's sarcoma may appear as a solitary nodule or papule localized to the feet or ankles. These lesions may vary in size and may coalesce into plaques, nodules, ulcerations, or even polypoid growths (Fig. 36-10).[1] In the epidemic form lesions may be multiple and are seen on the trunk, arms, head, and neck. These lesions are occasionally symmetric and follow the path of a superficial vein. They may be tender, painful, pruritic, and associated with edema. Over 90% of all cases involve men. An increased association with second malignancies including lymphomas, leukemia, Hodgkin's disease, melanoma, and multiple myeloma is reported.[103-105]

Visceral involvement is unusual in the classic form, but dissemination to the gastrointestinal tract, lungs, bone, liver, lymph nodes, and virtually every organ system is possible in the other types. Hemorrhages into the pulmonary or gastrointestinal tract may occur and can cause difficult management problems. Pulmonary involvement may lead to diffusion capacity abnormalities. Central nervous system involvement is rare.

Classic Kaposi's sarcoma usually behaves in an indolent

fashion, and a conservative approach to treatment may be warranted. In the classic form the prognosis is usually good, although chemotherapy or extended field radiation is needed when the tumor is more aggressive.

In the other forms of Kaposi's sarcoma a wide range of chemotherapeutic agents have been tried. These include both single agents and combined therapy using bleomycin, adriamycin, dactinomycin, vincristine, and vinblastine.[106] In the immunosuppressive form, discontinuing the drugs is necessary. In Kaposi's sarcoma associated with AIDS the use of interferon therapy is also advocated.[107] Local therapy will benefit some patients with Kaposi's sarcoma in this setting. This includes liquid nitrogen cryotherapy and intralesional vinblastine or vincristine. The prognosis is much worse in this group. Patients die less frequently from the tumor, however, than from the wasting, cachexia, and opportunistic infections.[106]

HEMANGIOPERICYTOMA. Hemangiopericytoma is an uncommon tumor comprising only 1% of all blood vessel–related neoplasms, with a spectrum of clinical manifestations from benign to overtly malignant.[108] Hemangiopericytomas are thought to arise from pericytes, mesenchymal cells that underlie the basement membrane of capillaries.[109,110] At one time hemangiopericytomas were thought to be related to glomus tumors, but subsequent studies have revealed the two to be separate entities.[111]

Hemangiopericytomas may occur at any age but are most common in the fifth and sixth decades.[112,113] Rare cases have been described in infants and children,[114] although these generally behave in a benign fashion. Hemangiopericytomas are most often located in the lower extremities or retroperitoneum[108,110,112] and involve deep soft tissues or muscle. Symptoms usually are related to a painless mass, which has been enlarging slowly. Apart from the lower extremities, hemangiopericytomas can be found intracranially, where distinction from angioblastic meningiomas may be problematic.[115] Sinonasal,[116] pulmonary,[117] cardiac,[118] and pelvic or uterine hemangiopericytomas[119] have also been reported. Hemangiopericytomas rarely have been described to involve large vessels such as the aorta.[120,121] Paraneoplastic syndromes, including hypoglycemia and gynecomastia, occasionally have been associated with hemangiopericytoma.[122] There is one report of a familial hemangiopericytoma occurring in three members of one family.[123]

X-ray and CT studies of hemangiopericytomas show a radiopaque soft tissue mass that may rarely be calcified.[113] Pelvic tumors often have associated hydronephrosis and hydroureter.[113,119] Because of the richly vascular nature of the hemangiopericytoma, contrast-enhanced CT and angiography will show a dense, well-circumscribed stain resulting from contrast agent accumulation in the tumor vascular bed.[113,124] MRI will also demonstrate a well-circumscribed vascular tumor and assist in defining the boundaries of the tumor, thus assisting in surgical evaluation.[125] These radiologic findings are not specific for hemangiopericytoma and must be differentiated from the more common soft tissue sarcomas, such as MFH, liposarcoma, and synovial sarcoma. MFH can also be hypervascular like hemangiopericytomas, but liposarcomas are often hypovascular, and synovial sarcomas often contain calcified foci.[113,124] Grossly hemangiopericytomas are usually solitary, well-circumscribed masses with dilated vascular spaces and areas of cystic degeneration.[110,112] Histologically hemangiopericytomas have a rich network of dilated vascular spaces, characteristically assuming a branching, or "staghorn," morphology. These vascular spaces are lined by a layer of attenuated endothelial cells. Features predictive of malignant behavior are not well defined, but the presence of increased mitotic rate (greater than 4 mitoses per 10 high-power fields) and the presence of hemorrhage and necrosis have been suggested as helpful.[110,112] The presence of metastases is the only absolute criterion for malignancy, however.

Benign hemangiopericytomas are more frequent than those with malignant behavior.[110] In the literature the rate of metastases varies from 11.7%[126] to 56.5%,[127] with most being blood-borne to bone or lung. The infantile and sinonasal hemangiopericytomas, in contrast to their soft tissue counterparts, rarely recur or metastasize, regardless of histologic appearance.[114,116] Treatment for well-differentiated hemangiopericytomas is usually complete excision, but more radical surgery may be required for tumors that display malignant features. Preoperative embolization has been employed to reduce tumor blood flow and facilitate resection.[126] Adjuvant radiation therapy and chemotherapy both have been tried, with relatively poor results.[112,125,126,128,129]

HEMANGIOENDOTHELIOMA. Although hemangiomas are benign vascular tumors, and angiosarcomas behave in a malignant fashion, there is a group of uncommon vascular tumors of intermediate malignancy, namely the hemangioendotheliomas. Three subtypes of hemangioendothelioma have been described including epithelioid hemangioendothelioma (EH), spindle cell hemangioendothelioma, and malignant endovascular papillary angioendothelioma, or Dabska tumor.[130-132] These three subtypes are histologically distinct, yet all have a similar, relatively benign clinical course.

The EH is perhaps the best characterized and most frequent of the hemangioendotheliomas. It is a tumor composed of plump, epithelioid cells and is often vasocentric, most often involving a vein.[133] Originally described as a tumor of superficial and deep soft tissue,[130] it has become clear that EH may involve parenchymal sites, namely lung and liver.[134,135] Thus the intravascular bronchioloalveolar tumor of the lung is now recognized to be an EH on the basis of ultrastructural and immunohistochemical studies. Likewise, EH has also been described in conjunction with large vessels,[136,137] as an osseous primary[138] and as a pleural neoplasm, grossly mimicking a mesothelioma.[139]

EHs can arise at any age but do not often occur in children.[133] The soft tissue type of EH may begin as a solitary, painful subcutaneous mass, whereas those EHs associated with larger vessels may appear with obstructive vascular symptoms such as claudication or peripheral edema.[130,136,137] EHs of the lung characteristically arise in young women, with chest x-ray films typically showing bilateral noncalcified parenchymal nodules.[134,139] In EH of the liver the initial symptoms are often abdominal pain and jaundice[135,140] but may also include venoocclusive symptoms. Grossly EHs may resemble organizing thrombi, except for their tenacious attachment to the surrounding tissue[130] or may be gray or white and fibrous.[130] In the lung and liver EHs often consist of multiple bulging tumor masses with central necrosis.[134,135]

Histologically EHs are composed of solid nests or sheets of plump cells with abundant eosinophilic cytoplasm resembling epithelioid cells seen in carcinoma.[130,133] Frequently these tumors can be mistaken for a carcinoma or melanoma on a histologic basis, but immunohistochemical stains with factor VIII–related antigen or Ulex europaeus lectin will usually identify the endothelial nature of these tumors.[133]

The overall prognosis of soft tissue EH is quite favorable, with recurrences developing in 13% of patients and lymph node metastases in 31% of patients in one series.[133] Of those patients who develop metastases, less than half will be expected to die of disease. Because of the low-grade nature of these tumors, recommended treatment includes complete excision without adjuvant chemotherapy or radiotherapy.[133] EHs of the lung and liver behave in a more aggressive manner than similar tumors confined to soft tissue, with a mortality of up to 65% from disease.[134,140] Liver transplantation has been successfully used as a treatment for hepatic EH, even in the presence of extrahepatic metastases.[140]

Brief mention will be made of the two other hemangioendotheliomas. A spindle cell hemangioendothelioma has recently been described by Weiss and Enzinger,[131] which appears as a slow-growing, painless nodule of the extremities or chest wall in patients of different ages. To differentiate it from EH, spindle cell hemangioendotheliomas are composed of two distinct histologic patterns: cavernous spaces resembling a hemangioma alternating with cellular areas of spindled cells with slitlike vascular spaces, resembling Kaposi's sarcoma.[131] Clinically over 50% of patients with spindle hemangioendothelioma experience local recurrence, but lymph node metastases and death from the disease are rare.

The malignant papillary angioendothelioma, or Dabska tumor, is a rare, low-grade angiosarcoma that appears as solitary, subcutaneous nodules in children.[132] Histologically the Dabska tumor is distinctive, having cavernous spaces filled with tiny papillae lined by endothelial cells, some of which may display intracytoplasmic vacuolization.[141] Similar to other hemangioendotheliomas, the prognosis of the Dabska tumor appears to be good, despite the frequent presence of lymph node metastases.

REFERENCES

1. Enzinger FM and Weiss SW: Soft tissue tumors, ed 2, St Louis, 1988, The CV Mosby Co.
2. Fenoglio JJ Jr and Virmani R: Primary malignant tumors of the great vessels. In Waller BF, ed: Pathology of the heart and great vessels, vol 12, Contemporary issues in surgical pathology, New York, 1988, Churchill Livingstone.
3. McAllister HA Jr and Fenoglio JJ Jr: Tumors of the cardiovascular system, atlas of tumor pathology, Armed Forces Institute of Pathology, 1978, Fascical 15, 2nd series.
4. Burke AP and Virmani R: Sarcomas of the great vessels, Cancer 71:1761, 1993.
5. Kevorkian J and Cento DP: Leiomyosarcoma of large arteries and veins, Surgery 73:390, 1973.
6. Altman NH and Shelley WM: Primary intimal sarcoma of the pulmonary artery, Johns Hopkins Med J 133:214, 1973.
7. Burke AP and Virmani R: Neoplasms of large arteries and veins, and tumor angiogenesis. In Stehbens WE and Lie JT, eds: Vascular pathology, London, 1995, Chapman and Hall.
8. Wray RC and Dawkins H: Primary smooth muscle tumors of the inferior vena cava, Ann Surg 174:1009, 1971.
9. Cacoub P et al: Leiomyosarcoma of the inferior vena cava, Medicine 70:293, 1991.
10. Goertler U et al: Cava Verschluss syndrome durch ein Leiomyosarkem der vena cava inferior, Radiologe 17:350, 1977.
11. Gutierez O and Desai S: Leiomyosarcoma of the inferior vena cava with intracardiac extension, Eur J Radiol 6:153, 1986.
12. Pollanen M, Butany J, and Chiasson D: Leiomyosarcoma of the inferior vena cava, Arch Pathol Lab Med 111:1085, 1987.
13. Brewster DC, Athanasoulis A, and Darling RC: Leiomyosarcoma of the inferior vena cava, Arch Surg 111:1081, 1976.
14. Bailey RV et al: Leiomyosarcomas of the inferior vena cava, Ann Surg 184:169, 1976.
15. Stringer BD: Leiomyosarcoma of artery and vein, Am J Surg 134:90, 1977.
16. Shmookler BM, Marsh HB, and Roberts WC: Primary sarcoma of the pulmonary trunk and/or right or left main pulmonary artery: a rare cause of obstruction to right ventricular outflow, Am J Med 63:263, 1977.
17. Smith WS et al: MR and CT findings in pulmonary artery sarcoma, J Comput Assist Tomogr 13:906, 1989.
18. Britton PD: Primary pulmonary artery sarcoma—a report of two cases, with special emphasis on the diagnostic problems, Clin Radiol 41:92, 1990.
19. Kruger I et al: Symptoms, diagnosis and therapy of primary sarcomas of the pulmonary artery, Thorac Cardiovasc Surg 38:91, 1990.
20. Birkenstock WE and Lipper S: Leiomyosarcoma of the right common iliac artery: a case report, Br J Surg 63:81, 1976.
21. Davis GL: Tumor and inflammatory conditions of the ear. In Gnepp DR, ed: Pathology of the head and neck, vol 10, Contemporary issues in surgical pathology, New York, 1988, Churchill Livingstone.
22. Tsuneyoshi M and Enjoji M: Glomus tumor: a clinicopathologic and electron microscopic study, Cancer 50:1601, 1982.
23. Shugart RR, Soule EH, and Johnson EW Jr: Glomus tumors, Surg Gynecol Obstet 117:334, 1963.
24. Chase WH: Familial and bilateral tumors of the carotid body, J Pathol and Bacteriol 36:1, 1933.
25. Lack EE, Cubilla AL, and Woodruff JM: Paragangliomas of the head and neck region: a pathologic study of tumors from 71 patients, Hum Pathol 10:191, 1979.
26. Saldana MJ, Salem LE, and Travezan R: High altitude hypoxia and chemodectomas, Hum Pathol 4:251, 1973.
27. Duke WW et al: A norepinephrine-secreting glomus jugulare tumor presenting as a pheochromocytoma, Ann Intern Med 60:1040, 1964.
28. Matsuguchi H et al: Noradrenaline-secreting glomus jugulare tumor with cyclic change of blood pressure, Arch Intern Med 135:1110, 1975.
29. Merino MJ and Livolsi VA: Malignant carotid body tumors: report of two cases and review of the literature, Cancer 47:1403, 1981.

30. Robertson DI and Cooney TP: Malignant carotid body paraganglioma: light and electron microscopic study of the tumor and its metastases, Cancer 46:2623, 1980.

31. Nora JD et al: Surgical resection of carotid body tumors: long-term survival, recurrence, and metastasis, Mayo Clin Proc 63:348, 1988.

32. Shamblin WR et al: Carotid body tumor (chemodectoma): clinicopathologic analysis of ninety cases, Am J Surg 122:732, 1971.

33. Meyer FB, Sundt TM Jr, and Pearson BW: Carotid body tumors: a subject review and suggested surgical approach, J Neurosurg 64:377, 1986.

34. Borges LF, Heros RC, and DeBrun G: Carotid body tumors managed with preoperative embolization, J Neurosurg 59:867, 1983.

35. Brismar J and Cronqvist S: Therapeutic embolization in the external carotid artery region, Acta Radiol Diagn 19: 715, 1978.

36. Olson JL and Salyer WR: Mediastinal paragangliomas (aortic body tumor): a report of 4 cases and a review of the literature, Cancer 41:2405, 1978.

37. Pachter MR: Mediastinal nonchromaffin paraganglioma: a clinicopathologic study based on 8 cases, J Thorac Cardiovasc Surg 45:152, 1963.

38. Surakiatchanukul S, Goodsitt E, and Storer J: Chemodectoma of the aortic body, Chest 60:464, 1971.

39. D'Altorio RA, Rishi US, and Bhagwanani DG: Arteriographic findings in mediastinal chemodectoma, J Thorac Cardiovasc Surg 67:963, 1974.

40. Hashimoto H, Daimaru Y, and Enjoji M: Intravascular papillary endothelial hyperplasia: a clinicopathologic study of 91 cases, Am J Dermatopathol 5:539, 1984.

41. Pins MR et al: Florid extravascular papillary endothelial hyperplasia (Masson's pseudoangiosarcoma) presenting as a soft-tissue sarcoma, Arch Pathol Lab Med 117:259, 1993.

42. Hart WR and Yoonessi M: Endometrial stromatosis of the uterus, Obstet Gynecol 49:393, 1977.

43. Yoonessi M and Hart WR: Endometrial stromal sarcomas, Cancer 40:898, 1977.

44. Phillips MR et al: Intracardiac extension of an intracaval sarcoma of endometrial origin, Ann Thorac Surg 59:742, 1995.

45. Kronzon I et al: Right atrial and right ventricular obstruction by recurrent stromomyoma, J Am Soc Echocardiogr 7:528, 1994.

46. Norris HJ and Parmley T: Mesenchymal tumors of the uterus v. intravenous leiomyomatosis: a clinical and pathologic study of 14 cases, Cancer 36:2164, 1975.

47. Harper RS and Scully RE: Intravenous leiomyomatosis of the uterus: a report of 4 cases, Obstet Gynecol 18:519, 1961.

48. Grella L et al: Intravenous leiomyomatosis, J Vasc Surg 20:987, 1994.

49. Politzer F et al: Intracardiac leiomyomatosis: diagnosis and treatment, J Am Coll Cardiol 4:629, 1984.

50. Tierney WM et al: Intravenous leiomyomatosis of the uterus with extension into the heart, Am J Med 69:471, 1980.

51. Suggs WD et al: Renal cell carcinoma with inferior vena caval involvement, J Vasc Surg 14:413, 1991.

52. Bennington JL: Tumors of the kidney. In Javadpor N and Barsky SH, eds: Surgical pathology of urologic disease, Baltimore, 1987, Williams & Wilkins.

53. Brenner DW et al: Suprarenal Greenfield placement to prevent pulmonary embolus in patients with vena caval tumor thrombi, J Urol 147:19, 1992.

54. Vekemans KM and Schroder FH: Prosthetic replacement of the inferior vena cava in renal cell carcinoma surgery, Eur Urol 19:262, 1991.

55. Montie JE et al: Renal cell carcinoma with inferior vena cava tumor thrombi, Surg Gynecol Obstet 173:107, 1991.

56. Stocker JT and Ishak KG: Undifferentiated (embryonal) sarcoma of the liver: report of 31 cases, Cancer 42:336, 1978.

57. Zornig C et al: Primary sarcoma of the liver in the adult. Report of five surgically treated patients, Hepatogastroenterology 39:319, 1992.

58. Symbas PN, Hatcher CR, and Gravanis MB: Myxoma of the heart: clinical and experimental observations, Ann Surg 183:470, 1976.

59. Shah AA et al: Malignant fibrous histiocytoma of the heart presenting as an atrial myxoma, Cancer 42:2466, 1978.

60. Harris LS and Adelson L: Fatal coronary embolism from a myxomatous polyp of the aortic valve: an unusual cause of death, Am J Clin Pathol 43:61, 1965.

61. Anderson KR, Fiddler GI, and Lie JT: Congenital papillary tumor of the tricuspid valve: an unusual cause of right ventricular outflow obstruction in a neonate with trisomy E, Mayo Clin Proc 52:665, 1977.

62. Reichmann H et al: Neurological long-term follow-up in left atrial myxoma: are late complications frequent or rare? J Neurol 239:170, 1992.

63. Budzilovich G, Aleksic S, and Greco A: Malignant cardiac myxoma with cerebral metastases, Surg Neurol 11:462, 1979.

64. Floriano de Morais C et al: Myocardial infarct due to a unique atrial myxoma with epithelial-like cells and systemic metastases, Arch Pathol Lab Med 112:185, 1988.

65. Kevebtgak KJ et al: Antiphospholipid antibody syndrome with right atrial thrombosis mimicking an atrial myxoma, Am J Med 87:111, 1989.

66. Carney JA: Differences between nonfamilial and familial cardiac myxoma, Am J Surg Pathol 9:53, 1985.

67. Carney JA et al: The complex of myxomas, spotty pigmentation and endocrine overactivity, Medicine 64:270, 1985.

68. Alles JU and Bosslet K: Immunocytochemistry of angiosarcomas: a study of 19 cases with special emphasis on the applicability of endothelial cell specific markers to routinely prepared tissues, Am J Clin Pathol 89:463, 1988.

69. Bardioil JM et al: Angiosarcomas of the head and neck region, Am J Surg 116:548, 1968.

70. Fisher JH: Postmastectomy lymphangiosarcoma in the lymphedematous arm: a review of 4 cases, Can J Surg 8:350, 1965.

71. Maddox JC and Evans HL: Angiosarcoma of skin and soft tissue: a study of 44 cases, Cancer 48:1907, 1981.

72. Donnell RM et al: Angiosarcoma and other vascular tumors of the breast: pathologic analysis as a guide to prognosis, Am J Surg Pathol 5:629, 1981.

73. Mark L et al: Clinical and morphologic features of hepatic angiosarcoma in vinyl chloride workers, Cancer 37:149, 1976.

74. Popper H et al: Development of hepatic angiosarcoma in man induced by vinyl chloride: thorotrast and arsenic, Am J Pathol 92:349, 1978.

75. Kanno J, Takemura T, and Kasaga T: Malignant endothelioma of the aorta, Virchows Arch A Pathol Anat Histopathol 412:183, 1987.

76. Adachi K et al: Right atrial angiosarcoma diagnosed by cardiac biopsy, Am Heart J 115:482, 1988.

77. Abratt RP et al: Angiosarcoma of the superior vena cava, Cancer 52:740, 1983.

78. Alosco T et al: Angiosarcoma of the axillary vein, Cancer 64:1301, 1989.

79. Holden CA, Spittle MF, and Jones EW: Angiosarcoma of the face and scalp, prognosis and treatment, Cancer 59: 1046, 1987.

80. Borgdorf WHC, Mukai K, and Rosai J: Immunohistochemical identification of factor VIII–related antigen in endothelial cells of cutaneous lesions of alleged vascular nature, Am J Clin Pathol 75:167, 1981.

81. Stewart F and Treves N: Lymphangiosarcoma in post mastectomy lymphedema, Cancer 1:64, 1948.

82. McConnell EM and Haslam P: Angiosarcoma in postmastectomy lymphoedema: a report of five cases and a review of the literature, Br J Surg 46:322, 1959.

83. Woodward AH, Ivins JC, and Soule EH: Lymphangiosarcoma arising in chronic lymphedematous extremities, Cancer 30:562, 1972.

84. Eby CS, Brennan MJ, and Fine G: Lymphangiosarcoma: a lethal complication of chronic lymphedema—report of two cases and review of the literature, Arch Surg 94:223, 1967.

85. Merrick TA, Erlandson RA, and Hajdu SI: Lymphangiosarcoma of a congenitally lymphedematous arm, Arch Pathol 91:365, 1971.

86. MacKenzie DH: Lymphangiosarcoma arising in chronic congenital and idiopathic lymphoedema, J Clin Pathol 24:524, 1971.

87. Sordillo PP et al: Lymphangiosarcoma, Cancer 48:1674, 1981.

88. Gajarj H et al: Lymphangiosarcoma complicating chronic primary lymphoedema, Br J Surg 74:1180, 1987.

89. Andersson HC, Parry DM, Mulvihill JJ: Lymphangiosarcoma in late-onset hereditary lymphedema: case report and nosological implications, Am J Med Genet 56:72, 1995.

90. Schreiber H et al: Stewart-Treves syndrome: a lethal complication of post mastectomy lymphedema and regional immune deficiency, Arch Surg 114:82, 1979.

91. Tomita K et al: Lymphangiosarcoma in post-mastectomy lymphedema (Stewart-Treves syndrome): ultrastructural and immunohistologic characteristics, J Surg Oncol 38:275, 1988.

92. Yap BS et al: Chemotherapy for post-mastectomy lymphangiosarcoma, Cancer 47:853, 1981.

93. Kaufmann T, Chu F, Kaufman R: Post-mastectomy lymphangiosarcoma (Stewart-Treves syndrome): report of two long term survivals, Br J Radiol 64:857, 1991.

94. Borel Rinkes IHM and de Jongste AB: Lymphangiosarcoma in chronic lymphedema, Acta Chir Scand 152:227, 1986.

95. Kaposi M: Idiopathisches multiples pigment-sarkom der haut, Arch Dermatol Syph 4:265, 1872.

96. Niemi M and Mustakallio KK: The fine structure of the spindle cell in Kaposi's sarcoma, Acta Pathol Microbiol Scand 63:567, 1965.

97. Armes J: A review of Kaposi's sarcoma, Adv Cancer Res 53:73, 1989.

98. Taylor JF et al: Kaposi's sarcoma in Uganda: a clinico-pathological study, Int J Cancer 8:122, 1971.

99. DeJarlais DC et al: Kaposi's sarcoma among four different AIDS risk groups, N Engl J Med 310:1119, 1984.

100. Cohn DL and Judson FN: Absence of Kaposi's sarcoma in hemophiliacs with the acquired immune deficiency syndrome, Ann Intern Med 101:401, 1984.

101. Padilla S, Rivera-Perlman Z, and Solomon L: Kaposi's sarcoma in transfusion-associated acquired immunodeficiency syndrome, Arch Pathol Lab Med 114:40, 1990.

102. Harwood AR et al: Kaposi's sarcoma in recipients of renal transplants, Am J Med 67:759, 1979.

103. Safai B et al: Association of Kaposi's sarcoma with second primary malignancies: possible etiopathogenic implications, Cancer 45:1472, 1980.

104. Law IP: Kaposi's sarcoma and plasma cell dyscrasia, JAMA 229:1329, 1974.

105. Gilbert TT, Evjy JT, and Edelstein L: Hodgkin's disease associated with Kaposi's sarcoma and malignant melanoma, Cancer 28:293, 1971.

106. Fauci AS et al: Acquired immunodeficiency syndrome: epidemiologic, clinical, immunologic, and therapeutic considerations, Ann Intern Med 100:92, 1984.

107. Groopman JE and Scadden DT: Interferon therapy for Kaposi sarcoma associated with the acquired immunodeficiency syndrome (AIDS), Ann Intern Med 110:335, 1989.

108. Stout AP and Murray MR: Hemangiopericytoma: a vascular tumor featuring Zimmerman's pericytes, Ann Surg 116:26, 1942.

109. Battifora H: Hemangiopericytoma: ultrastructural study of five cases, Cancer 31:1418, 1973.

110. Enzinger FM and Smith BH: Hemangiopericytoma: an analysis of 106 cases, Hum Pathol 7:61, 1976.

111. Stout AP: Tumors featuring pericytes: glomus tumor and hemangiopericytoma, Lab Invest 5:217, 1956.

112. McMaster MJ, Soule EH, and Ivins JC: Hemangiopericytoma: clinicopathologic study and long-term follow-up of 60 patients, Cancer 36:2232, 1975.

113. Lorigan JG et al: The clinical and radiologic manifestations of hemangiopericytoma, AJR 153:345, 1989.

114. Atkinson JB et al: Hemangiopericytoma in infants and children: a report of six patients, Am J Surg 148:372, 1984.

115. D'Amore ESG, Manivel JC, and Sung JH: Soft-tissue and meningeal hemangiopericytomas: an immunohistochemical and ultrastructural study, Hum Pathol 21:414, 1990.

116. Abdel-Fattah HM, Adams GL, and Wick MR: Hemangiopericytoma of the maxillary sinus and skull base, Head Neck Surg 12:77, 1990.

117. Rusch VW et al: Massive pulmonary hemangiopericytoma: an innovative approach to evaluation and treatment, Cancer 64:1928, 1989.

118. Fujii B et al: Primary cardiac hemangiopericytoma causing rupture of the right atrium and chronic cardiac tamponade, Jpn Circ J 55:1206, 1991.

119. Munoz AK et al: Pelvic hemangiopericytomas: a report of five cases and literature review, Gynecol Oncol 36:380, 1990.

120. Bowles LT, Ring EM, and Hill WT: Hemangiopericytoma in a resected thoracic aortic aneurysm, Ann Thorac Surg 1:746, 1965.

121. Blenkinsopp WK and Hobs JT: Pedunculated hemangiopericytoma attached to the thoracic aorta, Thorax 21:193, 1966.

122. Howard JW and Davis PL: Retroperitoneal hemangiopericytoma associated with hypoglycemia and masculinization, Del Med J 31:29, 1959.

123. Plukker JT et al: Malignant hemangiopericytomas in three kindred members of one family, Cancer 61:841, 1988.

124. Goldman SM, Davidson AJ, and Neal J: Retroperitoneal and pelvic hemangiopericytomas: clinical, radiologic and pathologic correlation, Radiology 168:13, 1988.

125. Craven J, Quigley TM, Bolen JW: Current management and clinical outcome of hemangiopericytoma, Am J Surg 163:490, 1992.

126. Smullens SN et al: Preoperative embolization of retroperitoneal hemangiopericytomas as an aid in their removal, Cancer 50:1870, 1982.

127. O'Brien P and Brasfield RO: Hemangiopericytoma, Cancer 18:249, 1965.

128. Bredt AB and Serpick AH: Metastatic hemangiopericytoma treated with vincristine and actinomycin D, Cancer 24:266, 1969.

129. Mira JG, Chu FC, and Forner JG: The role of radiotherapy in the management of malignant hemangiopericytoma: report of 11 new cases and review of the literature, Cancer 39:1254, 1977.

130. Weiss SW and Enzinger FM: Epithelioid hemangioendothelioma: a vascular tumor often mistaken for a carcinoma, Cancer 50:970, 1982.

131. Weiss SW and Enzinger FM: Spindle cell hemangioendothelioma: a low grade angiosarcoma resembling a cavernous hemangioma and Kaposi's sarcoma, Am J Surg Pathol 10:521, 1986.

132. Dabska M: Malignant endovascular papillary angioendothelioma of the skin in childhood, Cancer 24:503, 1969.

133. Weiss SW et al: Epithelioid hemangioendothelioma and related lesions, Semin Diagn Pathol 3:259, 1986.

134. Dial D et al: Intravascular bronchiolar and alveolar tumor of the lung (IVBAT): an analysis of twenty cases of a peculiar sclerosing endothelial tumor, Cancer 51:451, 1983.

135. Ishak KG et al: Epithelioid hemangioendothelioma of the liver: a clinicopathologic and follow-up study of 32 cases, Hum Pathol 15:839, 1984.

136. Toursarkissian B, O'Connor WN, and Dillon ML: Mediastinal epithelioid hemangioendothelioma, Ann Thorac Surg 49:680, 1990.

137. Harris EJ Jr, Taylor LM Jr, and Porter JM: Epithelioid hemangioendothelioma of the external iliac vein: a primary vascular tumor presenting as traumatic venous obstruction, J Vasc Surg 10:693, 1989.

138. Dorfman HD, Tsuneyoshi M, and Bauer T: Epithelioid hemangioendothelioma of bone, Lab Invest 54:17, 1986.

139. Yousem SA and Hochholzer L: Unusual thoracic manifestations of epithelioid hemangioendothelioma, Arch Pathol Lab Med 111:459, 1987.

140. Marino IR et al: Treatment of hepatic epithelioid hemangioendothelioma with liver transplantation, Cancer 62:2079, 1988.

141. Manivel JC et al: Endovascular papillary endothelioma of childhood: a vascular lesion possibly characterized by high endothelial differentiation, Hum Pathol 17:1240, 1986.

CHAPTER THIRTY-SEVEN

LEG ULCERS

Henry H. Roenigk, Jr.
Jess R. Young

Ulcerations of the lower extremity are fairly common and can present both a diagnostic and therapeutic problem to the physician. Leg ulcers are seen by both the general practitioner and the specialist. Because of the many problems involved in arriving at a proper diagnosis and course of treatment for leg ulcers, a comprehensive classification, diagnostic evaluation, and treatment program are needed for the patient who complains to the physician, "Doctor, what can you do about this ulcer I have on my lower leg?"

DIAGNOSIS OF LEG ULCERS

History

Since many leg ulcers have certain characteristic historic features, a comprehensive history of the ulcer, obtained through the following questions, is often necessary to establish a proper diagnosis:

1. What did the ulcer look like at first?
   Leg ulcers often change their appearance after secondary infection or after the application of many types of local medication, which may have been used in an attempt to heal the ulcer.
2. What started the ulcer?
   Local injury, strong medication, infection, thrombophlebitis, cold and factitial (self-induced) injury may be factors in precipitating the ulceration. Sometimes this is difficult to elicit. Neurotrophic ulcers are often unnoticed.
3. What is the family history?
   This is particularly helpful in certain hematologic disorders (e.g., sickle cell anemia or thalassemia) and certain connective tissue disorders (e.g., systemic lupus erythematosus or rheumatoid arthritis). Varicose veins, and eventually stasis ulcers, tend to be familial.
4. How quickly did the ulcer develop?
   Rapidly developing ulcers suggest venous insufficiency, or pyoderma gangrenosum; slowly developing ulcers suggest arterial insufficiency or malignancy.

5. How painful is the ulcer?
   Stasis ulcerations are often painless, whereas ulcers due to arterial insufficiency, livedoid vasculitis, and cutaneous polyarteritis nodosum are very painful. The patient with ischemic ulceration caused by arterial insufficiency often will sit in a chair all night and not elevate his legs because the dependent position gives him the best possible blood supply to his painful ulcers. Venous ulceration, on the other hand, often improves with elevation because this position relieves the edema of the surrounding tissues. Hypertensive ischemic ulcers and atrophie blanche vasculitis ulcers are very painful. Neurotrophic ulcers are often painless but the patient may experience paresthesias or burning pain in the leg.
6. What drugs has the patient taken?
   It is important to obtain a complete list of all medications taken by the patient. Specific questions concerning nonprescription medications such as sedatives, sleeping pills, analgesic, and antacid medications should be included since these drugs can cause leg ulcers or lead to vasculitis with secondary ulceration.
7. Is there a history of other systemic disorders?
   A current or past history of anemia, rheumatoid arthritis, diabetes mellitus, inflammatory bowel disease, ischemic heart disease or stroke, and collagen diseases often gives a clue to the cause of the leg ulcer.

Physical Examination

1. Where is the ulcer?
   Ulcers resulting from venous stasis are often located over the medial malleolus because this area is drained by the saphenous venous system and the perforating veins. These ulcers will usually be located over the inner aspect of the ankle but can be posterior, anterior, or lateral on occasion. Ischemic ulcers occur on areas farthest from the occluded vessel. The common location of ischemic ulcers caused by arteriosclerosis is the toes or dorsum of the foot. Hypertensive ischemic ulcers tend to occur on

the lateral malleolus. Neurotrophic ulcers occur on pressure points on the sole of the foot.

2. What is the condition of the surrounding skin?
The surrounding skin should be closely examined for stasis pigmentation, edema, varicose veins, evidence of scleroderma, petechia, or hemorrhage. The color of the skin is important. A pale color indicates poor arterial blood supply, as in ischemic ulcers.

3. Are there signs of other systemic diseases?
These will be discussed in detail later in this chapter, but a heart murmur of cardiovascular syphilis, arthritis caused by systemic lupus erythematosus, or other signs of diabetes mellitus (e.g., eyeground changes) are helpful in determining the cause of the leg ulcer.

Laboratory Tests

The tests in the box on this page are divided into three groups. Group I should be done for any leg ulcer. Groups II and III are specifically for the more unusual types of leg ulcers.

CLASSIFICATION OF LEG ULCERS

There are many classifications of leg ulcers.[1] Some are purely clinical and are mainly concerned with subdivision of the two major causes, arterial and venous. Some are purely histopathologic with various subdivisions of the histology of vasculitis or inflammatory skin lesions. The classifications in the box on pages 639 and 640 are a combination of clinical and histologic findings with emphasis on the clinical.

VASCULAR LEG ULCERS

Arterial Leg Ulcers
LEG ULCERS SECONDARY TO ARTERIOSCLEROSIS OBLITERANS. Arteriosclerosis obliterans (ASO), which is discussed in detail in Chapter 11, is a progressive disease that is becoming a more frequent cause of ischemic ulcers of the leg and foot. They may be associated with ischemic heart disease, strokes, diabetes, or hypertension. Ulceration in ASO usually appears in the terminal portions of the digits, often around the nails or in a nailbed following infection (Fig. 37-1). The ulcers are also common over bony prominences such as the first and fifth metatarsal heads, the heel, and the malleoli (Fig. 37-2). They may result from the normal pressures of shoes or may develop in corns or bunions as the result of infection or too vigorous treatment. If the ulcer is on the leg, it is usually the result of mechanical or thermal trauma.

Ischemic ulcers are usually small and shallow initially, gradually increasing in size. The base of the ulcer is often gray, yellow, or black (Fig. 37-2) and may be covered by necrotic debris and crusted exudates. Granulation tissue is minimal or absent. The rim of the ulcer is indolent, showing no tendency for proliferation or epithelialization. There may be secondary infection, especially in diabetics. This infection usually inhibits healing and produces a chronic purulent drainage. Osteomyelitis or suppurative arthritis may complicate deep ulcerations. Common associated findings in patients with ulcerations secondary to

LABORATORY TESTS

I. Routine Laboratory Studies
  A. CBC and differential
  B. Urinalysis
  C. SMA-20
  D. Chest x-ray
  E. Bacterial culture
  F. Serologic test for syphilis (VDRL, FTA abs)

II. Special Laboratory Test
  A. Antinuclear factor/anti-DNA
  B. Serum complement (Total, C_3, C_4)
  C. Special antibody studies (ENA, SSM, SSA)
  D. Latex fixation for rheumatoid arthritis
  E. Sickle cell preparation
  F. Special hematologic tests (serum protein electrophoresis, erythrocyte sedimentation rate)
  G. Hypercoagulation screen (protein S, protein C, antithrombin III, antiphopholipid antibodies)
  H. X-rays: chest CT scans for malignancy, colon (ulcerative colitis), local x-rays to rule out osteomyelitis, and others as indicated
  I. Skin biopsy culture for
    1. Bacteria
    2. Fungi
    3. Mycobacteria
  J. Skin tests: PPD
  K. Urinary porphyrins
  L. Skin biopsy and special stains: H & E, I-F, acid-fast
  M. Muscle biopsy
  N. Colonoscopy

III. Vascular
  A. Arterial noninvasive
    1. Doppler waveforms
    2. Segmental pressures
    3. Pulse volume recordings
    4. Doppler ultrasound
  B. Venous noninvasive
    1. Photoplethysmography
    2. Duplex ultrasound
  C. Invasive
    1. Angiography

ASO are the lack or decrease of leg pulses and atrophy of leg muscles with loss of muscle tone. Edema of the foot and leg may occur if the patient has been sitting up nightly in an attempt to relieve the pain of the ulcer.

Diagnosis. To determine the presence and severity of

CLASSIFICATIONS OF LEG ULCERS

I. Vascular
A. Arterial
  1. Arteriosclerosis obliterans
  2. Thromboangiitis obliterans
  3. Livedo reticularis
  4. Hypertension
  5. Chronic pernio (chronic chilblains)
  6. AV malformations
B. Venous: chronic venous insufficiency (stasis)
C. Lymphatic: elephantiasis nostras (lymphedema)

II. Vasculitis
A. Small vessel
  1. Hypersensitivity vasculitis (leukocytoclasis)
    a. Drug
    b. Cryoglobulinemia
    c. Infection
    d. Henoch-Schönlein purpura
    e. Malignancy
    f. Idiopathic
  2. Autoimmune disease
    a. Rheumatoid arthritis
    b. Systemic lupus erythematosus
    c. Scleroderma
    d. Sjögren's syndrome
    e. Behçet's disease
  3. Livedoid vasculitis
    a. Atrophie blanche vasculitis
B. Medium and large vessel
  1. Polyarteritis nodosa
  2. Cutaneous polyarteritis nodosa
  3. Wegener's granulomatosis
  4. Churg-Strauss granulomatosis
  5. Giant cell arteritis
  6. Malignant atrophic papulosis (Degos' disease)

III. Hematologic Diseases
A. Red blood cell disorders
  1. Sickle cell anemia
  2. Thalassemia
  3. Polycythemia rubra vera
B. Leukemia
C. Thrombocythemia
D. Dysproteinemias
  1. Cryoglobulinemia
  2. Cryofibrinogenemia
  3. Macroglobulinemia

E. Coagulation defects
  1. Protein S and C deficiencies
  2. Antithrombin III deficiency
  3. Antiphospholipid antibody syndromes

IV. Infectious
A. Fungus
  1. Blastomycosis
  2. Coccidiomycosis
  3. Histoplasmosis
  4. Sporotrichosis
  5. Maduromycosis
  6. Majocchi granuloma
B. Syphilis: secondary and tertiary
C. Bacterial infections: primary, secondary
D. Tuberculosis
  1. Erythema induratum
  2. Lupus vulgaris
  3. Papulonecrotic tuberculid
E. Leprosy
F. Atypical mycobacterial
G. Leishmaniasis
H. Infestations and bites

V. Neurotrophic
A. Diabetes mellitus
B. Tabes dorsalis
C. Poliomyelitis
D. Leprosy
E. Traumatic and toxic neuropathies
F. Inherited sensory deficiency

VI. Metabolic Disorders
A. Diabetic neurotrophic ulcer
B. Necrobiosis lipoidica diabeticorum
C. Pyoderma gangrenosum
D. Gaucher's disease
E. Gout
F. Porphyria cutanea tarda

VII. Tumors
A. Basal cell carcinoma
B. Squamous cell carcinoma
C. Kaposi's hemorrhagic sarcoma (classic type)
D. Lymphoma
  1. Lymphoma: B cell, Primary cutaneous B cell
  2. Cutaneous T cell lymphoma
E. Melanoma

Continued.

CLASSIFICATIONS OF LEG ULCERS—cont'd

VIII. Drugs
A. Halogens
B. Ergotism
C. Methotrexate
D. Illicit drug use
E. Vasopressors
F. Hydroxyurea
G. Coumadin

IX. Miscellaneous
A. Burns (thermal, chemical)
B. Lichen planus

C. Weber-Christian disease (panniculitis)
D. Acrodermatitis chronica atrophicans
E. Radiation
F. Frostbite
G. Factitial (self-induced)
H. Pressure

X. Panniculitis
A. Pancreatic fat necrosis
B. Lupus panniculitis
C. Alpha$_1$ antitrypsin deficiency
D. Weber-Christian disease

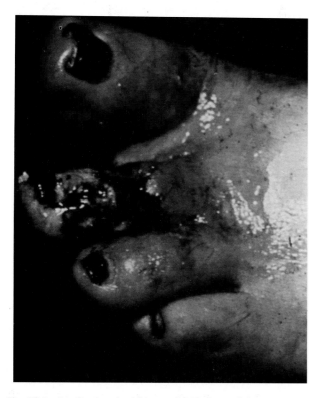

Fig. 37-1. Arteriosclerosis obliterans (ASO) ulcers of the terminal portions of the digits with necrosis of the skin.

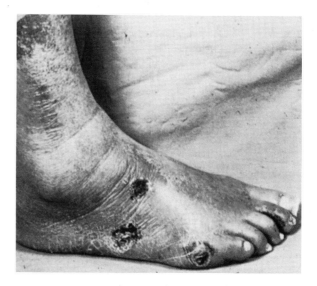

Fig. 37-2. ASO ulcers, gray or black, with poor granulation tissue in the base.

arterial insufficiency, no unusual or elaborate equipment is necessary although noninvasive Doppler and plethysmographic techniques are common today. An adequate evaluation may be accomplished in any physician's office. The most important finding from a physical examination is an absence or a decrease in amplitude of arterial pulsations. A good index for the severity of ischemia is a change in color of the feet with alterations in positions of the limb. After elevating the limb for about one minute, an abnormal pallor in the foot and leg will appear when there is significant ischemia. On subsequent dependence there is

delay in filling of the veins beyond the normal 10- to 15-second period. When the color does return, it may be bright red, the rubor of dependency.

Doppler measurement of ankle blood pressure will provide additional data on the severity of arterial disease. A useful ratio is a comparison of the ankle pressure to the brachial arm pressure, or ankle-brachial index. A normal ratio is 1.0 or greater.

Arteriograms are not necessary unless nonsurgical angioplasty or arterial surgical repair of major peripheral vessels is contemplated. They then give valuable information as to the site, extent, and operability of the occlusive arterial lesions. For a more complete discussion regarding the diagnosis of ASO, see Chapter 11.

Differential Diagnosis. In chronic venous insufficiency the ulcers are rarely as painful as ischemic ulcers. Dependency usually relieves the pain of ischemic ulcers while it increases the discomfort of stasis ulcers. The typical locations of the stasis ulcers in the region of the ankle, particularly just behind the medial malleolus, would be unusual sites for ischemic ulcers. The area around the stasis ulcer shows typical changes of pigmentation and induration. The base of the stasis ulcer is usually weeping and has extensive granulation tissue, while ischemic ulcers are dry with little or no granulations. Pulses are usually present in patients with stasis ulcers, but even if they are absent, the other features mentioned above should be sufficient to make the diagnosis.

Hypertensive ischemic ulcers are very painful, are most commonly seen on the lateral or posterior aspect of the legs, and are usually surrounded by a bluish-red ischemic rim of tissue. The patient is hypertensive and has normal pulses.

Treatment. Patients in bed with severe ischemia should be watched carefully and protected from pressure on heels or other bony prominences by the use of padded boots, sheepskin, or a flotation mattress. Pressure from bed clothes should be prevented by the use of a foot cradle. The head of the bed should be elevated 4 to 6 inches to increase the blood flow to the feet. A warm environmental temperature helps produce reflex vasodilation.

All patients should be asked to refrain from smoking. Repeated use of analgesics may be necessary for temporary relief of ischemic pain. A tranquilizer may be helpful in alleviating the anxiety often associated with severe pain, and may potentiate the effect of the analgesics. Narcotics should be used with caution because the chronicity of the pain may lead to addiction. Systemic antibiotics are usually not necessary unless the ulcer is associated with obvious cellulitis or lymphangitis or unless there is evidence of a systemic infection with chills or fever.

The precipitating cause of many severely ischemic ulcers is trauma from mechanical, chemical, or thermal sources. Patients should therefore be given detailed instructions concerning the care of their extremities and the avoidance of further trauma. They should be carefully advised regarding care of nails, avoidance of extremes of hot and cold temperatures, and proper treatment of athlete's foot. Ingrown toenails, corns, and calluses should be treated by a physician or a podiatrist who is aware of the fact that the patient has ischemic extremities.

The value of oral vasodilator drugs is a controversial subject. Most authorities have not found them to be effective. Pentoxifylline, a hemorrheologic agent, may be helpful to some patients.

Strong chemical solutions should be avoided as applications to ischemic ulcers. Lukewarm wet dressings, or intermittent soaks using 0.9% sodium chloride, 5% boric acid solution, or Burow's compresses may promote drainage and loosen sloughs and crusts. The temperature of the solutions applied to ischemic lesions should never exceed 35°C. Maceration of viable tissue should be avoided. Culture and sensitivity studies should be made for all ulcerations, although healing is usually not promoted by antibiotic ointments unless the ulcer is grossly infected. To remove adherent necrotic crusts or eschars from ischemic ulcers, enzymatic debridement has limited value. Surgical debridement, done carefully, may help. Hydrocolloid dressings (see *Leg ulcers secondary to chronic venous insufficiency*) may also help.

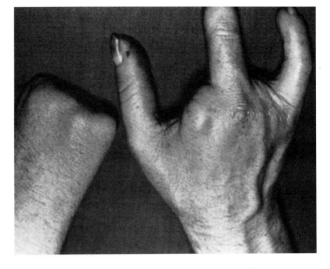

Fig. 37-3. Gangrene of the fingers resulted in multiple amputations in this man with thromboangiitis obliterans.

Ointments containing anesthetic agents often increase tissue necrosis even though they help relieve pain, and their use should be discouraged. At no time should adhesive tape for dressings be applied directly to ischemic skin.

Skin grafting for indolent ulcers is occasionally of value, but the ulcer should be as clean as possible and should have some granulation tissue in its base before grafting is attempted.

Surgical and nonsurgical approaches to improve arterial circulation are discussed in Chapter 11.

LEG ULCERS SECONDARY TO THROMBOANGIITIS OBLITERANS. Thromboangiitis obliterans (TAO) is a disease of the arteries and veins of the extremities and rarely of the viscera, which develops predominantly in young men and women who smoke. It is discussed in detail in Chapter 21.

Clinical Features. The typical patient with TAO is a young person less than 40 years of age, who smokes, who has occlusive arterial disease distal to the popliteal artery or in the hand, and who has a history of, or presence of, thrombophlebitis.

Severe ischemic changes of ulceration and gangrene are frequent manifestations of TAO and may develop early in the disease. The toes are most commonly affected, especially around the margins of the nails. Ischemic symptoms in the upper extremities occur in about 40% of patients, especially ulcerations around the fingertips and gangrene of the fingers (Fig. 37-3). Thrombophlebitis, usually superficial thrombophlebitis, also occurs at some stage in the disease in about 40% of patients with TAO.

Treatment. All patients with TAO should abstain from using tobacco in all forms. This abstinence should be complete and permanent, and there can be no compromise. The patient should be warned that even an occasional cigarette may be enough to cause a relapse in the disease.

Ischemic ulcers should be treated in the same manner as the ischemic ulcer of ASO. Many patients will improve markedly after the cessation of smoking, and no further measures will be needed. If significant improvement is not noted within 2 to 3 months after the patient has stopped smoking, regional sympathetic ganglionectomy should be considered. However, this sympathectomy will not be successful if the patient continues to smoke or resumes smoking.

LEG ULCERS SECONDARY TO LIVEDO RETICULARIS. Livedo reticularis is one of a relatively uncommon group of arteriospastic disorders that may cause ischemic ulcers of the extremity because of prolonged spasm and subsequent occlusion of the arteries and arterioles. These arteriospastic disorders also include acrocyanosis and Raynaud's phenomenon. Since acrocyanosis causes no significant ischemia and no ulcerations, and since the ulcerations in Raynaud's phenomenon are usually limited to distal fingers, these two conditions will not be included in this discussion.

Pathology and Pathogenesis. The changes that accompany livedo reticularis are brought about by narrowing of the arterioles that pierce the cutis from below. The narrowing can be either spastic or organic with secondary dilation of the capillaries and venules. This results in a marked slowing of blood flow. Pathologic studies may reveal no changes in the arterioles or may show proliferation of the intima and occasionally complete occlusion of some arteries.

Livedo reticularis is usually idiopathic but occasionally is associated with such diseases as atheromatous embolization, periarteritis nodosa, disseminated lupus erythematosus, antiphospholipid antibody syndrome, and cryoglobulinemia.

Clinical Features. Patients with livedo reticularis notice a persistent, bluish-red "fishnet" pattern of cyanotic mottling of the skin of the extremities. The majority are women whose symptoms are first noted between 20 and 40 years of age. The mottling may extend to the thighs and involve the arms to a lesser degree than the legs. Occasionally, it may involve the trunk, especially over the buttocks and lower abdomen. The mottling is more intense in cooler weather but never disappears entirely even in warm weather.

Many patients with livedo reticularis have no symptoms at all, while others complain of coldness, numbness, aching, or paresthesias of the feet and legs. In a few patients ulcerations of the lower legs and feet occur and continue to recur. The ulcers begin as bluish-red infarcted areas, which then break down to form irregular ulcerations from 1 to 2 cm in diameter. The ulcers are painful and resist healing.

Treatment. Since most patients with livedo reticularis are completely asymptomatic, no treatment is necessary other than reassurance. Patients with mild symptoms or patients who object to the unattractive appearance of the skin need only protect the involved areas from cold as much as possible. Vasodilating drugs such as phenoxybenzamine hydrochloride (Dibenzyline) in doses of 10 mg three or four times daily may be tried. Calcium channel blockers such as nifedipine may also be helpful. Pentoxifylline can help some patients. If ulcerations are present, they should be treated in the same manner as the ischemic ulcers of ASO. Sympathetic ganglionectomy may help resistant ulcers. Treatment of an underlying disease (i.e.,

systemic lupus erythematosus) can result in improvement of ulcerations.

HYPERTENSIVE LEG ULCERS

Pathology and Pathogenesis. In severe hypertension generalized arteriolar disease occurs. There is an increase in thickness in the arteriolar wall and decrease in the diameter of the lumen. Occasionally the lumen is obstructed with thrombosis. These changes in the arterioles can result in an area of decreased blood supply to the skin. If the decrease is severe enough, or if mild trauma occurs, an area of skin infarction results, which breaks down and forms an ischemic ulcer.

Clinical Features. Patients with hypertensive ulcers most often have had essential hypertension for a long time and have vascular changes in the fundi. Women in their fifth and sixth decades are most affected, although ulcers occur in men also.

Hypertensive ulcers usually originate on the lateral surface of the ankle, but may occur posteriorly or higher on the lateral calf (Fig. 37-4). An ulcer usually starts as a painful, reddish-blue plaque or as a small purpuric lesion. A hemorrhagic bleb then develops, which breaks down into a superficial ulcer. The ulcer frequently is surrounded by a cyanotic or purpuric halo, representing ischemic tissue that has not yet broken down. The ulcer may extend gradually in a serpiginous manner into this ischemic area and reach the size of 5 to 10 cm. It usually has the typical appearance of an ischemic ulcer with little granulation tissue and minimal drainage. The pain is severe, out of proportion to the size of the ulcer, and is usually the reason for seeking medical attention. There may be involvement of both legs, either simultaneously or sequentially. All lesions heal slowly, requiring weeks or months of treatment.

Treatment. It is most important that the patient's blood pressure be adequately controlled to try to retard or

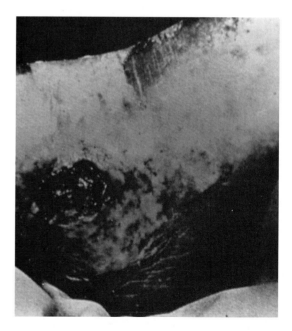

Fig. 37-4. Hypertensive ulcer over the lateral malleolus with a purplish hue around the ulcer.

arrest the underlying disease process. Healing of hypertensive ulcers is slow at best, but may be impossible without adequate treatment of the blood pressure.

Since the hypertensive ulcer is secondary to ischemia, the same plan of treatment outlined for the treatment of the arteriosclerotic ulcer applies. Treatment should be directed at increasing the blood supply, relieving pain, clearing up any local infection, and protecting the leg from any further injury. The patient should not smoke. Early skin grafting may be necessary to control the pain.

LEG ULCERS SECONDARY TO CHRONIC PERNIO (CHRONIC CHILBLAINS). When a person susceptible to chronic pernio is exposed repeatedly to cold, severe arteriospasm can result in ulcerative cutaneous lesions on the toes and lower legs. These ulcers tend to heal during the warm season and to recur during the cool months.

Pathology and Pathogenesis. The vascular changes in chronic pernio are most likely caused by repeated episodes of arteriospasm that occur on cold exposure. Intimal proliferation, thickening of arterial walls, and periarterial and perivenous infiltrations of lymphocytes, monocytes, and neutrophilic leukocytes may be seen. Arteriospasm also produces ischemic changes in the tissues with varying degrees of chronic inflammatory reactions.

Clinical Features. The typical patient with chronic pernio is a young man or woman with recurring, painful ulcerations of the toes, feet, or legs. Early in the disease the ulcers appear at the onset of cold weather and disappear in the summer, but later these seasonal effects may not be so prominent. Following cold exposure, small (5 to 15 mm), red, elevated lesions can be seen on the toes and occasionally on the dorsum of the feet and toes. Blisters then form on these lesions within a few days, and the color changes to a blue or violet hue. The blisters then form a superficial, painful ulcer with a hemorrhagic base. Often 15 to 20 ulcers are present at a time. After 3 to 5 weeks, these lesions heal spontaneously, leaving permanent pigmented and scarred areas. Successive crops of lesions may appear.

Treatment. The most important feature of treatment in chronic pernio is the avoidance of exposure to cold. If cold cannot be avoided, adequate protection should be sought by dressing warmly and by not exposing the affected areas to the cold. Oral vasodilators may be tried, but usually are not effective. Calcium channel blockers such as nifedipine are the treatment of choice. The use of ultraviolet-B (UVB) phototherapy before cold exposure may prevent the development of chronic pernio lesions. Sympathectomy should be done for lesions that do not respond to conservative measures, but it will not give permanent protection from recurrence of the lesions.

LEG ULCERS SECONDARY TO CHRONIC VENOUS INSUFFICIENCY. Stasis dermatitis and ulceration are the most frequent complications of chronic venous insufficiency. The stasis ulcer is the most common type of leg ulcer. Chronic venous insufficiency accounts for approximately 10% of admissions to large general hospitals; much time has been lost from work and large sums of money have been spent every year for treatment, and many of these persons become totally disabled from their diseases.

Pathology and Pathogenesis. An understanding of the pathogenesis of the stasis ulcer will help in planning more effective treatment for the patient.[2,3] Normal venous anatomy, as well as the pathophysiology of chronic venous insufficiency, are detailed in Chapter 28.

Clinical Features. Stasis ulcerations usually occur in the region of the ankle over the medial malleolus (Fig. 37-5). They rarely occur on the feet, upper leg, or thigh and often develop in areas of indurated cellulitis or dermatitis. There is usually brown pigmentation in the surrounding skin, and the affected leg is often edematous. The ulcers may develop spontaneously or may be secondary to minor trauma such as bumping, scratching, or kicking. The size of the ulcer varies greatly, and if neglected, the ulcer may extend until most of the circumference of the leg is involved. The base of the ulcer is usually moist with extensive granulations, and is often secondarily infected. The ulcers may or may not be painful and are never as painful as ischemic ulcers. The discomfort is often much relieved by rest and elevation, which is in contrast to the marked increase of pain of ischemic ulcerations on elevation. After an ulceration has healed, there is a tendency to recurrence in the same area.

Differential Diagnosis. In any type of ulcer the presence of a history of thrombophlebitis or edema, the presence of varicose or dilated veins, and the presence of stasis pigmentation, induration, and dermatitis will make chronic venous insufficiency the chief suspect in the search for the cause of the ulcer.

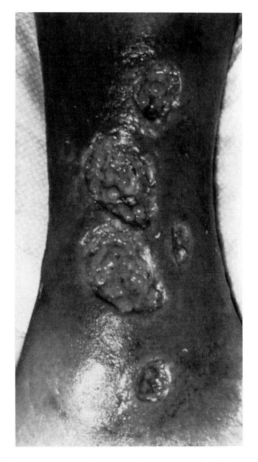

Fig. 37-5. Severe generalized chronic venous stasis with eczematous changes, edema, and ulcerations.

Arteriovenous fistula should be considered in all cases of chronic venous insufficiency. The history of a penetrating injury and the presence of a thrill and bruit may indicate a traumatic arteriovenous fistula. Increased length and circumference of the limb, the presence of hemangiomas and other vascular anomalies, and dilated veins in unusual places may indicate a congenital arteriovenous fistula.

It is important to differentiate between ischemic ulcers caused by ASO or TAO and stasis ulcers. Ischemic ulcers usually develop more distally on the feet and toes; they are more painful, and some relief is obtained by dependency. If ischemic ulcers do develop on the leg, they are usually the result of trauma. Pulses are absent in ischemic ulcers, and there are no signs of chronic venous insufficiency.

Hypertensive ischemic ulcers are usually found on the lateral or posterior aspect of the lower leg, are very painful, and often are surrounded by a purplish, cyanotic rim of ischemic tissue.

In lymphedema there is diffuse thickening and prominence of the skin and subcutaneous tissue that is not a feature of the edema of chronic venous insufficiency. On elevation the edema of lymphedema may not change at all, while chronic venous insufficiency edema usually subsides promptly with rest and elevation of the extremities. The typical stasis changes of dilated veins, pigmentation, dermatitis, and ulceration almost never occur as complications of lymphedema.

Treatment of Acute Dermatitis. If weeping acute dermatitis accompanies the stasis ulcer, the leg is best treated by bed rest and wet compresses. The compresses should be changed every 2 to 3 hours. The wet dressings should not be enclosed in a plastic covering since this will result in maceration of tissues and will prevent the evaporation necessary to promote the healing process. The following solutions are suggested for compresses: (1) aluminum acetate (Burow's solution) 0.5%, (2) isotonic saline solution 0.9%, or (3) acetic acid solution 1%. Between compresses a drying antiinflammatory topical steroid or steroid/antibiotic ointment or cream will help clear the dermatitis.

If any evidence of acute infection such as cellulitis, lymphangitis or purulent drainage is seen, treatment with systemic antibiotics, oral or IV, is necessary. Cultures and sensitivity studies should be done. Fungal cultures should also be done and appropriate antifungals used.

Treatment of Subacute Stasis Dermatitis. When the acute phase of the dermatitis has subsided and the patient becomes more ambulatory, recurrence of edema after prolonged standing must be prevented. If this is not done, acute dermatitis may promptly recur. The use of a modified Unna paste boot dressing is ideal in this situation. Prepackaged zinc paste wraps are available (e.g., Unna Pak, Medicopaste).[4] These flesh-colored roll bandages are impregnated with a uniformly spread paste of zinc oxide, calamine, glycerin, and gelatin. Their use eliminates the need for bed rest or extensive hospital care.

To apply the Unna boot the leg is first cleansed with lukewarm water or mineral oil to remove any debris or previous medication (Figs. 37-6 and 37-7). Any of the following topical medications may then be applied to the leg: (1) gentian violet 1% (Fig. 37-8), (2) fluocinolone

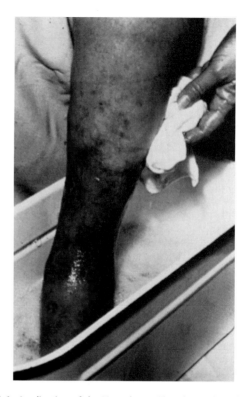

Fig. 37-6. Application of the Unna boot. The ulcer is first cleansed of previous medication.

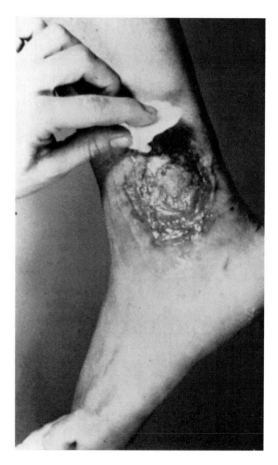

Fig. 37-7. Mineral oil cleansing of the ulcer.

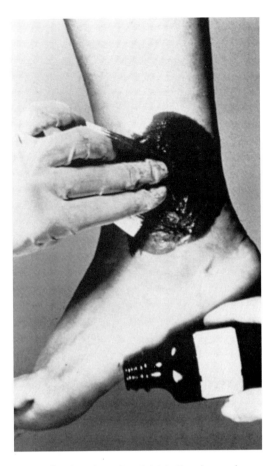

Fig. 37-8. Application of gentian violet to the ulcer and surrounding skin.

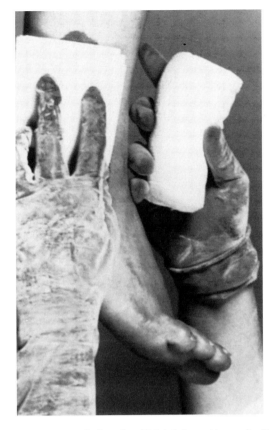

Fig. 37-9. Gauze applied to ulcer. This is followed by applications of Unna paste boot.

acetonide (Synalar) cream or ointment 0.025% (or any other topical corticosteroid preparation) to surrounding skin if there is an acute dermatitis, or (3) topical antibiotics alone, such as ointments containing polymyxin B, bacitracin, and neomycin (Polysporin, Neosporin), erythromycin (Ilotycin), or gentamicin sulfate (Garamycin).

The modified Unna boot is applied from an area just proximal to the toes to just below the popliteal space (Figs. 37-9 to 37-12). The foot should be kept at a right angle to minimize chafing. A circular turn is made with the bandage around the foot, and it is then directed obliquely over the heel as would be done in applying an elastic bandage. This is repeated until the calf has been adequately covered. The first layers of the boot should be snug, and the bandage roll should be cut frequently during its application to ensure a flat surface. It should be applied in a "pressure gradient manner" with the greatest pressure applied at the ankle and lower third of the leg with progressively diminishing pressure over the upper two thirds of the leg. At no time should the bandage be given any reverse turns because the resulting ridges may cause discomfort and skin irritation as the bandage hardens. Care should be taken not to apply the bandage too loosely or too tightly, and each turn should overlap the preceding turn. A double layer of tubegauze is placed over the Unna boot and secured at the upper and lower limits with tape (Figs. 37-13 to 37-15). The tape should not be placed directly on the skin. This dressing is

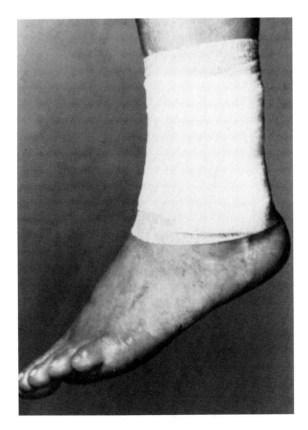

Fig. 37-10. Initial application of Unna paste boot.

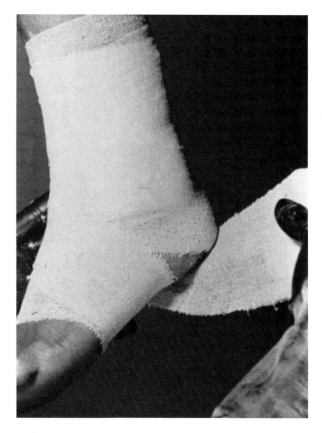

Fig. 37-11. Applications of Unna paste boot with increased pressure over ankle and foot.

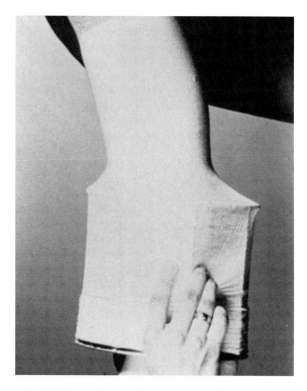

Fig. 37-13. Application of tubegauze over the Unna boot.

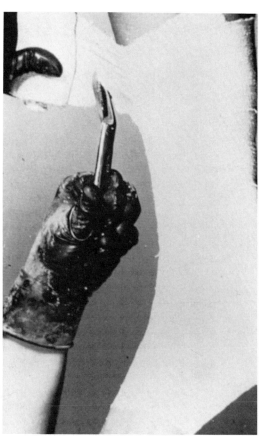

Fig. 37-12. Completion of the Unna paste boot up to the knee.

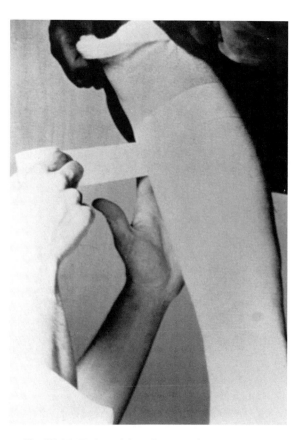

Fig. 37-14. Taping of the tubegauze dressing in place.

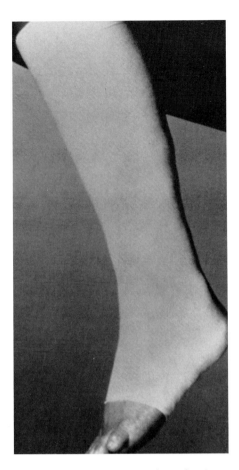

Fig. 37-15. Completed Unna boot dressing.

usually changed at weekly intervals unless excessive drainage necessitates changing every 3 to 5 days.

The use of hydrocolloid gel placed directly on the wound with a secondary zinc paste gauze wrap and then a tertiary compressive layer (Coban) has been referred to as a "Duke boot" (Figs. 37-16 and 37-17).

Even though the Unna boot is effective, there are problems associated with it including a long learning curve for correctly applying the cast, maceration of the skin when drainage is excessive, and inability to observe or bathe the leg while the cast is on.

Another approach to the problem is to apply wet-to-dry saline dressings (or boric acid dressings if the area appears infected) to the affected area (Figs. 37-18 and 37-19). The dressings are changed two to three times in a 24-hour period, depending on the amount of secretions. The dressings are held in place by a light white compression liner (Fig. 37-20). The changes of the dressings may be facilitated if the stocking comes with a zipper (Fig. 37-21). During the day, when the patient is active, the liner is covered by a heavy elastic support stocking (Fig. 37-22). This appears to be a simple, easy-to-learn, and effective option to the Unna boot. The patients like it because the dressing is less bulky and the dressing can be removed nightly to bathe the leg.

Treatment of Stasis Ulcers. The general principles of management of a stasis ulcer are the same as those for subacute stasis dermatitis.[5] The ulcer is cleansed and gently debrided. If there is considerable secondary infection, an occlusive dressing should not be applied. Bed rest and compresses are recommended as mentioned previously until the infection subsides. Pyogenic crusts should be removed, and any drainage should be cultured before antibiotic therapy. Topical antibiotic ointments may be used between the compresses. If cellulitis, lymphangitis, or septicemia are present, systemic antibiotic therapy is indi-

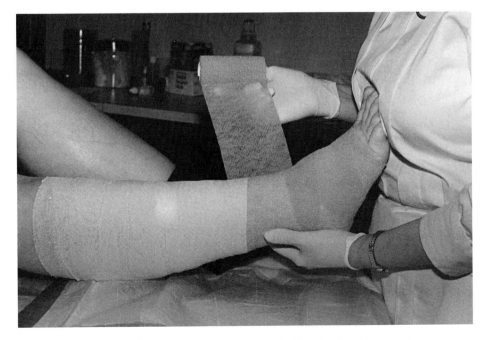

Fig. 37-16. The application of Coban over the Unna boot ("Duke boot").

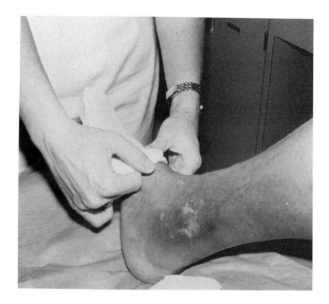

Fig. 37-18. A light white compression liner is being applied to the foot of a patient with a stasis ulcer.

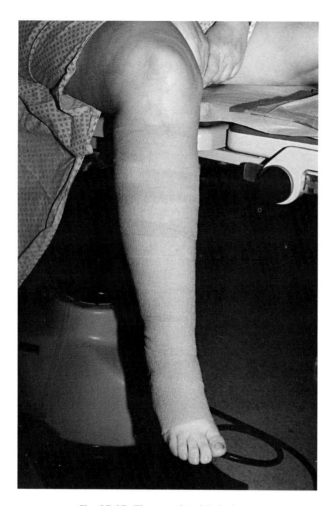

Fig. 37-17. The completed Duke boot.

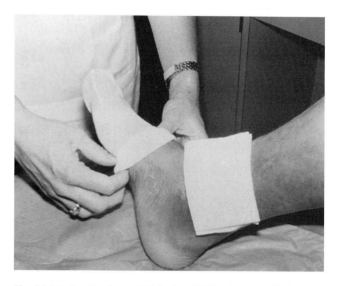

Fig. 37-19. A wet saline or 3% boric acid dressing is applied over the ulcer.

cated. The choice of antibiotics should be dictated by the culture and sensitivity reports. The Unna boot or compression stocking dressings are used in the manner outlined in the section on subacute stasis dermatitis.

Debridement of Ulcers. Topical enzymes,[6] antibiotics, and other agents are often used to debride leg ulcers and develop a healthy granulation tissue. Another excellent method of local debridement is the application of topical viscous lidocaine (Xylocaine) and the use of a small, sharp curet to remove the eschar that adheres to the granulation tissue and inhibits reepithelialization of the ulcer. Occasionally, forceps and small scissors can be used to cut away thicker eschar that cannot be removed by the curet.

Hydrocolloid Wound Dressings. In the past several years, new dressings have been developed that do more than just cover the wound and keep it clean.[7,8] These occlusive or semiocclusive dressings vary in the degree of debridement, cleansing, and wound granulation that speed the healing process.[9-11] It is well accepted that epithelial migration occurs more readily in a moist environment such as that created by occlusive dressings. Some examples are Op-Site, Tegaderm (polyrethan) Bioclusive, Vigilon (polyethylene oxidihydrogel with polyethylene film backing, thicker hydrogel films on both sides, and gel in

the middle), and DuoDerm (hydrocolloid material surrounded by an inert, hydrophobic polymer that is adhesive).[12-15]

Most of these dressings, except DuoDerm and Vigilon, will transport water,[16] and all except DuoDerm will transport oxygen. They all absorb bacteria, except Vigilon, and only DuoDerm is not transparent. All except Vigilon are self-adhesive to the skin. There is excessive accumulation of fluid under some of these dressings, especially Op-Site. There can be exacerbation of infection and cellulitis if these dressings are used on an infected leg ulcer.[17] They are best used when all infection is cleared, and there is good granulation tissue and reepithelialization is sought. Although these new dressings are physiologically better for wound healing, some clinical trials have indicated that ulcer healing is equally effective with the older elastic

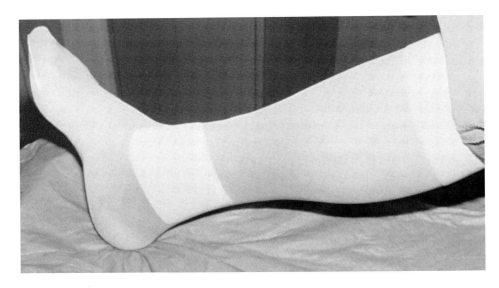

Fig. 37-20. The dressing is held in place by the liner.

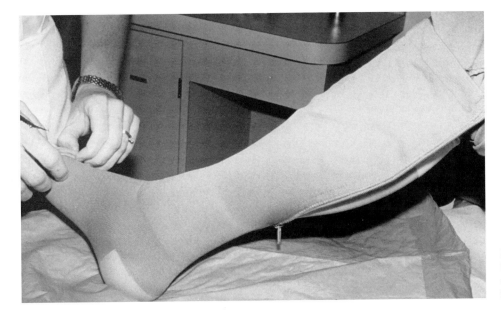

Fig. 37-21. A heavy support stocking is worn over the liner. The change of dressings is facilitated if the stocking has a zipper.

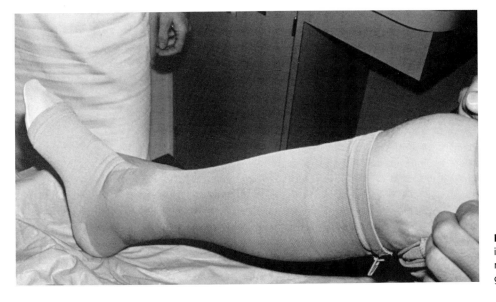

Fig. 37-22. The heavy support stocking is worn during the day and is removed at night when the patient goes to bed.

compressive dressing. These agents can be used under an Unna boot but should be changed every 2 to 3 days. Patients can also be instructed in the use of DuoDerm dressings at home, which can be changed every 2 to 3 days and compressed with an Ace bandage or elastic stockings.

Once the edema is gone and the infection has cleared, new granulation tissue will start to appear with the above techniques. Continued bed rest with elevation is recommended unless an Unna boot or heavy support stocking is used over the dressing, in which case the patient can ambulate normally. Once the granulation tissue fills the ulcer, then reepithelialization will start from the edges of the ulcer and occasionally from islands of granulation tissue in the center of the ulcer. The use of Vigilon dressing will enhance reepithelialization. If rapid reepithelialization is occurring, continued use of wound dressings and Unna boot will result in complete healing of the ulcer with a combination of scar tissue and new epithelium.

Cultured Epidermal Grafts. Human epidermal keratinocytes can now be grown reliably in vitro to form large sheets of epithelium that can be grafted onto cutaneous ulcers or surgical defects. The procedure can be performed using autografts (skin biopsy from patient) or allografts (biopsy from donor). Cultured keratinocyte grafts can be cultivated by digesting whole skin with trypsin and grown on irradiated 3T3 mouse fibroblasts, which support rapid keratinocyte proliferation. Within several weeks a 1 cm^2 skin sample can be expanded to generate a cultured epithelium to cover leg ulcers.[18]

Autografts. Autografts were first used successfully in 1981 on two men with third-degree burns using cultured keratinocyte autograft.[19] Subsequently, cultured keratinocyte autografts have gained moderate acceptance with varying success rates. The graft "take" rate varies from 30% to 80% and depends on such variables as host factors, postoperative care, and depth of cutaneous defect. The patient must remain immobilized for several days postoperatively to facilitate graft "take." Grafts that survive beyond 6 months have long-term durability and texture that is equivalent to split-thickness skin grafts.[20] There is evidence that the epidermis differentiates into basal, spinous, granular, and cornified layers. Rete ridges may not form for many years after grafting. Within 3 weeks of transplant, grafts develop basal lamina, hemidesmosomes, and anchoring fibrils. The major disadvantages of autologous keratinocyte grafts are the time required for the production (approximately 3 weeks), intensive postoperative care, and expense.

Allografts. Allografts are prepared by a technique of cultured epithelium derived from an unrelated donor, a cultured allograft. Leigh et al,[21] using skin obtained during mammoplasty as a source of donor keratinocytes, grafted chronic ulcers. Twenty-nine percent of the ulcers healed completely with improvement in an additional forty-four percent.

This procedure is limited by the fact that keratinocytes of older donors grow more slowly and are more senescent.[22] With this knowledge, Phillips et al[23] treated 36 chronic ulcers with cultured epidermal sheets derived from neonatal foreskin. In 73% of ulcers there was complete healing within 8 weeks. In the remaining ulcers there was marked reduction in size within 8 weeks. Pain was relieved within 24 hours after grafting.

Although initially believed to survive permanently, cultured keratinocyte allografts are now believed not to "take"[24] because they are rapidly rejected by the host. Using monoclonal antibodies against major histocompatibility complex (MHC) specificities that differ between host and donor keratinocytes, replacement of grafted keratinocytes by host cells is observed within 2 weeks following cultured allografting.[25] Nevertheless, allografts improve healing of cutaneous wounds, perhaps by the production of growth factors. Keratinocytes in culture are known to elaborate soluble mediators that enhance cell proliferation and differentiation.[26] The cytokines potentially relevant to wound healing after autologous grafting include interleukins 1 and 3,[27,28] fibronectin,[29] and transforming growth factor alpha.[30]

Allografting is more convenient than autografts because it obviates the need for biopsy and cultivation 3 weeks before the grafting procedure. Additionally these grafts could be harvested and stored for future use.

Surgical Management. The final goal in the treatment of all leg ulcers is to provide adequate skin coverage to the ulcer. With ulcers that have poor granulation tissue, with necrotic or fibrotic tissue at the border that shows no sign of epithelial ingrowth after conservative measures, more aggressive surgical approaches to growing skin over the ulcers must be considered.

When healthy granulation tissue has become established in the ulcer base and the surrounding inflammation has subsided, the patient is ready for pinch grafting if this is the planned surgical procedure. The donor area (usually on the anterior thigh) is prepared by shaving, if necessary, and washing with Betadine soap. Sterile technique is maintained when working in the donor area, but strict sterile technique is not necessary in the recipient site.

Circular areas of 5 to 10 mm are marked in parallel rows on the upper thigh with gentian violet. These areas are elevated by intradermal injections of 1% lidocaine beneath each circle. This serves two purposes: anesthesia and elevation of the skin for easy removal of small epidermal or dermal grafts. Anesthesia can also be produced by using a field block. In such a case, elevations should be produced by injection of sterile saline under each circle. A curved needle or tip of a 30-gauge needle is placed at the center of a circle and is used to further tent up the skin. A single-edged razor blade or No. 15 scalpel blade is used to cut a split-thickness graft. The depth of the pinch graft should be 1 to 2 mm or to middermis. Subcutaneous fat taken with the graft interfaces with the "take" and may produce undue scarring in the donor area. It is wise to take grafts first from the most dependent area of the donor site so that blood does not obscure the operative field.

As grafts are removed, they are placed in a Petri dish containing gauze moistened with saline. When an assistant is available, these can be transferred to him or her for placement on the ulcer. When performing the procedure without an assistant, the practitioner cuts all grafts first and then moves them to the recipient area to avoid contaminating the donor area by to and from movement with each graft. The recipient site is cleaned, and a curette is used to stimulate mild bleeding.

With a 25-gauge needle or forceps, the grafts are placed on the ulcer bed next to, but not touching, each other until the defect is covered. The placement of the pinch grafts can be facilitated by their marking with gentian violet on the epidermal side. After placement of the grafts, the practitioner must allow 1 to 2 mm at the margins of the ulcer because epithelium growing in from the edges of the ulcer may prevent the border grafts from taking.

Bioclusive dressings are ideal for pinch grafts since they adhere to the surrounding skin and are clear, so that the area can be observed for infection and graft viability.

The donor area should first be sponged free of blood, and covered with a semipermeable dressing and a bandage. Alternatively, each removed site in the donor area can be sutured with a 4-0 nylon stitch.

The patient should be kept strictly at bed rest for 72 hours with limited ambulation in a wheelchair with the leg elevated.

The ulcer is examined through the bioclusive dressing daily thereafter. If fluid collects beneath the membrane it may be punctured and the fluid drained. If infection develops, the membrane should be removed. However, with an adequate pressure dressing, any fluid that forms tends to drain from under the edges of the membrane. The membrane is removed from the ulcer 7 to 10 days after grafting. Should any of the grafts become dislodged, they are repositioned and the wound is redressed. Once the biocclusive dressing is removed, the wound is dressed by applying a 4 × 4 inch gauze pad and elastic bandage. This dressing is changed three times a day. Periods of ambulation may be started a week after grafting; however, elevation of the leg should be continued until healing is complete—usually a matter of 2 to 4 weeks.

If the donor sites are sutured, then the sutures should be removed 10 to 14 days after grafting. This area usually heals with minimal scarring.

Ceilley, Rink, and Zueklhe[31] treated 75 patients with a total of 130 ulcers of various causes by pinch grafting and found that most patients had better than 75% of graft "takes" by the fifth postoperative day. The most impressive results were seen in the stasis and posttraumatic groups. The least impressive results were seen in the group with ischemia; however, even in this group 50% of the ulcers were successfully grafted. Of the 75 patients, 15 had recurrences of ulceration in the grafted area in less than 12 months. Most of these recurrences were in the group with ischemia, and they usually took place within 1 month of grafting. They found no significant correlation of recurrence with age, duration of ulceration, or size of the ulcer. Gilmore and Wheeland[32] and Wheeland[33] found similar results with pinch grafts.

When there is adequate granulation tissue in the ulcer bed, an alternative to pinch grafting is the split-thickness skin graft (Fig. 37-23). The technique is similar to grafts placed in other areas of the body. The anterior thigh is usually chosen as the donor site.

The response to porcine xenografts has proved to be a reliable guide to successful autografting.[34] Other types of

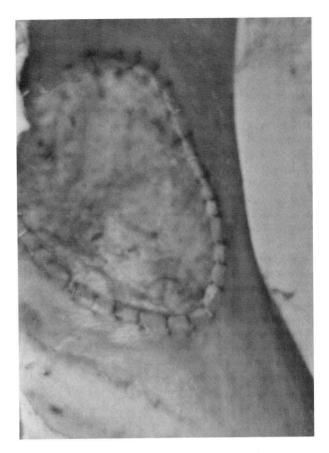

Fig. 37-23. Split-thickness skin graft to leg ulcer.

dressings have also been useful in preparing the graft bed including DuoDerm.[35] Lyophilized porcine skin, commercially available in sterile packages, is reconstituted in normal saline and applied to the wound. Adherence or loss of the xenograft is obvious within 24 hours. If the graft adheres, it is allowed to remain for 1 to 3 days. Autografting is undertaken within 72 hours of successful adherence. If the xenograft does not adhere, it is removed, and topical measures to improve the bed of the ulcer are reinstituted. A trial of the xenograft can be done again 2 to 3 days later.

For ulcers with exposed bone or tendon, fully vascularized full-thickness skin and subcutaneous tissue must be applied. Split-thickness skin grafts do not become revascularized when placed upon exposed bone denuded of its periosteum, or on tendon denuded of paratendon. This situation is not too common with leg ulcers, but when it does occur, it is usually over an exposed tibia. Full-thickness vascularized tissue may be provided by local flaps (Fig. 37-24), cross-leg pedicle flaps, or by the application of distant tissue in the form of a free flap transfer revascularized by microvascular technique. Such procedures require a skilled surgeon experienced in flap surgery.

Treatment of Generalized Eczematization. In patients with severe stasis dermatitis and ulceration, a generalized eczematous eruption may develop as a sensitization or id reaction. This can often be controlled by topical corticosteroids and antihistamines such as cyproheptadine (Periactin), 4 mg four times daily, or other

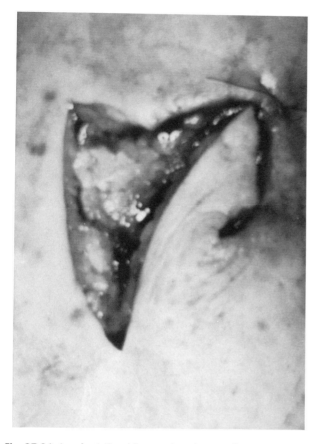

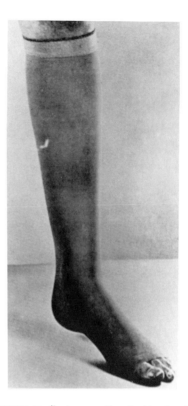

Fig. 37-25. Pressure gradient supportive stocking for chronic venous stasis problems.

Fig. 37-24. Local rotational flap used to close an ulcer and anterior tibial surface.

antihistamines. It may be necessary in severe cases to give systemic corticosteroids orally or intramuscularly.

Treatment of Neurodermatitis. Because of lichenification of "habit scratching," an associated neurodermatitis of the legs may develop. If this occurs, the application of fluocinolone acetonide (Synalar) or other potent topical corticosteroids under plastic food wrap at bedtime may be helpful. Intralesional injection of triamcinolone acetonide (Kenalog Parenteral) suspension (10 mg/ml) into localized neurodermatitis may bring more prompt relief of the pruritus.

Treatment of Chronic Venous Insufficiency. After the acute and subacute stages of dermatitis have subsided and the cellulitis and ulcerations have healed, the treatment of chronic venous insufficiency is not finished. The patient must be impressed with the fact that he or she has a lifelong problem and that continuous supportive measures will be necessary to prevent future complications.

Elastic bandages and proprietary elastic stockings are usually not satisfactory for most of these patients. Individually measured, "pressure-gradient" supportive stockings, such as the Jobst stocking,* are preferred (Fig. 37-25). Directions for Jobst stocking measurements are furnished by the company (Fig. 37-26). Measurement should be made only after all edema has subsided or after the

*Jobst Institute, Box 653, Toledo, Ohio 43601.

patient's legs have been mechanically pumped to make them edema free. There are other types of good supportive stockings such as Camp, Sigvaris 902 series, Medi-Strumpf, Bauer and Block, and Juzo stockings.

The patient should put on the supportive stockings before arising and remove them just before retiring. It is usually necessary to purchase new stockings every 3 to 4 months because the stockings will stretch out.

LYMPHATIC LEG ULCERS. Lymphedema of an extremity is a swelling of the soft tissues caused by an accumulation of tissue fluid. This condition is described in detail in Chapter 29. True, uncomplicated lymphedema, regardless of its cause, is not usually associated with ulcerations. When ulcers do occur, they are usually the result of trauma (Fig. 37-27). In rare patients lymphangiosarcoma may develop in a lymphedematous limb, and this tumor may ulcerate. For this reason any unusual appearing ulcer in a patient with lymphedema should be biopsied. The treatment of ulcerations in lymphedema is similar to that described for stasis ulcers. These ulcers are usually resistant to treatment, and often must be treated by skin grafts. The treatment of lymphedema is outlined in Chapter 29.

LEG ULCERS SECONDARY TO VASCULITIS

Vasculitis is an ill-defined term and if used alone includes all inflammatory reactions around and within all blood vessels. Vasculitis as used here, or angiitis, refers to the hypersensitivity vasculitis group with the primary inflammatory processes involving small- and medium-size

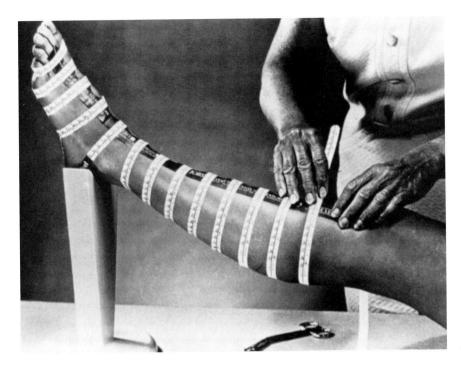

Fig. 37-26. Measurement for the Jobst stocking.

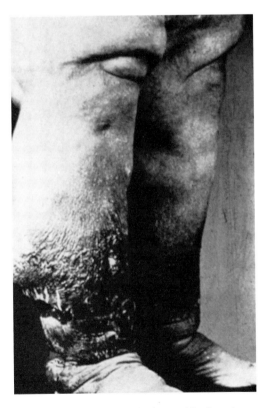

Fig. 37-27. Chronic lymphedema with ulceration.

blood vessels. This results in necrosis, fibrinoid degeneration, hyalinization, and a granulomatous reaction. Those vascular inflammations secondary to embolus or inflammation in neighboring tissues are not included. Vasculitis of the skin is usually the cutaneous sign of a complex benign or malignant pathologic process, which may herald

a systemic disorder. The vasculitis lesion that ulcerates may thus be the initial sign of a severe systemic disease.

Many different terms have been applied to the entity of vasculitis, including polyarteritis nodosa, hypersensitivity angiitis, Wegener's granulomatosis, allergic granulomatosis, and necrotizing vasculitis. The term vasculitis is often used to refer to a hypersensitivity or allergic reaction to drugs. The reaction is primarily in the small blood vessels of the skin. Leg ulcers resulting from a vasculitis may be associated with other generalized disorders such as systemic lupus erythematosus or rheumatoid arthritis.

The different types of vasculitis are based primarily on histopathologic criteria. The size of the blood vessel involved (small or large), the types of inflammatory cells (polymorphonuclear leukocytes, lymphocytes, or granulomatous lesions), and the evidence of or lack of necrosis of blood vessel walls determine the category of the lesion. Thus the skin biopsy becomes essential in the diagnosis of vasculitis. Biopsies are best taken from fresh, early (less than 24 hours old) papular purpuric lesions. It is often necessary to biopsy two or three different lesions to get the proper diagnosis. It is also important that the biopsy be deep and that the specimen have good subcutaneous fat and even muscle. Excision biopsy rather than punch biopsy is preferred. For a classification of vasculitis see Chapter 22.

Cutaneous Features of Vasculitis

Cutaneous lesions of vasculitis vary from erythematous macules to purpura, to hemorrhagic vesicles, and to urticarial, nodular, and eventually necrotic lesions and ulceration. The lower extremities are most often involved, but any portion of the skin may develop lesions, which may or may not be painful (Figs. 37-28 to 37-30).

Although the specific types of vasculitis have certain distinguishing clinical and histologic features, some types

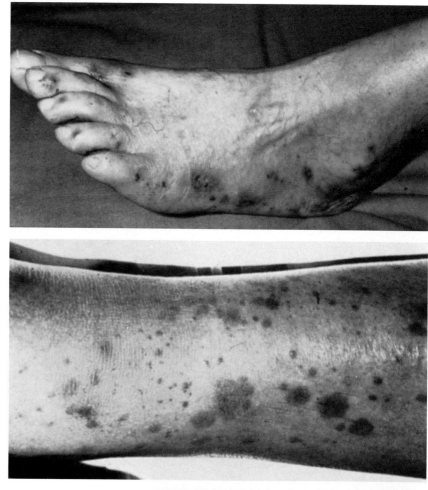

Fig. 37-28. Vasculitis with purpura and small ulcerations on the feet.

Fig. 37-29. Cutaneous vasculitis with palpable purpura on lower legs.

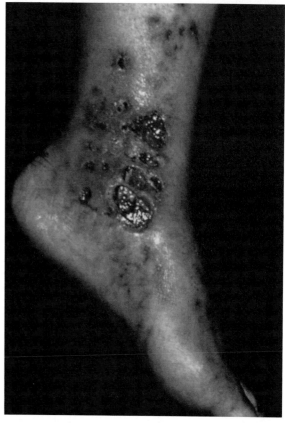

Fig. 37-30. Vasculitis with larger ulcerations, which simulate chronic venous stasis ulcers.

of cutaneous vasculitis are identified by the presence of many palpable purpuric lesions. The number of these depends on the stage of destruction and the size of blood vessels involved.

When the arterioles of the superficial dermis are affected, as in hypersensitivity angiitis, the skin manifestations begin as small urticarial or erythematous maculopapular lesions, which usually become petechial but in which brown pigmentation may develop as they evolve. The petechiae are almost always palpable. The raised lesions are indicative of more exudative and inflammatory response than is produced by simple vascular or thrombocytopenic purpura. The petechiae of bacterial endocarditis are also palpable but usually show a halo of erythema. The hemorrhagic lesions vary from pinpoint size to several centimeters in diameter and may result in blood-filled bullae or extensive areas of superficial hemorrhage or gangrene. The overlying damaged epidermis will usually break down and ulcerate at this point.

The site where most of these lesions occur is the lower extremities, concentrated around the ankles and dorsa of the feet (Figs. 37-28 to 37-30). Other areas of the body are more rarely affected.

Systemic Features of Vasculitis

Systemic manifestations are common in vasculitis. Fever is a common but nonspecific symptom in up to 75% of patients. Musculoskeletal pain and symptoms of peripheral neuropathy occur early in the majority of patients. Renal disease occurs in most patients and is a common cause of death. The pathologic manifestations may be varied in the kidney, but a needle biopsy, including direct immunofluorescence studies, is often helpful in establishing a diagnosis of systemic vasculitis. Gastrointestinal symptoms also vary depending on the size of the vessel affected. Abdominal pain, steatorrhea, or acute cholecystitis may lead to abnormal liver function tests or a picture of hepatitis. Pancreatitis and diabetes may appear as a manifestation of pancreatic vasculitis. Myocardial infarction is one of the more common causes of death from systemic vasculitis, but individual episodes are often clinically silent. Asymptomatic pericarditis may be present. Hypertension may be severe and probably caused by renal cortical ischemia. Pulmonary infiltrations are more often found in the granulomatous forms of vasculitis and may be associated with a blood eosinophilia. Almost any manifestation of brain involvement may be found when central nervous vasculitis is present. The multifocal nature of the neurologic signs is a clue to their cause, cranial nerve and cortical hemisphere involvement predominating.

Patients with lupus anticoagulant and antiphospholipid antibodies are at greater risk of ulceration; ulcers are usually of a thrombotic occlussive nature and not due to vasculitis.

Cutaneous polyarteritis nodosa and systemic polyarteritis nodosa can both cause leg ulceration. In the cutaneous group, findings are limited to the skin and lesions tend to have a chronic, recurrent course. Both diseases present with punched-out painful ulcerations of the legs associated with tender, erythematous deep dermal and subcutaneous nodules. Often there is a "starburst" or linear irregular "lightning bolt" livedoid pattern radiating from the ulcerated areas. Biopsy of a nodule will often reveal necrotizing vasculitis of a small- to medium-sized artery at the dermal-pannicular junction.

The granulomatous vasculitis seen on leg ulcer biopsies can be due to chronic infection (fungal, acid-fast), Wegener's granulomatosis, or Churg-Strauss vasculitis. In Wegener's granulomatosis, a necrotizing granulomatous vasculitis is noted in the upper respiratory tract and lungs. Glomerulonephritis is seen in the kidney and antineutrophil cytoplasmic antibodies are detected in the plasma. In Churg-Strauss granulomatosis, patients have a history of asthma, peripheral blood and tissue eosinophilia, necrotizing granulomatous vasculitis of the lung and other organs, and extravascular granulomas in the lung and skin.

Scleroderma Leg Ulcers

Scleroderma (progressive systemic sclerosis) is a chronic disease that often begins in the skin or small blood vessels. It progresses to form diffuse, hard, ivory-colored areas, in addition to a hidebound appearance of the hands and face. Internal organs (esophagus, heart, kidneys) may also become involved, and death may ensue.

Skin biopsy is often diagnostic of scleroderma with edema, homogenization, fibrosis, and sclerosis of the collagen. The glandular structures (sweat glands) in the dermis become atrophic and are bound down by the sclerosis of the collagen.

Digital ischemia is a prominent feature of scleroderma, especially of the fingertips, but painful ulcerations may also occur on the lower extremity over the medial and lateral malleolus.

Leg Ulceration in Rheumatoid Arthritis

Necrotizing vasculitis may occur in rheumatoid arthritis as it does in other autoimmune diseases; ischemic ulcerations may occur, primarily on the lower legs. Rheumatoid ulcers tend to be associated with subcutaneous rheumatoid nodules, which also may undergo necrosis and ulcerate (Fig. 37-31). Avoidance of high-dose corticosteroids or rapid withdrawal of corticosteroid is important

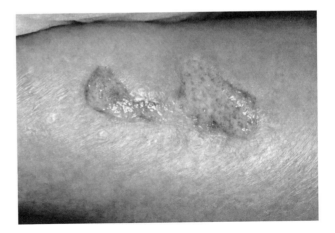

Fig. 37-31. Rheumatoid arthritis with severe ulceration of the lower leg.

in these patients. Surgical excision of the rheumatoid nodule that has ulcerated is indicated. Control of the rheumatoid arthritis with corticosteroids and immuno-suppressants, such as methotrexate,[36] may help the ulceration heal. Skin grafting is often needed, but failure of a skin graft to take is not uncommon.

For a more detailed account of the clinical features, diagnosis, and treatment of the various vasculitides, see Chapter 22.

HEMATOLOGIC LEG ULCERS

Leg Ulcers Secondary to Sickle Cell Anemia

Chronic leg ulcers are very common in sickle cell anemia (homozygous hemoglobin S disease) (Fig. 37-32). The incidence ranges between 25% and 75% and is more common in older patients. The ulcers usually have sharply defined edges and are single, but they may be multiple and bilateral. They most often occur in the lower leg around the malleoli. The ulcers are usually sharply marginated, round or oval, and may be shallow or deep. The borders may be elevated or irregular. The base usually shows granulation tissue and is occasionally covered with dried serous or seropurulent crust.

The mechanism leading to the development of sickle cell ulceration is the lowered oxygen tension and/or the low pH that is present in areas of stasis. This causes

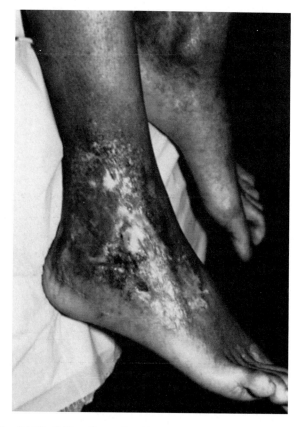

Fig. 37-32. Sickle cell anemia with scarring and ulceration around the ankle.

erythrocytes containing hemoglobin S to form intracellular hemoglobin tactoids that change the shape of the red cells to the sickle form. These sickled cells are more rigid, or less deformable, than normal cells. Increased viscosity results, and microthrombosis may occur. This in turn aggravates the stasis, setting up a vicious circle, which may result in ulceration.

The diagnosis of sickle cell anemia is readily confirmed by complete blood count, including a reticulocyte count and hemoglobin electrophoresis. There is no normal adult hemoglobin; there is an 80% to 90% hemoglobin S with the remainder fetal hemoglobin.

These ulcers are very resistant to healing. Unless the patient receives multiple transfusions of normal blood, maintaining the hemoglobin at about 10 g or above, the ulcers will not heal. Skin grafting has been successful if the hemoglobin is maintained at a near-normal level, but unfortunately the graft often breaks down when the transfusions are discontinued.

Similar types of leg ulcers are uncommon but may occur in the older age group of patients who have a combination of abnormal hemoglobins, such as hemoglobin SC disease or hemoglobin S-thalassemia disease. As a general rule, these leg ulcers do not occur in patients who maintain a hemoglobin above 9 g.

Leg Ulcers Secondary to Hereditary Spherocytosis

In hereditary spherocytosis it is the red cell membrane and not the hemoglobin molecule that is abnormal. The exact nature of this membrane defect is obscure, but the increased tendency to sphere and the increased viscosity seen with normal red cells at a low pH are exaggerated in hereditary spherocytosis. Furthermore, the defective cells are spheroidal even at a normal pH. Trapping occurs in the spleen because of lower pH that occurs in that organ, and a similar effect can be presumed for areas of stasis such as the lower legs.

In most patients with a severe form of hereditary spherocytosis, leg ulcers are uncommon because many of the patients have had a splenectomy before reaching middle age. Leg ulcers are common in patients who have a moderately severe degree of hereditary spherocytosis that has persisted for many years.

Leg Ulcers Secondary to Thalassemia

Thalassemia, sometimes referred to as *Mediterranean anemia,* occurs in both homozygous and heterozygous forms and with varying degrees of severity. In thalassemia major (Cooley's anemia) leg ulcers have been reported but are uncommon. In the very mildest forms of thalassemia minor, that is, in those patients who are totally asymptomatic and have no hemolytic process, leg ulcers do not occur. In the intermediate forms of thalassemia minor, however, leg ulcers may occur in a small percentage of patients (less than 5%). In these patients the hemoglobin is usually 9 g or less. The mechanism of leg ulcers is probably inadequate tissue oxygenation caused by the lower than normal concentration of hemoglobin A that characterizes this disorder.

Leg Ulcers Secondary to Polycythemia Vera, Leukemia, and Dysproteinemia

Other hematologic disorders such as polycythemia vera, chronic leukemia, and dysproteinemia (cryoglobulinemia and cryofibrinogenemia) occasionally produce thrombotic or vasculitic ulcers.

In patients with polycythemia vera there is an increase in the viscosity of the blood and usually an increase in the number of platelets. Venous stasis and venous thromboses are not uncommon in these patients, and stasis ulcers may occur. Deep venous thromboses of the lower extremities may render treatment of the stasis ulcer more difficult.

Leg ulcers are uncommon in patients with either acute or chronic leukemia, and when present, are usually caused by trauma with secondary infection. The leukemic cells do not combat infection as well as normal white blood cells.

Various types of dysproteinemia may be associated with leg ulcers. Patients with cryoglobulinemia of moderate or marked severity may have stasis pigmentation, superficial skin ulceration, and necrosis. Gangrene of the digits may also be present. Serum viscosity is markedly increased and aggravated by coldness of the extremities. The most effective immediate therapy is plasmapheresis, which will reduce the viscosity. The extremities can be provided with a warm environment by using an electric blanket and a heat cradle.

Leg ulcers are uncommon in patients with Waldenström's macroglobulinemia even though the serum viscosity is high. In those patients with cryomacroglobulinemia, leg ulcers are more frequent. Patients with the usual type of multiple myeloma, such as IgG and IgA, rarely have leg ulceration. Even those with myeloma kidney and/or amyloidosis have no problems with leg ulcers.

LEG ULCERS SECONDARY TO INFECTIONS

Whatever their original cause, leg ulcers usually become infected secondarily because of exposure to pathogenic bacteria on the surface of the skin. It must be remembered, however, that infection may be the primary etiologic factor as well as a secondary invader.

Leg Ulcers Secondary to Fungal Infections

Pathogenic fungus infections are categorized as superficial or deep. The superficial infections usually invade only the stratum corneum and epidermis and produce macerations or pustules in the groin or feet. Ulcerations are not a feature of these superficial infections except in Majocchi granuloma (dermatophyte). The deep fungal infections may produce granulomatous ulcerative lesions on the skin, but they are also responsible for more serious internal infections involving the lungs, brain, and other vital organs. Deep fungal infections should be suspected in HIV patients with skin ulcerations.

There are two distinct types of deep fungal infections of the skin. The rarer form, the chancriform syndrome, is an example of primary cutaneous inoculation. It usually follows trauma to the skin with an introduction of pathogenic organisms into the tissues. At the site of inoculation an area of erythema and induration develops. In 1 to 2 weeks a chancre appears followed by lymphangitis and lymphedema of the involved limb. The more common form of the deep fungal infections is associated with systemic involvement. The appearance of the lesion is usually a papular pustular nodule that enlarges peripherally to form an elevated ulcerated verrucous granuloma. The greatest activity of the infection occurs at the periphery, which is clearly demarcated from normal skin. The deep fungi, which may produce a lower extremity ulceration, include blastomycosis (Fig. 37-33), coccidioidomycosis, histoplasmosis, and sporotrichosis. These can be differentiated by direct examination (smear), fungal culture characteristics, identification of the organism on biopsy of the lesion with periodic acid-Schiff (PAS) stain, and cultures of tissue on agar. Treatment is with systemic antifungal therapy such as amphotericin B or ketoconazole (Nizoral).

Leg Ulcers Secondary to Syphilis

Even today syphilis in all its stages must be considered the "great masquerader," as it was 50 years ago. Although primary and secondary lesions of syphilis do not often appear as leg ulcers, the tertiary stage has several clinical forms that may present as leg ulcers. With the advent of AIDS, syphilis is increasing again.

Syphilitic gumma (Fig. 37-34), a late form of syphilis,

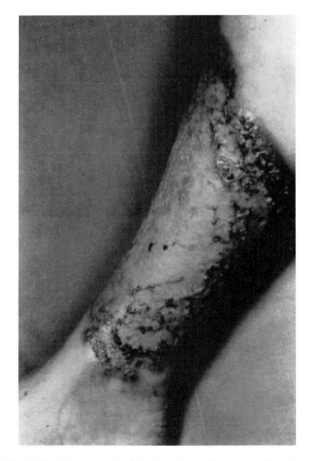

Fig. 37-33. Blastomycosis of the lower leg with an expanding ulceration with a verrucous border.

develops as a deep subcutaneous fixed nodule or plaque that may be singular or multiple. The lesions often ulcerate and extrude a thick sanguinous secretion. The ulcers are clearly demarcated, deep, and have a purulent base. They heal from the base and leave a contracted scar.

The causative organism, *Treponema pallidum,* is not identified on direct examination of the tissue. Serologic tests for syphilis usually show high titers. The fluorescent treponemal antibody (FTA) absorption test is positive. A tissue biopsy of the nodule or ulcer shows a granulomatous process that extends from the dermis into the subcutaneous tissue. Epithelial cells and giant cells are numerous and there is a plasma cell infiltrate. Massive caseation necrosis appears, typically in the center of the granulomatous lesion. The U.S. Public Health Service recommends treatment of this disorder with 6.0 to 9.0 million units of benzathine penicillin.

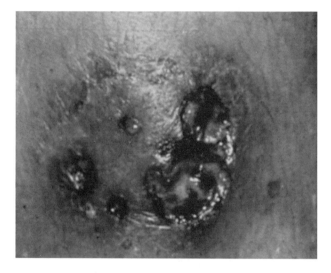

Fig. 37-34. Syphilitic gumma of the leg with ulceration.

Leg Ulcers Secondary to Bacterial Infections

Bacterial infections of the lower extremities are not often the primary cause of leg ulcers (Fig. 37-35) but often are secondary contaminants. The recognition of these organisms is important, because eradication is at times necessary before other medical or surgical management of the leg ulcer can be accomplished.

Ulcers of the leg often become secondarily infected and produce an increased inflammation of the ulcer and surrounding tissue. The clinical signs are erythema, edema, and either a purulent exudate or a heavy eschar with pronounced peripheral inflammation. The bacterial flora of the vascular ulcers can be polymicrobial. The most common significant bacteria are *Staphylococcus aureus* and *Escherichia coli.* Appropriate cultures and antibiotic sensitivity testing are indicated.

Treatment of secondary bacterial infection usually consists of local measures. Wet compresses with one of the following agents are helpful: (1) Burow's solution, (2) potassium permanganate solution 1:10,000 in saline, (3) 3% silver nitrate, (4) 1% acetic acid solution, and (5) 3% boric acid solution.

Local debridement of the ulcer with curette is helpful in removing the thick eschar and infection. This is often very painful and may have to be done with the patient under general anesthesia. Prior application of viscous Xylocaine may make the procedure more tolerable to the patient.

Systemic antibiotics (IV) are indicated after appropriate cultures have been taken if cellulitis or evidence of systemic infection is present.

Leg Ulcers Secondary to Tuberculosis

Primary lesions of tuberculosis are quite rare today but can be a cause of leg ulcers. Secondary forms of tuberculosis, or so-called tuberculids, can also cause leg ulcers.

PRIMARY TUBERCULOSIS. Lupus vulgaris of the lower extremity is rare. It appears as a well-demarcated

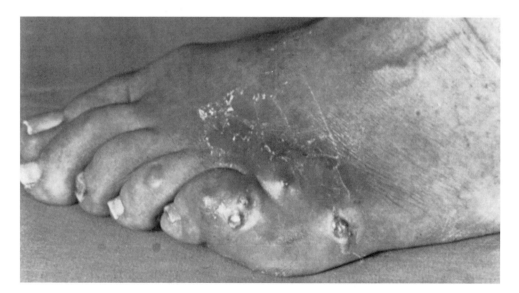

Fig. 37-35. Bacterial infection of the foot with cellulitis and ulceration caused by intraarticular injection of cortisone.

reddish-brown patch or patches containing small papules (Fig. 37-36). The papules show positive dioscopy (a yellow-brown color when a glass slide is pressed against them). These yellow lesions gradually become atrophic and show multiple areas of ulceration. Occasionally the borders develop a verrucal growth. A biopsy shows a typical tubercle with moderate caseation in the upper dermis. Acid-fast stains reveal the presence of small numbers of tubercle bacilli. Squamous cell carcinomas may occur in these chronic lesions.

The initial signs of tuberculosis verrucosa cutis usually are a single verrucous plaque with an inflammatory border and superficial pustules. The histologic pattern shows inflammatory reaction with caseation necrosis. Acid-fast stains reveal more tuberculosis bacilli than are seen in lesions of lupus vulgaris. The treatment of these two disorders is generally with the systemic antituberculosis drugs.

SECONDARY FORMS OF TUBERCULOSIS (TU-BERCULIDS). In the past tuberculids were thought to represent hematogenous dissemination of tubercle bacilli from a visceral focus into the skin. Over the years four disorders have been classified as tuberculids: erythema induratum (Fig. 37-37), papulonecrotic tuberculid (Fig. 37-38), lichen scrofulosorum, and lupus miliaris disseminatus faciei. These disorders are now thought to represent different diseases and are not necessarily secondary to tuberculosis, although they have histologic features similar to tuberculosis and some do respond to antituberculous drug therapies.

NEUROTROPHIC ULCERS

In a setting of sensory neuropathy, neurotrophic ulcers arise from frequent trauma or persistent pressure, leading

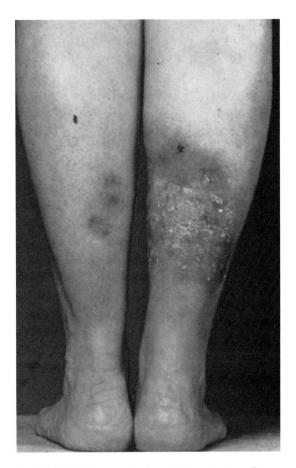

Fig. 37-37. Erythema induratum of the posterior calf area.

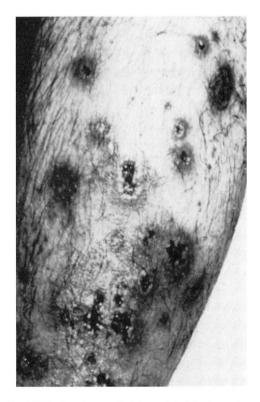

Fig. 37-38. Papulonecrotic tuberculid of the lower legs.

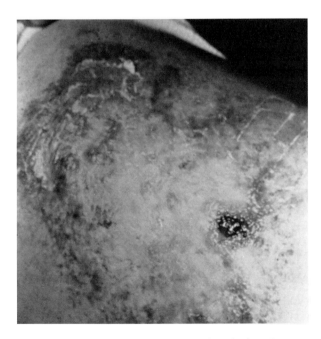

Fig. 37-36. Lupus vulgaris of the thigh with ulceration.

to tissue ischemia, necrosis, and ulceration. Concurrent autonomic neuropathy may lead to the absence of vasodilator reflexes, and this, in turn, contributes to ischemia. Diabetes mellitus is a common cause of neurotrophic ulcers, but leprosy, tabes dorsalis (syphilis), and traumatic neuropathy are also possible causes.

Neurotrophic ulcers are usually located over points of pressure, especially on the plantar foot surfaces under the metatarsal heads or heel. Footwear may contribute to the trauma of the ulcer. The ulcers are usually painless, with a necrotic or purulent base and are surrounded by a rim of thick callus. Deep ulcers with extension to tendon or bone are common. There are often signs of infection with surrounding erythema, cellulitis, or purulent drainage. The ulcers can proceed to osteomyelitis, gangrene, and amputation.

Treatment of neurotrophic ulcers is difficult and healing is slow. For a detailed description of diabetic neurotrophic ulcers and their treatment, see Chapter 40.

LEG ULCERS SECONDARY TO METABOLIC DISEASES

Leg Ulcers Secondary to Pretibial Myxedema

Pretibial myxedema typically occurs in about 3% of patients with toxic diffuse goiters. The characteristic lesions are firm, nonpitting, and irregular swellings, nodules, or plaques that are flesh colored and waxy and have a "pigskin" appearance. They may appear during the hyperthyroid stage, but often first appear following iodine-131 or surgical treatment of thyrotoxicosis.

The soft tissue lesions of pretibial myxedema ulcerate infrequently. Treatment with Cordran tape or intralesional triamcinolone suspension often produces resolution of the lesions.

Leg Ulcers Secondary to Lichen Amyloidosis

Amyloid may be deposited in the skin in patients with more serious underlying conditions. Lichen amyloidosis, however, is a benign localized deposition of amyloid, usually in the lower extremity, which rarely ulcerates. The eruption consists of discrete, firm papules that vary in color from red to reddish brown, and which may coalesce to form plaques.

Differential diagnosis includes lichen planus and lichen simplex chronicus. Skin biopsy confirms the diagnosis by using special stains (crystal violet, methyl violet, Thioflavin-T) that demonstrate the fibrous glycoprotein of amyloid in the upper dermis. Treatment of the lesions can be with intralesional steroids or dermabrasion destruction of the papules. The lesions are difficult to treat.

Leg Ulcers Secondary to Pyoderma Gangrenosum

Acute necrotizing ulcerations of the lower extremity with a rolled vegetating border are suggestive of pyoderma gangrenosum (Fig. 37-39), and investigation for possible gastrointestinal disease often discloses chronic ulcerative colitis.

The skin lesions usually begin as erythematous papulonodules that enlarge rapidly into plaques up to 12 cm or

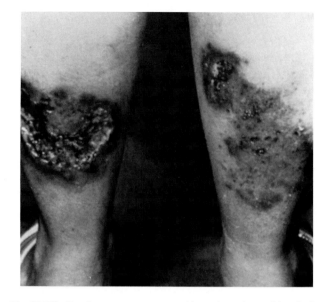

Fig. 37-39. Pyoderma gangrenosum. Note ulcerations with rolled granulomatous borders on lower legs.

more in diameter. The active border is deeply violaceous red and the central portion is necrotic and ulcerated. A halo of erythema surrounds the lesion. Lesions of pyoderma gangrenosum are often extremely painful, and although they usually occur on the lower part of the leg, they may occur anywhere on the body.

Bacteriologic cultures of the ulceration often are sterile or grow contaminant organisms. Skin biopsy from the edge of the ulcer shows considerable proliferation of the epidermis (pseudocarcinomatous hyperplasia) and necrosis with chronic inflammatory cells in the dermis. The biopsy is not diagnostic of pyoderma gangrenosum, but helps to exclude other causes. Special stains (e.g., PAS, Giemsa) should be done to rule out deep fungus or other infectious source.

Although pyoderma gangrenosum was considered at one time pathognomonic of an underlying chronic ulcerative colitis, today other conditions such as regional enteritis, gastric ulcer, empyema, diabetes mellitus, and chronic debilitating infections may be associated with it.[37] Therapy is directed primarily at the underlying systemic disorder.

Leg Ulcers Secondary to Porphyria Cutanea Tarda

Porphyria cutanea tarda (PCT) is an abnormality of porphyrin metabolism that results in cutaneous lesions and increased urinary excretion of uroporphyrins and coproporphyrins. The majority of patients have abnormal liver functions because of an excessive use of alcohol, toxins, or drugs.

The clinical features include fragility of the skin and bulla formation of the sun-exposed areas, especially the hands. Healing of bullae results in scar formation and milia. Hyperpigmentation, hypertrichosis, and morphea-like plaques are other features.

Ulcerations of the hands are common but ulcers of the lower extremity are an uncommon feature of PCT.

Leg Ulcers Secondary to Gaucher's Disease

Skin changes in the chronic form of Gaucher's disease are usually a brownish or brownish-yellow pigmentation on the face, body, or legs. The lesions usually do not ulcerate but resemble Schamberg's pigmented purpura.

Leg Ulcers Secondary to Gout

Gout is a form of recurrent arthritis associated with hyperuricemia that results in deposits of crystals of monosodium urate in joints and subcutaneous tissue. These will occasionally develop on the leg, especially around the malleolus, and may ulcerate and simulate a stasis ulcer or a rheumatoid nodule that can ulcerate. The more common locations of tophaceous deposits are the helix of the ear, hands, and elbows.

Skin biopsy may be necessary to identify the crystals of monosodium urate. Formalin fixation will dissolve away most urate crystals; therefore, fixation of skin biopsies in absolute ethanol is required for the preservation of crystals in histologic material.

Leg Ulcers Secondary to Diabetes Mellitus

Cutaneous disorders often found in diabetics include pruritus, bacterial and fungal infections, pigmentation, xanthomatous lesions, and dermal changes secondary to vascular disease and neurotrophic disorders. These skin clues are important because they may help detect unsuspected diabetes mellitus in its early stages. Many of these lesions are impossible to treat effectively unless the underlying diabetes is detected and treated.

Leg Ulcers Secondary to Necrobiosis Lipoidica Diabeticorum

Necrobiosis lipoidica diabeticorum (NLD) is a rare but almost certain diagnostic sign of underlying diabetes mellitus. NLD occurs in approximately 0.3% of all diabetics. It is somewhat more frequent in females under the age of 40. If the glucose tolerance test is normal, a cortisone glucose tolerance test may detect latent diabetes mellitus.

The clinical lesions are usually located on the anterior surface of the legs (Fig. 37-40), but they may be located on any portion of the skin, including the scalp. They are atrophic yellow or orange depressed areas with telangiectatic blood vessels coursing through them. They vary in number from one to several and are usually asymptomatic and present only a cosmetic problem. Occasionally trauma or therapy that is too vigorous causes ulceration of the NLD lesion. Degeneration of the dermal connective tissue is probably caused by proliferative angiitis and obliterative changes in the arterioles.

Treatment of NLD is difficult and often not necessary. The lesions are only of cosmetic concern. Control of diabetes mellitus does not prevent the extension of lesions of NLD. Topical corticosteroids with occlusion or Cordran tape may produce some improvement. Intralesional corticosteroids may also prevent extension of the lesion. Caution must be taken with the use of vasoconstrictive corticosteroids in a lesion with impaired circulation. Often the NLD lesions may ulcerate after intralesional steroids. Ulcerated NLD lesions, if they are small, will heal with good local wound care. Large ulcerations usually require exci-

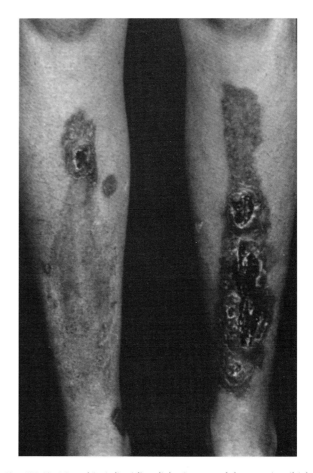

Fig. 37-40. Necrobiosis lipoidica diabeticorum of the anterior tibial areas with ulcerations in a diabetic.

sion of the entire lesion and split-thickness skin grafting. Lesions may persist for years and result in fibrosis and involution.

Leg Ulcers Secondary to Diabetic Dermopathy

Multiple, discrete, atrophic, pigmented macular lesions can occur on the anterior tibial surface of the lower extremities of a diabetic patient (Fig. 37-41). The lesions are usually asymptomatic but have been known to ulcerate and resemble areas of trauma.

The histopathologic features include proliferation and thickening of small blood vessels in the upper dermis and may be analogous to those vessel changes in neuropathy, nephropathy, and retinopathy. There is no specific treatment except local measures such as compresses, topical antibiotics, and good local wound care to heal the ulcerated lesions.

Leg Ulcers Secondary to Bullosis Diabeticorum

Blisters and bullae that appear mainly on the legs have been described in diabetics.[38] The bullae are predominantly sub-epidermal and histologically contain proteinaceous fluid, fibrin threads, and scanty polymorphonuclear cells. The lesions are probably multifactorial in origin, but diabetic microangiopathy and edemas appear to be contributing factors. Local care will heal the lesion.

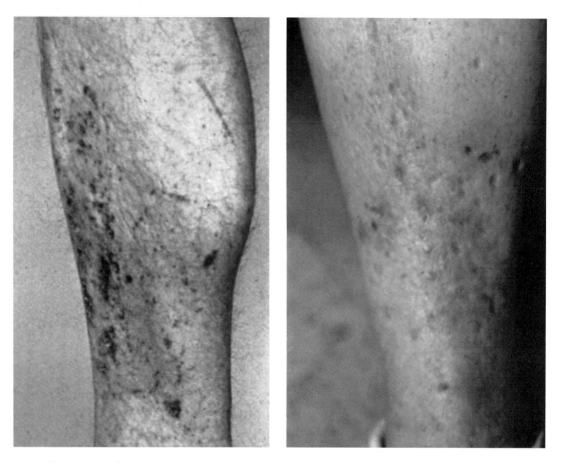

Fig. 37-41. Diabetic dermopathy on the anterior tibial surfaces with indentation and ulcerations.

LEG ULCERS SECONDARY TO TUMORS

Almost any type of tumor, whether primary in the skin or metastatic, may occur on the lower extremities. The tumors may ulcerate and have the appearance of a stasis ulcer that fails to respond to the usual modes of treatment. The importance of the history, especially a history of previous radiation therapy to the leg, is important.

Biopsy is always indicated when a tumor is suspected. If the lesion is ulcerated, the advancing border may be more revealing than the atrophic and possibly infected center of the scar. A deep wedge biopsy is preferred over a punch biopsy.

Leg Ulcers Secondary to Basal Cell Carcinoma

Basal cell carcinoma of the lower extremity is a relatively rare and frequently misdiagnosed skin lesion. Because the most common sites for basal cell carcinoma are the exposed areas of the head and neck, the clinical index of suspicion is low when it occurs on the legs.

The lesions may vary in size from a 1 to 2 mm skin-colored papule with slight telangiectasia to a large, eroded, and ulcerating lesion several centimeters in diameter.

The treatment of choice for small basal cell carcinomas (less than 1 cm in diameter) is surgical electrocautery and curettement. Because lesions on the legs may be larger and healing may be a problem, primary excision or excision and grafting may be the treatment of choice.

Leg Ulcers Secondary to Keratoacanthoma

Keratoacanthoma is a benign skin tumor that clinically and histologically resembles a squamous cell carcinoma. There are two types of keratoacanthomas—localized and generalized (rare).

The lesion consists of a firm, hemispheric nodule, 1 to 2 cm in diameter, which in its center has a horn-filled crater. The sites of predilection are exposed areas such as the face and the dorsa of the hands, but the lesions may occur on the legs as ulcerative tumor lesions. These ulcerative lesions are especially seen in patients who have recurrent longstanding phototherapy or PUVA for treatment of psoriasis (Fig. 37-42).

A true keratoacanthoma, if left untreated, will usually undergo spontaneous involution within several months and leave an atrophic scar. Because there is often a problem in clinical differentiation from squamous cell carcinoma, the treatment of choice is usually complete primary excision of the lesion. This gives the best cosmetic results and leaves a good specimen for the pathologist to evaluate. Intralesional 5-fluorouracil or methotrexate will also cause regression of lesions that are not suitable for surgery.

Leg Ulcers Secondary to Squamous Cell Carcinoma

Squamous cell carcinoma may occur anywhere on the skin as well as on mucous membranes. It may begin to

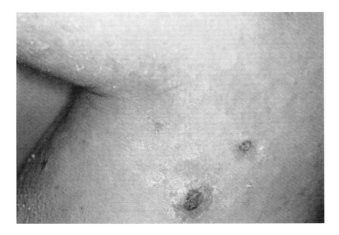

Fig. 37-42. Keratoacanthoma of the leg of a patient with chronic changes due to long-term PUVA therapy.

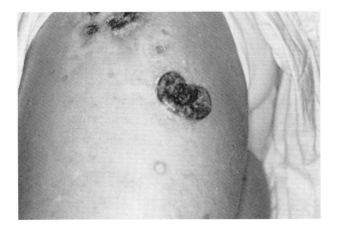

Fig. 37-43. Squamous cell carcinoma in a patient with long-standing PUVA therapy to the legs.

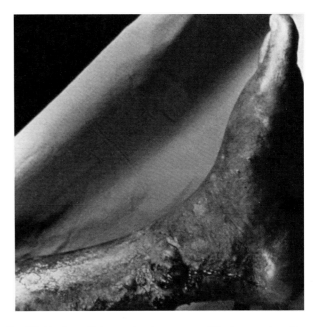

Fig. 37-44. Kaposi's hemorrhagic sarcoma of the lower extremity with fungating and ulcerating tumors.

develop as a senile keratosis or leukoplakia and is most common on the face, neck, and hands.

Most commonly, the lesion consists of a shallow ulcer surrounded by a wide, elevated, and indurated border. Occasionally, raised, fungoid, verrucous lesions without ulceration occur. The lesions are more common on exposed areas such as the face, hands, and arms, and are related to the total amount of solar exposure to the skin. Radiation therapy to the face for acne often predisposes the patient to squamous cell carcinoma. It is also a common complication of excessive radiation on the leg or foot, which may have been given years earlier for a neurodermatitis or a plantar wart. It is also common in patients with longstanding phototherapy and PUVA to the legs (Fig. 37-43). Squamous cell carcinoma can also occur in old injuries such as scars, burn wounds, or chronic ulcers.

Verrucous carcinoma frequently occurs on the foot or leg and appears as a persistent wart. Deep histologic sections show this malignant tumor. Mohs' chemosurgery is the treatment of choice. Complete excision of the primary lesion is necessary. Occasionally, amputation of a portion of the leg is necessary. Lymph node dissection of local and distal nodes is sometimes indicated. Recurrent

lesions are treated with chemotherapy and sometimes with deep x-ray therapy.

Leg Ulcers Secondary to Kaposi's Hemorrhagic Sarcoma

The cutaneous lesions of classic type Kaposi's sarcoma (not AIDS related) most frequently begin on the lower extremity, especially the feet (Fig. 37-44). Later lesions may spread to involve any area of the body. The earliest lesion may be a reddish-brown nodule or groups of nodules that resemble a dermatofibroma. The lesions may be unilateral, but usually they are bilateral and symmetrical. There is an associated brawny edema of the legs. The process tends to extend along veins and lymphatic vessels. Purpura and eventual ulceration of lesions often result. Chronic lymphedema is frequently present.

Treatment includes superficial x-ray therapy, injections of cytotoxic agents, and local treatment with laser or electrodesiccation and cautery.

Leg Ulcers Secondary to Lymphoma

The term *lymphoma* designates a group of malignant disorders that arise from the lymphoreticular system and appear with both cutaneous and visceral infiltration of these abnormal cells. Lymphomas may start from a solitary lesion, but usually the lesions are multiple from the beginning. The lesions may first develop as ulcerations of the lower extremities.

The proper diagnosis is established by an adequate skin or lymph node biopsy, hemogram, bone marrow biopsy, chest x-ray, and CT scans.

The histologic classification varies depending on the predominant cell patterns (T or B cell) and immaturity of cell types. Hodgkin's disease rarely produces skin lesions, but there are skin manifestations of other types of lymphoma. The most common type affecting the skin is

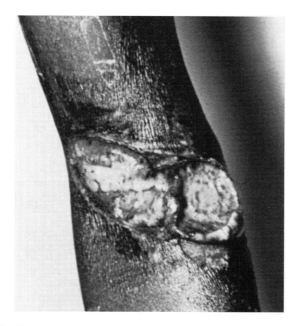

Fig. 37-45. Ulcerative tumor lesion of mycosis fungoides lymphoma.

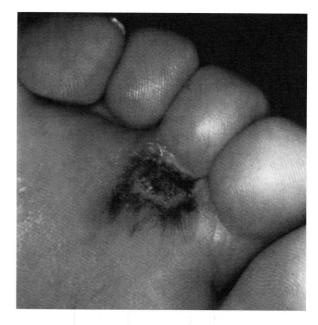

Fig. 37-46. Malignant melanoma of the sole of the foot with early ulceration.

mycosis fungoides, also known as cutaneous T cell lymphoma (CTCL). CTCL primarily involves the skin, but in the late stages it may invade lymph nodes and other internal organs.

CTCL is usually divided into three stages: the eczematous or premycotic stage, the infiltrative stage, and the tumor stage. The erythroderma or exfoliative type may be associated with abnormal cells in the peripheral blood called Sézary cells.

The eczematous stage of CTCL is very similar to eczema, neurodermatitis, psoriasis, parapsoriasis varigata, or parapsoriasis en plaques and may go undiagnosed for 10 to 20 years. There may be scaling patches with variable colors from red to purple. The plaque, or infiltrative stage, shows irregularly shaped, well-demarcated, slightly indurated plaques. There may be some central clearing, and lesions may resemble tinea corporis. The tumor stage consists of tumors of various sizes and round or lobulated brownish-red tumors. These tumors often undergo ulceration (Fig. 37-45).

In the rare form of mycosis fungoides d'emblée, the tumors of the skin develop without previous presence of erythematous or plaque lesions.

Treatment of CTCL depends on the stage of the disease. Early eczematous lesions respond to topical corticosteroids and UVB (ultraviolet B) phototherapy. The plaque stage responds well to photochemotherapy such as PUVA (psoralen and ultraviolet A) or to topical nitrogen mustard. Combination therapy with PUVA and interferon also works well. Total body electron beam therapy has a high cure rate but also results in considerable morbidity. Late stages are treated with various combinations of chemotherapeutic agents and newer experimental agents.

Hemangiolymphangioma Leg Ulcers

This form of tumor is composed largely of dilated and cystic lymphatic vessels combined with dilated blood vessels. The lesions are superficial or deep. The superficial lesions are called *lymphangioma circumscriptum* and are characterized by the presence of groups of small, thick-walled vesicles resembling frog's spawn. The vesicles may have a dark blue color because of red cells mixed in with lymph. The deep type of lesion is called *lymphangioma cavernosum,* and the lesions are more nodular and tumor-like. They also are a deeper reddish-blue. The lesions may ulcerate and drain lymph fluid to the skin.

Treatment is primary excision if the lesions are small or CO_2 laser to larger lesions. They need not be removed.

Malignant Melanoma Leg Ulcers

Malignant melanoma is a vicious tumor that often arises from the skin, occasionally having its origin in a junctional or compound nevus. It often develops in a nevus that the patient has had for many years. There is a sudden increase in size of the lesion, elevation, change in pigmentation, bleeding, or ulceration (Fig. 37-46). The majority of malignant melanomas begin on the lower extremities. The tumor may also appear in the skin as a metastatic melanoma and no primary lesion may ever be discovered.

Melanomas are divided into three clinicopathologic categories, which correlate fairly well with prognosis. The flat, spreading lesions have been designated as superficial spreading melanoma, the nodular lesions as nodular melanoma, and those arising in the melanotic freckles of Hutchinson (lentigo maligna) as lentigo maligna melanoma. Nodular melanoma appears to have the poorest prognosis, whereas lentigo maligna melanoma has the best. All deeply pigmented lesions that could possibly be malignant melanoma must have a biopsy. If the suspicion of melanoma is strong, a wide excision should be done as the initial diagnostic biopsy. If the diagnosis of melanoma is doubtful, a 4 mm punch biopsy is adequate.

The histologic depth of the melanoma (Levels I-V or

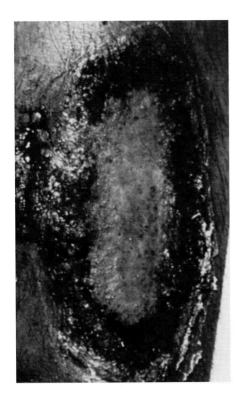

Fig. 37-47. Bromoderma with ulceration of the leg that simulates a deep fungal infection.

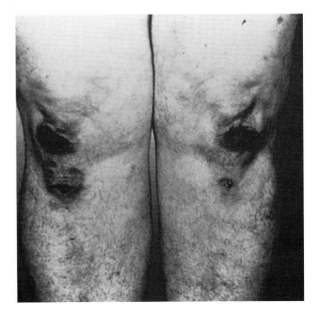

Fig. 37-48. Ulceration of psoriatic plaques on both knees caused by an overdose of methotrexate.

Breslow measurements) also correlates well with the prognosis and dictates the extent of treatment needed. Initial treatment is wide excision with primary closure with a skin graft. Lymph node removal is done in Level IV and V melanomas. Immunotherapy, chemotherapy, x-ray, and other experimental forms of therapy are used for late-stage melanoma, but prognosis is poor. Early recognition, public education about early signs, and avoidance of sunlight has improved the prognosis in recent years.

LEG ULCERS SECONDARY TO MISCELLANEOUS CAUSES

Leg Ulcers Secondary to Drugs

Many sedatives and analgesic medications contain bromide compounds. These were used much more commonly 30 years ago, but are still available in some nonprescription medications. Both bromide and iodide compounds can produce similar types of leg ulcers, although iodides tend to produce an acneform or follicular, pustular, bullous, and later fungating hemorrhagic ulcer (Fig. 37-47). The bromide and iodide lesions may also resemble erythema nodosum or the lesions of tertiary syphilis. One characteristic of these lesions, which are often found on the anterior tibial surface, is extreme local pain. Serum bromide or iodide levels in the blood are increased. Treatment consists of discontinuing the bromide or iodide and substituting another halogen such as sodium chloride. Granulomatous bromodermas are usually very slow to heal.

Ergot occasionally, particularly in America, may cause eruptions that result from ergoted grain. The lesions are bullous and pustular and may become gangrenous ulcers.

Similar conditions may be produced by ergotamine tartrate.

Methotrexate and hydroxyurea have become accepted drugs in the treatment of various neoplastic disorders and for many years have been used to manage severe treatment-resistant psoriasis vulgaris. Well-recognized adverse effects occur in the rapidly dividing organ systems of the body (bone marrow, gastrointestinal tract). In patients who take an overdose of methotrexate or hydroxyurea, severe painful oral mucosal ulcerations and spontaneous, painful ulcerations of plaques or psoriasis often develop on their skin (Fig. 37-48). Laboratory studies may show a leukopenia, thrombocytopenia, and anemia. Leukovoran factor may be effective if given within a few hours after an overdose of methotrexate. Ulcerations of the psoriatic plaques will heal slowly with conservative topical therapy.

Levophed and other vasopressor drugs are used for restoring blood pressure in controlling certain acute hypotensive states. These drugs are powerful peripheral vasoconstrictors, and it is usually recommended that they be administered in a large antecubital vein. When there is extravasation of the solution into the tissue, which might happen if given into a smaller vein in the legs, local necrosis of tissue can result in ulceration (Fig. 37-49). These ulcers usually require grafting to heal.

Several other drugs such as radiopaque dyes used for arteriograms and nitrogen mustard can produce similar local tissue necrosis and ulceration.

Leg Ulcers Secondary to Burns

Thermal and chemical burns, which are third degree, extending to full skin thickness, should be treated by skin grafting. Small ulcerations may heal with conservative management.

Leg Ulcers Secondary to Radiation

Ionizing radiation has been used for years to treat both benign and malignant lesions of the skin. In previous years

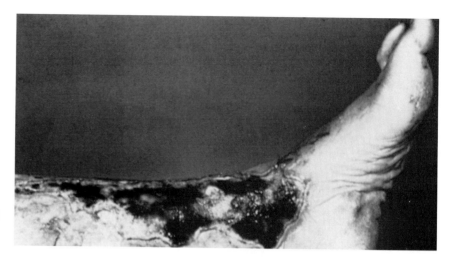

Fig. 37-49. Large necrotic ulcer of leg caused by an infiltration of Levophed into subcutaneous tissue.

many benign disorders such as acne, warts, and hypertrichosis in young individuals were treated with large doses of ionizing radiation. These patients began to show the cumulative effects of the radiation 20 years later. Some of the ulcerations may turn into basal cell or squamous cell carcinomas.

After a single exposure of the skin to a dose of 1000 R or above an acute dermatitis with erythema followed by blistering, pain, edema, necrosis, and ulceration may develop. The roentgen ulcer may take 6 to 8 weeks to develop after the acute phase subsides. The ulcer is characterized by a punched-out appearance, dirty granulating base, undermining of the borders, and extreme pain. The ulcers may enlarge for a time, then heal partially, break down intermittently, and finally heal with deforming scarring.

Chronic radiation dermatitis shows progressive hypopigmentation, loss of appendages, and atrophy of the epidermis and dermis. Later hyperpigmentation and hypopigmentation and superficial telangiectasia develop. The skin is very susceptible to minor trauma, and ulceration of chronic radiation dermatitis is quite common (Fig. 37-50).

Radiation carcinoma of the skin can occur many years after ionizing radiation. These cancers may first appear as hyperkeratotic plaques or as a chronic nonhealing ulcer. Skin biopsy to make the proper diagnosis and then aggressive destruction or excision and grafting of the tumor is the best treatment.

Leg Ulcers Secondary to Lichen Planus

Lichen planus is a papulosquamous dermatitis of unknown cause that usually appears as a generalized eruption. The diagnostic lesion is a small, flat-topped, polygonal, violaceous papule that later becomes brownish and may leave hyperpigmentation. Histopathology of a typical skin lesion confirms the diagnosis.

Hypertrophic lichen planus most commonly affects the shins and ankles. The lesions are thickened, warty hypertrophic plaques covered with fine adherent scales. Lichen planus may appear with bullae and ulceration confined to the feet and toes, permanent loss of toenails, and a

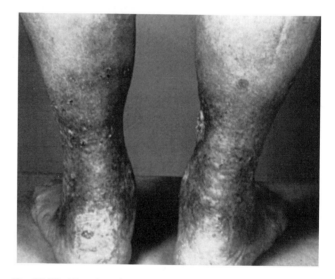

Fig. 37-50. Chronic radiation dermatitis of the legs with ulceration.

cicatricial alopecia of the scalp. The chronic, painful ulceration of the feet is often a diagnostic problem and may have a surrounding area of atrophic depigmented skin. Treatment consists of either systemic or intralesional corticosteroids.

Leg Ulcers Secondary to Erythema Nodosum

Erythema nodosum is a common cause of nodules on the lower leg and often is mistaken for superficial thrombophlebitis. It usually does not ulcerate, but if the lesions do ulcerate, a diagnosis of erythema induratum should be considered. The cause of erythema nodosum is variable, with streptococcal infections and drug sensitivity (iodides, sulfonamides, and penicillin) being the most common causes. Other diseases that may underlie the eruption are tuberculosis, sarcoidosis, deep fungal infections, ulcerative colitis, rheumatic fever, lymphogranuloma venereum, leprosy, and syphilis. Very often no underlying cause of the nodosum lesions is found, and symptomatic therapy with aspirin, antihistamines, or corticosteroids may be indicated.

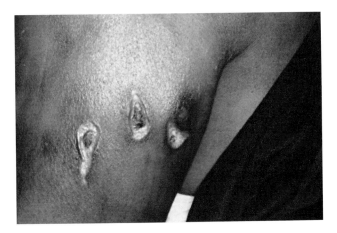

Fig. 37-51. Ulcerative lesions due to lupus panniculitis.

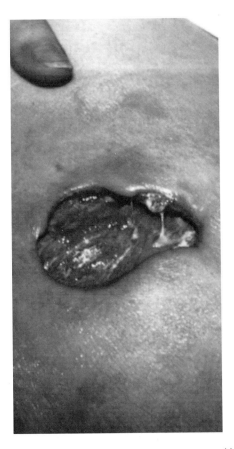

Fig. 37-52. Facticial ulcers of the legs caused by repeated burns by the patient with a cigarette.

Leg Ulcers Secondary to Panniculitis (Weber-Christian Disease)

Relapsing febrile nodular nonsuppurative panniculitis consists of crops of painful subcutaneous nodules, usually occurring on the thighs and buttocks. Fever and generalized malaise may accompany the attacks, and occasionally severe leukopenia may also be present. The lesions usually do not ulcerate, but there have been cases of ulceration on thighs from the fat necrosis (Fig. 37-51). Skin biopsy shows a nonspecific fat necrosis, depending on the stage of the disease when the biopsy is taken. There are numerous lymphocytes throughout the fat and also a secondary vascular inflammatory reaction. There are many other forms of panniculitis, which are subdivided mainly on histologic changes. They all produce nodules and ulcer-like lesions on the lower legs.

Factitial Leg Ulceration

Ulceration of the lower extremity that is caused by the patient may be one of the most difficult types of leg ulcer to diagnose correctly. The ulcerations may develop many bizarre patterns, mainly because of the multiple methods of producing the ulcerations. Many patients produce the ulcers by picking or probing with their fingers, but more commonly some device is used, including a syringe and needle (containing medicine or sputum), probes, scissors, sticks, acids, chemicals, or cigarettes (Fig. 37-52). Once the diagnosis is suspected the acceptance of the diagnosis by the patient and/or the family is at times even more difficult than is proving the diagnosis.

One method of proving a factitial cause is to have the ulcerations completely occluded with a nonremovable type of dressing (Unna boot) for several weeks. The factitial ulcer will usually heal, only to reoccur once the patient can get at the skin. A laissez-faire attitude toward the disease on the part of the patient and any peculiar affects that have been noticed will reinforce the suspected diagnosis.

These patients tend to go to many doctors and may be difficult patients to handle. Psychiatric consultation is only partially helpful.

REFERENCES

1. Roenigk HH Jr and Young JR: Leg ulcers: medical and surgical management, Hagerstown, Md, 1975, Harper & Row.
2. Krull EA: Chronic cutaneous ulcerations and impaired healing in human skin, J Am Acad Dermatol 12:394, 1985.
3. Lottie T et al: The pathogenesis of venous ulcers, J Am Acad Dermatol 16:877, 1987.
4. Hendricks WM and Swallow RT: Management of stasis leg ulcers with Unna boots versus elastic support stockings, J Am Acad Dermatol 12:90, 1985.
5. Witkowski JA and Parish LC: Cutaneous ulcer therapy, Int J Dermatol 25:420, 1986.
6. Westerhof W et al: Controlled double-blind trial of fibrinolysin-desoxyribonuclease (Elase) solution in patients with chronic leg ulcers who are treated before autologous skin grafting, J Am Acad Dermatol 17:32, 1987.
7. Falanga V: Occlusive wound dressings, Arch Dermatol 124:872, 1988.
8. Falanga V, Zitelli JA, and Eaglstein WH: Wound healing, J Am Acad Dermatol 19:559, 1988.
9. Freidman S and Su D: Hydrocolloid occlusive dressing management of leg ulcers, Arch Dermatol 120:1329, 1984.
10. Varghese MC et al: Local environment of chronic wounds under synthetic dressings, Arch Dermatol 122:52, 1986.
11. Katz S et al: Semipermeable occlusive dressings, Arch Dermatol 122:58, 1986.
12. Alper JC et al: Moist wound healing under a vapor-permeable membrane, J Am Acad Dermatol 8:347, 1983.
13. Alper JC et al: Use of the vapor permeable membrane for cutaneous ulcers: details of application and side effects, J Am Acad Dermatol 11:858, 1984.

14. Eaglstein WH: Experiences with biosynthetic dressings, J Am Acad Dermatol 12:434, 1985.

15. Eaglstein WH et al: Optimal use of an occlusive dressing to enhance healing, Arch Dermatol 124:392, 1988.

16. Angermeier MC, Alper JC, and Urbaniak HS Jr: Vapor-permeable membrane therapy for ulcers or osteomyelitis, J Dermatol Surg Oncol 10:384, 1984.

17. Marshal DA, Mertz PM, and Eaglstein WH: Occlusive dressings—does dressing type influence the growth of common bacterial pathogens, Arch Surg 125:1136, 1990.

18. Phillips TJ and Gilchrist BA: Cultured epidermal grafts in the treatment of leg ulcers, Adv Dermatol 5:33, 1990.

19. O'Connor NE et al: Grafting of burns with cultured epithelium prepared from autologous epidermal cells, Lancet 1:25, 1981.

20. Compton CG et al: Skin regenerated from cultured epithelial autografts on acute burn wounds: a light, electron microscopic and immunohistochemical study, Lab Invest 60:600, 1989.

21. Leigh IM et al: Treatment of chronic venous stasis ulcers with sheets of cultured allogeneic keratinocytes, Br J Dermatol 117:591, 1987.

22. Barrandon Y and Green H: Three clonal types of keratinocytes with different capacities for multiplication, Proc Natl Acad Sci U S A 84:2303, 1987.

23. Phillips T et al: Treatment of skin ulcers with cultured epidermal allografts, J Am Acad Dermatol 21:191, 1989.

24. Jonker M et al: The influence of matching for HLA-DR antigens on skin graft survival, Transplantation 27:91, 1979.

25. Gielen V et al: Progressive replacement of human cultured epithelial allografts as evidenced by HLA class I antigen expression, Dermatologica 175:166, 1987.

26. Gilchrest BA et al: Autocrine and paracrine growth stimulation of cells derived from human skin, J Cell Physiol 117:235, 1983.

27. Luger TA, Wirth U, and Kock A: Epidermal cells synthesize a cytokine with interleukin 3 like properties, J Immunol 134:915, 1985.

28. Kupper TS et al: Human keratinocytes contain mRNA indistinguishable from monocyte interleukin 1 alpha and beta mRNA: keratinocyte epidermal cell-derived thymocyte-activating factor is identical to interleukin 1, J Exp Med 164L:2095, 1986.

29. Wickner NE et al: Transforming growth factor beta stimulates the expression of fibronectin by human keratinocytes, J Invest Dermatol 91:207, 1988.

30. Coffey RJ et al: Production and autoinduction of transforming growth factor alpha in human keratinocytes, Nature 328:817, 1987.

31. Ceilley RI, Rink MA, and Zueklhe RL: Pinch grafting for chronic ulcers of liver extremities, J Dermatol Surg Oncol 3:303, 1977.

32. Gilmore WA and Wheeland RG: Treatment of ulcers on legs by pinch grafts and a supportive dressing of polyurethane, J Dermatol Surg Oncol 8:177, 1982.

33. Wheeland RG: The technique and current status of pinch grafting, J Dermatol Surg Oncol 13:873, 1986.

34. Dinner MI and Peters CR: Surgical management of ulcers on the lower limbs, J Dermatol Surg Oncol 4:696, 1978.

35. Jon ST, Roberts RH, and Sinclair SW: A comparison of Lessoderm with DuoDerm in the treatment of split skin graft donor site, Br J Plast Surg 46:82, 1993.

36. Espinoza LR et al: Oral methotrexate therapy for chronic rheumatoid arthritic ulcerations, J Am Acad Dermatol 15:508, 1986.

37. Perry HO and Brunsting LA: Pyoderma gangrenosum, Arch Dermatol 75:380, 1957.

38. Cantwell AR and Marty W: Idiopathic bullae in diabetics, Arch Dermatol 96:42, 1967.

CHAPTER THIRTY-EIGHT

THE SWOLLEN LIMB

William F. Ruschhaupt III
Bernardo B. Fernandez, Jr.

The patient with a swollen limb is a common problem for the practicing physician.[1] Swelling, like fever, should not be considered a disease in itself, but rather a sign of an underlying disorder. Although the disorder is often minor, at times edema may indicate a serious disease process. It is important to recognize, though, that all swelling is not edema. The finding of swelling or edema should alert the physician to seek the cause.

PHYSIOLOGIC PRINCIPLES

The process that leads to finding the correct cause of a swollen limb must be built on an understanding of all of the factors affecting edema formation.[2] Edema represents an increase in the interstitial (extravascular) component of the extracellular fluid volume. There are many systemic influences, such as renal salt and water balance, and physiologic concepts, such as effective blood volume or adequacy of arterial vascular filling, which will not be discussed in this chapter, but do affect edema formation systemically. However, there is a need to review six factors affecting edema formation in an extremity. Four of the factors are major physiologic principles: capillary blood pressure, plasma colloid oncotic pressure, tissue colloid oncotic pressure, and tissue pressure itself. The other two factors are changes in capillary permeability and obstruction of lymphatic flow, either of which can occur uniquely in the affected limb. None of the six factors is routinely measured or quantified for the clinician.

Interstitial fluid contains all the components found in blood plasma except the amount of protein. The principal physiologic processes that account for the dynamics of interstitial fluid within any extremity are filtration and reabsorption. Filtration is the process that occurs on the arterial end of the capillary system, while reabsorption is thought to occur on the venous side of the capillary system.[3] Changes in any of the six physiologic factors affecting the extracellular fluid volume can result in edema formation in the affected limb.

Capillary Blood Pressure

Arterial blood pressure is the driving force for filtration in the arterial portion of the capillary system. As blood passes through the normal arterial bed and begins to enter the venous side, the effects of arterial blood pressure are diminished. Working in conjunction with the one-way valve system of the deep veins of an extremity, the muscles of that extremity are the pump for the venous side of the circulation. Normal capillary venous pressure is therefore physiologically lower than normal capillary arterial pressure, facilitating reabsorption of interstitial fluid, if all other factors are static. However, a static state is never achieved in the dynamics of human physiology. At any given time, either filtration or reabsorption is occurring predominantly. If local venous pressure increases, as with a deep vein occlusion, then the localized central venous pressure in that extremity would be increased and transmitted in a retrograde fashion. An increase in capillary venous blood pressure would occur. In this setting reabsorption would then be decreased, and an increase in the interstitial fluid (edema) would follow.

Colloid Oncotic Pressure

Oncotic pressure in the extracellular fluid compartments is created by the concentration of electrolytes, glucose, urea, and proteins within the extracellular fluid. The relatively large protein molecules of the plasma exert their osmotic influence within the capillary system because of their inability to pass through the capillary walls. Plasma has a relatively high concentration of the osmotically active proteins, whereas interstital fluid has a relatively low concentration. In the normal state, low concentrations of osmotically active proteins in the interstitial fluid rarely favor an increase in the interstitial fluid volume at either side of the capillary bed. Therefore in the normal state, if there is no change in the number of protein molecules within the interstitial fluid, the concentration of proteins in the plasma would be highest on the venous side of the capillary bed. Reabsorption of the interstitial fluid on the venous side would again be favored.

Interstitial Tissue Pressure

The area available within the tissues of an extremity for interstital fluid volume is limited. When the volume increases above its normal level, the pressure within the space increases. Obviously, this increasing pressure must be overcome by the forces favoring filtration if any further accumulation of interstitial fluid is to continue. However, in the normal state, tissue pressure is not high in any of the extremities and can be easily exceeded by the dynamics of capillary arterial pressure.

Capillary Permeability

The permeability of the capillary walls to plasma proteins has already been mentioned. The capillary membrane is semipermeable, but any change in this condition would allow for a variation in flow of fluid from the normal pathways. Increasing capillary permeability to proteins would allow plasma proteins to exit the intravascular space for the extravascular space, thus critically changing colloid oncotic pressures in the plasma and interstitial fluid. Plasma colloid oncotic pressure is the major driving force for reabsorption of interstitial fluid. An increase in plasma protein concentration in the interstitial fluid would critically favor edema formation.

Lymphatic Flow

The lymphatic system is a direct outflow system for the interstitial fluid. However, lymphatic fluid contains large amounts of protein. The walls of the lymphatic system are permeable to protein, but the capillary walls are not. When the flow of lymph from an extremity is obstructed or inadequate, there are several factors that favor edema. Not only is edema caused by the direct obstruction of the lymphatic flow, but also the protein content of the interstitial fluid increases. This gives rise to an increase in interstitial colloid oncotic pressure, thus decreasing the pressure gradient favoring reabsorption on the venous side of the capillary bed.

CLINICAL APPROACH

The history and physical examination remain the cornerstones for the diagnosis of the swollen limb. The findings are important in determining what additional tests are necessary to confirm the diagnosis.

History

The acuity of onset of swelling in an extremity is a strong clue to its cause. Sudden onset of swelling over several hours or days suggests an acute process such as deep vein thrombophlebitis, cellulitis, compartment syndrome, or gastrocnemius muscle rupture. A gradual, progressive onset over several weeks to months suggests lymphedema, chronic venous insufficiency, some systemic process, or exposure to particular medications. Edema that occurs intermittently and then resolves, but continues to recur is typical for the limb swelling seen with recurrent episodes of lymphangitis and cellulitis.

Edema is usually worse at the end of the day and improved by morning. Redistribution occurs as a result of the recumbent position during sleep. If the patient is unable to sleep or rest horizontally, this diurnal variation may be lost. As the duration of the edema continues and the cause persists, daily variation will tend to diminish over time.

The presence or absence of pain can be helpful in arriving at the correct diagnosis. Painful swelling of a limb suggests thrombophlebitis, cellulitis, compartment syndrome, muscle rupture, or reflex sympathetic dystrophy. The swelling caused by lymphedema and the swelling from systemic causes should be painless.

Systemic symptoms are important. A history of swelling associated with a high fever and shaking chills directs the clinician to an infectious source such as recurrent cellulitis, lymphangitis, or septic phlebitis. Nonseptic deep vein thrombophlebitis may be associated with a low-grade fever, but it does not produce a high fever or chills.

The patient should be questioned regarding predisposing conditions that may have contributed to the development of the swollen leg such as prolonged plane flights, automobile trips, any period of prolonged immobility, trauma, accidents, prior radiation therapy, operations, or childbirth.

Physical Examination

One of the most obvious findings on physical examination is whether swelling involves one limb or both. The division of the causes of limb swelling into causes for unilateral or bilateral swelling forms the basis for the discussion of specific causes in subsequent portions of this chapter.

The appearance of the skin of the involved limb gives many clues to the underlying causes. Frequently, comparison with the opposite extremity is helpful in determining the change from normal appearance. A reddened area, perhaps with red tender streaks leading away from the area, is highly suggestive of cellulitis with lymphangitis. A more elongated raised area of redness with a palpable cord is suggestive of a superficial thrombophlebitis. A reddish-blue hue to the extremity suggests the presence of a proximal deep vein thrombophlebitis. Ecchymoses would indicate trauma or a ruptured muscle.

The location of the swelling is of particular importance. Swelling in the calf or thigh in the absence of ankle or foot edema indicates a local process within those muscle groups or regions and not a true edematous process. A ruptured medial head of the gastrocnemius, traumatic hematoma, or an osteogenic sarcoma can develop in this way. Involvement of the foot, resulting in a typical dorsal hump, and involvement of the toes is a sign of lymphedema. An enlarged limb that spares the foot and toes suggests lipedema.

Edema of the upper extremity versus edema of the lower extremity helps to create some interesting contrasts. Acute deep vein thrombophlebitis of the upper extremity is usually secondary to thoracic outlet syndrome or to iatrogenic causes from the use of intravenous catheters. Swelling is usually the first manifestation of the problem. By contrast acute deep vein thrombophlebitis in the lower extremity is variable in terms of its frequency of producing edema, not only at the time of onset but also through its course. The lower extremity is frequently the site of chronic venous insufficiency as a result of prior deep vein thrombophlebitis, yet venous insufficiency and stasis symptoms are unusual sequelae in the upper extremity. Lymphedema in the lower extremity is about equally distributed between primary and secondary causes, whereas in the upper extremity, lymphedema is almost always secondary in nature.

Diagnostic Tests

Following a thorough history and physical examination, the noninvasive vascular laboratory can play a critical role in the differential diagnosis of various causes of the swollen extremity. Negative as well as positive studies can be significant to the clinician. The diagnosis of proximal deep vein thrombophlebitis can be firmly established in an accredited noninvasive vascular laboratory with the use of duplex ultrasonography. In the lower extremities, this noninvasive study can accurately identify the presence or absence of deep vein thrombophlebitis in the popliteal, superficial femoral, common femoral, and iliac veins. The technique can also detect the presence of a Baker's cyst or popliteal artery aneurysm. While this technique is not as accurate for consistent demonstration of a calf vein thrombus, if the patient has a swollen leg from at least the knee distally, then a negative study implies that proximal deep vein thrombophlebitis is not the cause of that swelling.

If the noninvasive laboratory does not have duplex ultrasonography, then various plethysmographic techniques can be accurate in the diagnosis of proximal deep vein thrombophlebitis. It is important, however, that an ongoing quality control program exists in those laboratories, since these techniques are technician dependent for accuracy.

If the noninvasive vascular laboratory is unavailable, then standard radiographic contrast venography should be used to establish the presence or absence of acute deep vein thrombophlebitis.

Other studies are also used for assessing the swollen limb. Computerized tomography (CT) scanning and magnetic resonance imaging (MRI) are particularly useful in evaluating localized masses or unusual causes. When looking for systemic causes, electrocardiogram, chest x-ray, urinalysis, complete blood cell count, electrolytes, renal function tests, and hepatic function tests are necessary.

CAUSES OF UNILATERAL SWOLLEN LIMB
(see the accompanying box)

Acute Deep Vein Thrombophlebitis
(see Chapter 26)

Of the three most common vascular causes of the swollen limb (deep vein thrombophlebitis, chronic venous insufficiency, and lymphedema), acute deep vein thrombophlebitis can have the most dramatic onset. Swelling, bluish-red discoloration, and prominent veins may be associated with acute deep vein thrombophlebitis and may or may not be accompanied by or preceded by pain.

Chronic Venous Insufficiency (see Chapter 28)

One of the results of an acute deep vein thrombophlebitis can be the development of chronic venous insuffi-

---

CAUSES OF UNILATERAL SWOLLEN LIMB

Acute deep vein thrombophlebitis
Chronic venous insufficiency
Lymphedema
Cellulitis
Abscess
Osteomyelitis
Charcot's joint
Popliteal cyst
Popliteal artery aneurysm
Trauma
Compartment syndrome
Vascular anomalies
Thermal injury
Tumors
Dependency
Disuse
Gastrocnemius rupture
Revascularization
Retroperitoneal fibrosis
Hemihypertrophy
Factitial

---

ciency. Damage to the valves in the venous system can cause a stasis syndrome to develop with pigmentation, dermatitis, edema, cellulitis, and ulceration. It is important to note that stasis cellulitis is a nonbacterial inflammatory process.

Lymphedema (see Chapter 29)

The third most common vascular cause of limb swelling is lymphedema. Lymphedema has a slow, insidious onset, unless it is related to an acute surgical or traumatic disruption of the lymphatic system. Lymphedema should be categorized into either primary or secondary types. Depending on the age of the patient at the onset of the lymphedema and its duration, an aggressive search for the underlying cause may be necessary. It is important to recognize that lymphedema always begins in the most distal portion of the extremity; therefore careful observation of the hand or foot is important in discovering this entity early.

Cellulitis

Cellulitis is the most common infectious cause of limb swelling (Fig. 38-1). Cellulitis can occur as a single isolated event or a series of recurrent events and is regularly misdiagnosed (usually as recurrent thrombophlebitis or worsening chronic venous insufficiency). Cellulitis occurs when there is a portal through the normal skin barriers for bacteria to enter and to release their toxins in the subcutaneous tissues. The acute onset with swelling, localized

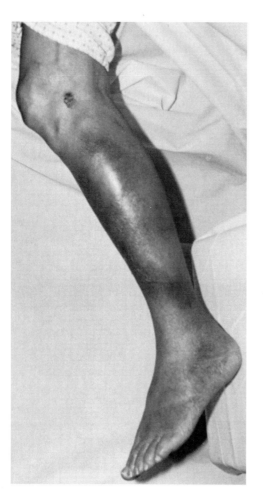

Fig. 38-1. Cellulitis. Notice the skip areas of involvement in the foot and leg.

redness, and pain is also frequently associated with systemic signs of high fever, shaking chills, and sweats. The redness does not have to be uniform and often does have skip areas. Regional lymph nodes can also be tender and enlarged.

Cellulitis generally responds well to antibiotic therapy, and improvement can be quite rapid, especially with intravenous therapy. The key to preventing recurrent attacks of cellulitis lies in adequate antibiotic therapy for the initial event, as well as in the recognition and appropriate management of the portal of entry through the skin.

Of all the portals of entry, the most commonly overlooked are the skin cracks and fissures that occur in the skin between the toes as a result of tinea pedis. Without recognition and treatment of this fungal infection of the skin, recurrent episodes of cellulitis will occur. Recurrent episodes of cellulitis and accompanying lymphangitis can produce severe secondary lymphedema as a result of the destruction and scarring of the lymphatic vessels in the involved extremity. Other portals of entry for recurrent cellulitis include the sites of drug abuse, contusions, abrasions, ulcerations, ingrown toenails, and hangnails.

Unfortunately, many episodes of cellulitis go unrecognized because a diagnosis of deep vein thrombophlebitis is erroneously made. Because many physicians in the past have treated deep vein thrombophlebitis not only with anticoagulants but also with antibiotics, the "phlebitis" responds to this therapy, and the cellulitis is not recognized. The problem with this approach is that episodes recur because the portal of entry has not been eliminated.

Abscess

Abscesses rarely develop from a cellulitic process, but instead they follow a deep-seated infection, which can occur as a result of some sort of puncture wound. Swelling of the involved limb is most frequently localized with early abscess formation but can be significant enough to give the appearance of a generalized edematous process. The principles of management of this entity are recognition of the problem, obtaining adequate cultures, adequate incision and drainage of the abscess, and appropriate antibiotic therapy.

Osteomyelitis

Osteomyelitis is the third infectious process that can produce limb swelling. Again the swelling occurs usually in the distal portion of an extremity. The diabetic patient with diabetic neuropathy and neurotrophic ulcers represents an ideal setting for this infection to occur, but any patient with a severe peripheral neuropathy is susceptible. Patients with sickle cell anemia are also prone to develop osteomyelitis, particularly from *Salmonella* organisms. With hematogenous osteomyelitis, any of the long bones of the extremity are common targets.

Charcot's Joints (see Chapter 40)

In Charcot's neuropathic arthropathy, the joints are not only swollen, but they are also usually deformed. The swelling can be easily noticed and is initially accompanied by localized warmth. The swelling and warmth can extend proximally from the involved joint and can produce localized tenderness on examination in an otherwise neuropathic distal portion of an extremity. Such a picture is not only frequently clinically confusing but also radiographically confusing. On plain films it is often difficult, if not impossible, to separate the early Charcot's joint from osteomyelitis since the neuropathic extremity is a prime setting for either process. Further radiographic investigations may be necessary, including various nuclear medicine scanning techniques, which may or may not shed further light on the matter. MRI also holds some promise for resolving these diagnostic conflicts before proceeding with exploratory surgical intervention.

Popliteal Cysts

Popliteal cysts (Baker's cysts) may produce localized swelling in an extremity behind the knee or swelling distally with the signs and symptoms of deep vein thrombosis.[4] The latter occurs when there is compression of the popliteal vein. Dissection of a Baker's cyst, without rupture, into the muscles of the lower extremities can also produce swelling. If a popliteal cyst ruptures, the signs and symptoms are difficult to distinguish from a deep vein thrombosis. Indeed, an acute deep vein thrombophlebitis can result from compression by a large popliteal cyst. Physical examination should suggest the presence of a popliteal cyst in either the swollen leg or the nonswollen leg, particularly in a patient with either rheumatoid arthritis or longstanding degenerative joint disease involving the knee. A popliteal cyst can be accurately diagnosed by ultrasound examination in the vascular laboratory, but occasionally arthrography may be needed to solidify the diagnosis. This is especially true if the cyst has ruptured.

Popliteal Artery Aneurysm (see Chapter 19)

Just as large popliteal cysts can cause venous compression, so can large popliteal artery aneurysms produce increased venous hypertension by this same mechanism. Persistent restriction of outflow of the venous system in an extremity will create the factors that favor distal edema formation and in some cases be the initial manifestation of this significant arterial problem.

Trauma

Severe trauma leading to fractures and even disruption of skin integrity is an obvious cause of a swollen limb. In such a setting the clinician is faced with the task of determining whether or not thrombophlebitis or cellulitis might be associated with the trauma. Incidental or unnoticed trauma can also produce limb swelling (Fig. 38-2). In most instances this is more localized and may or may not be accompanied by ecchymoses.

Compartment Syndrome (see Chapter 15)

Sudden occlusion of an artery by thrombosis or embolism can lead to severe pain, induration, and edema. Compartment syndromes can occur because of the local tissue response to severe hypoxemia or to restoration of blood flow to an ischemic extremity. In a relatively fixed, enclosed area, the compartment's ability to accommodate a sudden increase in volume is limited. This is particularly true if there are other mechanical factors such as trauma or encasement in bandages or dressings. These syndromes are most commonly seen in the lower extremity but can occur in the arms as well. Fasciotomy, either prophylactic or therapeutic, is occasionally necessary in the management of the compartment syndrome.

Vascular Anomalies (see Chapter 33)

The principle that not all swelling is edema is clearly demonstrated in patients with vascular anomalies. Hyperthophied extremities or muscle groups caused by either congenital or acquired arteriovenous fistulas are typical examples (Fig. 38-3). Physical findings of a thrill or bruit in the area can suggest the presence of an arteriovenous fistula. Increased temperature locally may also occur, and occasionally congestive heart failure and cardiac enlargement may be found.

Klippel-Trenaunay syndrome is a distinct clinical triad of varicose veins, port-wine stain (nevus flammeus), and muscular hypertrophy (Fig. 38-4). This syndrome has been associated with the occurrence of arteriovenous fistulas, as well as the agenesis of the deep venous system.[5] It is important to recognize the latter since surgical ligation and stripping of varicose veins in these patients can result in severe chronic venous insufficiency.

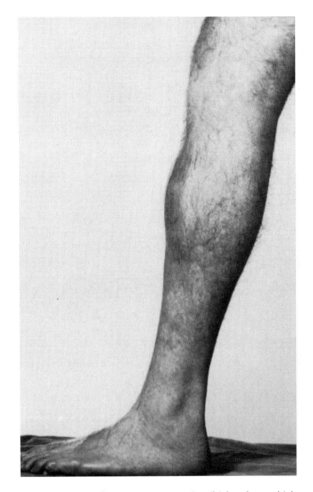

Fig. 38-2. Traumatic hematoma on anterior tibial surface, which did not produce compartment syndrome, but which did require drainage.

Thermal Injury

Exposure to severe heat, as well as cold, can produce a swollen limb. There is a common mechanism for edema formation in heat or cold injury. The major change occurs as a result of damage to the capillary membrane. Thermal injury increases capillary permeability, resulting in greater flow of plasma proteins from the intravascular space into the interstitial fluid. With severe cold exposure, edema does not occur until rewarming takes place.

Tumors

Limb swelling can be produced by a variety of tumors, both benign and malignant. Cavernous hemangiomas and others vascular tumors are discussed in Chapter 36. Any tumor of bone, muscle, tendon, cartilage, nerve, blood, or lymphatic vessel can produce a swollen extremity.[6]

Dependency

Both unilateral and bilateral limb swelling can be caused by dependency. Unilateral leg swelling secondary to dependency is frequently seen with severe arterial insufficiency. The patient will have rest pain and/or ischemic ulcerations and will be unable to sleep lying flat. The patient will dangle one foot over the side of the bed

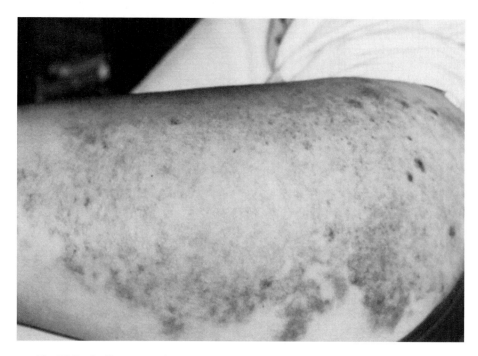

Fig. 38-3. Capillary venous hemangioma involving lateral proximal thigh and hip region.

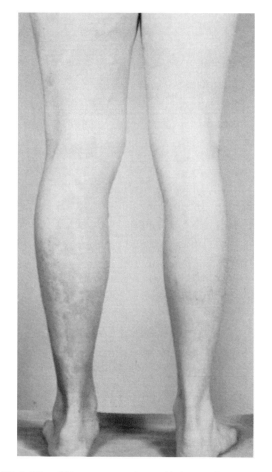

Fig. 38-4. Klippel-Trenaunay syndrome. Varicose veins, cutaneous hemangioma (port-wine stain), and muscular hypertrophy.

throughout the night, resulting in prolonged dependency and edema. Similarly, prolonged use of crutches with one leg dependent or a prolonged disuse of an extremity will result in limb swelling.

Gastrocnemius Rupture

The weekend athlete who has a history of sudden onset of pain in the calf and subsequent leg swelling is a classic example of a patient with a rupture of the medial head of the gastrocnemius muscle. However, this injury can occur by stepping off a curb or down a step. There is usually a history of a specific event. Some patients describe hearing a "snap" or "pop" with a sudden onset of severe pain in the calf and an inability to bear weight on the involved leg. The tear in the medial head of the gastrocnemius causes swelling to develop promptly, and within several days ecchymosis can occur around both the medial and lateral sides of the ankle and foot (Fig. 38-5). The ecchymosis is the result of gravitational dissection of blood from the torn muscle through the muscle tissue planes and can take a characteristic crescent shape beneath the malleoli.

It is important to recognize the clinical picture and to treat appropriately. This syndrome in the past has been confused with acute deep vein thrombophlebitis and treated with anticoagulants. This leads to further hemorrhage into the calf. Treatment with casting for this problem promotes the development of acute deep venous thrombophlebitis. The appropriate treatment consists of the application of ice packs to the calf during the first 24 to 48 hours and elevation. This should be followed with avoidance of all weight bearing on the leg for a few days and later progressive ambulation. Gradual stretching exercises in a physical therapy program may be helpful. As the patient returns to weight bearing, a lift in the heel of the shoe of the involved leg avoids severe stretching of the gastrocnemius.

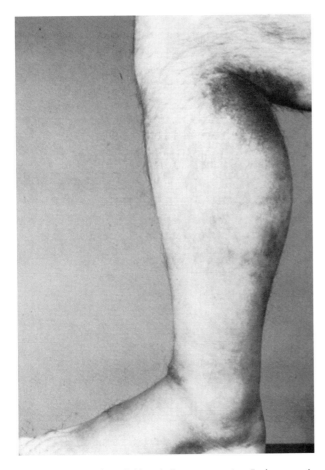

Fig. 38-5. Ruptured medial head of gastrocnemius. Ecchymoses in popliteal fossa and malleoli (below).

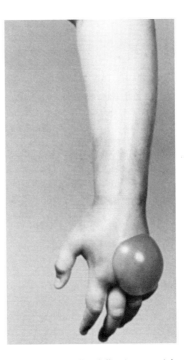

Fig. 38-6. Revascularization bullae following arterial revascularization.

The patient is advised to avoid physical activity with quick stop-and-go actions for the duration of the recovery process. Following recovery, an ongoing stretching program before and after any exercise is critical.

Revascularization

There are several mechanisms for limb swelling following revascularization of an extremity. Besides the trauma of surgical incisions, revascularization creates a pathophysiology similar to that discussed in the section on thermal injury. In the presence of severe, usually chronic, ischemia in an extremity the capillary membrane is damaged and permeability to plasma proteins is altered. Once revascularization occurs, not only is there increased intravascular pressure affecting a damaged capillary membrane, but also the increased permeability allows greater egress of the plasma proteins from the intravascular space. Occasionally, the factors favoring edema formation are so strong that in addition to generalized leg swelling, actual bullous formation occurs (Figs. 38-6 and 38-7).[2] These bullae can resolve quietly and require only clean dressings following spontaneous rupture.

Retroperitoneal Fibrosis

In retroperitoneal fibrosis, involvement of the venous and lymphatic vessels in the retroperitoneal space can

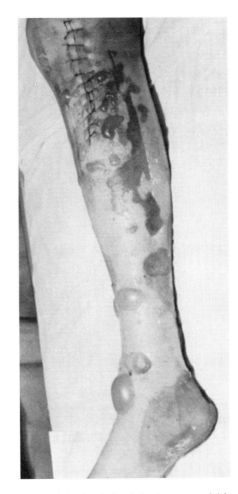

Fig. 38-7. Revascularization bullae following successful femoral-popliteal bypass.

produce lower extremity swelling. Lower extremity swelling can be either unilateral or bilateral. Retroperitoneal fibrosis can be idiopathic or can occur secondary to the use of methysergide (Sansert) for the treatment of migraine headache. Occasionally a positive response can be obtained with the use of steroids for retroperitoneal fibrosis.

Hemihypertrophy

Patients with hemihypertrophy usually know that one side of their body is larger than the other since birth. A size difference is present not only in the legs but also in the arms, and trunk, and occasionally there is a size difference in the face.[7]

Factitial Limb Swelling

Factitial limb swelling can be very difficult to diagnose and treat. Factitial edema is self-induced by a constrictive garment, strap, or device. The history is confusing because the edema has a fluctuating pattern in terms of its occurrence and its relationship to activity or time of day. The problem can continue for many months or years before being suspected. The most helpful clue on physical examination is a distinct, sharp demarcation at the edge of the edema and evidence of skin marks correlating with the type and location of constricting device used to produce the swelling (Fig. 38-8). Treatment of this entity requires the involvement of multiple clinical disciplines including psychiatry and the building of support networks for the patient.

CAUSES OF BILATERAL SWOLLEN LIMB
(see the accompanying box)

Bilateral development of any of the listed unilateral causes of limb swelling can occur and give the picture of bilateral swelling. For example, deep vein thrombophlebitis can occur in both legs, or a patient could have lymphedema in one leg and a deep vein thrombophlebitis in the other leg.

Congestive Heart Failure

Limb edema can be associated with congestive heart failure, may be very subtle, and may not be associated with the typical findings of dyspnea on exertion, orthopnea, or paroxysmal nocturnal dyspnea. In older people limb edema frequently occurs concurrently with chronic obstructive pulmonary disease and congestive heart failure. In this setting, edema can be an early manifestation.

Cirrhosis

Because of many dilated venous tributaries and multiple small arterial venous fistulas, hepatic cirrhosis is commonly associated with an increased total blood volume with decreased effective blood volume. When combined with alterations in serum albumin levels there is further activation of the salt and water retaining mechanisms of the body. Peripheral edema is usually seen in this condition only when both mechanisms are present and hypoalbuminemia is readily detected.[3]

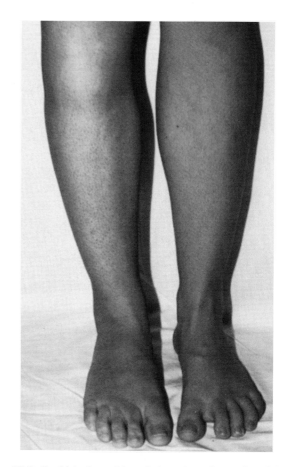

Fig. 38-8. Factitial edema. Note distinct circumferential mark from tourniquet constriction on proximal right calf.

CAUSES OF BILATERAL SWOLLEN LIMB

Congestive heart failure

Cirrhosis

Protein deficient states

Acute glomerulonephritis

Cushing's syndrome

Vena caval obstruction

Pregnancy

Obesity

Lipedema

Dependency

Pretibial myxedema

Drug-induced

Idiopathic cyclic edema

Protein Deficiency States

In protein deficiency states such as severe malnutrition or protein-losing gastroenteropathy, the marked decrease of plasma proteins results in a decrease in the plasma colloid oncotic pressure. These changes in plasma colloid oncotic pressure significantly enhance the increase in interstitial fluid accumulation. Nephrotic syndrome results in edema through the same changes in plasma proteins. However, the cause of the hypoproteinemic state is the markedly increased renal loss of protein in the urine, not secondary to decreased synthesis or intake.

Acute Glomerulonephritis

In the presence of abnormal renal function, not only are there hemodynamic factors causing edematous states but also intrinsic changes in the kidney that favor edema formation. Acute glomerulonephritis appears to create a primary renal avidity for sodium and water, in addition to changes in capillary permeability and their secondary hemodynamic changes.[3] Hematuria, proteinuria, and hypertension are usually also present with the edema.

Cushing's Syndrome

Cushing's syndrome is the result of increased production of cortisol (hydrocortisone) by the adrenal gland. The syndrome can also be produced by ingestion of hydrocortisone-containing or producing drugs. Although cortisol normally increases solute free water clearance, at high concentrations cortisol favors tubular sodium reabsorption. It is this mineralocorticoid activity of high levels of cortisol that leads to edema formation.

Vena Caval Obstruction

Superior and inferior vena caval syndromes are seen more frequently with the increasing use of indwelling catheters and devices. Both malignant and nonmalignant processes can compromise either caval system, resulting in bilateral edema.[8]

Idiopathic Cyclic Edema

Idiopathic cyclic edema is poorly understood and not well recognized. The diagnosis is made after other causes of edema have been excluded. It affects almost exclusively women who are usually 20 to 40 years of age. They may be mildly obese and may have associated psychosomatic complaints or disorders. The typical location for the edema is in both the upper and lower extremities as well as the face. The edema appears to be directly related to the upright position, and a 2- to 4-pound weight gain throughout the day can occur. This syndrome is not to be confused with the fluid retention associated with the menstrual cycle. There are no definitive pathophysiologic mechanisms to explain idiopathic edema. Several mechanisms have been proposed including secondary hyperaldosteronism, excessive secretion of antidiuretic hormone, orthostatic change in capillary membrane permeability, estrogen/progesterone hormone imbalance, abnormal albumin metabolism, and even defects in the vasomotor tone of the capillary venous system. The number of treatments suggested is greater than the number of explanations for this syndrome. Suggested treatments have included restrictive salt and water intake, bed rest, weight loss, the use of elastic support stockings, and modified psychotherapy. Numerous medications have been reported to be effective, including progesterone, spironolactone, thiazide, other diuretics, propranolol, captopril, and dextroamphetamine. With such a wide array of suggested pathophysiology and treatments, it is fortunate that idiopathic cyclic edema tends to subside in a self-limiting course from a few months to several years.[9]

Pregnancy

In contrast to disease processes that create swollen extremities, pregnancy causes peripheral vasodilation, which creates a decrease in the effective blood volume. This, in turn, leads to sodium and fluid retention. There appears to be some compensatory mechanism that does not allow the sodium retention to progress to the same degree as seen in individuals with abnormal disease states and similar pathophysiology.[10] In addition, during pregnancy the gravid uterus can compress the lower venous collecting system, thus increasing distal venous pressure.

Obesity

Obesity appears to be associated with sodium and fluid retention. Multiple mechanisms have been suggested for this including increased peripheral vasodilation with increased surface area of the interstitial spaces. Obesity also creates bilateral "swelling," with the deposition of fat in the subcutaneous tissues, giving the appearance of enlargement to the extremity.

Lipedema

Lipedema is a bilateral and symmetric deposition of fat in the lower extremities in a very characteristic pattern (Fig. 38-9). The excess fat deposits are noted in the buttocks and legs, but they stop at the ankles; the feet are spared. The enlargement of the extremities is nonpitting unless there is an associated fluid retention syndrome. This was first described by Allen and Hines in 1940, with little additional description or information written about this distinct entity since that time.[11] Lipedema occurs almost exclusively in women, and there may be a familial tendency. Patients complain of swelling, pain, and tenderness in the involved areas, especially if they have mistakenly been told to wear heavy elastic support stockings.

Dependency

Dependency warrants mentioning again as a mechanism for bilateral edema formation. Prolonged sitting or standing will result in some degree of edema in almost everyone. Patients with severe rheumatoid or osteoarthritis and patients confined to a wheelchair or chair because of a stroke, amputation, or paraplegia are especially prone to develop dependent edema. Dependency because of ischemic pain can cause marked swelling. These tendencies are aggravated by excessive salt intake or warm weather and can occur before or during menstruation or during pregnancy.

The recognition of dependent edema is important not only to avoid unnecessary testing or invasive procedures but also to focus on the treatment of the underlying cause of the dependency.

Pretibial Myxedema

Hyperthyroidism may be associated with the development of pretibial myxedema. Skin changes occur on the

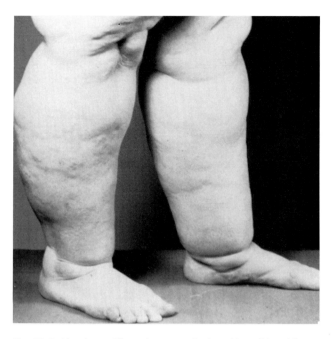

Fig. 38-9. Lipedema. Bilateral, symmetric deposition of fat with no involvement of the feet.

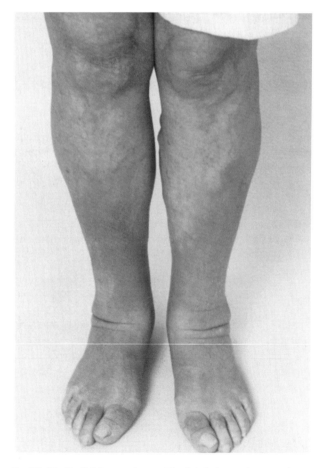

Fig. 38-10. Pretibial myxedema with slightly hyperpigmented, thickened skin over distal portion of lower legs and feet.

pretibial regions or on the dorsa of the feet (Fig. 38-10). The tissue appears to be raised, thickened, or infiltrated but without true pitting. Evidence of pretibial myxedema can occur during active hyperthyroidism after treatment, or even in the absence of thyroid disease.[12] The process appears self-limited, and spontaneous resolution can occur.

Drug-Induced Edema

Drugs can cause bilateral soft, pitting edema in the dependent portions of the extremities. The edema resolves after the drug is withdrawn. Many hormonal drugs including corticosteroids, estrogens, progesterones, and testosterone can cause edema. The nonsteroidal antiinflammatory drugs have also been implicated. For example phenylbutazone (Butazolidin), ibuprofen (i.e., Advil or Motrin), sulindac (Clinoril), and most of the other nonsteroidal antiinflammatory drugs. Antihypertensive drugs can also cause this syndrome, including methyldopa (Aldomet), hydralazine (Apresoline), diazoxide (Hyperstat), clonidine (Catapres), reserpine (Serpasil), and the calcium channel blockers. The antibiotics with a high-sodium content have also been reported to produce edema, especially carbenicillin. Edema can also result from taking antidepressants, especially the monoamine oxidase inhibitors.

CONCLUSION

Although the seemingly simple segregation of causes by bilateral versus unilateral involvement might be the most obvious of divisions, clinicians, particularly those who see patients with vascular diseases regularly, are presented with challenging situations that overlap any arbitrary categorization. Patients who have undergone an amputation can only develop unilateral lower extremity swelling, although the cause is one that ordinarily would cause bilateral swelling.

Patients who develop bilateral swelling may have simultaneous or concurrent processes of two normally unilateral causes. An example of simultaneous processes would be the patient who develops bilateral leg swelling caused by a deep vein thrombosis involving the inferior vena cava or the deep veins of both legs. This is not an uncommon occurrence in patients who have underlying cancers. Another example of concurrent activity of related processes is the presence of chronic venous insufficiency in one extremity and the new onset of acute deep vein thrombophlebitis in the other.

Separate causes for limb swelling can occur both simultaneously as well as concurrently. An example of this is the patient with a pelvic cancer that results in secondary lymphedema in one leg and a deep vein thrombophlebitis in the other. These types of unfortunate events do occur and challenge the clinician, not only in terms of diagnosis, but also in terms of management.

The patient with a swollen limb is not only a common problem for the practicing clinician but is also a diagnostic challenge. To accept the challenge and to properly care for the patient, the clinician must have an understanding of the many causes of leg swelling. With this foundation, a thorough history and complete physical examination along with certain tests will allow the clinician to arrive at the correct diagnosis.

REFERENCES

1. Dale WA: The swollen leg. In Ravitch MM, ed: Current problems in surgery, Chicago, 1973, Yearbook Publishers.
2. Ruschhaupt WF: Differential diagnosis of edema of the lower extremities. In Spittell JA: Clinical vascular disease, Philadelphia, 1983, FA Davis Co.
3. Braunwald E: Edema. In Isselacher KJ et al, eds: Harrison's principles of internal medicine, ed 13, New York, 1994, McGraw-Hill.
4. Lofgren KA: Varicose veins. In Juergens JL, Spittell JA, and Fairbairn JF, eds: Peripheral vascular disease, ed 5, Philadelphia, 1980, WB Saunders.
5. Fairbairn JF: Clinical manifestations of peripheral vascular disease. In Juergens JL, Spittell JA, and Fairbairn JF, eds: Peripheral vascular disease, ed 5, Philadelphia, 1980, WB Saunders.
6. Taylor JS and Young JR: The swollen limb: cutaneous clues to diagnosis and treatment, Cutis 21:553, 1978.
7. Young JR: The swollen leg, Cardiol Clin 9:443, 1991.
8. Browman MW et al: Pancreatic pseudocyst that compressed the inferior vena cava and resulted in edema of the lower extremities, Mayo Clinic Proc 67:1085, 1992.
9. Feldman HA, Jayakumar S, and Puschett JB: Idiopathic edema: a review of etiologic concepts and management, Cardiovasc Med 3:475, 1978.
10. Schrier RW: Body fluid volume regulation in health and disease. A unifying hypothesis, Ann Intern Med 113:155, 1990.
11. Allen EV and Hines EA Jr: Lipedema of the legs: a syndrome characterized by fat legs and orthostatic edema, Proc Staff Meet Mayo Clinic 15:184, 1940.
12. Somach SC et al: Pretibial mucin, Arch Dermatol 129:1152, 1993.

CHAPTER THIRTY-NINE

VASCULAR DISEASES OF THE UPPER LIMB

Thom W. Rooke
Anthony W. Stanson

A wide variety of pathologic conditions can affect the arteries, veins, and lymphatic vessels of the upper limb. Although the overall incidence of vascular disease is less in the upper limb than it is in the lower limb (largely because of the lower incidence of atherosclerosis and venous thrombosis), the frequency of certain conditions (i.e., cold-induced vasospasm or occupational occlusive disease) is substantially higher in the upper limb. The clinical spectrum of upper limb vascular disease is diverse. Some conditions cause symptoms that are minimal and little more than a nuisance, while others may result in limb loss or severe disability.

ARTERIOSCLEROSIS AND ARTERIAL OBSTRUCTIVE DISEASES

Atherosclerosis

Atherosclerosis affects the arteries of the upper limb less frequently than it does those of the lower limbs. Exact figures for the incidence of upper extremity atherosclerosis are difficult to obtain. One report from Cincinnati described a 20-year experience with 6149 limbs affected by arterial occlusive disease. Of these only 288 (4.7%) were upper limbs.[1] In most of these cases the occlusive process was thought to be atherosclerosis, although documentation of this was usually unavailable. A similar low incidence of clinically significant upper extremity atherosclerosis was also observed during a 20-year series from the Mayo Clinic.[2] Based upon these studies and others it is reasonable to estimate that serious atherosclerosis is at least 20 times less frequent in the upper extremity than in the lower extremity. The reasons for the lower incidence in the upper limbs is unknown.

The mechanisms underlying atherosclerosis formation are complex and have been discussed in Chapter 8. Risk factors for upper extremity atherosclerosis are probably the same as those for atherosclerosis elsewhere—namely family history of atherosclerosis, male gender, smoking, hypertension, diabetes, and increased lipids. Some forms of trauma may also predispose to the formation of atherosclerosis-like lesions. The relative contribution made by each of these factors remains uncertain.

Atherosclerosis in the upper limb occurs more frequently (and severely) in proximal than in distal vessels. The subclavian (or innominate) and axillary arteries are most commonly affected (Fig. 39-1), whereas disease development distally is unusual.[3] Atherosclerosis of the aortic arch may also limit blood flow to the upper extremities, particularly if it (1) involves the orifice of the vessels coming off the arch or (2) results in aortic aneurysm formation or dissection (the latter may cause subsequent obstruction of the brachiocephalic vessels). Other complications of atherosclerosis include *atheroemboli* (which typically originate from fragmenting plaques and ulcers) and thrombosis (which may occur spontaneously at sites where plaques rupture or cause vessel stenosis).

SYMPTOMS. The symptoms of upper extremity atherosclerosis are similar to those produced by atherosclerosis in the leg and are influenced not only by the level and severity of the arterial occlusion but also by the extent of arterial collateralization. *Claudication** occurs when arm exercise increases the muscular demand for blood beyond that which can be supplied via the diseased arteries and collaterals. The limb is asymptomatic at rest, but muscle fatigue, pain, or cramping develop during exercise. *Rest pain* occurs when the blood supply is insufficient to meet the resting metabolic demands of the limb (i.e., *ischemia*). If untreated, rest pain may lead to subsequent tissue breakdown, ulceration, and gangrene. *Atheroemboli* may cause small areas of infarction, particularly in the distal

*This is actually a misnomer, since the Latin root from which it is derived refers to a limping gait.

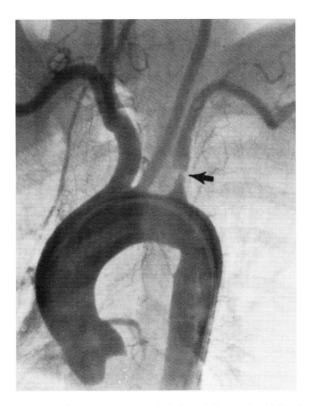

Fig. 39-1. Arch aortogram. Stenotic lesion of the proximal left sub-clavian artery *(arrow)* is atheromatous disease.

portion of the fingers. The *subclavian steal syndrome* occurs when subclavian obstruction develops proximal to the origin of the carotid or vertebral artery, thus creating a situation in which the arm may be perfused by retrograde carotid or vertebral flow. Physical activity involving the affected limb increases the demand for limb blood flow and in doing so augments the "steal" from the neural circulation, which may lead to the development of central nervous system symptoms.

EVALUATION. When upper extremity atherosclerosis is suspected, the history and physical examination should include an assessment of (1) the presence of atherosclerosis in other vessels, especially the coronary and renal arteries and the arteries of the lower extremities, (2) cardiovascular risk factors that can be potentially modified such as smoking, hypertension, hyperlipidemia, and poor control of diabetes, and (3) the degree of disability or discomfort produced by the occlusive disease. Each of these factors (along with other aspects of the patient's overall health status) will influence therapeutic decisions.

Functional testing plays an important role in the assessment of obstructive lesions (see Chapter 3). Segmental pressures (obtained from inflatable cuffs placed at various levels along the arm) can be measured and compared with the pressure in the contralateral arm or in the legs; this provides information about the location and severity of the disease. In situations where the degree of obstruction is insufficient to affect resting blood pressure, a drop in pressure may be observed following exercise of the limb. Other standard noninvasive vascular laboratory studies (e.g., pulse volume recordings, Doppler waveform analysis,

transcutaneous oxygen tension measurements, and skin temperature recordings) can provide variable degrees of potentially useful information and may be performed if available.

Arteriography remains the gold standard for imaging the arteries of the upper extremity and should be used to evaluate atherosclerosis when indicated. Angiographic studies must include an arch aortogram with additional selective injections and filming. Duplex scanning (two-dimensional real-time ultrasound and Doppler technology) and magnetic resonance imaging are becoming increasingly attractive as alternatives in certain situations, especially for screening purposes.

THERAPY. Significant atherosclerotic disease has traditionally been treated surgically. *Bypass operations*, using conduits such as saphenous veins, hypogastric artery, or synthetic grafts, can be performed.[4,5] Local endarterectomy may be useful in situations where focal disease is present.[6,7] *Stellate ganglion sympathectomy* is occasionally a useful adjunct to revascularization, especially when ischemia is severe and the small, more distal vessels of the hands or arms are also obstructed.[8] Balloon *angioplasty* (with or without stent placement),[9] mechanical *atherectomy*, and recanalization using urokinase or other means may be employed in some situations, although the potential for embolization into the cerebral arteries makes work with these methods dangerous when used on lesions proximal to the carotid or vertebral arteries.[10] Conservative therapy involving risk factor reduction and regular upper extremity exercise is an option in most cases and should be considered whenever possible. Except for the long-term benefits derived from the use of drugs that help to reduce such risk factors as hyperlipidemia, hypertension, and elevated blood sugar, there has been little success using medical pharmacology (such as vasodilators) in the treatment of upper extremity atherosclerosis.

Emboli

Clinically significant emboli to the upper extremities occur 5 to 10 times less frequently than emboli to the lower extremity.[11] Thrombotic material originating within the heart accounts for most (up to 90%) of these emboli[12]; conditions predisposing to embolization include atrial fibrillation, myocardial infarction, cardiomyopathy, congestive heart failure, rheumatic valvular disease, cardioversion, prosthetic valves, cardiac surgery or catheterization, and others.[13] Vegetations associated with endocarditis and atrial myxoma are other potential causes of cardiac-derived emboli, and may give rise to mycotic aneurysms (Fig. 39-2). Noncardiac sources of emboli include aneurysms of the aorta (or major branch vessels) and complicated arterial plaques (Fig. 39-3). These lesions frequently give rise to microemboli composed largely of platelets and plaque components such as cholesterol. Rarely, paradoxical emboli may pass from the venous circulation across a patent foramen ovale and lodge in the upper extremity.[14]

Emboli to large- or medium-size vessels usually manifest themselves as acute arterial occlusion. Typically, there is a discrete point beyond which pulsations are diminished or lost. The extremity becomes cool, painful, pale, mottled, or discolored, and both sensation and motor function may

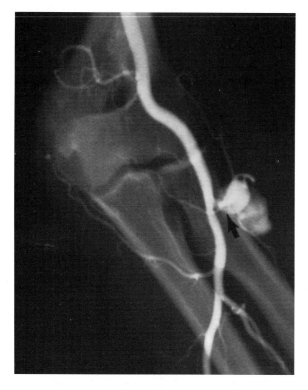

Fig. 39-2. Arm arteriogram. Mycotic aneurysm at the proximal radial artery *(arrow)* in a patient with bacterial endocarditis.

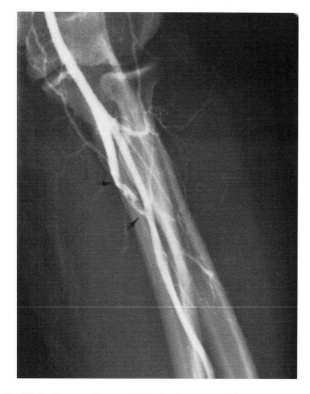

Fig. 39-3. Arm arteriogram. Embolus in proximal ulnar artery *(arrows)*. This was a complication from a proximal subclavian atheromatous stenosis.

become impaired. Acute arterial occlusion may constitute a true medical emergency that can lead to limb loss. However, if collateral vessels around the obstructed site are present, acute arterial occlusion may be relatively asymptomatic. Microemboli tend to shower the distal extremity and cause skin discoloration, pain, and small areas of cutaneous infarction. Repeated episodes of microembolization to the same area are common. Although often serious, microemboli are less likely than large emboli to cause limb loss.

EVALUATION. The diagnosis of acute arterial embolic occlusion can usually be made on clinical grounds alone, especially when there is sudden onset of ischemia in a patient known (or found on subsequent examination) to have a cardiac problem predisposing to emboli. It is essential to assess the severity of limb ischemia since this dictates the course and speed of therapy. Noninvasive vascular laboratory studies are rarely necessary. Angiography may be indicated, especially when a structural problem with the artery (such as aneurysm or stenosis) is suspected at or above the level of the occlusion. A thorough cardiac examination is required when emboli may have originated in the heart. Two-dimensional real-time echocardiography (either transthoracic or transesophageal) appears to be the best technique for identifying potential cardiac sources in these patients.[15,16]

THERAPY. The patient with acute arterial occlusion should be heparinized immediately if no contraindications are present. Steps to diagnose and localize the embolus should be performed promptly because of the potential seriousness of the situation. If ischemia is severe, and the embolus appears to be relatively proximal in location, balloon catheter embolectomy should be attempted as soon as possible (flow must be restored within 6 to 12 hours to prevent or minimize permanent damage). In cases of suspected embolism, this can be done without preceding angiography.[17] If embolectomy fails or if the artery has underlying structural problems, arteriography and revascularization surgery can be performed. Lysis of the emboli, using lytic agents such as streptokinase, urokinase, or tissue plasminogen activator (administered systemically or via a catheter placed in the artery), is also an option in certain patients.[18] The restoration of flow following a period of ischemia may be accompanied by muscle swelling and the development of compartment syndrome in up to 10% of patients.[11,19] When embolization is not limb threatening, conservative measures may be employed initially. These include anticoagulation, positioning of the limb into a slightly dependent position, protection of the limb from trauma, and prevention of heat loss. Spontaneous lysis, recanalization, or the development of collateral vessels may occur from hours to weeks and result in significant clinical improvement.

Microemboli are usually best treated by immediate anticoagulation and conservative measures. The cardiac or vascular source of emboli must be identified and treated appropriately to prevent recurrences. Depending on their etiology and the response to treatment, long-term therapy with warfarin or antiplatelet agents may be indicated.[20]

Despite the institution of therapeutic measures, upper extremity embolization often necessitates a minor (46%

incidence in one series) or major (16%) amputation.[21] Even when the limb has been successfully treated, there is a high (approximately 25%) mortality rate in these patients resulting from emboli affecting other organs.[21]

Inflammatory Disorders

The vasculitides (conditions in which blood vessel inflammation is the primary process) comprise a large group of systemic disorders that encompass an extremely broad spectrum of causes, pathologies, and clinical manifestations. Involvement of the upper extremity with arteritis, either as an isolated finding or as part of the systemic disorder, is a relatively infrequent occurrence. Unfortunately, the vasculitides of the upper extremity are a difficult group of diseases to classify or discuss for several reasons: (1) Most types of vasculitides are rare, and it is unusual for those investigating them to obtain a large series. Many conclusions about specific forms of vasculitides are therefore based upon findings from small series or even case reports. (2) For virtually all types of vasculitides, the underlying cause is unknown. (3) Diseases with different clinical pictures may have nearly identical pathologic findings. (4) The criteria used to diagnose many forms of vasculitides are often poorly defined and unclear. (5) Vasculitis terminology is nonuniform and confusing; in many situations different names are used by various authorities to describe the same diseases.

The histopathologic findings in vasculitis are highly variable. Inflammation is (by definition) present at some time in all types and includes such nonspecific findings as edema, deposition of fibrin and complement, and infiltration by various inflammatory cells.[22] Inflammation (which can be diffuse or focal) may involve the entire thickness of the vessel wall uniformly, or it may predominate in certain layers. Intraluminal thrombosis may occur. In some types granulomas form. When the integrity and structure of the vessel are destroyed by inflammation, the vasculitis is said to be *necrotizing*.

It is perhaps easiest to classify the vasculitides of the upper extremity according to the size of the involved vessel.

SMALL VESSELS. Many systemic disorders may have as part of their presentation a small vessel vasculitis involving the upper extremity. This type of vasculitis is frequently associated with rheumatic diseases such as systemic lupus erythematosus, rheumatoid arthritis, dermatomyositis, mixed connective tissue diseases, and scleroderma.[23] Other types such as erythema nodosum and hypersensitivity angiitis may be associated with various systemic disorders or can occur *de novo*. Circulating factors (such as cryoglobulins, hepatitis A antigen, myeloma proteins, macroglobulins, and others) and various drugs or medicines may also be associated with vasculitis.[24-26] Autoimmunity is thought to play an etiologic role in many, if not most, situations.[27] The tissues most frequently involved are the skin and joints, although damage to other structures can occur. Fingers and hands (Fig. 39-4) are usually affected but the entire upper limb may be involved. Clinical (primarily dermal) manifestations of disease include urticaria, rashes, livedo, purpura, Raynaud's phenomenon, hemorrhage, infarction, ulceration, and gangrene.

MEDIUM-SIZE VESSELS. Polyarteritis nodosa is the classic example of a vasculitis that affects medium-size vessels, although small vessels are frequently involved as well. The disease is idiopathic but resembles serum sickness in many ways, which suggests a possible autoimmune origin. A role for infective agents has also been postulated. Similar diseases that rarely affect medium and small vessels of the upper extremity (and which may be variants of polyarteritis nodosa) include such entities as Wegener's granulomatosis, lymphomatoid granulomatosis, Kawasaki

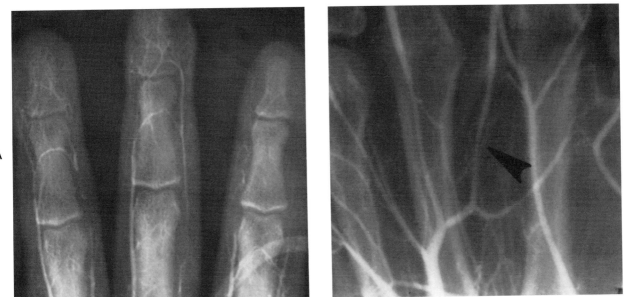

Fig. 39-4. Hand arteriogram. Vasculitis of an indeterminate type in a young female. **A,** Digital artery occlusions and segments of stenoses. **B,** Metacarpal artery with smooth-walled narrowing (*arrowhead*). A similar finding is present in two adjacent arteries.

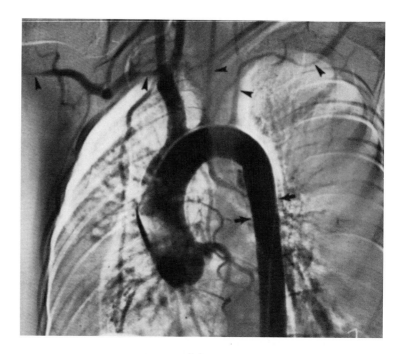

Fig. 39-5. Arch aortogram of patient with Takayasu's disease. The segments of stenoses *(arrowheads)* of the brachiocephalic arteries are typical for a giant cell type of arteritis. Because the left common carotid artery (and proximal left subclavian artery) is involved, the angiographic findings are specific for Takayasu's arteritis. Note also the irregularity of the aortic wall *(arrows)*.

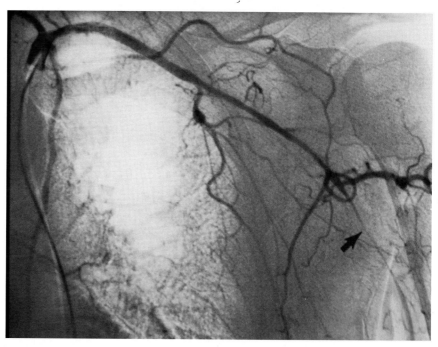

Fig. 39-6. Left subclavian arteriogram of patient with temporal arteritis. Axillary and proximal brachial *(arrow)* arteries have segments of smooth-wall narrowing and tapered stenosis.

disease,[28] and Churg-Strauss syndrome. These diseases typically involve the skin (necrosis or gangrene) and may produce neuropathy.

LARGE VESSELS. Large vessel vasculitides that affect the upper limb include Takayasu's arteritis (Fig. 39-5), temporal arteritis (Fig. 39-6), Behçet's syndrome, Cogan's syndrome, and the arteritis associated with relapsing polychondritis and various seronegative spondyloarthropathies. Takayasu's[29] and temporal arteritis are probably the most common and important of these. Both can affect the aorta and large branch vessels and appear pathologically similar, with granulomatous and nongranulomatous inflammation tending to involve the entire thickness of the

arterial wall. However, Takayasu's arteritis tends to affect patients who are younger (under 40 years of age) and frequently female (female-to-male ratio is 5:1), while temporal arteritis affects those who are older (over 55 years of age) and less often female (female-to-male ratio of 2:1). Takayasu's arteritis appears to affect the upper extremity more frequently than temporal arteritis does. The symptoms of these diseases are typically those of upper extremity arterial occlusive disease, namely arm claudication, rest pain, or tissue breakdown. Aneurysm formation involving the brachiocephalic vessels (and the associated complications of acute arterial occlusion or distal embolization) may also occur.

Buerger's Disease

Buerger's disease (thromboangiitis obliterans) is an unusual entity that is probably best classified as a vasculitis, although not all authorities agree.[10,30] Patients are usually male (80% to 90%) and young (under 50 years of age), suggesting that youth and male gender are important risk factors, although the incidence in women appears to be increasing as women smoke more.[31,32] Other factors such as heredity, race, and geography may also be involved. The cause of Buerger's disease is unknown, but tobacco abuse appears to play a critical role.

The disease affects the small- and medium-size arteries of the limbs early in its course and may progress to involve the large arteries (Fig. 39-7) as well as veins and nerves.[33-35] Pathologically, the disease is *panvasculitis* in which the lumen typically contains thrombus with organizing fibroblasts and other cellular elements (including giant cells), while the intima, media, and adventitia demonstrate various degrees of thickening and infiltration by inflammatory cells. Unlike other types of vasculitis, Buerger's disease rarely has systemic manifestations or involvement of blood vessels outside of the extremities. The clinical signs and symptoms are similar to those of occlusive disease from other causes, although often more severe. Gangrene with subsequent amputation (autoamputation or surgical) of fingers, hands, or arms is not unusual.

EVALUATION. The history and physical examination are helpful in assessing patients with vasculitis. Antecedent illness, smoking habits, a history of drug or medication use, and associated medical conditions (such as the presence of a rheumatic disease) should be sought. Vasculitis occurring elsewhere in the body must be identified and evaluated as necessary. The distribution and appearance of cutaneous findings may provide helpful clues. When large vessels are involved, pulses may be reduced and bruits heard. Laboratory tests, especially the erythrocyte sedimentation rate, can be very helpful. Abnormalities in hepatic or renal function may provide clues to the presence of vasculitis in these organs. In many cases, especially with small-vessel processes involving the skin, biopsy is the only way to confirm the diagnosis. Biopsy should be obtained from a clinically involved area when possible. When it is not possible, blind biopsy of the testicle, muscle, or nerve may be attempted but the diagnostic yield is low. Arteriography is indicated in many cases of large- and medium-size vessel disease, not only to make the diagnosis but also to plan surgery.

THERAPY. Treatment depends on the type of vasculitis present. In many situations the condition will resolve spontaneously and conservative measures are therefore all that is necessary. Discontinuation of tobacco use typically leads to improvement, especially in Buerger's disease.[36] Prednisone and various immunosuppressive agents are useful in a variety of disease types. The dosage and duration of therapy is largely determined by the clinical response, although changes in the erythrocyte sedimentation rate may also be used to guide treatment.[37] The occlusive symptoms of Takayasu's and temporal arteritis have been shown to stabilize and resolve following adequate steroid therapy. Some types of vasculitis are life-threatening because of their systemic effects, and balancing the therapeutic benefits of steroids or immunosuppressive agents against their toxicity can be difficult. Trimethoprim-sulfamethoxazole has been reported to be efficacious in patients with Wegener's granulomatosis,[38] but the role of antibiotics in other conditions is questionable. When aneurysms or fixed stenotic lesions have developed, surgical repair or revascularization is an option, especially after the inflammatory process is resolved or controlled.[39]

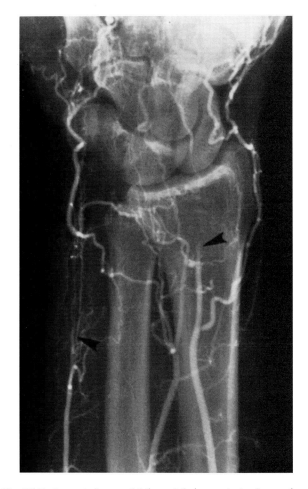

Fig. 39-7. Arm arteriogram (at the wrist) demonstrates Buerger's disease in a young male smoker. The tapered occlusions of the ulnar and radial arteries *(arrowheads)*, in conjunction with distal arterial occlusions and skip areas of normal arterial segments, are typical angiographic findings.

TRAUMATIC AND OCCUPATIONAL DISEASE

A significant amount of upper extremity vascular disease occurs as a result of trauma, which can be acute or chronic.

Acute Trauma

Of the 66,000 surgical procedures performed annually in the United States for the repair of damaged blood vessels, an appreciable number involve the upper extremity. *Penetrating wounds* caused by bullets, knives, and punctures predominate and may affect the blood vessels of the limb at any level. Vascular disruption usually causes obvious problems, but damage from penetrating wounds may be occult in up to 25% to 35% of injuries.[40] Secondary thrombosis or aneurysm (either true or false) formation[41] can complicate matters. *Blunt trauma* resulting from high-impact deceleration, crush injuries, or blows to the arm also occur frequently. Thrombosis is probably the most common sequela, but hemorrhage, spasm, stenosis, or aneurysm formation,[42,43] is possible. *Iatrogenic injuries* are seen with increasing frequency as medicine becomes more procedure-oriented. Catheterization procedures involving the arm[44] (especially those performed via a brachial or axillary vascular access site) and nonvascular surgical procedures on the upper extremity are the usual causes, but occasionally arterial punctures for blood gas determinations, direct pressure measurements, or even phlebotomy can produce significant vascular injury.[45] Vascular injuries related to intravascular drug use are also increasing in frequency.[46] *Miscellaneous* pathologic conditions caused by acute trauma include *fat embolization* (which follows injury to bones and adjacent blood vessels) and *compression syndromes* (which occur when edema or swelling cause extrinsic compression of blood vessels sufficient enough to impair flow). Fasciotomy may be required to relieve a compression syndrome and restore circulation.

Chronic Trauma

Repeated episodes of trauma may also injure arteries. Arterial occlusive complications related to intermittent periods of arterial compression caused by the thoracic outlet syndrome are common. Exposure to *chronic vibration* (which occurs in workers using chain saws, jack hammers, and drills) provides another example of ischemia caused by recurrent low-level trauma.[47-51] Histopathologic changes in the small arteries of affected individuals include hypertrophy of smooth muscle cells, periarterial fibrosis, demyelination and loss of periarterial nerve fibers, increases in collagen-containing connective tissues, and loss of elastic fibers. These changes (and others) result in arterial narrowing, luminal obstruction, vasospasm, and thrombosis (Fig. 39-8). For reasons that are not well understood, patients with vibratory-induced disease may also have increased blood viscosity. The use of antifibrin agents to reduce the viscosity has been investigated.[52] Generalized abnormalities in sympathetic nerve function also occur. The *hypothenar hammer syndrome*, in which the hands develop ulnar arterial irregularities (Fig. 39-9) or occlusion (Fig. 39-10) as a result of excessive vibration[53] or use in activities such as squeezing or pounding, represents another syndrome produced by chronic trauma.[54,55] Similar types of small vessel arterial occlusive, thrombotic, and vasospastic problems have also been observed in typists, piano players, baseball and hockey players, and in virtually every occupation or hobby wherein strenuous use of the hands occurs.[56]

The evaluation of patients with vascular trauma involving the upper extremity should include both functional and imaging studies when necessary. Noninvasive functional testing, described earlier in this chapter, is especially important in those patients for whom disability is an issue.[57-59] The liberal use of arteriography has been recommended for ruling out or evaluating vascular injury.[40,60] The roles of duplex scanning,[61] computerized tomography, and magnetic resonance imaging in the diagnosis and

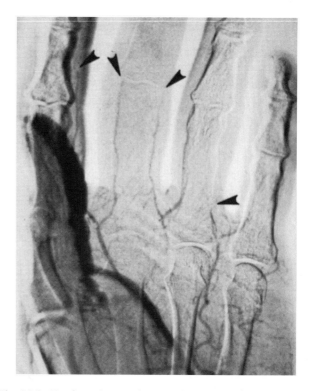

Fig. 39-8. Hand arteriogram showing chronic vibration injury. Multiple digital artery occlusions *(arrow)* and preceding irregular, stenotic segments indicate a long exposure to vibration tools.

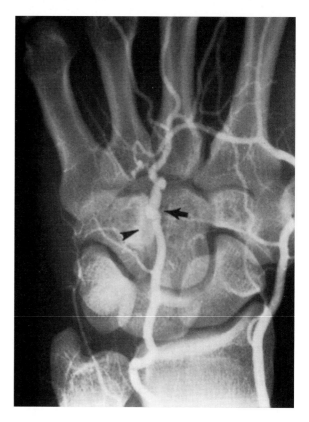

Fig. 39-9. Hand arteriogram. Ulnar artery injury from using the hand as a "hammer." The irregularities *(arrow)* of the short arterial zone over the hook of the hamate bone *(arrowhead)* are the result of repeated trauma.

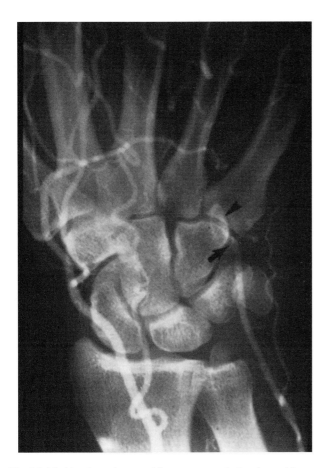

Fig. 39-10. Hand arteriogram. Ulnar artery occlusion *(arrow)* from trauma (hammer-hand) occurs over the hamate bone hook *(arrowhead)*.

evaluation of vascular trauma are expanding and may soon replace arteriography in many situations.

The treatment of traumatic and occupational diseases involves several steps. The most important is to eliminate the source of vibration or trauma. Structural repair or bypass of the affected arteries using microsurgical techniques may be indicated.[62] The use of vasodilators to combat spasm may offer some therapeutic benefit in selected patients (see the upcoming section on vasospasm).

Miscellaneous Conditions

A variety of miscellaneous pathologic processes can obstruct the arteries of the upper limb. For example, *degenerative arteriopathies* (as occur with diseases such as the Marfan syndrome, Ehlers-Danlos syndrome, so-called "cystic medial necrosis," and a multitude of congenital or acquired conditions involving abnormalities in collagen or elastic tissue composition) may result in aneurysm formation or dissection involving the upper extremity. Arteries such as the brachial artery may rarely be subject to *entrapment*.[63] *Fibromuscular dysplasia* occasionally occurs in the arteries of the upper limb, especially the axillary artery.[64] *Medial calcification*, although seldom a clinical problem, is sometimes incidentally noted on x-ray films of the arm.[65] *Coagulopathies* (including thrombocytosis and the various platelet disorders) may complicate certain systemic illnesses or can appear as isolated entities. Either

way they may contribute to thrombosis and subsequent occlusion of large or small arteries. *Malignancy* can cause thrombosis through unexplained mechanisms.[66-68]

VENOUS DISEASE

In comparison to the lower limbs, the upper limbs are rarely affected by venous disease. The most common venous problem is *thrombosis*, which may be superficial or deep. Usual causes of *superficial venous thrombosis* include systemic illnesses such as malignancy or inflammatory bowel disease, intravenous infusion or injection of irritating drugs, and direct (usually blunt) trauma. *Deep venous thrombosis* may also be caused by any of the factors that produce superficial venous thrombosis. In addition, venous compression (as occurs with any form of thoracic outlet obstruction), indwelling catheters,[69] pacemaker leads,[70] or vigorous use of the upper extremity[71,72] can contribute to thrombosis. Clotting abnormalities may play a role in the cause of either superficial or deep venous thrombosis.

Significant upper extremity deep venous clotting occurs most commonly in the axillary and subclavian veins, although thrombosis of the superior vena cava may also produce symptoms in the upper limb. The clinical manifestations of venous thrombosis include pain and/or swelling at (and distal to) the site of venous occlusion; tender, palpable veins; and cyanotic discoloration of the skin. The severity of symptoms depends on how acute and extensive the thrombosis is. When it is massive, there may be extreme swelling, skin breakdown, and gangrene. Pulmonary embolism from upper extremity deep venous thrombosis may occur in up to 12% of patients,[44] and may be more common in patients with catheter-related thrombosis.[73]

The diagnosis of upper extremity deep venous thrombosis has traditionally required venography, but recent advances in ultrasonic imaging combined with Doppler (i.e., duplex scanning) have made this the preferred test in many situations.[74,75] Treatment of venous thrombosis depends on the severity and location of the clot. As with cases of superficial venous thrombosis that occur elsewhere in the body, superficial venous thrombosis of the upper limb usually responds well to topical heat and antiinflammatory drugs. On the other hand, acute deep venous thrombosis is usually treated with anticoagulants (heparin initially and then warfarin for 6 to 12 weeks). Thrombolysis using any of the currently available lytic agents is also an option.[70,76] For chronic occlusion surgical venous bypass or balloon venoplasty[77] is a potential option.

Occasionally *extrinsic compression* of the brachial veins will mimic venous thrombosis. Tumors, aneurysms of the brachiocephalic arteries, and structural abnormalities of the thoracic outlet do this most commonly. Eliminating the cause of compression is usually sufficient to treat this condition.

NEUROVASCULAR COMPRESSION

The so-called "thoracic outlet syndrome" actually refers to a group of clinical conditions that result from compression of the neurovascular bundle supplying the upper extremity. Symptoms may vary, depending on whether the artery, vein, or nerve is the major affected structure. In many subjects two or even all three components are involved to some degree, thereby complicating the clinical picture. It is estimated by some that 97% of all symptoms in patients with thoracic outlet syndrome are related to compression of the nerves within the brachial plexus, while 2% are caused by venous compression and 1% by arterial compression.[78] Others[79] argue that mild vascular compression may mimic the symptoms of nerve compression. They cite a low incidence of positive electromyographic findings as evidence against significant primary neurologic involvement in most cases (Roos[80] offers opposing arguments as to why nerve involvement might not produce electromyographic changes). Matters are further confused by the fact that 50% to 60% of asymptomatic normal subjects (especially those who are young or athletic) have evidence of intermittent, positional arterial compression.[81] Thus while neurovascular compression appears well established as the cause of thoracic outlet syndrome, the exact pathophysiologic mechanisms by which signs and symptoms are produced remain unclear.

The neurovascular bundle is especially susceptible to compression at three sites along its exit path from the thorax.[79] These sites (costoscalene, costoclavicular, and retropectal) usually provide minimal room for the neurovascular bundle even in normal individuals. Minor anatomic variations can subsequently reduce these routes further and cause neurovascular impingement. Most authorities agree that the costoclavicular position is the most frequent site of compression.[79] Cervical ribs (Fig. 39-11) are common in patients with thoracic outlet syndrome. They occur in up to 1% of the population but cause symptoms in only 5% to 10% of subjects having them.[82] In 50% of cases cervical ribs occur unilaterally.[79] The ribs may be complete (i.e., they have a bony articulation with the first rib), but in most cases they are incomplete and connect to the first rib via a dense fibromuscular band; however, the ability to cause compression may be similar in both situations.

Other forms of congenital fibrous bands can also occur and cause compression, with nine separate types de-

scribed.[80] Other factors responsible for compression include hypertrophic muscles (especially the scalenus anterior); congenital variations in the origin and insertion of various muscles; clavicle or first rib bony abnormalities; trauma, including fractures and "whiplash"-type cervical injuries; poor posture[83,84]; scoliosis; tumors; changes after surgery; muscular dystrophy; and a host of others.[81] Minimal trauma or strain involving the head, neck, or shoulder precipitates the initial appearance of thoracic outlet syndrome in up to 60% of patients.[78]

Symptoms

Because neurovascular compression may affect arteries, veins, or nerves, it is not surprising that the clinical manifestations of thoracic outlet syndrome are extremely diverse. Symptoms of *nerve compression* include numbness, pain, and paresthesias that usually affect the hands and fingers but may involve the entire arm. Weakness is seen less frequently and may be difficult to separate from pain. Symptoms of *arterial compression and obstruction* include cold hands or fingers, arm claudication, aching pain, pallor or cyanosis, Raynaud's phenomenon (in up to 15% of patients), distal embolization, and skin breakdown or ulceration.[79] Symptoms of *venous compression and obstruction* (Fig. 39-12) include swelling, edema, pain, and cyanosis. The fact that certain symptoms (e.g., pain, swelling, or Raynaud's syndrome) can be caused by compression of either nerves or blood vessels makes it difficult to identify the involved structure on the basis of symptoms alone. Some symptoms may be intermittent, positional, and mild

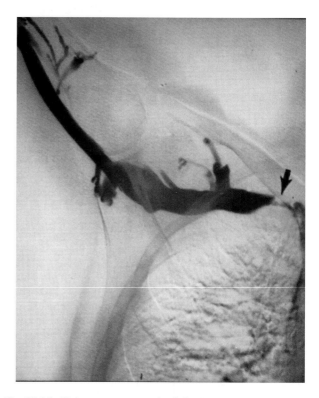

Fig. 39-12. Right arm venogram in abduction. Stenosis *(arrow)* at the junction of the axillary and subclavian segments. A cervical rib had been resected several months earlier. Venous obstruction resulted from postoperative fibrosis.

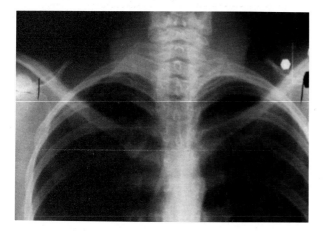

Fig. 39-11. Cervical rib on the right compromises the thoracic outlet.

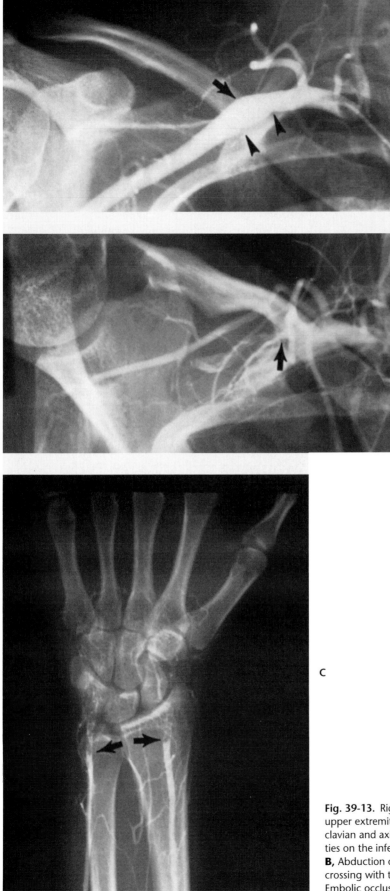

Fig. 39-13. Right subclavian arteriogram. **A,** Neutral position of the upper extremity. Fusiform aneurysm *(arrow)* at the junction of the subclavian and axillary artery segments over a cervical rib. The irregularities on the inferior border of the aneurysm are thrombus *(arrowheads)*. **B,** Abduction of the arm. The subclavian artery occludes *(arrow)* at its crossing with the cervical rib. **C,** Hand arteriogram of the same patient. Embolic occlusions of the radial and ulnar arteries *(arrows)*.

(reflecting compression that occurs in certain positions only) while others may be constant and debilitating (suggesting either chronic compression or failure to recover fully between episodes of intermittent compression).

Several complications appear to be directly related to neurovascular compression (Fig. 39-13).[85] The arterial wall can become inflamed, thickened, and adherent to surrounding structures at the site of compression.[81] Atherosclerosis development is possible. The vessel may also dilate and become ectatic or aneurysmal. These aneurysms are typically fusiform in shape and may be lined by mural thrombus. Complications of these aneurysms include embolization of thrombotic materials, thrombosis causing acute arterial occlusion, or rarely spontaneous rupture. The major venous complication caused by thoracic outlet compression is thrombosis with subsequent limb swelling. As previously noted, nerve dysfunction (documented by electromyography) is an unusual complication of chronic or intermittent compression.

Evaluation

There is universal agreement about the importance of a good history and physical examination in the workup of the patient with suspected thoracic outlet syndrome. The history should include a careful review of (1) the symptoms involved and the circumstances under which they occur (such as which limb position causes symptoms), (2) how long the symptoms have been present and what factor(s) such as strain or trauma precipitated the initial appearance, (3) the degree of disability or discomfort caused by the problem, and (4) other medical conditions that could be factors. The physical examination should include a search for cervical ribs, hypertrophied muscles, subclavian artery aneurysm, distal emboli, and hand or digital ischemia. A good neurologic examination is essential to search for problems such as cervical disk disease or carpal tunnel syndrome. The role of maneuvers designed to demonstrate the positional loss or attenuation of pulses (such as hyperabduction or Adson's maneuver) is controversial. Some authorities feel that many of these are totally unreliable, being falsely negative or positive in too many patients to be of clinical value.[80] Others assign high importance to their use.[79] The key fact on interpreting these tests is the association between a limb position and the development of the patient's usual symptoms. When present, this association is generally significant. Because of the difficulty in proving its presence, thoracic outlet syndrome is frequently a diagnosis of exclusion. One first demonstrates that the disease is consistent with thoracic outlet syndrome and then rules out other potential causes.

The role of many laboratory and imaging tests in the evaluation of thoracic outlet syndrome is often minimal. A chest or cervical x-ray film may be useful for identifying cervical ribs. Most authorities suggest arteriograms only for selected patients, such as those with bony abnormalities, neurologic involvement, arterial insufficiency (with possible atherosclerosis), subclavian aneurysm, or evidence of emboli. Arteriography should not be used to make the diagnosis of thoracic outlet syndrome but rather to identify a fixed vascular abnormality or emboli. Noninvasive laboratory tests are also of limited value, although duplex (ultrasound/Doppler) scanning may have some utility, especially for documenting or assessing stenosis, poststenotic dilation, aneurysm formation, and mural thrombus. The roles of electromyography[86] and somatosensory evoked potentials[87] in diagnosing brachial plexus involvement remain unclear.

Therapy

Conservative measures such as stretching exercises (or other forms of physical therapy), analgesics, and avoidance of positions that cause neurovascular compression may be all that is necessary in mild cases of thoracic outlet syndrome. When this fails or the symptoms are severe, surgery is usually indicated. A variety of operations designed to relieve the compression or to repair damaged blood vessels can be performed, depending on the exact problems present. The surgical details are beyond the scope of this work (see Chapter 31). Resection of ribs (first or cervical) or fibrous bands is usually performed.[79] If subclavian aneurysm formation has occurred, the aneurysm should be resected and replaced by a graft.[81] Nonaneurysmal poststenotic dilation may resolve following the repair of the stenosis or rib resection. However, at what point a reversible poststenotic dilation becomes an irreversible aneurysm is uncertain. Sympathectomy is sometimes performed along with rib resection or other corrective procedure.[88] Venous obstruction can be treated with thrombectomy[89] or thrombolysis.[90] This may be done as an isolated procedure or in conjunction with thoracic outlet decompression.[91]

VASOSPASM

Cutaneous vasoconstriction occurring in response to ambient temperature changes is a normal physiologic mechanism necessary for thermal regulation. When it occurs inappropriately or is excessively intense, it may become pathologic, causing a condition referred to as *Raynaud's syndrome* or *phenomenon*.* Raynaud's syndrome most often affects the upper limb. It may be caused by or associated with a systemic disorder (secondary Raynaud's syndrome), or it can occur as an isolated entity (primary Raynaud's syndrome).

In both the primary and secondary forms of Raynaud's syndrome, females are affected more often than males. Attacks are usually triggered by exposure to the cold or emotional stress.[92] Episodes are most often bilateral, but in some situations (usually with secondary disease) they may be unilateral or even confined to a single digit. During an attack the affected skin typically turns white and may

---

*Various authorities have attempted to differentiate between the terms *Raynaud's syndrome*, *Raynaud's phenomenon*, and *Raynaud's disease*, using Raynaud's disease to describe the primary condition and Raynaud's syndrome or phenomenon to describe secondary conditions. We prefer to use Raynaud's syndrome or phenomenon for any episodic, inappropriate, or severe episode of cutaneous vasoconstriction. Whenever possible, secondary Raynaud's syndrome should be described in terms of the causative or associated condition such as "posttraumatic Raynaud's syndrome," or "Raynaud's syndrome secondary to scleroderma."

become numb or painful. As the episode progresses the discolored areas may become cyanotic and develop rubor before returning to normal. Digital ulcerations are rare in the primary form but occur frequently and can be severe in the secondary disease. The clinical manifestations and consequences of the disease are often determined by the associated conditions. In primary Raynaud's syndrome the symptoms are usually stable and may be little more than a nuisance, while in some forms of secondary Raynaud's syndrome (e.g., scleroderma) severe and debilitating sequelae may evolve.

The pathophysiology of Raynaud's syndrome is poorly understood (see Chapter 23). Many patients appear to have abnormalities in adrenergic function that cause increased vasomotor tone and sensitivity to cold,[93] but the nature of these abnormalities remains obscure. Blood viscosity may also be elevated in some subjects.[94,95] Patients with primary Raynaud's syndrome usually have patent large and small arteries, although those with longstanding disease often demonstrate some evidence of intimal thickening and occasionally show fixed digital artery obstruction.[96] In contrast, patients with secondary disease may have considerable vascular obstruction in the involved extremities. This reflects the fact that vascular occlusive processes related to atherosclerosis, arteritis, thoracic outlet syndrome, embolic occlusions, or rheumatic or occupational diseases are often associated with Raynaud's syndrome. Certain drugs, especially β-blockers, nicotine,[97] and ergotamine-containing compounds[98] may also predispose to vasospasm.

Diagnosis

The diagnosis of Raynaud's syndrome is made largely on clinical grounds. Laboratory study of these patients has traditionally been unsatisfying. Tests to screen for the possibility of large vessel occlusive disease should be performed on all patients. Provocative testing to document and assess abnormal vasoconstriction is often of limited value because of the difficulty in reliably reproducing symptoms in a laboratory setting. In our noninvasive vascular laboratory we immerse the patient's hands in ice water for 30 seconds and document the time required for digital temperature to recover. Normal individuals usually do this in 10 minutes or less, while more prolonged rewarming periods are typically required for patients with clinical evidence of Raynaud's syndrome. Other investigators have used different forms of cold challenge including total-body cooling[99] and have also explored alternative methods for studying the changes in blood flow such as venous occlusion plethysmography,[100] laser-Doppler velocimetry,[101,102] pulse volume recordings, xenon-131 washout,[103] photoplethysmography,[104] and thermography.[105,106] No laboratory method of assessment has emerged as clearly superior at this time.

Therapy

The treatment of Raynaud's syndrome remains a difficult problem. In cases of secondary Raynaud's syndrome, treatment of the underlying condition should be attempted whenever possible. Simple conservative measures such as dressing warmly, avoiding unnecessary exposure to the cold, and intermittently warming the hands[107] may improve matters substantially. Occasionally, moving to a warmer climate may be necessary. Biofeedback is effective in a number of cases.[108] Avoiding drugs with a potential for causing vasoconstriction (e.g., β-blockers, nicotine, and ergotamine) is important. Certain vasodilators may help, especially nifedipine,[109-111] prazosin,[112,113] and possibly ketanserin.[114,115] Interruption of sympathetic nerves to the upper extremity, either through ganglionic injection or surgical sympathectomy, is an option for patients with severe and debilitating symptoms.[116]

ARTERIOVENOUS FISTULAS, MALFORMATIONS, AND VASCULAR TUMORS

Upper extremity arteriovenous fistulas may be *acquired* or *congenital* (see Chapter 33). Acquired arteriovenous fistulas usually result when trauma to the arm disrupts an artery and adjacent vein, allowing blood to flow between the two. These abnormal communications are often occult at first but tend to enlarge from weeks to months and may eventually carry a significant amount of blood. Symptoms of arteriovenous fistulas depend on the blood flow. They may be totally asymptomatic, or they can produce pain, swelling, discoloration, abnormal pulsations of the affected arms, increased limb growth, ischemia distal to the fistula, and elevated skin temperatures. Common types of injury that lead to fistula formation include gunshot and knife wounds, bone fractures, catheterization procedures involving the arm, and surgery.[117] One of the most common forms of upper extremity arteriovenous fistula are those created intentionally for use in hemodialysis.[118]

Congenital arteriovenous malformations (Fig. 39-14) encompass a wide spectrum of lesions in which abnormal arteriovenous shunting may be present. These include *arteriovenous fistulas*, certain tumorlike growths such as *hemangiomas* (which may be arterial, venous, capillary, or mixed, depending on which type of vessel the lesion developed from*), and various forms of *angiodysplasias*. Other benign and malignant tumors (such as hemangiosarcomas, lymphosarcomas, or any large vascular tumor) may be associated with abnormal arteriovenous shunting of blood. Numerous schemes have been developed for naming and categorizing these anomalies, none of which are totally satisfactory. The term *arteriovenous malformation* can therefore be used generically to include all significant congenital vascular lesions, with additional modifying terms affixed as needed.

The diagnosis of arteriovenous fistula or malformation is usually suspected on the basis of the above-mentioned physical findings. Arteriography may be necessary to define the extent of the fistula, especially if surgery or embolotherapy is contemplated. In arteriovenous malformations involving small vessels (especially those that grow rapidly) biopsy may be necessary to ensure that the malformation is not caused by a malignancy. Treatment is by surgical ligation or removal of the fistula (or tumor) when possible.[119] Traumatic arteriovenous fistulas can

---

*Some authors prefer to group all large vessel hemangiomas under the term "cavernous hemangioma."

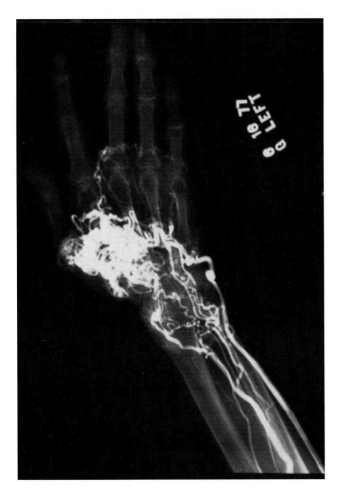

Fig. 39-14. Hand arteriogram. Arteriovenous malformation diffusely involving the wrist and radial aspect of the hand. The lesion involves bones and soft tissues. There is also venous shunting.

usually be repaired surgically without undue difficulty. However, in many cases of congenital malformation the lesion is too extensive to remove. Various embolization techniques have been tried. Unfortunately, while these procedures may temporarily reduce fistula flow, the lesions tend to recur or enlarge, making them difficult to eliminate completely.

LYMPHATIC DISEASE

Upper extremity lymphatic disorders include *lymphangitis* and *lymphatic obstruction.* Lymphangitis (i.e., lymphatic inflammation) usually results from bacterial or fungal entry into the lymphatic vessels via sites of localized infection in the hands or fingers, but it may also be triggered by the direct injection of irritants (such as contrast material for radiologic studies) into the lymphatic vessels. Lymphangitis manifests itself clinically with fever, localized pain and tenderness, and signs of lymphatic inflammation such as red streaks extending up the skin of the arm. In cases of infective lymphangitis, streptococcus is the usual cause and the use of penicillin or other antibiotics with an appropriate spectrum of activity is

therefore indicated.[120] Repeated episodes of lymphangitis may lead to loss or blockage of the lymphatic vessels.

Lymphatic obstruction in the upper extremity may occur secondary to a wide variety of disorders. In the United States the leading cause has been surgical disruption of lymphatic vessels or radiation-induced lymphatic fibrosis occurring as a result of surgical mastectomy and adjuvant radiation therapy for breast cancer.[121] Other common causes of lymphatic obstruction include congenital abnormalities or deficiencies of lymph vessels, recurrent episodes of lymphangitis, and blockage by various types of tumors (local or metastatic). In many tropical countries lymphatic infiltration with various parasites is the leading cause of lymphatic obstruction.[122] The swelling that develops throughout the arm as the result of lymphatic obstruction is referred to as *lymphedema.* The diagnosis of lymphedema is made by (1) ruling out other causes of upper limb swelling and (2) radionuclide lymphatic scanning *(lymphoscintigraphy)* to confirm the lack of vessel patency.[123,124] *Lymphangiography* is probably best avoided because of the potential for causing lymphangitis with additional loss of lymphatic vessels. The treatment of lymphatic obstruction in lymphedema can be difficult. Conservative measures include periodic limb elevation, protection of the involved arm from injury, use of prophylactic antibiotics to prevent infection, and the wearing of an elastic compression garment (sleeve) to reduce and control swelling.[125] Massage (manual lymphatic drainage) and externally applied intermittent compression devices ("lymphatic pumps") are of value in certain situations.[126,127] For patients with proximal obstruction of large lymphatic vessels, bypass operations are a possibility.

REFERENCES

1. Welling RE et al: Obliterative arterial disease of the upper extremity, Arch Surg 116:1593, 1981.
2. Laroche GP et al: Chronic arterial insufficiency of the upper extremity, Mayo Clin Proc 51:180, 1976.
3. Crawford ES et al: Thrombo-obliterative disease of the great vessels arising from the aortic arch, J Thorac Cardiovasc Surg 43:38, 1962.
4. Grant KC: Experience with distal in-situ vein grafts, Can J Surg 30:163, 1987.
5. Hallett JW: Trends in revascularization of the lower extremity, Mayo Clin Proc 61:369, 1986.
6. Carlson RE et al: Innominate endarterectomy: a 16-year experience, Arch Surg 112:1389, 1977.
7. Ekestrom S, Liljequist L, and Nordhus O: Surgical management of obliterative disease of the brachiocephalic trunk, Scand J Thorac Cardiovasc Surg 17:305, 1983.
8. Williams SJ: Chronic upper extremity ischemia: current concepts in management, Surg Clin North Am 66:355, 1986.
9. Bacharach M and Graor RA: Compromised lima graft secondary to proximal subclavian artery stenosis: treatment with endovascular stent placement, J Vasc Med Biol 4:213, 1993.
10. Gomes AS: Arteriography in the diagnosis and management of vascular disorders of the upper extremity. In Machleder HI, ed: Vascular disorders of the upper extremity, New York, 1983, Futura Publishing Co, Inc.
11. Fogarty TJ: Arterial embolism. In Dale A, ed: Management of arterial occlusive disease, Chicago, 1971, Year Book Medical Publishers, Inc.

12. Shoor PM and Fogarty TJ: Acute arterial insufficiency. In Miller DC and Roon AS, eds: Diagnosis and management of peripheral vascular disease, Menlo Park, Calif, 1982, Addison-Wesley Publishing Co, Inc.

13. Green RM, DeWeese JA, and Rob CG: Arterial embolectomy before and after the Fogarty catheter, Surgery 77:24, 1970.

14. Meister SG et al: Paradoxical embolism: diagnosis during life, Am J Med 53:292, 1972.

15. Seward JB et al: Transesophageal echocardiography: technique, anatomic correlations, implementation, and clinical applications, Mayo Clin Proc 63:649, 1988.

16. Shub C: The role of echocardiography in clinical practice. In Spittell JA, ed: Clinical medicine, Philadelphia, 1982, Harper & Row, Publishers, Inc.

17. Fairbairn JF, Joyce JW, and Pairolero PC: Acute arterial occlusion of the extremities. In Juergens JL, Spittell JA, and Fairbairn JF, eds: Peripheral vascular diseases, Philadelphia, 1980, WB Saunders Co.

18. Sullivan KL, Sminken SL, and White RI: Treatment of a case of thromboembolism resulting from thoracic outlet syndrome with intraarterial urokinase infusion, J Vasc Surg 7:568, 1988.

19. Savelyev VS, Zatevakhin II, and Stephanov NV: Artery embolism of the upper limbs, J Surg 81:367, 1977.

20. Hilton TC, Menke D, and Blackshear JL: Variable effect of anticoagulation in the treatment of severe protruding atherosclerotic aortic debris, Am Heart J 127:1645, 1994.

21. Machleder HI: Etiology and management of major arterial and venous occlusive processes involving the upper extremity. In Machleder HI, ed: Vascular disorders of the upper extremity, New York, 1983, Futura Publishing Co, Inc.

22. Sheps SG and McDuffie FC: Vasculitis. In Juergens JL, Spittell JA, and Fairbairn JF, eds: Peripheral vascular diseases, Philadelphia, 1980, WB Saunders Co.

23. Machleder HI: Vaso-occlusive disorders of the upper extremity, Curr Probl Surg 25:1, 1988.

24. Levo Y et al: Association between hepatitis B virus and essential mixed cryoglobulinemia, N Engl J Med 296:1501, 1977.

25. Brouet JC et al: Biologic and clinical significance of cryoglobulins: a report of 86 cases, Am J Med 57:775, 1974.

26. McDuffie FC et al: Hypocomplementemia with cutaneous vasculitis and arthritis: possible immune complex syndrome, Mayo Clin Proc 48:340, 1973.

27. Mills JL et al: Upper extremity ischemia caused by small artery disease, Ann Surg 206:521, 1987.

28. Ames EL et al: Bilateral hand necrosis in Kawasaki syndrome, J Hand Surg 10A:391, 1985.

29. Hall S et al: Takayasu arteritis, Medicine 64:89, 1985.

30. Juergens JL: Thromboangiitis obliterans. In Juergens JL, Spittell JA, and Fairbairn JF, eds: Peripheral vascular diseases, Philadelphia, 1980, WB Saunders Co.

31. Yorukogly Y et al: Thromboangiitis obliterans (Buerger's disease) in women (reevaluation), Angiology 44:527, 1993.

32. Olin JW et al: The changing clinical spectrum of thromboangiitis obliterans (Buerger's disease), Circulation 82 (Suppl 5):IV3, 1990.

33. McKusick VA et al: Buerger's disease: a distinct clinical and pathological entity, JAMA 181:5, 1962.

34. Lambeth J and Yong NK: Arteriographic findings in thromboangiitis obliterans, AJR 109:553, 1970.

35. Rivera R: Roentgenographic diagnosis of Buerger's disease, J Cardiovasc Surg 14:40, 1973.

36. Shionoya S: Buerger's disease: diagnosis and management, Cardiovasc Surg 1:207, 1993.

37. Kerr GS et al: Takayasu arteritis, Ann Intern Med 120:919, 1994.

38. DeRemee RA, McDonald TJ, and Weiland LH: Wegener's granulomatosis: observations on treatment with antimicrobial agents, Mayo Clin Proc 60:27, 1985.

39. Leitner DW, Ross JS, and Neary JR: Granulomatous radial arteritis with bilateral, nontraumatic, true arterial aneurysms within the anatomic snuffbox, J Hand Surg 10A:131, 1985.

40. Trunkey DD and Lim RC: Vascular trauma. In Miller DC and Roon AJ, eds: Diagnosis and management of peripheral vascular disease, Menlo Park, Calif, 1982, Addison-Wesley Publishing Company, Inc.

41. Kutsal A and Kivanc O: A case of ulnar aneurysm: clinical and surgical considerations, J Cardiovasc Surg 29:326, 1988.

42. Ho PK et al: Aneurysms of the upper extremity, J Hand Surg 12A:39, 1987.

43. Ho PK, Dellon AL, and Wilgis EF: True aneurysms of the hand resulting from athletic injury: report of two cases, Am J Sports Med 13:136, 1985.

44. Horattas MC et al: Changing concepts of deep venous thrombosis of the upper extremity: report of a series and review of the literature, Surgery 104:561, 1988.

45. Rooke TW: Vascular complications of interventional procedures. In Holmes DR Jr and Vlietstra RE, eds: Interventional cardiology, Philadelphia, 1989, FA Davis Co.

46. Benitez PR and Newell MA: Vascular trauma in drug abuse: patterns of injury, Ann Vasc Surg 1:175, 1986.

47. Nasu Y and Ishida K: Follow-up study of patients with vibration syndrome in Japan, Scand J Work Environ Health 12:313, 1986.

48. Pyykko I et al: Vibration syndrome among Finnish forest workers: a follow-up from 1972 to 1983, Scand J Work Environ Health 12:307, 1986.

49. Brubaker RL, Mackenzie CJ, and Hutton SG: Vibration-induced white finger among selected underground rock drillers in British Columbia, Scand J Work Environ Health 12:296, 1986.

50. Engstrom K and Dandanell R: Exposure conditions and Raynaud's phenomenon among riveters in the aircraft industry, Scand J Work Environ Health 12:293, 1986.

51. Yu ZS et al: Epidemiologic survey of vibration syndrome among riveters, chippers and grinders in the railroad system of the People's Republic of China, Scand J Work Environ Health 12:289, 1986.

52. Nasu Y: Defibrinogating therapy for peripheral circulatory disturbance in patients with vibration syndrome, Scand J Work Environ Health 12:272, 1986.

53. Kaji H et al: Hypothenar hammar syndrome in workers occupationally exposed to vibrating tools, Hand Surg (Br) 18:761, 1993.

54. Pineda CJ et al: Hypothenar hammer syndrome: form of reversible Raynaud's phenomenon, Am J Med 79:561, 1985.

55. Savader SJ, Savader BL, and Drewry GR: Hypothenar hammer syndrome with embolic occlusion of digital arteries, Clin Radiol 39:324, 1988.

56. McCarthy WJ et al: Upper extremity arterial injury in athletes, J Vasc Surg 9:317, 1989.

57. Bovenzi M: Finger thermometry in the assessment of subjects with vibration-induced white finger, Scand J Work Environ Health 13:348, 1987.

58. Ekenvall L: Clinical assessment of suspected damage from hand-held vibrating tools, Scand J Work Environ Health 13:271, 1987.

59. Paterson C: Canadian compensation law and vibration-induced white finger. A revised description, Scand J Work Environ Health 12:402, 1986.

60. McCready RA, Procter CD, and Hyde GL: Subclavian-axillary vascular trauma, J Vasc Surg 3:24, 1986.

61. Gooding GA: Sonography of the radial artery at the wrist, AJR 150:629, 1988.

62. Slavin SA: Microvascular reconstruction of the hand, Clin Plast Surg 10:139, 1983.

63. Talha H et al: Brachial artery entrapment: compression by the supracondylar process, Ann Vasc Surg 1:479, 1986.

64. Garrett HE, Hodosh S, and DeBakey ME: Fibromuscular hyperplasia of the left axillary artery, Arch Surg 94:737, 1967.

65. Lie JT and Juergens JL: Degenerative arterial diseases other than atherosclerosis. In Juergens JL, Spittell JA, and Fairbairn JF, eds: Peripheral vascular diseases, Philadelphia, 1980, WB Saunders Co.

66. Albin G et al: Paraneoplastic digital thrombosis: a case report, Angiology 37:203, 1986.

67. Petri M and Fye KH: Digital necrosis: a paraneoplastic syndrome, J Rheumatol 12:800, 1985.

68. Taylor LM Jr et al: Digital ischemia as a manifestation of malignancy, Ann Surg 206:62, 1987.

69. Curelaru I et al: Dynamics of thrombophlebitis in central venous catheterization via basilic and cephalic veins, Acta Chir Scand 150:285, 1984.

70. Bradof J, Sands MJ Jr, and Lakin PC: Symptomatic venous thrombosis of the upper extremity complicating permanent transvenous pacing: reversal with streptokinase infusion, Am Heart J 104:190, 1982.

71. Stevenson IM and Parry EWA: Radiological study of the aetiological factors in venous obstruction of the upper limb, J Cardiovasc Surg (Torino) 16:580, 1975.

72. Campbell CB et al: Axillary, subclavian, and brachiocephalic vein obstruction, J Surg 82:816, 1977.

73. Monreal M et al: Upper-extremity deep venous thrombosis and pulmonary embolism. A prospective study, Chest 99: 280, 1991.

74. Falk RL and Smith DF: Thrombosis of the upper extremity thoracic inlet veins: diagnosis with duplex Doppler sonography, AJR 149:677, 1987.

75. Sullivan ED, Peter DJ, and Cranley JJ: Real-time B-mode venous ultrasound, J Vasc Surg 1:465, 1984.

76. Drury EM et al: Lytic therapy in the treatment of axillary and subclavian vein thrombosis, J Vasc Surg 2:821, 1985.

77. Spittell PC et al: Venous obstruction due to permanent transvenous pacemaker electrodes: treatment with percutaneous transluminal balloon venoplasty, PACE 13:271, 1990.

78. Roos DB: Thoracic outlet syndromes. In Machleder HI, ed: Vascular disorders of the upper extremity, New York, 1983, Futura Publishing Co, Inc.

79. Fairbairn JF, Campbell JK, and Payne WS: Neurovascular compression syndromes of the thoracic outlet. In Juergens JL, Spittell JA, and Fairbairn JF, eds: Peripheral vascular diseases, Philadelphia, 1980, WB Saunders Co.

80. Roos DB: Thoracic outlet and carpal tunnel syndromes. In Management of neurovascular diseases involving the upper extremity, Philadelphia, 1984, WB Saunders Co.

81. Kieffer E: Arterial complications of thoracic outlet syndrome. In Bergen Y, ed: Evaluation and treatment of upper and lower extremity circulatory disorders, Orlando, Fla, 1984, Grune & Stratton, Inc.

82. Roos DB: Congenital anomalies associated with thoracic outlet syndrome, Am J Surg 132:771, 1976.

83. Priest JD: The shoulder of the tennis player, Clin Sports Med 7:387, 1988.

84. Bouhoutsos J, Morris T, and Martin P: Unilateral Raynaud's phenomenon in the hand and its significance, Surgery 82:547, 1977.

85. Scher LA et al: Vascular complications of thoracic outlet syndrome, J Vasc Surg 3:565, 1986.

86. Daube JR: Nerve conduction studies in the thoracic outlet syndrome, Neurology 25:347, 1962.

87. Machleder HI et al: Somatosensory evoked potentials in the assessment of thoracic outlet compression syndrome, J Vasc Surg 6:177, 1987.

88. Dunant JH: Thoracic outlet syndrome: treatment of vascular complications, Vasa 14:51, 1985.

89. DeWeese JA, Adams JT, and Gaiser DL: Subclavian venous thrombectomy, Circulation XLI, XLII (II): 158, 1970.

90. Steed DL et al: Streptokinase in the treatment of subclavian vein thrombosis, J Vasc Surg 4:28, 1986.

91. Machleder HI: Evaluation of a new treatment strategy for Paget-Schrötter syndrome: spontaneous thrombosis of the axillary-subclavian vein, Vasc Surg 17:305, 1993.

92. Freedman RR and Ianni P: Role of cold and emotional stress in Raynaud's disease and scleroderma, Br Med J 287:1499, 1983.

93. Freedman RR et al: Increased alpha-adrenergic responsiveness in idiopathic Raynaud's disease, Arthritis Rheum 32: 61, 1989.

94. Okada A et al: Usefulness of blood parameters, especially viscosity, for the diagnosis and elucidation of pathogenic mechanisms of the hand-arm vibration syndrome, Scand J Work Environ Health 13:358, 1987.

95. Sandhagen B and Wegener T: Blood viscosity and finger systolic pressure in primary and traumatic vasospastic disease, Ups J Med Sci 90:55, 1985.

96. Lewis T: The pathological changes in the arteries supplying the fingers in warm-handed people and in cases of so-called Raynaud's disease, Clin Sci 3:287, 1938.

97. Bovenzi M: Finger systolic pressure during local cooling in normal subjects aged 20 to 60 years: reference values for the assessment of digital vasospasm in Raynaud's phenomenon of occupational origin, Int Arch Occup Environ Health 61:179, 1988.

98. Siefert KB et al: Bilateral upper extremity ischemia after administration of dihydroergotamine-heparin for prophylaxis of deep venous thrombosis, J Vasc Surg 8:410, 1988.

99. Engelhart M, Nielsen HV, and Kristensen JK: The blood supply to fingers during Raynaud's attack: a comparison of laser-Doppler flowmetry with other techniques, Clin Physiol 5:447, 1985.

100. Halperin JL, Cohen RA, and Coffman JD: Digital vasodilatation during mental stress in patients with Raynaud's disease, Cardiovasc Res 17:671, 1983.

101. Goodfield MJ, Hume A, and Rowell NR: The effect of simple warming procedures on finger blood flow in systemic sclerosis, Br J Dermatol 118:661, 1988.

102. Wollersheim H, Reyenga J, and Thien T: Laser Doppler velocimetry of fingertips during heat provocation in normals and in patients with Raynaud's phenomenon, Scand J Clin Lab Invest 48:91, 1988.

103. Olsen N and Petring OU: Vibration elicited vasoconstrictor reflex in Raynaud's phenomena, Br J Ind Med 45:415, 1988.

104. Cooke ED, Bowcock SA, and Smith AT: Photoplethysmography of the distal pulp in the assessment of vasospastic hand, Angiology 36:33, 1985.

105. Dupuis H: Thermographic assessment of skin temperature

during a cold provocation test, Scand J Work Environ Health 13:352, 1987.

106. Belcaro G et al: Infrared and ELC thermography in the assessment of the digital rewarming curve after a finger-cooling test: a preliminary report, Panminerva Med 27:33, 1985.

107. Goodfield MJ and Rowell NR: Hand warming as a treatment for Raynaud's phenomenon in systemic sclerosis, Br J Dermatol 119:643, 1988.

108. Freedman RR: Long-term effectiveness of behavioral treatments for Raynaud's disease, Behav Res Ther 18:387, 1987.

109. Nilsson H et al: The effect of the calcium-entry blocker nifedipine on cold-induced digital vasospasm: a double-blind crossover study versus placebo, Acta Med Scand 221:53, 1982.

110. Rodeheffer RJ et al: Controlled double-blind trial of nifedipine in the treatment of Raynaud's phenomenon, N Engl J Med 308:880, 1983.

111. Pin PG, Sicard GA, and Weeks PM: Digital ischemia of the upper extremity: a systematic approach for evaluation and treatment, Plast Reconstr Surg 82:653, 1988.

112. Lewis P et al: Nifedipine in patients with Raynaud's syndrome: effects on radial artery blood flow, Eur Heart J 8:83, 1987.

113. Waldo R: Prazosin relieves Raynaud's vasospasm, JAMA 241:1037, 1979.

114. Arneklo-Nobin B, Elmer O, and Akesson A: Effect of long-term ketanserin treatment on 5-HT levels, platelet aggregation and peripheral circulation in patients with Raynaud's phenomenon: a double-blind, placebo-controlled crossover study, Int Angiol 7:19, 1988.

115. Lagerkvist BE and Linderholm H: Cold hands after exposure to arsenic or vibrating tools: effects of ketanserin on finger blood pressure and skin temperature, Acta Pharmacol Toxicol (Copenh) 58:327, 1986.

116. van de Wal HJ et al: Thoracic sympathectomy as a therapy for upper extremity ischemia: a long-term follow-up study, Thorac Cardiovasc Surg 33:181, 1985.

117. Miller DR and Malki A: Large saccular aneurysm and A-V fistula of the brachial vessels, J Cardiovasc Surg (Torino) 26:605, 1985.

118. Kherlakian GM et al: Comparison of autogenous fistula versus expanded polytetrafluoroethylene graft fistula for angioaccess in hemodialysis, Am J Surg 152:238, 1986.

119. Wilgis EFS: Tumors. In Vascular injuries and diseases of the upper limb, Boston, 1983, Little, Brown & Co, Inc.

120. Schirger A: Lymphedema, Cardiovasc Clin 13:293, 1983.

121. Kobayashi MR and Miller TA: Lymphedema, Clin Plast Surg 14:303, 1987.

122. Lymphatic filariasis—tropical medicine's origin will not go away, Lancet 1:1409, 1987.

123. Samuels LD: Lymphoscintigraphy, Lymphology 20:4, 1987.

124. Ohtake E and Matsui K: Lymphoscintigraphy in patients with lymphedema: a new approach using intradermal injections of technetium-99m human serum albumin, Clin Nucl Med 11:474, 1986.

125. Stillwell GK: Management of arm edema. In Stoll BA, ed: Breast cancer management: early and late, Chicago, 1977, Heinemann Medical and Year Book Medical.

126. Zanolla R et al: Evaluation of the results of three different methods of postmastectomy lymphedema treatment, J Surg Oncol 26:210, 1984.

127. Bunce IH et al: Post-mastectomy lymphedema treatment and measurement, Med J Aust 161:125, 1994.

CHAPTER FORTY

DIABETIC FOOT LESIONS

Marvin E. Levin

The human foot is a mechanical marvel. It consists of 26 bones, 29 joints, 42 muscles, and innumerable tendons and ligaments. The interplay among these bones, tendons, and ligaments cushions the body, allowing the foot to adapt to uneven surfaces. It provides traction for movement, awareness of joint and body position for balance, and leverage for propulsion.[1] Chan and Rudins have written an excellent review on foot biomechanics during walking and running.[1] The toes are extremely important. They were present in the earliest tetrapods.[2] Toes provide traction, help maintain balance, and improve locomotor performance.[2] What a shame that diabetics are prone to lose their toes. In a lifetime this phenomenal machine, the foot, with its multiple moving parts, walks over 100,000 miles, four times around the world. It is exposed to significant pressures. The forefoot and hallux bear the stepping off, or dynamic pressure. The diabetic tends to have increased foot pressures, and this can be demonstrated even in diabetics with early sensory neuropathy.[3] In diabetics with ulceration there are significantly higher pressures.[4] Veves et al found that all patients who developed plantar ulcers had abnormally high foot pressures.[5] The explanation for these increased foot pressures has not been completely defined. One probable reason relates to glycosylation of tendons and ligaments. Glycosylation leads to an increased cross-linkage of collagen, which causes stiffness of the tendons and ligaments, resulting in decreased flexibility of the foot. This loss of flexibility can result in increased plantar foot pressure when walking.[6]

Most diabetic plantar ulcerations occur at the areas of maximum pressure, the metatarsal heads. Foot problems are common in the population at large; however, the diabetic is especially vulnerable because of increased plantar pressures, arteriosclerosis obliterans (ASO), and peripheral neuropathy. The combination of these factors compounded by infection can lead to gangrene and amputation.

Diabetic foot problems are one of the major reasons for hospital admissions. The percentage of hospital admissions for foot problems in the diabetic population in the United States has risen from 25% in the 1960s to more than 50% in the 1980s.[7] The most common cause of hospital admission for diabetics in Great Britain is for diabetic foot problems.[8] In a study of 6000 diabetic patients, Young et al[9] found 2% to have a foot ulcer.

Diabetes is one of the oldest diseases known. The *Papyrus Ebers* of 1500 BC mentions its symptoms and suggests treatment. However, the history of gangrene of the feet goes back to biblical times, where, in II Chronicles 16:12-14, the first case of gangrene, possibly caused by diabetes, is described: "In the 39th year of his reign King Asa became affected with gangrene of his feet; he did not seek guidance from the Lord but resorted to physicians. He rested with his forefathers in the 41st year of his reign."

Whether or not King Asa did indeed have diabetic gangrene is a moot point. Certainly in biblical times there was not much one could do for a foot lesion except to pray. Even in the late 1800s the famous surgeon, Ambroise Paré said, "I dressed [the wound] and God healed it." Today, however, the skills of multiple medical disciplines are significantly reducing amputation rates. With increasing awareness of diabetic foot problems and improved treatment, amputation rates will continue to decrease.

This chapter is devoted to describing the pathogenesis of diabetic foot lesions and providing information on management so that the goal of decreasing amputation can be realized.

EPIDEMIOLOGY

Today there are approximately 16 million diabetics in the United States. We can expect to see this number increase since the diabetic population is increasing by 6% per year and doubling every 15 years.[10] By the turn of the century there will be 20 million diabetics in this country. This increasing diabetic population is caused by a decrease in fetal mortality and a prolonged life span, which has been increased by the discovery of insulin, antibiotics, and antihypertensives. Of these, antibiotics are probably the most significant. McDermott and Rogers stated that curing all cancers would add 2 years to the life expectancy for Americans, but the introduction of antibiotics has added 10 years.[11] However, these added years have not always been quality years for the diabetic since they have resulted in a multitude of complications, not the least of which are foot problems. The diabetic who is most likely to develop a foot lesion is over age 40. Today 90% of the diabetics in this country are over age 40.[12] Of all diabetics, 15% will develop a foot ulcer during their lifetime.[13] Most of these are the result of peripheral neuropathy and the insensate foot. Peripheral neuropathy is extremely common in the diabetic type I patients with the incidence gradually increasing with age and duration. After 20 years of diabetes 42% of diabetics have evidence of peripheral neuropathy.[14]

Of diabetics, 8% have ASO at the time of diagnosis, 15% after 10 years, and 45% after 20 years.[15] Kreines et al reviewed the natural history of ASO in type II diabetics.[16] Of diabetics, 20% will enter the hospital because of foot problems.[17] Of these patients, 30% have symptomatic ASO, and 7% will require vascular surgery or amputation.[17]

Race

Race may play a significant role in the number of amputations required by the diabetic population. After adjusting for age, the U.S. hospital discharge rates show that despite the annual variation, a higher rate of amputation exists among blacks than in whites.[18] A 1.4 times greater incidence of amputation was found in nonwhites compared with whites, in New Jersey.[19] One study suggested that the increased prevalence of hypertension and smoking in blacks may be a contributory factor.[20] The Pima Indians in the Southwest have shown an exceptionally high rate, a 3.7 times greater incidence than whites.[21]

Age

In comparing age groups researchers have found the amputation rate in the 45- to 64-year-old group is two to three times higher, compared with nondiabetics. In those over 65 it is seven times higher.[22] Of all lower extremity amputations, 96% occur in those over age 45 and 64% in those 65 years of age or older.[23] Younger diabetics may also undergo amputation. I have seen an above-knee amputation needed because of atherosclerosis in a 27-year-old type I diabetic.

Sex

Diabetes has been a great equalizer between the sexes when looking at ASO alone. The ratio of ASO in nondiabetic men as compared with women is significantly higher. However, in the diabetic the ratio of men to women is almost equal. The risk for lower extremity amputation has been found to be from 1.4 to 2.6 times greater for men than for women with diabetes.[19,21,22] In a series of 20 consecutive diabetic amputations performed in 1988 at our university hospital, there were an equal number of men and women. Sex per se may not be a factor. Men are more likely to traumatize their feet. They do more physical work than women, are on their feet more, thereby subjecting them to a greater degree of trauma.

Type of Diabetes

Amputation rates between type I and type II diabetics are comparable. In a study by Humphrey et al, it was found that cumulative risk of one lower extremity amputation was 11.2% in type I patients and 11% in type II patients.[24] When compared with lower extremity amputation rates for nondiabetics, patients with type II diabetes were 400 times more likely to undergo an initial transphalangeal amputation and 12 times more likely to have a below-the-knee amputation.[24]

AMPUTATION

Almost 50,000 major diabetic amputations were reported in 1985 in the United States.[23] The cost of an amputation can be very expensive. Mackey et al, at the University of Minnesota, reported an average cost of $40,000 per amputation.[25] In the 1988 review of 20 diabetics undergoing amputation at our university hospital, there was an average hospital stay of 22.85 days, with a range of 10 to 45, and an average in-hospital cost of $24,430, with a range of $7,000 to $44,800. The age of the patients undergoing amputation ranged from 40 to 82 years, with an average age of 63.7 years. Based on 50,000 plus amputations at an average cost of approximately $25,000 each, $1.2 billion is spent annually on amputations. This figure does not include the surgeon's fee, cost of rehabilitation, possible loss of job, disability and welfare payments, and Medicare payments for patients who go on Medicare before age 65 as a result of amputation. As the population ages and medical costs rise, these numbers will increase. It is difficult to establish the exact costs of an amputation because third party insurers and Medicare have established maximum reimbursement, which may vary with third party payees and in different areas of the country. However, the increasing numbers of educational programs in foot care and the use of therapeutic shoes have demonstrated a reduction in the number of amputations being performed annually. Several recent studies have shown a reduction of 50% in the amputation rate when special foot care programs are initiated. Davidson et al[26] and Edmonds et al[27] have decreased their amputation rate by 50% and Assal et al have decreased their center's amputation rate by 83%.[28] It is hoped that by the year 2000, there will be worldwide reduction in amputations by 50%.

Pathway To Diabetic Limb Amputation

Pecoraro, Reiber, and Burgess evaluated the pathways leading to amputation. They attributed 46% of the amputations to ischemia, 59% to infection, 61% to neuropathy, 81% to faulty wound healing, 84% to ulceration, 55% to gangrene, and 81% to initial minor trauma. The ulcerations attributed to minor trauma included ill-fitting shoes, leading to cutaneous ulceration in 36% of all cases.[29]

Another factor they felt contributed to many of the amputations was nutritional impairment believed to impede normal tissue repair. This was indicated by plasma ascorbic acid and zinc levels 2 standard deviations below the laboratory values and was found in over half their amputees. Other deficiencies included low levels of plasma albumin, carotene, and zinc-protoporphyrin heme ratio.[29] An important factor leading to amputation is a delay in aggressive treatment.

Delay in aggressive treatment of foot ulcers and/or delay in referral to a specialist frequently results in amputation. Mills et al found that delay in aggressive treatment or referral to a specialist in cases of diabetic foot ulcer frequently results in amputation. They reported delays of 2 weeks to 12 months. These delays led to more proximal levels of amputation in patients with limbs that were initially salvageable. Specific causes of delay were underestimation of the severity of the foot infection and lack of recognition of large-vessel occlusive disease.[30]

The long-term and short-term outlook for the diabetic undergoing amputation has always been poor. In the preantibiotic era the principal cause of in-hospital mortality in patients with diabetic gangrene was toxemia and infection.[31] With the availability of antibiotics and newer management techniques, a mortality rate of 50% in 1935[32] had fallen to 3% in the 1980s.[33] Bodily and Burgess reported that their in-hospital mortality had decreased to 1.5%.[34] They felt that this improvement was the result of better cardiovascular support and early rehabilitation.[34] The amputation site is also a critical factor in predicting mortality. Rosenberg and Shah found that midthigh amputations were twice as lethal as below-knee amputations.[35] Age was a factor after age 60, and obesity led to a somewhat increased mortality.[35] The high frequency of in-hospital mortality and the relative short-term survival rate in all these reports was the result of the high incidence of cardiac and renal disease. For example, in the series of Rosenberg and Shah 90% of those who died had associated heart disease.[35]

Fearon et al found local complication rates of 18% and systemic complication rates of 36%. Complications included such problems as gastrointestinal bleeding, myocardial infarction, congestive heart failure, and cerebral vascular accidents.[33] In the diabetic patient the major postoperative problem is not the operative site but the control of blood glucose and the management of medical problems such as cardiac and renal difficulties, which require the constant attention of trained medical personnel. Therefore any diabetic undergoing surgery should be seen daily by the endocrine team and the internist.

The long-term outlook for the diabetic amputee has not improved significantly since Silbert's report of 1952, when he found in a follow-up study of 294 cases a 65% survival rate for 3 years but only a 41% survival rate at the end of 5 years.[36] Eighteen years later Ecker and Jacobs found data similar to those of Silbert. In their series of 103 patients they found only a 61% survival rate 3 years after the first amputation.[37] As recently as 1993 Lee et al reported a 50% 5-year mortality among diabetic amputees.[38]

Because of the high mortality in this group of diabetics, many of them do not live long enough to undergo a second amputation. For those who do, the long-term outlook for the second leg is poor. This poor prognosis for the second leg is not new. Marchal de Calvi in 1864 stated that "often the opposite leg is affected, gangrene sets in and soon the

patient succumbs to horrible suffering. Having relieved him only of his local affliction (by amputation), I have done nothing but mutilate him."[39] This problem still exists. On the average, 42% of these patients will have amputation of the remaining leg in 1 to 3 years and 56% in 3 to 5 years. The dismal outlook for the contralateral leg reported in the 1960s has not improved over the past two decades. In the 1980 report of Ebskov and Josephsen,[40] the high risk of a contralateral amputation was still present with an incidence of 11.9% within 1 year, 17.8% after 2 years, 27.2% after 3 years, and 44.3% at 4 years. A contributing factor is the increased load pattern on the remaining foot. Larsen, Christiansen, and Ebskov[41] concluded that regulation of pedal load pattern on the remaining foot had a considerable curative and preventive effect in preventing and healing ulcerations. This redistribution of pressures is accomplished with shoes fitted with special insoles designed to redistribute pressure.

Infection is one of the major reasons for amputation in the contralateral leg. Kucan and Robson, in a 3-year follow-up study of 45 patients, found that 49% of the patients developed a severe infection involving the contralateral foot within 28 months.[42]

PATHOGENESIS

The foot of the diabetic is especially prone to atherosclerosis and neuropathy. The signs and symptoms of either ischemia or neuropathy may predominate; however, neither is ever present to the total exclusion of the other. The clinical picture is therefore the result of complications stemming from one or more of these factors (Fig. 40-1). Peripheral neuropathy is the leading cause of most diabetic foot lesions. Impaired blood flow to the injured or lacerated areas prevents healing and, in the presence of infection, limits the delivery of antibiotics. The most important effect of peripheral neuropathy on the diabetic foot is the loss of sensation, making the foot vulnerable even to trivial trauma. A break in the skin, though inconspicuous and minuscule, can become a portal of entry for bacteria. Once infection develops in the diabetic foot the final cataclysmic events of gangrene and the need for amputation result. Fig. 40-1 outlines the pathogenesis of diabetic foot lesions.

Peripheral Vascular Disease

ASO involves both large and small vessels. The pathogenesis of atherosclerosis in diabetes mellitus has been reviewed by Colwell et al.[43] The deposits of lipids, cholesterol, calcium, and smooth muscle cells and platelets in the plaques, are qualitatively the same in the diabetic and nondiabetic, although quantitatively much greater in the diabetic. There are, however, important differences. These are listed in Table 40-1. In the diabetic the vessels involved are primarily those below the knee, the tibial and peroneal arteries. In the series of Janka, Standl, and Mehnert the overall prevalence of isolated proximal vascular disease involving femoral and iliac vessels was 5.8% in the diabetic, the same percentage as in the general population.[44] They concluded that proximal vascular disease in the

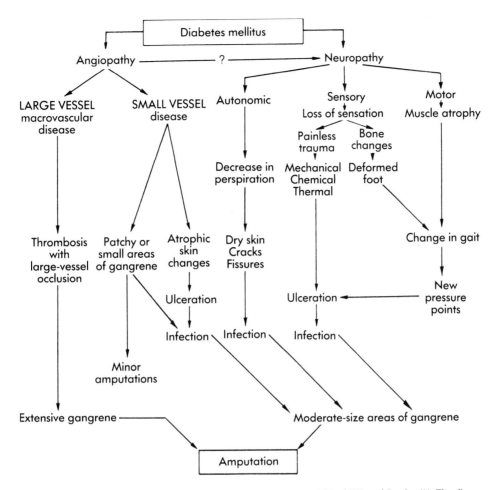

Fig. 40-1. Pathogenesis of diabetic foot lesions. *(From Levin ME, O'Neal LW, and Bowker JH: The diabetic foot, ed 5, St Louis, 1993, Mosby–Year Book.)*

Table 40-1. Differences in Diabetic and Nondiabetic Peripheral Arterial Disease

	Diabetic	**Nondiabetic**
Clinical	More common	Less common
	Younger patient	Older patient
	More rapid	Less rapid
Male/female	M = F	M >> F
Occlusion	Multisegmental	Single segment
Vessels adjacent to occlusion	Involved	Not involved
Collateral vessels	Involved	Usually normal
Lower extremities	Both	Unilateral
Vessels involved	Tibial	Aortic
	Peroneal	Iliac
		Femoral

(Modified from Levin ME: Pathogenesis and management of diabetic foot lesions. In Levin ME, O'Neal LW, and Bowker JH, eds: The diabetic foot, ed 5, St Louis, 1993, Mosby–Year Book.)

diabetic may represent the atherosclerotic process with co-existing diabetes but did not necessarily represent diabetogenic macroangiopathy.[44] While this may be true, it is my clinical impression that there is acceleration of this athero-sclerotic process, even in these larger vessels. Atherosclerotic involvement of the larger proximal vessels, iliac, and femoral vessels is definitely accelerated by smoking. For example, we recently saw a type I 27-year-old patient, diabetic since age 5, who had been a heavy smoker since age 13. At age 27 he developed intermittent claudication in his right leg. Vascular laboratory studies demonstrated a right superficial femoral artery obstruction (Fig. 40-2). It was felt that his prolonged heavy smoking had contributed significantly to his proximal artery atherosclerotic process.

Further evidence of which vessels are involved is demonstrated by the type of vascular surgery that is performed in these patients. While vascular surgery of all types is more common in the diabetic than in the nondiabetic, the procedure most frequently performed in the diabetic is tibioperoneal bypass surgery, involving the vessels below the knee. Vascular surgery performed on the diabetic lower extremity is approximately 10% aortofemoral bypass, 40% femoropopliteal bypass, and 70% tibioperoneal bypass.[45] The experience with percutaneous angioplasty is limited. It tends to be less applicable in the diabetic because the atherosclerotic process occurs most often in the smaller vessels. Large and small vessel disease do not necessarily progress at the same rate. It is not uncommon, for example, for small vessels in the toes to have evidence of ischemia, while the dorsalis pedis or posterior tibial pulses may be

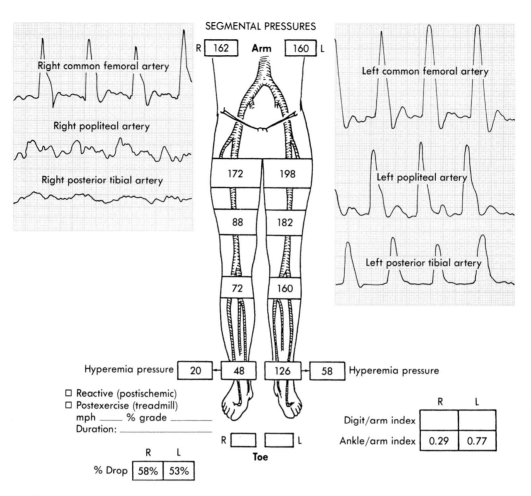

Fig. 40-2. Severe peripheral vascular disease in 27-year-old man. Doppler pressures reveal evidence of right superficial femoral artery obstruction. Note blunted waveforms in right popliteal and right posterior tibial arteries, with ankle/arm index of only 0.29. Patient had been diabetic since age 5 and was heavy smoker since early teens. He required right femoral-popliteal Gore-Tex bypass graft. *(From Levin ME, O'Neal LW, and Bowker JH, eds: The diabetic foot, ed 5, St Louis, 1993, Mosby–Year Book; courtesy Dr. Charles B. Anderson, Department of Surgery, Washington University School of Medicine, St Louis.)*

present and of adequate quality. Approximately one third of the diabetic population may have small areas of gangrene with palpable dorsalis pedis or posterior tibial pulses. Fig. 40-3 illustrates a significant decrease in toe pressure and ischemic changes in a patient with a normal ankle pressure.

Microangiopathy is not a significant factor in the pathogenesis of diabetic foot lesions. While there may be capillary basement membrane thickening, there is no evidence that this contributes to the foot lesions. This has been noted by LoGerfo and Coffman.[46] They stressed that in many instances there are enough patent vessels at the ankle to allow vascular surgery. This is usually a tibioperoneal bypass surgery with the bypass to the tibial vessels at the ankle.

Ischemia or gangrene of the toes can result from four possible causes: (1) atherosclerosis with thrombosis, (2) microthrombi formation resulting from infection (Fig. 40-4), (3) cholesterol emboli, and (4) drugs, which can decrease blood flow. Microthrombi secondary to infection can convert the small vessels in the toes to end-arteries

with resulting gangrene of the toes (Fig. 40-5). Cholesterol emboli that break off from atheromatous plaques in the proximal larger vessels can also cause cyanosis and gangrene of the toes. This results in the blue or purple toe syndrome. The toe takes on a deep purplish discoloration, and gangrene can develop. On occasion these toes can be revascularized. Cholesterol emboli to the foot also result in painful petechia and a livedo reticularis pattern (Fig. 40-6). The atheromatous plaques may be present in the aorta, iliac, or more distant vessels. The syndrome is characterized by the sudden onset of pain in the toe. Leg and thigh myalgias may be present if muscular arteries are involved. When digital artery blood flow becomes sluggish, the toe may become bluish-purple. A sharp demarcation frequently occurs between normally perfused skin and ischemic areas.

Many of these patients have received anticoagulation therapy with warfarin.[47] Thrombolytic therapy, streptokinase,[48] and tissue plasminogen activator[49] can also cause the blue toe syndrome. It is therefore extremely important to periodically check the toes and feet of patients receiving

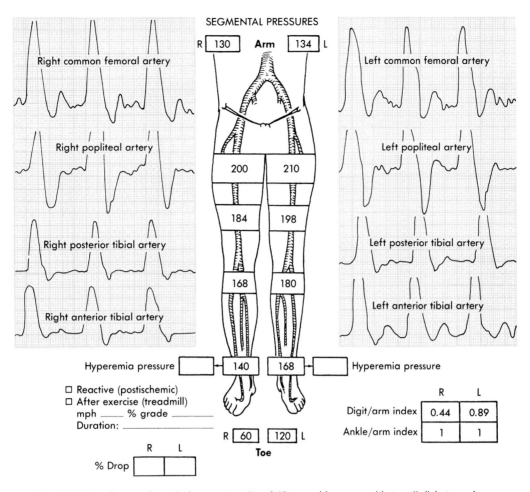

SEGMENTAL PRESSURES

R 130 Arm 134 L

Right common femoral artery

Right popliteal artery

Right posterior tibial artery

Right anterior tibial artery

Left common femoral artery

Left popliteal artery

Left posterior tibial artery

Left anterior tibial artery

	R	L
	200	210
	184	198
	168	180

Hyperemia pressure 140 | 168 Hyperemia pressure

□ Reactive (postischemic)
□ After exercise (treadmill)
mph _____ % grade _____
Duration: _____

	R	L
Digit/arm index	0.44	0.89
Ankle/arm index	1	1

R 60 | 120 L
Toe

	R	L
% Drop		

Fig. 40-3. Doppler waveforms in lower extremity of 62-year-old woman with type II diabetes, who had ischemic changes in right great toe. Note normal ankle/arm indexes but low pressure in right great toe. Low toe pressure and normal ankle pressure confirm small-vessel disease of great toe. *(From Levin ME, O'Neal LW, and Bowker JH, eds: The diabetic foot, ed 5, St Louis, 1993, Mosby–Year Book.)*

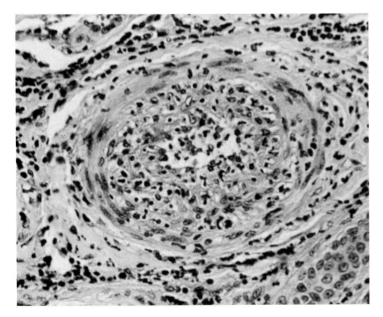

Fig. 40-4. Obliteration of lumen of small dermal arteriole by intimal hyperplasia and septic thrombus. Note cellular evidences of inflammation in areolar tissues near arteriole. This arteriole was about 1 mm from margin of area of dry gangrene. *(From Levin ME, O'Neal LW, and Bowker JH, eds: The diabetic foot, ed 5, St Louis, 1993, Mosby–Year Book.)*

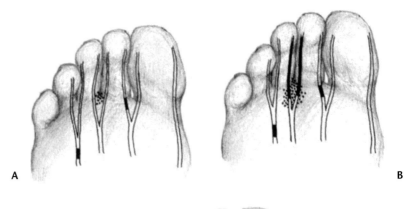

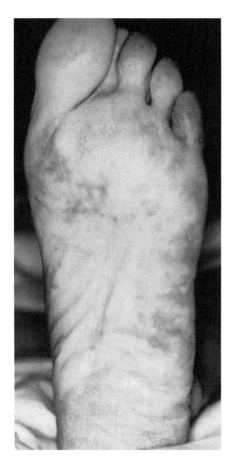

Fig. 40-5. Schematic drawings of mechanism whereby advancing infection causes obliteration of small arteries that have been converted into end-arteries by arteriosclerotic disease process, with resultant gangrene. **A,** Early web-space infection in foot with patchy segmental arteriosclerotic occlusion of digital and metatarsal vessels. **B,** Thrombosis of arteries adjacent to web-space infection. **C,** Gangrene of second and third toes. *(From Levin ME, O'Neal LW, and Bowker JH, eds: The diabetic foot, ed 5, St Louis, 1993, Mosby–Year Book.)*

Fig. 40-6. Cyanotic changes in the fifth toe and livedo reticularis pattern of the foot secondary to cholesterol emboli from atheroscleromatous plaque shown in Fig. 40-7. *(Courtesy Dr. Gregorio Sicard, Department of Surgery, Washington University School of Medicine, St Louis.)*

anticoagulants or thrombolytic therapy. Repeated attacks of acute ischemic changes, the development of painful cyanotic toes, petechiae, and a livedo reticularis pattern strongly suggest microemboli.

A 60-year-old man developed a painful, cyanotic fifth toe on his right foot and painful petechial lesions on both feet. These did not blanch on compression. He also complained of myalgias of the lower extremities. An angiogram (Fig. 40-7) showed a large atheromatous plaque in the left lateral wall of the infrarenal portion of the aorta with ulceration. Fig. 40-6 shows a purplish discoloration of his right fifth toe and a livedo reticularis pattern on the sole of the foot. The patient underwent successful removal of this ulcerated plaque. The treatment in such cases is vascular surgery with removal of the plaques, thereby preventing further embolization. In the study of Fisher et al[50] patients with multilevel atherosclerotic occlusive disease had their peripheral lesions treated first. In this small series the authors had no morbidity or mortality. Recurrent embolization did not occur during the follow-up period of 8 to 24 months.

Syphilis can present as the blue toe syndrome.[51] O'Keeffe, Woods, and Reslin have recently reviewed the various causes and management of the blue toe syndrome.[52]

Finally, certain drugs can affect ASO and cause gangrenous changes in the toes. Vasopressors such as dopamine (Intropin) frequently are used to treat shock. Because of the norepinephrine-like and vasoconstrictive effects of these agents, ischemic gangrene can develop in the toes and feet, particularly in diabetics who already have peripheral arterial insufficiency. Dopamine exerts positive inotropic effects by direct action on the adrenergic receptors. When sufficiently large doses of these inotropic drugs are administered, the predominant effect is vasoconstriction in all

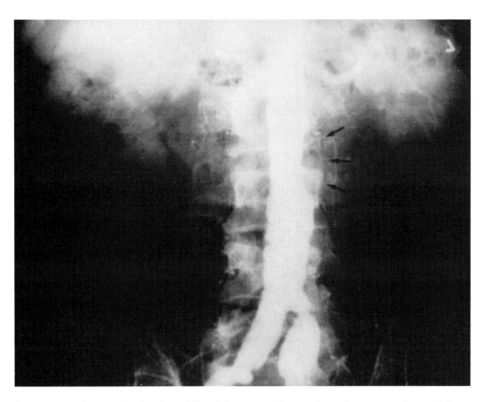

Fig. 40-7. Arteriogram showing large filling defect caused by an atheroscleromatous plaque of the aorta just inferior to the renal artery in a patient showing evidence of cholesterol emboli to the foot. *(Courtesy Dr. Gregorio Sicard, Department of Surgery, Washington University School of Medicine, St Louis.)*

vascular beds.[53] Dopamine should be used with caution and in as low a dose as possible. If a patient is in shock, the risk/benefit ratio would dictate the use of inotropic drugs despite the peripheral vascular risks; however, the feet of these patients must be observed daily. Peripheral circulation can also be impaired by the use of β-blockers, which are commonly used for treatment of angina and hypertension. Zacharias et al[54] found peripheral vascular complications to be a side effect in 22 of 305 patients treated with a β-blocker. This mechanism appears to result from unopposed α-vasoconstriction subsequent to β-blockade.

Diabetes is a hypercoagulable state resulting in increased blood viscosity[55] and impaired blood flow in the microvascular vessels. The increase in hypercoagulability or blood viscosity is caused by several factors. Increased platelet hyperactivity has been well documented.[43] Elevated levels of fibrinogen have been reported, and a decrease in fibrinolysis has been documented in diabetes mellitus and may play a role in the increased fibrinogen levels.[56] Small et al have shown that there is an increase in fibrinolysis in poorly controlled NIDD patients who are treated with insulin.[57] Von Willebrand's factor is elevated.[58] Increase in red cell rigidity has also been demonstrated.[59] An increased tendency toward hypercoagulability has been demonstrated in smokers, compared with control subjects.[60] All of these factors can lead to an increase in blood viscosity and a decrease in blood flow.

RISK FACTORS. Listed in the accompanying box are the risk factors in the development of diabetic arterial disease. Age, duration, and genetic factors may well be the most important factors, but unfortunately, they cannot be

RISK FACTORS FOR DIABETIC MACROVASCULAR ARTERIOSCLEROSIS

1. Genetic predisposition
2. Age
3. Duration of diabetes
4. Smoking
5. Hypertension
    a. Systolic blood pressure
    b. Diastolic blood pressure
6. Hypercholesterolemia
7. Hypertriglyceridemia
8. Hyperglycemia
9. Miscellaneous risk factors
    a. Hyperinsulinemia
    b. Obesity
    c. Truncal obesity

Modified from Levin ME: The diabetic foot: pathophysiology, evaluation and treatment. In Levin ME and O'Neal LW, eds: The diabetic foot, ed 4, St. Louis, 1988, The CV Mosby Co.

corrected. However, certain risk factors can be altered. Of the correctable risk factors, smoking tops the list. Pollin[61] has estimated that cigarette smoking causes an estimated 325,000 to 355,000 deaths annually in the United States.

This is more than all other drug and alcohol abuse deaths combined; seven times more than all automobile fatalities per year; more than eleven times all reported deaths caused by acquired immunodeficiency syndrome; and more than all American military fatalities in World War I, World War II, and Vietnam combined.[61] A clinical series from New Zealand found that cigarette smoking was 2.5 times as frequent in persons who were diabetic and had ischemia and gangrene as in a control series of persons without diabetes.[62] Kannel,[63] in a 26-year follow-up study of the Framingham study of 5209 subjects, found that cigarette smoking together with impaired glucose tolerance and hypertension were powerful predisposing factors in ASO. Cigarette smoking approximately doubled the risk in both sexes. The impact was discernible into advanced age and was dose related. Mortality was increased twofold to fourfold in men and women, respectively, predominantly because of coexisting cardiovascular disease.

Experience strongly confirms that patients who smoke and have chronic occlusive arterial disease affecting the extremities do not do well. A single cigarette can cause narrowing of the arteries and reduction of blood flow, which may last as long as one hour or more.[64]

The mechanisms by which smoking is atherogenic are unknown but may be related to intimal injury from increased levels of carboxyhemoglobin.[65] Smoking has been demonstrated to affect platelet function and increase the tendency toward thrombus formation.[66] The series of Beach and Strandness[67] on ASO and associated risk factors in diabetics showed a high correlation between smoking and atherosclerosis. They found this to be one of the most important risk factors and presented evidence to show that the cessation of smoking was associated with a decrease in the progression of atherosclerosis. Another effect of smoking is its possible influence on prostacyclin (PGI_2), an important prostaglandin that prevents platelet aggregation and promotes vasodilation. Nadler, Velasco, and Horton[68] have shown that cigarette smoking inhibits prostacyclin formation. In their study smoking tobacco with nicotine abolished the PGI_2 response to norepinephrine. Their observations suggest that inhalation of nicotine-containing tobacco smoke reduces vascular PGI_2 production and that this may be a factor in developing accelerated cardiovascular disease.

The nicotine and carbon monoxide content of cigarette smoke has been felt to be the major risk. However, Palmer, Rosenberg, and Shapiro found that smoking "low yield" cigarettes did not lower the risk of a first nonfatal myocardial infarction.[69]

Cigarette smoking may also contribute to the pathogenesis of atherosclerosis through its effect on lipid metabolism. The study of Brischetto et al showed the plasma lipid and lipoprotein profiles of cigarette smokers from randomly selected families to be abnormal.[70] The study demonstrated that those who smoked had higher plasma cholesterol, triglycerides and VLDL levels, and a lower HDL cholesterol concentration.[70]

An increased hypercoagulability has been found in chronic smokers, compared with nonsmokers.[60] It became pronounced immediately after smoking three cigarettes.[60] The group who smoked had higher plasma fibrinogen, lower plasminogen and plasminogen activator, and higher plasma viscosity.[60] After smoking three cigarettes there was an increase in platelet aggregation, von Willebrand's factor, and a decrease in red blood cell deformability.[60]

A possible miscellaneous effect of smoking is altered insulin absorption. Evidence suggests that the absorption of insulin in smokers may be impaired from subcutaneous sites because of the peripheral vasoconstriction caused by nicotine.[71] Smoking also has a deleterious effect on wound healing.[72] Cessation of cigarette smoking improves transcutaneous oxygen levels.[73] Nevertheless, every effort should be made to control the blood sugars because uncontrolled diabetes may result in increased triglycerides, which may adversely affect the endothelium. These deleterious effects of smoking on ASO apply to the diabetic as well as the nondiabetic. However, because of the many risk factors associated with diabetes, smoking is an even greater risk for ASO in the patient population. Despite this, the prevalence of smoking is 27% in the diabetic population and 26% in nondiabetics.[74] Black and Hispanic diabetic men had an insignificantly higher prevalence of smoking compared with white men with diabetes.[74]

Hypertension is also a risk factor that can be controlled. Control of both systolic and diastolic pressure is important. The treatment of hypertension is critically important to all patients, especially diabetics with microangiopathy and macroangiopathy. There is no question that a strong correlation exists between hypercholesterolemia and cardiovascular disease. However, not all authorities have found a correlation between peripheral ASO and hypercholesterolemia.[21,44] Nevertheless, any patient with elevated cholesterol values should be treated.

Hyperglycemia is an important factor in the pathogenesis of ASO. Nelson et al[21] have found a correlation between hyperglycemia and ASO. Experimentally, Lorenzi, Cagliero, and Toledo have shown glucose toxicity for human endothelial cells in culture.[75] The results of the recent Diabetes Control and Complications Trial has shown that tight control of diabetes decreases macrovascular events of cardiac and peripheral ASO.[76] Moss, Klein, and Klein have also shown a correlation of high hemoglobin A, C and lower extremity amputations.[77]

Hyperglycemia leads to increased glycosylation cross-linkage of collagen and stiffness in the arterial wall.[78] Binding of advanced glycosylation end products to macrophages results in increased synthesis and release of interleukin-1, which can also stimulate the arterial wall smooth muscle proliferation.[78]

Hyperinsulinemia can also be a risk factor in the pathogenesis of atherosclerosis. Hyperinsulinemia is common in type II patients who have insulin resistance. It is also common in type I patients because the insulin is administered subcutaneously and does not initially pass through the liver for removal. Of insulin secreted by the pancreas 50% is removed by one pass through the liver. Insulin is a growth–hormonelike factor and has been found by several investigators to stimulate the duplication of smooth muscles and their migration into the lumen.[79,80] This process plays a major role in the formation of the atherosclerotic plaque. Evidence of atherosclerosis caused by hyperinsulinemia has been reported to occur in the presence of normal glucose tolerance. Zavaroni et al[81] found that a group of "healthy persons" with hyperinsulinemia and normal glucose tolerance had an increase in vascular risk factors and triglycerides and lower HDL concentrations. In the experimental diabetic BB rat, Larson and Haudenschild found a genetic predilection, sensitivity of the vascular smooth muscle cells to insulin, and a dissociation of this effect from hyperglycemia.[82]

Adiposity, and especially the fat distribution, is a vascular risk factor. Distribution of body fat has been found to be an independent predictor of metabolic aberrations, including cardiovascular morbidity and mortality.[83] Abdominal or truncal obesity has been associated with hyperinsulinemia, hypertriglyceridemia, decreased HDLs, and hypertension.[84,85] Peiris et al measured intraabdominal fat, using computerized tomography.[86] They found that intraabdominal fat deposition constitutes greater cardiovascular risk than obesity alone. They also reached the conclusion that hyperinsulinemia may constitute an important component of increased vascular risk associated with abdominal obesity.[86]

Truncal obesity has been linked to smoking. Shimokata, Muller, and Andres[87] found the waist-hip ratio in smokers to be significantly higher than in nonsmokers, and that waist-hip ratio in patients who started smoking actually increased despite weight loss. Barrett-Connor and Khaw[88] also found that cigarette smokers have more central obesity than do nonsmokers. The explanation for this relation to cigarette smoking is not known. However, cigarette smoking is associated with increased adrenal androgens in both men and women, and androgens contribute to truncal obesity in women.[89,90]

Truncal obesity is also associated with insulin resistance and hyperinsulinemia, which has been shown to be correlated with atherosclerosis. A study by Facchini, Hollenbeck, and Jeppesen showed that chronic cigarette smokers have insulin resistance, hyperinsulinemia, and dyslipidemia compared with a matched group of nonsmokers.[91]

In summary, the development of ASO in the diabetic obviously stems from a wide combination of risk factors.

SIGNS AND SYMPTOMS OF ARTERIOSCLEROSIS OBLITERANS (ASO). The subjective (symptoms) and objective (signs) findings of ASO are listed in the accompanying box. Intermittent claudication is a common symptom associated with diabetic ASO. In the Framingham study diabetes was associated with twofold to threefold excess risk of intermittent claudication for both sexes.[92] An excess risk for intermittent claudication was observed in men receiving oral hypoglycemic therapy and in women receiving insulin or oral agents. Diabetics with intermittent claudication were at an especially high risk of cardiovascular events.[92] The word *claudication* comes from the Latin, meaning "to limp." The patient with claudication may limp; however, more characteristically he or she stops to rest. The pain or discomfort is usually localized in the calf, is characterized by pain associated with walking, and is relieved by cessation of walking without the need to sit down. The discomfort associated with intermittent claudication must be distinguished from pain in the leg

SIGNS AND SYMPTOMS OF ASO IN THE LOWER EXTREMITY

1. Intermittent claudication
2. Cold feet
3. Nocturnal pain
4. Rest pain
5. Nocturnal and rest pain relieved with dependency
6. Absent pulses
7. Blanching on elevation
8. Delayed venous filling after elevation
9. Dependent rubor
10. Atrophy of subcutaneous fatty tissues
11. Shiny appearance of skin
12. Loss of hair on foot and toes
13. Thickened nails, often with fungal infection
14. Gangrene
15. Miscellaneous
    a. Blue-toe syndrome
    b. Acute vascular occlusion

with walking, which can result from degenerative arthritic changes; disk disease; tumors of the spinal cord, particularly the cauda equina; thrombophlebitis; anemia; and even myxedema.

Pain with walking resulting from these causes is referred to as *pseudoclaudication*. Differentiation from ischemic claudication and pseudoclaudication can be made by history alone. Patients with claudication caused by ischemia simply need to stop walking and rest for a minute or two and then proceed. Patients with pseudoclaudication usually require 15 to 20 minutes of rest and frequently give a history of having to sit down, change position, flex or extend their back to get relief. The symptom of intermittent claudication depends on ischemia in the muscle. Because of the small-muscle mass in the foot some investigators believe that claudication is infrequent in the foot.

Some diabetics, despite significant ASO, may not have symptoms of intermittent claudication because of the loss of pain sensation. This stresses the need for routine examination of the diabetic's lower extremity for signs of ASO, even though the patient is not complaining of symptoms. Improvement in intermittent claudication can be achieved with cessation of smoking and supervised training and exercise programs.

Cold feet are a common complaint in patients with ASO. It is cold feet that prompt the diabetic to resort to using hot water bottles and heating pads. This can result in severe burns to a foot that has become insensitive to heat because of peripheral neuropathy.

Rest pain usually indicates at least two hemodynamically significant arterial blocks in a series. Rest pain is caused by nerve ischemia and is persistent with peaks of intensity. It is worse at night and may require the use of narcotics for relief. Rest pain is decreased by dependency of the legs. Therefore the patient often sleeps in a chair, and edema of the leg, secondary to constant dependency, is common.

Nocturnal ischemic pain is a form of neuritis that usually precedes rest pain. It occurs at night or during sleep because the circulation is essentially of the core variety, with very little perfusion of the lower extremity. Ischemic neuritis thus produced becomes intense and disrupts sleep. The patient invariably gains relief by standing up or dangling his or her feet over the edge of the bed and on occasion by walking a few steps. This activity increases the cardiac output, leading to improved perfusion of the lower extremities and relief of the ischemic neuritis. If vascular lesions that produce rest and nocturnal pain are not corrected by vascular surgery, gangrene almost always develops, necessitating amputation. Rest pain and nocturnal pain are therefore indications for angiography and, when possible, vascular surgery. Diabetics with severe ASO and ischemia may not experience rest pain or night pain because of peripheral neuropathy, again stressing the need for examining the lower extremity on a routine basis. Nocturnal leg pain may also be caused by peripheral neuropathy. The nocturnal pain of neuropathy can be differentiated from that of ischemia simply by history. The patient with nocturnal neuropathic pain will get up and walk to alleviate his or her discomfort, while the patient with ischemic pain sits up all night with the legs dependent. Absent pulses are significant evidence of ASO. Examination of the patient with intermittent claudication involving the calf muscle may reveal both a femoral and pedal pulse but no popliteal pulse. The pedal pulses are present because of the collateral vessels in these patients. After a brisk walk the foot will pale and become pulseless.

Further ischemic changes are characterized by shiny, atrophic cool skin. As vascular insufficiency progresses there is loss of hair on the dorsum of the foot. Thickening of the nails is also influenced by the arterial insufficiency. These nails frequently have fungal infections. In addition, the nails tend to grow more slowly when the blood supply is decreased. Ischemia leads to atrophy of the subcutaneous tissue. The skin appears to be tightly drawn over the foot, and ulceration can occur from minor trauma to this atrophic skin. Fig. 40-8 illustrates the typical diabetic foot afflicted with ASO and neuropathy.

In the diabetic most of the changes of ischemia occur slowly, although the possibility of sudden occlusion from emboli or complete thrombosis must always be considered. The signs and symptoms of a sudden arterial occlusion are usually called the *five p's* (see the box on this page). The extent of ischemia and the final outcome depend on the collateral circulation and the time elapsing from the onset of acute occlusion to treatment. Most sudden occlusions are the result of emboli, but they can occur from thrombosis at the site of an atherosclerotic plaque. These occlusions must be treated within 4 to 6 hours since peripheral nerves and skeletal muscle have less resistance to ischemia than skin and bone. Pain from embolism is usually more severe and sudden in onset than pain from thrombosis. Pallor is also more severe with embolism than

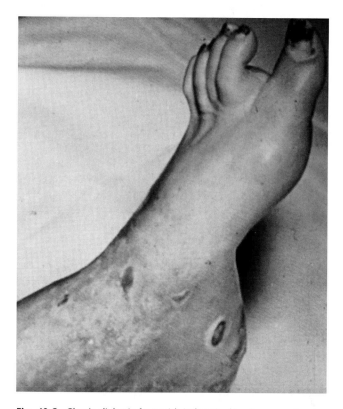

Fig. 40-8. Classic diabetic foot with ischemic skin changes: atrophy of subcutaneous tissues, hair loss on dorsum of foot, thickening of nails, atrophy of interosseus muscles resulting in cocked up toes, and commonly seen superficial ulcerations. *(From Levin ME, O'Neal LW, and Bowker JH, eds: The diabetic foot, ed 5, St Louis, 1993, Mosby–Year Book; courtesy John F. Fairbairn II, M.D., Mayo Clinic, Rochester, Minn, and The Upjohn Company, Kalamazoo, Mich.)*

THE FIVE *P*'s OF ACUTE ARTERIAL OCCLUSION IN THE LOWER EXTREMITY

1. Pain: sudden onset
2. Pallor: waxy
3. Paresthesias: numbness
4. Pulselessness: no pulse below block
5. Paralysis: sudden weakness

---

with thrombosis. With embolism the affected extremity is waxlike and lemon yellow. With thrombosis the extremity appears less cadaverous and tends to be somewhat cyanotic. The paresthesia is caused by peripheral nerve ischemia. The management of acute arterial occlusion is discussed in Chapter 15.

Peripheral Neuropathy

The first description of the manifestations of diabetic neuropathy was made by Marchal de Calvi in 1864.[39] Now over 100 years later, despite much research and many publications, the exact cause of diabetic neuropathy remains unexplained. The pathogenesis is undoubtedly multifactorial. A decreased blood flow in the vasonervorum caused by vascular narrowing of the vessel or increased blood viscosity is a factor. Another possible factor under investigation is the trapping of immunoglobulins on peripheral nerve myelin.[93] This does not occur in the brain and may account for the fact that there are rarely central nervous system neuropathies.[93]

Metabolic change is probably the most significant factor in the development of diabetic peripheral neuropathy.[94,95] Glucose enters the nerve without the need for insulin. It is then converted by the enzyme aldose reductase to the polyols, sorbitol, and fructose. It has been postulated that when high levels of polyols or glucose are present, there is a decrease of *myo*-inositol in the nerves. *Myo*-inositol appears to be important for nerve membrane function and nerve conduction.[94] The use of aldose reductase inhibitors to prevent the conversion of glucose to sorbitol and fructose has been shown to improve motor nerve conduction. Sural nerve biopsy specimens from patients with diabetic neuropathy treated the aldose reductase inhibitor, sorbinil, showed regeneration and repair of myelinated fibers.[96] Dyck et al biopsied the sural nerve of diabetic patients treated with sorbinil. Despite improved motor nerve conduction they did not find any significant change in levels of *myo*-inositol, casting doubt on its importance.[97]

Increased levels of polyols diffuse very poorly out of the nerve, resulting in a hyperosmotic effect, which causes edema of the nerve. Edema of sural nerves has been confirmed by Griffey et al.[98] This group, using magnetic resonance spectroscopy, found that the sural nerves of patients with peripheral neuropathy were edematous and treatment with sorbinil decreased this edema.[98] This was probably accomplished by a decrease in the levels of sorbitol and fructose, thus decreasing hyperosmolality and decreasing the influx of water.

There are a number of syndromes associated with diabetic neuropathy.[99] The most common of those involving the foot are distal symmetric sensorimotor polyneuropathies, resulting in pain; paresthesias; atrophy of the interosseous muscles; the loss of sensation; autonomic neuropathy with dry, scaly feet; radiculopathy; and entrapment syndromes. An important entrapment syndrome affecting the foot is the tarsal tunnel syndrome. This results from compression of the posterior tibial nerve at the tarsal tunnel or of the plantar nerves. This causes sensory impairment in the sole of the foot and weakness of the intrinsic pedal musculature. It usually occurs unilaterally. This differentiates it from the metabolic bilateral symmetric polyneuropathy. Its symptoms are burning pain and paresthesias at the ankle and plantar surface of the foot.[100]

Diabetic patients with peripheral neuropathy do not always have neuropathy because of diabetes. These patients, like any nondiabetic individual, may have neuropathy resulting from a number of other causes (see the accompanying box). Neoplastic effects may result from humoral causes or direct nerve compression. Recently we saw a woman with diabetes and peripheral neuropathy. Her neuropathy, being unilateral, was atypical. Further evaluation revealed a meningioma of the spinal cord. Treatment for diabetic peripheral neuropathy in this patient would have resulted in a misdiagnosis.

CAUSES OF PERIPHERAL NEUROPATHY

1. Diabetes mellitus
2. Alcoholism
3. Herniated nucleus pulposus
4. Heavy metals
5. Vitamin deficiencies
6. Collagen disease
7. Pernicious anemia
8. Malignancy
9. Pressure neuropathy
10. Uremia
11. Porphyria
12. Hansen's disease (leprosy)
13. Drugs

As noted in Fig. 40-1, neuropathy can ultimately result in amputation, through various pathways. These include the loss of autonomic, sensory, or motor nerve function. Autonomic involvement results in decreased perspiration. This leads to dryness, cracking, and fissuring of the skin, which can be portals of entry for bacteria. Autonomic dysfunction can also lead to the loss of the flare reaction. Any noxious stimuli to the skin results in an increased blood flow. In the diabetic with autonomic neuropathy, this effect can be blunted, thereby impeding wound healing. Orthostatic hypotension, a complication of autonomic involvement, may lead to a decrease in pressure and arterial perfusion with standing.

The most important neuropathic factor leading to foot lesions is the loss of pain and temperature sensation. The patient with nerve impairment develops an insensate foot that endures painless trauma from mechanical, chemical, or thermal sources, frequently resulting in ulceration and infection (Fig. 40-1). Symptoms of sensory neuropathy affect 30% to 40% of diabetic patients. Men and women are equally affected. Prevalence of symptoms increases with duration.[101] In this study, age, ethnicity, cigarette smoking, and height were not found to be contributing factors.[101]

Painless mechanical trauma can occur from a variety of causes. The most common injury is the classical plantar ulcer from walking on insensate feet. The repetitive stress of walking results in callus buildup and hot spots. Because there is no pain, the patient continues to walk. The callus builds up, and pressure necrosis and ulceration result. Abnormally high pressures, especially under the forefoot, have been found in such feet. Cavanagh and Ulbrecht have reviewed the biomechanics of the foot and the resulting pressures in the patient with diabetes.[102]

Trauma from painless puncture wounds is not rare. Fig. 40-9 shows a carpenter's nail deep in the tissues of the foot of a 45-year-old who required insulin for 10 years. He had a small, painless draining area on his foot for approximately 1 month and sought medical attention only be-

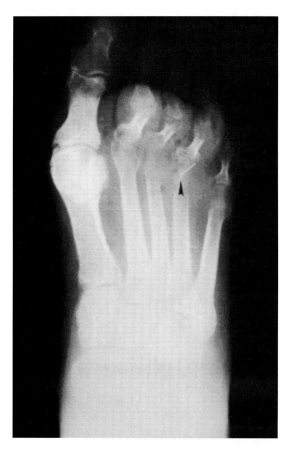

Fig. 40-9. Carpenter's nail present for approximately 1 month in tissues of foot of an insulin-requiring diabetic patient. He had no knowledge of having stepped on this nail, nor did he have any pain or discomfort. *(From Levin ME, O'Neal LW, and Bowker JH, eds: The diabetic foot, ed 5, St Louis, 1993, Mosby–Year Book; courtesy Dr. J. Joseph Marr, Sr. Vice President, Discovery Research Searle, Skokie, Ill.)*

cause the area had failed to heal. The dorsalis pedis and posterior tibial pulses were of good quality. However, vibratory sense and pain and touch sensation were markedly diminished. Radiographs of the foot revealed the carpenter's nail, which must have been present for at least a month without any discomfort to the patient. The area involved had caused severe osteomyelitis and was ultimately amputated.

I would agree with Dr. Paul Brand, who stated that "the diabetic who claims his shoes are killing him may well be right." Painless ulceration from ill-fitting shoes may become infected; gangrene may follow, and amputation may be necessary. Ulcers most often occur on the side of the foot (Fig. 40-10). The number of foreign objects found in patients' shoes that they have walked on without pain or awareness is legion. To mention only a few, there are pebbles, coins, and unbelievably large objects such as hearing aids and shoehorns (Figs. 40-11 and 40-12).

Another extreme example of painless trauma is noted in Fig. 40-13, *A*. This shows ulceration over the Achilles tendon of a patient who kept the back of his heel against a chair while on jury duty. Blisters developed, ulcerated, and penetrated to the Achilles tendon. The patient's physician advised using a Band-Aid and returning to work. Fortunately the patient sought a second opinion, and a skingraft flap procedure was done, and the ulceration healed (Fig. 40-13, *B* and *C*).

Another common cause of painless injury results from "home surgery." Because persons with diabetic neuropathy feel no pain, they frequently cut their calluses too deep and their nails too close, resulting in ulceration and infection. Fig. 40-14 shows an infected and gangrenous great toe that resulted from a patient practicing "home surgery." Even though she was partially blind, she attempted to cut the nail and in doing so, cut into the tissue.

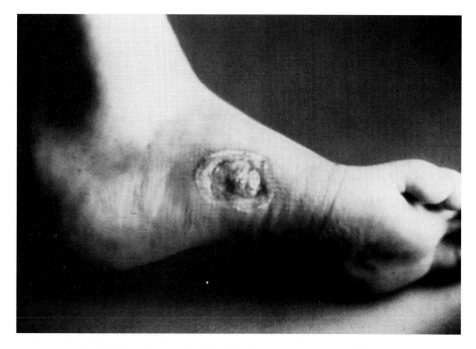

Fig. 40-10. Ulceration on the side of the foot, suggestive of an ill-fitting shoe.

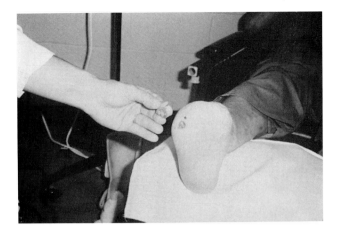

Fig. 40-11. Painless foot ulcer resulting from the patient inadvertently walking on his hearing aid, which he did not know had fallen into his shoe.

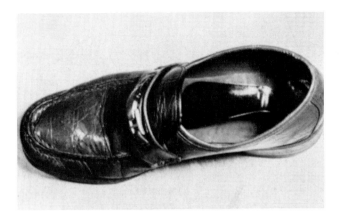

Fig. 40-12. Shoehorn in shoe worn by patient who, because of insensitive foot resulting from diabetic neuropathy, was unaware of its presence until removing shoe at end of day. *(From Levin ME, O'Neal LW, and Bowker JH, eds: The diabetic foot, ed 5, St Louis, 1993, Mosby–Year Book.)*

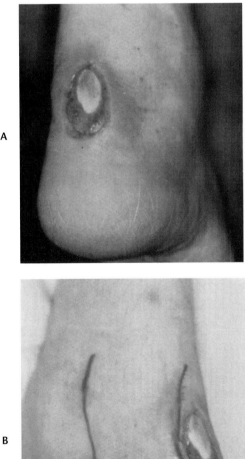

A

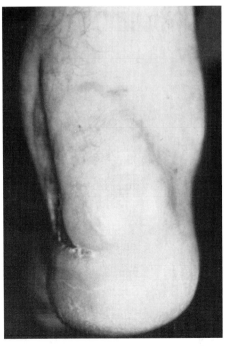

B

C

Fig. 40-13. A, Ulceration resulting from breakdown of painless blister that penetrated to Achilles tendon. **B,** Outline of skin flap for treatment of ulceration **(A). C,** Healed skin-flap graft for treatment of ulceration **(A).** *(From Levin ME, O'Neal LW, and Bowker JH, eds: The diabetic foot, ed 5, St Louis, 1993, Mosby–Year Book; courtesy Dr. Leroy Young, Department of Plastic Surgery, Washington University School of Medicine, St Louis.)*

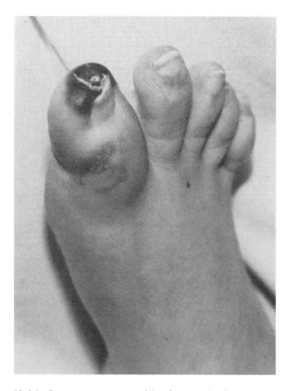

Fig. 40-14. Gangrenous toes resulting from patient's attempt at home surgery. Toenail was cut too deep, became infected, and gangrene developed. *(From Levin ME, O'Neal LW, and Bowker JH, eds: The diabetic foot, ed 5, St Louis, 1993, Mosby–Year Book.)*

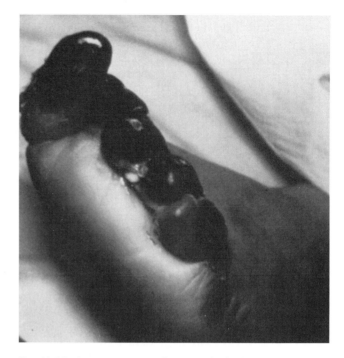

Fig. 40-15. Gangrene in toes of patient who had soaked his cold foot in hot water. *(From Levin ME, O'Neal LW, and Bowker JH, eds: The diabetic foot, ed 5, St Louis, 1993, Mosby–Year Book.)*

This resulted in infection, gangrene, and partial amputation.

Chemical trauma results from the use of callus and corn removers. It has also occurred from soaking the feet in chemical solutions and strong antiseptics.

Thermal injuries are quite common in the insensitive diabetic foot. Fig. 40-15 shows gangrene of the toes of a diabetic who had soaked his cold insensate foot in a bucket of hot water. Fortunately the patient had good dorsalis pedis and posterior tibial pulses and had a successful midtarsal amputation. The fact that only the toes became gangrenous is good evidence for the existence of small vessel disease. Severe burns have occurred in patients with insensitive feet who have walked on hot sandy beaches or other hot surfaces. We have seen a number of these patients ultimately require amputation. Diabetic patients going to the beach or to swimming pools should wear protective footwear. Patients who have placed their feet in front of the fireplace to warm them have sustained severe burns, not an uncommon occurrence. Perhaps the most dramatic case of painless thermal injury that I have encountered was in a diabetic patient who had a previous below-knee amputation. While mowing his lawn on a riding mower, he inadvertently placed his remaining foot on the manifold, which became extremely hot. Only when he smelled "something burning" did he look down to discover that his shoe and foot were on fire. Unfortunately, subsequent amputation of his remaining foot was necessary.

SIGNS AND SYMPTOMS OF NEUROPATHY IN THE DIABETIC FOOT AND LEG

1. Paresthesia
2. Hyperesthesia
3. Hypoesthesia
4. Radicular pain
5. Loss of deep tendon reflexes
6. Loss of vibratory and position sense
7. Anhidrosis
8. Heavy callus formation over pressure points
9. Trophic ulcers
10. Infection complicating trophic ulcers
11. Foot drop
12. Changes in shape of foot produced by:
    a. Muscle atrophy
    b. Changes in bone and joints
13. Radiographic signs:
    a. Demineralization
    b. Osteolysis
    c. Charcot's joint

SIGNS AND SYMPTOMS OF DIABETIC NEUROPATHY. The signs and symptoms of diabetic peripheral neuropathy are listed in the accompanying box. Diabetic neuropathy in the lower extremity is bilateral and tends to

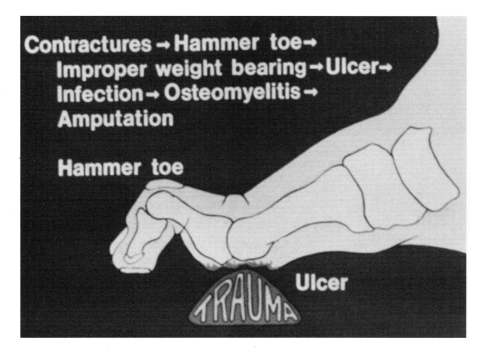

Fig. 40-16. Progression of contractures leading to hammer toes, ulceration, and infection. *(From Levin ME, O'Neal LW, and Bowker JH, eds: The diabetic foot, ed 5, St Louis, 1993, Mosby–Year Book; courtesy the Michigan Diabetes Research and Training Center, Ann Arbor, Mich, 1983, The University of Michigan.)*

be symmetric. The sensory involvement is characterized by two major system complexes. One consists of pain and paresthesias. The other, paradoxically, consists of a decreased or absent sensation of touch, pain, and temperature. The paresthesias may be manifested as tingling or burning. Many patients exhibit marked hyperesthesias of the feet and legs, which may be so great that they cannot stand even the lightest touch such as sheets or pajamas. Treatment for this extreme sensitivity, which may involve the entire trunk, other than control of the blood sugar and the use of pharmacologic agents, consists of wearing firmly fitting hose or even a body stocking. Putting these on is very uncomfortable but once they are applied, there is no longer any contact with movable clothing, and the patient is much more comfortable. The pain of peripheral neuropathies may be severe, knifelike, or shooting. It can be almost constant and frequently is more severe at night. The pain may be severe enough to require narcotics for relief. A great deal of caution must be observed in prescribing narcotics for these patients, since the treatment may be long, and drug habituation or addiction can develop. The decrease in sensory perception is not only manifested by loss of pain and temperature sensation, but can also be manifested by a "dead feeling" in the feet, giving the sensation of walking on an unusual surface such as cushions.

Radicular pain, or mononeuropathy, in the lower extremity is not uncommon. One example is the relatively frequent occurrence of diabetic femoral neuropathy, or L-3 radioculopathy, which is characterized by low back pain that may be of sudden onset. The pain extends into the anterior part of the thigh and is associated with paresthesias and sensory loss in that area. There may be weakness of

flexion at the hip, extension of the knee (quadriceps weakness), and adduction of the thigh. The knee jerk may be significantly decreased or absent. Radicular pain must always be differentiated from root pain produced by other causes, such as a ruptured disk, arthritis, or tumor. Although peripheral symmetric polyneuropathy is metabolic in origin, the mononeuropathies are most likely the result of thrombi in a vessel of the vasonervorum. Over a period of weeks or months this will recanalize, nerve function will return, and the pain will disappear.

In evaluating sensation in the foot, it is important not only to do the physical examination but also to take a careful history. For example, changes in shoe size can be a tip-off to the development of neuropathy. Dr. Paul Brand has pointed out that with loss of sensation a patient tends to purchase a smaller shoe size. The smaller size is no longer uncomfortable because the patient has lost sensation. In fact, the correct size feels too large to the patient. The patient should be asked, as part of the history, whether he or she has had a change in shoe size.

FOOT DEFORMITIES. Muscle atrophy caused by involvement of the motor nerves leads to an imbalance of the interosseous muscles in the foot. This frequently leads to cocked up toes. Ulceration may occur on the tips and tops of the toes, and because of thinning of the fat pad underneath the first metatarsal-phalangeal joint, ulceration may occur in this area (Fig. 40-16). Prevention of ulceration in these areas requires straightening out of these cocked up, or claw, toes at a time when circulation is good. However, if this cannot be done, then it is important to make sure the toe box of the shoe is large enough to accommodate the top of these deformed toes. Cushioned insoles should be worn to protect the tips of these toes.

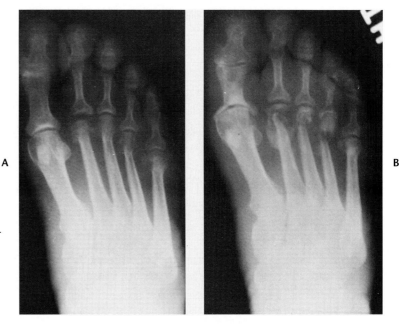

Fig. 40-17. A, Foot of 60-year-old man with known diabetes of 4 years' duration. **B,** Same foot, 3 months later, showing classic osteolytic bone changes of diabetic neuropathy involving distal segment of the metatarsals. *(From Levin ME, O'Neal LW, and Bowker JH, eds: The diabetic foot, ed 5, St Louis, 1993, Mosby–Year Book; courtesy Dr. Robert Karsh, Washington University School of Medicine, St Louis.)*

These insoles must be worn only in indepth therapeutic shoes that can accommodate the insoles.

The most extreme example of diabetic foot deformity is the Charcot's foot or neuroarthropathy. The incidence of Charcot's foot is most common in the fifth and sixth decades and increases with the duration of diabetes. It is essentially the same in both sexes and is bilateral in approximately one third of all cases. The average duration of diabetes before the development of this lesion is 12 years. In Boehm's series the duration of the disease ranged between 2 and 20 years.[103] However, it may occur in the younger diabetic patient and in the patient with diabetes of recent onset. It has even been reported as the initial clinical manifestation of diabetes. There appears to be no significant relationship between the development of Charcot's foot and the degree of blood glucose control. Radiographically, the sites most often affected in diabetic patients are the smaller joints of the foot, particularly the tarsometatarsal joints and, to a lesser extent, the joints of the metatarsophalangeal area, and the ankle.[104]

Classically, Charcot's foot develops as an acutely hot, erythematous, and swollen foot with bounding pulses and prominent veins. Despite what is written in some textbooks, patients with Charcot's foot frequently have moderate pain and discomfort. It may be difficult to differentiate the warm, red Charcot's foot from cellulitis. However, the patient with Charcot's foot is afebrile, and the white blood cell count is normal. The sedimentation rate may be slightly elevated. The neuropathic component to the development of Charcot's foot probably stems from involvement of the autonomic nervous system. The result is the equivalent of sympathectomy to the arteries in the foot. The arteries dilate and A-V shunts have been demonstrated in these feet.[105] X-ray examination in the acute stage usually reveals no bony abnormality (Fig. 40-17, A). If the patient continues to walk, there can be gradual dissolution and fragmentation of the distal ends of the metatarsals (Fig. 40-17, B) and the ankle bones. The distal ends of the metatarsals become pointed, the "peppermint stick sign," as if the ends of the bone were licked away.[106] The x-ray films also show the absence of calcification in the interosseous arteries, further evidence that there is no significant vascular insufficiency. It is felt that the increased circulation causes reabsorption of the bone. Evidence that increase in circulation contributes to the Charcot's foot has been suggested by the report of Edelman et al.[107] These authors reported three cases of Charcot's foot that developed following successful peripheral vascular surgery. These cases demonstrate the important role of increased blood flow in the absorption of calcium from the bones in the foot, their collapse, and the development of Charcot's foot. Because there is relative insensitivity in these feet, patients continue to walk, subsequently developing the so-called stress fractures and further bone destruction. Treatment for these patients in the acute stage is nonweight bearing, frequently with the aid of a contact cast. If the process is allowed to progress, the arch collapses and the foot becomes everted and shortened and takes on a clubfoot shape. The arch is lost and takes on a rocker bottom configuration (Fig. 40-18). It is the plantar area of the arch that breaks down and becomes ulcerated (Fig. 40-19). Ulceration on the plantar surface in the area of the arch is a classic sign of Charcot's foot.

Because of bone destruction in Charcot's foot, it is sometimes difficult to distinguish between osteoarthropathy and osteomyelitis. If there is no portal of entry or ulceration overlying the area of bone destruction and there are other findings compatible with Charcot's foot, the most likely diagnosis is neuroarthropathy. However, osteomyelitis must always be ruled out. Routine imaging techniques have not always been conclusive. Recently, the combined use of leukocyte and bone imaging has helped to make this distinction. Using this technique, Splittgerber et al[108] found that bone imaging frequently demonstrated increased activity in both osteoarthropathy and osteomyelitis. However, leukocyte imaging showed increased ac-

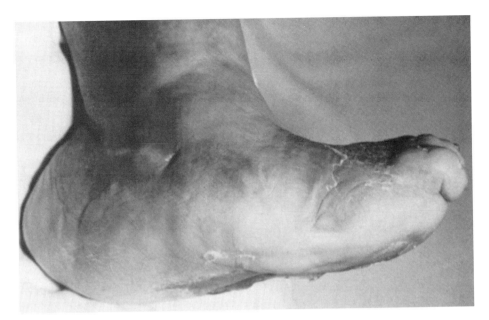

Fig. 40-18. Clubfoot appearance of Charcot's foot, with collapse of the tarso-metatarsal joints. *(From Levin ME and O'Neal LW: The diabetic foot, ed 5, St Louis, 1993, The CV Mosby Co.)*

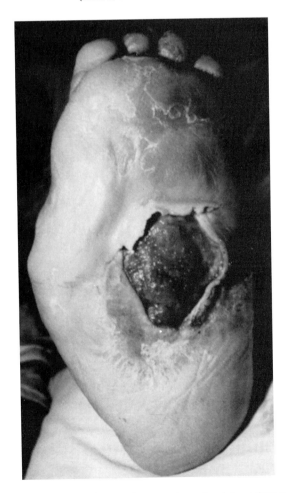

Fig. 40-19. Massive ulcer on plantar surface of arch in patient with Charcot's foot (Fig. 40-18). *(From Levin ME: Pathophysiology of diabetic foot lesions. Reprinted by permission from Clinical diabetes mellitus: a problem-oriented approach, J. Davidson, 1986, © 1986 by Thieme Medical Publishers, Inc., New York.)*

tivity in only the cases of osteomyelitis. There was minimal or no activity in the cases with osteoarthropathy.[108] In a larger series of 35 cases Schauwecker et al also found the use of leukocyte scanning useful for evaluating osteomyelitis in the presence of osteoarthropathy.[109]

Indium-labeled leukocytes localize to areas of active bone marrow. However, active bone marrow is not present in adult feet. Therefore any sequestration of indium-111–labeled leukocytes within the bones of adult feet is indicative of infection.[110]

Sanders and Frykberg have recently reviewed the multiple aspects of the Charcot foot.[111]

It is important to x-ray the diabetic foot of patients with significant peripheral neuropathy and especially those with a history of previous ulcer. Studies have shown that a significant number of patients with diabetic neuropathy had bone changes that were previously undiagnosed.[112]

Infection

Infection is the third major factor in the pathogenesis of diabetic foot lesions and when associated with ischemia, frequently leads to amputation.[113] Breaks in the skin, which may be almost imperceptible, such as cracks, fissures in calluses, and major wounds, such as neurotrophic foot ulcers, act as portals of entry for bacteria. A variety of factors contribute to the diabetic's difficulty in handling infection. In the nondiabetic, infection leads to increased blood flow. In the diabetic, however, infection frequently leads to microthrombi formation in the small arterioles, which further impairs circulation (Fig. 40-4).[114] When this occurs in the small arteries of the toes, it can convert the vessels into end-arteries, resulting in gangrene of the toes (Fig. 40-5). Vascular disease impairs the delivery of antibiotics and oxygen to the affected areas. Impaired autonomic neurogenic vascular responses have already been mentioned. Leukocyte function is frequently impaired with defective adherence, diapedesis, chemotaxis, phagocytosis, and microbicidal activity of leukocytes in diabetic patients, particularly in those with uncontrolled diabetes and ketosis.

In the infected diabetic foot, one cannot rely entirely on the white blood cell count. Mean total white blood cell counts may not be elevated even in the presence of significant infection.[115] A normal white blood cell count should not dissuade the initiation of early aggressive antibiotic therapy.

Most diabetic foot infections are polymicrobial.[116] It is not unusual to culture four to five organisms from these wounds. These may be gram-negative or gram-positive organisms, aerobes and anaerobes. The most common gram-positive aerobes are *Staphylococcus aureus,* group B streptococcus, and enterococcus. The most common gram-negative aerobes are *Escherichia coli, Proteus, Klebsiella, Enterobacter, Pseudomonas,* and other enteric bacilli. The most common gram-positive anaerobes are *Peptostreptococcus* and *Clostridium.* The most common gram-negative anaerobe is *Bacteroides fragilis.* Among the anaerobes, *B. fragilis* is extremely common. Finegold has found 95% of diabetic foot ulcers to be infected with it.[117] Based on our own experience, this figure is probably high. Nevertheless, anaerobes are found in a high percentage of all diabetic foot wounds. Many of the polymicrobial flora occurring in the diabetic foot are gas formers. Extensive gas formation frequently can be demonstrated by soft tissue x-rays. When gas is present it indicates virulent infection frequently caused by *E. coli, Proteus,* or *Bacteroides.* Gas formation does not necessarily indicate that a clostridial infection is present. However, if it is, the prognosis is extremely poor.

The culturing technique is extremely important.[118] Culturing for anaerobes is particularly difficult. Special bedside kits for the collection of specimens likely to contain anaerobes should be used, such as anaerobic transport vials.* Infected ulcers or open sinuses may appear to be only superficial, and simple swabbing of these areas may not reflect the nature of deeper tissue infection. Curettage or needle aspiration are the most reliable methods. If grossly necrotic tissue is present or there is eschar overlying the ulceration, the overlying tissue should be removed during debridement and the underlying necrotic tissue cultured both for anaerobes and aerobes. It is critically important in the treatment of infection that the necrotic material be vigorously removed, and debridement carried deep enough to identify all areas of infection. Superficial debridement will result only in delay and inaccurate evaluation of the extent of the infection, its degree, and the types of organisms involved.

On occasion, even in an obviously infected foot, the culture may be reported as negative.[115] This may be due to culture techniques and does not rule out infection, especially deep in the foot.

Osteomyelitis is extremely common in the diabetic foot but its presence may be difficult to detect on a clinical basis. Newman et al[119] showed that in biopsy-proven osteomyelitis only one third of the patients had clinically suspected osteomyelitis. If bone is visible or the ulcer can be probed to bone the probability of the presence of osteomyelitis is

almost 100%. Routine x-rays frequently miss osteomyelitis. Three-phase scanning techniques are also not always specific. Newman et al have found the use of labeled leukocyte indium techniques to be highly specific.[120] Magnetic resonance imaging (MRI) is proving to be a highly successful technique for the presence of osteomyelitis. The sensitivity of MRI to the presence of osteomyelitis has been reported to be between 90% and 100%, with a specificity of 80%.[121] McEnery et al have reviewed imaging of the diabetic foot.[122]

Excellent reviews of diabetic foot soft tissue and bone infection have been reviewed. Lipsky, Pecoraro, and Wheat[123] and Little[124] have reviewed soft tissue and bone infections in the diabetic foot.

TREATMENT. The use of a variety of oral antibiotics can be satisfactory in treating superficial infections. Effectiveness of ciprofloxacin in these infections has been demonstrated.[125] However, ciprofloxacin-resistant staphylococci have begun to appear. When a significant or deep infection is suspected, hospitalization and parenteral antibiotics are the treatments of choice. Because impaired circulation, which is so frequently present in these patients, limits the delivery of antibiotics, they should be given parenterally. In addition, the antibiotic of choice may be available only in a parenteral form.

Treatment should begin with broad-spectrum antibiotics, while waiting for the culture results. The definitive antibiotics of choice will depend on the nature of the infection and the organisms that are identified. Because of the difficulty in obtaining totally accurate cultures, clinical judgment may become important in the choice of antibiotics. In the face of severe infection, the use of a second- or third-generation cephalosporin is indicated. The presence of *Pseudomonas* may require an aminoglycoside. However, aminoglycosides can be associated with nephrotoxicity, and this becomes extremely important in the diabetic who frequently has impaired renal function. Daily peak and trough levels are critically important as are frequent measures of BUN and creatinine values. Ototoxicity may also occur. One of the best treatments for *Bacteroides* is metronidazole (Flagyl). Because the treatment of infection can be difficult and the numerous antibiotics available confusing, consultation with an expert in infectious disease should be considered.

An important factor in the successful treatment of infection is nutrition. Serum albumin is the most sensitive indicator of the nutritional state. Hypoalbuminuria may pose a significant risk for pedal infection.[126]

SPECIAL DIABETIC FOOT PROBLEMS

The Heel

The heel of the diabetic is particularly vulnerable to trauma. The heel is exposed to a great deal of pressure, resulting in callus buildup. As the callus becomes thicker it tends to crack and becomes a source of infection. When the heel is infected, the infection tends to penetrate deeply. The skin of the heel is tightly bound by numerous vertical septa extending through the subcutaneous tissue to the surface of the calcaneus. These septa result in formation of

*Gibco Laboratories, Lawrence, Massachusetts.

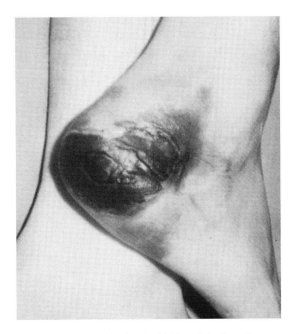

Fig. 40-20. Gangrene of heel of bedridden diabetic patient caused by weight of immobile neuropathic foot on mattress. *(From Levin ME, O'Neal LW, and Bowker JH, eds: The diabetic foot, ed 5, St Louis, 1993, Mosby–Year Book.)*

small cylinders that are packed with fatty tissue. These small fat-containing tubes act like shock absorbers on heel impact. With ischemic changes there is atrophy of the subcutaneous fatty tissue, thus decreasing the shock absorber-like effect. When the skin covering the heel is destroyed, much of the subcutaneous fat colliquates, and the septa are disrupted. If healing does occur, a tight scar will result, which makes the heel susceptible to further trauma.

When the diabetic is required to have bed rest for any length of time, such as when hospitalized, particular attention must be paid to the heel. Because of loss of sensation, the patient tends to keep the heels in the same position. This results in pressure necrosis, skin breakdown, infection, and gangrene (Fig. 40-20). Needless to say, prevention is the solution to this problem. The use of heel protectors or pressure-decreasing mattresses is essential. The available heel protectors may not always stay in place, therefore daily checks of the protector and the heel are necessary. The development of even slight erythema is a warning sign of impending pressure necrosis.

Painful Neuropathy

One of the most difficult therapeutic problems confronting the physician is the diabetic with painful neuropathy. Despite a long list of treatments none have proved totally successful. Some are totally ineffective, and those that have shown some benefit can have significant side effects. Fortunately in most patients with painful neuropathy, the pain and paresthesias disappear with time, months to years. The loss of sensation is permanent. The apparent success of some treatments in uncontrolled studies can be attributed to the coincidental disappearance of pain while taking the treatment. Injections of B_{12} and

megavitamins do not work. Phenytoin (Dilantin) is one of the oldest recommended treatments for painful neuropathy. However, controlled studies have not found phenytoin to be effective.[127] Furthermore, phenytoin can have significant side effects, not the least of which is severe exfoliative dermatitis. Carbamazepine (Tegretol) has been reported to help in some patients with painful peripheral neuropathy especially those with lancinating pain. However, this drug must be used with caution because of its many side effects. In the study of Rull et al[128] side effects occurred in 28 of 30 patients. Tricyclics, especially amitriptyline, alone or in combination with fluphenazine hydrochloride (Prolixin), have been a current treatment of choice.[129] Success with tricyclics can occur within several days. However, it may require several weeks to achieve the result. Because tricyclics may have some cardiac side effects, these drugs should be used cautiously and should be closely monitored in patients who have cardiac disease. Tricyclic drugs may also have an anticholinergic effect and should be used with caution in patients in whom anticholinergic drugs could be contraindicated, for example, patients with prostatism. Fluphenazine hydrochloride (Prolixin) may also cause signs and symptoms of parkinsonism, and its use should be carefully monitored.

The use of aldose reductase inhibitors to relieve pain is still experimental, and at present the Food and Drug Administration has not released them for clinical use. Feeding *myo*-inositol to a streptozotocin diabetic mouse improved motor nerve conduction.[130] However, there are no human studies using *myo*-inositol. Because *myo*-inositol has not been clearly evaluated in humans, I would not recommend its use at this time.

The use of topically applied capsaicin (Axsain) is a recent addition to the long list of drug treatments for painful peripheral neuropathy. Capsaicin is the pungent ingredient of hot peppers of the genus *Capsicum*.[131] While capsaicin is a new treatment for painful neuropathy, it has been in use for over a decade in neural science research to probe the function of unmyelinated and thinly myelinated afferent neurons. Capsaicin appears to be selective for type C nociceptive neurons and depletes them of the neural transmitter, substance P, thus preventing the transmission of pain impulses. A multicenter, double-blind, randomized, vehicle-controlled trial evaluating the safety and efficacy of topical capsaicin (0.075%) in patients with confirmed painful diabetic neuropathy has been carried out by Chad et al.[132] Seventy-one percent of the capsaicin-treated patients and 42% of the vehicle-alone patients showed an overall improvement in their pain. This drug is applied topically four times a day to the painful area. Skin irritations have been noted with the use of capsaicin.

Transcutaneous electrical nerve stimulation (TENS) has been postulated to relieve pain by stimulation of large myelinated afferent A fibers that, when properly stimulated, inhibit transmission of nociceptive impulses by the A-delta and C nerve fibers. Inhibition of the C fibers, which carry the pain impulses, could help relieve pain. This theory was first suggested by the classic paper of Melzack and Wall.[133]

The most important treatment of peripheral neuropathy is strict control of the blood sugar. The Diabetes

Control Complication Trial (DCCT) has conclusively shown that tight diabetic control can improve neurologic function in 60% of cases.[73] This improvement was in nerve conduction and clinical signs. How effective tight control would be in eliminating pain in patients who have progressed to this stage has not been established. Therefore tight control will, in all probability, be a preventive approach.

Toenails

Abnormalities of the toenails are common in the diabetic.[114] The nails are frequently thickened (Fig. 40-21). The markedly thickened nail, onychogryphosis, frequently occurring with fungal infection, is a potential hazard. This nail can get hooked in bedding or stockings, causing avulsion of the nail. Furthermore, the nail can cause severe pressure necrosis, subungual hemorrhage, ulceration, and infection of the nailbed. The patient may have nails that are markedly curved. These are particularly hazardous to the diabetic (Fig. 40-22). Older patients frequently neglect to trim their toenails or have them trimmed. Nails that curve in may cut into an adjacent toe

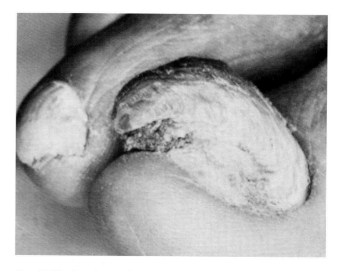

Fig. 40-21. Onychogryphosis. In diabetic patient infection may begin in debris covering nailbed. This type of nail easily hooks bedding, socks, or furniture, causing avulsion of nail and trauma to proximal nail fold. (From Levin ME, O'Neal LW, and Bowker JH, eds: The diabetic foot, ed 5, St Louis, 1993, Mosby–Year Book.)

A

B

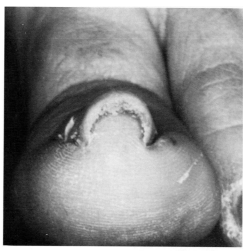
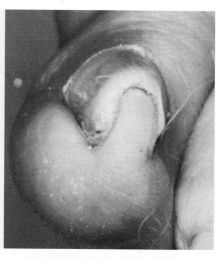

Fig. 40-22. Type of nail **(A)** that is particularly hazardous in diabetic patient. It starts from wide base at nail root and incurves distally, pinching nailbed **(B).** These two nails form arcs of greater than 200 degrees at distal toe. If neglected, medial and lateral nail margins may meet beyond distal toe, forming full circle and brittle claw. (From Levin ME, O'Neal LW, and Bowker JH, eds: The diabetic foot, ed 5, St Louis, 1993, Mosby–Year Book.)

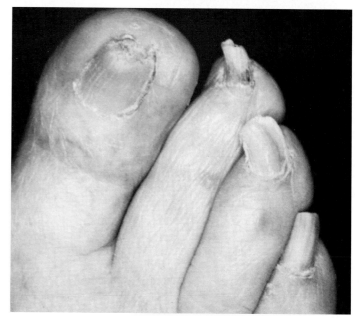

Fig. 40-23. Toes of obese diabetic patient with onychomycosis of nail of hallux and incurving distal growth of all nails. Nails have grown long because of neglect. Note that nail of third toe gouges skin of second toe. (From Levin ME, O'Neal LW, and Bowker JH, eds: The diabetic foot, ed 5, St Louis, 1993, Mosby–Year Book.)

with resulting ulceration (Fig. 40-23). Ingrown toenails are a potential source of infection, either by growing into the skin or because patients may attempt to do "home surgery" to remove the ingrown nail (Fig. 40-14). The resulting infection of the foot can make amputation necessary.

EXAMINATION OF THE DIABETIC FOOT

One of the most important aspects of the office or clinic visit is the examination of the diabetic's foot and leg. Despite the problems associated with the diabetic foot, it is frequently the most neglected part of the examination. The low rate of foot inspection in a clinic setting has been documented by Cohen, who found that only 15% to 19% of patients who entered the examining room had their feet inspected.[134] In the review of Bailey, Yu, and Rayfield only 12.3% of the diabetic patients' feet were examined.[135] The foot and lower extremity of the diabetic should be examined at every routine office visit at least three or four times a year and more often when indicated. This examination should include not only the removal of shoes and stockings but also the trousers or pantyhose as well. It is only in this setting that the lower extremity can be properly examined. Patients are reluctant to remove their shoes and stockings because they seldom feel pain or discomfort and therefore assume that all is well. Secondly, it is embarrassing to many of these patients to remove their shoes and stockings. However, if this is not done on a routine basis, lesions will be missed, treatment delayed, and amputation may be the result. Examination of the foot and lower extremity includes inspection, palpation, and a neurologic and vascular examination.

Inspection

Simply inspecting the legs and feet will give many clues to the vascular status. Evidence of significant ischemia in the foot includes the loss of hair on the dorsum of the foot and toes, skin that is shiny and atrophic and appears to be drawn tightly around the foot because of loss of the subcutaneous fat layers, and dependent rubor. All of these findings are indicative of severe peripheral arterial disease. One of the simplest evaluations for vascular insufficiency is to measure delayed capillary filling time. This is done by having the patient lie on his or her back, raising the legs to a 45-degree angle, and keeping them in this position until the feet blanch. Then have the patient sit upright, and dangle the legs. By measuring the time required for capillary filling one can estimate the degree of vascular insufficiency. Normal capillary filling time is 10 to 15 seconds. A filling time over 40 seconds indicates very severe ischemia. The extremity with severe ASO will develop dependent rubor. Patients with varicose veins may also have dependent rubor. Shiny atrophic skin, pallor on elevation, delayed filling time, and dependent rubor are the hallmarks of significant lower extremity vascular insufficiency. Details of the vascular examination can be found in Chapter 2.

Inspection between the toes is of the utmost importance. Soft corns and heloma molle, with ulceration occurring between the toes, usually the fourth and fifth, are caused by friction of the adjacent head of the proximal phalanx of the fifth toe (Fig. 40-24).

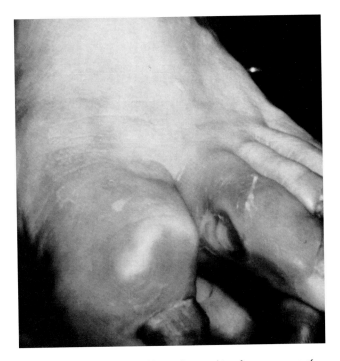

Fig. 40-24. Heloma molle of base of second toe from pressure of deformed adjacent interphalangeal joint of hallux. *(From Levin ME, O'Neal LW, and Bowker JH, eds: The diabetic foot, ed 5, St Louis, 1993, Mosby–Year Book.)*

Fig. 40-25 shows an example of a painless interdigital ulcer in an elderly woman. When this patient came into the office and was asked to remove her shoes and socks, she refused, saying that her feet felt fine and that she had no problems with them. After much insistence she removed her shoes and stockings, and the ulcer was identified. When asked how long she had the ulcer the patient looked down and with great surprise stated that she did not know that she had an ulcer because she had felt no pain. Foot inspection frequently will reveal interosseous muscle atrophy with resulting contractions, hammer and cocked up toes. Because ulcerations can occur at the tip and top of the toes (Fig. 40-16), I refer to this as the "tip-top toe ulcer syndrome." These patients need a special shoe with an insole to protect the tips of the toes and a toe box big enough to accommodate these cocked up toes.

Painless blisters may occur because of friction. However, other bullous lesions are peculiar to the diabetic. These are referred to as *bullosis diabeticorum,* which consists of two types, the acute superficial blister, which heals rapidly (Fig. 40-26) and a deeper hemorrhagic type, which tends to go on to superficial necrosis of the skin. The mechanism for the development of these lesions is unknown. Allen and Hadden[136] stress that the condition should be recognized because the treatment course and prognosis differ from those of ischemic and neuropathic lesions. However, bullosis diabeticorum is rare, with fewer than 100 cases reported up to 1991.[137] Jelinek has reviewed diabetic skin lesions.[138,139]

Palpation

Touching the skin is a simple and important part of the examination. The experienced hand and eye (see inspec-

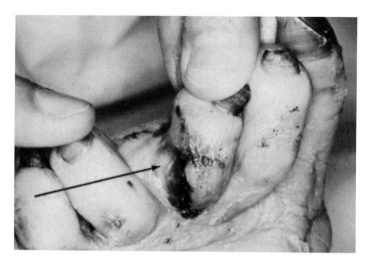

Fig. 40-25. Painless interdigital ulcer in elderly diabetic woman. Arrow points to exposed tendon, indicating depth of ulceration. This painless ulcer was found on routine foot examination. *(From Levin ME, O'Neal LW, and Bowker JH, eds: The diabetic foot, ed 5, St Louis, 1993, Mosby–Year Book.)*

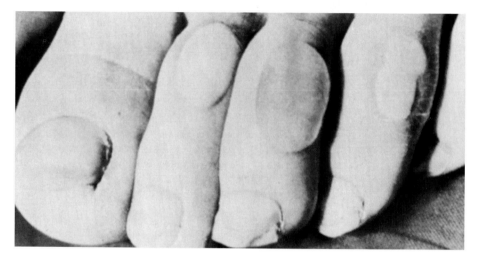

Fig. 40-26. Characteristic bullosis diabeticorum seen on toes of diabetic individual. *(From Allen GE and Hadden DR: Bullous lesions of the skin in diabetes [bullous diabeticorum], Br J Dermatol 82:216, 1970.)*

tion) are extremely important in the evaluation of ASO. Palpation consists of evaluating the pulses—the femorals, popliteals, dorsalis pedis, and posterior tibial. Auscultation for bruits will help identify the presence of atheromatous plaques and narrowing of the arterial lumen. One of the most important aspects of palpation is detecting whether the skin is warm or cool. Sophisticated instruments are available for quantitative measurements of skin temperature, for example, the Mikron digital infrared thermometer.* The approximate cost is $1800. This is a useful instrument for doing research but it is not necessary for routine examination of the foot. Palpation with the palm or back of the hand is sufficient. When indicated, a hand-held Doppler, relatively inexpensive and easy to use, should be employed in evaluating the peripheral vascular status. The use of Doppler and other laboratory techniques for evaluating ASO can be found in Chapter 3.

*Mikron Instrument Company, Box 211, Ridgeway, NJ 07451.

Sensory Examination

While a variety of sophisticated techniques are available for measurement of vibratory sense (large nerve fibers), such as the biothesiometer,† a simple tuning fork with a 128 cycle is sufficient. This examination should include vibratory sense, not only at the ankle and tibia but also at the tips of the toes. Once the patient can no longer feel the vibration, the examiner can apply the tuning fork to the same area of his or her own foot to see whether further vibrations can be detected. Young et al found that decreased vibratory sense was a predictor of subsequent foot ulceration.[140]

The examination to assess the ability to perceive temperature, a small nerve fiber modality, can also be carried out. Guy et al found the lateral aspect of the foot to be the most sensitive location for the measurement of thermal sensation.[141] These authors noted loss of thermal sensa-

†Biomedical Instruments, Newburg, Ohio.

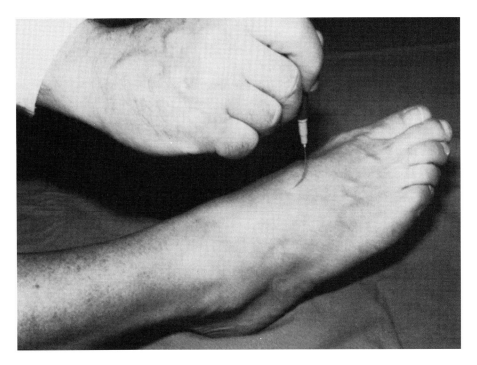

Fig. 40-27. Semmes-Weinstein monofilament being used to evaluate sensory perception. Patient should be able to detect sensation at the time the monofilament buckles. The 5.07 filament equals 10 grams of linear strength to buckle and represents the threshold for loss of touch sensation. *(From Levin ME: State of the art: on the evaluation, prevention, and treatment of diabetic foot lesions, J Diabet Complications 3:211, 1989.)*

tion in all feet with neuropathic ulcerations and in feet with Charcot's joint. When thermal sensitivity was compared with vibratory perception threshold, it was found that thermal sensitivity was sometimes selectively affected, especially in those patients with painful neuropathy, suggesting that the small fibers are more vulnerable in the diabetic.[141]

Sensory evaluation to perceive protective sensation is frequently carried out by using a pin. This is an inadequate way to evaluate sensation since it will vary with each investigator, depending on how forcefully one uses the pin. Today's state-of-the-art evaluation for the ability to perceive touch is done using the Semmes Weinstein monofilaments.* These filaments come in three different thicknesses, 4.17, 5.07, and 6.10. The monofilament is simply placed against the skin and pressure applied until the filament buckles (Fig. 40-27). The monofilament is usually applied to the bottom of the foot and to different areas. The patient should be able to identify the area being touched. The patient should also be able to detect the presence of the monofilament at the time it buckles. A thickness of 5.07 is equal to 10 g of linear pressure and is the limit used to determine protective sensations.

While there is variability from patient to patient, the natural history of loss of peripheral nerve function is as follows: Vibratory sense is usually the first to be lost, followed by loss of reflexes (the Achilles reflex is usually the first to go), and finally, loss of sensations of pain and touch.

*These may be obtained from the Gillis W. Long Hansen's Disease Center, Nylon Filament Project, Carville, Louisiana 70721.

MANAGEMENT OF DIABETIC FOOT ULCERS

Treatment of Diabetic Neurotrophic Foot Ulcers

Ulcers occur in the diabetic foot because of repetitive stress on insensitive feet. When repetitive stress continues, the foot develops hot spots, callus buildup, pressure necrosis, and ultimately ulceration. Patients with high plantar foot temperatures are at increased risk for neuropathic foot ulceration.[142] This occurs most often at the site of the most pressure and excessive callus buildup, usually over the metatarsal heads, especially the first, and on the plantar surface of the hallux. Patients who develop ulcers have increased foot pressures. Fig. 40-28 illustrates the classic diabetic foot ulcer, sometimes referred to as a malperforans ulcer. Note the marked callus buildup surrounding the ulcer. Ulceration on the dorsum of the foot is caused by trauma. Ulceration on the side of the foot is most likely caused by an ill-fitting shoe. Persistent ulceration in the diabetic foot leads to lower limb amputation in 84% of cases.[143]

The accompanying box outlines the management of diabetic foot ulcers. X-ray films are necessary to rule out osteomyelitis, gas formation, and the possibility of the presence of foreign objects. I believe a radiograph should be taken of any foot with a diabetic foot ulcer or infection.

Treatment of diabetic foot ulcers requires the establishment of depth and degree of ulceration. What appears to be a superficial ulceration may in fact penetrate deep into the tissues. Fig. 40-29, *A* shows what appears to be a relatively small ulcer on the plantar surface of the foot in a 60-year-

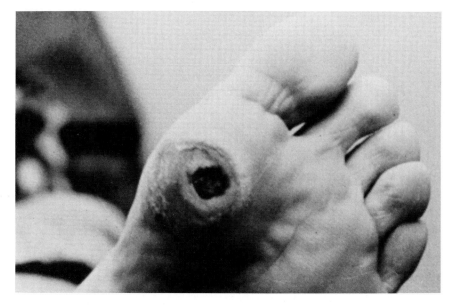

Fig. 40-28. Classic neuropathic diabetic foot ulcer. Note ulceration in callus is well circumscribed. Lesion is painless. *(From Levin ME, O'Neal LW, and Bowker JH, eds: The diabetic foot, ed 5, St Louis, 1993, Mosby–Year Book; courtesy the Michigan Diabetes Research and Training Center, Ann Arbor, Mich, 1983, The University of Michigan.)*

PRIMARY TREATMENT OF DIABETIC FOOT ULCERS

1. Evaluation
   a. Clinical appearance
   b. Depth of penetration
   c. X-rays to detect
      (1) Foreign body
      (2) Osteomyelitis
      (3) Subcutaneous gas
   d. Location
   e. Biopsy
   f. Blood supply (noninvasive vascular studies)
2. Debridement, radical
3. Bacterial cultures (aerobic and anaerobic)
4. Metabolic control
5. Antibiotics
   a. Oral
   b. Parenteral
6. Do not soak feet
7. Decrease of edema
8. Non–weight bearing
   a. Bed rest
   b. Crutches
   c. Wheelchair
   d. Special sandals
   e. Contact casting
9. Improvement of circulation (vascular surgery)

Modified from Levin ME: Pathogenesis and management of diabetic foot lesions. In Levin ME, O'Neal LW, and Bowker JH, eds: The diabetic foot, ed 5, St Louis, 1993, Mosby–Year Book.

old woman. She had been diabetic for 20 years and had severe peripheral neuropathy with an insensate foot. While walking barefoot, she stepped on a nail and developed a painless ulceration on her instep, which she treated with a variety of "home remedies." When the wound failed to heal after several weeks, she sought medical attention. The wound appeared to be a small superficial ulcer with minimal infection. However, extensive debridement revealed the infection to have penetrated deep into the interfascial spaces (Fig. 40-29, *B*). Because this patient's circulation was good, she responded to parenteral antibiotic therapy, and a skin graft was successful. Multiple lessons can be learned from this case. First, patients should not go barefoot. Second, the physician should not assume that what appears to be a superficial ulceration is simply that, and treat it only with topical agents. Finally, vigorous debridement of the ulcer must be done to establish the degree of penetration and to remove all necrotic material. It is currently believed that debridement should be taken down to healthy tissue. The ulcer after debridement in all probability will be larger than it was at manifestation. Eschars should be completely removed. Whirlpool is not the method of choice for debridement. When the foot is insensitive, minor debridement can be carried out at the bedside; however, frequently the patient must be taken to the operating room for adequate debridement under anesthesia.

Biopsy should be considered when the ulcer appears at the atypical location—for example, not over the metatarsal heads or the plantar surface of the hallux, when it cannot be explained by trauma, and when it is unresponsive to aggressive therapy. On numerous occasions biopsies of atypical ulcers have revealed malignancies.

Evaluation should include testing for peripheral neuropathy and status of the blood supply by noninvasive vascular studies. Cultures should be taken aerobically and anaerobically. However, Wheat,[144] commenting on the report of Lipsky et al,[145] believed that baseline cultures were not always required, especially when the lesion was not septic and there was no extensive infection, cellulitis,

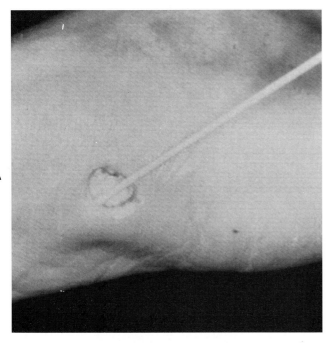

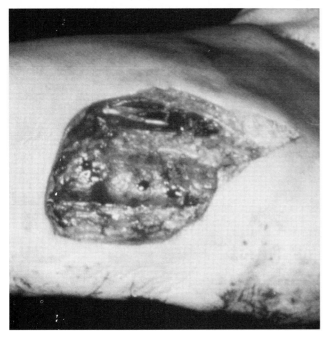

Fig. 40-29. A, Ulcer appears to be small and superficial on plantar surface of foot. **B,** Exploration of ulcer reveals infection to penetrated tissues and interfascial plane. *(From Levin ME, O'Neal LW, and Bowker JH, eds: The diabetic foot, ed 5, St Louis, 1993, Mosby–Year Book.)*

INDICATIONS OF WORSENING INFECTION

1. Signs and symptoms
   a. ↑ Drainage
   b. ↑ Erythema
   c. ↑ Pain
   d. ↑ Temperature
   e. Foul odor
   f. Lymphangitis
   g. Lymphadenopathy
   h. Gangrene
2. Laboratory results
   a. ↑ Blood glucose level
   b. ↑ WBC level
   c. ↑ Sedimentation rate

Modified from Levin ME: Pathogenesis and management of diabetic foot lesions. In Levin ME, O'Neal LW, and Bowker JH, eds: The diabetic foot, ed 5, St Louis, 1993, Mosby–Year Book.

lymphangitis, soft tissue necrosis, gangrene, crepitus, or gas in the tissues and when baseline x-ray films did not show focal erosive changes suggestive of osteomyelitis. The patient should have adequate local care, including debridement, toenail removal if indicated, and incision and drainage of abscesses. The patient must keep the legs elevated, minimize ambulation, and use protective shoes. The patient and/or family member must be able to assist in home management. Wheat[144] believed that if these criteria were met, the following approaches were reasonable:

(1) obtain x-ray films, and (2) initiate oral treatment with an antibiotic with good activity against gram-positive organisms. If the lesion does not improve, appropriate curettage cultures should be obtained on which to base proper antibiotic therapy, and the patient should be hospitalized for additional workup and treatment. Parenteral antibiotics are necessary when significant infection is present.

It should be kept in mind that many of these diabetic foot infections contain gram-negative organisms. Consideration therefore should be given to choosing an oral antibiotic effective against both gram-positive and gram-negative organisms.

The selection of an oral antibiotic or parenteral antibiotic for the treatment of a diabetic foot infection is based on medical judgment. However, certain criteria strongly suggest the need for hospitalization and the use of parenteral antibiotics. These include patients who are septic or febrile or have leukocytosis, cellulitis, or deep infection. Patients with what appears to be a minor infection on the plantar surface of the foot, but with evidence of infection on the dorsum of the foot suggested by erythema, should be hospitalized. Although sepsis may not be present, there is a high probability of severe infection deep in the tissues. Patients with severe ASO should be hospitalized and given parenteral antibiotics to achieve higher concentration of antibiotics in the peripheral tissues than frequently can be achieved by oral therapy alone. Furthermore, the antibiotic of choice can be given only parenterally.

Infection in the diabetic foot can deteriorate within 24 hours. If an oral antibiotic is selected, I believe the patient should be seen every 2 to 3 days until the infection is under control. The patient must be carefully instructed to notify the physician at once should any of the signs or symptoms listed in the accompanying box develop. It is very important that patients with infection monitor their blood glucose levels closely. A rising blood glucose level strongly suggests worsening infection. Blood glucose levels may rise, indicative of worsening infection even though other signs or symptoms of infection have not occurred. Although many of these patients have insensate feet, the development of pain is indicative of deep infection and requires immediate attention. The development of odor also indicates worsening infection and frequently the presence of anaerobes. The fact that these instructions have been given to the patient should be documented in the patient's chart.

When infection does not respond to aggressive debridement and antibiotic therapy, the wound should be debrided again and another culture done, because the flora may have changed. Chronic recurrent or resistant infection suggests the presence of osteomyelitis. Vascular status should be evaluated carefully, and vascular surgery considered when indicated. Impending or developing gangrene also suggests possible progression of infection.

Edema frequently is present. Elevation of the feet, no more than the thickness of one pillow, can be beneficial. Higher elevation may impede circulation.

Soaking the feet has no benefit, although it has been a traditional approach.[146] Soaking can lead to maceration and further infection. Because of insensitivity of the foot, the patient may soak it in water that is too hot (Fig 40-15), resulting in severe burns. Chemical soaks can result in chemical burns.

Non–weight bearing is essential. Because the feet are insensitive and the ulcer does not hurt, patients continue to walk. The result is increased pressure necrosis, forcing bacteria deeper into the tissues, and failure to heal. The use of crutches and wheelchairs is seldom successful in achieving total and consistent non–weight bearing. Many patients with neuropathy have ataxia, making the use of crutches potentially dangerous. The best method for non–weight bearing in appropriately selected patients is the use of a contact cast. This cast allows the patient to be ambulatory by redistributing the weight, thereby decreasing the pressure on the ulcer area. Contraindications for total contact casting include active or acute infection, excessive edema, blindness or obesity, patients with Doppler indexes less than 0.45, and noncompliance.[147]

When an ulcer does not heal despite good metabolic control, adequate debridement, parenteral antibiotic therapy, and non–weight bearing, underlying osteomyelitis, changes in bacterial flora, and inadequate blood supply should be considered. In the presence of ischemia in cases of impaired healing, vascular surgery should be considered. Ankle/brachial indexes of less than 0.45 or $tcPo_2$ less than 30 mm Hg (and certainly less than 20 mm Hg) is highly predictive that the infection will not resolve and the ulcer will not heal. Fig. 40-30, *A* shows an ulceration on the plantar surface of the heel. The patient had an insensitive foot and had worn a shoe with a rough area in the heel. He was hospitalized, and aggressive therapy was carried out. Debridement was continued to the periosteum of the calcaneus, but 4 weeks later there had been no progress in healing. Vascular surgery was considered. Arteriograms revealed a previously transplanted kidney in the left iliac fossa, and good aortic and iliac vessels (Fig. 40-30, *B*); and

---

IMPEDIMENTS TO WOUND HEALING

1. Vascular
   a. Atherosclerosis
   b. Increased viscosity
2. Neurologic
   a. Insensate foot
   b. Deformed foot
3. Infection
   a. Inadequate debridement
   b. Poor blood supply
   c. Microthrombi
   d. Hyperglycemia
   e. Decreased polymorphonuclear neutrophil function
   f. Polymicrobial infection
   g. Changing bacterial flora
   h. Osteomyelitis
4. Mechanical
   a. Edema
   b. Weight bearing
5. Poor nutrition
   a. Low serum albumin level
6. ? Decreased growth factors
7. Poor patient compliance

Modified from Levin ME: Pathogenesis and management of diabetic foot lesions. In Levin ME, O'Neal LW, and Bowker JH, eds: The diabetic foot, ed 5, St Louis, 1993, Mosby–Year Book.

---

slight atherosclerosis in both superficial femoral arteries but occlusion of both left and right tibial and peroneal vessels at their origins (Fig. 40-30, *C*). The patient underwent a left posterior tibial bypass (Fig. 40-30, *D*). The initial left ankle Doppler index, 0.66 preoperatively, probably an erroneously high reading because of noncompressible vessels, had now risen to 0.95. Within 3 weeks the plantar ulcer had completely healed (Fig. 40-30, *E*). The importance of treating diabetic foot ulcers by improving circulation has been noted by Sage and Doyle.[148] They believe, and I agree, that the degree of ischemia and not necessarily the extent of the ulcer is the most significant factor in predicting the potential outcome of treatment. Their success rate in the ischemic group was 25%, and in the nonischemic group 83%. Impediments to wound healing are noted in the box. One of the most overlooked factors is poor nutrition. A serum albumin level of less than 3.0 g or a lymphocyte count of less than 1500 mm^3 is evidence of preexisting malnutrition.[149] A good nutritional state with particular attention to protein intake is essential for wound healing. Although there is suggestive evidence that increase in vitamin intake can be helpful, there is no conclusive evidence that supplemental vitamins will play a significant role. In addition, in a well-balanced diet,

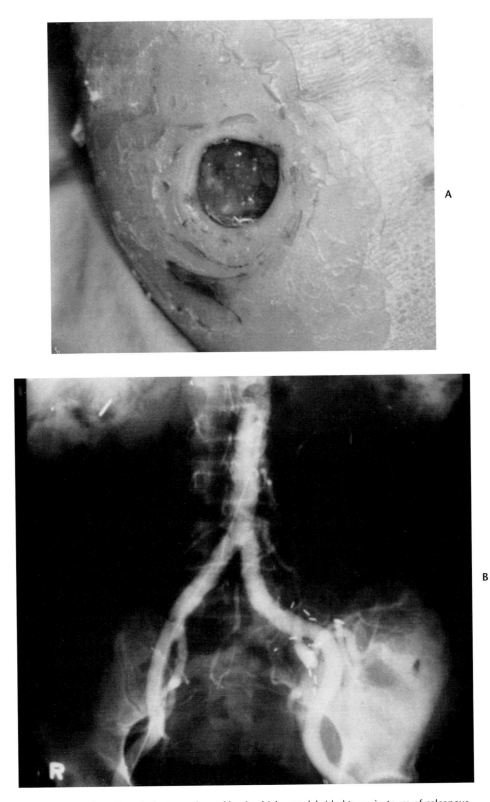

Fig. 40-30. A, Ulceration of plantar surface of heel, which was debrided to periosteum of calcaneus. **B,** Arteriogram of patient with ulcer **(A).** Arteriogram revealed normal aorta and iliac arteries. Previously transplanted kidney is noted on left side of pelvis. *(From Levin ME, O'Neal LW, and Bowker JH, eds: The diabetic foot, ed 5, St Louis, 1993, Mosby–Year Book; courtesy Dr. Gregorio Sicard, Department of Surgery, Washington University School of Medicine, St Louis.)*

Continued.

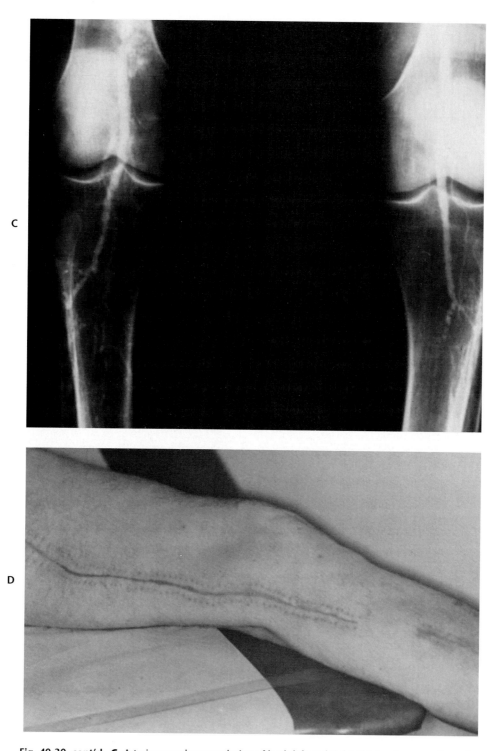

Fig. 40-30, cont'd. C, Arteriogram shows occlusion of both left and right tibial and peroneal vessels at their origin. **D,** Extent of surgery for popliteal posterior tibial bypass.

adequate amounts of these vitamins are available.[150] There is some evidence to support supplementation with zinc. Magnesium supplementation has been suggested as magnesium has been reported by some to be deficient in 25% of the population with diabetes.[151] However, magnesium is also well distributed in a normal balanced diet. Although there are suggestions that supplements may play a role,

adequate vitamin and mineral intake can be achieved by a well-balanced diet.

The efficacy of hyperbaric oxygen in treating diabetic foot ulcers continues to be investigated. The use of topical hyperbaric oxygen is of no benefit. Leslie et al[152] conducted a prospective and randomized study of 28 diabetic patients treated with topical hyperbaric oxygen. These

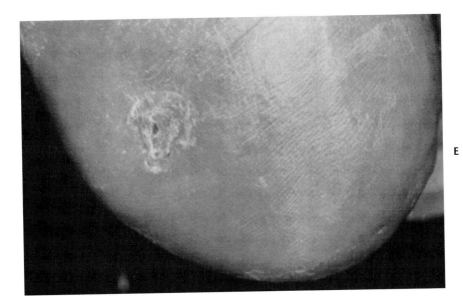

E

Fig. 40-30, cont'd. E, Healed ulcer 3 weeks after vascular surgery.

patients were followed for 14 days. At 7 days and 14 days there were no differences in the type of microorganisms isolated by curettage. Changes in ulcer size did not differ between the control group and the topical hyperbaric oxygen group. It was their conclusion that the healing of diabetic foot ulcers was not accelerated by topical hyperbaric oxygen.[152] Results obtained from the use of the hyperbaric oxygen chamber are more encouraging. Baroni et al[153] treated 18 hospitalized adult diabetic patients with gangrenous lesions of the foot. These patients were compared with a group of 10 diabetic patients with comparable foot lesions who were not treated in the hyperbaric chamber.[153] They found that hyperbaric oxygen treatment greatly reduced leg amputations. However, confirmation that the hyperbaric oxygen chamber for treatment of diabetic foot ulcers is a beneficial modality will require a study that has a larger patient population and is better controlled. It must be kept in mind that no degree of hyperbaric oxygen breathing will elevate tissue oxygen tension in a nonperfused wound. The benefit of hyperbaric oxygen in healing diabetic foot ulcers has been demonstrated by Cianci and Hunt.[154]

Topical Treatment

The use of topical therapy goes back to ancient times, when an unbelievable number of substances, ranging from wine to human excreta, were used to treat wounds. Today the list of topically applied agents remains long and is growing. Like various weight-loss diets, if one of these treatments was specifically effective, we would not see a continuing stream of new topical preparations being advocated. The use of resins and enzyme therapy to help debride is advocated by some. Although these are of some benefit, they represent adjunct therapy and should not be substituted for total aggressive surgical debridement. It remains traditional to use povidone-iodine (Betadine), acetic acid, hydrogen peroxide, and sodium hypochlorite (Dakin's solution). Although these substances will destroy

surface bacteria, they are cytotoxic to granulation tissue.[155] Oberg and Lindsey[156] also have cautioned against the use of hydrogen peroxide and povidone-iodine in wounds. Rodeheaver has reviewed the controversies in topical wound management.[157,158] Other topical antibiotics such as silver sulfadiazine (Silvadene) or topical triple antibiotic therapy can be used but are beneficial only for removing surface bacteria. Using topical preparations and allowing these patients to bear weight puts them at great jeopardy for amputation.

The latest addition to topical therapy is topically applied wound-healing growth factors. Current investigation suggests that the use of platelet-derived growth factor is an important adjunct to wound healing.[159,160] A wound-healing formula derived from platelets consists of a variety of factors. The most important function of the growth factors is chemoattractive, which attracts the neutrophils and monocytes; fibroblast growth factor, which promotes matrix formation by stimulating fibroblasts; angiogenesis factor, which stimulates endothelial cells to form granulation tissue; and epidermal growth factor to promote skin growth. Bentkover and Champion[161] have shown the use of platelet-derived growth factors, platelet releasate, to be cost-effective.[161]

There are a wide variety of dressings suggested for wounds. Each has a special applicability for the type of wound. This has been reviewed by Alvarez, Gilson, and Auletta.[162]

Treatment After Diabetic Neurotrophic Foot Ulcers Are Healed

Even though a neurotrophic foot ulcer has healed, the job has not been completed. The underlying causes of the ulceration, such as foot deformities, calluses, and increased pressure, are still present. Therefore special measures are necessary to protect the vulnerable sites of previous breakdown. This requires reeducation of the patient in walking, teaching him or her to take shorter steps, and frequently a change in jobs is necessary. Special shoes are very important.

SPECIAL SHOES. Special shoes for patients who have cocked up toes have been discussed. The patient with a markedly deformed foot, such as Charcot's foot, needs a specially molded shoe. The use of special therapeutic shoes is critically important in preventing ulcerations or recurrence of ulcers. This frequently requires an extra-depth shoe with a plasticlike material, frequently a Plastizote insert, to redistribute the weight and to prevent recurrence of ulceration. This was clearly demonstrated at a study at King's College in London, which showed an 83% recurrence of ulcers when patients returned to wearing their regular shoes. However, with the use of special shoes there was only a 17% recurrence.[27] The importance of therapeutic shoes is being recognized with increasing frequency. A recent demonstration study that supplied therapeutic shoes to diabetic patients with severe foot problems showed no increased cost to Medicare.[163] As a result, Medicare now covers shoes for diabetics with specific foot problems. Footwear management has been reviewed by Coleman[164] and Janesse.[165]

TEAMWORK. Teamwork in the management of the diabetic foot is not that depicted in Fig. 40-31. The goal of teamwork is to save the diabetic foot and leg, not to remove it. It is obvious that treatment of diabetic foot problems can be quite complex, requiring many medical disciplines (see the accompanying box).

The primary physician's most important task is examining the foot at every visit and educating the patient in foot care. Unfortunately, this is done infrequently. Foot inspection can save many feet and prevent multiple hospitalizations. Because diabetic neuropathy or ASO cannot be totally prevented, the best approach toward saving the diabetic foot is patient education. The primary physician who does not do this loses the advantage of the adage, "an ounce of prevention is worth a pound of cure."

The nurse educator and trained assistant are important members of the team. They not only educate the patient about the various aspects of diabetes, but they also examine the feet and teach foot care. Many times the podiatrist is the first to detect a neurotrophic foot lesion and occasionally the first to diagnose the patient's diabetes. The podiatrist may be able to correct the presenting foot lesion, such as cocked up toes or chronic recurrent ingrown toenails. The podiatrist's role in patient education in foot care is paramount. The frequency of neuropathic syndromes and their differential diagnoses may require a neurologist. The vascular surgeon's role in revascularizing feet and legs has saved many a patient from amputation. The orthopedist frequently sees the patient because of foot deformities. The expertise of the orthopedist in prophylactic or other corrective surgery is of the utmost importance. Other important members of the team treating diabetic foot deformities consist of the certified pedorthist and orthotist. These specialists in fitting prophylactic shoes are extremely important. The physical therapist may have two roles. In medical centers where contact casting is practiced, it is frequently the physical therapist who is trained to apply these special casts. When amputations occur, the physical therapist's skills, together with those of

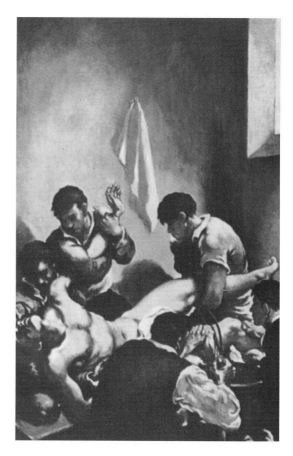

Fig. 40-31. Painting depicts agonies of patient undergoing amputation in ancient time. Formerly amputations were performed only with alcohol as an anesthetic. Many people died during this guillotine operation, some even died of shock and terror before the operation began! *(Painting by Italian Count Gregorio Calvi de Bergolo in 1953. From the International Museum of Surgical Sciences and Hall of Fame. International College of Surgeons, Chicago.)*

TEAM MEMBERS INVOLVED IN THE CARE OF THE DIABETIC FOOT

1. Primary physician
2. Endocrinologist
3. Diabetologist
4. Nurse educator
5. Podiatrist
6. Infectious disease specialist
7. Radiologist
8. Neurologist
9. Vascular surgeon
10. Orthopedist
11. Pedorthist
12. Orthotist
13. Social worker
14. Home care nurse

PATIENT INSTRUCTIONS FOR THE CARE OF THE DIABETIC FOOT

1. Do not smoke.
2. Inspect the feet daily for blisters, cuts, and scratches. The use of a mirror can aid in seeing the bottom of the feet. Always check between the toes.
3. Wash feet daily and dry carefully, especially between the toes.
4. Avoid extremes of temperature. Test water with hand or elbow before bathing.
5. If feet feel cold at night, wear socks. Do not apply hot water bottles or heating pads. Do not soak feet in hot water.
6. Do not walk on hot surfaces such as sandy beaches or on the cement around swimming pools.
7. Do not walk barefoot.
8. Do not use chemical agents for the removal of corns and calluses. Do not use corn plasters. Do not use strong antiseptic solutions on the feet.
9. Do not use adhesive tape on the feet.
10. Inspect the inside of shoes daily for foreign objects, nail points, torn linings, and rough areas.
11. If your vision is impaired, have a family member inspect feet daily, trim nails, and buff down calluses.
12. Do not soak feet.
13. For dry feet use a very thin coat of a lubricating oil or cream. Apply this after bathing and drying the feet. Do not put the oil or cream between the toes. Consult your physician for detailed instructions.
14. Wear properly fitting stockings. Do not wear mended stockings. Avoid stockings with seams. Change stockings daily.
15. Do not wear garters.
16. Shoes should be comfortable at time of purchase. Do not depend on them to stretch out. Shoes should be made of leather. Running or special walking shoes may be worn after checking with your physician.
17. Do not wear shoes without stockings.
18. Do not wear sandals with thongs between the toes.
19. In wintertime take special precautions. Wear wool socks and protective foot gear, such as fleece-lined boots.
20. Cut nails straight across.
21. Do not cut corns and calluses. Follow instructions from your physician or podiatrist.
22. Avoid crossing your legs since this can cause pressure on the nerves.
23. See your physician regularly and be sure that your feet are examined at each visit.
24. Notify your physician or podiatrist at once should you develop a blister or sore on your feet.
25. Be sure to inform your podiatrist that you are a diabetic.

Modified from Levin ME: Pathogenesis and management of diabetic foot lesions. In Levin ME, O'Neal LW, and Bowker JH, eds: The diabetic foot, ed 5, St Louis, 1993, Mosby–Year Book.

---

the specialist in physical medicine, are required for rehabilitation. Treatment of diabetic neuropathic lesions can be prolonged, and since hospital stays must be shortened, many patients require home nursing care services. The home care nurse may be needed to carry out prolonged parenteral antibiotic therapy, change dressings, and observe the clinical course of the patient at home, thus shortening the hospital stay.

Financial problems resulting from loss of a job can be monumental. The social worker becomes an important team member in these cases.

The importance of teamwork in reducing lower extremity clinical abnormalities in patients with type II diabetes has been demonstrated by Litzelman et al.[166] The odds ratio in decreasing the number of foot lesions in this study was 0.41, $P = 0.05$. The program also resulted in the patients being more likely to report appropriate self-foot care behaviors, to have foot examinations, and to receive foot care education.

PATIENT EDUCATION. Of all the approaches to saving the diabetic foot, the most important is patient education. Despite our current knowledge and good diabetic control, physicians cannot totally prevent atherosclerosis and peripheral neuropathy. However, the patient can be educated in proper foot care, learning how to prevent injury to insensitive feet and detect foot lesions as early as possible.

At the time of the office visit, and while the shoes and socks are off, the nurse and physician should review the *do's* and *don't's* of foot care with the patient. This cannot be done by simply handing the patient a sheet of instructions. The instructions must be explained and questions encouraged and answered. If this is done, the patient will have a better understanding of the importance of foot care. The list of instructions that I use for patient education is given in the accompanying box. Patients should be instructed to look not only at their feet but also to inspect between the toes. Patients with impaired vision, extreme obesity, or arthritis cannot inspect their feet adequately. These inspections can be carried out by a family member. For patients who cannot see their feet because of obesity or arthritis, a mirror can be placed on the floor, allowing them to inspect the bottom of the foot. The feet should be kept clean and the patient should be cautioned to dry carefully between the toes. Moisture left in these areas can lead to maceration and infection.

Because autonomic neuropathy leads to the inability of the foot to perspire, the skin becomes dry, flaky, and cracked. The application of a very thin coat of lubricating material to the foot after bathing helps to seal in the moisture. It is moisture rather than the oil itself that keeps the skin pliable and decreases the dryness. Any type of cream can be used. Each practitioner has his or her favorite. It is very important that lubricants not be placed between the toes where extra moisture can accumulate and lead to maceration.

Extremes of temperature should be avoided. Many patients with cold insensitive feet caused by ASO or peripheral neuropathy have incurred severe burns by soaking them in water that is too hot (Fig. 40-15) and using heating pads or hot water bottles. The water temperature should be tested before bathing. This should be done with the elbow, not with the hand, which may also have developed insensitivity because of peripheral neuropathy. Cement around swimming pools and hot, sandy beaches are other areas frequently not suspected of being extremely hot and potentially disastrous for the diabetic. Many diabetic patients with insensitive feet have suffered severe burns secondary to walking on these surfaces. Patients should be advised to wear protective footwear at the beach and pool.

Chemical burns can occur from chemical agents used to remove corns and calluses. The use of these substances should be avoided. The diabetic should inspect the inside of the shoes daily for foreign objects, nail points that have protruded through, and torn linings. Some of the unusual items found in shoes resulting in foot trauma are discussed in this chapter.

A critically important part of the diabetic's educational program is instruction in proper footwear. The shoes should be comfortable at the time of purchase and the patient should not depend on them to "stretch out." However, shoes that feel comfortable at the time of purchase may actually be too small since the patient with an insensitive foot cannot detect discomfort. New shoes should be worn only a few hours a day. The shoes should be made of leather and not synthetic materials. However, running or walking shoes may reduce the rate of callus buildup.[167] Patients with foot deformities should wear special therapeutic or molded shoes. The patient should be instructed not to wear thongs. Fig. 40-32 shows an ulceration between the first and second toes of a patient who had worn thonged sandals.

The patient should be taught the proper method of cutting nails straight across or following the curve of the nails but never to cut deep into the corners. Improper trimming can result in an ingrown toenail. Recurring ingrown toenails may be treated conservatively, but they are always a potential source of infection and, when indicated, should receive definitive therapy, usually surgical intervention by either the patient's surgeon or podiatrist. Patients must be instructed repeatedly not to do "home surgery." Serious complications can result when the patient cuts on insensitive feet (Fig. 40-14).

Calluses should not be cut by the patient. Pumice stones, emery boards, and callus files can be used, but if the calluses are particularly thick, they should be trimmed by a physician, surgeon, or podiatrist.

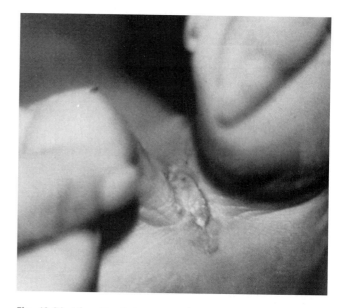

Fig. 40-32. Ulceration between toes from wearing thongs. *(From Levin ME, O'Neal LW, and Bowker JH, eds: The diabetic foot, ed 5, St Louis, 1993, Mosby–Year Book.)*

Patients should be reminded to inform any physician working with their feet that they are diabetic so that the physician can take the necessary precautions.

The effectiveness of total foot care programs has been previously noted.[26-28] Lippmann has reduced the amputation rate of 8 to 15 cases a year to zero with a special foot care program implemented in nursing homes.[168]

PATIENT ADHERENCE

Despite the most detailed and repeated instructions, many patients will not adhere to a good foot care program. For instance, it is very difficult to convince some women to forego wearing fashionable high-heeled shoes despite their lament that "these shoes are killing me," which in fact may be more truth than cliche. And, as previously noted, despite warnings, many patients succumb to that irresistible urge to do "home surgery." For many patients going barefoot "feels too good to give up," or they are simply not motivated enough to put on their shoes for their own protection. Cessation of smoking is almost impossible for many patients. It is not unusual for a physician to visit a patient after amputation and find him or her lying in bed, smoking. When the danger and risk to the remaining limb is explained for the "hundredth time," the response is usually "You're right, Doc. I know smoking can cause the loss of the other leg. I am going to quit smoking—some day."

For all the reasons listed, and despite the constant efforts of health care professionals, patient adherence is difficult to accomplish. The problem is compounded even further by patients who do not keep their clinic appointments. Miller found that an intensified foot care program resulted in approximately two-thirds fewer hospital admissions of those patients with diabetic foot problems who faithfully participated in the program, compared with patients who did not attend the clinic on a regular basis.[169] Without patient cooperation, adherence to good foot care cannot be achieved; but with the continued efforts of the physician and assistants, patient adherence can be greatly improved.

Rehabilitation Following Lower Limb Amputation In the Diabetic

Unfortunately all amputations cannot be prevented. Therefore rehabilitation becomes an important facet in the overall management of the diabetic amputee. If we achieve our goal of reducing the amputation rate by 50%, we will still have 25,000 plus diabetic amputations per year. A significant number of these patients can benefit from a prosthetic rehabilitation program.

Following amputation, the goal is to furnish and train a diabetic amputee with a prosthesis, and most importantly, to return the patient to his or her previous life-style. However, not all amputees are candidates for a prosthesis. General contraindications for prosthetic fitting are: (1) chronic and progressive mental deterioration; (2) advancing neurologic disorders such as parkinsonism or stroke; (3) chronic pulmonary obstructive disease; (4) a patient who has not walked for long periods before amputation; (5) when the other extremity is affected by impending gangrene, ulceration, and infection; (6) when there is irreducible pronounced knee flexion contractures in below-knee amputees and hip flexion contractures in above-knee amputees; and (7) when cardiac disease with congestive heart failure or angina is present.[170]

It must be kept in mind that diabetic patients with ASO also have a high incidence of coronary artery disease. The use of a prosthesis increases energy requirements and work load. For example, a normal patient, when walking, requires 0.16 ml of oxygen per meter per kilogram. The individual with a below-knee amputation requires 0.26 ml of oxygen, and an above-knee amputee requires 0.35. A bilateral above-knee amputee requires 0.72.[170] Many diabetics cannot handle this increased work load and some only with extreme difficulty, even taking into account the fact that patients with amputations tend to walk at a much slower rate. A nonamputee will walk at 82 meters per minute, approximately 3 miles per hour, a below-knee amputee at 45 meters per hour, an above-knee amputee at 36 meters per hour, and a bilateral above-knee amputee at 22 meters per hour.[170] Careful evaluation of the cardiac status therefore becomes critically important.

Advanced age is not necessarily a contraindication to prosthetic fitting nor is a history of myocardial infarction from which the patient has recovered. However, special consideration must be given to these patients.

In general if the patient has walked before amputation and has learned to walk with a walker after the operation, he or she should be able to manage a below-knee prosthesis. The use of an above-knee prosthesis presents a more difficult problem since the energy cost is higher and control of the prosthetic knee requires neuromuscular coordination, which is often beyond the ability of the elderly amputee. The decision as to whether the amputee can be fitted with a prosthesis or not can often be made early in the postoperative period.

While there may be some variability in techniques for fitting prostheses, they are basically the same in all institutions. To prepare the stump for a prosthesis, a balloon

REHABILITATION TEAM

Primary physician

Surgeon

Physiatrist

Physical therapist

Prosthetist

Psychologist

Sex therapist

Occupational therapist

Social worker

pressure device is applied to decrease edema and promote healing for early fitting. The techniques of prosthetic fitting are not covered in this chapter since they are basically the same in most physical therapy departments. However, there are different types of prostheses, and the choice of a prosthesis depends on the patient's life-style. Amputees can resume many of their previous physical activities, such as bicycle riding and playing golf; even competitive golf can be accomplished.*

An important part of the rehabilitation program is the patient's understanding of the prosthesis, its capabilities and limitations. Use of the prosthesis depends to a significant degree on the patient's motivation. However, motivation alone is not enough. Many patients feel that an artificial limb will restore normal gait. They must understand that a prosthesis will feel heavy, walking will require more energy, and there will be some physical discomfort. They must learn the skill of prosthetic walking before a gait becomes automatic. Dispelling the unrealistic expectations and proper psychologic preparation are vital to prevent disappointment and rejection.

It is obvious that the total rehabilitation of the diabetic amputee requires a coordinated team (see the box on this page). The team required for successful rehabilitation consists initially of physicians; surgeons; diabetologists; and internists, or primary physicians, whose role must be to prepare the patient physically and emotionally for the amputation. Thus rehabilitation must begin before the amputation. Time may be a limiting factor in this preparation. Because of the emotional state associated with an impending amputation, the disturbed patient and family may be limited in their ability to understand the initial information. The surgeon must also prepare the patient and family for the amputation. The surgeon must be knowledgeable regarding future prosthetic fitting so that the bone and skin flaps will be appropriate. A psychologist, when necessary, should see these patients during the rehabilitation period to help with their emotional state and to provide reassurance and training. A physiatrist, physical therapist, and prosthetist are essential members of the team. An often neglected part of the patient's rehabili-

*Information on the proper prosthesis for the golfer can be obtained from the National Amputee Golf Association (NAGA), P.O. Box 1228, Amherst, NH 03031.

tation is instruction in how to manage sex following an amputation. A sex therapist can be a very important member of the team since emotional, esthetic, and functional difficulties related to the amputation can result. Finally, a social worker may be necessary since an amputation has a major socioeconomic impact on the patient's life-style.

SUMMARY

The pathogenesis of diabetic foot lesions is multifactorial. Physicians involved in the management of the diabetic foot must understand the pathogenesis and risk factors involved so that whenever possible the development of foot problems can be prevented or delayed. Management is complicated and consultation can help save the foot. The physician who does not seek help is not being fair to himself or herself or to the patient. Aggressive treatment of foot ulcers, the use of special shoes, and patient education have been stressed. Taking all of these factors into consideration, the goal of all physicians and clinics managing the diabetic foot should be to reduce their amputation rate by at least 50%. This goal is a realistic one and can be achieved.

REFERENCES

1. Chan CW and Rudins A: Subject review: foot biomechanics during walking and running, Mayo Clin Proc 69:448, 1994.
2. Coates MI and Clack JA: Polydactyly in the earliest known petrapod limbs, Nature 347:66, 1990.
3. Boulton AJM et al: Abnormalities of foot pressure in early diabetic neuropathy, Diabetic Med 4:225, 1987.
4. Boulton AJM et al: Dynamic foot pressure and other studies as diagnostic and management aids in diabetic neuropathy, Diabetes Care 6:26, 1983.
5. Veves A et al: The risk of foot ulceration in diabetic patients with high foot pressure: a prospective study, Diabetologia 35:660, 1992.
6. Fu MX et al: Glycation, glycoxidation, and cross-linking of collagen by glucose; kinetics, mechanisms, and inhibition of late stages of the Maillard reaction, Diabetes 43:676, 1994.
7. Fletcher F, Ain M, and Jacobs R: Renal transplant patients, Clin Orthop Rel Res 296:37, 1993.
8. Williams DR: Hospital admissions of diabetic patients: information from hospital activity analysis, Diabetic Med 2:27, 1985.
9. Young MJ et al: A multicentre study of the prevalence of diabetic peripheral neuropathy in the United Kingdom hospital clinic population, Diabetologia 36:150, 1993.
10. Crofford OB: Report of the National Commission on Diabetes to the Congress of the United States, U.S. Department of Health, Education and Welfare Publication NIH pub. no. 67-1018, Washington, D.C., 1975, U.S. Government Printing Office.
11. McDermott W and Rogers DE: Social ramifications of control of microbial disease, Johns Hopkins Med J 151:302, 1982.
12. Drury TF, Danchik KM, and Harris MI: Chapter VII. Sociodemographic characteristics of adult diabetes. In Harris MI and Hammer RF, eds: Diabetes in America, Bethesda, Maryland, 1985, NIH pub. no. 85-1468, p. 1.
13. Palumbo PJ and Melton LJ III: Chapter XV. Peripheral vascular disease and diabetes. In Diabetes in America: Diabetes data compiled in 1984, Washington, D.C., U.S. Government Printing Office, 1985, NIH pub. no. 85-1468, p. 1.
14. O'Brien IAD and Corrall RJM: Epidemiology of diabetes and its complications, N Engl J Med 318:1619, 1988.
15. Melton LJ III et al: Incidence and prevalence of clinical peripheral vascular disease in a population-based cohort of diabetic patients, Diabetes Care 3:650, 1980.
16. Kreines K et al: The course of peripheral vascular disease in non-insulin dependent diabetes, Diabetes Care 8:235, 1985.
17. Block P: The diabetic foot ulcer: a complex problem with a simple treatment approach, Mil Med 146:644, 1981.
18. Diabetes surveillance. Atlanta, 1991, Centers for Disease Control, Division of Diabetes Translation.
19. Miller AD et al: Diabetes related lower extremity amputations in New Jersey: 1979-1981, J Med Soc N J 82:723, 1985.
20. Ogbuawa B, Williams JT, and Henry WL: Diabetic gangrene in black patients, South Med J 75:285, 1982.
21. Nelson RG et al: Lower-extremity amputation in NIDDM: 12 year follow-up study in Pima Indians, Diabetes Care 11:8, 1988.
22. Most RS and Sinnock P: The epidemiology of lower extremity amputations in diabetic individuals, Diabetes Care 6:87, 1983.
23. Bild DE et al: Lower-extremity amputation in people with diabetes: Epidemiology and prevention, Diabetes Care 12:24, 1989.
24. Humphrey LL et al: The contribution of non-insulin-dependent diabetes to lower-extremity amputation in the community, Arch Intern Med 154:885, 1994.
25. Mackey WC et al: The costs of surgery for limb-threatening ischemia, Surgery 99:26, 1986.
26. Davidson JK et al: Assessment of program effectiveness at Grady Memorial Hospital-Atlanta. In Steiner G and Lawrence PA, eds: Educating diabetic patients, New York, 1981, Springer-Verlag.
27. Edmonds ME et al: Improved survival of the diabetic foot: The role of a specialized foot clinic, Q J Med 60:763, 1986.
28. Assal JP et al: Patient education as the basis for diabetes care in clinical practices, Diabetologia 28:602, 1985.
29. Pecoraro RE, Reiber GE, and Burgess EM: Pathways to diabetic limb amputation: basis for prevention, Diabetes Care 13:513, 1990.
30. Mills JL, Beckett WC, and Taylor SM: The diabetic foot: consequences of delayed treatment and referral, South Med J 84:970, 1991.
31. Mandelberg A and Sheinfeld W: Diabetic amputations: amputation of lower extremity in diabetes—analysis of one hundred twenty-eight cases, Am J Surg 71:70, 1944.
32. Levin CM and Dealy FN: The surgical diabetic: a five year survey, Ann Surg 102:1029, 1935.
33. Fearon J et al: Improved results with diabetic below-knee amputations, Arch Surg 120:777, 1985.
34. Bodily KC and Burgess EM: Contralateral limb and patient survival after leg amputation, Am J Surg 146:280, 1983.
35. Rosenberg MW and Shah DM: Bilateral blue toe syndrome: a case report, JAMA 243:365, 1980.
36. Silbert S: Amputation of the lower extremity in diabetes mellitus: a follow-up study of 294 cases, Diabetes 1:297, 1952.
37. Ecker LM and Jacobs BS: Lower extremity amputation in diabetic patients, Diabetes 19:189, 1970.
38. Lee JS et al: Lower-extremity amputation. Incidence, risk factors, and mortality in the Oklahoma Indian Diabetes Study, Diabetes 42:876, 1993.

39. Marchal de Calvi CJ: Recherches sur les accidents diabeques, Paris, 1864, P. Asselin.

40. Ebskov B and Josephsen P: Incidence of reamputation and death after gangrene of the lower extremity, Prosthet Orthot Int 4:77, 1980.

41. Larsen K, Christiansen JS, and Ebskov B: Prevention and treatment of ulcerations of the foot in unilaterally amputated diabetic patients, Acta Orthop Scand 53:481, 1982.

42. Kucan JO and Robson MC: Diabetic foot infections: fate of the contralateral foot, Plast Reconstr Surg 77:439, 1986.

43. Colwell JA et al: New concepts about the pathogenesis of atherosclerosis in diabetes mellitus. In Levin ME and O'Neal LW, eds: The diabetic foot, ed 4, St Louis, 1988, The CV Mosby Co.

44. Janka HU, Standl E, and Mehnert H: Peripheral vascular disease in diabetes mellitus and its relation to cardiovascular risk factors: screening with Doppler ultrasonic technique, Diabetes Care 3:207, 1980.

45. Levin ME and Sicard GA: Evaluating and treating diabetic peripheral vascular disease. Part I, Clin Diab 5:62, 1987.

46. LoGerfo FW and Coffman JD: Vascular and microvascular disease of the foot in diabetes, N Engl J Med 311:1615, 1984.

47. Moldveen-Geromimus M and Merriam JC Jr: Cholesterol embolization: from pathologic curiosity to clinical entity, Circulation 35:946, 1967.

48. Queen M, Biem HJ, and Moe GW: Development of cholesterol embolization syndrome after intravenous streptokinase for acute myocardial infarction, Am J Cardiol 6:1042, 1990.

49. Shapiro LS: Cholesterol embolization after treatment with tissue plasminogen activators, N Engl J Med 321:2370, 1989.

50. Fisher DF et al: Dilemmas in dealing with the blue toe syndrome: aortic versus peripheral source, Am J Surg 148:863, 1984.

51. Federman DG, Valdivia M, and Kirsner RS: Syphilis presenting as the "blue toe syndrome," Arch Intern Med 154:1029, 1994.

52. O'Keeffe ST, Woods BB, and Reslin DJ: Blue toe syndrome: causes and management, Arch Intern Med 152:2197, 1992.

53. Golbranson FL et al: Multiple extremity amputations in hypotensive patients treated with dopamine, JAMA 243:1145, 1980.

54. Zacharias FJ et al: Propranolol in hypertension: a study of long-term therapy, 1964-1970, Am Heart J 83:755, 1972.

55. Prentice CRM and Lowe GDO: Blood viscosity and the complications of diabetes, Adv Exp Med Biol 164:99, 1984.

56. Geiger M and Binder BR: Plasminogen activation in diabetes mellitus, J Biol Chem 259:2976, 1984.

57. Small M et al: Enhancement of fibrinolysis after insulin administration in NIDDM, Diabetes Care 9:216, 1989.

58. Borkenstein MH and Muntean WE: Elevated factor VIII activity and factor VIII-related antigen in diabetic children without vascular disease, Diabetes 31:1006, 1982.

59. Sargent WQ: Hemorheology. In Levin ME and O'Neal LW, eds: The diabetic foot, ed 4, St. Louis, 1988, The CV Mosby Co.

60. Belch JJF et al: The effects of acute smoking on platelet behavior, fibrinolysis and haemorheology in habitual smokers, Thromb Haemost 51:6, 1984.

61. Pollin W: The role of the addictive process as a key step in causation of all tobacco-related disease, JAMA 252:2874, 1984.

62. Delbridge L, Appleburg M, and Reeve TS: Factors associated with the development of foot lesions in the diabetic, Surgery 93:78, 1983.

63. Kannel WB: Cigarette smoking and peripheral arterial disease, Prim Cardiol 12:13, 1986.

64. Fairbairn JH II and Juergens JL: The principles of medical treatment. In Juergens JL et al, eds: Peripheral vascular disease, Philadelphia, 1980, WB Saunders Co.

65. Wald N et al: Association between atherosclerotic disease and carboxy-hemoglobin levels in tobacco smokers, Br Med J 1:761, 1973.

66. Levine PH: An acute effect of cigarette smoking on platelet function: a possible link between smoking and arterial thrombosis, Circulation 48:619, 1973.

67. Beach KW and Strandness DE Jr: Arteriosclerosis obliterans and associated risk factors in insulin dependent diabetics, Diabetes 29:882, 1980.

68. Nadler JL, Velasco JS, and Horton R: Cigarette smoking inhibits prostacyclin formation, Lancet 1:1248, 1983.

69. Palmer JR, Rosenberg L, and Shapiro MB: "Low yield" cigarettes and the risk of nonfatal myocardial infarction in women, N Engl J Med 320:1569, 1989.

70. Brischetto CS et al: Plasma lipid and lipoprotein profiles of cigarette smokers from randomly selected families: enhancement of hyperlipidemia and depression of high-density lipoprotein, Am J Cardiol 52:675, 1983.

71. Klemp P and Stagbert B: Smoking reduces insulin absorption from subcutaneous tissue, Br Med J 284:237, 1982.

72. Sherwin MA and Gastwirth CM: Detrimental effects of cigarette smoking on lower extremity wound healing, J Foot Surg 29:84, 1990.

73. Ricci MA, Fleishman C, and Gerstein N: The effects of cigarette smoking and smoking cessation aids on transcutaneous oxygen levels, J Vas Med Biol 4:260, 1993.

74. Ford ES et al: Diabetes mellitus and cigarette smoking—findings from the 1989 National Health Interview Survey, Diabetes Care 17:688, 1994.

75. Lorenzi M, Cagliero E, and Toledo S: Glucose toxicity for human endothelial cells in culture: delayed replication, disturbed cell cycle, and accelerated death, Diabetes 34:621, 1985.

76. The Diabetes Control and Complications Trial Research Group: The effect of intensive treatment of diabetes on the development and progression of long-term complications in insulin-dependent diabetes mellitus, N Engl J Med 329:976, 1993.

77. Moss SE, Klein R, and Klein BE: The prevalence and incidence of lower extremity amputation in a diabetic population, Arch Intern Med 152:610, 1992.

78. Brownlee M, Cerami A, and Vlassara H: Advanced glycosylation end products in tissue and the biochemical basis of diabetic complications, N Engl J Med 318:1315, 1988.

79. Capron L et al: Growth-promoting effects of diabetes and insulin on arteries: an in-vivo study of rat aorta, Diabetes 35:973, 1986.

80. Sato Y et al: Experimental atherosclerosis-like lesions induced by hyperinsulinism in Wistar rats, Diabetes 38:91, 1989.

81. Zavaroni I et al: Risk factors for coronary artery disease in healthy persons with hyperinsulinemia and normal glucose tolerance, N Engl J Med 320:702, 1989.

82. Larson DM and Haudenschild CC: Activation of smooth muscle cell outgrowth from BB/Wor rat aortas, Diabetes 37:1380, 1988.

83. Lapidus L et al: Distribution of adipose tissue and risk of cardiovascular disease and death: a 12 year follow-up of participants in the population study of women in Gothenburg, Sweden, Br Med J (Clin Res) 289:1257, 1984.

84. Haffner SM et al: Hyperinsulinemia, upper body adiposity and cardiovascular risk factors in non-diabetics, Metabolism 37:333, 1988.

85. Anderson AJ et al: Body fat distribution, plasma lipids, and lipoproteins, Arteriosclerosis 8:88, 1988.

86. Peiris AN et al: Adiposity, fat distribution, and cardiovascular risk, Ann Intern Med 110:867, 1989.

87. Shimokata H, Muller DC, and Andres R: Studies in the distribution of body fat. III. Effects of smoking, JAMA 261:1169, 1989.

88. Barrett-Connor E and Khaw KT: Cigarette smoking and increased central adiposity, Ann Intern Med 111:783, 1989.

89. Dai WS, Gutai JP, and Kuller LH: Cigarette smoking and serum sex hormones in men, Am J Epidemiol 128:796, 1988.

90. Evans DJ, Barth JH, and Burke CW: Body fat topography in women with androgen excess, Int J Obes 12:157, 1988.

91. Facchini FS, Hollenbeek CB, and Jeppesen J: Insulin resistance and cigarette smoking, Lancet 339:1128, 1992.

92. Brand FN, Abbott RD, and Kannel WB: Diabetes, intermittent claudication, and risk of cardiovascular events: the Framingham Study, Diabetes 38:504, 1989.

93. Brownlee M, Vlassara H, and Cerami A: Trapped immunoglobulins on peripheral nerve myelin from patients with diabetes mellitus, Diabetes 35:999, 1986.

94. Greene DA, Lattimer SA, and Sima AAF: Sorbitol, phosphoinositides, and sodium-potassium-ATPase in the pathogenesis of diabetic complications, N Engl J Med 316:599, 1987.

95. Harati Y: Diabetic peripheral neuropathies, Ann Intern Med 107:546, 1987.

96. Sima AAF et al: Regeneration and repair of myelinated fibers in sural-nerve biopsy specimens from patients with diabetic neuropathy treated with sorbinil, N Engl J Med 319:548, 1988.

97. Dyck PJ et al: Nerve glucose, fructose, sorbitol, myo-inositol, and fiber degeneration and regeneration in diabetic neuropathy, N Engl J Med 319:542, 1988.

98. Griffey RH et al: Diabetic neuropathy: structural analysis of nerve hydration by magnetic resonance spectroscopy, JAMA 260:2872, 1988.

99. Greene DA: Neuropathy in the diabetic foot: new concepts in etiology and treatment. In Levin ME and O'Neal LW, eds: The diabetic foot, ed 4, St Louis, 1988, The CV Mosby Co.

100. Aguayo AJ: Neuropathy due to compression and entrapment. In Dyck PJ, Thomas PK, and Lambert EH, eds: Peripheral neuropathy, Philadelphia, 1975, WB Saunders Co.

101. Harris M, Eastman R, Cowie C: Symptoms of sensory neuropathy in adults with NIDDM in the U.S. population, Diabetes Care 16:1446, 1993.

102. Cavanagh PR and Ulbrecht JS: Biomechanics of the foot in diabetes mellitus. In Levin ME, O'Neal LW, and Bowker JH, eds: The diabetic foot, ed 5, St Louis, 1993, Mosby–Year Book.

103. Boehm JJ: Diabetic Charcot's joint, N Engl J Med 267:185, 1962.

104. Sinha SK, Frykberg RG, and Kozak GP: Neuroarthropathy in the diabetic foot. In Kozak GP, ed: Clinical diabetes mellitus, Philadelphia, 1982, WB Saunders Co.

105. Boulton AJM, Scarpello JHB, and Ward JD: Venous oxygenation in the diabetic neuropathic foot: evidence of arterial venous shunting, Diabetologia 22:6, 1981.

106. Robillard R, Gagnon P, and Alaries R: Diabetic neuroarthropathy: a report of four cases, Can Med Assoc J 91:795, 1964.

107. Edelman SV et al: Neuroosteoarthropathy (Charcot's joint) in diabetes mellitus following revascularization surgery: three case reports and a review of the literature, Arch Intern Med 147:1504, 1987.

108. Splittgerber GF et al: Combined leukocyte and bone imaging used to evaluate diabetic osteoarthropathy and osteomyelitis, Clin Nucl Med 14:156, 1989.

109. Schauwecker DS et al: Combined bone scintigraphy and Indium-III leukocyte scans in neuropathic foot disease, J Nucl Med 29:1651, 1988.

110. Maurer AH et al: Infection in diabetic osteoarthropathy: use of indium-labeled leukocytes for diagnosis, Radiology 161:221, 1986.

111. Sanders LJ and Frykberg RG: Charcot foot. In Levin ME, O'Neal LW, and Bowker JH, eds: The diabetic foot, ed 5, St Louis, 1993, Mosby–Year Book.

112. Nguyen VD: The radiographic spectrum of abnormalities of the foot in diabetic patients, Can Assoc Radiol J 43:333, 1992.

113. Klamer TW et al: The influence of sepsis and ischemia on the natural history of the diabetic foot, Am Surg 53:490, 1987.

114. O'Neal LW: Debridement and amputation. In Levin ME and O'Neal LW, eds: The diabetic foot, ed 4, St Louis, 1988, The CV Mosby Co.

115. Leichter SB et al: Clinical characteristics of diabetic patients with serious pedal infections, Metabolism 37:22, 1998.

116. Sapico FL et al: The infected foot of the diabetic patient: quantitative microbiology and analysis of clinical features, Rev Infect Dis 6(suppl 1):S171, 1984.

117. Finegold SM: Anaerobic bacteria: their role in infection and their management, Postgrad Med 81:141, 1987.

118. Little JR and Kobayashi GS: Infection of the diabetic foot. In Levin ME and O'Neal LW, eds: The diabetic foot, ed 4, St. Louis, 1988, The CV Mosby Co.

119. Newman LG et al: Unsuspected osteomyelitis in diabetic foot ulcers, JAMA 266:1246, 1991.

120. Newman LG et al: Leukocyte scanning with 111 IN is superior to magnetic resonance imaging in diagnosis of clinically unsuspected osteomyelitis in diabetic foot ulcers, Diabetes Care 15:1527, 1992.

121. Yuh WTC et al: Osteomyelitis of the foot in diabetic patients: evaluation with plain film, 99m-Te-MDP bone scintigraphy, and MR imaging, AJR 152:795, 1989.

122. McEnery KW et al: Imaging of the diabetic foot. In Levin ME, O'Neal LW, and Bowker JH, eds: The diabetic foot, ed 5, St Louis, 1993, Mosby–Year Book.

123. Lipsky BA, Pecoraro RE, and Wheat LJ: The diabetic foot: soft tissue and bone infection, Infect Dis Clin North Am 4:409, 1990.

124. Little JR, Kobayashi GS, and Bailey TC: Infection of the diabetic foot. In Levin ME, O'Neal LW, and Bowker JH, eds: The diabetic foot, ed 5, St Louis, 1993, Mosby–Year Book.

125. Peterson LR et al: Therapy of lower extremity infections with ciprofloxacin in patients with diabetes mellitus, peripheral vascular disease, or both, Am J Med 86:801, 1989.

126. Leichter SB and O'Brian JT: Reduced nutritional competency at presentation in diabetic patients with pedal infection, Diabetes 43:157A, 1994 (abstract).

127. Saudek CD, Werns S, and Reidenberg MM: Phenytoin in the treatment of diabetic symmetrical polyneuropathy, Clin Pharmacol Ther 22:196, 1977.

128. Rull JA et al: Symptomatic treatment of peripheral diabetic neuropathy with carbamazepine (Tegretol): double blind crossover trial, Diabetologia 5:215, 1969.

129. Davis JL et al: Peripheral diabetic neuropathy treated with amitriptyline and fluphenazine, JAMA 238:2291, 1977.

130. Winegard AI and Greene DA: Diabetic polyneuropathy: the importance of insulin deficiency, hyperglycemia and alterations in myoinositol metabolism in its pathogenesis, N Engl J Med 295:1416, 1976.

131. Holzer P: Peppers, capsaicin and the gastric mucosa: Letter to the editor, JAMA 261:3244, 1989.

132. Chad DA et al: Treatment of painful diabetic neuropathy with topical capsaicin: a double-blind multicenter investigation, Diab. Program of the 49th Annual Meeting of The American Diabetes Association 38(suppl 2):26A, 1989 (abstract 104).

133. Melzack R and Wall PD: Pain mechanisms: a new theory, Science 150:971, 1965.

134. Cohen SJ: Potential barriers to diabetes care, Diabetes Care 6:499, 1983.

135. Bailey TS, Yu HM, and Rayfield EJ: Patterns of foot examination in a diabetes clinic, Am J Med 78:371, 1985.

136. Allen GE and Hadden DR: Bullous lesions of the skin in diabetes (bullous diabeticorum), Br J Dermatol 82:216, 1970.

137. Oursler JR, Goldblum OM: Blistering eruption in a diabetic, Arch Dermatol 127:247, 1991.

138. Jelinek JE, ed: Diabetes and the skin, Philadelphia, 1985, Lea & Febiger.

139. Jelinek JE: Dermatology. In Levin ME, O'Neal LW, and Bowker JH, eds: The diabetic foot, ed 5, St Louis, 1993, Mosby–Year Book.

140. Young MJ et al: The prediction of diabetic neuropathic foot ulceration using vibration perception thresholds: a prospective study, Diabetes Care 17:557, 1994.

141. Guy RJC et al: Evaluation of thermal and vibration sensation in diabetic neuropathy, Diabetologia 28:131, 1985.

142. Benbow SJ et al: The prediction of diabetic neuropathic plantar foot ulceration by liquid-crystal contact thermography, Diabetes Care 17:835, 1994.

143. Pecoraro RE, Reiber GE, and Burgess EM: Pathways to diabetic limb amputation: basis for prevention, Diabetes Care 13:513, 1990.

144. Wheat LJ: Commentary on Lipsky et al: outpatient management of uncomplicated lower-extremity infections in diabetic patients, Diabetes Spect 4:78, 1991.

145. Lipsky BA et al: Outpatient management of uncomplicated lower-extremity infections in diabetic patients, Arch Intern Med 150:790, 1990.

146. Levin ME and Spratt IL: To soak or not to soak, Clin Diabetes 4:44, 1986.

147. Sinacore DR and Mueller MJ: Total-contact casting in the treatment of neuropathic ulcers. In Levin ME, O'Neal LW, and Bowker JH, eds: The diabetic foot, ed 5, St Louis, 1993, Mosby–Year Book.

148. Sage R and Doyle D: Surgical treatment of diabetic foot ulcers: a review of forty-eight cases, J Foot Surg 23:102, 1984.

149. Dickhaut SC, Delee JC, and Page CP: Nutritional status: importance in predicting wound-healing after amputation, J Bone Joint Surg 66:71, 1984.

150. Liszewski RF: The effects of zinc on wound healing: a collective review, J Am Osteopath Assoc 81:104, 1981.

151. Campbell RK and Nadler J: Magnesium deficiency and diabetes, Diabetes Educator 18:17, 1992.

152. Leslie CA et al: Randomized controlled trial of topical hyperbaric oxygen for treatment of diabetic foot ulcers, Diabetes Care 11:115, 1988.

153. Baroni G et al: Hyperbaric oxygen in diabetic gangrene treatment, Diabetes Care 10:81, 1987.

154. Cianci P and Hunt TK: Adjunctive hyperbaric oxygen therapy in treatment of diabetic foot wounds. In Levin ME, O'Neal LW, and Bowker JH, eds: The diabetic foot, ed 5, St Louis, 1993, Mosby–Year Book.

155. Lineaweaver W et al: Topical antimicrobial toxicity, Arch Surg 120:267, 1985.

156. Oberg MS and Lindsey D: Do not put hydrogen peroxide or povidone iodine into wounds! Am J Dis Child 141:27, 1987 (editorial).

157. Rodeheaver G et al: Bacteriocidal activity and toxicity of iodine-containing solutions in wounds, Arch Surg 117:181, 1982.

158. Rodeheaver G: Controversies in topical wound management, Ostomy Wound Manage 20:58, 1988.

159. Knighton DR et al: Stimulation of repair in chronic, non-healing, cutaneous ulcers using platelet-derived wound healing formula, Surg Gynecol Obstet 170:56, 1990.

160. Poucher RL, Leahy JD, and Howells G: Active healing of diabetic wounds utilizing growth factor therapy, Wounds Compend Clin Res Pract 3:65, 1991.

161. Bentkover JD and Champion AH: Economic evaluation of alternative methods of treatment for diabetic foot ulcer patients: cost-effectiveness of platelet releasate and wound care clinics, Wounds Compend Clin Res Pract 5:207, 1993.

162. Alvarez OM, Gilson G, and Auletta MJ: Local aspects of diabetic foot ulcer care: assessment, dressings, and topical agents. In Levin ME, O'Neal LW, and Bowker JH, eds: The diabetic foot, ed 5, St Louis, 1993, Mosby–Year Book.

163. Wooldridge J and Moreno L: Evaluation of the costs to Medicare of covering therapeutic shoes for diabetic patients, Diabetes Care 17:541, 1994.

164. Coleman WC: Footwear in a management program for injury prevention. In Levin ME, O'Neal LW, and Bowker JH, eds: The diabetic foot, ed 5, St Louis, 1993, Mosby–Year Book.

165. Janisse DJ: Pedorthic care of the diabetic foot. In Levin ME, O'Neal LW, and Bowker JH, eds: The diabetic foot, ed 5, St Louis, 1993, Mosby–Year Book.

166. Litzelman DK et al: Reduction of lower extremity clinical abnormalities in patients with non-insulin-dependent diabetes mellitus, Ann Intern Med 119:35, 1993.

167. Soulier SM: The use of running shoes in the prevention of plantar diabetic ulcers, J Am Podiatr Med Assoc 76:395, 1986.

168. Lippmann HI: Must loss of limb be a consequence of diabetes mellitus, Diabetes Care 2:432, 1979.

169. Miller LV: Evaluation of patient education: Los Angeles County Hospital experience, report of National Commission on diabetes to the Congress of the United States, U.S. Department of Health, Education and Welfare, NIH pub. no. 76-1021, Vol 3, Part V, Washington, DC, 1975.

170. Steinberg FU: Rehabilitation of the diabetic amputee and neuropathic disabilities. In Levin ME and O'Neal LW, eds: The diabetic foot, ed 4, St Louis, 1988, The CV Mosby Co.

INDEX

Program on Surgical Control of Hyperlipidemia, 169, 170t, 171f-172f
Promthrombinase complex, formation
of, inhibitors of, 121
Propranolol, 194t
Prostacyclin; see Prostaglandin I₂
Prostaglandin I₂, for platelet inhibition,
117, 118f
Prostaglandins
for Raynaud's phenomenon, 417
for thromboangiitis obliterans, 378
Prostheses, for lower extremity amputations, 229
Protein C
activated
resistance to, 96-97
as thrombin inhibitor, 121
in primary hypercoagulable disorders,
95-97, 96f
Protein deficiency, bilateral swollen limb
from, 676-677
Proteins, in coagulation, 91-93, 92f
Protein S, in hypercoagulable disorders,
97, 97f
Proteoglycans, and binding of low-density
lipoproteins, 154, 156f-157f, 161
Prothrombin time, 108, 110
Prourokinase, 132
Pseudoaneurysms
from catheter-based angiography, 68f
from coronary artery bypass graft, arch
aortogram of, 71f
intravascular stents for, 242f
Pseudoclaudication
with cauda equina syndrome, 6
vs. intermittent claudication, 213, 213t
Pseudoxanthoma elasticum, vs.
thromboangiitis obliterans, 377
PT; see Prothrombin time
PTA; see Percutaneous transluminal angioplasty
Pulmonary angiography, 75, 75f
in pulmonary embolism, 478-479, 479f
Pulmonary arterial mean pressure, in pulmonary embolism, 472f
Pulmonary artery, sarcomas of, 622-623
Pulmonary closure sound, in pulmonary
embolism, 470, 470t
Pulmonary disease
in polyarteritis nodosa, 383-384
in Wegener's granulomatosis, 391, 392f
Pulmonary embolism, 468-488
adjunctive therapy for, 487-488
angiography of, 75f
anticoagulants for, INR ranges for, 110t
cardiac index in, and systemic arterial
hypoxemia, 472f, 472-473
in children, 547, 547t
clinical syndromes in, 469
diagnosis of, 475-481, 476t, 478f-479f,
479t, 481f
angiography in, 478-479, 479f
arterial oxygen tension in, 477
echocardiography in, 480
electrical impedance plethysmography in, 479-480
electrocardiography in, 476t, 476-477
laboratory tests in, 475-476

perfusion lung scan in, 477-478,
478f, 479t
radiography in, 476, 476t
filling defects in, 479f
heart sounds in, 470, 470t
hemodynamic responses in, with prior
cardiovascular disease, 473, 474f,
475
hemodynamic responses to, 470-475,
471f-472f, 474f
without prior cardiopulmonary disease, 470-473, 471f-472f
incidence of, 468
in Klippel-Trenaunay syndrome, 543
mortality in, 468
phlebitis in, 470, 470t
pulmonary arterial mean pressure in,
472f
pulmonary closure sound in, 470, 470t
right atrial mean pressure in, 472f
right ventricular filling pressure in,
471-472, 472f
risk factors for, 468-469
symptoms and signs of, 469t-470t,
469-470
systemic arterial hypoxemia in, and
cardiac index, 472f
thrombolytic therapy for, 133t, 134
treatment of, 481-484, 483f-484f
heparin in, 481-482
pulmonary microcirculation after,
484f, 484-485
surgical, 486-487, 487f
thrombolysis in, 482, 483f-484f,
484-487
efficacy of, 482, 483f-484f, 484
Pulmonary hypertension
in pulmonary embolism, 471, 472f
Raynaud's phenomenon in, 416
Pulmonary microcirculation, after resolution of pulmonary embolism, 484f,
484-485
Pulse-volume, recording,
plethysmographic, penile, in vasculogenic impotence, 443-444, 444f
Pulse-volume recording, in limbs, in peripheral arterial disease, 36
Pulse waveform analysis, in atherosclerosis of lower extremities, 216
Purple toe syndrome, in atheromatous
embolization, 262, 263f
Purpura
Henoch-Schönlein, 388
in true hypersensitivity vasculitis, 387,
387f
in vasculitis, 654f
Purpura fulminans, 96
Purpuric lesions, in chilblains, 612-613
PVD; see Peripheral vascular disease
Pyoderma gangrenosum, leg ulcers in,
660, 660f
Pyogenic granuloma, 583, 584f

Q

Quinapril, 195t
Quinethazone, 194t

R

Radial artery, embolism of, 682f
Radial pulse, palpation for, 23f
Radiation, leg ulcers from, 665-666, 666f
Radiography
in aortic dissection, 360, 361f
in atherosclerosis of lower extremities,
217
in pulmonary embolism, 476, 476t
Rales, in pulmonary embolism, 470, 470t
Ramipril, 195t
Rauwolfia alkaloids, 195t, 198-199
Raynaud's phenomenon, 10, 11f, 407-
418
with arteriovenous fistulas, 415
in biliary cirrhosis, 416
in carpal tunnel syndrome, 414
clinical manifestations of, 409, 409f
cold agglutinins in, 414-415
conditioning and biofeedback for, 417
in connective tissue diseases, 411-413,
412f
in cryoproteinemia, 414
diagnosis of, 410
drugs and, 411
drug therapy for, 416-417
in erythromelalgia, 616
heavy metals and, 416
in hypothenar hammer syndrome,
413-414
in hypothyroidism, 415
in obstructive arterial disease, 415
pathophysiology of, 407-409
plasmaphersis for, 417
in polymyositis and dermatomyositis,
413
primary, 407-411, 409f
prognosis in, 410-411
in pulmonary hypertension, 416
in reflex sympathetic dystrophy, 415
in renal disease, 415
in rheumatoid arthritis, 413
in scleroderma, 411-413, 412f
secondary causes of, 411-416, 412f
Sjögren's syndrome in, 413
sympathectomy for, 417-418
in systemic lupus erythematosus, 412-
413
in thromboangiitis obliterans, 375
in tumors, 415-416
vascular imaging in, 58-59
in vasculitis, 415
in vinyl chloride disease, 415
α₁-Receptor blockers, 194t, 198
Recombinant tissue plasminogen activator, for frostbite, 611
Reflex sympathetic dystrophy
in children, 571
clinical features of, 569, 570t, 571
definition of, 567
diagnosis of, 571-572
differential diagnosis of, 572
disorders associated with, 567t-568t
epidemiology of, 568-569
etiology of, 568, 568t
osteoporosis in, 571
pathophysiology of, 569, 569f